The Textbook of Pharmaceutical Medicine

The Textbook of Pharmaceutical Medicine

EDITED BY

John P. Griffin

BSc, PhD, FRCP, FRCPath, FFPM
Director, Asklepieion Consultancy Ltd.
Formerly Director of the Association of the British Pharmaceutical Industry, London
Formerly Professional Head of the Medicines Division, DOH, London (now MHRA)

6TH EDITION

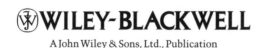

WILEY-BLACKWELL

A John Wiley & Sons, Ltd., Publication

BMJ | Books

This edition first published 1993 by The Queen's University Belfast © 1994, 1998 by
The Queen's University Belfast; 2002, 2006, 2009 by Blackwell Publishing Ltd

BMJ Books is an imprint of BMJ Publishing Group Limited, used under licence by Blackwell Publishing which
was acquired by John Wiley & Sons in February 2007. Blackwell's publishing programme has been merged with
Wiley's global Scientific, Technical and Medical business to form Wiley-Blackwell.

Registered office: John Wiley & Sons Ltd, The Atrium, Southern Gate, Chichester, West Sussex, PO19 8SQ, UK
Editorial offices: 9600 Garsington Road, Oxford, OX4 2DQ, UK
       The Atrium, Southern Gate, Chichester, West Sussex, PO19 8SQ, UK
       111 River Street, Hoboken, NJ 07030-5774, USA

For details of our global editorial offices, for customer services and for information about how to apply for
permission to reuse the copyright material in this book please see our website at www.wiley.com/wiley-blackwell

Library of Congress Cataloging-in-Publication Data
The textbook of pharmaceutical medicine / [edited by] John Parry Griffin. – 6th ed.
    p. ; cm.
  "BMJ Books."
  Includes bibliographical references and index.
  ISBN 978-1-4051-8035-1
  1. Pharmacology, Experimental. I. Griffin, J. P. (John Parry)
  [DNLM: 1. Drug Approval. 2. Clinical Trials as Topic. 3. Pharmacology.
QV771 T3445 2009]
  RM301.25.T49 2009
  615'.1–dc22

                      2009024878

ISBN: 9781405180351
A catalogue record for this book is available from the British Library.

Set in 8.5/11pt Minion by Graphicraft Limited, Hong Kong
Printed and bound in Singapore by Fabulous Printers Pte Ltd

1 2009

Contents

Contributors

Geoffrey R. Barker, TD, BSc, MSc, FDSRCD, FRCS, FFPM
Adj. Professor Immunology, Duke University Medical Center, NC, USA
Executive and Limited Partner, Pappas Ventures, NC, USA
Consultant to EGeen (USA), Abingworth LLP (UK), Reuters Insight Community of Experts
Trustee Member of the Board of the Faculty of Pharmaceutical Physicians of The Royal Colleges of Physicians UK

Nick Beckett. BSc(Hons)
Partner, CMS Cameron McKenna LLP
London, UK

Bensita Bernard, BPharm, MPharm, MClin Pharm
Clinical Research Associate
Cytosystems Ltd, Aberdeen, Scotland

Susan Bews, BSc, MBBS, FRCP, PFPM
President of the Faculty of Pharmaceutical
Medicine of the Royal Colleges of Physicians, London UK

Carole A. Bradley MSc
Boehringer Ingelheim Canada Ltd
Burlington, ON
Canada

Kate Darwin, BA, Dphi, CSci, MRQA, MICR
Hammersmith Medicines Research Ltd,
Park Royal, London, UK

Charles de Wet, MBChB, MPharm Med, FFPM
Medical Director
Boehring Ingelheim Limited
Bracknell
Berkshire, UK

Ian C. Dodds-Smith, MA(Cantab)
Arnold & Porter (UK) LLP
London, UK

Anand S. Dutta, PhD
Pharmaceutical Consultant
Hazel Grove
Stockport, UK

A. Peter Fletcher, MBBS, PhD, MFPM
Independent Consultant Little Maplestead
Essex formerly Senior Principal Medical Officer, DOH

David Galloway, MB, ChB, DRCOG, FRCP, FRCPE, FFPM
Medical & Scientific Director, Cytosystems Ltd, Aberdeen, Scotland

David Gillen, BSc, MBBS, MRCGP, MFPM
Head of Medical Teams
Primary Care BU Europe Canada Australia and NZ
Pfizer, Walton Oaks, UK

Andrew P. Grieve, PhD
Formerly at Pfizer Global Research and Development,
Sandwich, UK

Jane R. Griffin, BA(Hons), MSc
Director, Market Access, Pricing and Oucomes Research,
Boehringer Ingelheim Ltd
Bracknell, Berks, UK

John P. Griffin, BSc, PhD, FRCP, FRCPath, FFPM
Director, Asklepieion Consultancy Ltd, Herts, UK
Formerly Director of the Association of the British
Pharmaceutical Industry, London
Formerly Professional Head of the Medicines Division, DOH,
London (now MHRA)

Gavin Halbert, BSc, PhD, CChem, MRSC, MRPharmS
Director, Cancer Research UK Formulation Unit
Department of Pharmaceutical Sciences
University of Strathclyde
Glasgow, Scotland, UK

Sarah Hanson, MA
Partner, CMS Cameron McKenna LLP
London, UK

Dean W.G. Harron, BSc, PhD, FRPharmS, MPSNI
Professor, School of Pharmacy
Medical Biology Centre, Belfast,
Northern Ireland, UK

Janice Hirshorn, BSc(Hons), PhD, FSALS
Consultant, Rose Bay, NSW, Australia

Christopher J.S. Hodges, MA(Oxon), PhD, FSALS
Head of the CMS Research Programme on Civil Justice Systems,
Centre for Socio-Legal Studies, University of Oxford, Oxford, UK

Peter Barton Hutt, BA(Yale), LLB(Harvard), LLM(Nyu)
Senior Counsel
Covington & Burling LLP
Washington, DC, USA. Formerly Chief Counsel to the US Food
and Drug Administration

Huw Jones, MA, MD, MSc, FRCP, FRCR, FFPM(Hon)
Dean of Postgraduate Medical and Dental Education for the East
of England
Lead Dean for the Faculty of Pharmaceutical Medicine, UK

Judith K. Jones, MD, PhD
President, The Degge Group
President, The Pharmaceutical Education and
Research Institute;
Adjunct Professor of Pharmacology, Georgetown University
Washington, DC, USA

Yuichi Kubo, MSc
Vice President, Traslational Medicine and Clinical Pharmacology
Daiichi Sankyo Co. Ltd,
Tokyo, Japan

Anke Lühe Dr. phil. nat.
Toxicology Project Leader
F. Hoffmann-La Roche Ltd.
Non-clinical Drug Safety
Basel, Switzerland

Shuna Mason, BA(Hons)
Head of Regulatory, CMS Cameron McKenna LLP,
London, UK

Valèria Molnár, MScPharm
Director
Clinical Pharmacology Consulting Ltd
Beaumont, Australia

Deborah Monk, B Pharm Dip Hosp BA
Director, Innovation and Industry Policy
Medicines Australia, Deakin, ACT, Australia

Lutz Müller Dr. rer. nat.
Toxicology Project Leader
Scientific Expert
F. Hoffmann-La Roche Ltd.
Non-clinical Drug Safety
Basel, Switzerland

Heike Rabe, State Exam, MD, Habilitation, FRCPCH
Consultant Neonatologist
Honorary Senior Clinical Lecturer
Brighton and Sussex Medical School
Brighton, UK
Honorary Assistant Professor Medical Faculty
Westphalian Wilhelms-University Münster
Germany

John Posner, BSc, PhD, MBBS, FRCP, FFPM
Independent Consultant in Pharmaceutical medicine
John Posner Consulting
Beckenham, Kent, UK

Paul Rolan, MB, BS, MD, FRACP, FFPM, DCPSA
Professor of Clinical and Experimental Pharmacology
Medical School
University of Adelaide
Adelaide, Australia

Agnès Saint Raymond, MD
Head of Sector
Scientific Advice, Orphan Drugs and Paediatric
Medicinal Products
European Medicines Agency (EMEA)
London, UK

Rashmi R. Shah, BSc, MBBS, MD, FRCP, FFPM
Pharmaceutical Consultant
Former Senior Clinical Assessor
Medicines and Healthcare Products
Regulatory Agency (MHRA)
London, UK

Susan Shaw, MBBS, BSc, MRCPsych
Consultant Psychiatrist
Chelsea and Westminster Hospital
London, UK

Richard N. Spivey, Pharm, D PhD
Senior Vice President
Corporate Technology Policy
Pharmacia, Peapack, New Jersey, USA

Nadarajah Sreeharan, MD, PhD, FRCP, FACP, FFPM
Consultant & Senior Partner
TRANSCRIP LLP
Visiting Professor, University of Surrey, UK
Senior Visiting Professor, UITM
Medical School, Malaysia

Peter D. Stonier, BA BSc PhD MB ChB MRCPsych FRCP FRCPE FFPM
Medical Director
Amdipharm plc
Essex, UK

Jennie A. Sykes, MBChB, MRCP, FFPM
Vice President and Medical Director Asia Pacific,
Japan and Emerging Markets,
GlaxoSmithKline, UK

Silvia Valverde, LLM
Arnold & Porter (UK) LLP
London, UK

Duncan Vere, MD, FRCP, FFPM
Professor (Emeritus) of Therapeutics,
University of London, UK.
Formerly Chair Tower Hamlets Research Ethics Committee

William Vodra, JD
Senior Counsel to Arnold & Porter LLP,
Washington, DC, USA

William Wardell, MA(Oxon), MD, PhD
President, Wardell Associates International
Princeton, New Jersey, USA

Steve Warrington, FRCP, FFPM
Hammersmith Medicines Research Ltd,
London, UK

The editor

Professor John P Griffin BSc PhD MBBS FRCP MRCS FRCPath FFPM graduated in medicine at the Royal London Hospital, where he was also in clinical practice. He was a lecturer in Physiology at King's College, London and held the post of Head of Clinical Research at Riker Laboratories from 1967 to 1971. Professor Griffin joined the then Medicines Division of the Department of Health, now Medicines Healthcare Agency (MHRA) London, as a Senior Medical Officer, in 1971, and was subsequently appointed Medical Assessor to the Committee on Safety of Medicines. From 1977 to 1984, Professor Griffin was Senior Principal Medical Officer and Professional Head of Medicines Division in addition to being Medical Assessor to the Medicines Commission. As the Professional Head of Medicines Division he also attended the Scientific Sub-Committee of the Veterinary Products Committee of the Ministry of Agriculture, Food and Fisheries. During this time he was a member of the EC committee on Proprietary Medicinal Products and Chairman of the CPMP's Working Party on Safety Requirements.

From 1976 to 1984 John P. Griffin served on the Joint Formulary Committee of the British National Formulary, during which period the first eight issues of the current format were produced.

John P. Griffin was the director of the Association of the British Pharmaceutical Industry from 1984 to 1994. During this time he was a member of the Executive Board of the European Federation of the Pharmaceutical Industries' Associations and IFPMA. He chaired the ICH Safety Working Group from 1988 to 1994 and presented papers at ICH1 and ICH2 in the plenary sessions.

Since June 1994, John P. Griffin has run his own independent consultancy company, which has provided independent and impartial advice to governments on the development of a pharmaceutical policy, and to national trade associations and individual companies. John P. Griffin was Visiting Professor in Pharmaceutical Medicine at the University of Surrey, for 6 years and was also Honorary Consultant Clinical Pharmacologist at the Lister Hospital in Hertfordshire, UK.

Professor Griffin was on the Board of the Faculty of Pharmaceutical Medicine for 12 years, was Chairman of the Board of Examiners of the Faculty of Pharmaceutical Medicine of the Royal College of Physicians for 7 years, and was Academic Registrar and served on the Task Force on Specialist Medical Training in Pharmaceutical Medicine. He has served on a number of Royal College of Physicians, London Working Parties including that on the 'Development of Clinical Pharmacology and Therapeutics in a Changing World'.

Professor Griffin is the author and co-author of over 250 publications on adverse drug reactions and iatrogenic disease, aspects of neurophysiology and clinical pharmacology and toxicology and drug regulation. Notable among his publications are the following four standard texts:

• *Iatrogenic Diseases*. Oxford University Press, 1st edn 1972, 3rd edn 1986; jointly with Professor PF D'Arcy.

• *A Manual of Adverse. Drug Interactions*. John Wright, Bristol, 1st edn 1975; Elsevier Press, Amsterdam, 5th edn. 1997; jointly with Professor PF D'Arcy.

• *The Textbook of Pharmaceutical Medicine*. The Queen's University of Belfast Press, 1st edn 1993, 2nd edn 1994, 3rd edn 1998, 4th edn 2002 published by the BMJ Publishing Group in 2002, 5th edn. 2006 Blackwell.

• *Medicines, Research, Regulation and Risk*. The Queen's University of Belfast Press, 1st edn 1989, 2nd edn 1992.

From 1991 to 2003 he served as Editor in Chief of *Adverse Drug Reactions and Toxicological Reviews*, a peer-reviewed journal produced quarterly by Oxford University Press.

In 2005 he was awarded the Faculty of Pharmaceutical Medicines Commemorative Medal for outstanding services to the Faculty.

John Griffin
London
2009

Acknowledgements

First, I would wish to thank all those who have contributed so generously of their time to the preparation of their contributions to the 6th Edition of this book, especially those who have contributed to earlier editions. In particular, a very special thanks to those who with incredible loyalty and dedication have contributed to all six editions. The contributors have made the current edition of this book through the comprehensiveness of the revised chapters an encyclopaedic overview of the speciality of Pharmaceutical Medicine invaluable for anyone in the field.

Secondly, I would like to record my appreciation to Mary Banks who has steered this book through its 4th, 5th and 6th Editions. Special thanks are due to Simone Heaton and Rebecca Huxley for their dedication and unstinting help in the preparation of the 6th Edition, without them it would have been an impossible task. The help of Kathy Auger of Graphicraft is also gratefully acknowledged.

Finally, thanks are due to the World Medical Association (WMA), and the European Medicines Evaluation Agency (EMEA) for permission to publish key documents as Appendices. Others have allowed us to quote or use their material and this generosity is acknowledged in the text; however, a general thanks is appropriate at this point.

Preface: the development of pharmaceutical medicine as a specialty in the UK

The UK is at the forefront in the recognition of pharmaceutical medicine as a fulfilling career for physicians, enabling them to make a major contribution to patient and public welfare, both in terms of bringing new medicines to market and of ensuring their safe and effective use. The Faculty of Pharmaceutical Medicine has been instrumental in supporting pharmaceutical physicians and in achieving specialty recognition in the UK in order to achieve and ensure the practice of the highest standards for the benefit of patients. As with all other recognised medical specialties in the UK, achievement of specialist registration confers a comparable standard of professional competence. As such, speciality training in pharmaceutical medicine will continue to evolve in line with other UK specialties.

Compared with the history of many other medical and surgical specialties, pharmaceutical medicine is a relative newcomer. Despite having only a relatively short history it has made major strides and, in the UK, has overtaken certain other medical specialties in terms of trainee numbers and viability.

Pharmaceutical medicine is a medical specialty concerned with the discovery, evaluation, licensing and monitoring of medicines and the medical aspects of their marketing. Physicians practising in pharmaceutical medicine have, in the past, mainly worked for pharmaceutical companies although more recently there has been a shift towards a greater number working in the regulatory agencies, contract research organisations and, now, a substantial proportion being independent contractors. The pharmaceutical industry itself has a rather longer history. Its formal beginnings were in 1891 when the Drug Club was set up. The members were not companies as would be recognised today but were certainly the forerunners. The members of the Drug Club had to be principals of wholesale druggists and at the time of the first meeting in February 1892 there were 50 members. In 1929 the Wholesale Drug Trade Association was formed and the Drug Club was wound up. This organisation was renamed the Association of the British Pharmaceutical Industry (ABPI) in 1948. It was probably around this time that physicians started to provide advice to pharmaceutical companies on medical matters although there were few who did so and for those who did it was usually in addition to their other medical work rather than as a full-time employee of a company. It may have been lucrative but it would certainly not have been considered prestigious.

However, the 1950s saw the introduction of a large number of therapeutic agents and in parallel there was a need for informed medical advice to the pharmaceutical companies. As a consequence, there was a rapid expansion of doctors employed by those companies to advise on drug development and medico-marketing. Inevitably, these doctors were breaking new ground and the need for peer support and a forum in which to share issues and ideas resulted in the formation, in October 1957, of the first pharmaceutical physicians' association, the Association of Medical Advisers in the Pharmaceutical Industry (AMAPI). AMAPI also provided some training.

The term 'pharmaceutical physician' came into use in the mid-1970s and, in 1986, AMAPI changed its name to BrAPP – British Association of Pharmaceutical Physicians – to reflect this new nomenclature.

The Textbook of Pharmaceutical Medicine. Edited by John P. Griffin. © 2009, ISBN: 978-1-4051-8035-1.

AMAPI grew rapidly from its original 20 or so members to about 700 in the mid-1980s of whom around one-quarter were from overseas. An enlightened group of physicians from within this fraternity realised that if pharmaceutical physicians were to develop further their chosen career paths within medicine, they needed to establish an organisation alongside the medical Royal Colleges which would set and continually develop high ethical and professional standards in the practice of pharmaceutical medicine. The primary aim of this charitable organisation would be to promote the science of, and knowledge in, the field of pharmaceutical medicine for the benefit of patients and the public – a different remit from that of the AMAPI.

Thus, with very considerable support and advice from the Royal College of Physicians of London, the Royal College of Physicians of Edinburgh and the Royal College of Physicians and Surgeons of Glasgow, the Faculty of Pharmaceutical Medicine was established in 1989 as a Faculty of all three colleges and as a registered charity. The Faculty now has a membership of over 1300 pharmaceutical physicians with almost 40% working overseas in nearly 40 countries. The membership is primarily physicians who work within the pharmaceutical industry, contract research organisations and regulatory agencies or who are self-employed.

Back in the mid-1970s, AMAPI and ABPI, in collaboration with the University of Wales Institute of Science and Technology (later Cardiff University), set up a 2-year modular postgraduate course to prepare physicians for the examination in pharmaceutical medicine – the Diploma in Pharmaceutical Medicine. Originally, the responsibility for the examination rested with the three parent medical Royal Colleges. With the establishment of the Faculty as the standard setting body, it was entirely appropriate that in 1994 responsibility for the setting, conduct and adjudication of the examination, together with awarding the Diploma, passed to the Faculty. The syllabus has been updated regularly and has acted as a template for other diplomas in pharmaceutical medicine in other countries. The format of the examination has evolved such that it now includes a multichoice question paper but, as from the outset, comprises written and oral components. A Board of Examiners, comprised of over 40 of the Faculty membership and around 10 external medical and scientific colleagues, are responsible for all aspects of the examination, including question setting, conduct of the examination and marking. The pass rate is comparable to that of the Membership examination for the Royal College of Physicians.

Some 10 years after the formation of the Faculty, towards the end of the century, the Trustee Board of the Faculty took the decision to work to establish pharmaceutical medicine as a recognised speciality. In the late 1990s, in conformance with the European Specialist Medical Qualifications Order 1995, the UK introduced specialist medical training for clinical specialties leading to the granting of a Certificate of Completion of Specialist Training (CCST). The introduction of specialist training afforded pharmaceutical medicine, through the Faculty, the opportunity to seek equivalent recognition as a listed specialty and for pharmaceutical physicians to gain a CCST-UK and then apply to be listed on the General Medical Council (GMC) Specialist Register. If the Faculty could put in place all the requisite processes and documentation to achieve this, pharmaceutical physicians would be able to undertake Higher Medical Training (HMT) in this specialty as with other medical specialties in order to be recognised for entry onto the GMC Specialist Register. [The CCST became the CCT (Certificate of Completion of Training) in 2005.]

There was a very considerable amount of work for the Faculty to do to prepare the requisite documents and define its procedures in compliance with the requirements of the Specialist Training Authority (STA) of the medical Royal Colleges in order to apply to become a recognised specialty. A curriculum had to be prepared for approval and a system had to be set up to ensure each trainee had a Senior Specialty Adviser (SSA) as well as an Educational Supervisor (ES) – all of whom would have to be trained by the Faculty. The SSA is a joint appointment by the Faculty and the Lead Dean for Pharmaceutical Medicine who is also a Dean of Postgraduate Medical and Dental Education. The Lead Dean is responsible for quality managing the training programme across the UK. The role of the SSA is to oversee the delivery of the training programme in a specified number of approved training sites – usually determined geographically or, for the larger ones, by company or institution. It is a role of considerable responsibility as the Specialty Advisory Committee (SAC) of the Joint Royal Colleges of Physicians Training Board (JRCPTB) on Pharmaceutical Medicine relies very heavily on these committed individuals, who are usually Fellows of the Faculty, to assure ongoing quality of the training sites. The Educational Supervisor role also carries considerable responsibility. It is a mandatory requirement that the ES must be a registered doctor and an experienced pharmaceutical physician, normally a Member or Fellow of the Faculty, and must be familiar with the trainee's work and able to oversee the medical work of the trainee. The ES is normally the trainee's medical manager working in the same organisation. The ES carries overall responsibility for the supervision of training for the trainee including the conduct of educational and performance appraisals, assessments of performance and competency and ensuring availability of and access to the components of the curriculum.

It was also a requirement that the Faculty establish a process for reviewing progress throughout the period of HMT in Pharmaceutical Medicine in the form of the annual Review of In-Training Assessments (RITAs). This process was set up in line with that established for clinical trainees within NHS bodies except that evidence of experience would be documented in the context of work-related modules rather than clinical ward-based practice.

Hard work and patience were eventually rewarded and in 2002 the Secretary of State signed his agreement to pharmaceutical medicine becoming a recognised specialty. The first National Training Numbers (NTNs) were issued in March 2003, and 73 pharmaceutical physicians had started their specialist training by the end of that year. No doubt these first trainees entered the programme with some trepidation as they were stepping into unchartered waters. This recognition of pharmaceutical medicine as a specialty was a major milestone for pharmaceutical physicians. No longer could they be considered outside of mainstream medicine. Their training programme and standards achieved had been externally validated and recognised to be at least equal to that of any other medical or surgical specialty. Pharmaceutical medicine was truly born even if it did still have some further steps to take to achieve complete independence. Between 2002 and 2007 pharmaceutical medicine existed as a specialty under the umbrella of Clinical Pharmacology and Therapeutics, but as the specialty rapidly expanded it became clear that it needed its own separate identity in line with all the other medical specialties that constituted the Joint Committee of Higher Medical Training (JCHMT) and its successor, the JRCPTB. This independence was achieved in 2007 with the establishment of the Specialty Advisory Committee on Pharmaceutical Medicine of the JRCPTB and pharmaceutical medicine 'became of age'.

The regulatory work of the STA was transferred to the newly formed Postgraduate Medical Education and Training Board (PMETB) in 2005. One of the roles of this body is responsibility for approving both the training site and the individualised (*ad personam*) training programme. At about this time, agreement was gained for the training to be approved across a group of company sites, such approval remaining appropriate for whatever individual might be in post (if they were registered for training). This change in arrangements allows trainees to move more easily within a company within the UK, or even across Europe and beyond, provided that the company's programme is approved for training, that the curriculum can be delivered in its entirety and that appropriate named supervisors are available. The Faculty of Pharmaceutical Medicine, in conjunction with the Lead Postgraduate Dean for the specialty, monitors the training programmes approved within companies, and it provides, on an annual basis, the regulatory body with evidence gathered from trainees, trainers and from on-site visits, evidence of appropriate quality management.

The growth in trainee numbers is a major success story reflecting the commitment of those entering pharmaceutical medicine to their chosen specialty and to working to achieve the highest standard of professional competence for the benefit of both patients and the public. Around 40 new trainees enter the training programme each year. As of mid-2009, there are approximately 195 pharmaceutical physicians who have NTNs and are actively undertaking specialty training and 90 who have completed their training and are on the GMC Specialist Register as a consequence of undertaking specialty training in pharmaceutical medicine.

Structured training in pharmaceutical medicine, whether through the old curriculum of basic and higher specialist training, or the new (from 2007) Pharmaceutical Medicine Specialty Training (PMST) programme, requires commitment, enthusiasm and application. In preparation for training, doctors must have completed 4 years of clinical medicine following qualification (or 3 years for those qualifying prior to August 2005).

The revised (2007) curriculum for PMST sets out six specialty specific modules: Medicines Regulation, Clinical Pharmacology, Statistics and Data Management, Clinical Development, Healthcare Marketplace and Drug Safety Surveillance. Each module comprises up to 10 items and the trainee must attain a specified level of competence for each item. In addition, there is a generic module, in line with all UK specialty training programmes, encompassing Interpersonal and Management Skills and, for pharmaceutical medicine, the tenets of Good Pharmaceutical Medical Practice as approved by the GMC. Trainees are required to produce a portfolio of validated documented evidence to demonstrate that this level of competence has been achieved and each item has to be authenticated and signed off by the ES trained and approved by the Faculty. The trainee must identify a minimum of at least two modules which must be undertaken in their entirety in the workplace in addition to the generic module. The other modules can be undertaken in their entirety by attendance and completion of assignments at Faculty approved courses or can be achieved by a mixture of work-based assessments and attendance at other courses. The majority of trainees complete considerably more than the required minimum number of courses through in-house experience.

To facilitate appropriate and adequate collection of information as evidence of satisfactory achievement of competencies, trainees require the self-discipline and rigour of integrating their programme with their day-to-day work and it is this evidence that is reviewed by a panel of assessors at the Annual Review of Competence Progression (ARCP), formerly the RITA process. As a guide, the volume of documentation required is likely to be a full Lever Arch File for each module although frequently a piece of work can be used to fulfil the requirements for items within two or more different modules. All evidence within a Training Record can be appropriately anonymised with respect to confidential matters but it has to be clear that the work submitted is that of the trainee personally, whether by their name appearing on, for example, the front sheet of the protocol or by authentication as such by the ES. In future, it is likely that such authentication will be supported by a related entry of 'reflective learning' which will summarise what the trainee will have learnt from that particular experience. Original records may be archived within company records but they must be available for inspection in the event of an audit by the PMETB. In line with the requirements of the PMETB, the specialty is developing a set of tools to support workplace-based assessments. These will be validated

tools which will align with the curricular requirements and they will enable the ES to document the trainees' progress through their daily work. In addition to satisfactory completion of all the modules of the programme, success in the Diploma of Pharmaceutical Medicine is an absolute requirement prior to the issue of a CCT.

For UK pharmaceutical physicians, revalidation, involving relicensing as a physician, and recertification for those who are on the specialist register, will be mandatory within the next few years if those physicians want to remain licensed to practise with the GMC. It will be the responsibility of the Faculty to put in place for its physicians a system for recertification whose processes and standards are acceptable to the GMC. The Faculty will also be working with the GMC to enable all pharmaceutical physicians to relicense and remain on the general medical register.

Pharmaceutical medicine has come a long way and would not be recognisable, in terms of its acceptance as a specialty and the consequent high standards it demands, to those physicians who gave advice to drug wholesalers and companies while undertaking their main medical practice some 60 years ago. But it still has a long way to go. It is recognised as a specialty in only a very few countries other than the UK (Mexico, Switzerland, Eire) and few countries hold examinations of an equivalent standard to the UK Diploma of Pharmaceutical Medicine. Yet it is a global specialty and, in the interests of patient and public safety and benefit, there needs to be an extension of the standards set by the Faculty of Pharmaceutical Medicine in the UK and similar bodies elsewhere, so that pharmaceutical medicine becomes recognised as a medical specialty in all countries where it is practised.

Susan Bews and Huw Jones
2009

The contributions provided by the authors and any opinions or views expressed therein are their personal views and do not necessarily reflect the views or opinions of the companies for which they work or their employees.

Part I Research and development

1 Discovery of new medicines

Anand S. Dutta

Pharmaceutical Consultant, Stockport, Cheshire, UK

1.1 Introduction

Ancient civilisations, like modern society, had a keen interest in the health of man and other animals. Continuation of this interest over a period of time led to the discovery of a large number of therapeutic agents primarily from the natural sources; many of the natural sources are still being used as lead structures for the discovery of new drugs. In more recent times (~50 years), with the involvement of a large number of pharmaceutical companies and many academic institutions, progress in the understanding of the disease processes and mechanisms to control or eliminate the disease has accelerated. Similarly, despite the advances and achievements of the last 50 years, the need to discover treatments for existing and evolving diseases has also increased. This is primarily because of the inadequacies of current medicines. In many cases treatment only leads to symptom relief or cure is associated with undesirable side effects. In infectious diseases such as tuberculosis, malaria and HIV, resistance or tolerance may develop to existing treatments, thus making them ineffective against the infecting bacteria, parasite or virus.[1–3] New infectious agents such as severe acute respiratory syndrome (SARS), hepatitis C, human herpes virus-6, -7 and -8 and bird flu (H5N1 virus) are also appearing.[4] In addition, with changing environmental factors, lifestyle and increasing lifespan, more pathological abnormalities that require new treatments are being identified. Obesity and a number of cardiovascular diseases have their origins in altered (more prosperous?) lifestyle habits including environmental and psychosocial factors and diet. Prevalence of obesity is rising worldwide and

there are few drugs currently available for treatment. Obesity appears to be a risk factor for other diseases such as cardiovascular disease, diabetes, some forms of cancer and severe asthma.[5,6] Changing social attitudes are also creating markets for the so-called 'lifestyle' drugs. Although the term 'lifestyle' drug is applied currently to drugs such as sildenafil for erectile dysfunction[7] and minoxidil or finasteride for baldness, the precise definition of 'lifestyle' drugs is a subject of debate.[8] Designer steroids also have the potential to produce various agents that can be useful as lifestyle drugs and drugs of abuse.[9] Treatment of erectile dysfunction is currently based on oral phosphodiesterase-5 inhibitors (e.g. sildenafil, vardenafil, udenafil (1) and tadalafil). Increasing use of drugs for illicit purposes (substance abuse), such as opiates, cannabis, cocaine and amphetamines, is creating a need for additional treatments to manage and treat drug addiction and mental disorders associated with many of the illicit drugs.[10,11] Addiction is broadly defined as a chronic brain disease that involves complex interactions between repeated exposure to drugs along with biological (i.e. genetic and developmental) and environmental (i.e. drug availability, social and economic variables) factors. Although some agents such as methadone, buprenorphine (Subutex) and naloxone are available to control opiate addiction, treatments

The Textbook of Pharmaceutical Medicine. Edited by John P. Griffin. © 2009, ISBN: 978-1-4051-8035-1.

1 Udenafil

2 Varenicline

for addictive substances are generally lacking.[12] In addition to these illicit drugs, treatments are also required for tobacco and alcohol addiction.[13,14] Nicotine patches are available as nicotine replacement therapy for tobacco addiction and recently a nicotinic $\alpha_4\beta_2$ partial agonist varenicline (Champix) (2) has been launched as a non-nicotine therapy. Varenicline partially activates the nicotinic receptors and reduces the severity of craving for nicotine as well as withdrawal symptoms. Approved medicines for the treatment of alcohol abuse include the aldehyde dehydrogenase blocker disulfiram, the opioid antagonist naltrexone, the functional glutamate antagonist acamprosate and topiramate.[15]

Increasing knowledge about the underlying causes of diseases is enabling the discovery of more selective and less toxic drugs. Progress in molecular biology (e.g. sequencing of the human genome, proteomics, pharmacogenomics and protein engineering) is creating new avenues for understanding precise disease mechanisms (biochemical pathways) and the discovery of new targets based on new disease pathways. Advances in the field are expected to lead to highly selective and efficacious medicines. Recombinant technologies are now enabling the synthesis of larger biologically active proteins in sufficient quantities. Proteins and monoclonal antibodies are therefore becoming more important and common as therapeutic agents. More vaccines are being developed against infectious diseases.

Equally important is the progress being made in the fields of combinatorial chemistry, enabling the synthesis of millions of compounds. High-throughput screening technologies and other automation techniques are facilitating more rapid drug discovery. In the longer term, a combination of all these new developments is likely to generate safer and more effective medicines, not only for the existing diseases, but also for the diseases of the future which may become more important as a consequence of lifestyle changes and increasing age.

Malaria (caused in humans by single-celled *Plasmodium* protozoa parasites), tuberculosis (caused by *Mycobacterium tuberculosis*) and leprosy (caused by *Mycobacterium leprae*) can be considered examples of 'older' diseases still in need of more effective and cheaper treatments. Each year, 300–500 million people contract malaria and about 2–3 million die. A number of medicines, including chloroquine, 4-aminoquinolines, atovaquone, malarone, halofantrine, mefloquine, proguanil and artemisinin derivatives, are available for treatment.[16,17] Three main types of vaccines, based on the three major phases of the parasite life cycle, are being developed: antisporozoite vaccines designed to prevent infection (pre-erythrocytic vaccines); anti-asexual blood stage vaccines (anti-invasion and anticomplication) designed to reduce severe and complicated manifestations of the disease; and transmission-blocking vaccines aimed at arresting the development of the parasite in the mosquito itself.[18] A number of vaccines are in phase I and II clinical trials. Monoclonal antibodies against specific malarial antigens are being explored for diagnostic and potential therapeutic purposes. In addition, efforts are beginning to be made to shed light on the origin of the development of resistance in specific cases. Discovery of complete genome sequences of the human malaria parasite *Plasmodium falciparum* and the malaria-transmitting mosquito *Anopheles gambiae* is likely to enhance the discovery of antimalarial drug candidates.

Like malaria, tuberculosis and leprosy are more common in less developed countries. Tuberculosis is the second leading cause of death worldwide, killing nearly 2 million people each year. Multidrug-resistant tuberculosis continues to be a serious problem, particularly among some countries of Eastern Europe, China and Iran. Currently available drugs for tuberculosis include isoniazid, rifampicin, pyrazinamide and ethambutol. Further work is ongoing to discover new tuberculosis targets and drugs.[19–22] Several vaccines, including subunit vaccines and live vaccines such as recombinant bacille Calmette–Guérin (BCG) and other attenuated live vaccines, are currently in development for the prevention and treatment of tuberculosis.[23] The goal is to obtain a new generation of vaccines (superior to BCG), effective against more transmissible forms of tuberculosis. The first-line drugs against leprosy are rifampicin, clofazimine and dapsone. Other drugs such as minocycline, the macrolide clarithromycin and the fluoroquinolones pefloxacin and ofloxacin are all highly active against *M. leprae* but because of their cost are rarely used in field programmes.

Bone disorders such as arthritis, osteoporosis and Paget's disease are examples of diseases that are becoming increasingly important with the ageing population.[24,25] Anti-inflammatory glucocorticoids such as prednisolone and methylprednisolone, and

H$_2$NSO$_2$

CF$_3$

Me

3 Celecoxib

Me

OH

O

NH

Cl

F

4 Lumiracoxib

H$_2$NO$_2$S

Me

O

N

5 Valdecoxib

immunosuppressants such as ciclosporin and dexame-thasone are used for treatment. Although the treatment options have increased recently, most of these therapies focus on addressing the symptoms rather than the underlying causes of the disease. For example, cyclo-oxygenase-2 (COX-2) inhibitors such as celecoxib (3), lumiracoxib (4), etoricoxib,[26] valdecoxib[27] (5) and parecoxib (prodrug of valdecoxib) are being marketed as safer non-steroidal anti-inflammatory drugs (NSAIDs).[28,29] Although the older NSAIDs are highly effective as analgesic, antipyretic and anti-inflammatory agents, long-term ingestion causes gastric lesions. The discovery that the COX enzyme, which catalyses the conversion of arachidonic acid to prostaglandin H$_2$ (common biosynthetic precursor to prostaglandins and thromboxane – mediators of physiological and pathological processes, including pain, fever and inflammation),[30] exists in two isoforms, with COX-2 being the primary isoform at sites of inflammation, led to a suggestion that inhibition of this isoform accounts for the therapeutic benefit of NSAIDs whereas inhibition of COX-1 results in adverse effects. The newer COX-2 selective agents appear to have a superior gastrointestinal safety profile. COX-2 inhibitors are also being investigated for the prevention

and treatment of colorectal cancer. In addition to COX-2 inhibitors, inhibitors of matrix metalloproteinases (MMPs) are emerging for the treatment of many diseases including arthritis. Enzymes that degrade the extracellular matrix are normally controlled by a set of tissue inhibitors that, if disrupted, will allow the enzymes to work unchecked, degrading the matrix and promoting not only arthritis but also tumour growth and metastasis. Another treatment option is inhibition of tumour necrosis factor α (TNFα), an inflammation-promoting cytokine associated with multiple inflammatory events, including arthritis. Anti-TNFα therapies are already on the market.

Recently, the process of drug discovery has been expanded to cover a range of molecular biology, biotechnology and medicinal chemistry (including combinatorial chemistry) techniques. The newer disciplines such as genome analysis, proteomics and bioinformatics are likely to lead to many new targets (e.g. receptors, enzymes) and therapeutically important proteins. Techniques such as combinatorial chemistry and high-throughput screening are expected to identify hits/leads against various therapeutically important receptors and enzymes. Depending upon the knowledge available on the receptor or the enzyme of interest, the hits/leads can then be modified in a random, semi-rational or rational manner to generate drug candidates. From the commercial point of view, this progress is essential as the discovery process becomes more expensive and more generic drugs become available.[31] Some of the best-selling drugs of today that have either come off patent recently or are near the end of their patent-protected life include alendronate, cetirizine, interferon β-1b, risperidone, lansoprazole, atorvastatin, docetaxel, donepezil, pioglitazone, clopidogrel, enoxaparin and sildenafil.

As in earlier chapters in the 4th and 5th Editions of the book,[32] this chapter includes a short account of the historical aspects[33] and a short introduction to some of the newer disciplines. The main objective of the chapter is to give an idea about the changing disease patterns which may be reflected in the discovery process, examples of receptor agonists and antagonists, enzyme inhibitors (including signal transduction inhibitors) and inhibitors of protein–protein interaction that have been discovered by random and 'semi-rational/rational' approaches, antibody, vaccine and protein therapeutics and currently available drugs for more widespread diseases. This enables one to understand actual drug discovery procedures and the science that has led to many drugs currently on the market and also gives an idea about the currently

available drugs for the treatment/prevention of various diseases. Examples of some of the commonly used drugs to treat various diseases (acting by different mechanisms) include:
- COX inhibitors (3–5);
- Angiotensin-converting enzyme (ACE) inhibitors (antihypertensives such as captopril and lisinopril);
- Histamine H_1 receptor antagonists [anti-allergic compounds such as fexofenadine (6)];
- Histamine H_2 receptor antagonists [acid secretion inhibitors such as cimetidine and ranitidine (7)];
- Proton pump inhibitors [acid secretion inhibitors such as omeprazole and esomeprazole (8);[34]
- Nuclear peroxisome proliferator activated receptor-γ activators such as pioglitazone (9) and troglitazone (type 2 diabetes mellitus treatments);
- Lipid-lowering agents such as atorvastatin (10) and rosuvastatin and cholesterol absorption inhibitor ezetimibe (11);[35]
- Anti-influenza treatments such as zanamivir (12);[36]
- Acetylcholinesterase inhibitors such as donepezil (13) for the treatment of Alzheimer's disease;

6 Fexofenadine

7 Ranitidine

8 Esomeprazole

9 Pioglitazone

10 Atorvastatin

11 Ezetimibe

12 Zanamivir

13 Donepezil

- Selective and competitive inhibitor of the cysteinyl leukotrienes (LTC_4, LTD_4 and LTE_4) such as zafirlukast and montelukast (14) for the treatment of asthma;
- Sildenafil (15) and udenafil (1) (inhibitors of phosphodiesterase type 5 used for erectile dysfunction);
- Antiobesity drugs such as orlistat (16);
- Atypical antipsychotic agents such as quetiapine (17) and olanzapine (18); and
- Immunosuppressant drugs such as tacrolimus (FK506) (19), ciclosporin (calcineurin inhibitors)[37] and everolimus.[38]

It may be useful to mention at this stage that many of the highly successful drugs launched in the last

14 Montelukast

15 Sildenafil

16 Orlistat

17 Quetiapine

18 Olanzapine

19 Tacrolimus

in the clinic as an anti-anginal drug when its beneficial effects in improving erectile function were observed.

1.2 Market needs and changing disease patterns

From the point of view of the discovery of new medicines, it is important to project changing disease patterns and markets so that the new drugs may become available early. Currently, the industrialised world accounts for 11–12% of the global burden from all causes of death and disability but >90% of health expenditure; most of the remainder is spent in the form of public health aid. The Global Burden of Disease Study initiated in 1992 by the World Bank in collaboration with the World Health Organization (WHO) has sought to quantify mortality, life expectancy and risk factors for different regions of the world, and to project trends in mortality and disability in 2020. Of the 10 leading causes of death and disability in 1990 (Table 1.1), those from ischaemic heart disease, cerebrovascular disease, cancer and lower respiratory infections are in the established market economies, whereas most deaths brought about by diarrhoea, communicable diseases, maternal and perinatal conditions and nutritional deficiencies are in the developing world. Overall, in the industrialised regions, only 6.1% deaths were brought about by communicable (infectious and parasitic diseases), maternal, perinatal and nutritional conditions, and deaths from non-communicable diseases (e.g. cardiovascular, cancer) and injuries accounted for 86.2% and 7.6%, respectively. Considering disability alone in the industrialised regions, the leading causes in 1990 were unipolar major depression, iron deficiency anaemia, falls, alcohol abuse, chronic obstructive pulmonary disease,

25 years were discovered in the pre-genomic era and the real contribution of all the new technologies mentioned above remains to be proven. In some cases the drug was initially investigated for different indications. For example, sildenafil was being investigated

Table 1.1 Leading causes of death and disability worldwide (1990–2020)

Rank	1990	2020
1	Ischaemic heart disease	Ischaemic heart disease
2	Cerebrovascular disease	Unipolar major depression
3	Lower respiratory infections	Road traffic accidents
4	Diarrhoeal diseases	Cerebrovascular disease
5	Perinatal disorders	Chronic obstructive pulmonary disease
6	Chronic obstructive pulmonary disease	Lower respiratory infections
7	Tuberculosis (HIV excluded)	Tuberculosis
8	Measles	War injuries
9	Road traffic accidents	Diarrhoeal diseases
10	Lung, tracheal and bronchial cancer	HIV

In 1990, just over 50 million died worldwide (53% males); 10.912 million in the industrialised world and 39.554 million in the developing regions.

bipolar disorder, congenital anomalies, osteoarthritis, schizophrenia and obsessive-compulsive disorder. Absence of cancer from the top 10 killers of 2020 reflects use of a disability-adjusted measure used in the study rather than discovery of a magical cure, although new medicines and regimens have increased survival rates in cancer patients. Indeed, the fact that the analysis of gastrointestinal cancer is organ-based while cancers affecting the respiratory system are lumped together also distorts the above analysis. Thus, deaths from all cancers affecting the respiratory system (lung, trachea and bronchi) have been aggregated to make this the tenth leading cause of mortality. Aggregating all the data for the bowel (oesophageal, stomach and colorectal tumours) would elevate gastrointestinal cancer to eighth place. Similarly, liver disease (cirrhosis plus cancer) at 1.38 million would rank as the ninth leading cause of death.

Health trends over the next 20 years will be largely determined by ageing of the world's (female) population, a 40% fall in developing world deaths from communicable, perinatal and nutritional causes, and a 77% increase in non-communicable diseases, including a 180% increase in tobacco-attributable mortality. The potential for so-called 'lifestyle' drugs (e.g. anti-smoking treatments) is also apparent. While the drug industry may not be quite so aware of opportunities in relation to trauma, it has recognized the threats posed both by psychotic illness and AIDS. The prediction that depression will rank second in terms of disability-adjusted life-years creates opportunity for drugs directed at peripheral as well as central sites such as those targeting the brain–gut axis.

1.3 Medicines marketed in the years 2004–2007

The issue of productivity in drug discovery using all the new technologies is currently being debated.[39–41] Looking at the drugs marketed during 2004–2007 (approximately 250 in total) it is clear that very few are medicines with a new mechanism of action (first-in-the-class) and the remaining are follow-up compounds based on the initial discovery, new formulations of existing drugs, new indications for existing medicines or combination products incorporating existing medicines.[42–44] In fact, over the last 30 years (1997–2006) only about 70 first-in-class drugs were launched.[45] The best-known examples of these include cimetidine (1977), captopril (1980), lovastatin (1987), omeprazole (1987), enoxaparin (1987), ondansetron (1990), losartan (1994), saquinavir (1995), clopidogrel (1997), celecoxib (1998), trastuzumab (1998), ezetimibe (2002), enfuvirtide (2003), natalizumab (2004), rimonabant (2006) and sitagliptin (2006). Many of the new formulations (Table 1.2) were transdermal formulations (ease of administration) or depot formulations allowing the drug to be released over an extended period of time. In some cases, such as albumin-bound paclitaxel (Abraxane), the new formulation was designed to increase solubility and to increase drug delivery to tumour cells.[46] Drugs marketed for new indications (Table 1.3) included many drugs such as aripiprazole, quetiapine, risperidone, duloxetine and pregabalin, initially licensed for neurological diseases such as schizophrenia, depression and epilepsy and then expanded

Table 1.2 Examples of new drug formulations

Drug	Constituent	New formulation, indication
Veramyst	Fluticasone furoate	Nasal spray, seasonal and year round allergy symptoms
Omnaris	Ciclesonide	Nasal spray formulation, allergic rhinitis symptoms
AzaSite	Azithromycin	DuraSite drug delivery vehicle – synthetic polymer-based formulation (ophthalmic solution), bacterial conjunctivitis
Relestat	Epinastine HCl	Ophthalmic solution formulation – prevention of itching associated with allergic conjunctivitis
Retisert	Fluocinolone acetonide	Drug reservoir to deliver sustained levels of the drug for 30 months (intravitreal implant), chronic non-infectious uveitis affecting the posterior segment of the eye
Daytrana	Methylphenidate	Transdermal patch (adhesive-based matrix), once daily, attention deficit hyperactivity disorder
Emsam	Selegiline	Transdermal patch, major depressive disorder
Exelon	Rivastigmine	Transdermal patch, Alzheimer's disease
Reclast, Aclasta	Zoledronic acid	Once-yearly formulation (15-minute intravenous infusion) – reducing the risk of fractures (hip, spine and non-spine)
Synera	Lidocaine and tetracaine	Topical local anaesthetic patch, used to numb the skin before various medical procedures
Zingo	Lidocaine HCl monohydrate	Powder form incorporated in an intradermal delivery system – reduction of pain associated with venous access procedures
DepoDur	Morphine sulfate	Injectable depot formulation using lipid-based drug delivery technology (epidural injection) – 48 h of pain control in patients undergoing surgical procedures (e.g. hip and knee replacement, and lower abdominal surgery)
Abraxane	Paclitaxel	Protein-bound particles for injectable suspension (using nanoparticle albumin-bound technology), breast cancer
Lialda	Mesalamine	Oral once-daily formulation – active, mild to moderate ulcerative colitis
Roliflo OD	Tamsulosin HCl and tolterodine tartarate	Extended-release capsule formulation (once daily) – management of bladder outlet obstruction (men with benign prostatic hyperplasia, with concomitant over-active bladder)
Climara Pro	Tradiol/levonorgestrel	Transdermal patch (once-a-week) – moderate to severe symptoms of menopause such as hot flushes and night sweats
Estrasorb	Oestradiol	Topical emulsion (soya-based oil formulation) – moderate to severe symptoms in menopausal women
Menostar	Oestradiol	Transdermal patch (once-a-week), oestrogen therapy for post-menopausal osteoporosis
Intrinsa	Testosterone	Transdermal patch (twice a week) – low sexual desire in women who have experienced an early menopause
Tostrex	Testosterone	Transdermal gel (metered dose delivery system) – treatment of male hypogonadism
Nebido	Testosterone undecanoate	Depot injection formulation (four times a year) – testosterone replacement therapy for men with hypogonadism

Table 1.3 Existing drugs marketed for new indications

Drug	Old indication	New indication
Abilify (aripiprazole)	Schizophrenia	Acute manic and mixed episodes associated with bipolar disorder
Seroquel (quetiapine)	Schizophrenia	Bipolar disorder in patients experiencing acute mania (in combination with mood stabilisers)
Risperdal (risperidone)	Acute and chronic schizophrenia	Irritability associated with autistic disorder, including symptoms of aggression, deliberate self-injury, temper tantrums and quickly changing moods, in children and adolescents
Cymbalta (duloxetine)	Major depressive disorder, urinary incontinence	Pain associated with diabetic peripheral neuropathy, generalised anxiety disorder
Lyrica (pregabalin)	Epilepsy and neuropathic pain	Fibromyalgia syndrome, generalised anxiety disorder
CellCept (mycophenolate mofetil)	Immunosuppression (with ciclosporin and corticosteroids)	Induction and maintenance treatment of lupus nephritis, when used concomitantly with corticosteroids
Prograf (tacrolimus)	Prophylaxis of rejection (bone marrow and organ transplant), generalised myasthenia gravis	Treatment of lupus nephritis, rheumatoid arthritis in patients who respond insufficiently to current therapies
Tracleer, Actelion (bosenthan)	Treatment of PAH	Reduction of new digital ulcers in patients with systemic sclerosis and ongoing digital ulcer disease
Taxotere (docetaxel)	Breast and lung cancers	Hormone-refractory metastatic prostate cancer (in combination with prednisone)
Evista (raloxifene HCl)	Prevention and treatment of osteoporosis in postmenopausal women	Reducing the risk of invasive breast cancer in postmenopausal women with osteoporosis or at high risk for invasive breast cancer
Sigmart (nicorandil)	Unstable angina pectoris	Acute heart failure, including acute decompensation of chronic heart failure
Aceon (perindopril erbumine)	Hypertension	Treatment of patients with stable coronary disease to reduce the risk of cardiovascular mortality or non-fatal myocardial infarction
Yaz (drospirenone/ethinyl estradiol)	Oral contraceptive, emotional and physical symptoms of premenstrual dysphoric disorder	Treatment of moderate acne in women, oral contraceptive for birth control
EvaMist (estradiol)	Treatment of hot flushes in women	Treatment for vasomotor symptoms associated with menopause
Dinagest (dienogest)	Component in oral contraceptive and hormone replacement therapy agents	Endometriosis
Osonase (ciclesonide)	Asthma	Seasonal and perennial allergic rhinitis in adults and adolescents

PAH, pulmonary arterial hypertension.

to cover other neurological conditions. The combination products (Table 1.4) launched were primarily for cardiovascular and respiratory disorders and type 2 diabetes. Combinations of calcium-channel blockers such as amlodipine and lercanidipine, ACE inhibitors such as ramipril and enalapril, and angiotensin II receptor antagonists such as valsartan and olmesartan were launched for the treatment of hypertension.

Table 1.4 Drugs marketed as combination products

Drug	Components	Indication
Caduet	Amlodipine besylate and atorvastatin calcium	Simultaneous treatment of hypertension and high cholesterol
Exforge	Amlodipine besylate and valsartan	Hypertension
Azor	Amlodipine besylate and olmesartan medoxomil	Hypertension
Zanipress, Zaneril and Carmen ACE	Lercanidipine and enalapril	Hypertension
CVpill	Atorvastatin, ramipril, enteric-coated aspirin and metoprolol succinate (extended release)	Cardiovascular disease in patients with multiple risk factors (LDL cholesterol, hypertension, serum homocysteine and platelet function)
Vytorin, Zintrepid	Ezetimibe and simvastatin	Treatment of hypercholesterolaemia
BiDil	Hydralazine and isosorbide nitrate	Heart failure (black patients)
Pylera	Metronidazole, tetracycline and bismuth biskalcitrate	Eradication of *H. pylori*, gastric acid secretion
Janumet	Sitagliptin phosphate monohydrate and metformin	Type 2 diabetes – not adequately controlled on metformin or sitagliptin alone
Avandaryl	Rosiglitazone maleate and glimepiride	Type 2 diabetes in patients not adequately controlled on a sulphonylurea alone
Duetact	Pioglitazone and glimepiride	Type 2 diabetes
ACTOplus Met	Pioglitazone and metformin	Type-2 diabetes not adequately controlled with metformin or pioglitazone alone
Fosamax Plus D	Alendronate sodium and cholecalciferol	Osteoporosis in postmenopausal women
GEM-21S	Recombinant human platelet-derived growth factor and β-tricalcium phosphate	Periodontal bone defects and associated gingival recession
Symbyax	Olanzapine and fluoxetine	Depressive episodes associated with bipolar disorder
Ganfort	Bimatoprost and timolol maleate	Open-angle glaucoma and ocular hypertension
DuoTrav	Travoprost and timolol maleate	Open-angle glaucoma or ocular hypertension
Zylet	Loteprednol etabonate and tobramycin	Steroid-responsive inflammatory ocular conditions with superficial bacterial ocular infection or a risk of infection
Osovair	Ciclesonide and formoterol fumarate (dry powder inhaler)	Treatment of asthma
Avessa	Formoterol fumarate and fluticasone propionate	Treatment of asthma
Foster	Formoterol fumarate and beclometasone dipropionate	Treatment of asthma
Clarinex-D	Desloratadine and pseudoephedrine sulphate, extended release (24 h) tablet	Relief of the nasal and non-nasal symptoms of seasonal allergic rhinitis, including nasal congestion

ACE, angiotensin converting enzyme; LDL, low density lipoprotein.

A combination of amlodipine and atorvastatin was marketed for simultaneous treatment of hypertension and high cholesterol. Atorvastatin and ezetimibe were combined to reduce low-density lipoprotein (LDL) cholesterol in patients with high levels of cholesterol. In one case (CVpill), four drugs [atorvastatin, ramipril, enteric-coated aspirin and metoprolol succinate (extended release)] were combined to cover all major cardiovascular risk factors. Combination products for respiratory diseases such as asthma included established therapies with steroids (ciclesonide, fluticasone, beclometasone) and β-stimulants (formoterol). A new approach to design multi-target drugs, in place of combination drugs, has been suggested to be better against complex diseases.[47]

1.4 Historical aspects

1.4.1 Early discoveries
A number of early medicines, including morphine, atropine, salicylic acid and quinine, were isolated from plants. Over the years the search for therapeutic agents was widened to isolate compounds from natural products[48] including living agents such as bacteria, fungi,[49] sea animals and even humans. The important discoveries from this research not only include anti-infective agents such as penicillin and tetracyclin, but many other hormones and transmitters. Ivermectin (a drug used to treat tropical filariosis), amphotericin B, lovastatin (HMG-CoA reductase inhibitor), insulin, heparin (anticoagulant), paclitaxel (anticancer), artemisinin (antimalarial), ciclosporin, mycophenolate mofetil, tacrolimus and FK506 (immunosuppressants) and Xenical (anti-obesity) are other examples either originating from natural sources or modified versions of the natural products. One of the more recent examples of a natural product-derived medicine reaching the market is trabectedin (Yondelis) (20). This marine-derived antitumour compound, a DNA minor groove-binding agent, was approved for marketing for the treatment of advanced soft tissue sarcoma. Many of the biologically active peptides such as oxytocin, vasopressin, adrenocorticotrophic hormone, insulin, calcitonin, luteinising hormone releasing hormone, growth hormone and erythropoietin are important examples of compounds isolated from humans and other animals that have led to medicines currently used in clinical practice. In addition, discoveries of many other agents such as adrenaline, histamine, tyramine, tryptamine and γ-aminobutyric acid their receptors have led to extremely important medicines.

20 Trabectedin

21 Prontosil

22 Sulfanilamide

23 Furosemide

24 Tolbutamide

Many other early discoveries were primarily based on low-throughput random screening approaches. The mechanism of action was later rationalised when additional biochemical and pharmacological information became available. Examples of early drugs include sulfa drugs which led to the discoveries of several other classes of drugs.[33] For example, the active metabolite of the sulfonamide prontosil (21), inhibits the enzyme carbonic anhydrase, leading to an increase in natriuresis and the excretion of water. Sulfanilamide (22) gave rise to better carbonic anhydrase inhibitors such as acetazolamide and later led to more effective diuretics such as hydrochlorothiazide and furosemide (23). Further chemistry in the field led to the development of sulfonylureas such as tolbutamide (24), used in the treatment of type 2 diabetes.

1.5 Impact of new technology on drug discovery

1.5.1 Receptor subtypes

Since the idea of a receptor as a selective binding site for chemotherapeutic agents was developed, huge progress has been made in the identification, characterisation and classification of receptors and receptor subtypes. In addition, knowledge has been gained about the downstream signalling pathways, most often involving transcription factors that ultimately act on DNA and result in altered gene expression. Mapping the key signalling molecules in biochemical pathways and attempting to modulate their effects is resulting in new areas of drug discovery. The early assumption that a ligand acts at one receptor is no longer tenable and it is now well established that many endogenous ligands act at different receptor subtypes. The availability of more selective synthetic ligands, and cloning and amino acid sequencing technologies, have shown that different receptor subtypes exist for most of the receptors. The situation is further complicated by the existence of different receptor subtypes in different tissues in the same species, and by structural differences in receptor subtypes in different species of animals. Many recent studies have indicated that G-protein-coupled receptors form homo-oligomeric and hetero-oligomeric complexes and these complexes ('new receptors') have functional characteristics that differ from homogeneous populations of their constituent receptors.[50] Thus, the accumulated knowledge has not only provided many challenges for the drug discovery process, but has opened a way to many new drug discovery targets and much more selective treatments.

From the point of view of drug discovery, ligands acting at the G-protein-coupled receptors [at orthosteric sites (interacting with the same domain as the endogenous agonist) or allosteric sites (topographically distinct from the orthosteric site)] have resulted in most successful drug candidates and new drug targets.[51–55] Current work on nuclear receptors involved in the metabolism of glucose, fat, cholesterol and bile acid (e.g. peroxisome proliferator-activated receptors, the liver X receptors and the farnesoid X receptor in human diseases), including type 2 diabetes, dyslipidaemia, atherosclerosis and the metabolic syndrome, illustrates an example of receptors that have given some drugs (e.g. pioglitazone, rosiglitazone and ciglitazone) and provided new targets for additional drugs. Similarly, oestrogen receptors have provided many drugs (e.g. tamoxifen) and work is ongoing to establish the role of oestrogen receptors as new target

for the treatment of diabetes.[56] Some examples illustrating how receptor research has led to more selective drugs and enhanced our understanding of the roles of various receptor subtypes in disease processes are mentioned below. Early examples of different receptor subtypes that led to clinically useful drugs include α and β adrenergic receptors (cell-surface G-protein-coupled receptors for catecholamines) and histamine H_1 and H_2 receptor subtypes. One of the more complicated and extensively studied area of receptor subtypes is the field of 5-hydroxytryptamine (5-HT; serotonin) receptors.[57] The seven receptor subtypes, 5-HT_1 to 5-HT_7, have been characterised by using selective ligands (agonists and antagonists); cloning and amino acid sequencing techniques have been used to define molecular structures and intracellular transduction mechanisms. Several of the more selective compounds have reached the market for the treatment of various disorders of the nervous system. For example, several selective 5-HT_3 antagonists [e.g. ondansetron (25), granisetron, tropisetron, nazasetron (26) and ramosetron] are marketed for the management of nausea and vomiting induced by cancer chemotherapy and radiotherapy. Tryptamine $5\text{-HT}_{1B/1D}$ receptor agonists such as sumatriptan (27), almotriptan, frovatriptan, zomitriptan (28), rizatriptan, naratriptan and eletriptan are marketed for the treatment of migraine. The 5-HT_3 receptor antagonist alosetron (diarrhoea-predominant irritable bowel

25 Ondansetron

26 Nazasetron

27 Sumatriptan

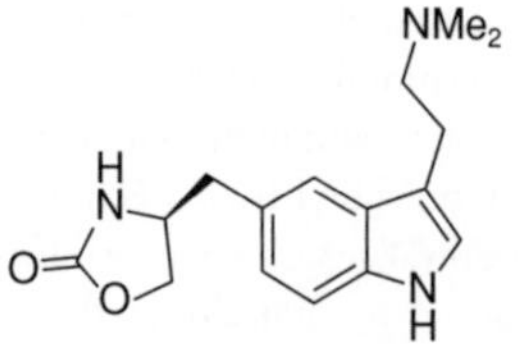

28 Zomitriptan

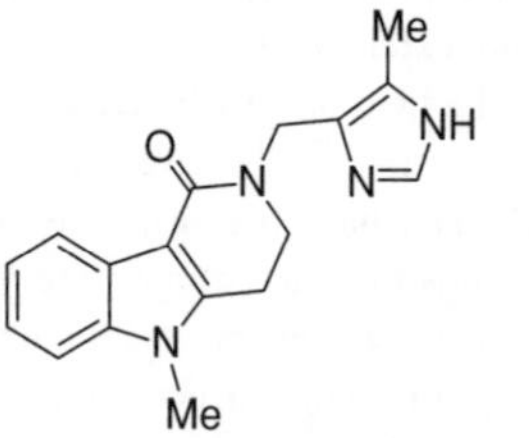

29 Alosetron

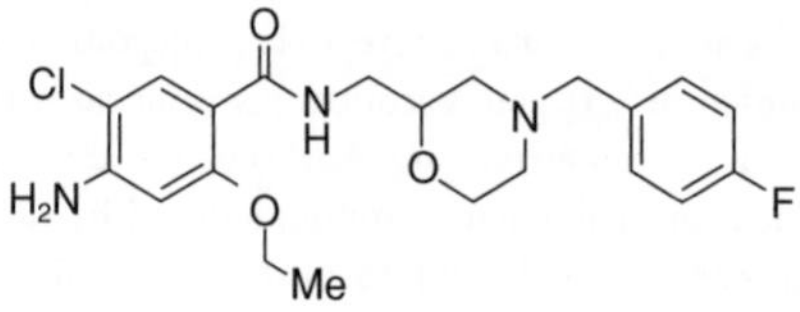

30 Mosapride

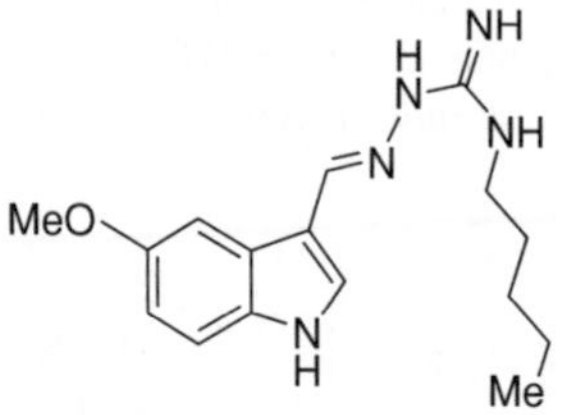

31 Tegaserod

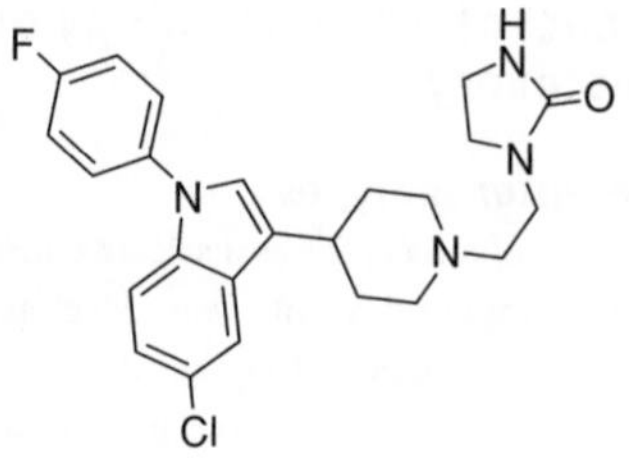

32 Sertindole

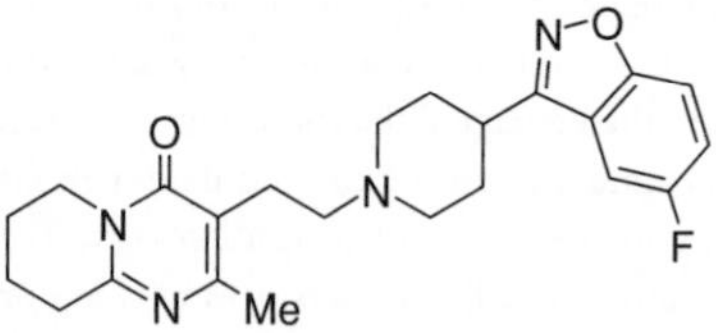

33 Risperidone

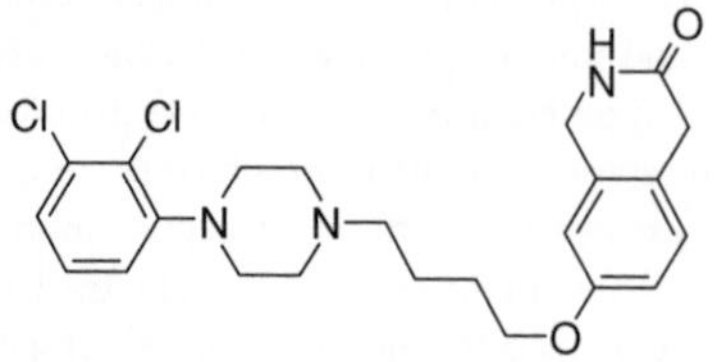

34 Aripiprazole

syndrome) (**29**) and the 5-HT$_4$ receptor partial agonists mosapride (**30**) (relief of gastrointestinal symptoms in patients with gastritis, gastro-oesophageal reflux, dyspepsia) and tegaserod (**31**) (constipation-predominant irritable bowel syndrome) are marketed for various gastrointestinal conditions. Many other 5-HT receptor ligands with dopamine receptor activity have been marketed as antipsychotic agents. Examples of this class of compounds include quetiapine (**17**), olanzapine (**18**), ziprasidone, sertindole (**32**), risperidone (**33**) and aripiprazole (**34**).

In case of the histamine receptor ligands, H$_1$ and H$_2$ receptor antagonists such as fexofenadine [(**6**), anti-allergic] and ranitidine [(**7**), acid secretion inhibitor] are highly successful drugs. However, two other receptor subtypes (H$_3$ and H$_4$) have only been

identified relatively recently and ligands to these receptor subtypes are currently being identified in order to explore the role of these subtypes in pathological processes. The role of histamine in atherosclerosis and brain is also under active consideration.[58–60] Like histamine receptors, new adrenoceptors have also been identified. Initially, β-adrenoceptors of the β$_1$ and β$_2$ subtypes were shown to mediate the effects of catecholamines on the force of contraction of cardiac muscle, and on the relaxation of vascular smooth muscle. However, characterization of a third β-adrenoceptor subtype (β$_3$) and its presence in human heart has changed the classically admitted paradigm on the regulation of heart function by the β-adrenergic system.[61] In blood vessels, β$_3$-AR, like β$_1$ and β$_2$, produced a relaxation. But, at the present time, the physiological role of β$_3$-AR is not clearly identified.

Other more recent examples of new receptor subtypes include neurokinin, melanocortin and somatostatin receptor subtypes. Neurokinins (substance P, neurokinin A and neurokinin B) act at three receptor subtypes: NK$_1$, NK$_2$ and NK$_3$. Selective ligands are being explored for the treatment of pain, asthma, depression, etc. The natural melanocortic peptides are derived from the precursor peptide pro-opiomelanocortin (expressed in the pituitary) by proteolytic cleavage in three regions of the protein generating adenocorticotrophic hormone (ACTH), and α-, β- and γ-melanocyte stimulating hormone (MSH) peptides. Pro-opiomelanocortin also generates a number of other peptides including enkephalin and β-endorphin. Five melanocortin receptor subtypes (MC_1–MC_5) belonging to the G-protein-coupled receptor family have been cloned (40–60% sequence identities) and selective ligands for the receptor subtypes have been synthesised.[62] Early pharmacological studies have indicated that drugs selective for the MC_1 receptor may be useful for the treatment of inflammatory conditions, whereas compounds selective for the MC_4 receptor may be useful for controlling eating behaviour and body weight.

Cloning studies have identified five receptor subtypes of somatostatin [Ala-Gly-Cys-Lys-Asn-Phe-Phe-Trp-Lys-Thr-Phe-Thr-Ser-Cys, a cyclic peptide with a disulphide bridge], a peptide discovered in 1971–1972 and shown to be an inhibitor of growth hormone, insulin, glucagon and gastric acid secretion. Library screening followed by studies of structure–activity relationships led to the development of compounds selective for the five human Somatostatin (hSST) receptor subtypes (35–39).[63,64] In vitro experiments using these selective compounds demonstrated

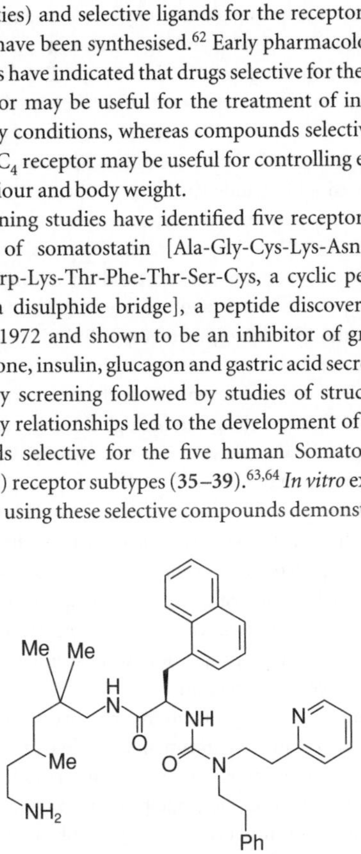

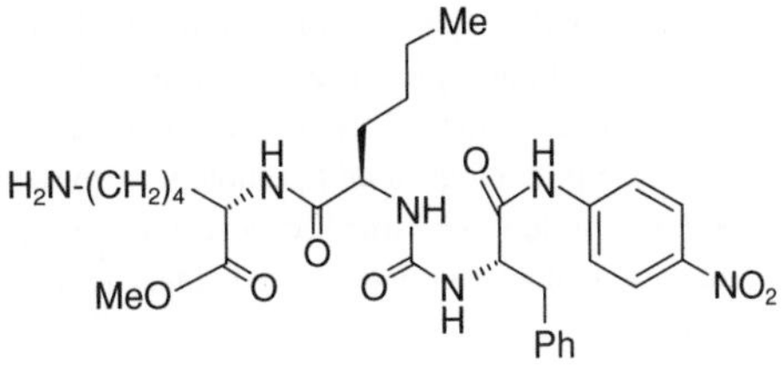

37 hSSTR₃ selective

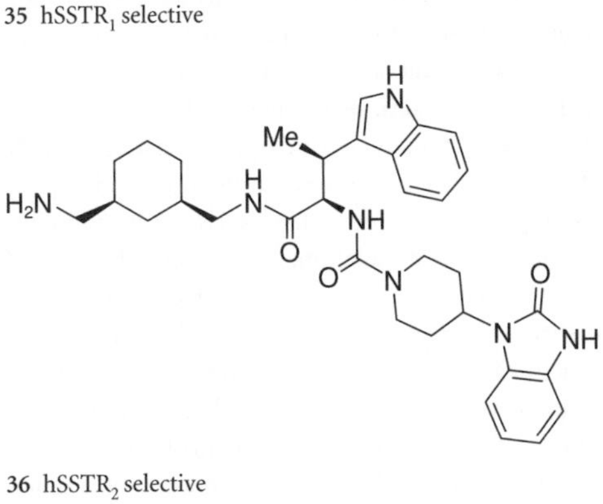

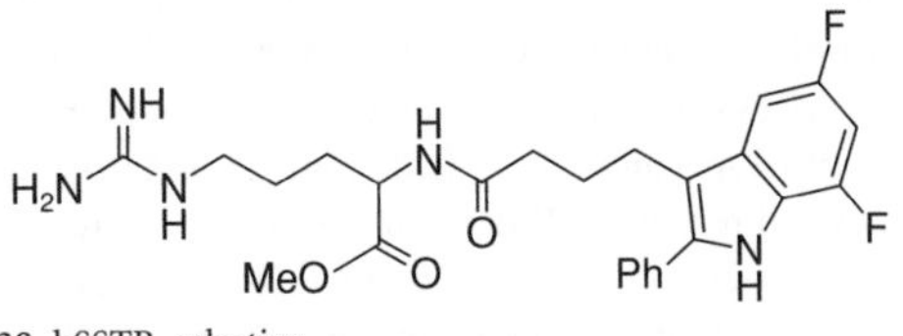

38 hSSTR₄ selective

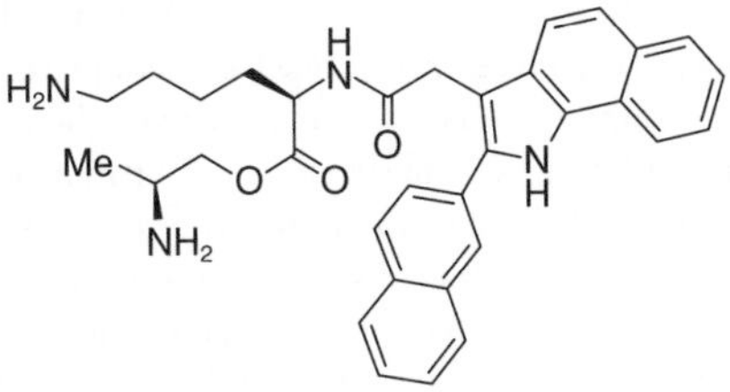

39 hSSTR₅ selective

35 hSSTR₁ selective

36 hSSTR₂ selective

the role of the $hSST_2$ receptor in inhibition of glucagon release from mouse pancreatic α-cells and the $hSST_5$ receptor as a mediator of insulin secretion from pancreatic β-cells. Both subtypes of receptors regulated release of growth hormone from the rat anterior pituitary gland. Some of the recent information has shown that the five receptor subtypes may fall into two classes or groups. One class ($SRIF_1$) appears to comprise SST_2, SST_3 and SST_5, and the other class ($SRIF_2$) consists of the other two recombinant receptor subtypes (SST_1 and SST_4).

More recently, attention has also been focused on orphan G-protein-coupled receptors, a family of plasma membrane proteins involved in a broad array of signalling pathways.[65] Novel members of the orphan G-protein-coupled receptors have continued to emerge through cloning activities as well as through bioinformatic analysis of sequence databases. Their ligands are unidentified and their physiological relevance remains to be defined. Methods are being developed to identify ligands acting at these receptors. One of these approaches identifies ligands by purification from biological fluids, cell supernatants or tissue extracts. The discoveries of endothelin (a vasoconstrictor peptide) and nociceptin (an orphan opioid-like receptor ligand) are examples of this type. It is also possible to identify ligands by screening orphan receptors against diverse chemical libraries. Once identified the ligand is used to clarify the physiological and pathological roles of the receptor, followed by the discovery of other agonist and antagonist analogues by medicinal chemistry approaches.

Proteinases (enzymes) have long been known for their degradation and catalytic properties and generating active enzymes from their inactive precursors. However, recent work has demonstrated the utility of enzymes in activating receptors. The discovery of receptors specifically activated by proteases, protease-activated receptors (PARs), has added to the concept that proteases are not only degradative enzymes, but also important signalling molecules. Proteases of the coagulation cascade, such as thrombin and factors Xa and VIIa, have been shown to activate PARs, which in turn have been recently identified as major players in innate immunity. The PARs may therefore be novel therapeutic targets for the treatment of inflammation, haemostasis, thrombosis and vascular dysfunctions.[66]

Currently, the drug discovery process has progressed beyond the receptor stage and various steps that result from the interaction of the receptor with a specific ligand have been characterised. One of the more important processes, signal transduction, converts the external signals induced by hormones, growth factors, neurotransmitters and cytokines into specific internal cellular responses (e.g. gene expression, cell division or even cell suicide). The process involves a cascade of enzyme-mediated reactions inside the cell which typically include phosphorylation and dephosphorylation of proteins (kinases and phosphatases) as mediators of downstream processes. Signal transduction inhibitors are currently being developed for the treatment of a number of diseases, including cancer and inflammation.

1.5.2 Genomics (including stem cell research)

The term genomics is applied to the study of genomes and the complete collection of genes that they contain. In addition to the protein-coding genes, it is now clear that many other elements have important functions in the genome, such as transcription factor binding domains, regions encoding microRNAs and antisense transcripts, and large, evolutionarily conserved regions. Genetic factors influence virtually every human disorder (e.g. Alzheimer's and Parkinson's diseases, diabetes, asthma and rheumatoid arthritis) by determining disease susceptibility[67] or resistance and interactions with environmental factors. Gene transfer research ('gene therapy') holds promise for treating disorders through the transfer and expression of DNA in the cells of patients. Initial concept of gene therapy was focused on the treatment of genetic diseases (e.g. cystic fibrosis, Duchenne's muscular dystrophy and Gaucher's disease) but the field has now been expanded and many more options such as cancer, cardiovascular diseases, arthritis, type 1 diabetes [e.g. non-insulin glucose lowering genes, gene(s) capable of restoring glucose-regulated production of insulin and neogenesis and regeneration of pancreatic islets],[68] neurodegenerative disorders, X-linked severe combined immunodeficiency[69] and infectious diseases, including acquired immunodeficiency syndrome, are being considered. Cancer treatment options are most advanced and include suicide gene therapy, tumour suppressor gene therapy, cytokine gene therapy and expression of 'prodrug activating enzymes' with the ability to convert a non-toxic 'prodrug' administered to the patient into a cytotoxic agent at the tumour site. Although many gene therapy clinical trials have started, several important issues, including efficient delivery of the genetic material to the required sites,[70] along with other chemical, biological, safety, toxicity and ethical issues, have not yet been fully resolved. From the point of view of drug discovery, mapping of the human genome is only the first step. It is likely that even when the human genomic sequencing has been fully completed and all genes have been identified, a substantial fraction of these, possibly up to 50%, will have complex biochemical or physiological functions. Therefore, only a proportion will be amenable to pharmacological exploitation.

Another major problem is the involvement of many genes and environmental factors in various diseases. For example, with the exception of some diseases or traits resulting principally from specific and relatively rare mutations (e.g. cystic fibrosis), most of the genetic disorders (e.g. cardiovascular diseases, diabetes, rheumatoid arthritis and schizophrenia) develop as a result of a network of genes failing to perform correctly, some of which might have a major disease effect but many of which have a relatively minor effect. Complex diseases and traits result principally from genetic variation that is relatively common in the general population. Along with the role of multiple genes and environmental factors in various diseases, problems exist with gene 'redundancy' at the functional level. Thus, completion of the human genome will not provide an immediate solution to the genetics of complex diseases. This can only be achieved by documenting the genetic variation of human genomes at the population level within and across ethnic groups and by characterising mutant genes. DNA microarray analysis is an important technique which is used as a means to probe the expression of thousands of genes simultaneously and to study a wide range of biologic processes. The technique could be used to compare two biologic classes in order to identify the differential expression of the genes in them, thus identifying genes with potential relevance to a wide range of diseases.[71] For further progress it is essential to identify the function of each gene in the normal and disease situation and establish a link with the expressed protein (before and after post-translational modification) and its role in physiological and disease pathways. Thus, structure and function of expressed proteins is likely to make an important contribution to the discovery of new drug targets – leading finally to new drugs.[72] This process (understanding the function of genes and proteins) and further phenotypic analysis through detailed biology will then lead to new validated targets for drug discovery by traditional methods or treatment options using gene therapy or protein products.[73,74]

Since the complete genome of *Haemophilus influenzae* was published, sequencing of genomes from a wide range of organisms, from bacteria to humans has continued apace. Initial sequencing and analysis of the human genome has been published.[75,76] Another more recent example includes the genome sequence of *Escherichia coli* O157 : H7, implicated in many outbreaks of haemorrhagic colitis.[77] The functional characterisation of microbial genomics will have a significant impact on genomic medicine (new antimicrobial targets and vaccine candidates) and on environmental (waste management, recycling), food and industrial biotechnology. In addition to the work on human and microbial genomes, progress is also being made on the sequencing of the mouse and rat genomes.[78] Data from rodent species should speed the discovery of genes and regulatory regions in the human genome and make it easier to determine their functions. In addition, these sequences may have significant impact on the disease models because these animal are most often used in the early discovery and preclinical testing of new drugs.[79] Comparative genomics and proteomics studies between various genomes may also lead to additional information useful for various stages of the drug discovery process.[80]

There are three main approaches to mapping the genetic variants involved in a disease: functional cloning, the candidate gene strategy and positional cloning. In functional cloning, identification of the underlying protein defect leads to localisation of the responsible gene (disease-function-gene-map). An example of functional cloning is the finding that individuals with sickle cell anaemia carried an amino acid substitution in the β chain of haemoglobin. Isolation of the mutant molecule led to the cloning of the gene encoding β-globin. In the candidate-gene approach, the most frequently used approach adopted to identify the predisposing or causal genes in the complex and multigenic and multifactorial diseases, genes with a known or proposed function with the potential to influence the disease phenotype are investigated for a direct role in disease. In a small number of cases of type 2 diabetes, candidate-gene studies have identified mutations in, for example, the genes encoding insulin and the insulin receptor. Marker genes not related to disease physiology and genome-wide screens are the starting points for mapping the genetic components of the disease. The aim is first to identify the genetic region within which a disease-predisposing gene lies and, once this is found, to localise the gene and determine its functional and biological role in the disease (disease-map-gene-function).

The introduction of functional genes for the restoration of normal function or the transfer of therapeutic genes to treat particular diseases such as cancer or viral infections is of growing interest. The hurdles to overcome in efficient gene therapy include successful transfer of the therapeutic genes, appropriate expression levels associated with sufficient duration of gene expression, and the specificity of gene transfer to achieve therapeutic effects in the patient. Viral vectors are still among the most efficient gene transfer vehicles.[81,82] Because of the comparatively long history of characterisation of particular viruses and their genomes, their valuable characteristics for target cell infectivity, transgene capacity and accessibility of established helper cell lines for the production of recombinant virus stocks to infect target cells, the most commonly used vectors are developed from retroviruses, lentiviruses, adenovirus, herpes simplex virus and adeno-associated virus. The advantages of retroviral vectors (stable integration into the host genome, generation of viral titres sufficient for efficient gene transfer, infectivity of the recombinant viral particles for a broad variety of target cell types and ability to carry foreign genes of reasonable size) are accompanied by several disadvantages (e.g. instability of some retroviral vectors, possible insertional mutagenesis by random viral integration into host DNA, the requirement of cell division for integration of Moloney murine leukaemia virus-derived retroviral vectors and targeting of retroviral infection and/or therapeutic gene expression). In addition to the viral transfection procedures, non-viral transfection procedures (e.g. liposomes, gene gun and DNA conjugates) are also being developed. In a recent example, human monocyte-derived dendritic cells were transfected with genes encoding tumour-associated antigens. The transfection was achieved by dimerisation of a 35 amino acid cationic peptide (Lys-Lys-Lys-Lys-Lys-Lys-Gly-Gly-Phe-Leu-Gly-Phe-Trp-Arg-Gly-Glu-Asn-Gly-Arg-Lys-Thr-Arg-Ser-Ala-Tyr-Glu-Arg-Met-Cys-Asn-Ile-Leu-Lys-Gly-Lys) and then using a complex of this dimeric peptide with plasmid DNA expression constructs. Injection of transfected dendritic cells expressing a tumour-associated antigen protected mice from lethal challenge with tumour cells in a model of melanoma.

Identification of the genes that provide structural and regulatory functions in an organism are likely to be useful in obtaining genetically modified (transgenic) animals using gene knock-out or knock-in strategies. The transgenic animals are useful in determining the physiological functions of genes, identification and validation of new molecular drug targets, generation of animal models of disease for the testing of novel therapeutic strategies, and early recognition of toxicological effects.[83] In a number of cases, a direct correlation between the gene knock-out phenotype and the efficacy of drugs that modulate that specific target has been demonstrated.[84] Using gene knock-out methodology and phenotypic studies, a number of new targets have been suggested in cancer and neurological, metabolic, cardiovascular, immunological and bone disorders.

The use of embryonic or adult stem cells (unspecialised cells capable of dividing, renewing themselves and generating specialised cells) to treat human diseases is currently being investigated along with various techniques to identify, isolate and grow stem cells to required tissues.[85,86] Molecular processes (including genes) underlying the differentiation of embryonic stem cells into specialised cells of a particular tissue are being studied along with mechanisms that maintain embryonic stem cells in their undifferentiated state. Stem cells are being widely investigated for the treatment of cardiovascular diseases (e.g. heart failure), metabolic diseases such as diabetes,[87,88] neurodegenerative diseases (including amyotrophic lateral sclerosis, multiple sclerosis, Huntington's disease, Parkinson's disease and stroke), haematological disease[89] and cancer. In the case of cancer, the stem cells (stationary cancer stem cells and mobile cancer stem cells) may also have a critical role in the development and spread (metastasis) of several forms of human tumours. Biologically distinct and relatively rare populations of 'tumour-initiating' cells have been identified in cancers of the haematopoietic system, brain and breast.[90–92] Cells of this type have the capacity for self-renewal, the potential to develop into any cell in the overall tumour population, and the proliferative ability to drive continued expansion of the population of malignant cells. Eradication of the stem-cell compartment of a tumour may also be essential to achieve stable long-lasting remission, and even a cure, of cancer.

1.5.3 Pharmacogenomics and toxicogenomics

Because different patients with the same disease symptoms respond differently to the same drug, both in terms of therapeutic benefits and side effects, understanding of the relationships between gene variations and the effect of such variations on drug responses within individuals is likely to lead to tailor-made therapies for specific population of patients. For example, a variety of antihypertensive and congestive heart failure drugs are now available, including calcium antagonists, ACE inhibitors, β-blockers, diuretics, α-blockers, centrally acting antihypertensives and, more recently, AT_1 receptor antagonists. Although all of these agents are effective in lowering blood pressure in most cases, there are significant differences between their therapeutic and side effect profiles. A better knowledge of the mechanisms that influence the efficiency of the drugs in different individuals and understanding why some patients can tolerate the drug better than others may lead to more efficacious drugs with a better side effect profile. The variation of the individual's response to such drugs may be caused by either the heterogeneity of the mechanisms underlying hypertension, inter-individual variations in the pharmacokinetics of drugs (genetic polymorphisms in drug metabolizing enzymes), or a combination of both.

The likely benefit of more efficacious tailor-made drugs with fewer side effects has led to the development of the science of pharmacogenomics, a name given to any drug-discovery platform that attempts to address the issues of efficacy and toxicity in individuals based on the influence of inheritance on variable drug response.[93] The concept of individual variation at the molecular level is not new. Proteins obtained from different individuals have been known to have different amino acid sequences. These protein isoforms originate either by genomic variation at the level of the actual gene sequence, or by variation in expression that results from changes in the promoter and control elements that regulate expression. Alleles differ from each other by structural features, such as single-base-pair changes, or as the result of rearrangements or deletions of entire gene portions. Depending on the structure of regulatory sequences, some alleles may be expressed at very high levels, while others may be repressed. Similarly, depending on variation at the critical points in the assembly of genes, splicing variants may result from alternative arrangement of building blocks. Technologies that enable the monitoring of gene expression under different circumstances (based on high-throughput sequencing and screening approaches) are currently being developed and will enable systematic investigations of the patterns of gene expression between normal and disease states in a statistically meaningful way along with the expression of the relevant proteins in different individuals. In addition, the potential of using single-nucleotide polymorphisms to correlate drug regimens and responses is also being investigated.[94] The availability of precisely located single-nucleotide polymorphic sites spanning the genome holds promise for the association of particular genetic loci with disease states. This information, together with high-throughput gene-chip technologies, will offer new opportunities for molecular diagnostics and monitoring of disease predisposition in large sections of the population. It will also allow much earlier preventive treatment in many slowly evolving diseases.

Toxicogenomics uses global gene expression analyses studies to detect expression changes that influence, predict or help define drug toxicity.[95] The principle behind the technique relies on the identification of toxicity-related gene expression signatures (fingerprints) of known compounds and comparing these to gene-expression profiles of new similar compounds. Similarities between the two sets of compounds may predict the toxic potential of unknown compounds. It is expected that toxicogenomics will reduce failure rates of drugs by helping select the right compounds for development early on and by accelerating toxicology testing and identifying suitable biomarkers amenable to screening using the generated data. Several toxicogenomics databases are currently being built. A substantial amount of data has already been generated in animal models with known toxicants, mainly hepatotoxins, proving that gene expression analysis can provide information to allow classification of compounds according to their mechanism of toxicity as well as identifying cellular pathways related

to the toxic event. More recently, this global gene expression analysis has been applied to the evaluation of nephrotoxicity, genotoxicity and testicular toxicity. In addition to the classification of compounds based on gene expression fingerprints obtained from tissue samples after exposure to toxicants, information has also been obtained about the underlying mechanisms of toxicity. Identification of genes and/or pathways that are modulated by certain toxicants provides insight into possible mechanisms of toxicity. Much further work such as quality of databases and relationship between gene expression and dose-dependent induction of toxicity still needs to be carried out before the techniques becomes fully acceptable.

1.5.4 Proteomics

The control mechanisms in health and disease are found at the protein level and, as mentioned above, genome sequencing does not provide sufficient information at the protein level. The tertiary structure and the type and extent of post-translational modifications (e.g. glycosylation and phosphorylation) of a protein is critical to its function and cellular localisation but this information is not encoded in the protein's corresponding DNA. An additional complication between genes and proteins is the existence of alternative splice variants of mRNA which give rise to isomeric proteins that might contribute to regulatory processes in the cell. The processing of proteins may also be different in various tissues under different conditions. Some proteins may give rise to biologically active fragments and some may exert diverse functions in collaboration with other proteins. Therefore, the complete structure and function of an individual protein cannot be determined by reference to its gene sequence alone. Thus, beyond genomics it is essential to compare the protein content of cells/tissues/organs in the normal and disease situation and to generate functional information on proteins required for various drug discovery processes. Proteomics is any protein-based approach that provides new information about proteins on a genome-wide scale and addresses these difficulties by enabling the protein levels of cellular organisation to be screened and characterised.[96,97] In a high-throughput manner, a large number of proteins from normal and disease samples (cells and tissue extracts) are separated on the basis of their charge and molecular weight by two-dimensional electrophoresis and the amino acid sequences of proteins and their post-translational modifications are identified by mass spectrometry. The separated proteins are then stained and the maps of protein expression are digitally scanned into databases. The protein expression maps can be used to study cellular pathways and the perturbation of these pathways by disease and drug action. Thus, an understanding of cellular pathways and protein changes resulting from the disease and drug actions can not only lead to new drug targets, but can also provide early markers for diseases and early indications of drug toxicity.[98] It should be emphasised, however, that characterisation of a different protein in a disease state does not necessarily means that it has a causal role or represents a potential therapeutic target. In many cases, the new protein may be a consequence of the disease rather than the cause. Further studies are required to check whether the activity of a candidate target eliminated by molecular/cellular techniques could reverse the disease phenotype. Moreover, even when a potential therapeutic target has been identified and a molecule capable of disrupting it has been obtained, we cannot assume it will constitute an effective treatment for the disease under investigation. Alternative metabolic routes may provide cells with ways of circumventing blocked pathways.

The potential benefit of proteomics in predicting toxicity at an early stage may lead to accelerated drug discovery programmes. A comparison of the protein profiles of normal tissue with those of tissue treated with the known toxic agent might give an indication of the drug's toxic activity. Similarly, identification of a known toxic protein in drug-treated tissues may give an idea about the toxicity of the drug. As a first approach, an examination of liver and kidney (major sites for metabolism and excretion of most drugs) before and after the drug administration may provide early indications about events that might result in toxicity. Proteomic analysis of the serum, where the majority of toxicity markers released from susceptible organs and tissues throughout the entire body collect, can be utilised to identify serum markers (and clusters thereof) as indicators of toxicity. The serum markers could subsequently be used to predict the response of each individual and allow tailoring of therapy whereby optimal efficacy is achieved while minimising adverse side effects. Surrogate markers for drug efficacy could also be detected by this procedure and could be used for identifying patient classes who will respond favourably to a drug.

There is currently some debate about the ability of the techniques being used to detect all the proteins present in a given sample. It is possible that global proteome displays based on two-dimensional gel electrophoresis are largely limited to the more abundantly expressed and stable proteins. Thus, important classes of regulatory proteins involved in signal transduction and gene expression, for example, and other proteins of lower abundance remain undetected by current methodologies. Proteins of lower abundance are more likely to be detected by separating these from high abundance proteins. The disadvantage of this strategy is that it requires much larger amounts of protein, and many additional separations, and therefore may be impractical for studies of small cell populations or tissue samples. Efforts are underway to develop advanced proteomic technologies that do not rely upon two-dimensional gel electrophoresis.

After the discovery of protein maps and characterisation of individual proteins, the most important aspect of proteomics is to define protein function. Although new proteins are likely to include receptors, ligands, enzymes, enzyme inhibitors, signalling molecules and pathways that may be therapeutic targets, precise functions of the individual proteins have to be identified. To discover and monitor the relevance of a protein to a disease-related process, it is also important to find where, when and to what extent a protein is expressed. Many approaches are being used to discover protein function.[99,100] Structural homology methods may be used to ascribe function to some proteins, because it is known that proteins of similar function often share structural homology (tertiary structure). Another approach to defining protein function is chemical proteomics (or chemical genomics),[101] the identification of small molecules that interact with the proteins by screening new proteins against diverse chemical libraries using methods such as nuclear magnetic resonance (NMR) spectroscopy, microcalorimetry or microarrays. Another method for identifying ligand-binding sites involves scanning the surface of a protein molecule for clefts. In many cases, the largest cleft is the known primary binding site for small ligands. Further information about the ligand structures that can be accommodated in the binding site can be obtained by various computational methods such as DOCK or HOOK. Some of the proteins likely to have known enzyme activity or enzyme inhibition properties can be identified by using screens for generic enzyme activities. Chemical proteomics techniques, which involve the use of chemical probes (synthetic small molecules) designed to covalently attach to proteins of interest and allow purification and/or identification, have also been used to identify new protease drug targets.[102] Along with the structural and chemical library methods, several 'non-homology' methods are being developed to identify protein functions.[103] These computational methods take advantage of the many properties shared among functionally related proteins, such as patterns of domain fusion, evolutionary co-inheritance, conservation of relative gene position and correlated expression patterns. Protein function is defined by these methods in terms of context (i.e. which cellular pathways or complexes the protein participates in), rather than by suggesting a specific biochemical activity. Large-scale functional analysis of new proteins can be accomplished by using peptide or protein arrays, ranging from synthetic peptide arrays to whole proteins expressed in living cells.[104] Comprehensive sets of purified peptides and proteins permit high-throughput screening for discrete biochemical properties, whereas formats involving living cells facilitate large-scale genetic screening for novel biological activities. Protein arrays can be engineered to suit the aims of a particular experiment. Thus, an array might contain all the combinatorial variants of a bioactive peptide or specific variants of a single protein species (splice variants, domains or mutants), a family of protein orthologs from different species, a protein pathway or even the entire protein complement of an organism.

Access to structural information on a proteome-wide scale is not only important for ascribing protein function, but may also be useful in target validation and medicinal chemistry on hits/leads requiring structural information for rational design processes. The most straightforward strategy for predicting structure is to search for sequence similarity to a protein with known three-dimensional structure.[105,106] Additional information can be obtained by identifying known and novel folds in a protein. There are databases of structural motifs in proteins which contain data relevant to helices, β-turns, γ-turns, β-hairpins, ψ-loops, β-α-β motifs, β-sheets, β-strands and disulphide bridges extracted from proteins, which can be used for comparison. Novel protein folds can be identified by employing *ab initio* approaches used for prediction of protein structure. With the aim of extracting further information from protein sequences, sequence motif libraries have been developed. Advances in X-ray crystallography, particularly the use of synchrotron radiation sources, and NMR spectroscopy also allow more rapid determination of protein structures. Using protein crystals in which methionine residue is replaced by selenomethionine and multi-wavelength synchrotron experiments, electron-density maps for proteins can be generated in less than an hour instead of the weeks of experimental

time required for a conventional crystallography-based structure determination.[107] Despite great improvements in X-ray crystallography techniques, the rate-limiting step in structure determination remains the expression, purification and crystallisation of the target protein.

Many problems still remain to be solved before protein function can be confidently assigned by using the above techniques. For example, the idea of 'one gene–one protein–one function' is not valid in many cases and increasing numbers of proteins are found to have two or more different functions.[108] The multiple functions of such moonlighting proteins can vary as a consequence of changes in cellular localisation, cell type, oligomeric state or the cellular concentration of a ligand, substrate, co-factor or product. Multidrug transporter P-glycoprotein (a large 170 kD cell-surface molecule encoded by the human *MDR1* gene) is an example of a protein with multiple functions. It is well established that P-glycoprotein can efflux xenobiotics from cells and is one mechanism that tumour cells use to escape death induced by chemotherapeutic drugs. Recent observations have raised the possibility that P-glycoprotein and related transporter molecules might have a fundamental role in regulating cell differentiation, proliferation and survival. P-glycoprotein encoded by *MDR1* in humans and *Mdr1a* in mice can regulate an endogenous chloride channel. This activity of P-glycoprotein can be inhibited by phosphorylation by protein kinase C. MDR1 P-glycoprotein has also been proposed to have a role in phospholipid translocation and cholesterol esterification. Functional P-glycoprotein has also been suggested to have a role in regulating programmed cell death (apoptosis).[109]

1.5.5 Bioinformatics and data mining technologies

The availability of genomic data and the corresponding protein sequences from humans and other organisms together with structure/function annotations, disease correlations and population variations requires sophisticated data management systems (databases) for analytical purposes. Proteomics-oriented databases include data on the two-dimensional gel electrophoresis maps of proteins from a variety of healthy and disease tissues. Bioinformatic systems (computer-assisted data management and analysis) are used to gather and analyse this information in order to attach biological knowledge to genes, assign genes to biological pathways, compare the gene sets of different species, understand processes in healthy and disease states, and find new or better drugs.[110] The currently available techniques have the capability to translate a given gene sequence into a protein structure, complete with prediction of secondary structure and database comparisons. Progress is being made in devising systems that provide information on biological function derived from sequencing and functional analysis. In addition to the gene–function analysis studies, the need for data mining techniques (defined as 'the non-trivial extraction of implicit, previously unknown, and potentially useful information from data') is becoming necessary in order to deal with the enormous amounts of information that the industry collects in individual databases (ranging from, for example, databases of disease profiles and molecular pathways to sequences, chemical and biological screening data, including structure–activity relationships, chemical structures of combinatorial libraries of compounds, individual and population clinical trial results). A large number of companies are developing data mining applications (software) that can identify cause–effect relationships between data sets and group together data points or sets based on different criterion. A time-delay data mining approach is used when a complete data set is not available immediately and in complete form, but is collected over time. The systems designed to handle such data look for patterns, which are confirmed or rejected as the data set increases and becomes more robust. This approach is geared toward analysis of long-term clinical trials and studies of multi-component modes of action. It is also possible to overlay large and complex data sets that are similar to each other and compare them. This is particularly useful in all forms of clinical trial meta-analyses, where data collected at different sites over different time periods, and perhaps under similar but not always identical conditions, need to be compared. Here, the emphasis is on finding dissimilarities, not similarities. Predictive data mining programmes are available for making simulations, predictions and forecasts based on the data sets analysed.

1.5.6 Combinatorial chemistry and high-throughput screening

One of the earliest approaches to drug discovery was the random screening process. More recently, significant efforts were directed towards rational and semi-rational approaches. However, recent advances in high-throughput screening and synthesis techniques, coupled with large-scale data analysis and data management methods, has shifted the balance towards testing libraries of 'diverse' chemical compounds in multiple screens (>20,000 compounds in a week) in the shortest possible time.[111] This approach is expected to provide leads much more quickly for optimisation using combinatorial synthesis methods (targeted libraries) to generate drug candidates. Starting from the solid phase peptide synthesis in the early 1960s, which opened the way to chemical synthesis on solid supports, automated synthesis of diverse organic compounds has now become routine in many laboratories. To cope with high-throughput synthesis, assays have been developed to generate biological results quickly and cheaply. Many assays make use of fluorescently labelled reagents (e.g. receptors, ligands and enzyme substrates) allowing rapid optical screening of large collections of compounds. Assays using microtitre plates (96–384 wells in each plate) are designed to enable small quantities of compounds to be tested at a much-reduced cost in terms of the reagent use. High-throughput cell-based assays are used for compound screening during hit identification and lead optimisation stages.[112] The emergence of 'high content screening' platforms (a high-throughput technology that applies sophisticated image processing algorithms to analyse cell images generated by automated fluorescence microscopy) is opening up new possibilities to study a range of cell biological parameters such as object localisation, intensity, texture or shape, thereby enabling the analysis of more subtle and physiologically relevant cellular events such as cell or protein movements, shape changes or protein modification. *In silico* screening (any computational technique that supports the lead discovery process) based on focused and sequential screening approaches is recommended as a substitute to testing large libraries and is likely to be less expensive. The technique minimises the number of compounds to be screened. Focused screening begins by screening a subset of the compound collection based on an *in silico* hypothesis (e.g. pharmacophore or docking models) of compounds that are active against a specific target. Sequential screening is carried out iteratively and begins by screening a small representative set of 'diverse' compounds. Analysis of the data enables the generation of an initial hypothesis that is used to create a subsequent and more focused subset of compounds for a second round of screening. Several cycles of testing and analysis can be performed until sufficient active molecules have been discovered.[113]

In the early phase of the work, combinatorial libraries and screening procedures had many problems, primarily because the main focus of the work was on the number of compounds produced in a mixture, with little regard for their quality. Over the years, many improvements have been made in the library design process.[114,115] The attention has now shifted to smaller high-quality libraries of discrete compounds, using various data mining technologies, new parallel and combinatorial approaches and filters for lead-like or drug-like properties,[116,117] as well as avoiding non-selective or promiscuous inhibitors. Because of the importance of natural products to early drug discovery process, many natural-product-like libraries containing natural product scaffolds, including carbohydrates, steroids, fatty acid derivatives, polyketides, peptides, terpenoids, flavonoids and alkaloids, have been prepared and investigated in various screens. Advances in analytical chemistry have enabled the routine high-throughput purification of compounds by mass-triggered preparative liquid chromatography. Although the quality of leads discovered directly from combinatorial libraries is steadily increasing, it is clear that parallel synthesis is even more powerful at the lead optimization phase, when a series of related compounds needs to be made and tested rapidly.

1.5.6.1 Combinatorial synthesis

Combinatorial chemistry is having a major impact in generating libraries containing large numbers of compounds in a relatively short period of time using solid phase synthesis technologies. In addition, it is possible to buy ready-made libraries built around specific molecular themes and consisting of many thousands of compounds, and to test these libraries in high-throughput screening systems using automated off-the-shelf instrumentation and reagents. The technique of combinatorial biocatalysis is also used to obtain diverse libraries.[118] This approach takes advantage of natural catalysts (enzymes and whole cells), as well as the rapidly growing supply of recombinant and engineered enzymes, for the direct derivatisation of many different synthetic compounds and natural products. The types of reactions catalysed by enzymes and micro-organisms include reactions which can introduce functional groups (e.g. carbon–carbon bond formation, hydroxylation, halogenation, cyclo additions, addition of amines), modify the existing functionalities (oxidation of alcohols to aldehydes and ketones, reduction of aldehydes or ketones to alcohols, oxidation of sulphides to sulphoxides, oxidation of amino groups to nitro groups, hydrolysis of nitriles to amides and carboxylic acids, replacements of amino groups by hydroxyl groups, lactonisation, isomerisation, epimerisation, dealkylation and

methyl transfer) or addition onto functional groups (esterification, carbonate formation, carbamate formation, glycosylation, amidation and phosphorylation). Currently available technologies allow these biocatalysis reactions to be carried out in aqueous and non-aqueous solvents.

Techniques are available to screen individual compounds or mixtures in solution or still attached to the solid support. The main advantage of screening single compounds in solution (the most commonly used technique in the past) is that activity can be directly correlated with chemical structure. Screening mixtures of compounds has the advantage that fewer assays need to be performed and at the same time fewer synthetic steps are required to generate mixtures. However, it is not possible to synthesise mixtures that contain entirely different structures without compromising synthetic efficiency. Screening of mixtures can lead to false positives as a result of additive or cooperative effects of weakly active compounds. Thus, the most active mixture may not contain the most potent compound. An additional disadvantage of testing mixtures is that once an active mixture has been identified, the exact structure of the active compound, in most cases, can only be obtained by extensive deconvolution studies. There are some procedures such as the positional scanning approach, which enable the active compound to be identified directly from screening. This method depends on the synthesis of a series of subset mixtures which contain a single building block (substituent) at one position and all the building blocks at the other positions. The structure of the most active compound is then assigned by selecting the building block from the most active subset at each position. The structure is confirmed by synthesis.

The most widely used solid phase method for the synthesis of libraries (originally used for peptides) has been termed the 'split-mix', 'divide, couple and recombine' and 'one bead–one compound' method. The resin beads display a linker to which building blocks are sequentially attached, to effectively grow molecules. As a first step, different batches of resin are reacted individually with a unique set of reagents (first set of building blocks); the resins are then combined and deprotected to liberate another reactive group. The resin is then divided into several components and each component is reacted individually by the second building block. This 'divide, couple, recombine' strategy is continued until all the building blocks have been added. The resin batches are not combined after the final building blocks have been added. This strategy results in a resin library in which a single compound is attached to an individual bead. When a synthesis is complete, cleavage at the linker releases the molecule(s) from the bead(s). The screening of single beads, or the compounds derived from single beads, corresponds to screening of single compounds. Screening of these libraries can quickly identify the preferred last building block in the most active set. The subset library is then resynthesised by keeping this preferred final building block constant and screened to identify the penultimate preferred building block in each set. This deconvolution process, or iterative resynthesis and screening, is repeated in order to define all of the positions. The deconvolution process has to be repeated each time the library is tested in a new screen. Several different approaches have been investigated to avoid this inconvenient and time-consuming deconvolution method. One of these, using tagging/encoding strategies, involves introduction of chemical tags at each stage of the 'split-mix' synthesis either before the addition of each building block during the synthesis or before the subsequent mixing step. At the end of the synthesis any individual bead will possess a compound made up from a single combination of building blocks and an associated tag sequence with a specific tag corresponding to each specific building block. The identity of the compound on a single bead can be determined simply by ana-lysing the tagging sequence. The original tagging methods, oligonucleotides [read by polymerase chain reaction (PCR) amplification and DNA sequencing] and peptides (read by Edman micro-sequencing), have now been replaced by using binary coding with chemical tags. This tagging strategy increases the number of steps in the synthesis of each library but allows more rapid identification of the active hits.

Another solid phase technique called small-molecule macroarrays is used for combinational library synthesis and screening.[119] This array platform originates from the SPOT-synthesis technique, or the spatially addressed synthesis of peptides on cellulose supports. Again, used initially for the synthesis of peptides, the technique is now being used for the synthesis of small molecules. Small-molecule macroarrays offer some advantages (e.g. hydrophilic support) over traditional combinatorial synthesis platforms – these focused 50–200 compound arrays are straightforward to syn-thesize and amenable to numerous screening applica-tions where the array compounds are either bound to or cleaved from the planar support. Newer synthetic techniques such as the use of microwave-assisted organic reactions, multi-component reactions and automated spotting methods can be used in the pre-paration of these libraries.

1.5.6.2 Library design

The design strategy may vary according to the informa-tion available on the target and the purpose of the library. For example, when the class of target is known (e.g. an enzyme with a known mechanism of action and/or structural information or a known or sim-ilar receptor type/subtype), library design may be started from a known pharmacophore. For example, compounds containing a statine residue, a known transition-state analogue, inhibit aspartyl proteinases such as renin, HIV and cathepsin D. Several libraries based on statine or a hydroxyethylamine core have been prepared and investigated against other aspartyl proteinases. The use of synthetic positional-scanning combinatorial libraries offers the ability to rapidly test and evaluate the extended substrate specificities of proteases.[120] For example, a fluorogenic tetrapeptide positional-scanning library (containing a 7-amino-4-methylcoumarin-derivatised lysine) in which the P_1 amino acid was held constant as a lysine and the P_4-P_3-P_2 positions were positionally randomised was used to investigate extended substrate specificities of plasmin and thrombin, two of the enzymes involved in the blood coagulation cascade. The optimal P_4 to P_2 substrate specificity for plasmin was P_4-Lys/Nle/Val/Ile/Phe, P_3-Xaa, and P_2-Tyr/Phe/Trp. The optimal P_4 to P_2 extended substrate sequence determined for thrombin was P_4-Nle/Leu/Ile/Phe/Val, P_3-Xaa and P_2-Pro. By three-dimensional structural modelling of the substrates into the active sites of plasmin and thrombin, it was possible to identify potential deter-minants of the defined substrate specificity. This method is amenable to the incorporation of diverse substituents at the P_1 position (all 20 proteinogenic and other non-proteinogenic amino acids) for explor-ing molecular recognition elements in various new uncharacterised proteolytic enzymes.

A similar approach can be adopted when random screening has identified a lead ligand. The structural template in the lead is then modified to generate a targeted library. Many libraries have been synthesised around the so-called 'privileged structures' which have shown activity against various targets. For example, compounds based on a benzodiazepine core have shown activity against a number of G-protein-coupled receptors. Similarly, poly-functionalised purine deriv-atives have been used in the design process of highly diverse purine libraries based on the known biological activities of this class of compounds.[121] Many purine derivatives have shown interesting activity against various receptors (e.g. ligands of corticotrophin-releasing hormone receptors). Moreover, many drugs already in the market, e.g. 6-mercaptopurine, aciclovir, ganciclovir, abacavir and azathioprine) are purine derivatives. However, when there is little information, or when entirely different structural leads are required, a larger diverse library is likely to be more suitable to increase the chance of success. The chemical diversity between the different members of the library is also very important to cover a wide chemical area and increase chances of success. In addition to some simple rules such as incorporating acidic, basic, hydrophilic and hydrophobic groups of different sizes, a large number of computer-based methods are available for diversity analysis. Information is also available on the so-called 'drug-like molecules' that tend to have certain properties. For example, log P, molecular weight, and the number of hydrogen bonding groups have been correlated with oral bioavailability.[122] Analysis of a large number of compounds from the World Drug Index establishment resulted in the 'rule of five' based on the assumption that compounds meeting these criteria have entered human clinical trials, and therefore must possess many of the desirable characteristics of drugs. A high percentage of compounds contained ≤5 hydrogen bond donors (expressed as the sum of OHs and NHs), ≤10 hydrogen bond acceptors, ≤500 relative molecular weight and log P of ≤5.[123] Along with these measures, it is also desirable to exclude functional groups that tend to be undesirable because of chemical reactivity (e.g. alkylating and acylating groups) and other unstable groups leading to metabolism (solvolysis or hydrolysis).[124]

The availability of complex large and diverse chemical libraries and ultra high-throughput screening technologies also provides an option whereby the biological pathways and proteins do not have to be fully characterised before starting the screening process. A number of preselected, incompletely characterised, disease-associated protein targets can be screened against many different libraries. Using the whole cell systems and libraries containing membrane-permeable compounds, it is possible to identify compounds that perturb a cellular process or system, followed by identification of proteins required in cell function. From the perspective of drug discovery, this approach offers the means for the simultaneous identification of proteins that can serve as targets for therapeutic intervention ('therapeutic target validation') and small molecules that can modulate the functions of these therapeutic targets ('chemical target validation'). The overall process differs from the traditional methods of drug discovery in which the biological methods are first used to select and characterise proteins targets for therapeutic intervention, followed by chemical efforts to determine whether the protein target can be modulated by small molecules.

1.5.6.3 Examples of compounds discovered by library approaches

Over the years, with improving design and screening processes, the success rate for the discovery of 'hits' and 'leads' from various high-throughput, project-directed and thematic libraries has increased significantly. A large number of examples are mentioned in two recent reviews.[125,126] Other examples include ligands for the five somatostatin receptor ligands (see section 1.3.1), fibrinogen receptor antagonist, PPARα, PPARδ and VLA4 antagonists (40–44).

40 5-HT$_6$ receptor ligand

41 Fibrinogen receptor antagonist

42 PPARα agonist

43 PPARδ agonist

44 VLA4 antagonist

1.5.7 Structure-based drug design

The entire process of structure-based drug design requires identification and characterisation of a suitable protein target, determination of the structure of the target protein, the availability of an easy and reliable high-throughput screening assay, identification of a lead compound, development of computer-assisted methods for estimating the affinity of new compounds and access to a synthetic route to produce the designed compounds. Progress has been made on many of these aspects. For example, expression systems are now available which allow the production of large amounts of naturally occurring proteins and modified proteins such as isotope labelled proteins required for NMR studies and proteins containing residues such as selenomethionine (in place of methionine) which simplify determination of X-ray structure. Advances in automation technologies have resulted in increasing the synthesis and screening capabilities. From the point of view of design, more important aspects of 'rational design' strategy involve methods of using the information contained in the three-dimensional structure of a macromolecular target and of related ligand–target complexes, and predicting novel lead compounds. A variety of 'docking' programmes now exist that can select from a large database of compounds a subset of molecules that usually includes some compounds that bind to the selected target protein.[127] One such programme, DOCK, systematically attempts to fit each compound from a database into the binding site of the target structure, such that three or more of the atoms in the database molecule overlap with a set of predefined site points in the target binding site. The newer computational methods are aimed at using the information contained in the three-dimensional structure of the unligated target to design entirely new lead compounds *de novo*, as well as to construct large virtual combinatorial libraries of compounds that can be screened computationally (virtual screening) before going to the effort and expense of actually synthesising and testing them.

The *de novo* design of structure-based ligands involves fragment positioning methods, molecule growth methods and fragment methods, coupled to database searches.[128] The fragment positioning methods determine energetically favourable binding site positions for various functional group types or chemical fragments. In the molecule growth methods, a seed atom (or fragment) is first placed in the binding site of the target structure. A ligand molecule is successively built by bonding another atom (or fragment) to it. Fragment positioning methods can also be coupled to database searching techniques either to extract from a database existing molecules that can be docked into the binding site with the desired fragments in their optimal positions or for *de novo* design. Once a lead compound has been found by some means, an iterative process begins that involves solving the three-dimensional structure of the lead compound bound to the target, examining that structure and characterising the types of interactions the bound ligand makes, and using the computational methods to design improvements to the compound. A large number of examples that demonstrate the utility of this approach (e.g. designing inhibitors of enzymes such as renin, HIV protease and thrombin) exist in the literature.

1.5.8 Virtual screening

The virtual screening strategy involves construction or 'synthesis' of molecules on the computer. The two approaches used in virtual screening may be classified as a ligand-based approach or a receptor-based approach. The ligand-based approach aims to identify molecules with physical and chemical similarities (pharmacophore-based, descriptor-based) to known ligands that are likely to interact with the target.[129] Ligand-based strategies limit the diversity of the hits as they are biased by the properties of known ligands. Receptor-based virtual screening (protein–ligand docking, active-site-directed pharmacophores), however, aims to exploit the molecular recognition between a ligand and a target protein to select out chemical entities that bind strongly to the active sites of biologically relevant targets for which the three-dimensional structures are known or inferred.[130] The number of 'synthesised' compounds is limited by synthesising focused libraries (e.g. a hydroxamate library of matrix MMP inhibitors) and concentrating on reactions that will work in high yield with reagents that are easily accessible and incorporating 'drug-like' properties. Synthetic accessibility can be checked using programs such as computer-aided organic synthesis or computer-aided estimation of synthetic accessibility.

As molecules are constructed, a variety of filters are applied to 'weed out' compounds that do not meet certain criteria (e.g. similarity and diversity analysis, presence of undesirable functional groups, molecular weight and lipophilicity). Once a virtual library has been created and the undesirable compounds removed, the next step is to generate three-dimensional conformations for each molecule. Because most molecules are quite flexible, a multi-conformer docking approach is adopted. In this strategy, a set of conformations (typically, 10–50) is generated and then each conformer is docked as a rigid molecule into the target enzyme or receptor, which is held fixed throughout. None of the docking approaches can take into account the important conformational changes that take place during the binding process of the ligand to its receptor. Before the three-dimensional conformational analysis, it is also useful to obtain two-dimensional 'shape' and 'distance' information, to remove molecules that cannot possibly match the active site.

The factors taken into account for searching the virtual library include:
• Knowledge about compounds that interact with the target (e.g. substrates, known classes of inhibitors, antagonists and agonists, SAR within various series, pharmacophores deduced from compound classes).
• Knowledge about receptor structure and receptor–ligand interactions (e.g. homology models, X-ray and/or NMR structures, thermodynamics of ligand binding, effect of point mutations and dynamic motions of receptor and ligands).
• Knowledge about drugs in general (e.g. chemical structures and properties of known drugs, rules of conformational analysis and thermodynamics of receptor–ligand interactions).

In the early stages of the project when leads do not exist, computational methods can be used to select a diverse set of compounds from a large virtual library. If a compound shows activity, then other similar compounds from the library are synthesised and tested. If a lead already exists at the start of the program, selecting a subset of compounds that are similar to the lead can reduce the size of the virtual library.

1.5.9 NMR, X-ray and mass spectroscopic techniques

As a first step in structure-based design, the three-dimensional structure of the target macromolecule (protein or nucleic acid) is determined by X-ray crystallography, NMR spectroscopy or homology modelling. Many examples of this type of research are well known in the literature.[131,132] However, it should

be emphasised that even after many cycles of the structure-based design process, when a compound that binds to the target with high affinity has been developed, it is still a long way from being a drug on the market. The compound may still fail in animal and clinical trials as a result of factors such as toxicity, bioavailability, poor pharmacokinetics (absorption, metabolism and half-life) and lack of efficacy.

In the lead generation phase, NMR methods are first used to detect weak binding of small-molecule scaffolds to a target protein.[133] The binding information is subsequently used to design much tighter binding inhibitors, or drug leads. Fragment-based information may be used to design combinatorial libraries (targeted libraries) to generate additional higher affinity binding fragments, which can then be linked to give leads.[134] SAR by NMR was the first NMR screening method disclosed in the literature.[135] This is a fragment-based approach wherein a large library of small molecules is screened using two-dimensional ^1H or ^{15}N spectra of the target protein as a readout. From spectral changes one can identify the compounds binding to the target. After deconvolution and identification of the active compound(s), a second screen of close analogues of the first 'hit' is performed to optimise binding affinity to the first subsite. In order to identify small molecules that bind to another site on the target molecule, the screen is then repeated with the first site saturated. If small-molecule fragments are identified that occupy several neighbouring subsites, one can then, based on the known structure, synthesise compounds that incorporate the small molecule fragments with various linking groups. If linked effectively, resulting compounds may have affinities for the target that are even stronger than the products of the binding constants of the individual unlinked fragments. As an example of the approach, several small fragments (**45**, **46**) were

45 Ki 2 μM

46 Ki 100 μM

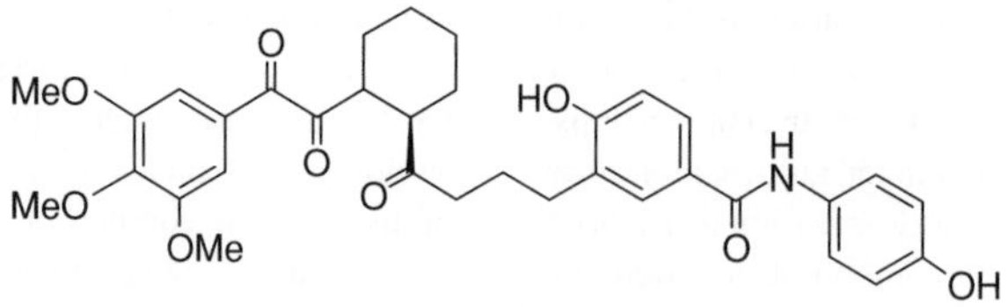

47 Ki 49 nM

discovered as ligands for the FK506 binding protein (Ki values 2–9500 µmol). Linking these fragments led to more potent compounds such as (47) (Ki 49 nmol).

The SHAPES strategy technique, like the above methods, relies on monitoring of ligand signals to determine which compounds in a mixture bind a drug target.[136] The method uses standard one-dimensional line broadening and two-dimensional transferred nuclear Overhauser effect measurements to detect binding of a limited (<200) but diverse library of soluble low molecular weight scaffolds to a potential drug target. The scaffolds are derived largely from shapes or frameworks, most commonly found in known therapeutic agents, and as such represent approximations to 'successful' regions of diversity space. This approach was used to identify p38 inhibitors. In the initial screen, the simple imidazole core did not appear to bind to p38. However, several tethered bicyclic compounds containing an imidazole (or close derivative) and an aryl moiety (pyridyl, phenyl or benzoic acid) (48–51) exhibited weak binding (200 µmol to 2 mmol). Because imidazole by itself did not bind, it was used as a core to fuse two of the tethered bicyclics or their derivatives, creating tricyclic molecules with aryl derivatives as side-chains and the imidazole as the binding core. Two such compounds (52, 53) showed improved binding. Further modifications resulted in

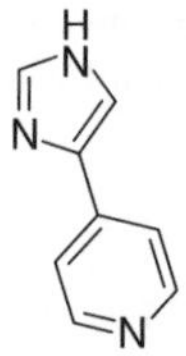

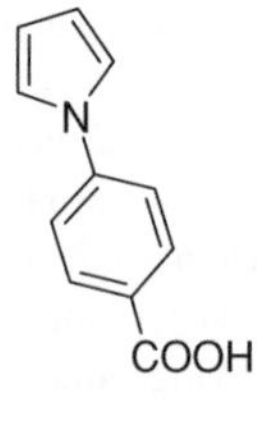

50

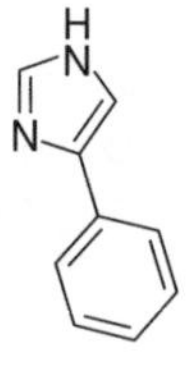

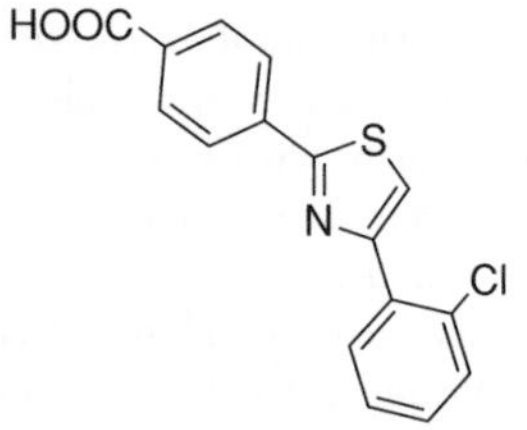

51

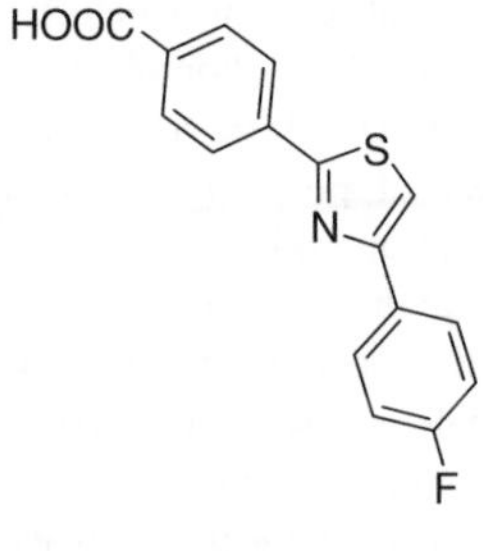

52 200 µM

48

49

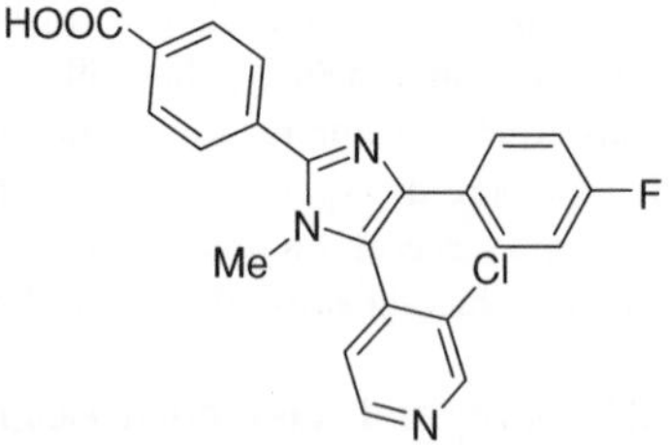

53 200 nM

more potent trisubstituted imidazoles such as **54** (Ki approximately 200 nmol in a p38 enzyme assay).

Unlike in the past when X-ray crystallography was used to study the structures of proteins and ligands, the technique is now being incorporated in all aspects

54

55

56

57

58

of drug discovery, including lead identification, structural assessment and optimisation. Crystallographic screening methods are being developed enabling experimental 'high-throughput' sampling of up to thousands of compounds per day. One such technique, CrystaLEAD, has been used to sample large (≥10,000) compound libraries and detect ligands by monitoring changes in the electron density map relative to the unbound form.[137] By careful design of the library, the technique leads to identification of the bound molecule from the primary data (electron density map) and eliminates the need for the deconvolution process. The electron density map yields a high-resolution picture of the ligand–protein complex and the resulting information on the ligand–target interactions can be used for structure-directed optimisation. As an example, the method was used for the discovery and optimisation of an orally active series of urokinase inhibitors for the treatment of cancer. The initially identified weaker 5-aminoindole and 2-aminoquinoline leads (55, 56; Ki values 50–200 μmol) were optimised. One of the 2-aminoquinoline inhibitor (57; Ki 0.37 μmol) demonstrated oral bioavailability (38%). The 2-naphthamidine derivative (58) did not show oral bioavailability.

In addition to its application in drug discovery, crystallographic screening may also be applied in the structural genomics field, where crystal structures will become available even in the absence of functional characterisation of the protein. In such cases, the ligands discovered could facilitate target validation, assay development and the assignment of function.

1.5.10 Pharmacokinetics

The issues related to pharmacokinetics – drug absorption, distribution, metabolism, excretion (ADME) – have always been important to the success of the drug discovery process. In many cases not enough attention was paid to these factors in the early stages of the discovery process, leading to failures in the late stages of development. To avoid expensive late stage failures and to cope with the high-throughput synthesis and screening technologies that result in many hits/leads, efforts are being directed to identify ADME problems at an early stage of the discovery process.[138] High-throughput ADME assays are being developed to differentiate between the large number of hits that are now routinely identified from screening compound collections and compound libraries.[139] The techniques making this possible include liquid chromatography/mass spectrometry and liquid chromatography/tandem mass spectrometry principally because of enhanced sensitivity, selectivity and ease of automation relative to traditional analytical methods. Many *in vitro* ADME screens (e.g. metabolic stability assays, plasma protein binding, solubility and log P screens) may be performed in microtiter plate format and it is at the time of biological screening that several daughter plates may also be generated for high-throughput ADME. It has become common practice to determine cytochrome P450 (responsible for >90% of the metabolism of all drugs) inhibition, blood levels after intravenous and oral administration, and identification of metabolites at an early stage.[140,141] In recent years, many *in vitro* techniques have emerged that attempt to elucidate drug toxicity and metabolism in high-throughput manner. These include the use of isolated liver slices, primary hepatocytes, transformed cultured human hepatoma cell lines (e.g. HepG2, Hep3B and BC2), as well as the human liver microsomes and isolated recombinant CYP450s. Hepatocytes, whether primary or transformed, provide a complete set of drug-metabolizing pathways and offer an appropriate system to test for toxicity, metabolite production and drug stability. The *in vitro* data available from the current methods is not always a reliable predictor for hepatotoxicity *in vivo* and some of the newer techniques, including new cell lines derived from stem cells, are expected to result in more predictive *in vitro* assays.[142] Some of this information may be useful for detecting hepatotoxicity[143] in the lead optimisation process so that chemistry can be directed to overcome the problems. Bioavailability studies may be particularly important for evaluating the significance of the *in vivo* biological results, especially if the results are negative or less convincing. Although the ADME studies may be valuable in highlighting the short-comings of the early hits/leads, these may sometimes result in inappropriate rejection of a lead. In many cases, the physicochemical and toxicological properties of the early hits/leads may be very different to those of the optimised drug candidates.

1.5.11 Imaging

Major advances have been made in imaging techniques such as magnetic resonance imaging (MRI), nuclear tomographic imaging, X-ray computed tomography, positron emission tomography (PET) and single photon emission computed tomography.[144] The entire body can now be imaged in exquisite anatomical detail leading to greatly improved capacity to detect pathological processes. The information generated by imaging techniques can be used not only for visualization of gross anatomy and detection of diseased tissue based on morphological alterations or abnormalities, but also to visualize gene expression, biochemical reactions, signal transduction, regulatory pathways and direct drug action in whole organisms *in vivo*.[145] The main advantages of imaging techniques include direct visualisation of disease processes, the ability to quantitate changes over time and the non-invasive nature of the techniques. For example, MRI allows the precise localisation of the site of vascular occlusion in several vascular beds such as the aorta, the carotid arteries and the coronary arteries. Most importantly, MRI can be used to characterize plaque composition

as it allows the discrimination of lipid core, fibrosis, calcification and intra-plaque haemorrhage deposits.[146] In stroke patients, MRI allows precise localisation of the site of vascular occlusion, quantification of ensuing perfusion and the oxygenation deficit. Cardiac MRI has become an important tool for the detection and characterization of myocardial viability in patients with coronary artery disease.[147] Similarly, MRI of tumours, including brain tumours, can provides anatomical detail and can also reveal the biology, cellular structure and vascular dynamics of a tumour.[148] Functional MRI has been used increasingly to map the modulatory effects of psychopharmacological agents on cognitive activation of large-scale networks in the human brain.[149] Such pharmacological MRI studies can be informative about pharmacodynamics, specific neurotransmitter mechanisms that underlie the adaptivity of neurocognitive systems to variation in task difficulty and familiarity, and changes in neurophysiological drug effects associated with genetic variation, neuropsychiatric disorders and normal ageing. Like MRI, PET has also been used in assessing the viability of myocardial tissue and detecting various tumours.[150,151] These imaging techniques have become essential tools for the diagnosis of central nervous system disorders and are used increasingly for the evaluation of a variety of diseases (e.g. cancer, vascular diseases, musculoskeletal diseases and developmental abnormalities). New tissue and antigen-specific contrast agents and radioligand tracer molecules are being developed. Discovery of improved therapies for neurological disorders and/or drugs acting on the brain is particularly likely to depend on access to imaging modalities to aid early clinical studies.[152]

In addition to the diagnostic uses mentioned above, imaging techniques are also helpful in patients during the treatment stage.[153] Imaging techniques are being used in cancer patients both for design of treatment plans and to localise the target for precise administration of radiation. At the planning stage, computerized tomography (CT) scanning undertaken with the patient immobilised in the treatment position is most frequently used before radiotherapy. Other imaging modalities such as MRI and magnetic resonance spectroscopy, and PET and single photon emission tomography can be registered to this scan to enhance tumour definition and to display functional data about the tumour or healthy tissues (including any movement caused by breathing or peristalsis). At the treatment stage, three-dimensional soft-tissue imaging can also be used to localise the target and tumour motion can be tracked using fluoroscopic imaging of radio-opaque markers implanted in or near the tumour. These developments allow changes in tumour position, size and shape that take place during radio-therapy to be measured and accounted for to boost geometric accuracy and precision of radiation delivery. This allows the radiation dose to tightly conform around tumours, enabling more healthy tissue to be spared than with two-dimensional non-CT-based radiotherapy. The improvement in precision radiation delivery allows doses to tumours to be escalated, with the potential for further clinical gains.

1.6 Examples of drug discovery

This section covers the discovery of many successful drugs on the market, together with some others that did not make it to the market for various reasons. Although medicinal chemistry, along with structural (e.g. X-ray and NMR spectroscopy) and modelling studies, has played a major part in all the cases, the starting leads and the final drugs were not always obtained by totally rational design processes. The structure activity studies in the most relevant *in vitro* and *in vivo* models have had a significant role in converting the initial lead into the final drug that reached the market. Even today, because of the complexities of the drug discovery process, a totally rational approach leading to a marketed drug is not possible.

In each of the examples discussed below, chosen to include different design strategies, an attempt has been made to highlight the origins of the starting leads and various rational/semi-rational discovery steps used in the optimisation process. Several interesting points emerge from the examples. One of the more interesting and recent developments has been the discovery of non-peptide antagonists and agonists acting at the peptide receptors. Although non-peptide antagonists have been obtained in many cases [e.g. ACTH, angiotensin, bradykinin, cholecystokinin, gastrin and luteinizing hormone releasing hormone (LHRH)], the agonists have only been obtained in a few cases (e.g. angiotensin and bradykinin). These agonist/antagonist discoveries show how small chemical changes can convert an antagonist to an agonist and thus highlight the importance of the screening process. In a chapter of this size it is not possible to cover the topics in detail and to include all the SAR and modelling data and original references. Recent references to reviews have been included. These can be used to trace original publications. Details of some of the peptide-based topics have been published previously.[154,155]

59 Morphine

1.6.1 Receptor ligands (agonists and antagonists)

1.6.1.1 Early examples

In the past, a number of discoveries have been made in the absence of any knowledge about the receptors or ligands. One of the earliest examples of this kind is morphine (**59**) which was used for many years as an analgesic agent (as a constituent of opium, extracted from the poppy plant, *Papaver somniferum*) without any knowledge about its mechanism of action. Only in the last 30 years have various opiate receptor subtypes (μ-, δ-, κ- and σ-receptors) been identified. In addition, endogenous opiate-like peptides, such as enkephalins (Tyr-Gly-Gly-Phe-Met and Tyr-Gly-Gly-Phe-Leu) and endorphins, have been isolated and characterised. Many other opiate-peptides have been isolated from different species, and enormous number of receptor-selective analogues (agonist and antagonist) have been synthesised in the hope of finding analgesic agents without the side effects associated with morphine. However, no such compound has yet reached the market. Although there are some reports about peptides acting at the benzodiazepine receptor, the story of morphine and enkephalins is the only example so far where a non-peptide ligand (morphine) acting at a peptide receptor was known before the peptide ligand (enkephalin) was isolated. In all the other examples (described below), the endogenous peptide ligand was isolated first from natural sources and the non-peptide ligands were obtained later by random screening or semi-rational approaches.

Another example of drug discovery without much knowledge of the receptor or the ligand is the discovery of benzodiazepines initially obtained by random (*in vivo*) screening of compounds for anxiolytic activity. The compounds were later found to act as modulators of γ-aminobutyric acid at its receptor. Many years later, the discovery and characterisation of benzodiazepine receptors from brain tissue led to the development of *in vitro* receptor binding assays and drugs such as diazepam (**60**). In a similar manner, histamine had been recognised as a chemical messenger and shown

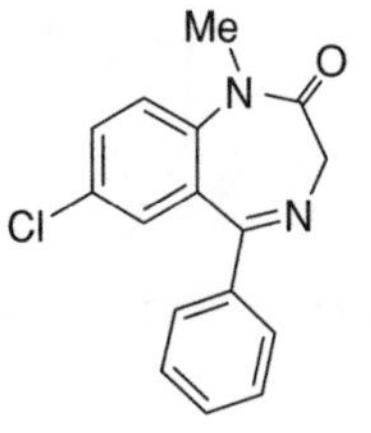

60 Diazepam

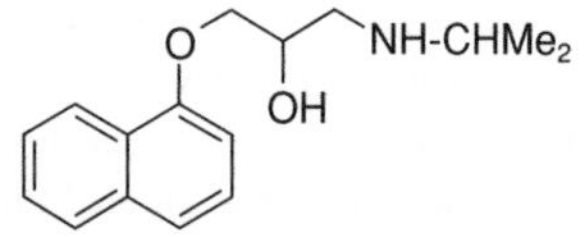

63 Propranolol

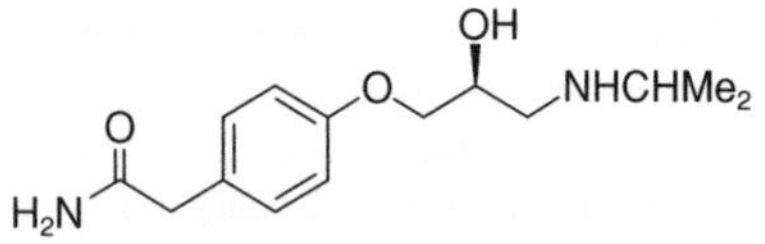

64 Atenolol

to stimulate acid secretion many years before the discovery of its receptors. Discovery of antihistamine compounds resulted in the classification of four receptor subtypes (H_1, H_2 H_3 and H_4). Histamine acting *via* H_1 receptors causes contraction in some smooth muscles (e.g. in the gut, the uterus and the bronchi) and relaxation in other smooth muscles (e.g. in some blood vessels) causing hypotension. Physiologically, histamine has a role in regulating the secretion of gastric acid by stimulating the parietal cells to produce the acid. This effect is mediated by H_2 receptors. The role of H_3 and H_4 receptor is much less defined. Extensive work on antihistamine compounds has resulted in many successful drugs such as fexofenadine (Allegra) (**6**), cimetidine and rantidine (**7**).

In many cases, including the adrenergic receptors, the nature of the ligand/transmitter [(**61**), dopamine R1=R2=H; epinephrine (adrenaline) R1=OH, R2=Me; norepinephrine (noradrenaline) R1=OH, R2=H] was known before starting the drug discovery programmes. The availability of many synthetic analogues led to receptor classification (α- and β-adrenergic receptors and other subtypes) and selective ligands. Many of these such as salbutamol [(**62**), a β_2-selective agonist used as a bronchodilator for the treatment of asthma], propranolol [(**63**), a non-selective β-antagonist] and atenolol [(**64**), a selective β_1-antagonist], used for the treatment of angina and hypertension, have been successful drugs.

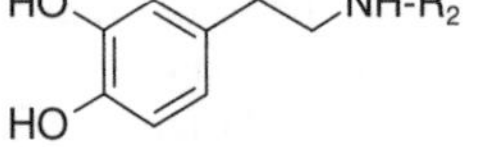

61 Dopamine, adrenaline and noradrenaline

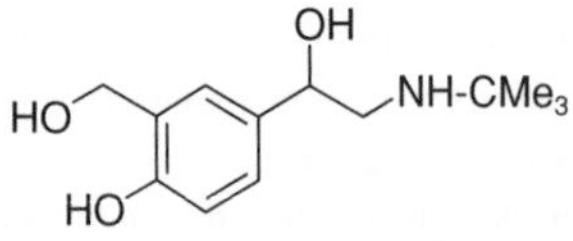

62 Salbutamol

1.6.1.2 Selective oestrogen receptor modulators (oestrogen antagonists and aromatase inhibitors)

Another example of drug discovery in the absence of any significant knowledge about the receptors has been the discovery of selective oestrogen receptor modulators. Like the above examples, the structures of the ligands were known and were utilised, in some cases, for the discovery of drugs on the market. The discovery of selective oestrogen receptor modulators (agonists and antagonists) highlights the impact of developing science in any area of drug discovery as new information emerges and new indications become obvious. In the case of oestrogens, over the years it has become clear that oestrogen is important not only in the growth, differentiation and function of tissues of the reproductive system, but it also has an important role in maintaining bone density and protecting against osteoporosis. It also has beneficial effects in the cardiovascular (cardioprotective) and central nervous systems (protecting against Alzheimer's disease). In addition, the two isoforms of oestrogen receptor (ERα and ERβ) belonging to a family of nuclear hormone receptors that function as transcription factors on binding to their respective ligands have been identified. Thus, tissue-selective oestrogen receptor modulators ranging from full agonist activity to pure anti-oestrogenic activity may be useful in the treatment and prevention of osteoporosis, treatment of breast cancer[156] and may reduce the risk of cardiac disease and Alzheimer's disease.

Tamoxifen (**65**), a non-steroidal anti-oestrogen, demonstrates antiproliferative effects in the breast and is widely used for the treatment of breast cancer.[157] However, it does not show anti-oestrogenic properties in all the tissues. For example, tamoxifen acts as an agonist on bone, liver and the endometrium. This mixed antagonist–agonist profile leads to many advantages in cancer patients. As an antagonist, tamoxifen

65 Tamoxifen

66 Toremifene

67 Droloxifene

68 Raloxifene

69 Fulvestrant

70 Formestane

71 Exemestane

72 Anastrozole

prevents oestrogen-induced proliferation of breast ductal epithelium and breast cancer, and as an agonist in bone and liver it prevents bone loss in post-menopausal women and reduces cholesterol levels. However, the oestrogenic effects in the endometrium in postmenopausal women can result in an increased risk of endometrial cancer. Many other tamoxifen analogues such as toremifene (**66**) and droloxifene (**67**) show similar selectivity profile. The activity of raloxifene (**68**) is also similar to that of tamoxifen, except on the endometrium where it possesses less agonist activity. Recent clinical trials showed that raloxifene reduced the risk of invasive breast cancer

and reduced the risk of clinical vertebral fractures but the drug was associated with an increased risk of fatal stroke.[158] In comparison to the above mixed agonist–antagonist compounds, the steroidal anti-oestrogen fulvestrant (**69**) demonstrates a pure anti-oestrogenic profile in all tissues.

As an alternative to blocking the actions of oestrogen by compounds such as tamoxifen, similar biological and/or clinical effects can be obtained by inhibiting aromatase, the enzyme that catalyses the final and rate-limiting step in oestrogen synthesis (conversion of androgens into oestrogens).[159] Steroidal compounds such as formestane (**70**) and exemestane (**71**) which are structurally related to the natural substrate of aromatase, and non-steroidal compounds such as anastrozole (**72**), letrozole (**73**), fadrozole and vorozole have been developed as aromatase inhibitors.

73 Letrozole

Many of these are currently in use for the treatment of breast cancer.

1.6.1.3 LHRH agonists and antagonists

In more recent times, efforts have been directed towards finding receptor agonists and antagonists acting at the peptidergic receptors. In most of these cases (including LHRH), naturally occurring ligands were first isolated from various animal species, including humans, and crude receptor preparations were then used to screen for other agonist and antagonist ligands. Extensive structure activity studies are carried out to identify the regions responsible for binding to the receptor and intrinsic activity. In general, SAR studies involve the synthesis of a large number of analogues by carrying out deletion studies (eliminating one or more amino acids from the chain), amino acid replacements by natural and unnatural amino acids, peptide bond replacements and synthesis of conformationally restricting cyclic peptides. These studies are often followed by conformational studies using various spectroscopic and modelling techniques. Based on the results, further modifications are carried out in a semi-rational manner to obtain compounds with desired properties.

LHRH (Pyr-His-Trp-Ser-Tyr-Gly-Leu-Arg-Pro-Gly-NH$_2$) is secreted from the hypothalamus and its action on the pituitary gland leads to the release of luteinising hormone and follicle-stimulating hormone. Both of these hormones then act on the ovaries and testes and are responsible for the release of steroidal hormones. Early studies indicated that chronic administration of potent agonist analogues leads to tachyphylaxis or desensitisation of the pituitary receptors, leading finally to a suppression (not stimulation) of oestrogen and testosterone. This finding has led to the use of potent LHRH agonists in the treatment of hormone-dependent tumours. The LHRH antagonists are also expected to be useful for the treatment of these tumours but progress in the antagonist field has been relatively slow. Potent antagonists have been obtained by multiple amino acid substitutions in various positions of the LHRH molecule and a number of the best antagonists have between 5 and 7 amino acid residues replaced by unnatural amino acids. These combinations of multiple substitutions were arrived at in a step-wise manner starting from the first antagonist, [des-His^2]-LHRH. Most of the peptide gonadotrophin-releasing hormone (GnRH) antagonists in various stages of clinical trials are shown in Table 1.5. Based on some of the recent animal data, degarelix (74) appears to have the best profile. In castrated male rats injected subcutaneously with degarelix (2 mg/kg), plasma concentrations of degarelix remained above 5 ng/mL until day 41. At a dose of 2 mg/kg, it maintained testosterone at castrate levels for 49 days. Rats sacrificed on day 45 had considerably reduced prostate, seminal vesicles and testes weights. Degarelix was less potent than other antagonists in histamine releasing assays.

For the discovery of potent LHRH agonist and antagonist analogues, a large number of analogues were synthesised by incorporating amino acid changes in single and multiple positions.[160,161] The most important structure-activity findings that led to these compounds were:

• Replacement of the C-terminal glycinamide residue (-NHCH$_2$CONH$_2$) by a number of alkyl amide (-NH-R) or aza-amino acid amide residues (-NH-N(R)-CONH$_2$) (two- to threefold improvement in potency).

Table 1.5 Luteinizing hormone-releasing hormone (LHRH) antagonists in various stages of clinical trials

Name	Chemical structure
Abarelix	Ac-D-Nal-D-Phe(p-Cl)-D-Pal-Ser-MeTyr-D-Asp-Leu-Lys(iPr)-Pro-D-Ala-NH$_2$
Acyline	Ac-D-Nal-D-Phe(p-Cl)-D-Pal-Ser-Aph(Ac)-D-Aph(Ac)-Leu-Lys(iPr)-Pro-D-Ala-NH$_2$
Antarelix	Ac-D-Nal-D-Phe(p-Cl)-D-Pal-Ser-Tyr-D-hCit-Leu-Lys(iPr)-Pro-D-Ala-NH$_2$
Cetrorelix	Ac-D-Nal-D-Phe(p-Cl)-D-Pal-Ser-Tyr-D-Cit-Leu-Arg-Pro-D-Ala-NH$_2$
Degarelix	Ac-D-Nal-D-Phe(p-Cl)-D-Pal-Ser-Aph(Hor)-D-Aph(Cbm)-Leu-Lys(iPr)-Pro-D-Ala-NH$_2$
Ganirelix	Ac-D-Nal-D-Phe(p-Cl)-D-Pal-Ser-Tyr-D-hArg(Et$_2$)-Leu-hArg(Et$_2$)-Pro-D-Ala-NH$_2$
Iturelix/Antide	Ac-D-Nal-D-Phe(p-Cl)-D-Pal-Ser-Lys(Nic)-D-Lys(Nic)-Leu-Lys(iPr)-Pro-D-Ala-NH$_2$
Ornirelix	Ac-D-Nal-D-Phe(p-Cl)-D-Pal-Ser-Lys(Pic)-D-Orn(6-Anic)-Leu-Lys(iPr)-Pro-D-Ala-NH$_2$

74 Degarelix

- Substitution of the glycine residue in position 6 by a D-amino-acid residues [e.g. D-Ala, D-Leu, D-Arg, D-Phe, D-Trp, D-Ser(Bu^t)] (two- to 100-fold improvement in potency).
- A combination of D-amino-acids in position 6 and an ethylamide or azaglycine amide in position 10.

The effects of multiple changes were not always additive. A combination of many of these changes has led to the discovery of potent agonists which are currently on the market for the treatment of prostate and breast cancer and some non-malignant conditions such as endometriosis and uterine fibroids. The marketed drugs include Zoladex {[D-Ser(Bu^t)^6, Azgly^{10}]-LHRH},[162,163] leuprolide {[D-Leu^6, des-Gly-NH$_2$^{10}]-LHRH(1-9)NHEt}, nafarelin {D-Nal(2)^6]-LHRH}, buserelin {[D-Ser(Bu^t)^6, des-Gly-NH$_2$^{10}]-LHRH(1-9) NHEt} and triptorelin {[D-Trp^6]-LHRH}.

The potential of LHRH agonists in human medicine has been greatly enhanced by the development of convenient formulations for the delivery of these peptides. The most successful of these have been the biodegradable poly(D,L-lactide-co-glycolide) depot formulations which release the drug over a period of 1–3 months. A biodegradable poly(D,L-lactide-co-glycolide) sustained release formulation of 'Zoladex' can deliver 3.6–10.5 mg of the peptide over a period of 1–3 months. The formulation consists of a homogeneous dispersion of the drug (20% w/w) in a rod of the polymer and is administered by subcutaneous injection.

Non-peptide antagonists of GnRH, discovered by random screening approaches, are further behind the peptide antagonists in term of clinical development. Takeda compound TK-013 (75) is most advanced. Other major companies have recently published data on their non-peptide antagonists (76). However, be-

75

76

cause of the availability of longer acting (1–4 months) depot formulations of GnRH agonists already in the market and the possibility of depot formulations of peptide antagonists and longer acting compounds such as degarelix, the need for orally active compounds is debatable.

1.6.1.4 Somatostatin agonists and antagonists

The cyclic peptide somatostatin [Ala-Gly-Cys-Lys-Asn-Phe-Phe-Trp-Lys-Thr-Phe-Thr-Ser-Cys, disulphide bridge between Cys[3] and Cys[14]] and the 28 amino acid precursor containing 14 additional amino acid residues (Ser-Ala-Asn-Ser-Asn-Pro-Ala-Met-Ala-Pro-Arg-Glu-Arg-Lys) at the N-terminus were isolated from the extracts of ovine and porcine hypothalamus, respectively. Both peptides are associated with a large number of biological activities, including the inhibition of growth hormone, insulin, glucagon and gastric acid secretion. Thus, somatostatin may have an important role in many physiological and pharmacological systems. Five human receptor subtypes (hSSTR$_1$–hSSTR$_5$) of somatostatin have been characterised. There is now emerging evidence for additional somatostatin receptor subtypes. The realisation that somatostatin acts through multiple receptors suggested the possibility that somatostatin may also achieve functional selectivity by acting through a specific receptor subtype to control a specific action. Large number of analogues have therefore been synthesised in the hope of finding drugs for various diseases. These analogues are being used to define specific functions of various receptor subtypes. However, the process of linking specific functions to receptor subtypes has proved to be much more difficult.[164,165] The task has been made more difficult by the finding that somatostatin and its receptor subtypes are widely distributed in the body.

Examples of compounds that have reached the market include octreotide [Sandostatin, D-Phe-cyclo(Cys-Phe-D-Trp-Lys-Thr-Cys)-Thr-ol], lanreo-tide [D-Nal-cyclo(Cys-Tyr-D-Trp-Lys-Val-Cys)-Thr-NH$_2$] and vapreotide (RC-160) [D-Phe-cyclo(Cys-Tyr-D-Trp-Lys-Val-Cys)-Trp-NH$_2$]. Daily and slow release depot formulation of octreotide are used for the treatment of growth-hormone secreting pituitary tumours, thyrotrophin secreting pituitary adenomas, pancreatic islet cell tumours and carcinoid tumours that express somatostatin receptors.[166] A long-acting formulation of octreotide administered to acromegalic patients for 18 months (once every 4 weeks) suppressed growth hormone and insulin-like growth factor levels in all the patients, and signs and symptoms of acromegaly improved during treatment. Reduction of the pituitary tumour was seen in all previously untreated patients.

Progress towards small cyclic peptides, equipotent or more potent than somatostatin, was made in several steps. Early SAR established that the Ala^1-Gly^2 residues and the disulphide bridge were not essential for biological activity. Amino acid substitution studies indicated that replacements of Lys^4 by Arg, Phe, Phe(F$_5$) or Phe(p-NH$_2$) residues, Asn^5 by Ala or D-Tyr, Phe^7

by Tyr, Trp^8 by D-Trp, D-Trp(5-F), D-Trp(6-F), D-Trp(5-Br), Phe^{11} by Phe(p-I) or Nal(2) and Cys^{14} by D-Cys gave compounds that were either equipotent or more potent than the parent peptide. Amino acid substitutions in other positions gave less potent analogues. For example, most of the analogues obtained by substituting the Phe^6 and Phe^7 residues, except by other aromatic amino acids such as Phe(p-Cl), Phe(p-I) and Tyr, were less potent (<10%) than somatostatin. Deletion of the C-terminal carboxyl group or its replacement by an ethylamide group also resulted in compounds equipotent to somatostatin. An equally important finding, useful in designing smaller peptides, emerged by deleting various amino acid residues. Compounds lacking Lys^4 and Asn^5 were found to retain significant biological activity whereas the compounds lacking Phe^6, Trp^8, Lys^9, Thr^{10}, Phe^{11}, Thr^{12} were relatively poor agonists. The deletion and substitution studies led to much smaller peptides such as cyclo(Aha-Phe-Phe-D-Trp-Lys-Thr-Phe), cyclo(Pro-Phe-D-Trp-Lys-Thr-Phe) and cyclo(Pro-Phe-D-Trp-Lys-Val-Phe). The most potent analogue cyclo(MeAla-Tyr-D-Trp-Lys-Val-Phe) was 20- to 50-fold more potent than somatostatin in inhibiting growth hormone, 70 times more potent in inhibiting insulin and >80 times more potent in inhibiting glucagon. Other more potent cyclic peptides containing a disulphide bridge, D-Phe-Cys-Phe-D-Trp-Lys-Thr-Cys-Thr(ol), D-Phe-Cys-Tyr-D-Trp-Lys-Val-Cys-Thr-NH$_2$, D-Phe-Cys-Tyr-D-Trp-Lys-Val-Cys-Trp-NH$_2$ and D-Phe-Cys-Tyr-D-Trp-Lys-Val-Cys-Thr-NH$_2$, were 80–200 times more potent than somatostatin. Since the discovery and availability of cloned multiple receptors, additional SAR studies have led to more receptor-selective agonist and antagonist analogues. For example, the cyclic peptide [Cys-Lys-Phe-Phe-D-Trp-Phe(p-CH$_2$NH-CH(CH$_3$)$_2$-Thr-Phe-Thr-Ser-Cys, disulphide bridge] was a potent agonist at hSSTR$_1$ receptors and the N(α-Me)benzylglycine containing analogue cyclo[(R)-βMeNphe-Phe-D-Trp-Lys-Thr-Phe] is an hSSTR$_2$ selective agonist. The hSSTR$_2$ agonist selectively inhibited the release of growth hormone in rats (equipotent to sandostatin) but had no effect on the inhibition of insulin at the same dose. Cyclo(Phe(N-aminoethyl)-Tyr-D-Trp-Lys-Val-Phe(N-carboxypropyl)-Thr-NH$_2$ – a backbone-cyclic somatostatin analogue displayed high selectivity for the SSTR$_5$ receptor.

In comparison with the agonist analogues, very few antagonists of somatostatin have been obtained by amino acid substitution. Two octapeptide derivatives, 4-NO$_2$-Phe-c(D-Cys-Tyr-D-Trp-Lys-Thr-Cys)-Tyr-

NH_2 and Ac-4-NO_2-Phe-c(D-Cys-Tyr-D-Trp-Lys-Thr-Cys)-D-Tyr-NH_2 (inactive at the SST_1 and SST_4 receptor subtypes; high affinity at the $SSTR_2$ and $SSTR_5$ receptor subtypes) inhibited somatostatin-mediated inhibition of cyclic adenosine monophosphate (cAMP) accumulation in a dose-dependent manner. The more potent antagonist [Ac-4-NO_2-Phe-c(D-Cys-Tyr-D-Trp-Lys-Thr-Cys)-D-Tyr-NH_2] displays a binding affinity to $SSTR_2$ comparable with that observed for the native hormone. H-Nal-c[D-Cys-Pal-D-Trp-Lys-Val-Cys]-Nal-NH_2 was also a more selective $hSST_2$ receptor antagonist.

1.6.1.5 Angiotensin agonists and antagonists (peptides and non-peptides)

The renin–angiotensin system has been one of the most active fields of research for antihypertensive drugs.[167] Angiotensin II and other members of the angiotensin family are produced by the processing of a protein called α_2-globulin or angiotensinogen which is synthesised in the liver and found in the blood. The protein is first cleaved by the enzyme renin to generate a decapeptide angiotensin I [Asp-Arg-Val-Tyr-Ile-His-Pro-Phe-His-Leu], which is further cleaved by ACE to produce octapeptide angiotensin II [Asp^1-Arg-Val-Tyr-Ile-His-Pro-Phe^8], which is a potent vasoconstrictor.

Angiotensin II acts at two receptor subtypes (AT_1 and AT_2). Drugs that inhibit the production of angiotensin II or its access to the type 1 receptor are prescribed to alleviate high blood pressure and its cardiovascular complications. Accordingly, much research has focused on the molecular pharmacology of AT_1R activation and signalling.[168] In the case of the agonist analogues, one of the most significant change has been the replacement of the N-terminal Asp by Sar (N-methylglycine) to give [Sar^1]-angiotensin II, which in a number of in vitro tissue preparations was 1.5–2.5 times more potent than the natural ligand. AT_2 receptor selective analogues were obtained by modifications at the N- and C-terminal ends of the peptide. The N-terminally modified compounds [Me_2Gly^1]-, [Me_3Gly^1]- and [Me_3Ser^1]-angiotensin II were >1000-fold more potent at the AT_2 receptor subtypes. The analogue modified at positions 1 and 8, [Sar^1, Phe^8]-angiotensin II was 345-fold more potent than angiotensin II at the AT_2 receptor. Modifications of the C-terminal dipeptide (Pro^7-Phe^8) of [Sar^1, Val^5]angiotensin II with constrained aromatic (Tic) and hydrophobic (Oic) amino acids led to analogues with negligible affinity for the AT_1 receptor, but nanomolar affinity for the AT_2 receptor. The most potent

and AT_2-selective analogue of the series was Sar-Arg-Val-Tyr-Val-His-Phe-Oic (IC_{50} 240 and 0.51 nmol at the AT_1 and AT_2 receptors, respectively). A conformationally restricted analogue of angiotensin II, [$hCys^3$, $hCys^5$]-angiotensin II, was equipotent to angiotensin II in displacing [^{125}I]-angiotensin II from rat uterus membranes and in inducing contractions in the rabbit aortic rings (pD_2 8.48). Conformational analysis studies indicated that the cyclic peptide-like analogues {e.g. c[$hCys^{3,5}$]-angiotensin II} may assume an inverse γ-turn conformation; thus, amino acid residues 3–5 in angiotensin II were substituted with different turn mimetic residues. Most of the analogues were either inactive or much less potent than angiotensin II.

Antagonists of angiotensin II were initially obtained by eliminating the side-chain from the C-terminal phenylalanine residue. Antagonist such as [Gly^8]-angiotensin II which competitively blocks the myotropic action of both angiotensin I and angiotensin II in in vitro test systems but did not antagonise the pressor response to angiotensin II in anaesthetised cats were further modified in position 8 to give more potent antagonists, for example [Ile^8]-angiotensin II. A combination of positions 5 and 8 changes along with the N-terminal changes (Sar^1) discovered in the case of agonist series of compounds gave more potent antagonists such as [Sar^1, Ala^8]-angiotensin II, [Sar^1, Ile^8]-angiotensin II (pA_2 9.48) and [Sar^1, $Pen(SMe)^5$, Ile^8]-angiotensin II. [Sar^1, $Thr(Me)^5$, Ile^8]-, [Sar^1, β-$MePhe^5$, Ile^8]- and [Sar^1, His^5, Ile^8]-angiotensin II were more potent than [Sar^1, Ile^8]-angiotensin II in the in vivo rat blood pressure test. In the cyclic series of antagonists, except [Sar^1, $hCys^3$, $hCys^5$, Ile^8]-angiotensin II, many other cyclic compounds, for example [$Cys^{1,5}$, Ile^8]-, [D-Cys^1, Cys^5, Ile^8]-, [Sar^1, $Cys^{5,8}$]-, [Sar^1, Cys^5, D-Cys^8]- and [Sar^1, $hCys^5$, D-Cys^8]-angiotensin II, were much less potent.

Non-peptide antagonists of angiotensin II were obtained by random screening approaches. Despite all the progress achieved in discovering potent agonist and antagonist analogues and the ligand receptor information derived from the above compounds, it was not possible to design non-peptidic molecules by this rational design procedure. The discovery from a random screening lead of DuP753 [(77), losartan] which is selective for AT_1, opened the way to non-peptide antagonists. The SAR studies indicated that a considerable variation was allowed in the chemical structures of the antagonists. The synthetic medicinal chemistry approaches identified various replacements for the imidazole and the biphenyl tetrazole groups

77 Losartan

78

79

80

Another interesting aspect of the non-peptide agonist–antagonist structure-activity studies has been the identification of both agonists and antagonists in the same series of compounds by minor structural modifications. For example, compound **81** was an agonist and a similar analogue that differs chemically by only a single methyl group (**78**) was an antagonist. At present, it is not possible to predict changes which lead to agonist–antagonist analogues by any rational design approaches. Only by screening the compounds in appropriate tests can selective compounds with the desired biological profile be identified. A large amount of chemical effort in the angiotensin antagonist field has led to the discovery of many successful drugs such as losartan (**77**), valsartan (**82**), candesartan (**83**) ibresartan (**84**), eprosartan, telmisartan and olmesartan for the treatment of high blood pressure and other cardiovascular complications.

81 Agonist

82 Valsartan

and highlighted chemical changes which led to AT$_1$- or AT$_2$-selective or mixed (AT$_1$ and AT$_2$) receptor antagonists. Compound **78** (L-162,389) is an example of a mixed antagonist (AT$_1$ and AT$_2$ binding affinities 2–4 nmol). In a macrocyclic series of analogues, **79** bound primarily to the AT$_1$ receptor (AT$_1$ and AT$_2$ receptor IC$_{50}$ values 23 and 4000 nmol, respectively) whereas a very similar analogue **80** bound to both the receptors with similar affinity (IC$_{50}$ 20–30 nmol).

83 Candesartan

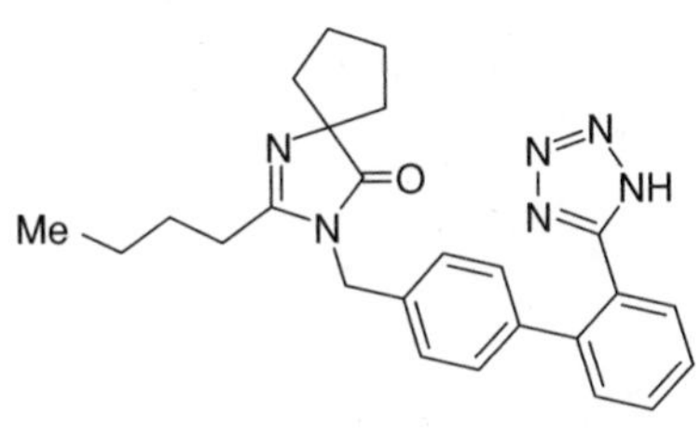

84 Ibresartan

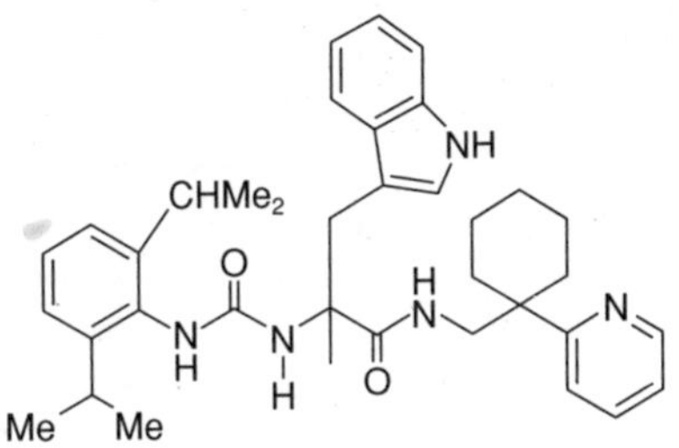

86

1.6.1.6 Bombesin/neuromedin agonists and antagonists

1.6.1.6.1 Semi-rational approaches Four subtypes of the bombesin receptor have been identified (gastrin releasing peptide [GRP] receptor, neuromedin B receptor, the orphan receptor bombesin receptor subtype 3 and bombesin receptor subtype 4). The roles of individual receptor subtypes are under investigation and selective ligands for these receptor subtypes are being synthesised. Systematic SAR studies have provided many receptor antagonists.[169] A semi-rational approach was used for the discovery of non-peptide antagonists of neuromedin B. The role of each amino acid side-chain was defined by alanine scanning in bombesin(7-14)-octapeptide, Ac-Gln-Trp-Ala-Val-Gly-His-Leu-Met-NH$_2$ (minimum active fragment), and indicated that Trp^8, Val^{10} and Leu^{13} were most important for the binding affinity to the receptors. A search within the company compound collection was then initiated for various templates containing Trp, Val/Leu types of side-chains. This led to a moderately active lead (85). Changes at the C-terminal end led to more potent (S) α-methyl-Trp derivative (86). Additional chemical modifications on 86 resulted in a series of 'balanced' neuromedin-B preferring (BB$_1$)/GRP preferring (BB$_2$) receptor ligands, as exemplified by PD 176252 (87). Compound 87 displaying a BB$_2$ receptor affinity of 1 nmol while retaining subnanomolar (0.17 nmol) BB$_1$ receptor affinity and is a competitive antagonist at both the receptor subtypes.

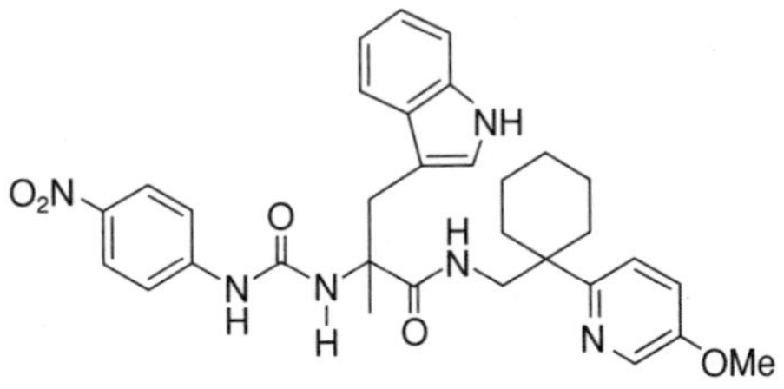

87

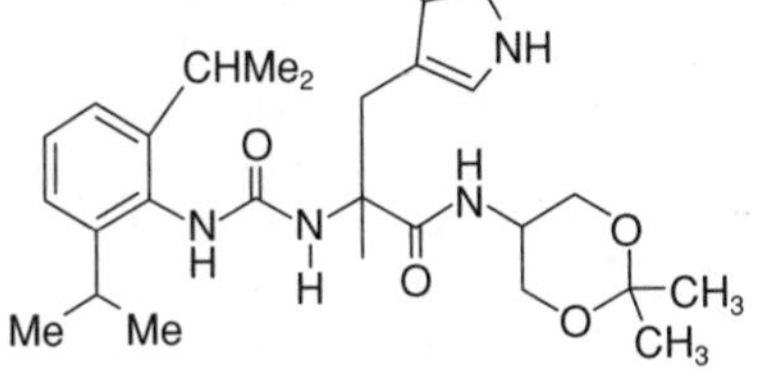

1.6.1.7 Bradykinin agonists and antagonists

Bradykinin (Arg-Pro-Pro-Gly-Phe-Ser-Pro-Phe-Arg) is a vasoactive peptide that mediates vasodilation, increase in vascular permeability, smooth muscle contraction, recruitment of inflammatory cells, induction of pain and hyperalgesia. The effects of bradykinin are mediated by the B$_2$ receptor. Because of its role in mediating pain and inflammation, a number of potent and selective non-peptide antagonists for the B$_2$ receptor have been identified in recent years.[170] Peptide SAR studies resulted in potent bradykinin B$_2$ receptor antagonists such as HOE 140 [D-Arg-Arg-Pro-Hyp-Gly-Thi-Ser-D-Tic-Oic-Arg]. Replacement of some of the amino acids by substituted 1,3,8-triazaspiro[4,5]decan-4-one-3-acetic acids in the B$_2$ receptor antagonist D-Arg-Arg-Pro-Pro-Gly-Phe-Ser-D-Tic-Oic-Arg gave potent B$_2$ receptor antagonists such as 88 (NPC 18521, Ki 0.15 nmol) which contains a phenethyl group at position 1 of the spirocyclic mimetic. Another example of a pseudopeptide analogue is compound NPC 18884 (89) which contains three arginine residues. Given intraperitoneally or

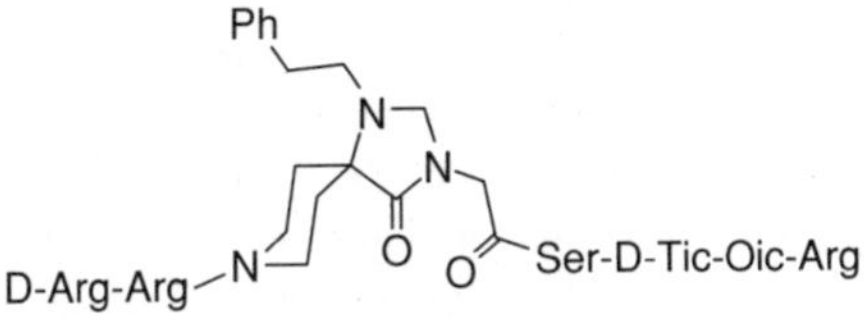

85

88

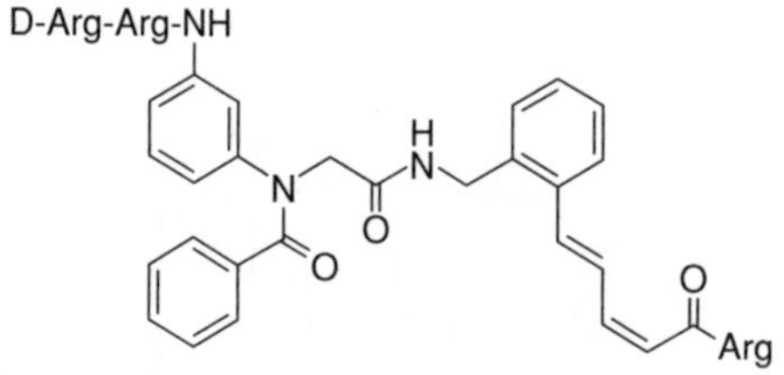

D-Arg-Arg-NH

89

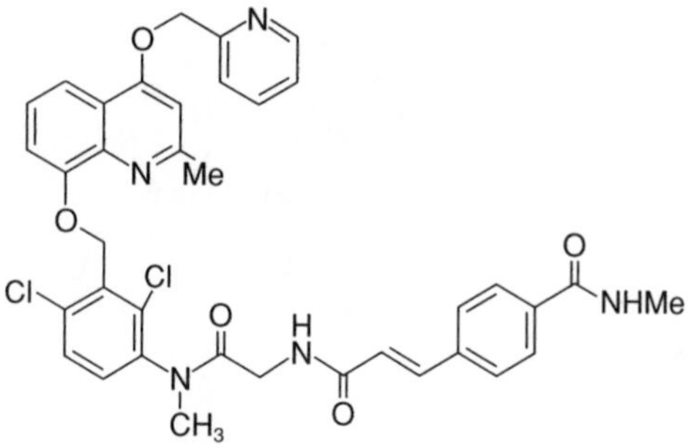

90

91 Antagonist

92 Agonist

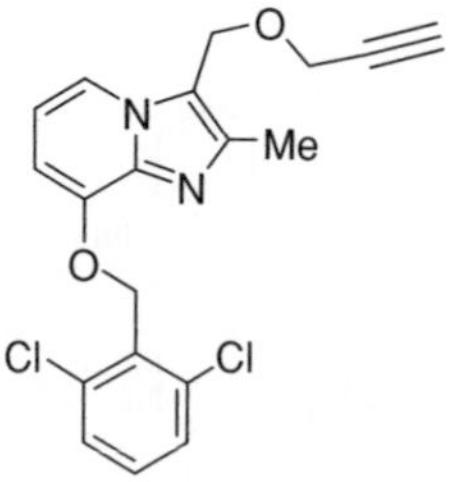

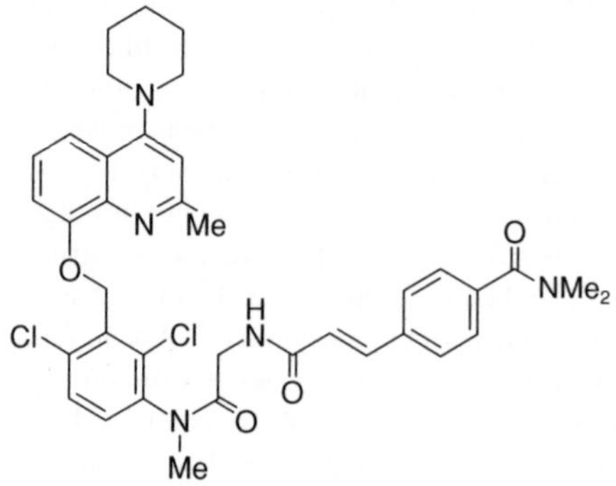

93 Partial agonist

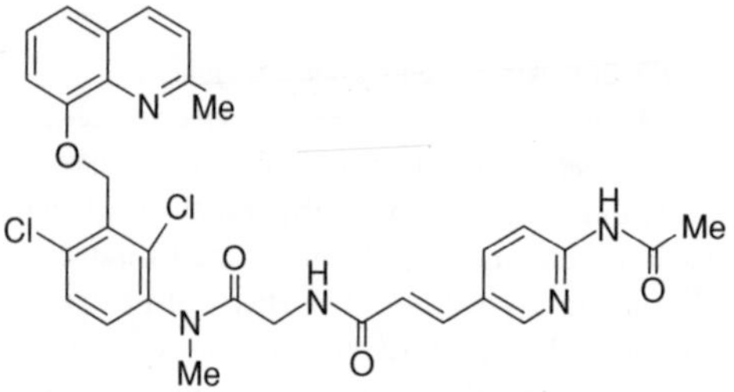

orally, compound **89** inhibited bradykinin-induced leucocytes influx and exudation. The effects lasted for up to 4 h and were selective for the bradykinin B_2 receptors. At similar doses compound **89** had no significant effect against the inflammatory responses induced by des-Arg^9-bradykinin, histamine or substance P.

Like angiotensin II, non-peptide B_2 receptor antagonists and agonists of bradykinin were obtained by random screening approaches. Chemical modifications on random screening leads such as **90** led to non-peptide antagonists such as **91** which were active in a number of *in vitro* and *in vivo* (e.g. bradykinin-induced bronchoconstriction and carrageenin-induced paw oedema) test systems.[171] The non-peptide agonist **92** bound with high affinity to the B_2 receptor (IC_{50} 5.3 nmol), had no binding affinity for the B_1 receptor, and at concentrations between 1 nmol/L and 1 μmol/L stimulated phosphatidylinositol hydrolysis in Chinese hamster ovary cells permanently

expressing the human bradykinin B_2 receptor. The response was antagonised by the B_2 receptor selective antagonist Hoe 140. Intravenous administration of bradykinin or the agonist **92** (both at 10 μg/kg) caused a fall in blood pressure. However, the duration of the hypotensive response to **92** was significantly longer than the response to bradykinin. Another non-peptide compound **93** was a partial agonist.

1.6.1.8 Cholecystokinin agonists and antagonists

Cholecystokinin (CCK), a 33-amino acid regulatory peptide hormone, regulates motility, pancreatic enzyme secretion, gastric emptying and gastric acid secretion in the gastrointestinal tract and is involved in anxiogenesis, satiety, nociception, and memory and learning processes in the nervous system.[172] Antagonists of CCK are being sought as therapeutic agents for various gastrointestinal disorders, anxiety and obesity. A number of peptide and non-peptide ligands acting at CCK_A and/or CCK_B receptors have been described. Peptidomimetic agonist and antagonist analogues of CCK were obtained from the C-terminal tetrapeptide of CCK/gastrin (Boc-Trp-Met-Asp-Phe-NH$_2$) and analogues such as Boc-Trp-MeNle-Asp-Phe-NH$_2$ and by synthesising conformationally constrained

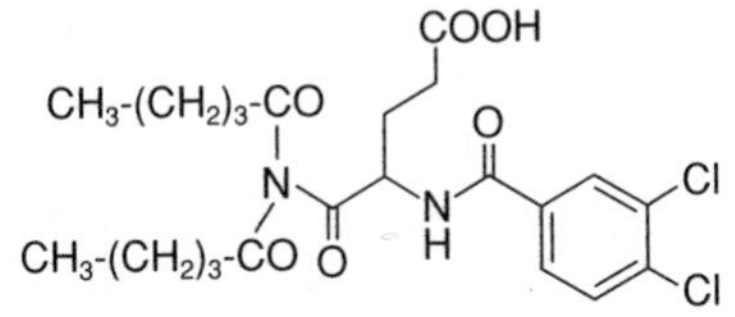

94 Lorglumide

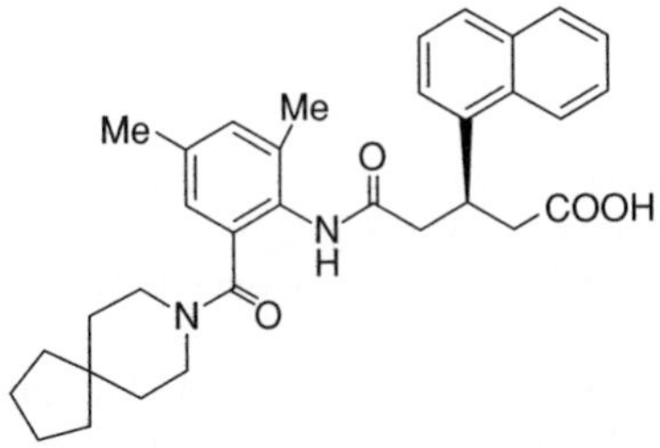

95 Itriglumide

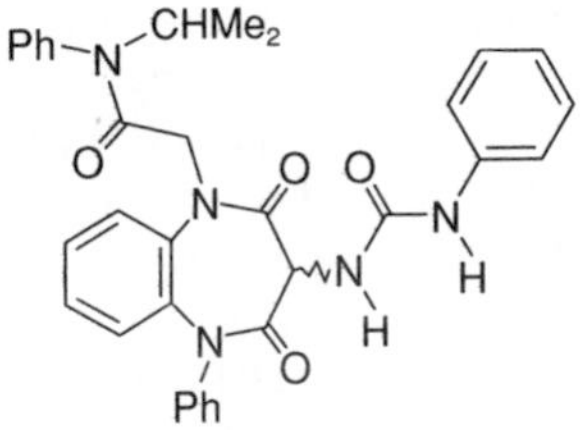

96

97

98

99

analogues by replacing the Trp-Met/Trp-MeNle dipeptides. Some of the early non-peptide antagonists of CCK$_A$ and CCK$_B$ receptors were glutamic acid derivatives. Benzoyl-glutamic acid dipropylamide (proglumide), a weak gastrin antagonist, was marketed for the treatment of ulcers. Further work on this series of compounds led to CCK$_A$ antagonists such as lorglumide (94) and CCK$_B$ receptor antagonists such as itriglumide (95). Non-peptide CCK agonists and antagonists based on a benzodiazepine skeleton were obtained by random screening and lead optimisation approaches. 1,5-Benzodiazepine derivatives such as 96 were shown to be agonists and antagonists of CCK$_A$ and CCK$_B$. The substitution pattern at the anilino-acetamide nitrogen had an important role for the activity. While compounds with a hydrogen or methyl substituent were weak antagonists of CCK-8, the ethyl, propyl (96), n-butyl and cyanoethyl derivatives were agonists. Compound 96 displayed 86% CCK-8 functional activity in the guinea pig gallbladder assay at 30 μmol (CCK-8 = 100% at 1 μmol) and showed similar affinity for CCK$_A$ and CCK$_B$ receptors. When given orally to rats, the CCK$_A$ agonist (97) (GW5823)

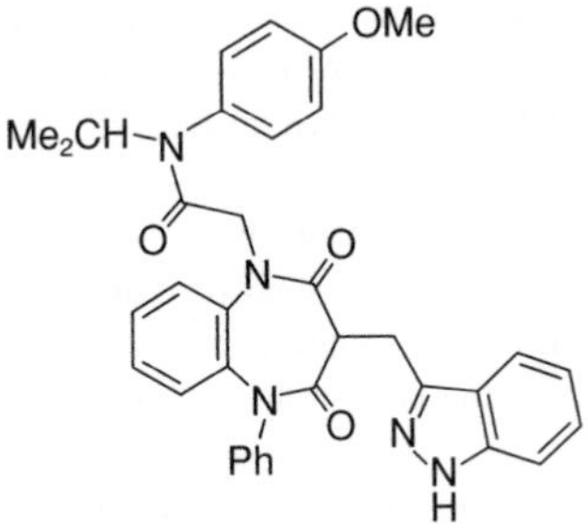

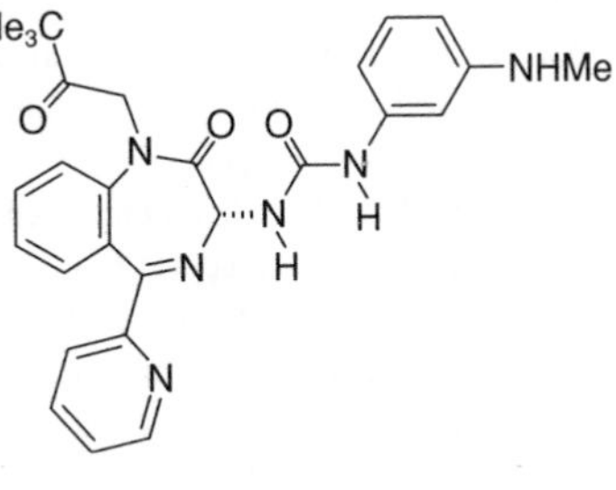

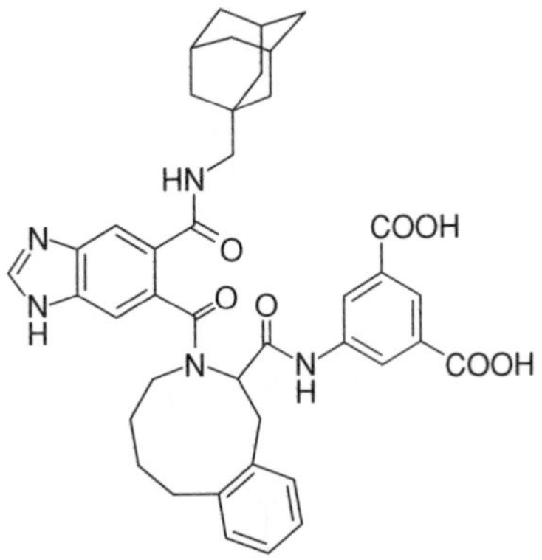

reduced food intake to 40% of that in vehicle-control treated animals. When administered orally, the CCK$_B$/gastrin antagonist YF476 (98) inhibited gastric acid secretion in a pentagastrin-induced acid secretion model and displayed a long duration of action (>6 h at a dose of 100 nmol/kg). In addition to the benzodiazepine derivatives, a number of other chemically distinct CCK antagonists have been prepared starting from the random screening leads. The 9-membered ring analogue (99) was a potent CCK$_B$/gastrin antagonist (rat stomach pK$_B$ 9.08, mouse cortex pIC$_{50}$ 8.3). In comparison, analogues containing 6-, 7- and 8-membered rings were poor CCK$_B$/gastrin receptor antagonists. Although, many of the compounds have reached various stages of clinical trials none of the compounds has yet reached the market.

1.6.1.9 Endothelin antagonists

Endothelin, a 21 amino acid peptide, is one of the most potent vasoconstrictor peptides that was isolated initially from the conditioned medium of cultured endothelial cells.[173] The peptide has been associated with many physiological and pathological functions, including chronic heart failure, ischemic heart diseases, hypertension, atherosclerosis, pulmonary hypertension, chronic renal failure, cerebrovascular spasm after subarachnoid haemorrhage and cancer.[174,175] Antagonists of endothelin-1 are, therefore, being sought for various cardiovascular disorders. Two receptor subtypes (ET_A and ET_B) have been identified for this family of peptides. The ET_A receptor binds ET-1 and ET-2 with greater affinity than it does ET-3, whereas the ET_B receptor binds all three isoforms with equal affinity. Leads for antagonist design have originated from natural sources, rational design approaches and by random screening. ET_A and ET_B receptor selective antagonists were obtained from cyclic pentapeptides of microbial origin such as the ET_A-selective peptide BQ 123 [c(D-Val-Leu-D-Trp-D-Asp-Pro)]. Linear tripeptide derivatives were subsequently developed as ET_A [BQ-485 (**100**)] or ET_B [BQ-788 (**101**)] receptor selective or non-selective [BQ-928 (**102**)] antagonists.

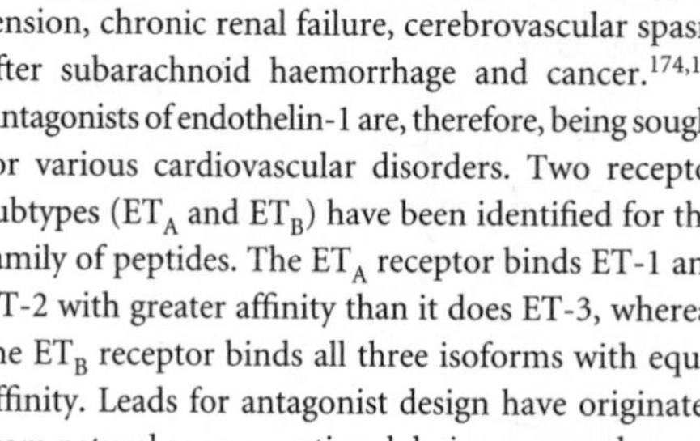

100

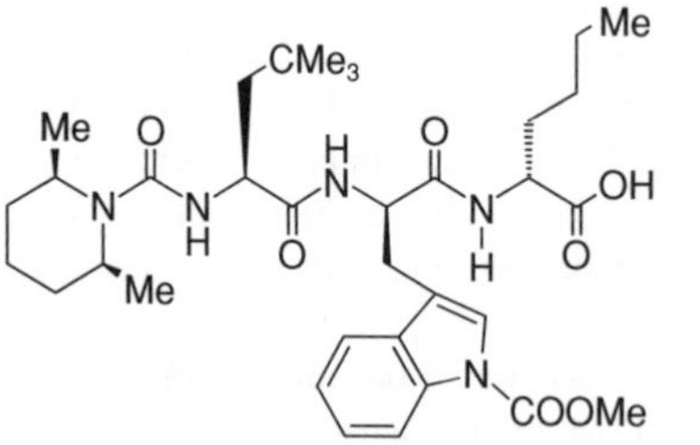

101

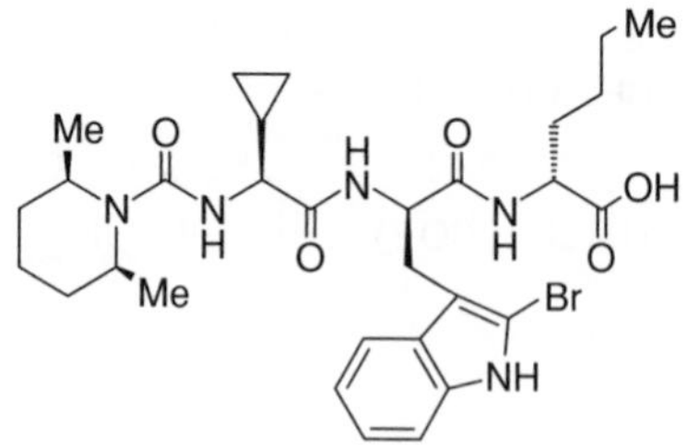

102

In the BQ-123 series, amino acid replacements converted the ET_A selective antagonist BQ-123 to ET_B selective and non-selective antagonists. For example, c(D-*t*-Leu-Leu-2-chloro-D-Trp-D-Asp-Pro)   and c[D-Pen(Me)-Leu-2-bromo-D-Trp-D-Asp-Pro] were nearly equipotent at both the receptors and c[D-Pen(Me)-Leu-2-cyano-D-Trp-D-Asp-Pro] was much more potent at the ET_B receptor. In the *cis*-(2,6-dimethylpiperidino)carbonyl-Leu-D-Trp-D-Nle series of analogues, the 2-bromo-D-Trp, 2-chloro-D-Trp and 2-methyl-D-Trp analogues were potent antagonists at both receptors while the 2-cyano-D-Trp and 2-ethyl-D-Trp analogues were more potent at the ET_B receptor.

Antagonists similar to compounds **100–102** were also discovered by using a rational approach starting from the endothelin C-terminal dodecapeptide derivative, succinyl-Glu-Ala-Val-Tyr-Phe-Ala-His-Leu-Asp-Ile-Ile-Trp. Replacing each of the amino acid in turn with glycine indicated that Phe[14], Ile[19,20] and Trp[21] were the most important residues. Based on this evidence, a series of compounds having an aromatic moiety attached through a spacer to the amino group of the Trp residue were synthesised. Further work around the initial weak antagonist lead, N-*trans*-2-phenylcyclopropanoyl-Trp, resulted in a 400-fold selective ET_B antagonist (**103**). Replacement of the biphenylalanine residue by 2-naphthylalanine, Met,

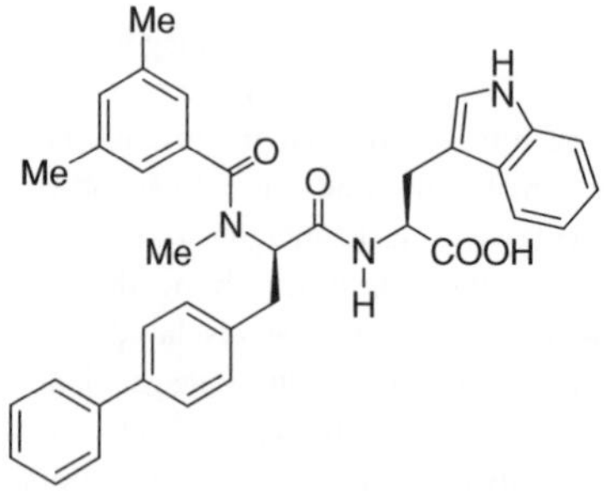

103

104

105

106

107 Bosentan

108 Sitaxsentan

109 Ambrisentan

Leu, Ile, Cha, Thr or ethylglycine gave antagonists that were two- to fourfold more potent at the ET_B receptor. The D-Phe-Val derivative (104) displayed similar affinity for ET_A and ET_B receptors (Ki 1–2 nM).

Non-peptide antagonists of endothelin were discovered by random screening approaches. Chemical modifications to the random screening leads led to receptor and selective and non-selective compounds. A series of ET_A-selective antagonists included a more selective (>25,000-fold) pyrrolidine carboxylic acid derivatives A-216546 (105). A-216546 was orally available in rat, dog and monkey and blocked endothelin-1-induced presser response in conscious rats. Replacement of the dialkylacetamide side-chain in 105 resulted in a complete reversal of receptor selectivity, preferring ET_B over ET_A. Compound 106 (A-308165) demonstrated over 27,000-fold selectivity favouring the ET_B receptor. Three endothelin ET_A-receptor antagonists, bosenthan (107), sitaxsentan (108) and ambrisentan (109), have reached the market for the treatment of pulmonary hypertension. Several other compounds have either failed in the clinic or are in various stages of development.

1.6.1.10 Cytokines and chemokines

Cytokines and chemokines (a family of small chemotactic cytokines interacting with G-protein-coupled receptors) are a family of proteins that have been implicated in many diseases. Cytokines are regulatory proteins produced by white blood cells and several other cell types in the body and released in response to a variety of inflammatory stimuli such as viruses, parasites, bacteria and their products, or in response to other cytokines and are responsible for the production of the final mediators involved in the induction of inflammatory signs and symptoms. Additionally, the cytokines can act on the receptors of the same cells that produced them (autocrine effect) or on the receptors of other cells (paracrine effect), and even circulate and act on distant tissues (hormonal effect). Cytokine actions include the regulation of innate and adaptive immune responses and the modulation of inflammatory responses, in addition to many other activities. Today, the number of known cytokine genes and proteins has reached several hundred, with new ones still being discovered.

Cytokine and chemokine research is one of the most active areas of medicinal research at present. In the case of cytokines, two very different strategies are being adopted to produce therapeutic agents. The first therapeutic strategy involves the administration of purified recombinant cytokines and the second relies on the administration of therapeutics that inhibit the harmful effects of upregulated endogenous cytokines. Examples of successful cytokine therapeutics include haematopoietic growth factors (colony stimulating factors such as granulocyte colony stimulating factor and granulocyte–macrophage colony stimulating factor), interferons [interferon-α for the treatment of chronic hepatitis C (often in combination with the nucleoside analog ribavirin), interferon-β or genetically engineered Cys[17]-interferon-β (interferon β-1b, Betaseron), Avonex (interferon β-1a, derived from Chinese hamster ovary cells) and Rebif (interferon β-1a) for the treatment of multiple sclerosis and recombinant interleukin-2 (IL-2) [Proleukin (aldesleukin)], licensed for the treatment of metastatic renal cancer and metastatic melanoma, and also used experimentally in AIDS patients to increase CD4[+] cell counts. Several other cytokines including IL-7 and IL-15 are currently being studied as immunostimulatory agents.[176,177] During an immune response, peripheral T-cell populations expand and then contract as the response subsides, thus maintaining a fairly constant number of CD4 and CD8 T cells throughout the life of the individual. IL-7 has emerged as a central regulator of the survival and homeostasis of CD4 and CD8 T cells. IL-24 has been shown to enhance radiation lethality and to inhibit tumour angiogenesis[178] and IL-10 and IL-12p40 appear to play an important part in human infectious diseases.[179,180]

Prime examples of cytokine antagonists that have profoundly altered the treatment of some inflammatory disorders are agents that inhibit the effects of TNF. These include monoclonal antibodies such as Remicade (infliximab) for the treatment of chronic inflammatory conditions such as Crohn's disease (a form of inflammatory bowel disease) and Humira (adalimumab) for the treatment of moderate to severely active Crohn's disease, rheumatoid arthritis, psoriatic arthritis, ankylosing spondylitis and moderate to severe plaque psoriasis. Other clinically useful anti-TNF and anti-IL-1 agents include the human p75 TNF receptor–IgG fusion protein, Enbrel (etanercept) and soluble IL-1 receptor antagonist, Kineret (anakinra), which prevents active IL-1 binding to its receptor. The development of other anticytokine therapies to treat several inflammatory disorders is based on blocking the effects of IL-6, IL-12, IL-15 and IL-17.[181,182] Tocilizumab is a humanized antihuman IL-6 receptor monoclonal antibody designed to block the actions of IL-6. The safety and efficacy of tocilizumab have been demonstrated in clinical trials conducted in patients with rheumatoid arthritis and other autoimmune inflammatory diseases, such as juvenile idiopathic arthritis and Crohn's disease.

Ongoing work on cytokine antagonists is being directed towards defining the role of various cytokines in a large number of diseases. In depression, the evidence includes the presence of higher levels of pro-inflammatory cytokines including IL-6 and/or C-reactive protein. Elevation in IL-1α and TNFα, acute phase proteins, chemokines and cellular adhesion molecules is also seen in depressed patients. In addition, therapeutic administration of the cytokine interferon-α leads to depression in up to 50% of patients.[183]Cytokines are also crucial mediators of neuroinflammation and acute and chronic neurodegeneration in various pathological conditions in the central nervous system. Among the candidate molecules, interferon (IFN)-γ, TNFα, lymphotoxin-α (formerly TNFβ) and the interleukins IL-1, IL-6, IL-8, IL-12 and IL-23 are important mediators of neuroinflammation under various conditions of neuropathology. These include acute insults from head injury, stroke, intracranial haemorrhage, perinatal hypoxia or iatrogenic perinatal hyperoxia, in addition to chronic autoimmune and neurodegenerative conditions such as Alzheimer's disease, multiple sclerosis[184] and experimental autoimmune encephalomyelitis (EAE; the animal model for MS). Recent studies have highlighted a crucial role for IL-18 (previously termed IFN-γ-inducing factor) in mediating neuroinflammation and neurodegeneration in the central nervous system under pathological conditions, such as bacterial and viral infection, autoimmune demyelinating disease, and hypoxic–ischemic, hyperoxic and traumatic brain injuries.[185] Activation of inflammatory cells within lesions associated with cardiovascular events (enriched in macrophages and other inflammatory cells) induces the release of cytokines which promotes more inflammation and associated tissue damage if cytokine signalling pathways remain unregulated. Thus, pathways capable of suppressing pro-inflammatory cytokine signalling hold the potential to limit life-threatening cardiovascular events caused by atherogenesis.[186]

Chemokines (chemotactic cytokines, chemotactic peptides) have diverse roles in controlling leucocyte (recruitment of white blood cells to the site of infection or injury) migration and their receptors have been shown to be upregulated in both acute and chronic inflammatory diseases. Chemokines also have an important role in the development of AIDS. The first chemokines to be identified included the neutrophil attractant IL-8, the monocyte chemoattractants MCP-1 (monocyte chemoattractant protein) and macrophage inflammatory protein 1α (MIP-1α) and MIP-1β. Currently, ~50 human and mouse chemokines and 18 chemokine receptors have been identified. Chemokine receptors are grouped into four sub-families (CXC, CC, C and CX$_3$C) on the basis of the arrangement of the two N-terminal cysteine residues. Individual chemokines are able to bind to more than one chemokine receptor and similarly multiple chemokines can bind to the same receptor. For example, CCL5 (RANTES) binds to and activates CCR1, CCR3 and CCR5 receptors. This apparent lack of specificity may have implications about the side effect profiles of drugs based on chemokines and their ligands. However, a large amount of work is ongoing to discover chemokine receptor antagonists (small molecule, protein products and antibodies)[187–189] that may be useful for the treatment of various inflammatory disorders such as allergic asthma,[190] chronic obstructive pulmonary disease,[191] rheumatoid arthritis, inflammatory and neuropathic pain,[192,193] multiple sclerosis (neuroinflammatory disease),[194] immunomodulation,[195] myocardial ischaemia,[196] host defence and other diseases.[197] From the point of view of drugs reaching to the market most progress in the area has been made in the treatment of HIV AIDS. Following the initial observation that the CXCR4 chemokine receptor acted as a co-receptor for HIV, it was found that CCR5 was a key receptor in the initial infection events for macrophage-trophic strains of the virus. This led to the discovery of CCR4 and CCR5 antagonists. One of these, maraviroc (CCR5 receptor antagonist – as measured by its ability to displace the endogenous radiolabelled protein MIP-1β from the receptor stably expressed in HEK-293 cells)[198] has already reached the market and others (e.g. vicriviroc) are in development. Genetic research in humans has provided evidence supporting a role for CCR5 in host defence against West Nile virus (a pathogen capable of causing fatal encephalitis). This receptor can function for or against the host, depending on the pathogen. Therefore, blocking CCR5 for the treatment of AIDS could carry an increased risk of West Nile virus disease in co-infected patients.[199]

Chemokine antagonist protein products have been synthesised by deleting amino acid residues from the N-terminal region or extending the N-terminus. Many such compounds retain binding affinity to the receptor and act as antagonists. For example, removal of the first seven or nine amino acids from the N-terminus of monocyte chemoattractant protein-1 resulted in antagonists. Extension of RANTES at the N-terminus by a methionine or an amino-oxypentane residue resulted in RANTES antagonists.

1.7 Enzymes and enzyme inhibitors

Although most of the enzyme-based drugs are inhibitors of enzymes, a number of enzyme preparations have also been developed as drugs for the treatment of a number of diseases.[200] The development of enzymes as therapeutics has been made easier by the advances in biotechnology. Most successful example of enzyme therapy includes various preparations of plasminogen activators (thrombolytic or fibrinolytic agents) such as a bacterial protein streptokinase and two plasminogen activators that occur naturally in blood, the tissue type (tPA) and the urokinase type (uPA) plasminogen activators. These plasminogen activators do not have a direct fibrinolytic activity and their therapeutic action is via limited proteolytic cleavage of the inactive plasminogen to fibrinolytic plasmin. In contrast, streptokinase possesses no enzymatic activity of its own but acquires its plasminogen activating property by complexing with circulatory plasminogen or plasmin. The resulting high-affinity 1 : 1 stoichiometric complex (i.e. the streptokinase–plasminogen activator complex) is a high-specificity protease that proteolytically activates other plasminogen molecules to plasmin. Examples of marketed fibrinolytic enzyme drugs that are used as antithrombolytic agents for the treatment of stroke and myocardial infarction[201,202] include anisoylated human plasminogen-streptokinase (eminase), single-chain tissue plasminogen activators (recombinant human tissue plasminogen activator alteplace and reteplase) and double-chain recombinant tissue-type plasminogen activator (duteplase).

Other successful examples of enzyme therapeutics include recombinant form of human α-galactosidase A (Agalsidase-β and Agalsidase-α) for the treatment of Fabry disease, a recombinant form of urate oxidase (rasburicase, a highly potent uricolytic agent that catalyses the oxidation of uric acid to allantoin, a water-soluble product which is readily excreted via the kidney) for the treatment and prophylaxis of acute hyperuricaemia (to prevent acute renal failure), modified version of glucocerebrosidase (alglucerase and imiglucerase) for the treatment of type I Gaucher's disease, recombinant human deoxyribonuclease I (dornase-α) for the treatment of cystic fibrosis, a polyethylene glycol conjugate of L-asparaginase (pegaspargase, Oncaspar) for combination therapy in acute lymphoblastic leukaemia, human α1-proteinase inhibitor (Aralast) for the treatment of emphysema and pegadamase bovine (Adagen; bovine adenosine deaminase) for the treatment of patients afflicted with a type of severe combined immunodeficiency disease. Antibody-directed enzyme prodrug therapy (ADEPT) illustrates a further application of enzymes as therapeutic agents in cancer. A monoclonal antibody carries an enzyme specifically to cancer cells where the enzyme activates a prodrug, destroying cancer cells but not normal cells.

1.7.1 Converting enzyme inhibitors

Many biologically active peptides are obtained from their precursors by the actions of converting enzymes (zinc metallopeptidases). For example, ACE cleaves a dipeptide from the C-terminus of angiotensin I to generate the pressor peptide angiotensin II. In addition, some of the biologically active peptides [e.g. bradykinin, atrial natriuretic peptide (ANP) and enkephalins] are degraded by the converting enzymes into inactive fragments. These enzymes are important in controlling many physiological and pathological processes. In the case of the peptides that, in some pathological conditions, produce undesirable effects (e.g. vasoconstriction in the case of angiotensin II and endothelin and inflammatory responses in case of TNFα), it is beneficial to prevent the formation of such peptides from their precursors by inhibiting the enzymes involved in the process (e.g. ACE, endothelin and TNFα converting enzyme). On the other hand, in the case of peptides producing therapeutically beneficial effects [e.g. enkephalins and atrial natriuretic factor (ANF)], inhibiting the enzymes that inactivate these peptides (e.g. enkephalinase and atriopeptidase) is likely to lead to an increased biological half-life of the peptide and thus extend the duration of action. From the point of view of drug discovery, ACE inhibitors, which prevent the formation of a pressor peptide angiotensin II, have been the most successful examples. From the point of view of medicinal chemistry, the lessons learned from the ACE story have been very useful in the design of inhibitors of many other metalloproteinases such as enkephalinase, atriopeptidase and MMPs.

ACE (peptidyl dipeptidase, EC 3.4.15.1), known to catalyse the hydrolysis of dipeptides from the C-terminus of polypeptides, belongs to a family of zinc metalloproteinases, which require a zinc atom in the active site. In these enzymes a combination of three His, Glu, Asp or Cys residues creates a zinc binding site. The first major step in the discovery of ACE inhibitors was the isolation of bradykinin potentiating peptides such as BPP5$_a$ (Pyr-Lys-Trp-Ala-Pro) and SQ 20881 (Pyr-Trp-Pro-Arg-Pro-Gln-Ile-Pro-Pro) from the venoms of the Brazilian snake, *Bothrops jaraca*, and the Japanese snake, *Agkistrodon halys blomhoffii*. SAR studies on these peptides indicated that a number of pentapeptide analogues of BPP5$_a$ (e.g. Pyr-Lys-Phe-Ala-Pro) were equipotent to the parent peptide in inhibiting ACE. However, smaller di- or tri-peptides (e.g. Gly-Trp, Val-Trp, Ile-Trp, Phe-Ala-Pro and Lys-Trp-Ala-Pro) were less potent. Although SQ 20881, was studied extensively in the clinic, it could not be used as a drug because of lack of oral activity. Progress towards the orally active ACE inhibitors was made after the discovery of D-benzylsuccinic acid as an inhibitor of another zinc metalloprotease, carboxypeptidase A. This led to the synthesis of proline derivatives by combining the features present in venom peptides and benzylsuccinic acid. One of the early compounds, succinylproline, was only a weak inhibitor of ACE (approximately 150-fold less potent than SQ 20881). Further modifications in this series led to 2-D-methylsuccinyl-proline and 2-D-methylglutaryl-proline (5- and 10-fold less potent, respectively, than SQ 20881). Replacement of the carboxyl group by a thiol group (a better zinc-ion ligand) resulted in potent ACE inhibitors such as captopril (2-D-methyl-3-mercaptopropanoyl-proline,   **110**), which produced dose-related inhibition of the pressor response to angiotensin I in normotensive male rats and produced marked antihypertensive effects in unanaesthetised Goldblatt two-kidney renal hypertensive rats. Captopril was the first ACE inhibitor to reach the market for the treatment of high blood pressure.

Since the discovery of captopril, a number of other analogues either containing a different chelating group

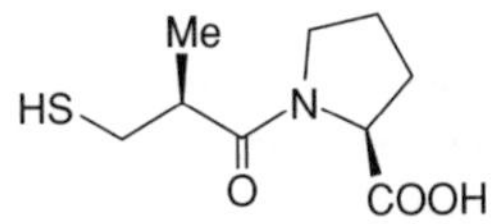

110 Captopril

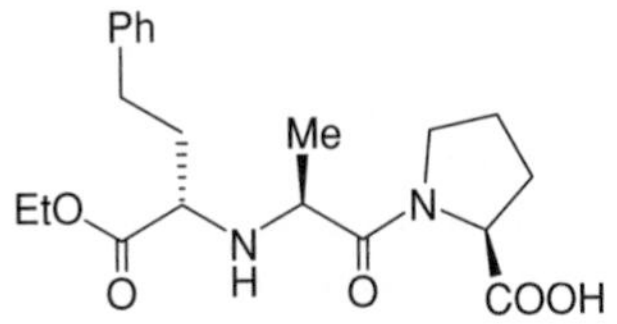

111 Enalapril

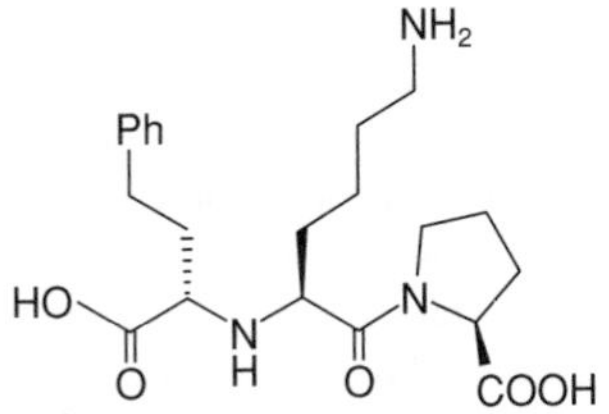

112 Lisinopril

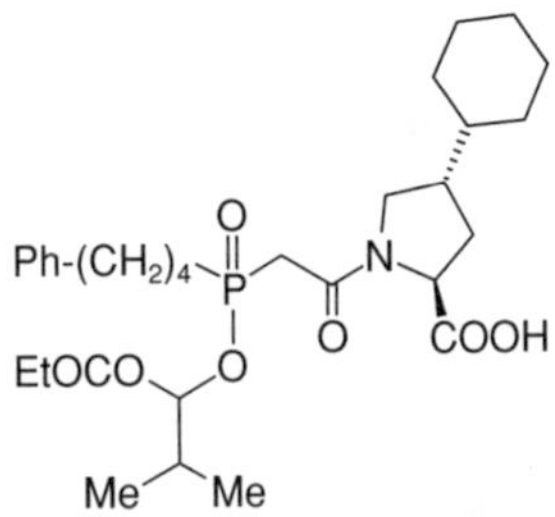

113 Fosinopril

or a proline replacement have been found to be potent inhibitors of ACE. Some of this work was based on a hypothetical model of the substrate (angiotensin I) binding at the active site of the enzyme. In the case of the ACE inhibitors containing a thiol function (e.g. captopril), the thiol group interacts with the zinc ion and the methyl group binds at the S_1' subsite. The proline residue binds at the S_2' subsite and the C-terminal carboxyl group of the proline residue interacts with a positively charged group present in the enzyme. Over the years, medicinal chemistry approaches involving modifications of the chelating group and different groups binding in the S_1' and S_2' subsites have resulted in many potent inhibitors of ACE, including captopril (110), enalapril (111) and lisinopril (112) that have become highly successful drugs for the treatment of hypertension and some other cardiovascular disorders. The design of phosphorus containing ACE inhibitors [e.g. fosinopril (113)] was based on the structure of phosphoramidon, [N-(α-L-rhamnopyranosyloxy-hydroxyphosphinyl)-Leu-Trp], an inhibitor of another zinc metalloproteinase (thermolysin) isolated from a culture filtrate of *Streptomyces tanashiensis*. In addition to the ACE inhibitors mentioned above, many others such as alacepril, perindopril, delapril, quinapril, ramipril, benazepril, cilazapril, imidapril, trandopril, temocapril, moexipril, spirapril and zofenopril are in

the market for the treatment of hypertension, heart failure, heart attack and kidney failure.

Since the discovery of early ACE inhibitors, additional information has become available indicating that ACE is a complex two-domain enzyme, comprising of an N- and a C-terminal domain, each containing an active site with similar but distinct substrate specificities and chloride-activation requirements. Currently available ACE inhibitors show some degree of selectivity for the C-terminal domain inhibition. High resolution crystal structure of human testis ACE (tACE; containing only the C-terminal domain with one catalytic site) has become available providing an opportunity for the discovery of N- and C-terminal domain-selective inhibitors.[203] The selective inhibitors may have much improved clinical profile. In addition to tACE, a human homologue of ACE (ACE2; cloned from a human heart failure cDNA library) has recently been identified with a more restricted distribution than ACE, and is found mainly in heart and kidney. In contrast to ACE, ACE2 has only one active enzymatic site and functions as a carboxypeptidase rather than a dipeptidyl carboxypeptidase. Instead of cleaving dipeptide residues from the C-terminal end of the peptide, ACE2 cleaves a single residue from angiotensin I to generate angiotensin(1–9), and degrades angiotensin II to the vasodilator angiotensin(1–7). ACE2 is insensitive to classic ACE inhibitors. The importance of ACE2 in normal physiology and pathophysiological states is currently under investigation.[204] It has been hypothesized that ACE2 might protect against increases in blood pressure and that ACE2 deficiency leads to hypertension.

In comparison to the effort required for the discovery of ACE inhibitors, the progress in identifying potent inhibitors of the enkephalin degrading dipeptidyl-carboxypeptidase (enkephalinase) (used as analgesics) and ANF degrading enzyme (used as antihypertensive agents) was more rapid because of similarities between the enzymes. However, the similarities resulted in problems in achieving selectivity.

114 Thiorphan

115 Kalatorphan

116 Glycoprilat

The differences in the S_1' and S_2' subsites of metalloproteinases were exploited to achieve selectivity. The first potent inhibitor of enkephalinase (thiorphan, 114) was about 30-fold more potent against enkephalinase (Ki ~4 nmol) than against ACE. Another inhibitor kelatorphan (115) was a potent inhibitor of enkephalinase and dipeptidylaminopeptidase and a weak inhibitor of aminopeptidase. Inhibitors such as glycoprilat (116) and their orally active prodrugs were potent inhibitors of ACE and enkephalinase; they prevented angiotensin I-induced pressor responses in rats and also increased urinary water and sodium excretion. Dual inhibitors of ACE and neutral endopeptidase were anticipated to provide additional benefits in cardiovascular diseases in comparison to ACE inhibitors alone because of the importance of the natriuretic peptide system in the pathogenesis of heart failure.[205] Recombinant B-type natriuretic peptide [nesiritide, Ser-Pro-Lys-Met-Val-Gln-Gly-Ser-Gly-Cys-Phe-Gly-Arg-Lys-Met-Asp-Arg-Ile-Ser-Ser-Ser-Ser-Gly-Leu-Gly-Cys-Lys-Val-Leu-Arg-Arg-His (disulphide bridge containing cyclic peptide)] is already approved for the treatment of acutely decompensated congestive heart failure in patients who have dyspnoea at rest or with minimal activity. The agent causes arteries and veins to dilate, alleviating symptoms by improving blood movement around the heart without a change in heart rate. Many dual inhibitors (vasopeptidase inhibitors) have been synthesised and investigated in cardiovascular disorders.[206] Until recently, omapatrilat (BMS 186716) was the most advanced ACE and neutral

endopeptidase (NEP) inhibitor in clinical trials. Although preclinical studies in experimental models of hypertension and heart failure and a few clinical trials demonstrated some pharmacological advantages, none of the vasopeptidase inhibitors, including omapatrilat have reached the market.

It has been much more difficult to achieve complete selectivity in the case of inhibitors of MMPs (e.g. collagenases, stromelysins and gelatinases), a family of zinc-containing proteinases involved in extracellular matrix remodelling and degradation. At least 20 members of this enzyme family, subdivided into collagenases (MMP-1, -8, -13 and -18), gelatinises (MMP-2 and -9), stromelysins (MMP-3, -10 and -11) and membrane-type (MMP-14, -15, -16 and -17) families, have been reported. These enzymes have been implicated in diseases such as rheumatoid arthritis, osteoarthritis, cancer, multiple sclerosis and other vascular and inflammatory disorders.[207-210] Work is also ongoing to discover novel antibacterial agents by designing inhibitors of bacterial metalloenzymes. This approach has been successfully applied to the discovery of in vivo active antibacterial agents that are inhibitors of bacterial peptide deformylase and UDP-3-O-(R-3-hydroxymyristoyl)-N-acetylglucosamine deacetylase.[211] Many inhibitors of matrix metalloproteinases were identified with different levels of selectivity against various MMPs. One of these inhibitors (marimastat) was extensively studied in the clinic for the treatment of pancreatic, lung, brain and stomach cancers but failed to demonstrate efficacy in humans. Despite the failure of marimastat in the clinic, new compounds continue to be designed and developed.

1.7.2 Aspartyl protease (renin and HIV protease) inhibitors

Aspartyl proteases are a family of enzymes that, in general, cleave peptide bonds between bulky hydrophobic amino acid residues. The cleavage of the peptide bond is mediated by a general acid–general base catalysis mechanism using the carboxyl groups of the aspartic acid residues at the active site. Enormous progress has been made in the discovery and optimisation of the pharmacokinetic properties of the inhibitors. Because the antihypertensive market is well served by a number of orally active agents such as β-blockers, ACE inhibitors and angiotensin II antagonists and the condition is chronic, requiring long-term treatment, it is essential to have orally active inhibitors for this indication. Many of the potent and selective renin inhibitors are now approaching the appropriate level of oral bioavailability after more than 25 years of research. In contrast, by using all the chemical information available in the case of renin inhibitors, it has been possible to discover potent orally bioavailable HIV protease inhibitors in a relatively short period of time, and many of these are already highly successful drugs.

1.7.2.1 Renin inhibitors

A number of chemical approaches have been used in the design of renin inhibitors. In the absence of the purified enzyme, most of the early search for inhibitors was carried out using crude renin preparations. The amino acid sequences of mouse, rat and human renin were obtained later on either by using the traditional isolation and sequencing techniques or by using cDNA methodology. Various three-dimensional models of renin were constructed in the early stages based on the X-ray structures of other similar aspartyl proteases (e.g. endothia-pepsin and penicillopepsin). Later on the X-ray crystal structure of recombinant human renin was reported. The inhibitor design process has been based on some of these models.

Initial design of the inhibitors was based on a rational design strategy using the renin substrate as a starting point. Some of the early studies indicated that the octapeptide of horse angiotensinogen (His-Pro-Phe-His-Leu-Leu-Val-Tyr), cleaved slowly by renin between the Leu-Leu residues, was a weak competitive inhibitor of renin. This led to the modifications in the P_1 and P_1' positions (Leu-Leu) of this peptide. The early work indicated that the two leucine residues could be replaced by other natural and unnatural amino acids (e.g. Phe, D-Leu). Many of the resulting analogues such as His-Pro-Phe-His-Leu-D-Leu-Val-Tyr, His-Pro-Phe-His-Phe-Phe-Val-Tyr and Pro-His-Pro-Phe-His-Phe-Phe-Val-Tyr-Lys although more potent than the original substrate based compounds were still weak inhibitors of renin. More potent inhibitors were obtained by replacing the peptide bond between the two leucine residues. Many of these peptides [e.g. Pro-His-Pro-Phe-His-Pheψ(CH$_2$NH)Phe-Val-Tyr-Lys, His-Pro-Phe-His-Leuψ(CH$_2$NH)Val-Ile-His and Pro-His-Pro-Phe-His-Leuψ(CH$_2$NH)Val-Ile-His-Lys (H-142)] were potent and selective inhibitors of human renin. The two peptides containing a reduced Leu-Val peptide bond were 800–1000 times more potent inhibitors of human renin (IC$_{50}$ 10–190 nmol) than of dog renin (IC$_{50}$ 10–150 mmol) and H-142 did not inhibit cathepsin D up to a concentration of approximately 700 mmol/L. One of the smaller peptides, Boc-Phe-His-Chaψ(CH$_2$NH)Val-NHCH$_2$CH(Me)-Et, approached the potency of H-142 in inhibiting

human renin and was effective in lowering blood pressure in salt-depleted cynomolgus monkeys at a dose of 0.1–0.5 mg/kg. Unlike the reduced peptide bond [-ψ(CH$_2$NH)-] analogues, replacement of the scissile peptide bond by –CH$_2$O–, –COCH$_2$–, –CH$_2$S– and –CH$_2$SO– did not lead to enhanced potency. The reduced peptide bond analogue, H-142, has been studied extensively in various animal and human models. At a dose of 1 and 2.5 mg/kg/h, H-142 produced a dose-related reduction in plasma renin activity and reduced the circulating levels of angiotensin I and II.

Another important step in the discovery of potent inhibitors of renin was the isolation of a naturally occurring aspartyl protease inhibitor pepstatin {Iva-Val-Val-Sta-Ala-Sta [Sta = (3S, 4S)-4-amino-3-hydroxy-6-methylheptanoic acid]}, which was a relatively poor inhibitor of human renin but a potent inhibitor of pepsin. Incorporation of the statine residue in the angiotensinogen octapeptide resulted in potent inhibitors of renin. His-Pro-Phe-His-Sta-Val-Ile-His and Iva-His-Pro-Phe-His-Sta-Leu-Phe-NH$_2$ were equipotent to H-142 as inhibitors of human plasma and kidney renin. Another similar compound, Iva-His-Pro-Phe-His-Sta-Ile-Phe-NH$_2$, was a fivefold more potent inhibitor of human plasma and kidney renin than was H-142. However, the statine analogue was much less selective. In comparison with H-142, the statine analogue was about 300-fold more potent inhibitor of dog renin. The statine residue [–NH–CH(CH$_2$CHMe$_2$)–CH(OH)–CH$_2$CO–] in the above transition-state analogues was modified in various ways to assess the importance of the side-chain isobutyl group, the hydroxyl group and the methylene group. In general, replacement of the isobutyl side-chain (occupying the P_1 position) by cyclohexylmethyl or benzyl groups resulted in more potent compounds. The hydroxyl and the methylene groups of statine were not essential for the renin inhibitory activity. Several analogues containing difluorostatine difluorostatone, norstatine [(2R, 3S)-3-amino-2-hydroxy-5-methylhexanoic acid], cyclohexylnorstatine [(2R, 3S)-3-amino-4-cyclohexyl-2-hydroxybutyric acid], aminostatine (3,4-diamino-6-methylheptanoic acid) and α,α-difluoro-β-aminodeoxystatine were potent inhibitors of human renin.

Incorporation of the hydroxyethylene, dihydroxyethylene and other statine-like residues in place of the scissile peptide bond in substrate-based analogues, along with other amino acid or non-peptide changes at the N- and C-termini, led to more potent, selective and relatively small molecular weight inhibitors of renin.[212] Examples of such compounds included

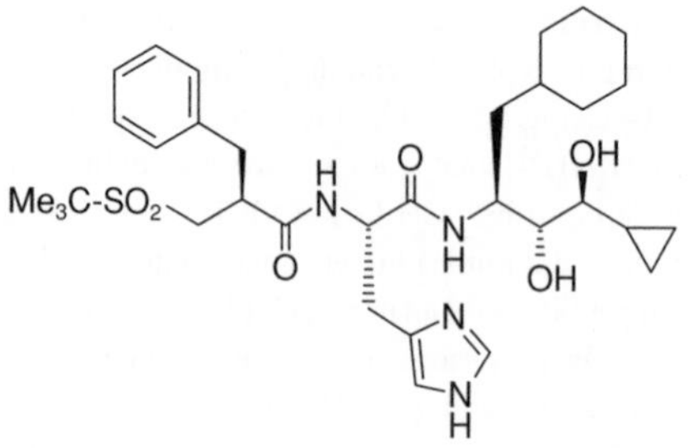

117 Remikiren

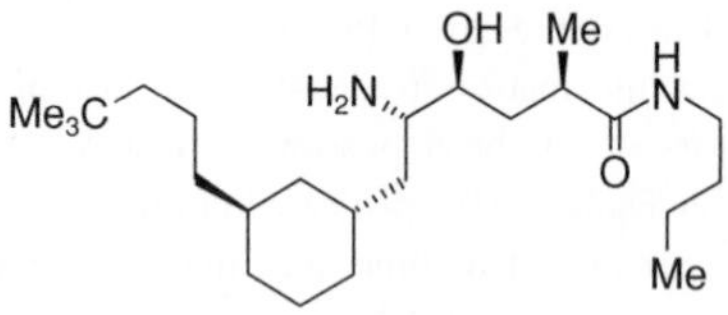

119

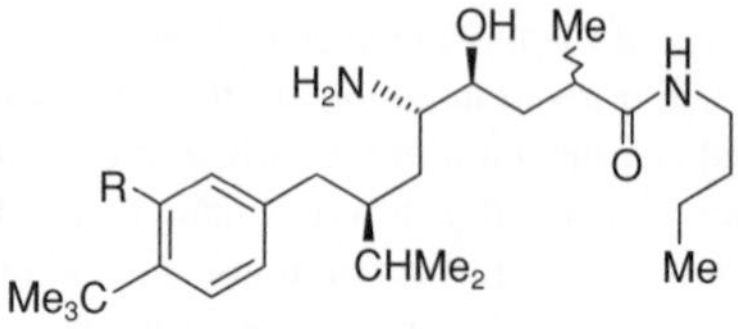

120

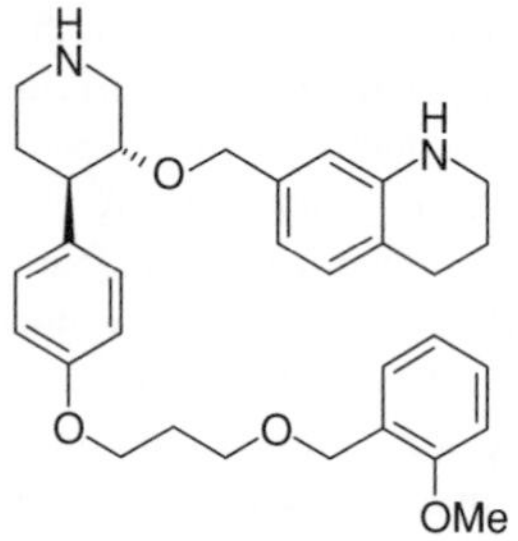

121

compound 117 [Ro 42-5892 (remikiren)] that was effective in lowering blood pressure in sodium-depleted marmosets and squirrel monkeys after oral administration (0.1–10 mg/kg). Further chemical modifications on similar types of compounds led to aliskirin (118). The once-daily oral direct renin inhibitor was approved for the treatment of hypertension as monotherapy or in combination with other antihypertensive medications. Aliskirin provided added efficacy when used in combination with other commonly used blood pressure-lowering medications.

Conformational analysis of the binding mode of one of the inhibitors indicated that the S_1 and S_3 pockets constitute a large contiguous, hydrophobic binding site accommodating the P_1 cyclohexyl and the P_3 phenyl groups in close proximity to each other. This led to the synthesis of δ-amino hydroxyethylene dipeptide isosteres lacking the P_4-P_2 peptide backbone. Compound 119 was a moderately potent inhibitor of human renin (IC_{50} 300 nmol). Non-peptide inhibitors such as compound 120 (R = –OCH$_2$COOCH$_3$, –OCH$_2$CONH$_2$ or –OCH$_2$SO$_2$CH$_3$) were 15- to 50-fold more potent inhibitors than 119. Random screening approaches led to non-peptide inhibitors such as the tetrahydroquinoline derivative 121 [IC_{50} 0.7 nmol (recombinant human renin) and 37 nmol (human plasma renin)], which displayed long-lasting (20 h) blood pressure lowering effects after oral administration (1 and 3 mg/kg) to sodium-depleted conscious marmosets. The piperidine derivative also inhibited plasmepsin I and II from *Plasmodium falciparum*.

1.7.2.2 HIV protease inhibitors

In comparison to the discovery of renin inhibitors, the task of discovering inhibitors of HIV protease has been relatively easy. This is primarily because many of the approaches used successfully in the design of renin inhibitors were also applicable in the design of HIV protease inhibitors. In addition, samples of both HIV-1 and HIV-2 proteases (99 residue peptides), obtained by chemical synthesis and recombinant technology, were available in the early stages of the programme, along with the three-dimensional structure of the HIV-1 protease. Like renin, HIV protease was found to prefer a hydrophobic amino acid (Leu, Ile, Tyr, Phe) in the P_1 position of the substrate and was inhibited by pepstatin. However, unlike renin, incorporation of

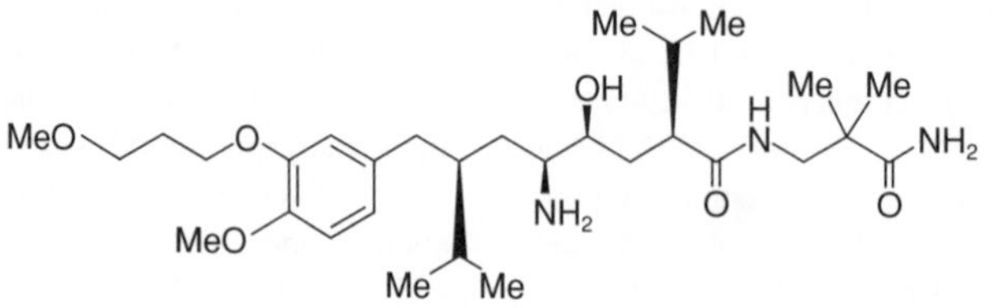

118 Aliskiren

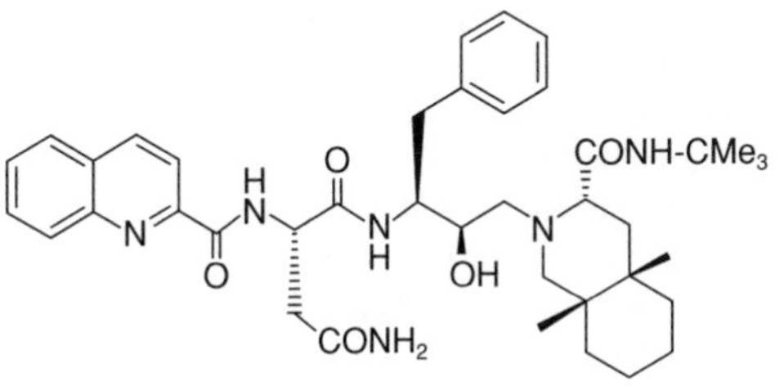

122 Saquinavir

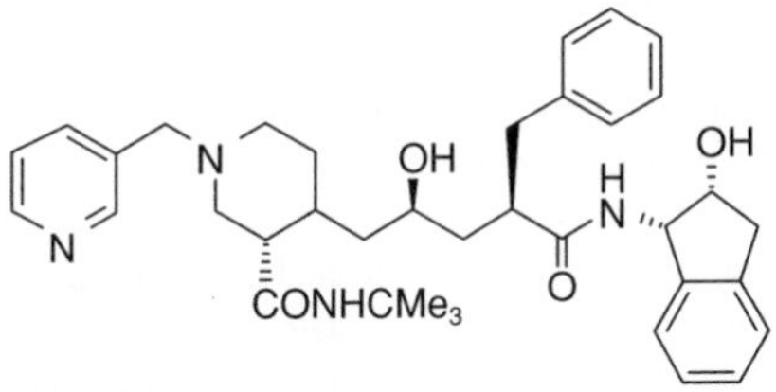

126 Palinavir

123 Indinavir

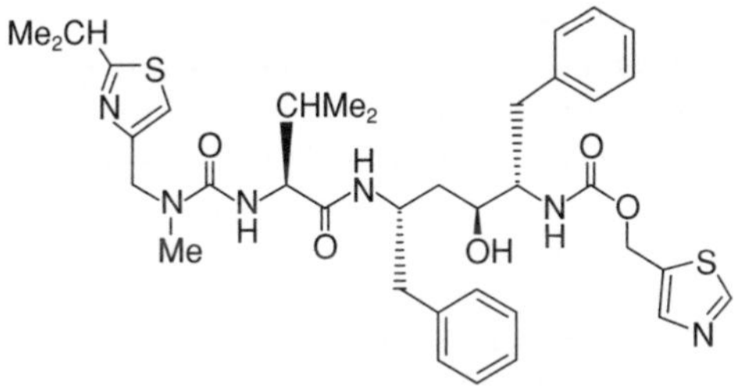

127 Atazanavir

124 Ritonavir

128 Darunavir

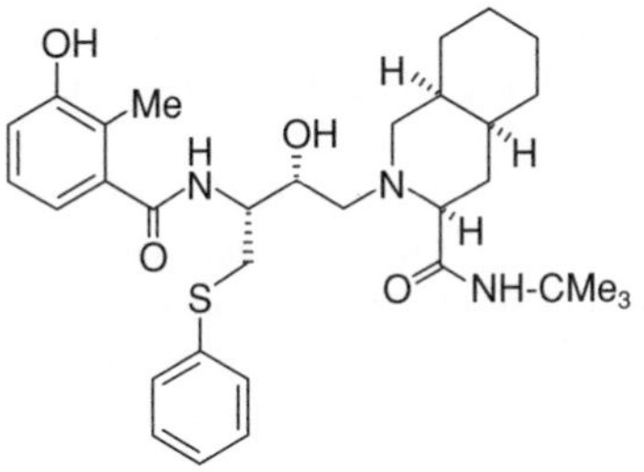

125 Neflinavir

the statine residue in the P_1 position of the substrate, or the replacement of the scissile peptide bond in the substrate-like peptides by a –CH$_2$NH– group, did not lead to potent inhibitors. Potent inhibitors of the enzyme were obtained by replacing the scissile peptide bond by a hydroxymethylcarbonyl, hydroxyethylamine hydroxyethylurea or a hydroxyethylene group. Many such compounds such as amprenavir, lopinavir, saquinavir (122), indinavir (123), ritonavir (124), nelfinavir (125) palinavir (126) and atazanavir (127)[213] have

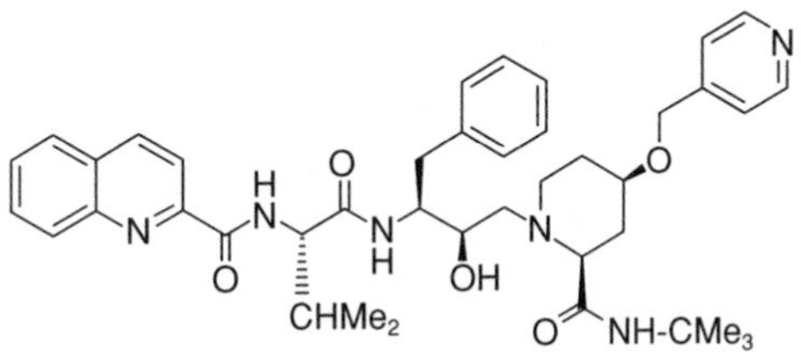

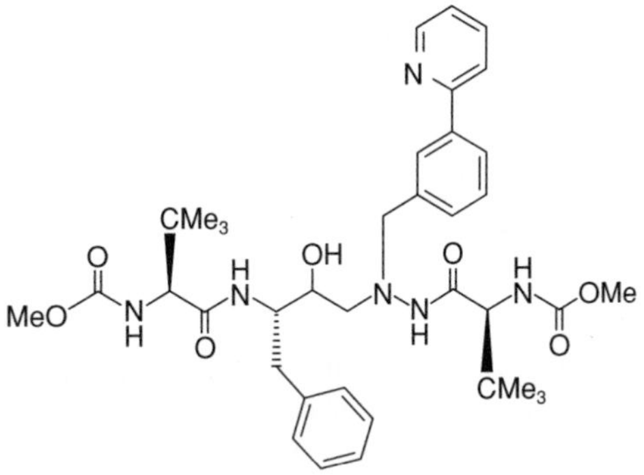

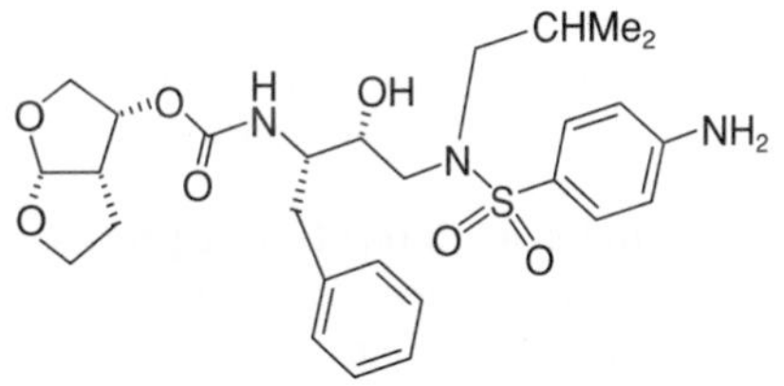

either reached the market or are in late stages of clinical trials. In order to overcome the problem of viral resistance, computational studies using HIV-1 protease mutants (Met[46]Ile, Leu[63]Pro, Val[82]Thr, Ile[84]Val, Met[46]Ile/Leu[63]Pro, Val[82]Thr/Ile[84]Val and Met[46]Ile/Leu[63]Pro/Val[82]Thr/Ile[84]Val) and known inhibitors of the enzyme were used to design inhibitors with better binding affinity towards both mutant and wild-type proteases. Several such compounds inhibited wild-type and mutant HIV protease, blocked the replication of laboratory and clinical strains of HIV type 1, and maintained high potency against mutant HIV selected by ritonavir *in vivo*. Two of the newer inhibitors darunavir (128) and tipranavir (129) are indicated for co-administration with ritonavir and with other antiretroviral agents, for the treatment of HIV infection in antiretroviral treatment-experienced

129 Tipranavir

130

patients, such as those with HIV-1 strains resistant to more than one protease inhibitor.

Non-peptide inhibitors of HIV protease (dihydropyrone, cyclic urea and sulfamide series of compounds) were obtained by modifications of random screening leads. Examples of these include compounds such as **130**, which showed activity against a variety of HIV type 1 laboratory strains, clinical isolates and other variants resistant to other protease inhibitors.

1.7.3 Thrombin inhibitors (serine protease)

Thrombin, a serine protease, cleaves fibrinogen into fibrin to create a fibrous plug and also amplifies its own production through the activation of factor XI and co-factors V and VIII. Thrombin also has a crucial role in the activation of platelets through the cleavage of the protease-activated receptors on the platelet surface. Antagonists of G-protein-coupled protease-activated receptor PAR_1 have been synthesised to study the role of thrombin PAR_1 receptor in thrombosis and vascular injury. Thrombosis is the most common cause of death in the industrialized world and, whether through venous thromboembolism, myocardial infarction or stroke, ultimately involves the inappropriate activity of thrombin. Although anticoagulants such as warfarin, heparin, low molecular weight heparin and hirudin are available for treating diseases such as deep vein thrombosis, these agents have significant disadvantages and their use has to be carefully monitored.[214–216] Orally available thrombin inhibitors may provide several advantages, and for this reason such agents have been sought from a long time for the treatment of venous

thromboembolism and for prophylactic prevention of venous thromboembolism after large-joint orthopedic surgery in high-risk patients.

Thrombin inhibitors such as D-Phe-Pro-Arg chloromethylketone and D-Phe-Pro-Arg aldehyde have been known for a long time. However, the compounds lacked oral bioavailability. A semi-rational approach was adopted to modify P_1 to P_3 positions to improve the potency, selectivity and pharmacokinetic properties. Changes in individual positions were followed by multiple changes and synthesis of conformationally restricted analogues. Substitution of the C-terminal arginine aldehyde moiety (P_1 position) in D-Phe-Pro-Arg aldehyde by p-amidinobenzylamine gave thrombin inhibitors comparable in potency to the transition-state aldehyde analogue and much less potent (130–400,000-fold) against trypsin, plasmin, tPA and urokinase. Incorporation of a conformationally restricted analogue of arginine in the P_1 position, along with a six- or a seven-membered lactam sulphonamide moiety at P_3 to P_4 positions, also resulted in inhibitors that showed much more selectivity against serine proteases such as factor Xa and trypsin. Inhibitor **131** containing conformationally restricting moieties in the P_3-P_2 region inhibited thrombus formation when administered orally (30 mg/kg; bioavailability 55%, 4 h duration) 1 h before induction of stasis.

A number of P_3 position modified thrombin inhibitors exhibited oral bioavailability in rats and dogs, and were efficacious in a rat $FeCl_3$-induced model of arterial thrombosis. Compounds such as **132** and the corresponding analogues with an unprotected amino group at the N-terminus showed selectivity (300- to 1500-fold selectivity for thrombin compared with trypsin) and oral bioavailability (40–76%) in rats or dogs. Compound **133** containing a Phe(p-CH_2NH_2) residue in the P_1 position was one of the more potent and selective inhibitor of thrombin (K_i values 6.6 and 14,200 nmol against thrombin and trypsin,

131

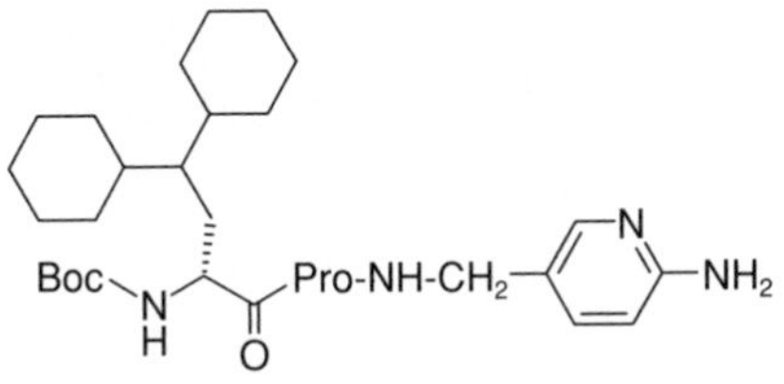

132

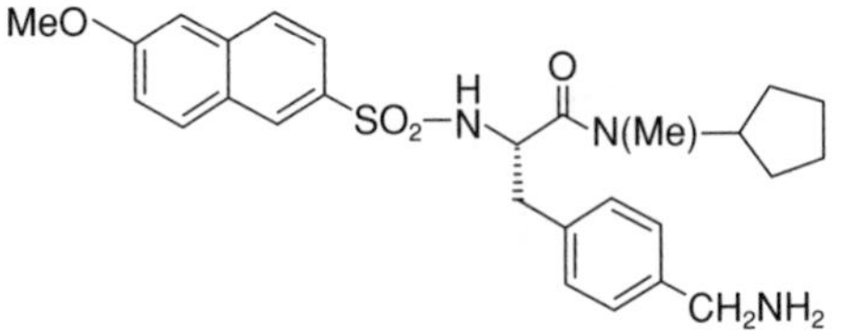

133

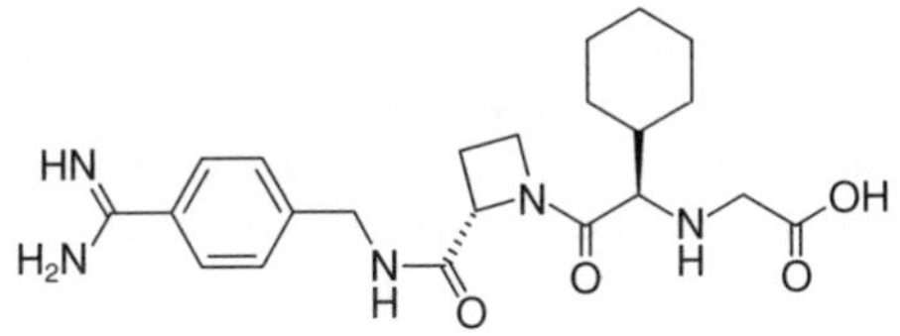

134 Melagatran

135

respectively) and showed good oral bioavailability in rats (approximately 70%) but low oral bioavailability in dogs (10–15%). One orally active thrombin inhibitor melagatran (ximelagatran, 134) reached the market but was later withdrawn because of side effects.

Non-peptide inhibitors of thrombin (obtained by random screening procedures) include compounds based around benzothiophene (e.g. 135) and other ring systems and cyclic and linear oligocarbamate derivatives (e.g. 136). The benzothiophene derivative 135 showed antithrombotic efficacy in a rat model of thrombosis after infusion (ED_{50} 2.3 mg/kg/h). The cyclic oligocarbamate tetramer 136 inhibited thrombin with an apparent Ki of 31 nmol.

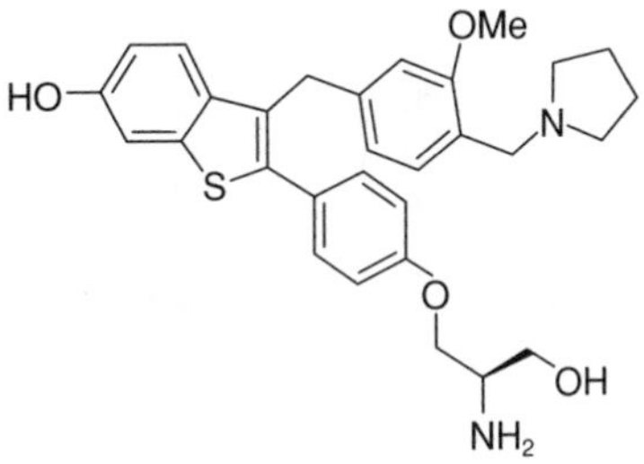

1.7.4 Ras protein farnesyltransferase inhibitors

Cysteine farnesylation of the ras oncogene product Ras is required for its transforming activity and is catalysed by the enzyme protein farnesyltransferase. The enzyme catalyses the transfer of a farnesyl group from farnesyl diphosphate to a cysteine residue of the protein substrate such as Ras. The enzyme recognises a tetrapeptide sequence [Cys-A-A-X (A is an aliphatic amino acid and X is Met, Ser, Ala, Cys or Gln)] at the C-terminus of the protein. A closely related enzyme, geranylgeranyltransferase, recognises the Cys-A-A-X motif when X is either Leu or Phe, but transfers a geranylgeranyl group from geranylgeranyl diphosphate. Inhibition of farnesyltransferase represents a possible method for preventing association of Ras p21 to the cell membrane, thereby blocking its cell-transforming capabilities. Such inhibitors may have therapeutic potential as anticancer agents.[217]

'Semi-rational' design approaches for the discovery of farnesyltransferase inhibitors were based on the tetrapeptide Cys-Val-Phe-Met. SAR studies, followed by the synthesis of conformationally restricted analogues, led to inhibitors such as 137, which was effective in prolonging the survival time in athymic mice implanted intraperitoneally with H-*ras*-transformed RAT-1 tumour cells. A non-thiol inhibitor incorporating an N-alkyl amino acid residue (138, methyl ester prodrug) showed activity in several *in vivo* tumour models. Further medicinal chemistry approaches on

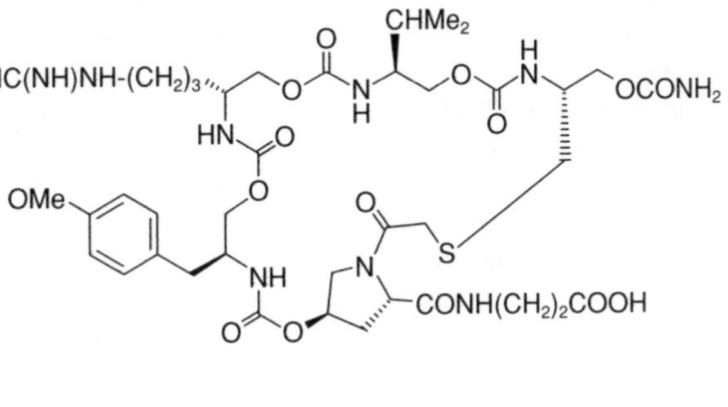

136

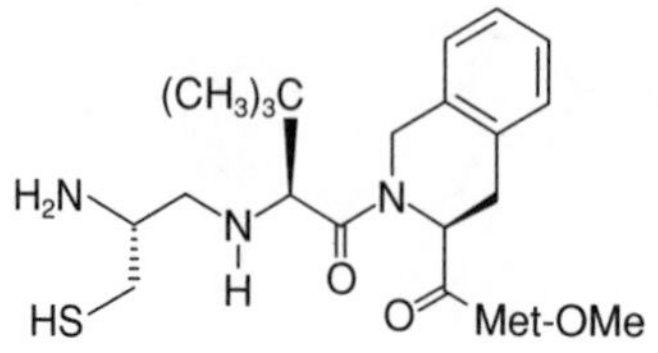

137

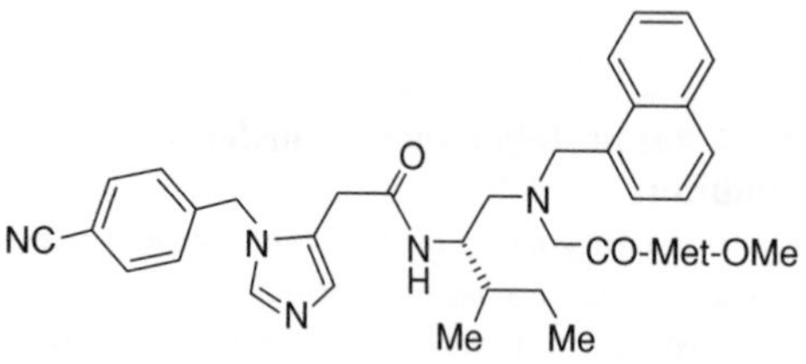

138

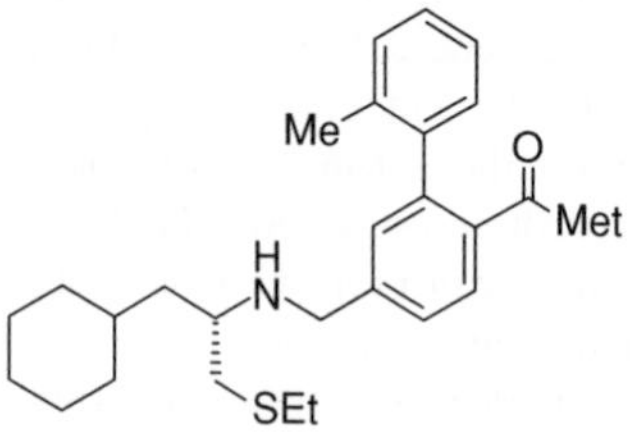

139

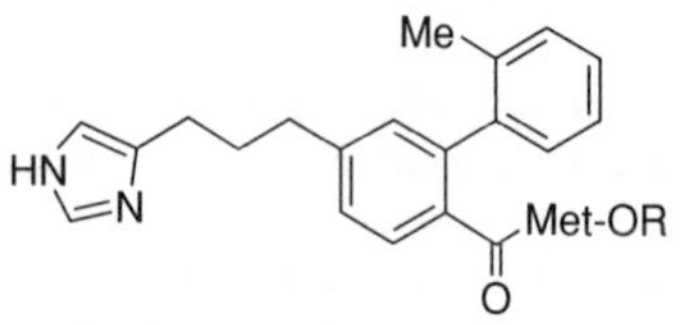

140

these modified peptides, including the synthesis of a library of secondary benzylic amines led to orally active methionine derivatives such as **139**, which attenuated tumour growth in a nude mouse xenograft model of human pancreatic cancer. The methyl ester prodrug (**140**) suppressed the growth of human lung adenocarcinoma A-549 cells in nude mice by 30–90% in a dose-dependent manner.

Random screening approaches also provided inhibitors of the enzyme. SAR studies on the random screening lead Z-His-Tyr(OBn)-Ser(OBn)-Trp-D-Ala-NH$_2$ (PD083176) (IC$_{50}$ 20 nmol), including the replacement of the N-terminal Z group and the histidine and Trp residues, led to less potent peptides. However, substitution of the Tyr(OBn) and Ser(OBn)

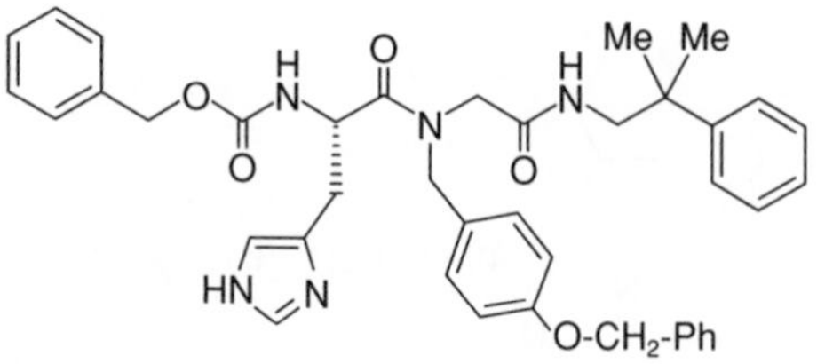

141

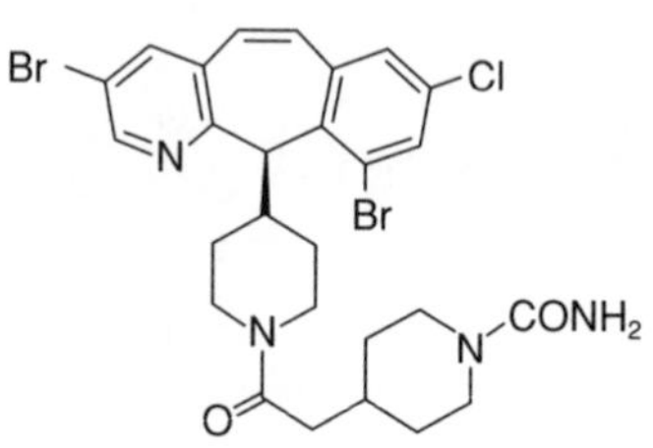

142

residues did not have much effect on the enzyme inhibitory activity. Based on the SAR and truncation studies, potent inhibitors of farnesyltransferase such as **141** were obtained. The Z-His derivative **141** inhibited isolated farnesyltransferase but was about 4000-fold less potent against geranylgeranyltransferase-1. Compound **141** was also active in athymic mice implanted with H-*ras*-F cells. When administered intraperitoneally (150 mg/kg/day once daily) for 14 consecutive days after tumour implantation, the tumour growth was inhibited by approximately 90%. Random screening approaches followed by medicinal chemistry also resulted in chemically distinct farnesyltransferase inhibitors. Examples include compounds such as **142** which was orally active in several human tumour xenograft models in the nude mouse, including tumours of colon, lung, pancreas, prostate and urinary bladder. Although many compounds such as **142** and others are in various stages of clinical trials, none of the farnesyltransferase inhibitors have yet reached the market.

1.7.5 Protein kinase (tyrosine and serine/threonine) inhibitors

The protein kinases are a family of proteins (serine/threonine and tyrosine kinases) involved in signalling pathways regulating a number of cellular functions, such as cell growth, metabolism, differentiation and death. Examples of protein tyrosine kinases include intracellular domains of transmembrane growth factor receptors, such as epidermal growth factor receptor (EGFR),[218] platelet derived growth factor receptor,[219] vascular endothelial growth factor (VEGF) receptor[220] and fibroblast growth factor receptor,[221] and cytosolic kinases, such as src, abl and lck. Examples of serine/threonine kinases include mitogen-activated protein kinase,[222,223] Jun kinase and cyclin-dependent kinases[224–226] and glycogen synthase kinase.[227,228] Signal transduction via these proteins occurs through selective and reversible phosphorylation of the substrates by the transfer of γ-phosphate of ATP (or GTP) to the hydroxyl group of serine, threonine and tyrosine residues.[229,230] A large number of protein kinases (>150) have been identified from mammalian sources, and the human genome is expected to provide many more in the future. Selective inhibitors of these enzymes are expected to be useful in a number of diseases such as cancer, inflammatory disorders, diabetes and neurodegenerative disorders and, for this reason, this is one of the most active areas of pharmaceutical research at the present time.[231–237] With approaches based on monoclonal antibodies and synthetic small molecules, inhibitors of kinases are being developed. Although many of the starting leads for small molecule kinase inhibitors were obtained by random screening approaches, further medicinal chemistry was aided by availability of a number of crystal structures and other modelling approaches.

A recent example of the antibody-based approach is the discovery of a monoclonal antibody against human EGFR2 (HER2), a family of EGFR tyrosine kinases, including the EGFR. Many epithelial tumours, including breast cancer, express excess amounts of these proteins, particularly HER2 – a tyrosine kinase receptor with extracellular, transmembrane and intracellular domains. Initially, several monoclonal antibodies against the extracellular domain of the HER2 protein were found to inhibit the proliferation of human cancer cells that over-expressed HER2. The antigen binding region of one of the more effective antibodies was fused to the framework region of human IgG to generate a 'humanised' monoclonal antibody. The antibody (trastuzumab, Herceptin) was investigated alone and in combination with chemotherapy in women with metastatic breast cancer that over-expressed HER2. Compared with chemotherapy alone, treatment with chemotherapy plus trastuzumab was associated with significantly higher rate of overall response and a longer time to treatment failure. Treatment with trastuzumab was associated with some side effects (chills, fever, infection and cardiac dysfunction). Two other EGFR antibodies cetuximab (a humanised monoclonal antibody) and panitumumab (Vectibix, a fully human immunoglobulin G2 monoclonal antibody) have demonstrated efficacy in patients with metastatic colorectal cancer.

In addition to the antibodies, a number of small molecule inhibitors of kinases (selective and non-selective) have been developed. Because kinases are expressed in normal cells and tumour cells, it was expected that interfering with their function in tumour cells is also likely to interfere with normal cell function. For this reason many of the kinase inhibitors that have reached the market (see below) are associated with a number of side effects. The most common side effects include skin toxicity, fatigue, dizziness, diarrhoea, superficial oedema, nausea, muscle cramps and various cardiovascular effects (e.g. hypertension, deep venous thrombosis, pulmonary embolism and arterial thromboembolism).[238,239] The first kinase inhibitor to reach the market was a selective EGFR kinase inhibitor gefitinib (143) which was approved for the treatment of locally advanced or metastatic non-small cell lung cancer (NSCLC) in patients who have undergone previous chemotherapy or who are not suitable for chemotherapy. However, because it failed to show an overall survival advantage, its use is now restricted to cancer patients who have already taken the medicine and who have benefited from it. The drug is only available in a limited number of countries.[240] By contrast, erlotinib (Tarceva) (144), another EGFR tyrosine-kinase inhibitor, showed an overall survival benefit, and was approval for treatment of patients with NSCLC who have progressed after treatment with chemotherapy. Both gefitinib and erlotinib are orally bioavailable synthetic anilinoquinazolines that selectively and reversibly prevent ATP binding and autophosphorylation of the EGFR tyrosine kinase. Another selective tyrosine kinase

143 Gefitinib

144 Erlotinib (Tarceva)

145 Imatinib

146 Nilotinib

147 Dasatinib

148 Sorafenib

149 Sunitinib

inhibitor, imatinib (Glivec) (145) is approved for the treatment of chronic myeloid leukaemia and gastrointestinal stromal tumours.[241] A complete cytogenetic response was achieved in 50–60% of patients treated in chronic phase after failure to respond to interferon-α and in more than 80% of those receiving imatinib as first-line therapy. Nilotinib (146, Tasigna), a selective inhibitor of Bcr-Abl tyrosine kinase, was approved for patients with a form of chronic myeloid leukaemia that is resistant or intolerant to imatinib mesylate.[242] Taken twice daily, nilotinib inhibits the production of cells containing the Philadelphia (Ph⁺) chromosome by targeting Bcr-Abl protein synthesis.

In addition to the above selective inhibitors, two multiple kinase inhibitors, dasatinib (147) and sorafenib (148), were also approved for cancer treatment. Dasatinib (Sprycel) was approved for two leukaemia indications: the treatment of chronic myeloid leukaemia (chronic, accelerated or myeloid or lymphoid blast phase) in patients with resistance or

intolerance to prior therapy including imatinib; and the treatment of Philadelphia chromosome-positive (Ph+) acute lymphoblastic leukaemia (ALL) with resistance or intolerance to prior therapy.[243] At nanomolar concentrations, dasatinib inhibits BCR-ABL, SRC family (SRC, LCK, YES, FYN), c-KIT, EPHA2 and PDGFR-B. By targeting these kinases, dasatinib inhibits the overproduction of leukaemia cells in the bone marrow of patients with chronic myeloid leukaemia and Ph+ ALL and allows normal red cell, white cell and blood platelet production to resume. Sorafenib (Nexavar), an oral multi-kinase inhibitor that targets serine/threonine and receptor tyrosine kinases (including RAF kinase, VEGFR-2, VEGFR-3, PDGRF-β, KIT and FLT-3) in both the tumour cell and tumour vasculature, is indicated for the treatment of patients with advanced renal cell carcinoma.[244] Sorafenib is involved in both tumour cell proliferation and tumour angiogenesis. Treatment with sorafenib resulted in approximately a doubling of progression-free survival in patients with renal cell carcinoma and tumour shrinkage was detected in 74% of sorafenib-treated patients and 20% of placebo-treated patients. A multiple tyrosine kinase inhibitor sunitinib (149, Sutent) was approved for the treatment of gastrointestinal stromal tumours in patients whose disease has progressed or who are unable to tolerate treatment with imatinib mesylate and for the treatment of patients with advanced renal cell carcinoma.[245] A dual kinase inhibitor (ErB1 and ErB2) lapatinib (150, Tyverb) was approved for the treatment, in combination with capecitabine, of advanced metastatic HER2 (ErbB2)-positive breast cancer in women who have received prior therapy

150 Lapatinib

including an anthracycline, a taxane and Herceptin (trastuzumab).[246]

In addition to receptor tyrosine kinases, which catalyse the formation of phosphate ester bond, protein phosphatases also have an important role in regulating signalling pathways by hydrolysing the phosphate ester bond on tyrosine and serine/threonine residues, thus creating a balance between the phosphorylated and non-phosphorylated states. Inhibitors of protein phosphatases are also being designed as treatment for various diseases mentioned above for protein receptor kinases.[247–251] Chemically, many protein phosphatase inhibitor leads were identified initially from natural products. Subsequently, combinatorial and other chemical approaches led to many compounds such as 151 and 152 which act as inhibitors, but so far, none of these agents has reached the clinic.

151

152

1.8 Protein–protein interaction inhibitors

Many physiological and pathological processes are mediated by protein–protein interactions. The proteins involved in cell adhesion have been most widely studied. The interactions between integrin (a family of at least 24 transmembrane glycoprotein heterodimers formed by the non-covalent associations between 18 α and eight β subunits) family of heterodimeric cell surface receptors and their protein ligands are fundamental for maintaining cell function (e.g. by tethering cells at a particular location), facilitating cell migration or providing survival signals to cells from their environment. Ligands recognised by integrins include extracellular matrix proteins (e.g. collagen and fibronectin), plasma proteins such as fibrinogen and cell surface molecules such as transmembrane proteins of the immunoglobulin family and cell-bound complement. A number of integrins and their ligands have been associated with many disease processes involved in cardiovascular (e.g. thrombosis involving platelet aggregation), inflammation, cancer (e.g. metastasis) and bone disorders.[252,253] The discovery of platelet aggregation inhibitors by blocking the interaction of platelet glycoprotein IIb/IIIa with its natural ligands fibrinogen and von Willebrand factor is described below as an example of protein–protein interaction inhibitors.

Novel inhibitors of glycoprotein IIb/IIIa and fibrinogen–van Willebrand interaction include injectable peptides (e.g. integrilin, 153) and orally active peptidomimetics that act as competitive inhibitors and a monoclonal antibody c7E3 (abciximab) that irreversibly binds to glycoprotein IIb/IIIa. Clinically, the antibody c7E3 has been shown to be effective in reducing 30-day and 6-month clinical events after high-risk coronary intervention. Administered intravenously, circulating abciximab has a plasma half-life of less than 10 min. However, the antibody binds tightly to platelets and provides receptor blockade up to a period of 15 days.

The design of peptide and non-peptide inhibitors of platelet aggregation was based on the early observations that the integrins recognise peptide sequences such as Arg-Gly-Asp present in the larger protein ligands such as fibronectin and vitronectin. This led to the synthesis of a large number of analogues containing the Arg-Gly-Asp tripeptide or the chemical features of the tripeptide side-chains (e.g. the guanidino function and the carboxyl group). SAR studies indicated that a basic functional group that mimics the side-chain of the arginine and a carboxylic acid group mimicking the Asp side-chain are critical to the receptor binding and platelet aggregation activities of these compounds. In addition, a lipophilic group near the carboxylic acid function was found to enhance the potency of the antagonists. These findings led to the synthesis of more stable cyclic peptides such as integrelin and many other compounds containing different non-peptide templates to hold the important functional groups in the proper spatial arrangements. All these approaches have resulted in potent, injectable or orally active platelet aggregation inhibitors. Examples of compounds that have reached the market include the antibody abciximab, the injectable peptides integrilin (153) and tirofiban (154). Many of the orally active compounds such as lamifiban,[254] sibrafiban,[255] xemilofiban, orbofiban and tirofiban have been studied extensively in the clinic. However, most of these have failed in the late stages of development.

In addition to the well known examples of glycoprotein IIb/IIIa, antagonists of other integrins such as αvβ3 (vitronectin receptor), αvβ5, αvβ6, α4β1 and α4β7 have been synthesised. The design of $\alpha_v\beta_3$ receptor antagonists was based on glycoprotein IIb/IIIa antagonists. Therefore some of the early compounds were antagonist of both $\alpha_v\beta_3$ and glycoprotein

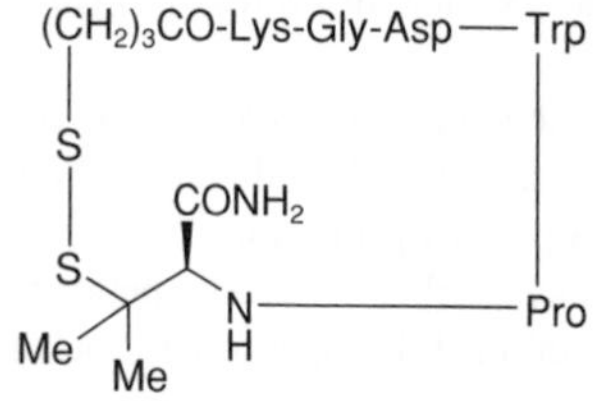

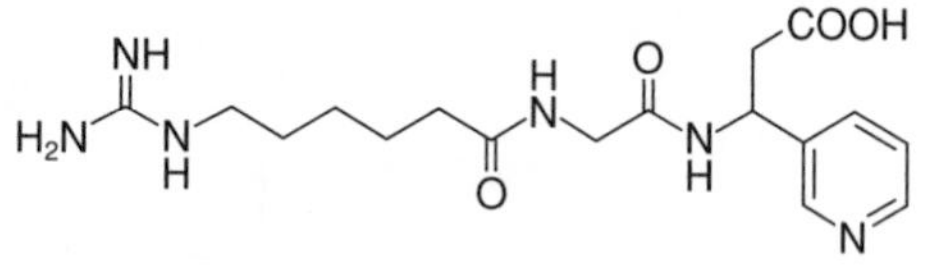

155

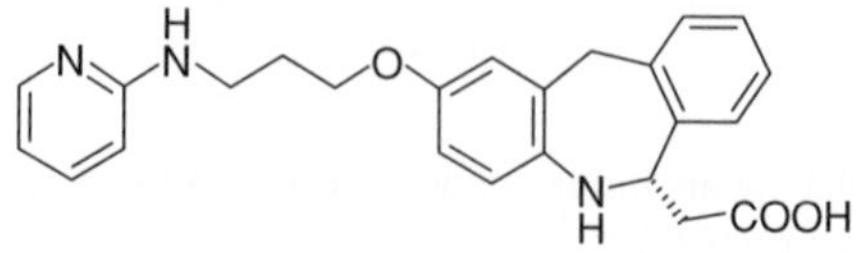

156

IIb/IIIa. Analogues such as 155 were more selective against $\alpha_v\beta_3$ receptor. Compound 155 blocked osteoclast-mediated bone particle degradation. Further medicinal chemistry led to non-peptide vitronectin receptor antagonists with oral activity. For example, compound (156) SB 265123 (Ki 4.1 nmol for $\alpha_v\beta_3$, 1.3 nmol for $\alpha_v\beta_5$, 18,000 nmol for $\alpha_5\beta_1$ and 9000 nmol for $\alpha_{IIb}\beta_3$) displayed 100% oral bioavailability in rats, and was active in vivo in the ovariectomized rat model of osteoporosis.

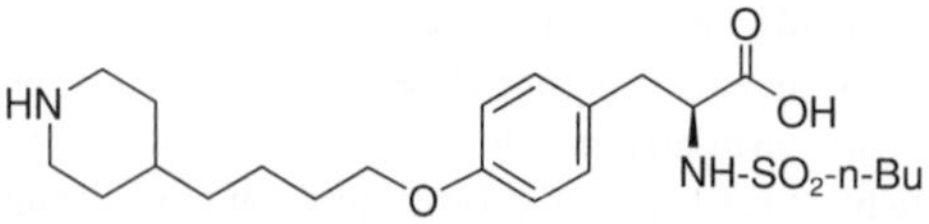

1.8.1 $\alpha_4\beta_1$ and $\alpha_5\beta_1$ antagonists

Cyclic peptide inhibitors of VLA-4 and fibronectin/VCAM-1 interaction, e.g. c[Ile-Leu-Asp-Val-NH(CH$_2$)$_5$CO] were reported. Several of these inhibitors such as c[Ile-Leu-Asp-Val-NH(CH$_2$)$_5$CO], c[Ile-Leu-Asp-Val-NH(CH$_2$)$_4$CO] and c(MePhe-Leu-Asp-Val-D-Arg-D-Arg) blocked VLA-4/VCAM-1 and VLA-4/fibronectin interaction in in vitro assays and inhibited oxazolone and ovalbumin-induced contact hypersensitivity responses in mice.[256–258] The compounds did not affect cell adhesion mediated by two other integrins [VLA-5 ($\alpha_5\beta_1$) and LFA-1 ($\alpha_L\beta_2$). p-Aminophenylacetyl-Leu-Asp-Val derivatives containing various non-peptide residues at the N-terminal end are reported as inhibitors of integrin $\alpha_4\beta_1$. In various integrin adhesion assay, compound 157 showed activity against $\alpha_4\beta_7$, $\alpha_1\beta_1$, $\alpha_5\beta_1$, $\alpha_6\beta_1$, $\alpha_L\beta_2$ and $\alpha_{IIb}\beta_3$ integrins at much higher concentrations. Other inhibitors of leucocyte function-associated antigen (LFA-1) and its ligand integrin-type cell adhesion

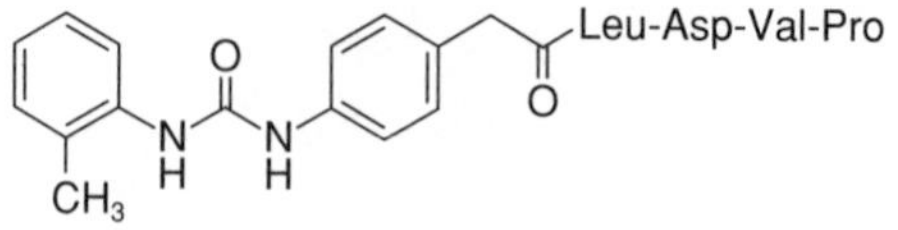

153 Integrilin

154 Tirofiban

157

158 SP-4206

159

160

molecule (ICAM-1) and vary late antigen (VLA-4) and endothelial vascular cell adhesion molecule (VCAM-1) were described in recent reviews.[259]

In addition to the inhibitors of integrins and their ligands, research is also ongoing to find small molecule compounds that are able to interfere interactions of other proteins and their receptors. Some success has been achieved in this field.[260] An example of this is the discovery of an inhibitor of cytokine IL-2 and its receptor. Extensive use of site-directed mutagenesis studies to identify IL-2 residues important for interaction with the receptor followed by modelling, X-ray crystallography and fragment-based discovery approach led to the conversion of a weak inhibitor Ro26-4550 (IC_{50} = 3–6 μmol) to a potent inhibitor SP-4206 (**158**, IC_{50} = 30 nmol) that binds to IL-2 and prevents its interaction with the IL-2 receptor. Random screening approaches have resulted in the discovery of reversible inhibitors (e.g. **159**) of cell-surface proteins B7-1 and B7-2 (found on antigen presenting cells) and CD28, found on the T cell, reducing T-cell activation. Several inhibitors of B-cell lymphoma (BCL2) and BCL-X_L (anti-apoptotic proteins) to the pro-apoptotic protein BAK have been discovered by various approaches such as virtual screening, high-throughput screening and ligand-based design techniques. Information about the binding of BCL-X_L to the 16 amino acid BH3 domain of BAK was obtained using NMR. Compound (**160**) represents one example of a BCL-X_L and BAK inhibitor.

1.9 Protein antibody and vaccine therapeutics

1.9.1 Protein therapeutics

Many successful protein products, including antibodies and vaccines, have been marketed over the years for the treatment of a number of diseases. In recent times, more biopharmaceuticals are entering the drug discovery and development pipelines and these agents are beginning to compete with traditional small molecule drugs.[261] This is despite the fact that peptide and protein products are complex molecules and expensive to manufacture. In 2005 alone, sales of biotechnology products were around $50 billion. One of the oldest examples of a protein product is insulin, still one of the most successful drugs after 70–80 years of its discovery. Early insulin preparations, derived from natural sources, are being replaced by recombinant human insulin preparations and new formulations are being marketed that provide a more gradual and continuous release profile and maximise glucose control in diabetic patients.[262]

The new genomic and proteomic discoveries will result in many more therapeutic protein products (including monoclonal antibodies and therapeutic vaccines) for the treatment of many diseases, including autoimmune, inflammatory and infectious diseases and cancer. These protein/antibody products pose different sets of problems than the traditional small molecular weight products. Many of these are highly glycosylated proteins and precise molecular structures, including secondary and tertiary protein structures, of these agents cannot be defined. Although many highly sophisticated analytical techniques are used for the characterisation of these protein products, it is still not possible to achieve the level of characterisation achieved with the small molecule products. The choice of expression systems and growth conditions for the production of these agents has a big impact on the quality of the final product. Safety and clinical testing in animals presents additional problems. Several biopharmaceuticals are species-specific in terms of their biological effects, and may induce immune reactions in animals. These agents, except orally active vaccines, are administered parenterally (subcutaneous injections or infusion) and it is often difficult to define precise pharmacokinetic–pharmacodynamic properties. Many problems associated with the development of protein products (e.g. production, characterisation, administration/formulation) are being overcome gradually. Various techniques such as pegylation[263] and N-glycosylation are used to increase biological half-life of protein products. Along with mammalian cell culture systems (currently the production system of choice for glycoproteins), several other expression systems, including yeast, plant and insect expression systems are currently being explored as alternatives to mammalian cell culture for the production of glycoproteins.[264] Methods are being developed to generate single proteins in cell-free and cell-based systems to enable the production of these proteins commercially viable.[265–268] Protein stability issues are being addressed by establishing high-throughput screening techniques.[269]

Successful protein products marketed in the last 15–20 years (listed in Table 1.6) include haematopoietic growth factors[270] such as erythropoietin (production of erythrocytes – involved in tissue oxygenation),[271] thrombopoietin (regulator of platelet production)[272] and granulocyte–macrophage colony stimulating factor

Table 1.6 Protein products in the market since 1987

Protein product	Treatment indication
Nesiritide – recombinant B-type natriuretic peptide	Heart failure
Carperitide – recombinant α-hANP	Congestive heart failure
Anact C – human plasma-derived activated protein C concentrate	Deep vein thrombosis, pulmonary thromboembolism due to congenital protein C deficiency
Plasma protein concentrate (Wilate) (human plasma-derived von Willebrand factor and coagulation factor VIII)	Haematological disorders in patients with von Willebrand disease and haemophilia A
Haemoglobin glutamer-250, bovine (Hemopure)	Eliminating, delaying or reducing the need for allogenic red blood cell transfusion in acutely anaemic adult surgical patients
Recombinant human antithrombin (ATryn)	Prophylaxis of venous thromboembolism in surgery of patients with congenital antithrombin deficiency
Thrombin, human plasma derived (Evithrom)	Stand-alone product – approved for haemostasis in surgery
Drotrecogin alfa (activated) – recombinant human activated protein C	Reducing mortality in patients with severe sepsis (sepsis associated with acute organ failure)
Protein C concentrate (human)	Purpura fulminans and coumarin-induced skin necrosis in congenital protein C deficiency patients
Anakinra – recombinant version of human IL-1 receptor antagonist	Rheumatoid arthritis patients failing to respond to disease-modifying anti-rheumatic drugs
Darbepoietin alfa – long-acting erythropoietin preparation	Anaemia in patients with chronic renal failure
Peginterferon alfa-2a – pegylated IFN derivative	Chronic hepatitis B and C; chronic HCV in patients co-infected with HCV and HIV (in combination with ribavirin)
Interferon Alfacon-1 – 30% identity with IFN-β and 60% identity with IFN-ω	Chronic hepatitis C

Table 1.6 *Continued*

Protein product	Treatment indication
IFN-β-1a	Relapsing form of multiple sclerosis
IFN-β-1b – recombinant, stable analogue of human IFN-β	Relapsing remitting multiple sclerosis
IFN-γ-1α – recombinant	Cutaneous T-cell lymphoma
IFN-γ-1b – recombinant	Chronic granulomatous disease
IFN-γ – recombinant	Rheumatoid arthritis
NovoMix 30 – combination of 30% soluble insulin aspart/70% insulin aspart protamine crystals	Diabetes
Insulin lispro – fast-acting, recombinant human insulin analogue	Diabetes
Insulin glulisine (Apidra) – rDNA human insulin analogue	Adult patients with diabetes mellitus (type 1 or 2) for the control of hyperglycaemia
Insulin detemir (Levemir) – a long-acting insulin analogue	Diabetes
Inhaled human insulin (Exubera) – fast-acting, dry powder formulation	Type 1 diabetes
Oral insulin (Oral-lyn) – oral spray formulation	Treatment of both type 1 and 2 diabetes
Human amylin – synthetic analogue (Symlin)	Type 1 and 2 and diabetes (in conjunction with insulin) for patients who have failed to achieve glucose control despite optimal insulin therapy
Amylin (exentide)	Type 2 diabetes (adjunctive treatment) – not controlled on metformin and/or a sulfonylurea
Recombinant glucagon	Insulin-induced hypoglycaemia; emergency treatment for severe hypogycaemic reactions
Secretin, (human, synthetically produced peptide)	Diagnostic of pancreatic exocrine dysfunction and gastrinoma in Zollinger–Ellison syndrome patients
OCT-43 (Octin) – recombinant variant of IL-1β (Cys^{71} replaced by Ser)	Mycosis fungoides and antitumour in malignant skin tumours and in the treatment of aplastic anaemia and myelodysplastic syndrome
IL-2 – Stable rDNA IL-2	Antineoplastic – renal cell carcinoma
Tasonermin – recombinant TNF	Soft tissue sarcoma of the limbs
Lepirudin – recombinant modified hirudin	Myocardial infarcts, unstable angina and cardiovascular events
Parnaparin – low MW heparin	Anticoagulant
Reviparin – low MW heparin	Prevention of deep vein thrombosis and pulmonary embolism following surgery
Enoxaparin – low MW heparin	Antithrombotic
Nartograstim – rGCSF derivative	Chemotherapy-induced leucopenia
Filgrastim – recombinant human GCSF	Adjunct to cancer chemotherapy for patients with non-myeloid malignancies
Pegfilgrastim – conjugate of recombinant methionyl-GCSF and monomethoxypolyethylene glycol	Decreasing infections in patients with non-myeloid malignancies receiving myelosuppressive anticancer drugs
Sargramostin – recombinant granulocyte–macrophage colony stimulating factor	Immunostimulant – cancer patients after autologous bone marrow transplant

Table 1.6 *Continued*

Protein product	Treatment indication
Recombinant human keratinocyte growth factor (palifermin)	Oral mucositis – in patients with haematologic malignancies receiving myelotoxic therapy requiring haematopoietic stem cell support
Somatomedin-1 – IGF-1	Growth disorders in children; hereditary Laron-type dwarfism
IGF-1 (Increlex) (recombinant)	Growth failure in children with IGF-1 deficiency, growth hormone gene deletion or with neutralising antibodies to growth hormone
Human IGF-1 and human IGF-binding protein-3 complex (iPlex), rDNA origin	Growth failure in children with IGF-deficiency, growth hormone gene deletion or with neutralising antibodies to growth hormone
Somatotropin – recombinant, modified human growth hormone	Growth failure in children due to a lack of endogenous growth hormone secretion
Somatropin – recombinant human growth hormone	Hypopituitary dwarfism and other disorders resulting from growth hormone deficiencies; Treatment of short bowel syndrome (impaired absorption of nutrition from food)
Epoetin delta, gene-activated human erythropoietin	Anaemia related to renal disease in dialysis patients and in patients not yet undergone dialysis (to elevate and maintain red blood cell production)
Erythropoietin – recombinant erythropoietin	Anaemia associated with renal transplant or end stage renal disease
Methoxy-polyethylene glycol-epoetin β (Mircera)	A continuous erythropoietin receptor activator – treatment of anaemia associated with chronic kidney disease (administered every 2 or 4 weeks)
EGF – recombinant	Healing of the corneal epithelium following various corneal diseases
Parathyroid hormone (PTH 1–84), rDNA origin (Preotact)	Treatment of postmenopausal women with osteoporosis at high risk for fractures
Recombinant thyroid stimulating hormone (Thyrogen)	Detection of recurrence of well-differentiated thyroid cancer and treatment of thyroid cancer when used in combination with radioiodine
Alglucosidase-α (recombinant, human) (Myozyme). Enzyme that breaks down glycogen in the body	Long-term enzyme replacement therapy in patients with Pompe's disease (a disorder that affects the heart and muscles)
Iduronate-2-sulfatase (human, purified) (Elaprase) (breaks down mucopolysaccharides)	Hunter syndrome (also known as mucopolysaccharidosis II)
Follitropin α/lutropin α (Pergoveris)	Stimulation of follicular development in women with severe LH and FSH deficiency
Follicle stimulating hormone (Follitrope), recombinant, human	Ovulation-inducing agent with high purity and efficacy
Abatacept (Orencia)	Treatment of rheumatoid arthritis – a selective co-stimulation modulator inhibiting T-cell activation by binding to CD80 and CD86

ANP, atrial natriuretic peptide; EGF, epithelial growth factor; FSH, follicle stimulating hormone; GCSF, granulocyte colony stimulating factor; HCV, hepatitis C virus; IFN, interferon; IGF, insulin-like growth factor; IL, interleukin; LH, luteinizing hormone; MW, molecular weight; TNF, tumour necrosis factor.

(e.g. production of neutrophils, eosinophils, basophils, monocytes), interferones, parathyroid hormone,[273] recombinant human parathyroid hormone N-terminal fragment (1–34) (teriparatide),[274] tinzaparin (a low molecular weight heparin formed by the enzymatic degradation of porcine unfractionated heparin),[275] etanercept and several others listed in Table 1.6. In patients receiving fibrinolysis for ST-elevation myocardial infarction, treatment with enoxaparin (a low molecular weight heparin) throughout the index hospitalisation was superior to treatment with unfractionated heparin for 48 h but was associated with an increase in major bleeding episodes.[276] Etanercept is a soluble dimeric fusion protein consisting of the two copies of the extracellular ligand-binding portion of the human TNF p75 receptor linked to the constant portion of human immunoglobulin G_1. It binds to TNFα, thereby blocking its interaction with cell surface receptors and attenuating its pro-inflammatory effects in rheumatoid arthritis and psoriasis.[277,278] Etancercept appears to have greater affinity for TNFα than infiximab (a monoclonal antibody against TNF). Etanercept is administered subcutaneously twice a week to rheumatoid arthritis patients. A 36-amino acid peptide (enfuvirtide) has recently been marketed for the treatment of HIV AIDS. The peptide binds to a region of the envelope glycoprotein 41 of HIV-1 that is involved in the fusion of the virus with host cell membrane and specifically prevents the fusion of the virus gp41 glycoprotein with the CD4 receptor of the host cell.[279,280] Like other therapeutics, protein therapeutics also have some side effects. For example, various interferones, used for the treatment of infectious diseases such as hepatitis and inflammatory diseases such as arthritis, can precipitate immune-mediated abnormalities.[281]

1.9.2 Antibody therapeutics

Along with the protein products mentioned above, significant progress has also been made in the discovery and marketing of antibodies.[282,283] Development of the hybridoma technology has allowed the production of rodent monoclonal antibodies that are the product of single clone of antibody producing cells and have only one antigen binding specificity. However, the therapeutic use of rodent monoclonal antibodies in humans is limited by their immunogenecity. Using genetic engineering and expression systems, it is now possible to produce chimeric, humanised and totally human antibodies as well as antibodies with novel structures and functional properties.[284] Although clinically used humanised and

human antibodies are safe and effective, many (like other therapeutics) suffer side effects.[285] In addition to the risk of infusion-related side effects (including the possibility of anaphylaxis), haematological toxicity is also frequent, especially if the antibodies are associated with chemotherapy; the resulting neutropenia – and with some agents lymphopenia – is associated with an increased risk of infection. Cardiac failure and pulmonary complications have been reported with some of these agents. Like other therapeutic agents, antibodies have also suffered from post-marketing problems. A humanised $α_4$ integrin monoclonal antibody natalizumab that had shown efficacy in multiple sclerosis and Crohn's disease was implicated in three cases of progressive multifocal leucoencephalopathy, two fatal and one disabling, and this resulted in the voluntary suspension of the antibody.[286–288] Natalizumab reduced the risk of the sustained progression of disability and the rate of clinical relapse in patients with relapsing multiple sclerosis. When added to interferon β-1a in patients with relapsing multiple sclerosis, natalizumab was significantly more effective than interferon β-1a alone.

Phage and ribosome display technologies are currently being used, in conjunction with targeted, random or semi-rational mutagenesis strategies, for potency optimisation and generating new antibody drug candidates.[289] Phage display technology was used successfully to isolate and optimise antibody molecules such as the human anti-TNFα antibody [marketed as Humira (adalimumab)]. Progress is also being made in developing methods (e.g. antigen arrays)[290] for antibody profiling and understanding the elimination mechanisms of therapeutic monoclonal antibodies.[291] Recent work is being directed towards producing recombinant polyclonal antibodies that have the potential to tackle complex and highly mutagenic targets.[292] In addition, immunostimulatory monoclonal antibodies (directed to immune-receptor molecules) are being developed to increase immune responses in cancer patients.[293] These antibodies are expected to act on target receptors and enhance ongoing immune responses, either by antagonizing the receptors that suppress immune responses or by activating others that amplify immune responses. However, this approach may suffer from toxicity problems such as autoimmunity and systemic inflammation by generating organ-specific autoimmunity and releasing pro-inflammatory cytokines.

Like protein products mentioned above, production, formulation and characterisation of antibodies also presents significant challenges.[294] Currently available antibodies are used for the treatment of many diseases such as cancer,[295] rheumatoid arthritis,[296] Crohn's disease, spondyloarthropathies, psoriasis, allograft rejection and respiratory diseases.[297] Compared with small molecule drugs, antibodies are very specific and are less likely to cause toxicity based on factors other than the mechanism of action. Bound to a target, therapeutic antibodies can deliver a toxic payload, act as agonists or antagonists of receptors, or as neutralizers of ligands. All of the antibodies that are currently on the market are produced in mammalian cell cultures. Chimeric, humanized and phage-display-derived monoclonal antibodies need to be produced from recombinant genes reintroduced into mammalian cells to enable proper folding and glycosylation. These time-consuming steps are not required for human antibodies from genetically engineered mice, as these can be produced directly from the original hybridomas. Development of transgenic animals such as goats or cows, which are engineered to produce monoclonal antibodies in their milk may offer an economical alternative.[298]

Examples of antibodies currently in the market (Table 1.7) include trastuzumab (Herceptin, anti-HER2 monoclonal antibody), rituximab, natalizumab (α_4-integrin antibody), abciximab, infiximab (targets TNFα in Crohn's disease and rheumatoid arthritis), alemtuzumab, adalimumab (TNFα antibody for the treatment of rheumatoid arthritis), efalizumab (anti-CD11a monoclonal antibody for the treatment of psoriasis)[299] and eculizumab (treatment of patients with paroxysmal nocturnal haemoglobinuria to reduce haemolysis; binds to the terminal complement protein C5).[300] Trastuzumab (Herceptin) is one of the most successful antibody products of recent times. It is a humanised monoclonal antibody used in the treatment of breast cancer that over-expresses HER2, which is associated with clinically aggressive disease

and a poor prognosis.[301,302] The antibody is indicated both as monotherapy for use in patients with HER2-positive metastatic breast cancer who have previously received chemotherapy for their metastatic disease and in combination with paclitaxel or docetaxel. Addition of intravenous trastuzumab to first-line chemotherapy improved the time to disease progression, objective response rate, duration of response and overall survival in randomised multicentre trials in women with HER2-positive metastatic breast cancer. Minor side effects associated with trastuzumab include fever, chills, abdominal pain, headache, diarrhoea, nausea and rash. Serious side effects associated with the antibody include cardiac events, severe hypersensitivity reactions (including anaphylaxis) and pulmonary events. Risk of ventricular dysfunction and congestive heart failure in patients treated with trastuzumab alone or in combination with paclitaxel or docetaxel is particularly increased if administered in combination with anthracycline-containing chemotherapy.

In addition to trastuzumab (Herceptin), several other growth factor-related antibodies such as panitumumab and cetuximab have also been developed. An EGFR selective antibody panitumumab (Vectibix, a fully human immunoglobulin G2 monoclonal antibody) demonstrated efficacy in patients with metastatic colorectal cancer and significantly improved progression-free survival.[303] The antibody, indicated for the treatment of patients with EGFR-expressing metastatic colorectal cancer after disease progression on, or following, fluoropyrimidine-, oxaliplatin- and irinotecan-containing chemotherapy regimens, may also be useful as first-line therapy in combination with fluorouracil, folinic acid and irinotecan in patients with metastatic colorectal cancer. Cetuximab is a chimeric monoclonal antibody highly selective for the EGFR that induces a broad range of cellular responses

Table 1.7 Examples of antibodies currently on the market

Antibody (trade name)	Indication (target)
Rituximab (Rituxan), chimeric antibody	Non-Hodgkin's lymphoma, rheumatoid arthritis in patients with an inadequate response to TNFα inhibitors (anti-CD20 antibody that selectively targets B cells)
Ibritumomab	Non-Hodgkin's lymphoma (CD20)
Tositumomab	Non-Hodgkin's lymphoma (CD20)
Trastuzumab (Herceptin), humanised monoclonal antibody	Metastatic breast cancer, non-small-cell lung cancer, pancreatic cancer [binds selectively and with high affinity to the extracellular domain of HER-2/neu (p183^{neu})]

Table 1.7 *Continued*

Antibody (trade name)	Indication (target)
Gemtuzumab Ozogamicin	Acute myelogenous leukaemia (CD33)
Alemtuzumab	Chronic lymphocytic leukaemia, multiple sclerosis (CDw52)
Cetuximab	Colorectal cancer (IgG1 chimeric human-murine monoclonal antibody directed at the EGFR)
Bevacizumab (Avastin)	Metastatic colon or rectum cancer – in combination with 5-fluorouracil-based chemotherapy (vascular endothelial growth factor)
Ranibizumab (Lucentis), recombinant humanised IgG1 κ isotype monoclonal antibody fragment	Treatment of neovascular (wet) age-related macular degeneration (human vascular endothelial growth factor A)
Panitumumab (Vectibix), human monoclonal antibody	Treatment of EGF receptor-expressing metastatic colorectal cancer after disease progression on, or following, fluoropyrimidine-, oxaliplatin- and irinotecan-containing chemotherapy regimens
Nimotuzumab, monoclonal antibody	Head and neck cancer (anti-EGFR)
Endrecolomab	Colorectal cancer (17-A1)
Adrecolomab	Colorectal cancer (EpCAM)
Infiximab	Crohn's disease, rheumatoid arthritis (TNFα)
Adalimumab (Humira), recombinant human monoclonal antibody	Moderate to severely active Crohn's disease, rheumatoid arthritis, psoriatic arthritis, ankylosing spondylitis, moderate to severe plaque psoriasis (human IgG1 antibody targeting TNFα)
Certolizumab (Cimzia)	Treatment of Crohn's disease (PEGylated anti-TNFα monoclonal antibody)
Etanercept (Enbrel), fully human anti-TNF therapy	Treatment of adult patients with chronic moderate to severe plaque psoriasis, rheumatoid arthritis, polyarticular-course juvenile rheumatoid arthritis and psoriatic arthritis (anti-TNFα therapy)
Efalizumab (Raptiva), recombinant humanised monoclonal antibody	Treatment of psoriasis (anti-CD11 monoclonal antibody that inhibits the binding of LFA-1 to ICAM-1)
CDP-870	Crohn's disease, rheumatoid arthritis (TNFα)
Natalizumab (humanised monoclonal antibody)	Crohn's disease, relapsing form of multiple sclerosis (VLA4β1)
Omalizumab	Allergic asthma (IgE)
Muromonab	Organ transplant rejection (CD3)
Daclizumab	Kidney transplant rejection (CD25), leukaemia
Basiliximab	Kidney transplant rejection (CD25)
Epratuzumab	Autoimmune diseases (CD22)
Tocilizumab (Actemra), humanised monoclonal antibody	Treatment for Castlemen's disease (non-cancerous growth in the lymph node tissues throughout the body) (antihuman IL-6 receptor)
Eculizumab (Soliris), humanized monoclonal antibody	Paroxysmal nocturnal hemoglobinurea (characterised by breakdown of the red blood cells) (anti-CD88, C5aR) – binds to complement protein C5, preventing its cleavage into C5a and C5b)

EGFR, endothelial growth factor receptor; Ig, immunoglobulin; ICAM, integrin-type cell adhesion molecule; LFA, leucocyte function-associated antigen; TNF, tumour necrosis factor.

(e.g. inhibits cell cycle progression, apoptosis, reduction in growth factors such as EGF, transforming growth factor α and VEGF) that enhance tumour sensitivity to radiotherapy and chemotherapeutic agents. The antibody has a longer half-life (79–129 h) and is administered once a week by intravenous infusion. It is indicated for the treatment of colorectal cancer in combination with irinotecan.[304,305] Ranibizumab (Lucentis, a recombinant humanized monoclonal antibody Fab that neutralizes all active forms of VEGF-A) prevented vision loss and improved mean visual acuity, with low rates of serious adverse events, in patients with minimally classic or occult (with no classic lesions) choroidal neovascularization secondary to age-related macular degeneration.[306]

Infliximab (Remicade), the chimeric monoclonal antibody directed against TNFα, has profoundly changed therapy for Crohn's disease.[307,308] It is used as a remission-inducing agent in patients who have moderate to severe ulcerative colitis and are either refractory to or intolerant of mesalazine (5-ASA) products and immunomodulators; infliximab may be an alternative to ciclosporin in hospitalised patients with severe to moderately severe but not fulminant ulcerative colitis who do not respond to intravenous corticosteroids. Adalimumab (Humira, TNFα antibody approved for the treatment of rheumatoid arthritis) demonstrated efficacy in psoriatic arthritis patients when used as monotherapy. The arthritis response was similar for recipients of adalimumab alone or adalimumab plus methotrexate.[309]

Rituximab (MabThera, Rituxan) is another commercially successful mouse/human chimeric anti-CD20 monoclonal antibody used for the treatment of various lymphoid malignancies.[310–312] The antibody that induces lysis and apoptosis of normal and malignant human B cells, and sensitises malignant B cells to the cytotoxic effect of chemotherapy. As CD20 antigen is found on the surface of malignant and normal B lymphocytes, treatment with rituximab induces lymphopenia in most patients, but the effects are reversible (6–9 months after therapy). Administered once a week by intravenous infusion, rituximab is approved for the treatment of aggressive non-Hodgkin's lymphoma in combination with cyclophosphamide, doxorubicin, vincristine and prednisone chemotherapy. Rituximab is also approved for the treatment of rheumatoid arthritis. Recent studies have demonstrated the efficacy of rituximab in several refractory autoimmune disorders including systemic lupus erythematosus, immune thrombocytopenic purpura, chronic cold agglutinin disease, IgM-mediated neuropathies and mixed cryoglobulinaemia. In clinical trials in patients with indolent or aggressive B-cell non-Hodgkin's lymphoma or chronic lymphocytic leukaemia, intravenous rituximab in combination with chemotherapy was more effective as first- or second-line therapy than chemotherapy alone in providing tumour remission and patient survival. In addition, rituximab maintenance therapy was shown to significantly prolong tumour remission and patient survival in these patients. The combination of rituximab with cyclophosphamide, doxorubicin, vincristine and prednisone was cost effective as first-line therapy for advanced-stage diffuse large B-cell non-Hodgkin's lymphoma.

Omalizumab (Xolair) is an IgE-neutralizing antibody and can block binding of IgE immunoglobulin to the high-affinity IgE receptor (FcεRI) on mast cells and basophils, rendering the mediator-packed inflammatory cells insensitive to allergen stimulation. This recombinant humanized monoclonal antibody is recommended for allergic asthma.[313] Side effects associated with the anti-IgE antibody included risks of the development of cancer and anaphylaxis. Cancer developed (predominantly epithelial or solid-organ cancers) in more patients exposed to omalizumab than in those who received placebo. Alemtuzumab is an unconjugated humanised monoclonal antibody directed against the cell surface antigen CD52 on lyphocytes and monocytes. Administered by intravenous infusion (three times a week) for 12 weeks for the treatment of B-cell chronic lymphocytic leukaemia in patients previously treated with alkylating agents and refractory to fludarabine.[314]

Basiliximab is a mouse/human chimeric monoclonal antibody with specificity and high affinity for the α-subunit of the IL-2 receptor. The antibody acts as an IL-2Rα antagonist and inhibits IL-2-mediated activation and proliferation of T lymphocytes. It is indicated for the prevention of acute organ rejection in adult and paediatric renal transplant recipients in combination with other immunosuppressive agents such as ciclosporin, azathioprine, mycophenolate mofetil and corticosteroids.[315] Abciximab is an antibody fragment that inhibits platelet aggregation and leucocyte adhesion by binding to the glycoprotein IIb/IIIa, vitronectin and Mac-1 receptors. It reduces the short- and long-term risk of ischaemic complications in patients with ischaemic heart disease undergoing percutaneous coronary intervention. It is administered by intravenous infusion for 12 h.[316]

An example of targeted delivery of cytotoxic agents to tumours is gemtuzumab. In this case, calicheamicin, a potent cytotoxic agent that causes double-strand DNA breaks, resulting in cell death, is conjugated to monoclonal antibodies specific for tumour-associated antigens. The tumour-specific antibody directs the cytotoxic agent to the tumour cells, thereby reducing damage to other cells in the body.[317] Examples of many other therapeutic antibodies are listed in Table 1.7 along with their clinical indications.

1.9.3 Vaccine therapeutics

Like some of the antibodies mentioned above, vaccines have also been used in clinical practice for a long time. Many of the currently available vaccines (Table 1.8), including diphtheria, tetanus, measles, mumps and rubella (MMR), meningococcal and pneumococcal, are directed against microbes that cause mostly acute rather than chronic infections. These vaccines rely on the production of memory T-cell responses to recognise the infective agent. In recent times, vaccines have been developed that combine the antibody-based responses with cell-based immunity.[318] Some recently used vaccines against hepatitis A, hepatitis B, tuberculosis and influenza are examples of these types of vaccines. Work is currently ongoing to develop DNA-based vaccines.[318] Although vaccines against hepatitis A and B have been available for the last 20 years, work is still ongoing to develop triple antigen vaccines and polyvalent vaccines that can be effective against several diseases.[319] Tuberculosis remains an area of interest because of some problems associated with the BCG vaccine, primarily its lack of effectiveness against pulmonary tuberculosis in children and adults.[320,321] A number of vaccines such as rBCG30 (live, recombinant BCG-Tice, over-expressing Ag85B from *M. tuberculosis*), MVA-85A (live recombinant replication-deficient vaccinia virus, expressing Ag85A from *M. tuberculosis*) and Ag85B-ESAT6 (recombinant protein, composed of a fusion of ESAT6 and Ag85B from *M. tuberculosis*) are currently in development for protection against tuberculosis.[322,323] Some recent data have indicated limited efficacy of the BCG vaccine in prevention of leprosy (a chronic infection caused by *Mycobacterium leprae*).[324] A new oral cholera vaccine has been developed by combining a killed whole cell cholera vaccine with the recombinant B subunit of cholera toxin (rCTB-WC). Because of the similarity between cholera toxin and the heat-labile toxin of *Escherichia coli*, a cause of travellers' diarrhoea, it has been proposed that the rCTB-WC vaccine may be used against travellers' diarrhoea. Although the vaccine shows some protection against cholera (4–6 months protection in 61–86%), protection against cases of travellers' diarrhoea was very poor (7% or less).[325] Attempts are being made to generate vaccines against bacterial pneumonia caused by *Streptococcus pneumoniae*.[326]

Recent outbreaks of highly pathogenic avian influenza A virus (H5N1 subtype) infections in poultry and some humans (through direct contact with infected birds) have raised concerns about an influenza pandemic in the near future. Person-to-person spread of current H5N1 strains appears to be unlikely. For immediate treatment, the currently available antiviral agents such as adamantanes and neuraminidase inhibitors such as oseltamivir and zanamivir may be useful in some patients and for this reason a number of health authorities have accumulated large stockpiles of these drugs. However, resistance may soon develop against these agents. Indeed, H5N1 isolates resistant to these agents have already

Table 1.8 Examples of vaccines currently on the market

Vaccine	Indication
Quadrivalent HPV (types 6, 11, 16, 18) recombinant vaccine (Gardasil)	Prevention of cervical cancer and vulvar and vagina precancers caused by HPV type 16 and 18 and low-grade and precancerous lesions and genital warts caused by HPA types 6, 11, 16 and 18 (for use in girls aged 9–26 years)
HPV vaccine (types 16 and 18), recombinant, AS04 adjuvanted (Cervarix)	Prevention of cervical cancer in girls and women aged 10–45 years of age, cytological abnormalities including atypical squamous cells of uncertain significance and cervical intraepithelial neoplasia and precancerous lesions caused by HPV types 16 and 18
Zoster vaccine live (Zostavax)	Prevention of herpes zoster (shingles) in individuals aged 60 years or older and herpes zoster-related post-herpetic neuralgia
Rotavirus vaccine (Rotarix) – oral, live attenuated vaccine	Protection against multiple rotavirus strains and prevention of gastroenteritis caused by rotavirus infection

Table 1.8 *Continued*

Vaccine	Indication
Rotavirus vaccine (RotaTeq), live, oral	Prevention of rotavirus gastroenteritis in infants and children caused by the serotypes G1, G2, G3 and G4 – administered as a three-dose series to infants between the ages of 6–32 weeks
Hepatitis B immune globulin, human (HepaGram B)	Treatment of acute exposure to blood containing HBsAg, perinatal exposure of infants born to HBsAg-positive mothers, sexual exposure to HBsAg-positive persons and household exposure to persons with acute HBV infection
Quinavaxem (liquid pentavalent vaccine)	Protection against five childhood diseases: diphtheria, tetanus, pertussis, hepatitis B and *Haemophilus influenzae* type B
Hepatitis B vaccine (Supervax) recombinant	Recombinant DNA hepatitis B vaccine combined with the fully synthetic adjuvant RC-529
Combined hepatitis A and B vaccine (Bilive) – inactivated hepatitis A virus antigen and recombinant HBsAg	Protection against hepatitis A and B, Bilive junior is for use in non-immune children and adolescents aged 1–15 years, and Bilive adult is for use in non-immune adults and adolescents 16 years of age and older
Hepatitis B rDNA vaccine (adjuvanted, adsorbed) (Fendrix)	Prevention of hepatitis B in patients with renal insufficiency including specific high-risk groups such as pre-haemodialysis and haemodialysis patients (15 years and older)
Meningococcal [groups A, C, Y and W-135] polysaccharide diphtheria toxoid conjugate vaccine (Menactra)	Quadrivalent conjugate vaccine for the prevention of meningococcal disease and to offer protection against four subgroups of *Neisserria meningitides* [A, C, Y and W-135] in adolescents and adults aged 11–55 years
Meningococcal B vaccine (MeNZB)	Prevention of meningococcal disease (B subgroup)
Measles, mumps, rubella and varicella virus vaccine live (ProQuad)	Simultaneous vaccination against measles, mumps, rubella (German measles) and varicella (chickenpox) in children 12 months to 12 years of age
Smallpox (vaccinia) vaccine, live (ACAM2000)	Protection against smallpox (a single dose vaccine), indicated for active immunisation against smallpox disease for persons determined to be at high risk of smallpox infection
Vaccinia immune globulin intravenous (DIGIV)	Approved for the treatment of certain rare complications of smallpox vaccination
Measles and rubella vaccine (Mearubik)	A combination vaccine (live attenuated) against measles and rubella into a single injection
Rabies vaccine (Rabirix)	Prevention and treatment of human rabies infection
Pandemic influenza vaccine (Daronrix), H5N1, inactivated whole viron	Prophylaxis of influenza infection – for use once a pandemic has been declared and would be modified to include the exact pandemic strain, once such a strain has been identified
Pandemic influenza vaccine (H5N1 vaccine)	Prophylaxis of influenza infection
Pandemic influenza vaccine (Focetria), surface antigen, inactivated, adjuvanted	Prophylaxis of influenza infection – to be manufactured to contain the influenza strain declared at the time of a pandemic
Influenza virus vaccine (Afluria)	Active immunisation to prevent influenza caused by influenza virus type A and B in adults 18 years and older
Influenza vaccine (Optaflu), surface antigen, inactivated	For vaccination against seasonal influenza

HBsAg, hepatitis B surface antigen; HBV, hepatitis B virus; HPV, human papillomavirus.

been isolated. There is currently a great deal of interest in developing safer and effective vaccines against this virus.[327] In one study, six inactivated split-viron influenza A/Vietnam/1194/2004 (H5N1 strain isolated from a person with H5N1 influenza) vaccine formulations (manufactured by Sanofi Pasteur) were investigated in human volunteers. All formulations were well tolerated, with no serious adverse events.[328]

In addition to the vaccines for infectious diseases such as tuberculosis, cholera, pneumonia and influenza, significant effort has been deployed towards discovering therapeutic and preventative vaccines for various cancers.[329–331] As micro-organisms are the cause of 10–20% of all human tumours, vaccines that reduce infection with viruses that cause cancer are likely to be useful in primary cancer prevention. Vaccination against hepatitis B virus, for example, has reduced the incidence of hepatocellular carcinoma whereas vaccines against human papillomaviruses (HPV) are expected to greatly reduce the incidence of cervical carcinoma. Although more than 100 different human papilloma genotypes have been defined, of which about 40 infect the genital mucosa, the low-risk HPV types (typified by HPV6 and HPV11) produce benign genital warts, condyloma accuminata and the high-risk types (most notably HPV16 and HPV18) are the aetiological agent of cervical cancer. Successful examples of recently discovered and marketed cancer vaccines include Gardasil [HPV quadrivalent (types 6, 11, 16, 18) recombinant vaccine][332] and Cervarix (HPV vaccine types 16 and 18, recombinant, AS04 adjuvanted). The discovery was based on the established link between HPV and cervical cancer (second most common type of cancer after breast cancer in women worldwide).[333] Gardasil is indicated for use in the prevention of cervical cancer, vulvar and vaginal precancer and cancers, precancerous lesions and genital warts associated with HPV types 6, 11, 16 or 18 infection in adolescents and young women. Similarly, Cervarix is indicated for the prevention of cervical cancer in girls and women aged 10–45 years of age, cytological abnormalities including atypical squamous cells of uncertain significance and cervical intraepithelial neoplasia and precancerous lesions caused by HPV types 16 and 18.

Another area of active interest for vaccination is development of vaccines against rotavirus – the most common cause of severe diarrhoea in children worldwide and diarrhoeal deaths in children in developing countries.[334] The first such vaccine (RotaShield – a tetravalent rhesus rotavirus vaccine) was initially shown to be safe and highly effective but was withdrawn later because of the complication of intussusception (infolding of one segment of the intestine within another). Two new vaccines, Rotarix and RotaTeq, have been licensed recently. These vaccines are based on slightly different principles to achieve broad immunity against the diverse strains of rotavirus in circulation. Rotarix was prepared from an individual human strain that replicates well in the intestine and is shed in the stool. RotaTeq is a combination of five bovine-human reassortants that replicate poorly in the gut, are administered in a 100-fold higher dose and are shed in the stool of only around 10% of infants. Each vaccine has proven highly effective in preventing severe rotavirus diarrhoea in children and is safe from the possible complication of intussusception.

An injectable seasonal allergy vaccine Pollinex, containing glutaraldehyde-modified allergens (grass pollen or tree pollen) and the adjuvants 3-deacylated monophosphoryl lipid A and L-tyrosine has been approved for the treatment of seasonal allergic rhinitis (hayfever), most commonly caused by allergy to pollen from trees, grasses or weeds.[335] In patients with seasonal allergic rhinitis and/or allergic asthma, pre-seasonal vaccination using the allergy vaccine showed significant reduction in symptoms and reduced medication use compared with the previous pollen season.

1.10 DNA and RNA based therapeutics

Since the discovery of human genome and its role in producing proteins of interest which regulate physiological/pathological functions, many other functions of DNA/RNA, including role in gene transcription have been discovered and research is ongoing to discover new medicines based on these new pathways.[336–338] The earlier concept that DNA ultimately leads to genes that give rise to proteins has changed with the discovery of non-coding transcripts. The topics of interest in DNA-based therapeutics include correction of genetic defects (e.g. to correct specific mutations), antisense therapeutics, aptamers (small RNAs), RNA interference using small interfering RNAs and microRNAs. The use of antisense oligonucleotides as therapeutic agents is currently the most advanced.[339–342] The interest in antisense was based on the discovery that antisense transcripts (non-coding) can regulate the expression of their partner sense transcripts (conventional protein-coding genes). The theory of antisense inhibition is that the synthetic DNA will hybridise to a gene or the messenger RNA carrying the information from that gene, and block the reading of that genetic information. In this way, the expression of the target protein thought to be critical to the disease in question is blocked, leaving other uninvolved proteins and cellular processes untouched. Unlike most current therapeutic approaches, the cellular target of the antisense drug is a nucleic acid that codes for a protein of interest, rather than the protein itself. Most of the current work on antisense therapeutics is directed towards cancer treatments by selectively modulating the expression of genes involved in the pathogenesis of malignancies. A variety of genes known to be key regulators of apoptosis, cell growth, metastasis and angiogenesis which are associated with the malignant phenotype of cancer cells rather than with normal cell physiology (e.g. Bcl-2, protein kinase C-α, c-raf or Ha-ras), have been validated as molecular targets for antisense therapy.

A large number of natural antisense transcripts (RNAs containing sequences that are complementary to other endogenous RNAs) have been found and some of these transcripts have been shown to regulate gene expression. It is therefore possible that antisense transcription might be a common mechanism of regulating gene expression in human cells, including genomic imprinting, RNA interference, translational regulation, alternative splicing, X-inactivation and RNA editing. Three general mechanisms by which antisense transcription can regulate gene expression have been suggested: transcriptional interference, RNA masking and double-stranded RNA-dependent mechanisms. There is growing evidence to suggest that antisense transcription might have a key role in a range of human diseases, including viral infections, cardiovascular, haematological and inflammatory disorders and cancer. Changes in antisense transcription can lead to abnormal patterns of gene expression, which in turn contribute to pathological phenotypes. Some examples of antisense transcripts that are implicated in human disease are already known but others remain to be identified.

Antisense oligonucleotides are short synthetic DNA molecules (usually 18–20 nucleotides in length) designed to bind strongly and specifically to complementary nucleic acids inside the cells of target tissues. Like other therapeutic products, antisense therapeutic agents also have several drawbacks. For example, oligodeoxynucleotides are vulnerable to nucleases in the serum and are rapidly degraded *in vivo*. Other issues include problems of cell penetration, non-specific binding, pharmacokinetics and toxicity. The 'first-generation' modified antisense molecules were phosphorothioate oligodeoxynucleotides (one

non-bridging oxygen atom is replaced with sulphur; nuclease resistant), the most frequently used oligonucleotide modification at present, but later modifications included modifications of the sugar residues, phosphodiester linkage or complete modification of the sugar phosphate backbone, including peptide nucleic acids (sugar-phosphate backbone replaced with N-(2-aminoethyl) glycine units). Most are extremely resistant to degradation and form tighter complexes with the target RNA or DNA than do unmodified or phosphorothioate oligodeoxynucleotides. However, first generation oligonucleotides have shown a variety of potentially toxic non-antisense effects, including complement activation, thrombocytopenia, inhibition of cell–matrix interaction and reduction of cell proliferation.

The first FDA-approved oligonucleotide-based drug, Vitravene (fomivirsen sodium), is a phosphorothioate oligodeoxynucleotide. It is licensed for the treatment of cytomegalovirus-induced retinitis (intraocular injection). However, uptake of phosphorothioate oligodeoxynucleotides by living cells is as poor as that of unmodified oligodeoxynucleotides. In addition, the complexes between phosphorothioate oligodeoxynucleotide and mRNA are less stable compared with those between the corresponding phosphodiester oligonucleotide and RNA. The main advantage of phosphorothioate oligodeoxynucleotides is that they are more stable to endo- and exonuclease cleavage than phosphodiesters. While phosphorothioate oligodeoxynucleotides have been shown to inhibit gene expression *in vitro* and *in vivo* in an antisense sequence-specific manner, they can also produce 'non-antisense' effects by enhanced binding to other proteins and stimulating mammalian immune system. It is this non-specific protein binding that is responsible for many of the 'non-antisense' effects associated with phosphorothioate oligodeoxynucleotides.

Rapid progress is also being made on aptamer (selected nucleic acid binding species with affinities and specificities for protein targets) therapeutics. Aptamers have definite advantages over antibodies in that they can be chemically synthesized and modifications can be introduced that improve their stabilities and pharmacokinetic properties.[343] In general, aptamers have proven to have high affinities (picomolar to nanomolar dissociation constants) for their cognate targets and specificities that are comparable to those of monoclonal antibodies. Work is ongoing to develop delivery methods for nucleic acid derivatives and chemical modifications that improve aptamer stability and efficacy. To date, the most successful therapeutic application of an aptamer has been the discovery of an antivascular endothelial growth factor (anti-VEGF) aptamer (Macugen) for the treatment of age-related macular degeneration. VEGF 165 participates in promoting the growth of abnormal new blood vessels in the eyes, which eventually leak blood and cause vision loss. The aptamer can be directly injected into the vitreous cavity (avoiding delivery problems) and it functions by binding to VEGF 165 and concomitantly inhibiting binding to its receptor. In clinical trials, more than 80% of patients who received the aptamer showed stable or improved vision 3 months after the treatment.

RNA interference, guided by small RNAs that include small interfering RNAs and microRNAs (derived from imperfectly paired non-coding hairpin RNA structures that are naturally transcribed by the genome), is another area of active interest for the discovery of medicines. This highly specific mechanism of sequence-specific gene silencing might result in drugs that interfere with disease-causing or disease-promoting genes.[344] The sequence-specific degradation of messenger RNA is elicited by the base pairing of complementary RNA strands, each approximately 22 nucleotides in length. These molecular complexes, which are termed small interfering RNA (siRNA) duplexes, are generated in the cytoplasm, either through the cleavage of endogenous long double-stranded RNA or from synthetic short hairpin RNA (shRNA). The production of the synthetic shRNA from gene-therapy vectors (either viral or non-viral) is an efficient means of experimentally eliciting RNAi *in vivo*.[345] A related endogenous pathway, involving microRNA (miRNA), also exists in mammalian cells. Hundreds of discrete regions within the genome encode atypical genes that give rise to miRNA. Although they are transcribed by RNA polymerase II, the enzyme that typically produces mRNA destined for translation into proteins, these atypical genes do not encode a protein. Instead, they produce RNA species that regulate the translation of other proteins.[346,347] Most endogenous miRNA functions as a sophisticated conductor of genetic pathways by manipulating the translational regulation of many genes at the same time. The specificity of this manipulation is relatively low, because target RNA species contain sequences that are only roughly related to the complementary miRNA sequence. Bioinformatics analyses suggest that up to 30% of human genes may be regulated by miRNA. In brief, RNAi and miRNA both result in decreased levels of functional protein within cells, but RNAi tends to affect steady-state mRNA levels, whereas miRNA usually affects the efficiency with which mRNA is translated into protein.

1.11 Conclusions

Drug discovery has been a continuously changing and evolving field of science over the years as a result of changing disease patterns, drug requirements and new targets and technologies.[348] More and more effective and safer treatments have been discovered. Although chemical and biological sciences have always played a major part in the discovery process, new scientific developments and technologies are altering the ways in which these sciences are applied to the discovery process. Advances in rapid DNA sequencing techniques have resulted in the discovery of the human genome sequence. Finding the disease-related genes, translating the gene sequences into biologically active proteins and evaluating their functions is likely to lead to new drug discovery targets based on new biochemical pathways. The genomic and proteomic studies may also lead to new therapeutic proteins and antibodies. Given the therapeutic success of the interferons, erythropoietin, granulocyte–macrophage colony stimulating factor, Herceptin (trastuzumab), rituximab and many others, protein drugs are likely to make many additional therapeutic contributions.

Combinatorial library techniques and natural product libraries are providing large numbers of new compounds for screening. Automated high-throughput screening techniques are being developed continuously to test large numbers of available compounds in multiple screens. A combination of these two technologies along with the discovery of new target proteins (e.g. receptors, enzymes) has the potential to generate leads for various drug discovery programmes. However, before the leads can be taken seriously, it is essential to appropriately validate the target. Otherwise, the optimised leads are likely to fail in the later stages of development. In many cases where some treatments exist along with some knowledge about the causes of the disease, the need for the target validation and development of the relevant biological models is less stringent. The discovery of new medicines in these fields becomes a continuous process of identifying medicines which are more efficacious and convenient to administer in a larger number of patients and display the best possible toxicity profile.

The availability of leads along with advances in multiple parallel solid phase synthetic and purification techniques would enable the lead optimisation procedure to be carried out in a relatively short period of time. The design strategies for the lead optimisation are likely to be a combination of the types of approaches highlighted in the examples mentioned above. Structure-activity studies along with structural and modelling studies using cloned proteins (e.g. receptors, enzymes) are likely to make the lead optimisation procedure somewhat more rational. Availability of cloned receptor subtypes and various members of the enzyme classes in the early stages of the programme can be used to build selectivity in the receptor ligands and enzyme inhibitors. Better understanding of the signalling processes will enable the cellular processes to be controlled in a more efficient manner.

References

1 Grundmann H, Aires-de-Sousa M, Boyce J et al. Emergence and resurgence of meticillin-resistant *Staphylococcus aureus* as a public-health threat. *Lancet* 2006;**368**:874–85.

2 Robicsek A, Jacoby GA, Hooper DC. The worldwide emergence of plasmid-mediated quinolone resistance. *Lancet Infec Dis* 2006;**6**:629–40.

3 Gerrits MM, van Vliet AHM, Kuipers EJ et al. *Helicobacter pylori* and antimicrobial resistance: molecular mechanisms and clinical implications. *Lancet Infect Dis* 2006;**6**:699–709.

4 The Writing Committee of the World Health Organization Consultation on Human Influenza A/H5. Avian influenza A (H5N1) infection in humans. *N Engl J Med* 2005;**353**:1374–85.

5 Shore SA, Johnston RA. Obesity and asthma. *Pharmacol Ther* 2006;**110**:83–102.

6 Shore SA. Obesity and asthma: cause for concern. *Curr Opinion Pharmacol* 2006;**6**:230–6.

7 Sivalingam S, Hashim H, Schwaibold H. An overview of the diagnosis and treatment of erectile dysfunction. *Drugs* 2006;**66**:2339–55.

8 Flower R. Lifestyle drugs: pharmacology and the social agenda. *Trends Pharmacol Sci* 2004;**25**:182–5.

9 Fourcroy J. Designer steroids: past, present and future. *Curr Opin Endocrinol Diabetes* 2006;**13**:306–9.

10 Thirthalli J, Benegal V. Psychosis among substance users. *Curr Opin Psychiatry* 2006;**19**:239–45.

11 van den Bosch LMC, Verheul R. Patients with addiction and personality disorder: treatment outcomes and clinical implications. *Curr Opin Psychiatry* 2007;**20**:67–71.

12 Fiellin DA, Pantalon MV, Chawarski MC et al. Counseling plus buprenorphine–naloxone maintenance therapy for opioid dependence. *N Engl J Med* 2006;**355**:365–74.

13 Moss M, Burnham EL. Alcohol abuse in the critically ill patient. *Lancet* 2007;**368**:2231–42.

14 Goldstein BI, Diamantouros, SAA, Naranjo CA. Pharmacotherapy of alcoholism in patients with co-morbid psychiatric disorders. *Drugs* 2006;**66**:1229–37.

15 Heilig M, Egli M. Pharmacological treatment of alcohol dependence: target symptoms and target mechanisms. *Pharmacol Ther* 2006;**111**:855–76.

16 Ashley EA, White NJ. Artemisinin-based combinations. *Curr Opin Infect Dis* 2005;**18**:531–6.

17 Franco-Paredes C, Santos-Preciado JI. Problem pathogens: prevention of malaria in travellers. *Lancet Infect Dis* 2006;**6**:139–49.

18 Matuschewski K. Vaccine development against malaria. *Curr Opin Immunol* 2006;**18**:449–57.

19 Mdluli K, Spigelman M. Novel targets for tuberculosis drug discovery. *Curr Opin Pharmacol* 2006;**6**:459–67.

20 Spigelman M, Gillespie S. Tuberculosis drug development pipeline: progress and hope. *Lancet* 2006;**367**:945–7.

21 de Souza MVN. Current status and future prospects for new therapies for pulmonary tuberculosis. *Curr Opin Pulm Med* 2006;**12**:167–71.

22 Zhang Y, Post-Martens K, Denkin S. New drug candidates and therapeutic targets for tuberculosis therapy. *Drug Discov Today* 2006;**11**:21–7.

23 Martin C. Tuberculosis vaccines: past, present and future. *Curr Opin Pulm Med* 2006;**12**:186–91.

24 Felson DT. Osteoarthritis of the knee. *N Engl J Med* 2006;**354**:841–8.

25 Henry G, Hosking D, Devogelaer J-P et al. Ten years' experience with alendronate for osteoporosis in post-menopausal women. *N Engl J Med* 2004;**350**:1189–99.

26 Cochrane DJ, Jarvis B, Keating GM. Etoricoxib. *Drugs* 2002;**62**:2637–61.

27 Fenton C, Keating GM, Wagstaff AJ. Valdecoxib. *Drugs* 2004;**64**:1231–61.

28 Ardoin SP, Sundy JS. Update on non-steriodal anti-inflammatory drugs. *Curr Opin Rheumatol* 2006;**18**:221–6.

29 Stichtenoth DO, Frolich JC. The second generation of COX-2 inhibitors: what advantage do the newest offer? *Drugs* 2003;**63**:33–45.

30 Kurumbail RG, Kiefer JR, Marnett LJ. Cyclooxygenase enzymes: catalysis and inhibition. *Curr Opin Struct Biol* 2001;**11**:752–60.

31 Graul AI, Prous JR. Overcoming the challenges in the Pharma/Biotech industry. *Drug News Perspect* 2007;**20**:57–72.

32 Dutta AS. Discovery of new medicines. In: Griffin JP, O'Grady J, eds. *Textbook of Pharmaceutical Medicine*, 5th edn. Oxford: BMJ Books, Blackwell Publishing, 2006;3–86.

33 Drews J. Drug discovery: a historical perspective. *Science* 2000;**287**:1960–4.

34 Olbe L, Carlsson E, Lindberg P. A proton-pump inhibitor expedition: the case histories of omeprazole and esomeprazole. *Nat Rev Drug Discov* 2003;**2**:132–9.

35 Clader JW. The discovery of ezetimibe: a view from outside the receptor. *J Med Chem* 2004;47:1–9.

36 Varghese JN. Development of neuraminidase inhibitors as anti-influenza virus drugs. *Drug Dev Res* 1999;46:176–96.

37 Masuda S, Inui K. An up-date review on individualized dosage adjustment of calcineurin inhibitors in organ transplant patients. *Pharmacol Ther* 2006;112;184–98.

38 Dunn C, Croom KF. Everolimus: a review of its use in renal and cardiac transplantation. *Drugs* 2006;66:547–70.

39 Schmid EF, Smith DA. R&D technology investments: misguided and expensive or a better way to discover medicines? *Drug Discov Today* 2006;11:775–84.

40 Federsel H-J. In search of sustainability: process R&D in light of current pharmaceutical industry challenges. *Drug Discov Today* 2006;11:966–74.

41 Coulie B, De Decker N, Maes V et al. Design and implementation of an activity-based costing system in a pharmaceutical drug discovery environment. *Drug Dev Res* 2006;67:107–18.

42 Graul AI, Prous JR. The year's new drugs. *Drug News Perspect* 2006;19:33–53.

43 Groul AI, Sorbera LA, Bozzo J et al. The year's new drugs and biologics – 2006. *Drug News Perspect* 2007;20:17–44.

44 Graul AI, Prous JR, Barrionuevo M et al. The year's new drugs and biologics – 2007. *Drug News Perspect* 2008;21:7–35.

45 Prous JR, Khurdayan VK. The story so far in R&D. *Drug News Perspect* 2007;20:7–15.

46 Robinson DM, Keating GM. Albumin-bound paclitaxel: in metastatic breast cancer. *Drugs* 2006;66:941–8.

47 Zimmermann GR, Lehár J, Keith CT. Multi-target therapeutics: when the whole is greater than the sum of the parts. *Drug Discov Today* 2007;12:34–42.

48 Koehn FE. Therapeutic potential of natural product signal transduction agents. *Curr Opin Biotechnol* 2006;17:631–7.

49 Lam KS. Discovery of novel metabolites from marine actinomycetes. *Curr Opin Microbiol* 2006;9:245–51.

50 George SR, O'Dowd BF, Lee SP. G-protein-coupled receptor oligomerization and its potential for drug discovery. *Nat Rev Drug Discov* 2002;1:808–20.

51 Dorsam RT, Gutkind JS. G-protein-coupled receptors and cancer. *Nat Rev Cancer* 2007;7:79–94.

52 Langmead CJ, Christopoulos A. Allosteric agonists of 7TM receptors: expanding the pharmacological toolbox. *Trends Pharmacol Sci* 2006;27:475–81.

53 Gao Z-G, Jacobson KA. Allosterism in membrane receptors. *Drug Discov Today* 2006;11:191–202.

54 Yasuda K, Matsunaga T, Adachi T et al. Adrenergic receptor polymorphisms and autonomic nervous system function in human obesity. *Trends Endocrinol Metab* 2006;17:269–75.

55 Tobin JF, Freedman LP. Nuclear receptors as drug targets in metabolic diseases: new approaches to therapy. *Trends Endocrinol Metab* 2006;17:284–90.

56 Barros RPA, Machado UF, Gustafsson J-A. Estrogen receptors: new players in diabetes mellitus. *Trends Mol Med* 2006;12:425–31.

57 Hoyer D, Clarke DE, Fozard JR et al. International union of pharmacology classification of receptors for 5-hydroxytryptamine (serotonin). *Pharmacol Rev* 1994;46:157–203.

58 Yanai K, Tashiro M. The physiological and pathophysiological roles of neuronal histamine: an insight from human positron emission tomography studies. *Pharmacol Ther* 2007;113:1–15.

59 Masaki T, Yoshimatsu H. The hypothalamic H_1 receptor: a novel therapeutic target for disrupting diurnal feeding rhythm and obesity. *Trends Pharmacol Sci* 2006;27:279–84.

60 Tanimoto A, Sasaguri Y, Ohtsu H. Histamine network in atherosclerosis. *Trends Cardiovasc Med* 2006;16:280–4.

61 Rozec B, Gauthier C. β_3-Adrenoceptors in the cardiovascular system: putative roles in human pathologies. *Pharmacol Ther* 2006;111:652–73.

62 Getting SJ. Targeting melanocortin receptors as potential novel therapeutics. *Pharmacol Ther* 2006;111:1–15.

63 Rohrer SP, Birzin ET, Mosley RT et al. Rapid identification of subtype-selective agonists of the somatostatin receptor through combinatorial chemistry. *Science* 1998;282:737–40.

64 Weckbecker G, Lewis I, Albert R et al. Opportunities in somatostatin research: biological, chemical and therapeutic aspects. *Nat Rev Drug Discov* 2003;2:999–1017.

65 Civelli O, Saito Y, Wang Z et al. Orphan GPCRs and their ligands. *Pharmacol Ther* 2006;110:525–32.

66 Cirino G, Vergnolle N. Proteinase-activated receptors (PARs): crossroads between innate immunity and coagulation. *Curr Opin Pharmacol* 2006;6:428–34.

67 Burgner D, Jamieson SE, Blackwell JM. Genetic susceptibility to infectious diseases: big is beautiful, but will bigger be even better? *Lancet Infect Dis* 2006;6:653–63.

68 Onengut-Gumuscu S, Concannon P. Recent advances in the immunogenetics of human type 1 diabetes. *Curr Opin Immunol* 2006;18:634–8.

69 McCormack MP, Rabbitts TH. Mechanisms of disease: activation of the T-cell oncogene LMO2 after gene therapy for X-linked severe combined immunodeficiency. *N Engl J Med* 2004;350:913–22.

70 Pack DW, Hoffman AS, Pun S et al. Design and development of polymers for gene delivery. *Nat Rev Drug Discov* 2005;4:581–93.

71 Quackenbush J. Microarray analysis and tumour classification. *N Engl J Med* 2006;354:2463–72.

72 Rigden DJ. Understanding the cell in terms of structure and function: insights from structural genomics. *Curr Opin Biotechnol* 2006;17:457–64.

73 Zheng C, Han L, Yap CW et al. Progress and problems in the exploration of therapeutic targets. *Drug Discov Today* 2006;11:412–20.

74 Ricke DO, Wang S, Cai R et al. Genomic approaches to drug discovery. *Curr Opin Chem Biol* 2006;10:303–8.

75 International Human Genome Sequencing Consortium. Initial sequencing and analysis of the human genome. *Nature* 2001;**409**:860–921.

76 The sequence of the human genome. *Science* 2001;**291**:1304–51.

77 Perna NT, Plunkett G III, Burland V et al. Genome sequence of enterohaemorrhagic *Escherichia coli* O157:H7. *Nature* 2001;**409**:529–33.

78 Pennisi E. Rat genome off to an early start. *Science* 2000;**289**:1267–69.

79 Prosser H, Rastan S. Manipulation of the mouse genome: a multiple impact resource for drug discovery and development. *Trends Biotechnol* 2003;**21**:224–32.

80 Karlin S, Mrázek J, Gentles AJ. Genome comparisons and analysis. *Curr Opin Struct Biol* 2003;**13**:344–52.

81 Kay MA, Glorioso JC, Naldini L. Viral vectors for gene therapy: the art of turning infectious agents into vehicles of therapeutics. *Nat Med* 2001;**7**:33–40.

82 McTaggart S, Al-Rubeai M. Retroviral vectors for human gene delivery. *Biotechnol Adv* 2002;**20**:1–31.

83 Zambrowicz BP, Turner CA, Sands AT. Predicting drug efficacy: knockouts model pipeline drugs of the pharmaceutical industry. *Curr Opin Pharmacol* 2003;**3**:563–70.

84 Zambrowicz BP, Sands AT. Knockouts model the 100 best-selling drugs: will they model the next 100? *Nat Rev Drug Discov* 2003;**2**:38–51.

85 Khurdayan VK. Stem cells: therapeutic present and future. *Drug News Perspect* 2007;**20**:119–28.

86 Huh WJ, Pan XO, Mysorekar IU et al. Location, allocation, relocation: isolating adult tissue stem cells in three dimensions. *Curr Opin Biotechnol* 2006;**17**:511–7.

87 Stainier D. No stem cell is an islet (yet). *N Engl J Med* 2006;**354**:521–3.

88 Roche E, Jones J, Arribas MI et al. Role of small bioorganic molecules in stem cell differentiation to insulin-producing cells. *Bioorg Med Chem* 2006;**14**:6466–74.

89 Copelan EA. Hematopoietic stem-cell transplantation. *N Engl J Med* 2006;**354**:1813–26.

90 Jordan CT, Guzman ML, Noble M. Cancer stem cells. *N Engl J Med* 2006;**355**:1253–61.

91 Brabletz T, Jung A, Spaderna S et al. Migrating cancer stem cells: an integrated concept of malignant tumour progression. *Nat Rev Cancer* 2005;**5**:744–9.

92 Vescovi AL, Galli R, Reynolds BA. Brain tumour stem cells. *Nat Rev Cancer* 2006;**6**:425–36.

93 Johnson JA. Pharmacogenetics: potential for individualized drug therapy through genetics. *Trends Genet* 2003;**19**:660–6.

94 McCarthy JM, Hilfiker R. The use of single-nucleotide polymorphism maps in pharmacogenomics. *Nat Biotechnol* 2000;**18**:505–8.

95 Suter L, Babiss LE, Wheeldon EB. Toxicogenomics in predictive toxicology in drug development. *Chem Biol* 2004;**11**:161–71.

96 Blackstock WP, Weir MP. Proteomics: quantitative and physical mapping of cellular proteins. *Trends Biotechnol* 1999;**17**:121–7.

97 Wang JH, Hewick RM. Proteomics in drug discovery. *Drug Discov Today* 1999;**4**:129–33.

98 Walgren JL, Thompson DC. Application of proteomic technologies in the drug development process. *Toxicol Lett* 2004;**149**:377–85.

99 Campbell SJ, Gold ND, Jackson RM et al. Ligand binding: functional site location, similarity and docking. *Curr Opin Struct Biol* 2003;**13**:389–95.

100 Kinoshita K, Nakamura H. Protein informatics towards function identification. *Curr Opin Struct Biol* 2003;**13**:396–400.

101 Mayer TU. Chemical genetics: tailoring tools for cell biology. *Trends Cell Biol* 2003;**13**:270–7.

102 Jeffery DA, Bogyo M. Chemical proteomics and its application to drug discovery. *Curr Opin Biotechnol* 2003;**14**:87–95.

103 Marcotte EM. Computational genetics: finding protein function by non-homology methods. *Curr Opin Struct Biol* 2000;**10**:359–65.

104 Qureshi EA, Cagney G. Large-scale functional analysis using peptide or protein arrays. *Nat Biotechnol* 2000;**18**:393–7.

105 Jones DT. Protein structure prediction in the postgenomic era. *Curr Opin Struct Biol* 2000;**10**:371–9.

106 Man O, Atarot T, Sadot A et al. From subgenome analysis to protein structure. *Curr Opin Struct Biol* 2003;**13**:353–8.

107 Sali A, Kuriyan J. Challenges at the frontiers of structural biology. *Trends Cell Biol* 2000;**9**:M20–4.

108 Jeffery CJ. Moonlighting proteins: old proteins learning new tricks. *Trends Genet* 2003;**19**:415–7.

109 Johnstone RW, Ruefli AA, Smyth MJ. Multiple physiological functions for multidrug transporter P-glycoprotein. *Trends Biochem Sci* 2000;**25**:1–6.

110 Andrade MA, Sander C. Bioinformatics: from genome data to biological knowledge, *Curr Opin Biotechnol* 1997;**8**:675–83.

111 Hergenrother PJ. Obtaining and screening compound collections: a user's guide and a call to chemists. *Curr Opin Chem Biol* 2006;**10**:213–8.

112 Rausch O. High content cellular screening. *Curr Opin Chem Biol* 2006;**10**:316–20.

113 Davies JW, Glick M, Jenkins JL. Streamlining lead discovery by aligning *in silico* and high-throughput screening. *Curr Opin Chem Biol* 2006;**10**:343–51.

114 Geysen HM, Schoenen WD, Wagner R. Combinatorial compound libraries for drug discovery: an ongoing challenge. *Nat Rev Drug Discov* 2003;**2**:222–30.

115 Irwin JJ. How good is your screening library? *Curr Opin Chem Biol* 2006;**10**:352–6.

116 Keller TH, Pichota A, Yin Z. A practical view of 'druggability'. *Curr Opin Chem Biol* 2006;**10**:357–61.

117 Hann MM, Oprea TI. Pursuing the leadlikeness concept in pharmaceutical research. *Curr Opin Chem Biol* 2004;**8**:255–63.

118 Michels PC, Khmelnitsky YL, Dordick JS et al. Combinatorial biocatalysis: a natural approach to drug discovery. *Trends Biotechnol* 1998;**16**:210–5.

119 Blackwell HE. Hitting the SPOT: small-molecule macroarrays advance combinatorial synthesis. *Curr Opin Chem Biol* 2006;10:203–12.

120 Backes BJ, Harris JL, Leonetti F et al. Synthesis of positional-scanning libraries of fluorogenic peptide substrates to define the extended substrate specificity of plasmin and thrombin. *Nat Biotechnol* 2000;18:187–93.

121 Legraverend M, Grierson DS. The purines: potent and versatile small molecule inhibitors and modulators of key biological targets. *Bioorg Med Chem* 2006;14:3987–4006.

122 Walters WP, Ajay, Murcko MA. Recognising molecules with drug-like properties. *Curr Opin Chem Biol* 1999;3:384–7.

123 Lipinski CA, Lombardo F, Dominy BW et al. Experimental and computational approaches to estimate solubility and permeability in drug discovery and development settings. *Adv Drug Deliv Rev* 1997;23:3–25.

124 Rishton GM. Reactive compounds and *in vitro* false positives in HTS. *Drug Discov Today* 1997;2:382–5.

125 Golebiowski A, Klopfenstein SR, Portlock DE. Lead compounds discovered from libraries. *Curr Opin Chem Biol* 2001;5:273–84.

126 Golebiowski A, Klopfenstein SR, Portlock DE. Lead compounds discovered from libraries: Part 2. *Curr Opin Chem Biol* 2003;7:308–25.

127 Ooms F. Molecular modelling and computer aided drug design: examples of their application in medicinal chemistry. *Curr Med Chem* 2000;7:141–58.

128 Erlanson DA, McDowell RS, O'Brien T. Fragment-based drug discovery. *J Med Chem* 2004;47:3463–82.

129 Klebe G. Virtual ligand screening: strategies, perspectives and limitations. *Drug Discov Today* 2006;11:580–94.

130 Ghosh S, Nie A, An J et al. Structure-based virtual screening of chemical libraries for drug discovery. *Curr Opin Chem Biol* 2006;10:194–202.

131 Homans SW. NMR spectroscopy tools for structure-aided drug design. *Angew Chem Int Ed Engl* 2004;43:290–300.

132 Kuhn P, Wilson K, Patch MG at al. The genesis of high-throughput structure-based drug discovery using protein crystallography. *Curr Opin Chem Biol* 2002;6:704–10.

133 Erlanson DA. Fragment-based lead discovery: a chemical update. *Curr Opin Biotechnol* 2006;17:643–52.

134 Rupasinghe CN, Spaller MR. The interplay between structure-based design and combinatorial chemistry. *Curr Opin Chem Biol* 2006;10:188–93.

135 Shuker SB, Hajduk PJ, Meadows RP et al. Discovering high affinity ligands for proteins: SAR by NMR. *Science* 1996;274:1531–4.

136 Fejzo J, Lepre CA, Peng JW et al. The SHAPES strategy: an NMR-based approach for lead generation in drug discovery. *Chem Biol* 1999;6:755–69.

137 Nienaber VL, Richardson PL, Klighofer V et al. Discovering novel ligands for macromolecules using X-ray crystallographic screening. *Nat Biotechnol* 2000;18:1105–9.

138 Eddershaw PJ, Beresford AP, Bayliss MK. ADME/PK as part of a rational approach to drug discovery. *Drug Discov Today* 2000;5:409–14.

139 Kassel DB. Applications of high-throughput ADME in drug discovery. *Curr Opin Chem Biol* 2004;8:339–45.

140 de Groot MJ. Designing better drugs: predicting cytochrome P450 metabolism. *Drug Discov Today* 2006;11:601–6.

141 Lee M-Y, Dordick JS. High-throughput human metabolism and toxicity analysis. *Curr Opin Biotechnol* 2006;17:619–27.

142 Suter W. Predictive value of *in vitro* safety studies. *Curr Opin Chem Biol* 2006;10:362–6.

143 Navarro VJ, Senior JR. Drug-related hepatotoxicity. *N Engl J Med* 2006;354:731–9.

144 Iglehart JK. The new era of medical imaging: progress and pitfalls. *N Engl J Med* 2006;354:2822–8.

145 Gross S, Piwnica-Worms D. Molecular imaging strategies for drug discovery and development. *Curr Opin Chem Biol* 2006;10:334–42.

146 Corti R. Non-invasive imaging of atherosclerotic vessels by MRI for clinical assessment of the effectiveness of therapy. *Pharmacol Ther* 2006;110:57–70.

147 Isbell DC, Kramer CM. Magnetic resonance for the assessment of myocardial viability. *Curr Opin Cardiol* 2006;21:469–72.

148 Kwock L, Smith JK, Castillo M et al. Clinical role of proton magnetic resonance spectroscopy in oncology: brain, breast, and prostate cancer. *Lancet Oncol* 2006;7:859–68.

149 Honey G, Bullmore E. Human pharmacological MRI. *Trends Pharmacol Sci* 2004;25:366–74.

150 Sawada SG. Positron emission tomography for assessment of viability. *Curr Opin Cardiol* 2006;21:464–8.

151 Malik E, Juweid M, Cheson BD. Positron-emission tomography and assessment of cancer therapy. *N Engl J Med* 2006;354:496–507.

152 Lee C-M, Farde L. Using positron emission tomography to facilitate CNS drug development. *Trends Pharmacol Sci* 2006;27:310–6.

153 Dawson LA, Sharpe MB. Image-guided radiotherapy: rationale, benefits, and limitations. *Lancet Oncol* 2006;7:848–58.

154 Dutta AS. *Small Peptides: Chemistry, Biology and Clinical Studies.* Elsevier Science Publishers, 1993.

155 Dutta AS. Design and therapeutic potential of peptides. *Adv Drug Res* 1991;21:145–286.

156 Jordan VC. Chemoprevention of breast cancer with selective oestrogen-receptor modulators. *Nat Rev Cancer* 2007;7:46–53.

157 Jordan VC. Tamoxifen: a most unlikely pioneering medicine. *Nat Rev Drug Discov* 2003;2:205–13.

158 Barrett-Connor E, Mosca L, Collins P et al. Effects of raloxifene on cardiovascular events and breast cancer in postmenopausal women. *N Engl J Med* 2006;355:125–37.

159 Johnston SRD, Dowsett M. Aromatase inhibitors for breast cancer: lessons from the laboratory. *Nat Rev Cancer* 2003;3:821–31.

160 Dutta AS. Luteinizing hormone-releasing hormone (LHRH) agonists. *Drugs Future* 1988;13:43–57.

161 Dutta AS. Luteinizing hormone-releasing hormone (LHRH) antagonists. *Drugs Future* 1988;13:761–87.

162 Dutta AS, Furr BJA, Hutchinson FG. The discovery and development of goserelin (Zoladex). *Pharm Med* 1993;7:9–28.

163 Dutta AS. Goserelin. *Drugs Today (Barc)* 1987;23:545–51.

164 Culler MD. Evolving concepts in the quest for advanced therapeutic analogues of somatostatin. *Dig Liver Dis* 2004;36(Suppl 1):S17–25.

165 Dasgupta P. Somatostatin analogues: multiple roles in cellular proliferation, neoplasia, and angiogenesis. *Pharmacol Ther* 2004;102:61–85

166 Lamberts SWJ, van der Lely A-J, de Herder WW et al. Drug therapy: octreotide. *N Engl J Med* 1996;334:246–54.

167 Zaman MA, Oparil S, Calhoun DA. Drugs targeting the renin–angiotensin–aldosterone system. *Nat Rev Drug Discov* 2002;1:621–36.

168 Oro C, Qian H, Thomas WG. Type 1 angiotensin receptor pharmacology: signaling beyond G proteins. *Pharmacol Ther* 2007;113:210–26.

169 Moody TW, Jensen RT. Bombesin receptor antagonists. *Drugs Future* 1998;23:1305–15.

170 Meini S, Cucchi P, Bellucci F et al. Site-directed mutagenesis at the human B_2 receptor and molecular modelling to define the pharmacophore of non-peptide bradykinin receptor antagonists. *Biochem Pharmacol* 2004;67:601–9.

171 Sawada Y, Kayakiri H, Abe Y et al. A new class of nonpeptide bradykinin B2 receptor ligands, incorporating a 4-aminoquinoline framework: identification of a key pharmacophore to determine species difference and agonist/antagonist profile. *J Med Chem* 2004;47:2667–77.

172 Herranz R. Cholecystokinin antagonists: pharmacological and therapeutic potential. *Med Res Rev* 2003;23:559–605.

173 Masaki T. Historical review: endothelin. *Trends Pharmacol Sci* 2004;25:219–24.

174 Ertl G. Endothelin receptor antagonists in heart failure. *Drugs* 2004;64:1029–40.

175 Motte S, McEntee K, Naeije R. Endothelin receptor antagonists. *Pharmacol Ther* 2006;110:386–414.

176 Alpdogan O, van den Brink MRM. IL-7 and IL-15: therapeutic cytokines for immunodeficiency. *Trends Immunol* 2005;15:241–50.

177 Bradley LM, Haynes L, Swain SL. IL-7: maintaining T-cell memory and achieving homeostasis. *Trends Immunol* 2005;26:172–6.

178 Gupta P, Su Z-zhong, Lebedeva IV et al. *mda-7*/IL-24: Multifunctional cancer-specific apoptosis-inducing cytokine. *Pharmacol Ther* 2006;111:596–628.

179 Mege J-L, Meghari S, Honstettre A et al. The two faces of interleukin 10 in human infectious diseases. *Lancet Infect Dis* 2006;6:557–69.

180 Cooper AM, Khader SA. IL-12p40: an inherently agonistic cytokine. *Trends Immunol* 2007;28:33–8.

181 Wells AF. Anticytokine therapies in rheumatoid arthritis: from the pipette to the patient. *Drug Discov Today Ther Strateg* 2004;1:293–7.

182 Norihiro N. Interleukin-6 in rheumatoid arthritis. *Curr Opin Rheumatol* 2006;18:277–81.

183 Raison CL, Capuron L, Miller AH. Cytokines sing the blues: inflammation and the pathogenesis of depression. *Trends Immunol* 2006;27:24–31.

184 Imitola J, Chitnis T, Khoury SJ. Cytokines in multiple sclerosis: from bench to bedside. *Pharmacol Ther* 2005;106:163–77.

185 Felderhoff-Mueser U, Schmidt OI, Oberholzer A et al. IL-18: a key player in neuroinflammation and neurodegeneration? *Trends Neurosci* 2005;28:487–93.

186 Tang J, Raines EW. Are suppressors of cytokine signaling proteins recently identified in atherosclerosis possible therapeutic targets? *Trends Cardiovasc Med* 2005;15:243–9.

187 Wells TNC, Power CA, Shaw JP et al. Chemokine blockers: therapeutics in the making? *Trends Pharmacol Sci* 2006;27:41–7.

188 Johnson Z, Schwarz M, Power CA et al. Multi-faceted strategies to combat disease by interference with the chemokine system. *Trends Immunol* 2005;26:268–74.

189 Ribeiro S, Horuk R. The clinical potential of chemokine receptor antagonists. *Pharmacol Ther* 2005;107:44–58.

190 Bisset LR, Schmid-Grendelmeier P. Chemokines and their receptors in the pathogenesis of allergic asthma: progress and perspective. *Curr Opin Pulm Med* 2005;11:35–42.

191 Donnelly LE, Barnes PJ. Chemokine receptors as therapeutic targets in chronic obstructive pulmonary disease. *Trends Pharmacol Sci* 2006;27:546–53.

192 Verri WA Jr, Cunha TM, Parada CA et al. Hypernociceptive role of cytokines and chemokines: targets for analgesic drug development? *Pharmacol Ther* 2006;112:116–38.

193 Abbadie C. Chemokines, chemokine receptors and pain. *Trends Immunol* 2005;26:529–34.

194 Ubogu EE, Cossoy MB, Ransohoff RM. The expression and function of chemokines involved in CNS inflammation. *Trends Pharmacol Sci* 2006;27:48–55.

195 Viola A, Contento RL, Molon B. T cells and their partners: the chemokine dating agency. *Trends Immunol* 2006;27:421–7.

196 Frangogiannis NG, Entman ML. Chemokines in myocardial ischemia. *Trends Cardiovasc Med* 2005;15:163–9.

197 Bizzarri C, Beccari AR, Bertini R et al. ELR+ CXC chemokines and their receptors (CXC chemokine receptor 1 and CXC chemokine receptor 2) as new therapeutic targets. *Pharmacol Ther* 2006;112:139–49.

198 Price DA, Armour D, de Groot M et al. Overcoming HERG affinity in the discovery of the CCR5 antagonist maraviroc. *Bioorg Med Chem Lett* 2006;16:4633–7.

199 Lim JK, Glass WG, McDermott DH et al. CCR5: no longer a 'good for nothing' gene–chemokine control of West Nile virus infection. *Trends Immunol* 2006;27:308–12.

200 Vellard M. The enzyme as drug: application of enzymes as pharmaceuticals. *Curr Opin Biotechnol* 2003;14:444–50.

201 Schellinger PD, Kaste M, Hacke W. An update on thrombolytic therapy for acute stroke. *Curr Opin Neurol* 2004;**17**:69–77.

202 Banerjee A, Chisti Y, Banerjee UC. Streptokinase: a clinically useful thrombolytic agent. *Biotechnol Adv* 2004;**22**:287–307.

203 Acharya KR, Sturrock ED, Riordan JF et al. ACE revisited: a new target for structure-based drug design. *Nat Rev Drug Discov* 2003;**2**:891–902.

204 Burrell LM, Johnston CI, Tikellis C et al. ACE2, a new regulator of the renin–angiotensin system. *Trends Endocrinol Metabol* 2004;**15**:166–9.

205 Abassi Z, Karram T, Ellaham S et al. Implications of the natriuretic peptide system in the pathogenesis of heart failure: diagnostic and therapeutic importance. *Pharmacol Ther* 2004;**102**:223–41.

206 Tabrizchi R. Dual ACE and neutral endopeptidase inhibitors. *Drugs* 2003;**63**:2185–202.

207 Heath EI, Grochow LB. Clinical potential of matrix metalloprotease inhibitors in cancer therapy. *Drugs* 2000;**59**:1043–55.

208 Martel-Pelletier J, Welsch DJ, Pelletier J-P. Metalloproteases and inhibitors in arthritic diseases. *Best Pract Res Clin Rheumatol* 2001;**15**:805–29.

209 Bigg HF, Rowan AD. The inhibition of metalloproteinases as a therapeutic target in rheumatoid arthritis and osteoarthritis. *Curr Opin Pharmacol* 2001;**1**:314–20.

210 Hu J, Van den Steen PE, Sang Q-XA et al. Matrix metalloproteinase inhibitors as therapy for inflammatory and vascular diseases. *Nat Rev Drug Discov* 2007;**6**:480–98.

211 White RJ, Margolis PS, Trias J et al. Targeting metalloenzymes: a strategy that works. *Curr Opin Pharmacol* 2003;**3**:502–7.

212 Staessen JA, Li Y, Richart T. Oral renin inhibitors. *Lancet* 2006;**368**:1449–56.

213 Goldsmith DR, Perry CM. Atazanavir. *Drugs* 2003;**63**:1679–93.

214 Desai UR. New antithrombin-based anticoagulants. *Med Res Rev* 2003;**24**:151–81.

215 Bates SM, Ginsberg JS. Treatment of deep-vein thrombosis. *N Engl J Med* 2004;**351**:268–77.

216 Reiffel JA. Will direct thrombin inhibitors replace warfarin for preventing embolic events in atrial fibrillation? *Curr Opin Cardiol* 2004;**19**:58–63.

217 Bell IM. Inhibitors of farnesyltransferase: a rational approach to cancer chemotherapy? *J Med Chem* 2004;**47**:1869–78.

218 Grandis JR, Sok JC. Signaling through the epidermal growth factor receptor during the development of malignancy. *Pharmacol Ther* 2004;**102**:37–46.

219 Levitzki A. PDGF receptor kinase inhibitors for the treatment of PDGF driven diseases. *Cytokine Growth Factor Rev* 2004;**15**:229–35.

220 Cross MJ, Dixelius J, Matsumoto T et al. VEGF-receptor signal transduction. *Trends Biochem Sci* 2003;**28**:488–94.

221 Khurana R, Simons M. Insights from angiogenesis trials using fibroblast growth factor for advanced arteriosclerotic disease. *Trends Cardiovasc Med* 2003;**13**:116–22.

222 Olson JM, Hallahan AR. p38 MAP kinase: a convergence point in cancer therapy. *Trends Mol Med* 2004;**10**:125–9.

223 Bogoyevitch MA, Boehm I, Oakley A et al. Targeting the JNK MAPK cascade for inhibition: basic science and therapeutic potential. *Biochim Biophys Acta* 2004;**1697**:89–101.

224 Cruz JC, Tsai L-H. Cdk5 deregulation in the pathogenesis of Alzheimer's disease. *Trends Mol Med* 2004;**10**:452–8.

225 Smith PD, O'Hare MJ, Park DS. CDKs: taking on a role as mediators of dopaminergic loss in Parkinson's disease. *Trends Mol Med* 2004;**10**:445–51.

226 Dai Y, Grant S. Cyclin-dependent kinase inhibitors. *Curr Opin Pharmacol* 2003;**3**:362–70.

227 Goedert M, Cohen P. GSK3 inhibitors: development and therapeutic potential. *Nat Rev Drug Discov* 2004;**3**:479–87.

228 Meijer L, Flajolet M, Greengard P. Pharmacological inhibitors of glycogen synthase kinase 3. *Trends Pharmacol Sci* 2004;**25**:471–80.

229 Bose R, Holbert MA, Pickin KA et al. Protein tyrosine kinase–substrate interactions. *Curr Opin Struct Biol* 2006;**16**:668–75.

230 Gold MG, Barford D, Komander D. Lining the pockets of kinases and phosphatases. *Curr Opin Struc Biol* 2006;**16**:693–701.

231 Matthews SA, Cantrell DA. The role of serine/threonine kinases in T-cell activation. *Curr Opin Immunol* 2006;**18**:314–20.

232 Mayer RJ, Callahan JF. p38 MAP kinase inhibitors: a future therapy for inflammatory diseases. *Drug Disc Today Ther Strateg* 2006;**3**:49–54.

233 McLean GW, Carragher NO, Avizienyte E et al. The role of focal-adhesion kinase in cancer: a new therapeutic opportunity. *Nat Rev Cancer* 2005;**5**:505–15.

234 Strebhardt K, Ullrich A. Targeting polo-like kinase 1 for cancer therapy. *Nat Rev Cancer* 2006;**6**:321–30.

235 Kumar R, Gururaj AE, Barnes CJ. p21-activated kinases in cancer. *Nat Rev Cancer* 2006;**6**:459–71.

236 Bader AG, Kang S, Zhao L et al. Oncogenic PI3K deregulates transcription and translation. *Nat Rev Cancer* 2005;**5**:921–9.

237 Patel JD, Pasche B, Argiris A. Targeting non-small cell lung cancer with epidermal growth factor tyrosine kinase inhibitors: where do we stand, where do we go. *Crit Rev Oncol Hematol* 2004;**50**:175–86.

238 de Castro G Jr, Awada A. Side effects of anti-cancer molecular-targeted therapies (not monoclonal antibodies). *Curr Opin Oncol* 2006;**18**:307–15.

239 Lacouture ME. Mechanisms of cutaneous toxicities to EGFR inhibitors. *Nat Rev Cancer* 2006;**6**:803–12.

240 Blackhall F, Ranson M, Thatcher N. Where next for gefitinib in patients with lung cancer? *Lancet Oncol* 2006;**7**:499–507.

241 Jabbour E, Cortes, J, Kantarjian H. Novel tyrosine kinase inhibitors in chronic myelogenous leukaemia. *Curr Opin Oncol* 2006;18:578–83.

242 Kantarjian H, Giles F, Wunderle L et al. Nilotinib in imatinib-resistant CML and Philadelphia chromosome-positive ALL. *N Engl J Med* 2006;354:2542–51.

243 Talpaz M, Shah NP, Kantarjian H et al. Dasatinib in imatinib-resistant Philadelphia chromosome-positive leukemias. *N Engl J Med* 2006;354:2531–41.

244 Hahn O, Stadler W. Sorafenib. *Curr Opin Oncol* 2006;18:615–21.

245 Deeks ED, Keating GM. Sunitinib. *Drugs* 2006;66:2255–66.

246 Moy B, Kirkpatrick P, Kar S et al. Lapatinib. *Nat Rev Drug Discov* 2007;6:431–2.

247 Ostman A, Hellberg C, Böhmer FD. Protein-tyrosine phosphatases and cancer. *Nat Rev Cancer* 2006;6:307–20.

248 Rudolph J. Inhibiting transient protein–protein interactions: lessons from the CDC25 protein tyrosine phosphatases. *Nat Rev Cancer* 2007;7:202–11.

249 Boutros R, Dozier C, Ducommun B. The when and wheres of CDC25 phosphatases. *Curr Opin Cell Biol* 2006;18:185–91.

250 Trinkle-Mulcahy L, Lamond AI. Mitotic phosphatases: no longer silent partners. *Curr Opin Cell Biol* 2006; 18:623–31.

251 Mansuy IM, Shenolikar S. Protein serine/threonine phosphatases in neuronal plasticity and disorders of learning and memory. *Trends Neurosci* 2006;29:679–86.

252 Shimaoka M, Springer TA. Therapeutic antagonists and conformational regulation of integrin function. *Nat Rev Drug Discov* 2003;2:703–16.

253 George SJ, Dwivedi A. MMPs, cadherins, and cell proliferation. *Trends Cardiovasc Med* 2004;14:100–5.

254 Dooley M, Goa KL. Lamifiban. *Drugs* 1999;57:215–21.

255 Dooley M, Goa KL. Sibrafiban. *Drugs* 1999;57:225–30.

256 Dutta AS, Gormley JJ, Coath M et al. Potent cyclic peptide inhibitors of VLA-4 (α4 β1 Integrin)-mediated cell adhesion. Discovery of compounds like cyclo(MePhe-Leu-Asp-Val-D-Arg-D-Arg) (ZD7349) compatible with depot formulation. *J Pept Sci* 2000;6:398–412.

257 Dutta AS, Crowther M, Gormley JJ et al. Potent cyclic monomeric and dimeric peptide inhibitors of VLA-4 ($\alpha_4\beta_1$ integrin)-mediated cell adhesion based on the Ile-Leu-Asp-Val tetrapeptide. *J Pept Sci* 2000;6:321–41.

258 Haworth D, Rees A, Dutta AS et al. Anti-inflammatory activity of c(ILDV-NH(CH$_2$)$_5$CO), a novel, selective, cyclic peptide inhibitor of VLA-4-mediated cell adhesion. *Br J Pharmacol* 1999;126:1751–60.

259 Yang GX, Hagmann WK. VLA-4 antagonists: potent inhibitors of lymphocyte migration. *Med Res Rev* 2003;23:369–92.

260 Arkin M, Wells JA. Small-molecule inhibitors of protein–protein interactions: progressing towards the dream. *Nat Rev Drug Discov* 2004;3:301–17.

261 Reichert JM. Trends in US approvals: new biopharmaceuticals and vaccines. *Trends Biotechnol* 2006;24:293–8.

262 David R, Owens DR. New horizons: alternative routes for insulin therapy. *Nat Rev Drug Discov* 2002;1:529–40.

263 Harris JM, Chess RB. Effect of pegylation on pharmaceuticals. *Nat Rev Drug Discov* 2003;2:214–21.

264 Sethuraman N, Stadheim TA. Challenges in therapeutic glycoprotein production. *Curr Opin Biotechnol* 2006;17:341–6.

265 Falzon L, Suzuki M, Inouye M. Finding one of a kind: advances in single-protein production. *Curr Opin Biotechnol* 2006;17:347–52.

266 Hartley JL. Cloning technologies for protein expression and purification. *Curr Opin Biotechnol* 2006;17:359–66.

267 Endo Y, Sawasaki T. Cell-free expression systems for eukaryotic protein production. *Curr Opin Biotechnol* 2006;17:373–80.

268 Barnes LM, Dickson AJ. Mammalian cell factories for efficient and stable protein expression. *Curr Opin Biotechnol* 2006;17:381–6.

269 Bommarius AS, Broering JM, Chaparro-Riggers JF et al. High-throughput screening for enhanced protein stability. *Curr Opin Biotechnol* 2006;17:606–10.

270 Kaushansky K. Lineage-specific hematopoietic growth factors. *N Engl J Med* 2006;354:2034–45.

271 Macdougall IC, Eckardt K-U. Novel strategies for stimulating erythropoiesis and potential new treatments for anaemia. *Lancet* 2006;368:947–53.

272 Kaushansky K. Drug therapy: thrombopoietin. *N Engl J Med* 1998;339:746–54.

273 Lane NE. Parathyroid hormone: evolving therapeutic concepts. *Curr Opin Rheumatol* 2004;16:457–63.

274 Fox J. Developments in parathyroid hormone and related peptides as bone-formation agents. *Curr Opin Pharmacol* 2002;2:338–44.

275 Cheer MC, Dunn CJ, Foster R. Tinzaparin sodium: a review of its pharmacology and clinical use in the prophylaxis and treatment of thromboembolic disease. *Drugs* 2004;64:1479–502.

276 Antman EM, Morrow DA, McCabe CH et al. Enoxaparin versus unfractionated heparin with fibrinolysis for ST-elevation myocardial infarction. *N Engl J Med* 2006;354:1477–88.

277 Tyring S, Gottlieb A, Papp K et al. Etanercept and clinical outcomes, fatigue, and depression in psoriasis: double-blind placebo-controlled randomised phase III trial. *Lancet* 2006;367:29–35.

278 Culy CR, Keating GM. Etanercept. An updated review of its use in rheumatoid arthritis, psoriatic arthritis and juvenile rheumatoid arthritis. *Drugs* 2002;62:2493–537.

279 Cooper DA, Lange JMA. Peptide inhibitors of virus–cell fusion: enfuvirtide as a case study in clinical discovery and development. *Lancet Infect Dis* 2004;4:426–36.

280 Dando TM, Perry CM. Enfuvirtide. *Drugs* 2003; 63:2755–66.

281 Borg FAY, Isenberg DA. Syndromes and complications of interferon therapy. *Curr Opin Rheumatol* 2007;19:61–6.

282 Roskos LK, Davis CG, Schwab GM. The clinical pharmacology of therapeutic monoclonal antibodies. *Drug Dev Res* 2004;**61**:108–20.

283 Brekke OH, Sandlie I. Therapeutic antibodies for human diseases at the dawn of the twenty-first century. *Nat Rev Drug Discov* 2003;**2**:52–62.

284 Penichet ML, Morrison SL. Design and engineering human forms of monoclonal antibodies. *Drug Dev Res* 2004;**61**:121–36.

285 Klastersky J. Adverse effects of the humanized antibodies used as cancer therapeutics. *Curr Opin Oncol* 2006;**18**:316–20.

286 Bartt RE. Multiple sclerosis, natalizumab therapy, and progressive multifocal leukoencephalopathy. *Curr Opin Neurol* 2006;**19**:341–9.

287 Polman CH, O'Connor PW, Havrdova E et al. A randomized, placebo-controlled trial of natalizumab for relapsing multiple sclerosis. *N Engl J Med* 2006;**354**:899–910.

288 Rudick RA, Stuart WH, Calabresi PA et al. Natalizumab plus interferon beta-1a for relapsing multiple sclerosis. *N Engl J Med* 2006;**354**:911–23.

289 Dufner P, Jermutus L, Minter RR. Harnessing phage and ribosome display for antibody optimisation. *Trends Biotechnol* 2006;**24**:523–9.

290 Robinson WH. Antigen arrays for antibody profiling. *Curr Opin Chem Biol* 2006;**10**:57–72.

291 Tabrizi MA, Tseng C-ML, Roskos LK. Elimination mechanisms of therapeutic monoclonal antibodies. *Drug Discov Today* 2006;**11**:81–8.

292 Haurum JS. Recombinant polyclonal antibodies: the next generation of antibody therapeutics? *Drug Discoc Today* 2006;**11**:655–60.

293 Melero I, Hervas-Stubbs S, Glennie M et al. Immunostimulatory monoclonal antibodies for cancer therapy. *Nat Rev Cancer* 2007;**7**:95–106.

294 Harris RJ, Shire SJ, Winter C. Commercial manufacturing scale formulation and analytical characterisation of therapeutic recombinant antibodies. *Drug Dev Res* 2004;**61**:137–54.

295 Bernard-Marty C, Lebrun F, Awada A et al. Monoclonal antibody-based targeted therapy in breast cancer: current status and future directions. *Drugs* 2006;**66**:1577–91.

296 Taylor PC. Antibody therapy for rheumatoid arthritis. *Curr Opin Phrmacol* 2003;**3**:323–8.

297 Owen CE. Immunoglobulin E: role in asthma and allergic disease. Lessons from the clinic. *Pharmacol Ther* 2007;**113**:121–33.

298 Kellermann S-A, Green LL. Antibody discovery: the use of transgenic mice to generate human monoclonal antibodies for therapeutics. *Curr Opin Biotechnol* 2002;**13**:593–7.

299 Lebwohl M, Tyring SK, Hamilton TK et al. A novel targeted T-cell modulator, efalizumab, for plaque psoriasis. *N Engl J Med* 2003;**349**:2004–13.

300 Parker CJ, Kar S, Kirkpatrick P. Eculizumab. *Nat Rev Drug Discov* 2007;**6**:515–6.

301 Smith I, Procter M, Gelber RD et al. 2-year follow-up of trastuzumab after adjuvant chemotherapy in HER2-positive breast cancer: a randomised controlled trial. *Lancet* 2007;**369**:29–36.

302 Plosker GL, Keam SJ. Trastuzumab: a review of its use in the management of HER2-positive metastatic and early-stage breast cancer. *Drugs* 2006;**66**:449–75.

303 Hoy SM, Wagstaff AJ. Panitumumab in the treatment of metastatic colorectal cancer. *Drugs* 2006;**66**:2005–14.

304 Reynolds NA, Wagstaff AJ. Cetuximab in the treatment of metastatic colorectal cancer. *Drugs* 2004;**64**:109–18.

305 Starling N, Cunningham D. Monoclonal antibodies against vascular endothelial growth factor and epidermal growth factor receptor in advanced colorectal cancers: present and future directions. *Curr Opin Oncol* 2004;**16**:385–90.

306 Rosenfeld PJ, Brown DM, Heier JS et al. (for the MARINA Study Group). Ranibizumab for neovascular age-related macular degeneration. *N Engl J Med* 2006;**355**:1419–31.

307 Thukral C, Cheifetz A, Peppercorn MA. Anti-tumour necrosis factor therapy for ulcerative colitis: evidence to date. *Drugs* 2006;**66**:2059–65.

308 Scott DL, Kingsley GH. Tumour necrosis factor inhibitors for rheumatoid arthritis. *N Engl J Med* 2006;**355**:704–12.

309 Simpson D, Scott LJ. Adalimumab in psoriatic arthritis. *Drugs* 2006;**66**:1487–96.

310 Cvetkovic RS, Perry CM. Rituximab: a review of its use in non-Hodgkin's lymphoma and chronic lymphocytic leukaemia. *Drugs* 2006;**66**:791–820.

311 Ferrer E, Moral MA. Rituximab for dermatomyositis and TPP. *Drug News Perspect* 2006;**19**:482–4.

312 Looney RJ. B cell-targeted therapy for rheumatoid arthritis: an update on the evidence. *Drugs* 2006;**66**:625–39.

313 Strunk RC, Bloomberg GR. Omalizumab for asthma. *N Engl J Med* 2006;**354**:2689–95.

314 Frampton JE, Wagstaff AJ. Alemtuzamab. *Drugs* 2003;**63**:1229–43.

315 Chapman TM, Keating GM. Basiliximab: a review of its use as induction therapy in renal transplantation. *Drugs* 2003;**63**:2803–35.

316 Ibbotson T, McGavin JK, Goa KL. Abciximab: an updated review of its therapeutic use in patients with ischaemic heart disease undergoing percutaneous coronary revascularisation. *Drugs* 2003;**63**:1121–63.

317 Damle NK, Frost P. Antibody-targeted chemotherapy with immunoconjugates of calicheamicin. *Curr Opin Pharmacol* 2003;**3**:386–90.

318 Salerno-Gonçalves R, Sztein MB. Cell-mediated immunity and the challenges for vaccine development. *Trends Microbiol* 2006;**14**:536–42.

319 Zuckerman JN. Vaccination against hepatitis A and B: developments, deployment and delusions. *Curr Opin Infect Dis* 2006;**19**:456–9.

320 Baumann S, Eddine AN, Kaufmann SHE. Progress in tuberculosis vaccine development. *Curr Opin Immunol* 2006;**18**:438–48.

321 Kaplan G. Rational vaccine development: a new trend in tuberculosis control. *N Engl J Med* 2005;**353**:1624–5.

322 Doherty TM, Rook G. Progress and hindrances in tuberculosis vaccine development. *Lancet* 2006;**367**:947–9.

323 Ibanga HB, Brookes RH, Hill PC et al. Early clinical trials with a new tuberculosis vaccine, MVA85A, in tuberculosis-endemic countries: issues in study design. *Lancet Infect Dis* 2006;**6**:522–8.

324 Setia MS, Steinmaus C, Ho CS et al. The role of BCG in prevention of leprosy: a meta-analysis. *Lancet Infect Dis* 2006;**6**:162–70.

325 Hill DR, Ford L, Lalloo DG. Oral cholera vaccines: use in clinical practice. *Lancet Infect Dis* 2006;**6**:361–73.

326 Obaro SK, Madhi SA. Bacterial pneumonia vaccines and childhood pneumonia: are we winning, refining, or redefining? *Lancet Infect Dis* 2006;**6**:150–61.

327 Horimoto T, Kawaoka Y. Strategies for developing vaccines against H5N1 influenza A viruses. *Trends Mol Med* 2006;**12**:506–14.

328 Bresson J-L, Perronne C, Launay O et al. Safety and immunogenicity of an inactivated split-virion influenza A/Vietnam/1194/2004 (H5N1) vaccine: phase I randomised trial. *Lancet* 2006;**367**:1657–64.

329 Srivastava PK. Therapeutic cancer vaccines. *Curr Opin Immunol* 2006;**18**:201–5.

330 Lollini P-L, Cavallo F, Nanni P et al. Vaccines for tumour prevention. *Nat Rev Cancer* 2006;**6**:204–16.

331 van der Bruggen P, Van den Eynde BJ. Processing and presentation of tumour antigens and vaccination strategies. *Curr Opin Immunol* 2006;**18**:98–104.

332 Siddiqui MAA, Perry CM. Human papillomavirus quadrivalent (types 6, 11, 16, 18) recombinant vaccine (*Gardasil*). *Drugs* 2006;**66**:1263–71.

333 Roden R, Wu T-C. How will HPV vaccines affect cervical cancer? *Nat Rev Cancer* 2006;**6**:753–63.

334 Glass RI, Parashar UD, Bresee JS et al. Rotavirus vaccines: current prospects and future challenges. *Lancet* 2006;**368**:323–32.

335 McCormack PL, Wagstaff AJ. Ultra-short-course seasonal allergy vaccine (*Pollinex* Quattro). *Drugs* 2006;**66**:931–8.

336 Fichou Y, Férec C. The potential of oligonucleotides for therapeutic applications. *Trends Biotechnol* 2006;**24**:563–70.

337 Wahlestedt C. Natural antisense and noncoding RNA transcripts as potential drug targets. *Drug Discov Today* 2006;**11**:503–8.

338 Foloppe N, Matassova N, Aboul-ela F. Towards the discovery of drug-like RNA ligands? *Drug Disc Today* 2006;**11**:1019–1027.

339 Pirollo KF, Rait A, Sleer LS et al. Antisense therapeutics: from theory to clinical practice. *Pharmacol Ther* 2003;**99**:55–77.

340 Lavorgna G, Dahary D, Lehner B et al. In search of antisense. *Trends Biochem Sci* 2004;**29**:88–94.

341 Stahel RA, Zangemeister-Wittke U. Antisense oligonucleotides for cancer therapy: an overview. *Lung Cancer* 2003;**41**(Suppl 1):81–8.

342 Wraight C J, White PJ. Antisense oligonucleotides in cutaneous therapy. *Pharmacol Ther* 2002;**90**:89–104.

343 Lee JF, Stovall GM, Ellington AD. Aptamer therapeutics advance. *Curr Opin Chem Biol* 2006;**10**:282–9.

344 de Fougerolles A, Vornlocher H-P, Maraganore J et al. Interfering with disease: a progress report on siRNA-based therapeutics. *Nat Rev Drug Discov* 2007;**6**:443–53.

345 Marsden PA. RNA interference as potential therapy: not so fast. *N Engl J Med* 2006;**355**:953–4.

346 Czech MP. MicroRNAs as therapeutic targets. *N Engl J Med* 2006;**354**:1194–5.

347 Esquela-Kercher A, Slack FJ. Oncomirs: microRNAs with a role in cancer. *Nat Rev Cancer* 2006;**6**:259–69.

348 Dutta AS, Garner A. The pharmaceutical industry and research in 2020 and beyond. *Drug News Perspect* 2003;**16**:637–48.

2 Pharmaceutical development

Gavin Halbert

Cancer Research UK Formulation Unit, University of Strathclyde, Glasgow, Scotland, UK

2.1 Introduction

The current vogue in drug discovery is the identification and validation of a pharmacological target, followed by high-throughput screening to identify suitable chemical motifs or lead molecules that interact with the target. These molecules may be further refined by combinatorial or traditional medicinal chemistry approaches linked with computer modelling of the target site. This will provide a compound, or series of compounds, that is designed to elicit a maximal response from a specific target receptor in *in vitro* tests. At this stage, the candidate drug exists only as a powder in a 'test tube', or even as a computer model, and is not in a state to benefit the ultimate end user, the patient. The drug is therefore formulated into a medicinal product that can be easily handled and administered by medical staff and patients. Such products may range from simple solutions through to transdermal patch delivery systems, the ultimate form depending on pharmacological, pharmaceutical and marketing considerations. All of these medicinal products or dosage forms will contain the drug plus a variety of additives or excipients whose role is to enhance product performance. Therefore, it is a general rule that patients are never administered a 'drug' *per se* but rather a medicinal product that contains the drug.

Pharmaceutical development of a medicinal product must retain the drug's promising *in vitro* pharmacological activity and provide a predictable *in vivo* response. The marketed product must be stable, correctly packaged, labelled and easily administered, preferably by self-administration. The product must also be economical to manufacture on a large scale by a method that ensures product quality. In addition, development and eventual production processes must comply with the regulatory requirements of proposed market countries, and all development studies must be performed to acceptable levels of quality assurance.

Pharmaceutical development involves multiple skills, processes and stages and is therefore a large undertaking requiring extensive resources. The earlier the pharmaceutical intervention occurs during development the better, to preclude, for example, the use of toxic solvents during manufacture or to employ computer models to determine potential bioavailability problems with candidate compounds. Changes introduced at later stages may necessitate costly retesting or delay product marketing and are best avoided. Development consists of several stages such as preformulation, formulation, toxicology and clinical trials, and, where possible, research is normally conducted in parallel in order to expedite the process. Because of drug diversity and the many possible approaches, there is no single optimum development model but the general stages presented in this chapter will be applied.

For the majority of drugs, the initial formulation will be an injectable solution for basic pharmacology, pharmacokinetic and toxicology studies in animals or humans to confirm *in vitro* activity. Other more complex formulations will follow as the research and pharmaceutical development programmes progress. The eventual range and type of formulations produced for a single drug will depend on the drug's pharmacology and whether a local systemic action is required (Table 2.1). Some drugs can be administered by a variety of routes, resulting in several diverse formulations. Salbutamol, for example, is currently available in 10 different formulations, excluding different doses and variations resulting from different manufacturers (Table 2.2).

The Textbook of Pharmaceutical Medicine. Edited by John P. Griffin. © 2009, ISBN: 978-1-4051-8035-1.

Table 2.1 Basic information on common routes of administration

Route	Advantages	Disadvantages	Product types
Parenteral suspensions[a] (injection)	Exact dose 100% compliance	Painful	Solutions, emulsions, implants[a]
	Suitable for unconscious patient	Self-administration unusual	
	Rapid onset, especially after intravenous administration	Requires trained personnel	Expensive production processes
Oral	Easy	Inappropriate during vomiting	Solutions, syrups, suspensions, emulsions, powders, granules, capsules, tablets
	Convenient	Potential drug-stability problems	
	Acceptable	Interactions with food	
	Painless	Possible low availability	
	Self-administration possible	Patient must be conscious	
Rectal	Avoids problems of stability in gastrointestinal tract. No first-pass metabolism. Useful if oral administration is not possible	Unpopular. Inconvenient. Erratic absorption. Irritation	Suppositories, enemas (solutions, suspensions, emulsions), foams, ointments, creams
Buccal	Rapid onset of action	Taste	Tablets, mouthwashes
	No first-pass metabolism	Only suitable for low dose (high potency) drugs	
	Dosage form recoverable Convenient		
Inhalation	Convenient	Irritation	Gases, aerosols (solutions, suspensions), powders
	Local or systemic effects	Embarrassing	
	No first-pass metabolism	Difficult technique	
Transdermal	Easy	Irritation	Solutions, lotions, sprays, gels, ointments, creams, powders, patches
	Convenient	Potent drugs only	
	No first-pass metabolism	Absorption affected by site of application	
	Local or systemic effects	Hard to administer	
Eye	Local action only	Inefficient	Solutions, ointments, injections
		Irritation	
		Poor retention of solutions	
Vaginal	Local or systemic effects (hormones)	Inconvenient	Creams, ointments, foams, tablets, pessaries
	No first-pass metabolism	Erratic absorption	
		Irritation	

[a] Not for intravenous administration.

Table 2.2 Salbutamol preparations available in the UK

Route	Form	Product	Manufacturer	Strength
Parenteral	Solution	Injection	Non-proprietary	100 µg/mL
		Ventolin injection	A&H	50 and 500 µg/mL
		Ventolin intravenous infusion	A&H	1 mg/mL
Oral	Solution	–	Non-proprietary	2 mg/5 mL
	Syrup	Ventolin	A&H	2 mg/5 mL
	Tablets	–	Non-proprietary[a]	2 and 4 mg
	Tablets (modified release)	Volmax	A&H	4 and 8 mg
	Capsules (modified release)	Ventmax	Trinity	4 and 8 mg
Inhalation	Metered dose inhaler	–	Non-proprietary[b]	100 µg/inhalation
		Aerolin Autohaler	3M	100 µg/inhalation
		Easi-Breathe	A&H	100 µg/inhalation
	Metered dose inhaler CFC free	–	Non-proprietary	100 µg/inhalation
		Airomir Autohaler	3M	100 µg/inhalation
		Evohaler	A&H	100 µg/inhalation
	Powder for inhalation	Ventodisks	A&H	200 and 400 µg/inhalation
		Accuhaler	A&H	200 µg/inhalation
		Rotacaps	A&H	200 and 400 µg/inhalation
		Asmasal Clickhaler	Medeva	95 µg/inhalation
	Nebuliser	Solution	Non-proprietary[c]	1 and 2 mg/mL
		Nebules	A&H	1 and 2 mg/mL
		Respirator solution	A&H	5 mg/mL

From *British National Formulary* 40, September 2000. Liquid, tablet and powder preparations contain salbutamol as the sulphate salt; aerosols contain the free base.
[a] Five manufacturer's preparations available.
[b] Six manufacturer's preparations available.
[c] Four manufacturer's preparations available.

2.2 Preformulation

Before product development studies are conducted, fundamental physicochemical information on the new chemical entity (NCE) or drug must be obtained.[1,2] This provides valuable data to guide future work and initiates a sequence of specification setting exercises that define the drug's boundaries for use. At early stages, only limited drug supplies will be available and there may be competition between continuing pharmacology and early *in vivo* testing and preformulation studies. The utilisation of material has to be balanced to ensure that adequate information is obtained to determine future progress. For example, chemical purity and stability are important in both pharmacology and preformulation studies.

2.2.1 Structure determination

After synthesis it is important to determine the drug's exact chemical structure. This will involve a variety of techniques such as mass spectrometry, nuclear magnetic resonance (H^1 and C^{13}), infrared and ultraviolet/visible spectrophotometry along with elemental analysis. This will confirm the medicinal chemist's proposed structure and provide information useful in later stages such as analytical development.

2.2.2 Analytical development

An initial priority is to develop analytical methodology that detects the drug (main component), intermediate compounds carried over from synthesis and degradation products from chemical breakdown or instability. Paradoxically, these latter contaminants are of greater importance because their quantification, identification and control affect the quality of drug batches. In addition, chemical instability is more easily detected through an increased concentration of degradants than through decreased concentration of the main component. Methods are also required for quantification of other impurities such as residual solvents, catalyst

Table 2.3 Characteristics of fenoprofen salts

Salt	Hydration	Form	Melting point (°C)	Aqueous solubility (mg/mL)	Weight change (%) Relative humidity (%)					
					10	20	40	60	70	93
Free acid	O		40	0.05	–	–	–	–	–	–
K$^+$	Unknown	C		>200	Extremely hygroscopic					
Mg^{2+}	Dihydrate	–		>200	–	–	–	–	–	–
Al(OH)$^{2+}$	Dihydrate	A		0.10	0	–	0	–	–	0
Na$^+$	Anhydrous	A		>200	−0.5	+10.7	+12.5	–	+15.8	+36.5
Na$^+$	Dihydrate	C	80	>200	−11.4	+0.3	+0.4	–	+2.5	+9.3
Ca^{2+}	Anhydrous	A		2.5	+0.5	+1.7	+2.9	+3.7	–	+6.3
Ca^{2+}	Dihydrate	C	110	2.5	0	0	0	–	0	0

A, amorphous; C, crystalline; O, oil.

residues and heavy-metal and microbial contamination. Further analytical tests will also be specified such as the general characteristics, colour, melting point, loss on drying and a basic identification method. The basic analysis of a new drug therefore necessitates the application of a full range of analytical techniques, all of which must be validated to a suitable level.[3]

Drug assays are usually conducted using a specific chromatography or separative technique such as high-performance (or pressure) liquid chromatography (HPLC)[4] or capillary zone electrophoresis (CZE).[5,6] These techniques ensure that the drug is separated from impurities and breakdown products, all of which can then be quantified. Development of these methods allows specifications to be set for the required percentage of the main component, usually 98–101% by weight, and limits for the tolerated level of impurities.[7] If required, identification of the impurities and degradants will also be conducted. A reference sample will be retained and used as a standard for subsequent analysis. Simple ultraviolet or visible spectrophotometric analysis may suffice for some experiments such as solubility testing.

It is common to find that early small-scale batches exhibit a higher or different purity or impurity profile to subsequent batches from large-scale production. As development progresses, the ability to synthesise the drug reproducibly must be determined so that impurity profiles are known and predictable, and can be maintained within predetermined limits.

2.2.3 Salt form

The majority of NCEs synthesised are organic molecules of low molecular weight which are either weak acids or weak bases. There is therefore a choice between the free acid or base and a salt, with further complexity imposed by salt selection. The free acid or base does not normally possess an adequate aqueous solubility for the majority of applications and so salts are required. Because salt formation will occur during synthesis, the correct choice of salt at an early stage is critical. The non-steroidal anti-inflammatory drug fenoprofen is a derivative of 2-phenylpropionic acid and the free acid exists as a viscous oil at room temperature.[8] The potassium salt was found to be hygroscopic, the magnesium salt did not crystallise and the aluminium salt was insoluble in water. Anhydrous sodium or calcium salts could not be obtained but the dihydrate salt was readily isolated. The sodium dihydrate was not stable and dehydrated at room temperature whereas the calcium dihydrate salt was stable up to 70°C (Table 2.3) and was therefore chosen for further development.

2.2.4 Chemical stability

The solid drug's chemical stability will be examined under a range of different storage conditions and over varying periods of time, using the stability indicating assays described above. Chemical degradation occurs through four main routes:

1. Hydrolysis resulting from the presence of H_2O, H^+ or OH^-;
2. Oxidation;
3. Photolysis; and
4. Catalysis by trace metals such as Fe^{2+}, Cu^{2+}.

Hydrolysis and oxidation are the two main routes of degradation for the majority of drugs. Harmonised guidelines are available for new drugs[9] but these specify only two conditions: long-term testing at 25 ± 2°C/60 ± 5% relative humidity and accelerated testing at $40 \pm 2°C/75 \pm 5\%$ relative humidity, which may not provide enough information to characterise degradation processes fully. To gain more information, testing at a range of temperatures from (depending upon stability) $-80°C$ to $70°C$, variable levels of relative humidity up to 90% and exposure to artificial or natural light (Table 2.4) may be conducted.[10] Elevated temperatures, humidity and light deliberately stress the drug and induce rapid degradation. Determination of the physical chemistry of the degradation process will allow the extrapolation of results from short tests under stressed condition to provide estimates of shelf life in ambient environments (Figure 2.1). This will provide basic information on the conditions, processes and packaging which can be used to manipulate and store the drug safely. For example, hygroscopic

drugs may require packaging with a desiccant in containers that prevent moisture ingress.

Chemical stability studies will also be conducted on aqueous solutions of the drug at varying pHs and temperatures and in a variety of solvents, experiments that may be coupled with determination of solubility. This information is important for determining the shelf life of stock solutions for pharmacology testing and analytical assays.

2.2.5 Physicochemical properties

The drug's physicochemical parameters are determined in order to provide essential information for interpreting subsequent studies and guiding formulation.[11] Solubility in aqueous media of differing composition (e.g. buffers, physiological saline) and pH will be

Table 2.4 Typical stress conditions used for stability testing

Test	Stress	Conditions
Solution, chemical stability	Heat and pH	pH 1, 3, 5, 7, 9, 11
Solution, chemical stability		Ambient and elevated temperature
Solution, chemical stability	Light Oxidation	Ultraviolet and white light Sparging with oxygen
Solid, chemical stability	Heat and humidity	4°C, 25°C (60% and 75% RH), 30°C (70% RH), 40°C (75% RH), 50°C, 70°C
Solid, moisture uptake	Humidity	RH[a]: 30%, 45%, 60%, 75%, 90% Ambient temperature

RH, relative humidity.

[a] Provided using saturated aqueous solutions of $MgBr_2$, KNO_2, NaBr, NaCl, KNO_3, respectively, or controlled humidity cabinets.

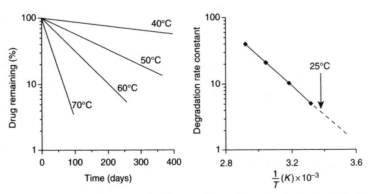

Figure 2.1 Accelerated stability testing. The percentage of drug remaining at elevated temperatures with time is measured (left) and the rate constants for the degradation reaction calculated. Using the Arrhenius relationship, a plot of the log of the rate constant against the reciprocal of absolute temperature of measurement yields a straight line (right). Extrapolation of the line permits calculation of the rate constant at lower temperatures and the prediction of shelf life.

determined, along with a range of biocompatible organic solvents (e.g. ethanol, propylene glycol, polyethylene glycol). Solubility is important in the formulation of liquid dosage forms and is also a critical parameter controlling a drug's biopharmaceutical properties. For example, absorption from administration sites can only occur if the drug is in solution in the biological milieu at the absorption site. Intrinsic dissolution rates in aqueous media at various pH values will also be measured; the magnitude of this parameter is directly related to solubility. Dissolution is only important when it is the rate-limiting step in drug absorption and can arise if drug solubility is below 1 mg/mL in aqueous media at pH 7.0. The bioavailability of drugs with low aqueous solubility can be controlled by this parameter, which is itself affected by the surface area available for dissolution (see below). The dissociation coefficient (pKa) will be measured because this also controls solubility in aqueous solutions. The partitioning of the drug between aqueous and organic solvents will be measured to determine the partition coefficient, although this parameter, along with pKa, can be assessed using computer programs.[12] This is useful for predicting drug absorption and distribution in vivo and for studies of structure–activity relationship, which may direct future synthesis.

2.2.6 Chiral properties

A large proportion of NCEs will have one or more chiral centres. Only single enantiomers can be used nowadays, whereas previously a racemic mixture would have been tested.[13] Different enantiomers produce different pharmacological responses, with one enantiomer usually being more active by at least an order of magnitude. There has been considerable debate on the administration of racemates versus the single active enantiomer or eutomer[14]; however, the current trend is to develop only the active optical isomer. The synthetic route employed will, if required, have to utilise chiral-specific reagents and catalysts or the compound will have to be purified after synthesis. With this type of compound, an additional specification or limit is required for the presence of the inactive enantiomer.[15]

2.2.7 Biopharmaceutical properties

Small-scale in vitro test systems may now be employed to assess biopharmaceutical properties or the drug's potential behaviour after in vivo administration. For example, drug penetration through monolayers of epithelial cells in tissue culture can be used to examine

bioavailability.[16] The drug's metabolism can be studied in vitro using hepatic microsomes and potentially toxic metabolites identified before problems arise in vivo.[17] Although not absolute, these tests provide useful indicators of potential problem areas and may eliminate problematical drug candidates early.

2.2.8 Physical properties of the solid drug

Basic physical properties of the solid drug such as melting point, particle or crystal size, distribution, shape and possible polymorphic variations are important in determining the performance of solid dosage forms. These parameters have profound effects on the drug's behaviour and subsequent formulation, and must be optimised. The bioavailability of drugs with low aqueous solubility and dissolution rate is inversely related to particle size distribution. For example, reduction of digoxin particle size from a diameter of 20–30 to 4 μm led to an increase in the rate and extent of absorption after oral administration.[18] For highly potent drugs, which may only form a small percentage of the formulation, a small particle size is essential to ensure homogeneity during mixing. Crystal shape will affect powder flow and mixing properties, and milling may be required to attain the desired characteristics. Crystal polymorphism can also have a profound effect on the bioavailability of solid dosage forms.[19] Chloramphenicol palmitate, for example, exists in three polymorphic forms: A, B and C. C is unstable under normal conditions; B is metastable and can be incorporated into dosage forms; A is the most stable polymorph. Orally, polymorph A has zero bioavailability whereas B is absorbed, a difference attributable to the slower dissolution of A compared with B. The British Pharmacopoeia (1988) sets a limit of 10% on the content of polymorph A. Amorphous forms may also exist, which are usually more soluble and dissolve more rapidly than crystalline structures.[20]

The powder's flow properties are also important because they control the physical processes that are used to manipulate the material. The Carr index, which is a measure of powder bulk density and angle of repose, provides information on flow properties, which are important when production utilises high-speed tableting machines.

Compression properties are important in determining the ability of the compound to form tablets, with or without the presence of excipients.

2.2.9 Excipient compatibility

Successful formulation depends on the careful selection of excipients that do not interact with the drug or with each other.[21] This phenomenon can be investigated before formulation commences by studying drug–excipient mixtures using differential scanning calorimetry up to typical processing temperatures. This requires only small samples of drugs and is normally conducted with analysis in order to correlate any chemical degradation with known pathways. It can be used to screen a range of excipients. No interaction indicates stability, but the method is not absolute.

Preformulation testing provides a basic dossier on the compound and has a significant role in identifying possible problems and suitable approaches to formulation. Such dossiers already exist for the common excipients.[22] The requirement for aqueous solubility is paramount and preformulation can identify salt forms that are appropriate for further development. Stability and solubility studies will indicate the feasibility of various types of formulation such as parenteral liquids and their probable shelf lives. Similar information can be garnered for solid products from the solid physical properties. By performing these studies on a series of candidate compounds, the optimum compound can be identified and further biological and chemical studies guided to provide the best results.

2.3 Formulation

The transformation of a drug into a medicinal product is a complex process that is controlled by a range of competing factors. The formulator must amalgamate the preformulation information and the clinical indication, which may suggest a particular route of administration (e.g. inhalation of salbutamol; Table 2.2), with toxicology and biopharmaceutical data determining the drug's required dose and frequency of administration. Dose is a major factor controlling the type of formulation and processing. Digoxin, for example, requires an oral dose of 125 µg, an amount too small to form a tablet on its own, so excipients are necessary; by contrast, a 500-mg paracetamol tablet requires minimal excipients in relation to the required dose. The regulatory requirements and local conditions of the proposed market countries also impinge on formulation. For example, the inclusion of alcohol may not be permitted in Muslim countries. Some excipients may also be excluded because of the incidence of adverse reactions[23] or insufficient data to warrant administration by a particular route. Different countries may demand varying specifications for product performance. For example, the test

for antimicrobial preservative efficacy varies between European pharmacopoeias and the US Pharmacopeia,[24] although attempts are being made to harmonise requirements (see International Conference on Harmonisation[3,7,9]). The formulation must therefore comply with the most stringent combination of regulations so that registration in all the proposed markets is possible. The formulation must also be suitable for rapid economical manufacture to provide a product of consistent performance and quality. The application of good pharmaceutical manufacturing practice (GMP)[25] during production will be useless unless similar quality principles are applied during formulation design. Even with all these strictures, there is still scope for variation in formulation: for example, the pharmacopoeias provide standards for the drug content of tablets but do not state the excipients or processing to be used.

Formulation is an experimental stage in development to set specifications for the final product that will be sold and administered to patients. Studies must therefore be conducted to provide production limits for the product. A solution may require a specific pH for drug stability, for example pH 7.0, so experiments will also be conducted at pH 6.5 and 7.5. If the drug is also stable at these two pH values, then the pH limits for the drug product can be set around the desired value of pH 7.0. Similar experiments will also be required with excipients to establish limits of variation in excipient properties that will not deleteriously affect product performance. An important element is that the formulation itself may alter the drug's biopharmaceutical behaviour, and *in vitro* and *in vivo* tests of formulation performance will be conducted to determine any relationship between formulation and response. For example, increasing compression pressure during tableting can alter disintegration and dissolution properties; *in vitro* dissolution tests can measure this effect and allow determination of compression pressure limits. Occasionally, the combination of drug, formulation and route of administration can lead to a product that produces adverse reactions, which are discovered only after administration to a large number of patients.[26] This is difficult to detect at an early stage but the formulator must be aware of this and aim for simple formulations that avoid potential problems.

The initial formulation for most drugs is to allow basic *in vivo* toxicology, pharmacology and biopharmaceutical assessments to be conducted. Aqueous solutions for injection are optimum for this application because the entire dose is administered at a single time point and the problem of bioavailability does not arise. It is important that these formulations are considered carefully, particularly for drugs that are poorly water-soluble, because potentially useful compounds may be rejected inadvertently. These early formulations are also crucial because they set an *in vivo* benchmark for the drug's future performance.

2.3.1 Liquid formulations

Liquid formulations account for about 30% of products in the UK market and, because they are easy to swallow, are favoured for paediatric and geriatric use. An aqueous solution is the simplest formulation to produce, but more complex suspensions or emulsion systems will be required if the drug is poorly soluble. Liquid formulations can be administered by all routes and are probably the most versatile systems. However, liquids are bulky, difficult to transport and container breakage can result in catastrophic loss. The ultimate aim is to provide the desired dose in a suitable liquid volume which, for oral products, is 5 mL.

Solution formulations require excipients to control their properties and improve performance; for example, buffers (such as citric acid) to adjust the pH, sugars or salts to alter the isotonicity of an injection, or flavourings to enhance organoleptic properties. Non-sterile aqueous liquids are liable to microbial colonisation and therefore require the addition of antimicrobial preservatives. If the drug is poorly soluble, solubility can be enhanced by utilising co-solvents (e.g. ethanol, propylene glycol), altering the pH or the use of solubilised systems (e.g. surfactants). If the drug is insoluble in aqueous media, then non-aqueous media (e.g. soya bean oil) can be employed; however, these solvents are not suitable for intravenous administration.

A special requirement for parenteral or injectable formulations is that they must be sterile, apyrogenic and free from visible particulate contamination.[27] Current requirements are that a sterilisation decision tree[28] is followed and, if possible, sterilisation is conducted using a terminal sterilisation method; for example, autoclaving at 121°C for 15 min for aqueous liquids. This is a severe challenge to the drug's chemical stability, and studies must be conducted to ensure that degradation does not occur. Thermolabile compounds may be sterilised by filtration but this route has implications for large-scale production, which requires specialised facilities,[29] and testing.

Suspensions contain a solid drug as a disperse phase in a normally aqueous-based liquid and are termed either coarse (particles >1 μm diameter) or colloidal (particles <1 μm diameter). The particle size of chloramphenicol palmitate suspension, for example, should not exceed a diameter of 45 μm. Because suspension systems are physically unstable, the solid sedimenting and caking under gravity, the formulation must be designed to limit this phenomenon. Rapid sedimentation or caking will prevent the withdrawal of consistent doses. Typical excipients include wetting agents (e.g. surfactants), thickeners to reduce sedimentation speed (e.g. methylcellulose) and flocculating agents (e.g. electrolytes, polymers) to control the degree of interparticulate interaction, which leads to caking. Suspension stability is also determined by the drug's particle size, and limits will be required because small variations can induce physical instability if the formulation is not robust. Antimicrobial preservatives are necessary and flavours may be required, although, because the drug is not in solution, texture rather than taste could be a problem.

Emulsions are a two-phase system consisting of water and oil.[30] Two types are available: the oil-in-water emulsion, which has oil droplets dispersed in a continuous aqueous phase; and the water-in-oil emulsion, which has water droplets in a continuous oil phase. The former is the most common pharmaceutical presentation with the oil as the therapeutic agent (e.g. liquid paraffin emulsion). An increasing use of emulsions is to solubilise water-insoluble drugs, particularly for intravenous administration. In this case, the oil is chosen for its ability to solubilise the drug and its compatibility with the route of administration. An oil-in-water emulsion is thermodynamically unstable and will tend to separate into two distinct liquid phases. The formulation must reduce the interfacial tension between the oil and water using emulsifying agents. Emulsifying agents can be natural (e.g. egg lecithin), synthetic (e.g. polysorbates) or semi-synthetic (e.g. methylcellulose), with the choice depending on the proposed application. Physical stability of the emulsion is paramount and the formulation must be designed to avoid coalescence by providing a large emulsifier layer around each droplet. Emulsions are particularly sensitive to adverse storage conditions such as changes in temperature and may require specialised storage. As with all aqueous-based preparations, an antimicrobial preservative will be required along with an antioxidant to prevent rancidification of the oil.

2.3.2 Semi-solid formulations

A diverse series of semi-solid formulations or vehicles exist and are normally employed for the topical application of drugs to the skin and mucous membranes in order to provide a local action. The drug can be either dissolved or suspended in the formulation, with the simplest system consisting of a single base, such as white soft paraffin, containing dissolved drug. More complex formulations consist of two-phase systems such as creams, which are oil-in-water emulsions, or ointments, which are anhydrous mixtures that can incorporate water to form water-in-oil emulsions. The emulsion systems have the same formulation constraints as the liquid formulations mentioned previously. Aqueous cream consists of emulsifying wax (cetostearyl alcohol and sodium lauryl sulphate in a ratio of 9 : 1), white soft paraffin and liquid paraffin dispersed in water.[31] When applied to skin, it 'vanishes' and is cosmetically acceptable, whereas white soft paraffin alone would form an occlusive hydrating layer. The vehicle can have a marked effect on the response after application, and several of the systems can be used alone for their emollient and protective actions. To exert its effect, the drug must partition from the formulation into the skin, a process that is controlled by the drug's relative solubility in skin and formulation. The balance must favour partitioning into skin, and special derivatives of the drug may be required. The anti-inflammatory steroids are incorporated into creams and ointments as esters in order to increase skin penetration and effect. Hydrocortisone is rated as mild when applied topically whereas the butyrate ester is described as potent. Other excipients are also added to these systems; for example, antimicrobial preservatives, buffering agents and perfumes to improve cosmetic acceptability.

2.3.3 Solid formulations

Tablet formulations account for about 45% of the formulations marketed in the UK, with capsules accounting for about 15%. These formulations have the advantage of providing the dose in a discrete unit form that is stable, easily produced, transported and, above all, easily administered. The tablet is favoured because it is marginally cheaper to produce and slightly more stable under in-use conditions. The simplest solid dosage form is the drug powder itself, a presentation mode that is still used for some antacid preparations. For modern drugs, the dose required is too small to be measured accurately by the patient and must therefore be presented preformed.

The tablet was introduced by Thomas Brockedon in 1843, and glyceryl trinitrate tablets appeared in the British Pharmacopoeia of 1885. Since that time, many variations have appeared but the basic process remains unchanged.[32] There are three main methods of tablet manufacture, with choice depending on the dose and the drug's physical properties such as compressibility and flow (Figure 2.2). A drug with a large dose (>100 mg) and good flow and compressibility properties may be directly compressed into a tablet after mixing with suitable excipients (Table 2.5).[33] Normally, however, the physical properties are not ideal and some form of pretreatment such as granulation is necessary.[34] In wet granulation, the drug is mixed with a diluent and then a solution of a polymeric binder is added during continuous mixing to form a wet powder mass. The mass is passed through a sieve with a mesh size of 1–2 mm to produce granules similar in nature to instant coffee. After drying in hot air and sieving to provide a homogeneous size, these granules are then further blended with a lubricant, disintegrant and maybe further diluents. The final granule mix should flow easily and is fed into a die and then compressed between two punches to produce the tablet. If the drug is not stable in aqueous systems, granulation using solvents, such as isopropyl alcohol, is possible although difficult because of the volatile and flammable properties of the solvent. Thermolabile drugs can be granulated by compressing a drug–diluent–lubricant mix with rollers to produce large slugs of solid material. This can then be broken down into granule-sized pieces and treated as described above.

The basic tablet can be varied in many ways simply by altering the excipients used or by further treatment after production using coatings. The initial formulation is usually a simple, rapidly disintegrating tablet, with modifications occurring only when further information is available. Dissolving tablets require water-soluble excipients; effervescent formulations utilise citric acid and sodium bicarbonate but require manufacture under dry conditions. A polymeric diluent without disintegrant produces a swelling tablet that will delay drug dissolution and provide a sustained release.

The traditional tablet coating is a sugar coat applied in stages. First, the tablet surface is sealed to prevent the ingress of water, then a subcoat of an aqueous polymeric or sucrose solution is added to smooth the surface of the tablet. This can be repeated until the desired size and shape is achieved. Finally, a coloured sugar coat is applied and wax polished, and the company logo may be printed on the tablets. This process is expensive and laborious and has largely been replaced by film coatings, which utilise a coat of a polymer dissolved in a suitable solvent.[35] The

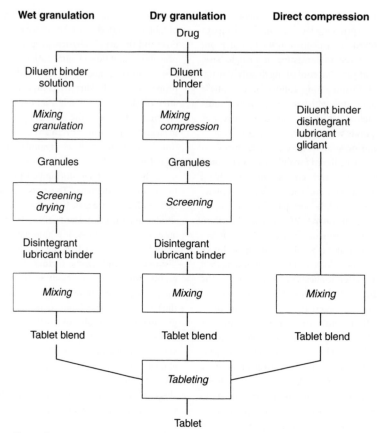

Figure 2.2 The tablet production process. Process stages are shown in boxes.

Table 2.5 Tablet excipients

Excipient	Functions	Examples
Diluent	Bulking agent to adjust tablet weight and ameliorate poor bulk drug properties	Lactose, crystalline cellulose, dicalcium phosphate
Binder	Adhesive to bind together diluent and drug during granulation and compaction	Starch, cellulose derivatives, polyvinylpyrrolidone
Glidant	Aids powder flow properties during manufacture	Colloidal silica, starch
Lubricant	Prevents powder/tablets sticking to punches	Stearic acid, magnesium stearate, sodium lauryl sulphate
	Aids punch movement	
Disintegrant	Aids tablet disintegration in aqueous environment	Starch, sodium starch glycollate, cross-linked polyvinylpyrrolidone
Coat	Physical protection of tablet	Sugar, methylcellulose, cellulose acetate phthalate (for enteric coatings)
	Taste masking	
	Control of drug release	

polymer characteristics can be modified by the addition of colours and plasticisers. The coat provides mechanical protection against chipping and also helps to mask the taste. The polymer coat can also be designed to provide a controlled release so that the tablet degrades only in the intestine (enteric coat) in order to protect either acid-labile drugs from the stomach or the stomach from irritant drugs. Unusual product specifications may be imposed by the marketing department in terms of tablet shape or colour. Usually, this does not affect the tablet performance but may induce manufacturing problems and is difficult to blind when comparative clinical trials are performed. Specialised tablet formulations can be used for vaginal administration to achieve a localised effect.

Capsules consist of a gelatin shell, which may be either hard or soft, enclosing, respectively, powders or non-aqueous liquids. The most common type is the hard gelatin shell, consisting of two halves which are formed separately but loosely fitted together after production.[36] A free-flowing formulation that can be filled into the bottom half before the top is completely pushed home is required. Powder formulations must flow, and a suitable powder blend containing a diluent and glidant will be required. Similar excipients to those employed in tablet formulations can be used, but the properties required of the powder are different because of variations in the filling machines. Hygroscopic materials can induce problems by drying the gelatin shell, producing brittle capsules or by drawing in water to soften the shell. Any flowing dry material can be placed into the hard shell, and a variation on powder blends is the spheronised formulation, which consists of small granulesized beads, which can be coated to control drug release. A novel technology for hard shell is the 'melt fill', which utilises a non-aqueous material, such as polyethylene glycol 6000, which is liquid at elevated temperatures but solidifies at room temperature after capsule filling. The drug is simply dissolved or suspended in the molten liquid, which reduces dust hazards normally associated with tablets or capsules. Soft gelatin capsules have to be formed at the point of fill from molten gelatin softened with glycerol or propylene glycol. The formulation is usually non-aqueous (e.g. a fish oil or lipid-vitamin mixture), although molten gel fills similar to those described above can be used.[37]

2.3.4 Contemporary formulations

The introduction of novel materials, polymers and delivery techniques has allowed a range of formulations to be developed that provide greater control over drug delivery to the body than traditional formulations.[38,39] These formulations are designed for a specific drug, drug delivery system or therapeutic application, although several of them have generic uses. The basis is to provide a constant drug level either in the body or at the site of use, which will provide a constant effect rather than the variable drug levels associated with conventional formulations. Two basic types of controlled-release system exist: one contains a reservoir of drug, which is released via a rate-controlling membrane; the other entraps the drug in a matrix, which controls release by restricting drug diffusion out of the matrix.

The transdermal patch looks like a standard sticking plaster of 2–3 cm, which is applied to the skin (Figure 2.3). Several methods of controlling drug release are available. Membrane moderated patches consist of a drug reservoir enclosed by an impermeable backing material sealed on to a rate-limiting membrane covered with adhesive that sticks to the skin.[40] Drug is released into the skin through the rate-controlling membrane and is then absorbed systemically to exert its pharmacological effect. The rate of drug transfer through the skin is dependent on its properties and this system is only suitable for drugs that meet specific physicochemical criteria.[41] The drug must also be sufficiently active (low dose) because the quantity absorbed by this route is minimal. Ocusert is a similar system for the prolonged release of drugs in the eye. A reservoir of pilocarpine is encased in a rate-limiting polymer membrane.[42] In the eye, pilocarpine diffuses through the membrane to deliver drug at a defined rate (20 or 40 μg/h) for periods of up to 1 week.

Spherical or pellet-based drug delivery formulations are possible, and range in diameter from millimetres down to nanometres. The larger systems are very useful for gastrointestinal administration,[43] especially where the system is enteric-coated to prevent drug release in the stomach. (The coating ensures that the tablet remains intact and does not disintegrate until it reaches the small intestine.) The passage of large enteric-coated tablets from the stomach is erratic, and pellet-based formulations of 1–2 mm diameter do not suffer from this problem.[44] Recent developments have extended this type of system to injectable (subcutaneous) formulations for labile peptide drugs that require a prolonged action (e.g. goserelin and leuprorelin). These drugs cannot be administered by the oral route, have very short plasma half-lives and would require repeated injections to be

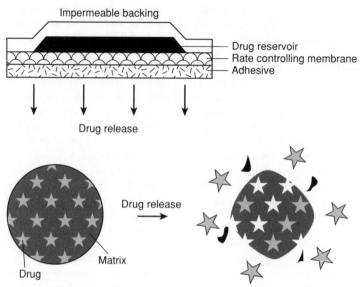

Figure 2.3 Reservoir (top) and matrix-based (bottom) drug delivery systems. The matrix system degrades during drug delivery, releasing the drug and matrix through either matrix erosion or degradation.

clinically effective. The drugs are therefore incorporated into the matrix of microspheres (tens of micrometres in diameter) of a biodegradable and biocompatible polymer (polylactide-co-glycolide).[45] The polymer degrades after injection, slowly releasing the drug to provide continuous therapy for 1–3 months, depending on the formulation. Even smaller systems, such as nanoparticles,[46] are under investigation as drug delivery, and also drug targeting, systems and future developments to 'formulate novel therapeutics, such as genes[47] and other biological molecules,[48–50] are undergoing concerted active research.

2.3.5 Packaging

The packaging of a medicinal product fulfils a variety of roles such as product presentation, identification, convenience and protection until administration or use. Selection of packaging requires a basic knowledge of packaging materials, the environmental conditions to which the product will be exposed and the characteristics of the formulation. Several types of packaging will be employed, the primary packaging around the product, and secondary packaging such as a carton and subsequent transit cases. The following discussion concerns primary packaging.

The packaging must physically protect the product from the mechanical stresses of warehousing, handling and distribution. Mechanical stress may take a variety of forms, from impact through to vibration in transit and compression forces on stacking. The

demands for mechanical protection will vary with product type: glass ampoules will require greater protection than plastic eye drop bottles, for example.

Other protection is required from environmental factors such as moisture, temperature changes, light, gases and biological agents such as micro-organisms and, importantly, humans. The global market for medicinal products requires that the products are stable over a wide range of temperatures ranging from subzero in polar regions, 15°C in temperate zones, up to 32°C in the tropics. Along with this temperature variation, relative humidity can vary from below 50% to up to 90%, a feature that the packaging should be able to resist if necessary. The majority of packaging materials (including plastics) is to some degree permeable to moisture and the type of closure employed, such as screw fittings, may also permit ingress of moisture. The susceptibility of the product to moisture and its hygroscopicity will have to be considered and may require packaging with a desiccant or the use of specialised strip packs using low permeability materials such as foil. Temperature fluctuations can lead to condensation of moisture on the product and, with liquids, formation of a condensate layer on top of the product. This latter problem is well known and can lead to microbiological spoilage as the condensate is preservative free. If the product is sensitive to photolysis, then opaque materials may be required. Most secondary packaging materials (e.g. cartons) do not transmit light but, in some cases, specialised primary packaging designed to limit light transmission is employed. The package must also prevent the entry of organisms; for example, packaging of sterile products must be absolutely micro-organism proof, hence the continued use of glass ampoules. For non-sterile products, the preservative provides some protection, but continual microbial challenge will diminish the efficacy of the preservative, and spoilage or disease transmission may occur.[51] Finally, the packaging material must not interact with the product either to adsorb substances from the product or to leach chemicals into the product. Plastics contain additives to enhance polymer performance. Polyvinyl chloride (PVC) may contain phthalate di-ester plasticiser, which can leach into infusion fluids from packaging.[52] Antimicrobial preservatives such as phenylmercuric acetate are known to partition into rubbers and plastics during storage, thus reducing the formulation concentration below effective antimicrobial levels.[53] A complication of modern packaging is the need for the application of security seals to protect against deliberate adulteration and maintain consumer confidence.

2.3.6 Stability testing

Once the optimal formulation and processing method have been determined and the most suitable packaging configuration decided, product stability tests may be commenced. The aim is to determine a shelf life and provide data that demonstrate the product's continued quality under the conditions of manufacture, storage, distribution and usage. Because time is a major parameter in stability testing, a large amount of resources is involved in conducting stability tests, and mishaps can be costly. To ensure commercial returns on an NCE, it must be marketed when only limited stability testing of 1–2 years has been performed. Accelerated stability studies are therefore carried out where the product is deliberately stressed using elevated temperatures and humidity (Table 2.6).[10] Extrapolation of the results to ambient conditions allows the prediction of a shelf life or expiration date (Figure 2.1). The study should monitor all the product's characteristics that may be affected by storage and this normally means testing to the full release specifications. For example, products containing antimicrobial preservatives must meet the specifications of pharmacopoeial microbial challenge tests at all times during the proposed shelf life. Some tests that are not part of the release specification may also be conducted to provide greater information on product behaviour, such as dissolution testing in tablets. The regulatory authorities expect these data to be presented for at least three different batches of the product, using three different batches of active ingredient, in the final marketing packaging.[54] Also, the batches used should, if possible, be manufactured at the same scale as production batches.

Table 2.6 Typical conditions and sampling profile for product stability tests

Sample time (months)	Storage conditions (temperature/relative humidity)							
	2–8°C		25°C/60%[a]		30°C/70%[a]		40°C/75%[a]	
	CT	Final	CT	Final	CT	Final	CT	Final
1	✓	✓	✓	✓	✓	✓	✓	✓
3	✓	✓	✓	✓	✓	✓	✓	✓
6	✓	✓	✓	✓	✓	✓	✓	✓
9	✓	✓	✓	✓	✓	✓		✓
12	✓	✓	✓	✓	✓	✓		✓
18	✓	✓	✓	✓	✓	✓		✓
24	✓	✓	✓	✓	✓	✓		✓
36		✓		✓		✓		
48		✓		✓		✓		
60		✓		✓				

The table shows one of a variety of possible test configurations; the EU requires at least 6 months of data before marketing. Clinical trial (CT) products do not require long shelf lives and therefore testing can be limited. For some thermolabile products, the temperature range may be lower, or testing at higher temperatures may be terminated quickly. A full analytical profile should be determined for all samples if possible.

✓ Sample analysed.

[a] May also be conducted with light exposure.

One interesting feature of stability is that a product may have two shelf lives, one for the manufactured material and another for the reconstituted or opened pack. Methyl prednisolone sodium succinate lyophilised injection, for example, is stable for up to 3 years in the dry state but the reconstituted injection must be used within 12 h.

2.3.7 Scale-up and manufacture

The evolution and optimisation of a formulation is an experimental stage that will be conducted on small batches of the material. For a drug with a tablet weight of 250 mg, test batches would typically be 0.5–1 kg, providing up to 4000 tablets for analysis, performance testing and initial stability studies. Similar scales will be used in the optimisation of the product's packaging.

The overall aim of pharmaceutical development is to transform the formulation into a product that can be manufactured on a large scale, which must be achieved without any deleterious alterations to the performance of the formulation. The complexity of scale-up is related to the proposed production batch size of the final product, typically around 2 million units, which for a 250-mg tablet is 500 kg of material. Additionally, the number of manufacturing sites to be employed must be considered, as ambient environmental conditions and equipment may vary, inducing variations in the final product. Several intermediate stages will be employed to gain experience with handling larger quantities of the formulation and ensure that no variations occur. Intermediate batches consuming 10–50 to 100 kg of material will be processed, and several problems may arise because of increases in batch size. Larger heating or mixing vessels have a smaller surface : volume ratio and may take longer to heat or cool, exposing the formulation to elevated temperatures and producing thermal degradation. Large-scale handling of powders in hoppers can induce separation of the constituents, leading to variation in tablet content during a production run. Development tablet machines produce about 100 tablets per minute, while a rotary tablet press (Figure 2.4) may produce up to 5000 tablets per minute. Regulatory authorities require that at least three full-scale production runs are conducted,[55] and that any of the processes employed (e.g. sterilisation) are fully validated.[56] This will allow manufacturing personnel to gain familiarity with the product and ensure that product quality can be guaranteed before full production commences. The increasing level of

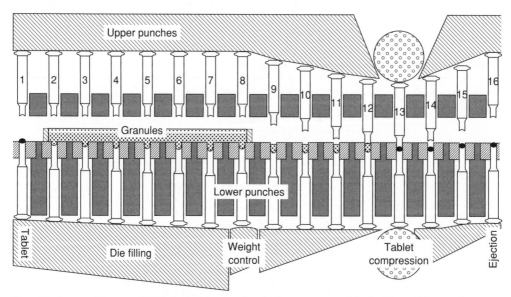

Figure 2.4 A rotary tablet press. The punches and dies move in a circular manner around the die filling, weight control, compression and ejection stages. At positions 2–7, the bottom punch drops and the space created in the die is filled with granules flowing under gravity. The tablet weight is set at position 8 by raising the bottom punch to a set height and skimming off the excess granulate. The tablet is compressed between the top and the bottom punches at position 13 and then ejected by removing the top punch and raising the bottom punch in positions 14–1. In this example, a single tablet is produced for each cycle but some presses may have two cycles per rotation and multiple punches and dies, thus increasing production rate.

product stocks that will be accumulated by this process can be employed in clinical trials and the latter batches may form part of the launch supplies.

Before the market launch of the product, regulatory authorities will inspect the production premises and processes to ensure that everything complies with the licence application and GMP.[25] GMP must be maintained throughout the production cycle, including, where required, suppliers and also the distribution chain. In fact, GMP (or its associated quality standards) should only end when the product is handed to the patient. At this stage, all control ceases.

Scale-up of drug synthesis will also be required, as initial manufacture will probably occur on a laboratory scale, providing only grams of material. The synthetic route may not be ideal for large-scale production and a new pathway may be required for the latter stages of development. Tests will have to be conducted to ensure that the active ingredient is not significantly different from the original material and that impurity levels are not increased. If different impurities arise from the new synthetic route, these will have to be studied.

2.3.8 Bioequivalence

Once a drug's patent protection has expired, it is common to find two or more products of the same strength and form produced by different manufacturers (Table 2.2). This is a consequence of financial pressures to reduce prescribing costs and has led to the development of a burgeoning generic industry. Products marketed under approved or brand names are classed as chemically or pharmaceutically equivalent because they contain the same dose of the same drug. However, chemical equivalence does not guarantee that the products will behave identically when administered to the patient because they may contain different excipients and may have been produced by widely differing techniques. An early example of the problem of bioequivalence occurred with the antiepileptic drug phenytoin. In 1970, it was reported that a change in capsule diluent from calcium sulphate dihydrate to lactose produced phenytoin overdosage in patients receiving chemically equivalent capsules.[57] Bioequivalence arises from extravascular routes of administration (e.g. oral, intramuscular, rectal) where absorption occurs before the drug appears in the blood (Figure 2.5). Absorption has two important pharmacokinetic features: the extent of absorption and the rate of absorption.[58] The former is measured by comparing the area under the plasma concentration–time curve (AUC) after administration of the formulation with the AUC of an intravenous injection. Intravenous injection provides an extent of absorption of one since the entire dose reaches the blood or systemic circulation. The rate of absorption may be measured by determining the maximum plasma concentration, C_{max}, and the time taken to reach C_{max}, t_{max}. The latter is a measure of the rate of absorption whereas the former is also dependent on the extent of absorption. Differences in either extent or rate of absorption can markedly alter the plasma concentration profile and produce different clinical effect (Figure 2.6).

There is extensive literature on this subject, mainly concentrated in the field of oral products.[59] However, bioequivalence is a potential problem with other routes of administration such as transdermal, topical[60] and intramuscular routes. The prescriber and patient expect that chemically equivalent products are therapeutically equivalent and this requires the generic formulation to mimic the marketed product's

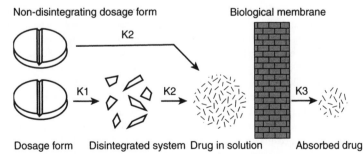

Figure 2.5 Stages in drug absorption from an extravascular administration site (stomach, small intestine, intramuscular injection). Only drug in solution is absorbed. If the rate of dissolution (K2) is less than the rate of absorption (K3), then the rate at which the drug is released from the dosage form controls absorption. This permits modified or sustained-release formulations, but can also lead to bioequivalence problems.

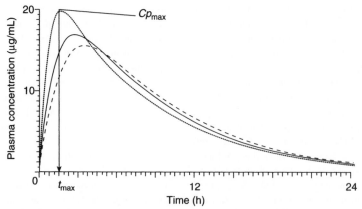

Figure 2.6 Effect of variation in absorption rate on plasma drug concentration. The graph shows simulated plasma concentration–time curves for theophylline after oral administration, illustrating a 20% difference in Cp_{max} values resulting from variation in the absorption rate constant. Absorption rate constants: top curve 2.2 per h (Cp_{max} 20 µg/mL); middle curve 1.0 per h (Cp_{max} 18 µg/mL); bottom curve 0.7 per h. Note that t_{max} also changes. The established therapeutic concentration of theophyllin is 10–20 µg/mL. The most rapidly absorbed formulation produces the highest concentration and greatest chance of side effects. Also, the duration for which the plasma concentration is within the therapeutic range also varies. Pharmacokinetic parameters: dose, 400 mg: bioavailability, 0.8; volume of distribution, 29 L; half-life, 5.5 h.

in vivo behaviour. The arbiters of bioequivalence are the regulatory authorities, and the regulations of various countries are not identical.[60,61] In general, bioequivalence is demonstrated if the mean difference between two products is within ±20% at the 95% confidence level. This is a statistical requirement, which may require a large number of samples (e.g. volunteers) if the drug exhibits variable absorption and disposition pharmacokinetics. For drugs for which there is a small therapeutic window or low therapeutic index, the ±20% limit may be reduced. The preferred test method is an *in vivo* crossover study and, because this occurs in the development phase, necessitates the employment of volunteers. These studies are therefore expensive and animal experiments may be substituted, or *in vitro* experiments if they have been correlated with *in vivo* studies.

Bioequivalence problems arise only when the formulation is the rate-limiting step in drug absorption. All formulations should be optimised to ensure maximal absorption equivalent to the administration of a solution, unless a controlled or sustained drug delivery is sought. In general, increasing formulation complexity and processing increases the risk of bioequivalence problems. Controlled-release preparations require proof of equivalence at steady state to already marketed rapid-release or sustained-release preparations. In addition, studies must prove the controlled-release characteristics claimed and rule

out the possibility of 'dose dumping'. Other problems associated with alternative formulations can be the inclusion of new excipients that induce adverse reactions, or changes in patient preferences resulting from differences in product colour or presentation.

2.4 Clinical trial supplies

Initial clinical trials will be conducted early in the drug's development simply to evaluate the pharmacological response, perform pharmacokinetic studies or determine the maximum tolerated dose in humans.[62] The formulations administered in these early trials should be as close as possible to the eventually marketed product to avoid costly retesting. These trials present no problems, other than those of quality and stability because there is no element of deceit or blinding because both volunteer and physician are aware of the administered product. Subsequent phase II, III and IV trials, however, may require blinding, particularly if some form of product comparison is undertaken. Blinding ensures that the patient (single blind) and maybe also the physician (double blind) do not know which treatment is administered[63] in order to eliminate any potential bias that may be introduced into the trial results. The trial protocol will be developed by the physician and the clinical research department of the sponsor; however, liaison with the pharmaceutical department should occur at an early stage to ensure that any proposed trial is pharmaceutically possible. The pharmaceutical challenge is to develop the appropriate manufacturing and packaging procedures that ensure the stability and quality of the trial supplies. In addition to this, blinding may be required by the clinical trial protocol. The simplest trial would be active product against matching placebo at a single dose level. Expanding the trial (e.g. by using multiple dose levels or comparisons with competitors' products) increases the complexity of supplies and pharmaceutical demands. The level of complexity is also controlled by the types of formulations or products that are employed in the trial.

2.4.1 Blinding

Clinical trial supplies can be blinded using several techniques depending on the availability of resources and the consideration of competitor companies. The ideal situation is to produce a placebo or comparator product that looks and behaves in an identical fashion to its active test counterpart (e.g. the same colour, weight, shape, size, markings, texture and taste). Colourless solutions or white tablets do not present a great problem, but if the drug is coloured, the placebo will have to match this. Production of in-house placebo formulations is relatively easy; however, if a competitor's product is involved, then difficulties can arise. The competitor can be asked to supply the drug in a form matching the product under test, but this may not always be possible for a variety of reasons. If a competitor's product cannot be matched, then it may be manipulated to eliminate differences between the two products. The ideal option is to reformulate the competitor's product to match the test product; however, great care must be taken to ensure that the two products (manipulated and original) are bioequivalent and exhibit the same stability, etc., as the original marketed product. Because this represents a new formulation, a great deal of time and effort would be required. To circumvent this, both products can be disguised, for example, by packaging small tablets in opaque, hard gelatin capsules or using rice paper cachets. Different tablets can be coated using either film or sugar coating to mask their distinguishing features and produce effectively similar products. Again, tests would be required to ensure that stability and bioequivalence were not compromised.

If products cannot be matched (e.g. a tablet versus an aerosol) or if the above techniques are not possible, then blinding can be performed using the double-

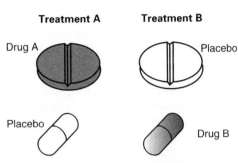

Figure 2.7 The double-dummy technique. The patient always takes a tablet and a capsule. In treatment A, the tablet contains the active drug and the capsule contains the placebo. In treatment B, the capsule contains the active drug and the tablet contains the placebo.

dummy technique, so-called because a matching placebo for both products is manufactured. The patient then has to administer two products at one time, only one of which contains the active drug (Figure 2.7). The advantage is that both products are used without manipulation, but it can be very confusing for the trial participants. In these cases, it is important that easily understood, explicit and comprehensive instructions are provided to the patient, possibly employing special packs to aid compliance. If different dose levels or dose escalations are required, then adaptations to the placebo and dummy techniques can be employed. For example, administration of three tablets three times daily would allow for doses ranging from nine placebo tablets through to nine active tablets daily. One drawback of complicated regimens is patient non-compliance or failure to take therapy as directed. This may have a capricious effect on trial results and a method to detect non-compliance should be employed, such as retrieval of the patient's supplies and determination of the number of doses administered. One feature of blinded clinical trials that has to be ascribed to human nature is the desire to break blinding, which may arise through a variety of routes. The active preparation will taste bitter, patients may prefer to crush or suck tablets before swallowing and the difference between placebo and active will be apparent.

2.4.2 Labelling of clinical trial materials

The UK Medicines Act 1968 regulations require that all medicinal products are properly labelled to certain minimum standards, but requirements vary from country to country. Clinical trial materials, however, cannot be labelled normally because if the trial is blind, nothing should reveal to the patient or physician the nature of the contents. The basic information on the label should provide the patient's name, study phase, study number, directions for use, any special warning or storage requirements, expiry date and the investigator's name and address, along with an indication that the drugs are 'for clinical trial use only'. The sponsoring company's name and address should also appear, together with a code that can be broken in the case of emergency to determine if the patient is receiving an active or placebo preparation.

2.4.3 Quality assurance of clinical trial supplies

European clinical trial products previously did not require manufacture to GMP; however, a new clinical trial directive will necessitate the manufacture to GMP in licensed premises.

The manufacture and packaging of clinical trial supplies present interesting quality assurance problems. The manufacture of placebo products, for example, must include testing to ensure freedom from any contaminating active drug. The active products used must also be stability tested in the proposed packaging because specialist packaging will be employed to aid blinding and meet the requirements of the trial protocol. The packaging exercise requires an ordered approach to meet the protocol requirements, including randomisation schedules, crossover, labelling and blinding with placebo or dummy techniques. A double-dummy trial comparing two products at one dose level with a crossover would require the packaging of two sets of supplies, one with active A/placebo B and one with placebo A/active B. These would then have to be combined and labelled following the requirements of the randomisation schedule and crossover. If the trial involves two dose levels for A, then the initial packaging will require three sets of supplies. Protocols that require dosage changes during the trial necessitate the packaging of extra supplies for each patient which can be called on when required by the protocol. However, if it is performed, the supplies must all look identical. It is hoped that the reader will realise that even simple trials can lead to incredible logistical problems in the provision of supplies. Once packaged, the supplies must be subjected to checking and quality control procedures (e.g. analysis for the active substance) to ensure that the packaging is correct. Because the trial is dependent on the supplies, packaging and analytical documentation form an integral part of the quality assurance for the trial.

2.5 Conclusions

The process of pharmaceutical development is the transformation of the chemist's compound through the pharmacist's formulation and production of the product to become marketable merchandise. This long involved process requires the input of large resources and a myriad of professional and technical expertise. Almost £3000 million[64] was spent on pharmaceutical research and development in the UK in 2000, with nominally about 60% spent on applied research and experimental development. The process consists of several distinct but overlapping and interlinked phases, which have a range of milestones to gauge progress: the initiation of preformulation studies, formulation of phase I clinical trial products, commencement of phase I trials in humans, full-scale production runs and, eventually, market launch. Careful coordination throughout the process is necessary to ensure that the development of any adverse results is acted upon and decisions to either progress or drop the compound are taken before expenditure is excessive. Once a drug is marketed, the pharmaceutical development process continues with ongoing stability studies, post-marketing surveillance and the development of new formulations and therapeutic uses as clinical experience with the drug expands. A complaint procedure must be established and reported incidences investigated to ensure that the product performs in the field as expected. This chapter has presented the reader with only a surface veneer of information regarding the pharmaceutical development process; it is hoped that this will stimulate interest and further reading on this extensive subject.

Further reading

Aulton ME, ed. Pharmaceutics. *The Science of Dosage Form Development, 2nd edn.* London: Churchill Livingstone, 2002.

Cartwright AC, Matthews BR, eds. *International Pharmaceutical Product Registration: Aspects of Quality, Safety and Efficacy.* London: Ellis Horwood, 1994.

References

1 Wells JI, ed. *Pharmaceutical Preformulation: The Physicochemical Properties of Drug Substances.* Chichester: Ellis Horwood, 1988.

2 Carstensen JT. Preformulation. In: Carstensen JT, Rhodes CT, eds. *Drug Stability Principles and Practices, 3rd edn.* New York: Marcel Dekker, 2000;237–60.

3 Anon. Text on validations of analytical procedures. In: *International Conference on Harmonisation of Technical Requirements for Registration of Pharmaceutical for Human Use*, 1994. http://www.ifpma.org/ich5q.html#Analytical.

4 Fong GW, Lam SK, eds. *HPLC in the Pharmaceutical Industry*. New York: Marcel Dekker, 1991.

5 Altria KD, Kelly MA, Clark BJ. Current applications in the analysis of pharmaceuticals by capillary electrophoresis. I. *Trends Anal Chem* 1998;**17**:204–14.

6 Altria KD, Kelly MA, Clark BJ. Current applications in the analysis of pharmaceuticals by capillary electrophoresis. II. *Trends Anal Chem* 1998;**17**:214–26.

7 Anon. Impurities in new drug substances (revised guideline) Q3AR. In: *International Conference on Harmonisation of Technical Requirements for Registration of Pharmaceutical for Human Use*, 1999. http://www.ifpma.org/ich5q.html#Impurity.

8 Hirsh CA, Messenger RJ, Brannon JL. Fenoprofen: drug form selection and preformulation stability studies. *J Pharm Sci* 1978;**67**:231–6.

9 Anon. Stability testing of new drugs and products. In: *International Conference on Harmonisation of Technical Requirements for Registration of Pharmaceutical for Human Use*, 2000. http://www.ifpma.org/ ich5q.html#Stability.

10 Grimm W. A rational approach to stability testing and analytical development for NCE, drug substance, and drug products: marketed product stability testing. In: Carstensen JT, Rhodes CT, eds. *Drug Stability Principles and Practices, 3rd edn*. New York: Marcel Dekker, 2000;415–81.

11 Florence AT, Attwood D. *Physicochemical Principles of Pharmacy, 2nd edn*. London: MacMillan Press, 1988.

12 Ooms F. Molecular modeling and computer aided drug design: examples of their applications in medicinal chemistry. *Curr Med Chem* 2000;**7**:141–58.

13 Cartwright AC. Introduction and history of pharmaceutical regulation. In: Cartwright AC, Matthews BR, eds. *Pharmaceutical Product Licensing. Requirements for Europe*. Chichester: Ellis Horwood, 1991;29–45.

14 Ariens EJ, Wuis EW, Veringa EJ. Stereoselectivity of bioactive xenobiotics: a pre-Pasteur attitude in medicinal chemistry, pharmacokinetics and clinical pharmacology. *Biochem Pharmacol* 1988;**37**:9–18.

15 Fanali S, Aturki Z, Desiderio C. Enantioresolution of pharmaceutical compounds by capillary electrophoresis: use of cyclodextrins and antibiotics. *Enantiomer* 1999; **4**:229–41.

16 Artursson P, Palm K, Luthman K. Caco-2 monolayers in experimental and theoretical predictions of drug transport. *Adv Drug Deliv Rev* 2001;**46**:27–43.

17 Li AP Screening for human ADME/Tox drug properties in drug discovery. *Drug Discov Today* 2001;**6**:357–66.

18 Shaw TRD, Carless JE. The effect of particle size on the absorption of digoxin. *Eur J Clin Pharmacol* 1974;**7**:269.

19 Borka L. Review on crystal polymorphism of substances in the European Pharmacopeia. *Pharm Acta Helv* 1991; **66**:16–22.

20 Yu L. Amorphous pharmaceutical solids: preparation, characterization and stabilization. *Adv Drug Deliv Rev* 2001;**48**:27–42.

21 Crowley P, Martini L. Drug–excipient interactions. *Pharm Technol Europe* 2001;**13**:26–34.

22 Anon. *Handbook of Pharmaceutical Excipients*. London: Pharmaceutical Press, 1986.

23 Weiner M, Bernstein IL. *Adverse Reactions to Drug Formulation Agents: A Handbook of Excipients*. New York: Marcel Dekker, 1989.

24 Akers MJ, Taylor CJ. Official methods of preservative evaluation and testing. In: Denyer SP, Baird RM, eds. *Guide to Microbiological Control in Pharmaceuticals*. London: Ellis Horwood, 1990;292–303.

25 Anon. *Rules and Guidance for Pharmaceutical Manufacturers and Distributors*. London: The Stationery Office, 1997.

26 Florence AT, Salole EG. *Formulation Factors in Adverse Reactions*. London: Wright, 1990.

27 Groves MJ. *Parenteral Technology Manual, 2nd edn*. Buffalo Grove: Interpharm Press, 1989.

28 Morris JM. Sterilisation decision trees and implementation. *PDA J Pharm Science Technol* 1999;**54**:64–8.

29 Walden MP. Clean rooms. In: Cole GC, ed. *Pharmaceutical Production Facilities*. Chichester: Ellis Horwood, 1990;79–126.

30 Eccleston GM. Emulsions. In: Swarbrick J, Boylan JC, eds. *Encyclopedia of Pharmaceutical Technology*. New York: Marcel Dekker, 1992;137–88.

31 Eccleston GM. Properties of fatty alcohol mixed emulsifiers and emulsifying waxes. In: Florence AT, ed. *Materials used in Pharmaceutical Formulation*. Oxford: Blackwell Scientific Publications, 1984;124–56.

32 Lieberman HA, Lachman L. *Pharmaceutical Dosage Forms: Tablets, 2nd edn*. New York: Marcel Dekker, 1992.

33 Murray M, Laohavichien A, Habib W, et al. Effect of process variables on roller-compacted ibuprofen tablets. *Pharm Ind* 1998;**60**:257–62.

34 Keleb EI, Vermeire A, Vervaet C, et al. Cold extrusion as a continuous single-step granulation and tableting process. *Eur J Pharm Biopharm* 2001;**52**:359–68.

35 Rowe RC. Defects in film-coated tablets: aetiology and solutions. In: Ganderton D, Jones T, eds. *Advances in Pharmaceutical Sciences*. London: Academic Press, 1992;65–100.

36 Ridgway K, ed. *Hard Capsules Development and Technology*. London: Pharmaceutical Press, 1987.

37 Jimerson RF, Hom FS. Capsules, soft. In: Swarbrick J, Boylan JC, eds. *Encyclopedia of Pharmaceutical Technology*. New York: Marcel Dekker, 1990;269–84.

38 Kydonieus A, ed. *Treatise on Controlled Drug Delivery: Fundamentals, Optimization, Applications*. New York: Marcel Dekker, 1992.

39 Dressman JB, Ridout G, Guy RH. Delivery system technology. In: Hansch C, ed. *Biopharmaceutics*. Oxford: Pergamon Press, 1990;615–60.

40 Govil SK. Transdermal drug delivery devices. In: Tyle P, ed. *Drug Delivery Devices: Fundamentals and Applications.* New York: Marcel Dekker, 1988;386–419.

41 Walters KA. Transdermal drug delivery. In: Florence AT, Salole EG, eds. *Routes of Drug Administration.* London: Wright, 1990;78–136.

42 Mitra AK. Ophthalmic drug delivery devices. In: Tyle P, ed. *Drug Delivery Devices: Fundamentals and Applications.* New York: Marcel Dekker, 1988;455–70.

43 Ghebre-Sellassie I. *Multiparticulate Oral Drug Delivery.* New York: Marcel Dekker, 1994.

44 Wilson CG, Washington N. *Physiological Pharmaceutics: Biological Barriers to Drug Absorption, 2nd edn.* Chichester: Ellis Horwood, 2001.

45 Sharifi R, Ratanawong C, Jung A, et al. Therapeutic effects of leuprorelin microspheres in prostate cancer. *Adv Drug Deliv Rev* 1997;**28**:121–38.

46 Kawashima Y. Preface nanoparticulate systems for improved drug delivery. *Adv Drug Deliv Rev* 2001;**47**:1–2.

47 Pouton CW, Seymour LW. Key issues in non-viral gene delivery. *Adv Drug Deliv Rev* 2001;**46**:187–203.

48 Oussoren C, Storm G. Liposomes to target the lymphatics by subcutaneous administration. *Adv Drug Deliv Rev* 2001;**50**:143–56.

49 Harashima H, Kiwada H. The pharmacokinetics of liposomes in tumor targeting. *Adv Drug Deliv Rev* 1999;**40**:1–2.

50 Clark MA, Jepson MA, Hirst BH. Exploiting M cells for drug and vaccine delivery. *Adv Drug Deliv Rev* 2001;**50**:81–106.

51 Bloomfield SR. Microbial contamination: spoilage and hazard. In: Denyer S, Baird R, eds. *Guide to Microbiological Control in Pharmaceuticals.* Chichester: Ellis Horwood, 1990;29–52.

52 Boruchoff SA. Hypotension and cardiac arrest in rats after infusion of mono(2-ethylhexyl)phthalate (MEHP), a contaminant of stored blood. *N Engl J Med* 1987; **316**:1218–9.

53 Aspinall JA, Duffy TD, Saunders MB, et al. The effect of low density polyethylene containers on some hospital-manufactured eye drop formulations. 1. Sorption of phenyl mercuric acetate. *J Clin Hosp Pharm* 1980;**5**:21–9.

54 Cartwright AC. Stability data. In: Cartwright AC, Matthews BR, eds. *International Pharmaceutical Product Registration: Aspects of Quality, Safety and Efficacy.* Chichester: Ellis Horwood, 1994;206–45.

55 Cartwright AC. New chemical active substance products: quality requirements. In: Cartwright AC, Matthews BR, eds. *Pharmaceutical Product Licensing: Requirements for Europe.* Chichester: Ellis Horwood, 1991;54–75.

56 Loftus BT, Nash RA, eds. *Pharmaceutical Process Validation.* New York: Marcel Dekker, 1984.

57 Bochner R. Factors involved in an outbreak of phenytoin intoxication. *J Neurol Sci* 1972;**16**:481.

58 Gibaldi M, Perrier D. *Pharmacokinetics, 2nd edn.* New York: Marcel Dekker, 1982.

59 Florence AT. Generic medicines: a question of quality. In: Wells FO, D'Arcy PF, Harron DWG, eds. *Medicines Responsible Prescribing.* Belfast: Queen's University, 1992;63–83.

60 Rauws AG. Bioequivalence: a European Community regulatory perspective. In: Welling PG, Tse FLS, Dighe SV, eds. *Pharmaceutical Bioequivalence.* New York: Marcel Dekker, 1991;419–42.

61 Dighe SV, Adams WP. Bioequivalence: a United States regulatory perspective. In: Welling PG, Tse FLS, Dighe SV, eds. *Pharmaceutical Bioequivalence.* New York: Marcel Dekker, 1991;347–80.

62 Monkhouse DC, Rhodes CT. *Drug Products for Clinical Trials: An International Guide to Formulation, Production, Quality Control.* New York: Marcel Dekker, 1998.

63 Pocock SJ. *Clinical Trials.* Chichester: John Wiley & Sons, 1983.

64 Anon. *Facts and Statistics for the Pharmaceutical Industry.* London: Association of the British Pharmaceutical Industry, 2001. http://www.abpi.org.uk/statistics.

3 Preclinical safety testing

Lutz Müller and Anke Lühe

F. Hoffmann-La Roche Ltd, Non-clinical Drug Safety, Basel, Switzerland

3.1 Introduction

When developing a potential new pharmaceutical compound, the primary objectives are to demonstrate that under the conditions of therapy, the potential new drug is of constant chemical quality, is effective in a significant proportion of patients and is safe. Concerning safety, regulatory agencies need to be assured that the benefits of a new medicine outweigh the risks of therapy. Thus, toxicologists have to assist clinicians in determining the likely range of safe exposures to the new pharmaceutical in appropriate animal and *in vitro* models and the possible consequences if these doses are exceeded. It is an advantage if biomarkers (early response surrogate markers for toxicity, ideally preceding toxicity at lower doses or earlier with regard to duration of treatment) can be identified to indicate when safety limits have been breached, but before significant damage has occurred. Such biomarkers allow monitoring of volunteers and patients in early controlled clinical trials to help identify safe exposures. Damage can be immediate and affect vital body functions, thus constituting concerns even for short-term human studies or use. Animal testing for such normally reversible damage is generally addressed in safety pharmacology and acute toxicity studies. Other types of damage include more complex disruption of body systems, often involving multiple organs, resulting in lost or impaired function. Such damage can be reversible or irreversible and it may only be observed after repeated and prolonged dosing; it may appear by degrees with slow onset or it may occur suddenly and precipitously. Toxicity can be observed in reproductive systems

and/or in the developing embryo/fetus, while other changes can result in the formation of tumours. In humans, such tumours can develop decades after the initial exposure – there can be a long latent period. Tumours can result from damage to specific genes involved in cell division (genotoxic carcinogens) or through a variety of mechanisms, such as prolonged hormonal disruption, which do not involve direct damage to genes (non-genotoxic). The risks to patients differ between these two types of mechanism in that genotoxic carcinogens are deemed to have no threshold for their effects, whereas most non-genotoxic carcinogens have an exposure threshold below which there is little risk, but risks increase once the threshold has been exceeded. Tumour development and changes to the developing embryo are typical examples for toxicities that are considered non-reversible in general and need to be avoided in volunteers and patients with rigid and highly sensitive animal testing even at the expense of dropping potentially valuable compounds if relevance of animal data for the human situation is not perfectly clear.

Clinicians and regulators need to be reassured that information concerning all of these aspects is available to enable clinical trials to start and progress to ultimately support regulatory decisions on whether a new drug can be approved for marketing. Preclinical studies of potential new medicines were relatively superficial until several disasters had occurred, in particular the thalidomide catastrophe in the 1960s, where exposure to this compound during early pregnancy resulted in limb deformities in developing embryos. Today there are national and international regulations that require manufacturers to provide information from a detailed package of preclinical studies. The timing and composition of these studies is linked to the type and extent of clinical trials that need to be supported. Thus, early clinical studies were

The Textbook of Pharmaceutical Medicine. Edited by John P. Griffin. © 2009, ISBN: 978-1-4051-8035-1.

considered very safe until in March 2006, when several volunteers experienced severe immunological reactions when being first treated with TGN1412, a CD28 antibody,[1] which, in hindsight, had been administered at too high a dose. Subsequently, the requirements for dose setting for first human trials were partly revised, in particular for investigational compounds for which severe side effects based on pharmacology can occur and for which there is limited ability to assess this pharmacology, in particular immunological properties, in animal models.

Most regulatory toxicity studies are conducted in animals to identify possible hazards from which an assessment of risk to humans is made by extrapolation with information on absorption, distribution, metabolism and elimination (ADME). Hazard in this context is regarded as the potential for a substance to cause harm, whereas risk is the likelihood that, under the conditions of use, it will cause harm. Comparison between the results of compound exposure in animals and humans has shown that such extrapolations, although by no means perfect, are credible in most cases.[2,3] In an attempt to offset some species differences, regulatory agencies request studies in a rodent (usually the rat, although mice are required for specific studies) and a non-rodent species. Dogs or non-human primates are most often used and rabbits are required for particular reproductive toxicology studies. In this context, the use of rabbits dates back to the thalidomide disaster, a case, in which only rabbits have been shown to be a sufficiently sensitive animal species to detect malformations that occurred in human embryos and children. Other rodents and non-rodents may be selected if deemed more appropriate for studying a specific compound. This choice may be based on the results of comparative metabolism, where metabolism in a particular species may more closely resemble that seen or predicted in humans, or the desired pharmacology in a particular species may be more applicable to humans than in other species. Often the choice by default has been limited to the rat and the dog, in the absence of data that would allow a more informed choice. However, it is hoped that the advent of new technologies such as toxicogenomics (differential gene expression)[4]; toxicoproteomics (protein expression profiles)[5]; metabonomics or metabolomics (study of endogenous metabolites in body fluids and tissues, using analytical techniques such as nuclear magnetic resonance)[6] together with characterization of receptors and receptor distribution, will allow better informed selection of possibly a single relevant species only in the future.

Jacobs[7] has recently published an interesting US Food and Drug Administration (FDA) perspective on the use of X-Omics technologies in the safety assessment of new drugs.

Adverse events affecting patients taking a medicine can occur with various degrees of frequency. For a serious adverse event, frequencies of greater than 1 patient affected per 10,000 treated or even 1 in 50,000 can be unacceptable. It is not possible or ethical to use animals in these sorts of numbers. In order to compensate for this it is assumed that increasing the dose and prolonging the duration of exposure will improve both the sensitivity and predictivity of these tests. Thus, a 6-month study at higher doses gives a greater comfort level to regulatory authorities than a 1-month study at lower doses. This is not necessarily based on scientific fact and again it is hoped that the new tools described above, plus a greater knowledge of genetics, will allow the identification of early events induced by lower doses that will be predictive of toxic events in human populations and thus reduce the reliance on animal testing. Nevertheless, it is clear that animal testing is not always capable of predicting human risk. This is important for sometimes serious human side effects that occur with a low incidence. In humans, such effects often occur independent of dose and very often involve the immune system. Because such events are hard to predict and a cause–effect relationship is not easy to determine, the term 'idiosyncratic' is generally used for these types of toxicities. Thus, it is self-evident that 'idiosyncratic' toxicities are major causes of late stage failures in drug development or post-marketing withdrawals. In this context, it may be useful to remind ourselves of evaluations that late stage and marketing failures of drugs because of rare human toxicities are highly significantly related to two aspects: cardiac ventricular arrhythmia[8] and liver toxicity.[9] Toxicologists have tried to devise useful models to better predict such toxicities with specific test approaches and regulatory agencies have issued draft guidance approaches to tackle this problem.

Toxicological evaluation of drug candidates is one of the most prominent areas of animal use nowadays. From an ethical point of view, toxicologists always have to bear animal rights in mind when designing appropriate safety testing programmes. Russell and Burch[10] propounded the concept of the three R's in relation to use of animals in research: reduction of animal use; refinement of testing that requires fewer animals; and replacement of animal studies by *in vitro* methods. This concept is becoming more integrated into mainstream research as better tools are now available to allow this approach to become much more of a reality. European regulatory law bans the use of animals if the required knowledge can be gained by other means.

Preclinical safety testing of pharmaceuticals is subject to thorough regulatory review. Regulatory agencies around the world have issued guidelines, which lay down their expectations of a thorough testing and assessment programme. In the past, these guidelines were very diverse and not necessarily consistent with each other. This often has led to repetition of animal experiments. This was recognized as a hindrance to innovation and animal rights. For more than 15 years now, the International Conference on Harmonization of Technical Requirements for Registration of Pharmaceuticals for Human Use (ICH) has issued guidelines, which are applicable for both industry and regulatory authorities. The process started in the three major economical regions (the EU, the USA and Japan), but many other countries and regions have either adopted the ICH guidelines or are following them. ICH guidelines in the preclinical safety areas are abbreviated as 'ICH S' guidelines. Multidisciplinary guidelines are termed 'ICH M' guidelines. When new scientific knowledge is generated, existing ICH guidelines undergo a so-called maintenance process. Revised ICH guidelines are recognizable by the letter 'R'. The ICH process of generating guidelines and ensuring their international acceptance has been a major international success story. The industry can rely on regulatory consistency and animal experiments can be conducted in a way that avoids unnecessary repetition. Important additional guidelines have been issued by the Committee on Human Medicinal Products (CHMP) of the EU and from the US FDA. The safety guidelines can be found on the respective ICH website or on the websites of the regional regulatory agencies (see references for their internet addresses). Most of the principles of preclinical safety testing that are laid down in this chapter are referring to ICH, CHMP and FDA guidelines.

3.1.1 The 'omic technologies

A brief description only of these emerging technologies is given below; the reader is referred to the referenced reviews for more details. A balanced view of the use of these technologies in toxicology is given by Lynch and Connelly.[11] At present these techniques are not part of mandatory regulatory toxicology, but are being used increasingly to provide supplementary

and supportive data alongside the required studies. The US FDA is strongly encouraging voluntary exploratory data submission (VXDS) of data generated using 'omic' technologies in order to build up and further develop the experience with techniques, analysis, interpretation and limitations of such data on both sides, the FDA as well as the sponsors. In case data derived from 'omic' technologies are used for supporting decisions pertaining to the conduct of pivotal non-clinical or clinical trials or to support scientific argumentation related to, for example, the dose selection, effectiveness or mechanism of action of a drug, the FDA requests submission of either full or abbreviated reports (FDA Guidance for Industry Pharmacogenomic Data Submissions, March 2005). Some useful aspects on how to implement this guidance have also been provided by the FDA.[12] In addition, helpful information on the submission of 'omic' data can also be found in another publication by the FDA where they shared their experiences in the review of three different 'mock submissions' provided by the pharmaceutical industry.[13] These 'mock submissions' were independent from any ongoing or future drug application and were used to evaluate quality, format and content of voluntary genomic data submissions especially on the basis of the MIAME (minimal information about a microarray experiment) and MINTox (minimum information needed for a toxicology experiment) principles as outlined in a proposal of the Microarray Gene Expression Data Society.[14]

3.1.1.1 Toxicogenomics or transcriptomics

This technology allows the simultaneous monitoring of either a small number of selected messenger RNAs (mRNA) from cells and tissues or assessment of transcriptional changes of essentially all genes in a genome. As mRNA expression reflects the rate of transcription of the corresponding gene, this gives insight to what genes or which pathways are being upregulated in expression, downregulated or whose expression is not changed following a given treatment or in a particular disease state. Thus, cells or tissues can be monitored before and after exposure to a toxin to determine the cells response to the toxin. From this information patterns of gene expression or, in rare cases, single gene changes can be linked to specific types of toxicity (e.g. liver toxicity, kidney toxicity, carcinogenicity), or to potential mechanisms of toxicity such as oxidative stress, apoptosis and necrosis.[15] In addition, biomarkers for specific toxicities may be identified which can be used for the purpose of monitoring for specific toxicities in upcoming preclinical or clinical studies. An overview of the possible applications and limitations of toxicogenomics in the development of a new drug candidate can be found in Lühe et al.[16]

3.1.1.2 Toxicoproteomics

Compared to the genome, the proteome (the entire diverse protein content of a cell) is a far more dynamic system. Proteins undergo post-translational modifications such as phosphorylation, glycosylation and sulphation, as well as cleavage for specific proteins.[17] These alterations determine protein activity, localisation and turnover. All are subject to change following a toxic insult and in some ways the study of proteins holds more promise than the study of gene expression as they are nearer to key activities in the cell.

Several techniques have been used to display protein profiles [e.g. the proteins can be separated by two-dimensional poly-acrylamide gel electrophoresis (2D-PAGE)]. Differentially expressed or modified proteins associated with treatment may be identified by their absence or by the appearance of new spots on the gel followed by isoelectric focusing in the first dimension and molecular weight separation in the second. Proteins can be identified from historical data or by excising the spots followed by peptide cleavage and sequencing. Matrix-assisted laser desorption/ionisation (MALDI) mass spectrometry is being used increasingly to identify the spectrum of peptides.[18] This area is developing quickly, but technical challenges remain to identify important low abundance proteins, which are often masked on gels by high abundance proteins.[19] Protein chips coated with specific surfaces to identify protein classes (e.g. Ciphergen's SELDI ProteinChip system) are also of interest. Recently, the first human protein arrays containing up to 8000 human proteins have been made available for the market (e.g. Invitrogen's ProtoArray Human Protein Microarray System). In contrast to 2D-PAGE technology, the application of these protein microarrays are slightly different. Whereas 2D-PAGE with subsequent MALDI or SELDI analysis allows the identification of unknown differentially expressed proteins, protein microarrays are used to study protein–protein interactions or for investigation of the specificity of antibodies.[20]

These 'omic technologies have yielded a wealth of new potential biomarkers for different types of toxicity over the last few years. One of the challenges now is to select the most promising biomarkers and to validate them appropriately in order to enable their application on a routine basis. One technique that is worth mentioning in this context are tissue micro-arrays (TMA). TMAs consist of up to several hundred tissue cores of approximately 1 mm in diameter that are positioned on an array. Specific changes in mRNA or protein expression in these tissue cores can subsequently be investigated by *in situ* hybridization or immunohistochemistry and intracellular localization of expression changes can be determined. Although representing a useful tool for the validation of biomarkers, major drawbacks of this technique remain: the successful application of TMAs depends on the availability of reliable antibodies and the selected tissue cores may not be representative for the remaining tissue or organ.[21]

3.1.1.3 Metabonomics

Metabonomics, in the context of this chapter, aims to define the status and dynamic changes of the endogenous metabolite profile in biofluids or tissues of animals or in *in vitro* systems in response to toxic insults. The most commonly applied methodology is ^{1}H nuclear magnetic resonance (NMR) spectroscopy, which yields a spectrum describing all relatively low molecular weight metabolites such as lipids, amino acids and carbohydrates (typically up to ~1000 kDa) in studied materials.[22] Study of biological fluids such as urine is attractive as it is non-invasive and can allow real time measurements to be made including those that can occur in recovery from a toxicity.

Successful applications of metabonomics include the identification of lyso-*bis*-phosphatidic acid in biofluids from rats treated with amiodarone (a cationic amphiphilic compound) as a potential biomarker for phospholipidosis as well as the identification of a 'metabolic fingerprint profile' in the urine of rats treated with different peroxisome proliferator-activated receptor (PPAR) agonists that mapped to the tryptophan pathway and may have potential as a biomarker for peroxisome proliferation.[23]

With all of these methods, understanding what is the 'normal' spectrum and also separating adaptive changes following changes in physiology brought about by dietary or diurnal changes, from true toxicity-related changes, is paramount.[24]

3.1.1.4 Bioinformatics

The 'omic technologies above produce massive amounts of data. The analysis of these data is a huge challenge and requires complex statistical analysis to identify key changes through pattern recognition and pathway analysis. In addition, large databases of historical data are needed to make the most of any findings. There are some major initiatives in progress to allow the integration of the data from these technologies together with biological networks and traditional fields such as pathology and clinical chemistry. These initiatives include efforts by regulatory authorities such as the ArrayTrack software developed at FDA's National Center for Toxicological Research (NCTR) and providing a means of management, analysis and interpretation of quality-checked microarray data.[25] In addition, the PredTox group of the InnoMed Initiative (IMI) has developed a database integrating 'omics', histopath, clinical pathology, TMAs and in-life data enabling queries across 'omic' and traditional toxicology study endpoints.[26] These projects are clearly a first step towards an integrated 'systems view' of toxicology and have the potential to revolutionise the field of preclinical safety assessment.

3.1.1.5 Current collaborative efforts to enhance predictivity of animal safety testing for humans

While animal safety testing has made the development of medicines for humans safe and effective, it has been recognized that important aspects of human toxicity are not fully covered yet. In this context, two recent collaborative efforts for the generation of more predictive data for human safety have to be mentioned. The FDA aims to increase the number of non-clinical biomarkers of safety through the Predictive Safety Testing Consortium, a public–private partnership led by the non-profit Critical Path Institute. In the EU, the joint industry and regulatory Predictive Toxicity consortium under the umbrella of the IMI is looking at what combination of 'omic' technologies deliver the best predictive results for hepatotoxicity and/or nephrotoxicity (http://www.innomed-predtox.com). Within the IMI, an important project is on *in silico* toxicity prediction (http://

imi.europa.eu/calls-01_en.html). In part, the IMI *in silico* prediction aims to address one of the biggest gaps in drug safety knowledge, that there is no single database with historical proprietary safety data for companies to predict the effect of a chemical structure based on what is already known. Companies will be able to compare their chemical structures with the database and make a prediction on various types of toxicity including hepatotoxicity or nephrotoxicity.

3.1.2 The drug development process

The usual sequence of events in the modern drug development process is shown in Figure 3.1. There is an increasing focus on trying to select more easily developable molecules at an early stage, so that the chance of failure at the very expensive later phases is minimised. Pharmaceutical companies therefore decide on which properties of a new molecule are key to faster development; for example, selection of soluble compounds or their salt forms for good oral bioavailability or to facilitate bioavailability of hardly soluble compounds by suitable formulation approaches including excipients. Amongst these is the selection of molecules with low or acceptable toxicity. Thus, a company may decide to develop high-throughput *in vitro* screens for cytotoxicity for use at the lead optimisation stage. Certainly by the 'candidate selection' stage, where there may be three or four possible candidates of which only one may go forward, there is a need for reassurance regarding toxicity to help in the selection process. Thus, companies may decide to screen for 'show-stopping' toxicities; for example, effects on cardiovascular parameters such as severe electrophysiology changes, genetic toxicity and also a preliminary screen for whole animal toxicology in the rat or mouse, in which three doses may be tested in five animals per group, dosing for a

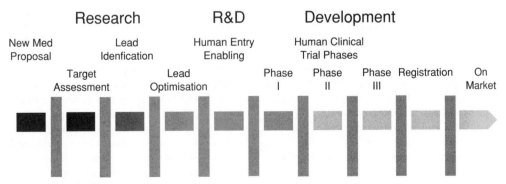

Figure 3.1 Drug development process.

short period of up to 14 days, depending on the target characteristics and compound availability. This would be expected to flag up marked toxicities and allow ranking or elimination of specific candidates. The same compounds would also go through screens in other preclinical functions (e.g. pharmacy, drug metabolism and pharmacokinetics) and the information pooled, along with the likely cost of manufacturing the compounds by the chemical synthesis routes identified. All of this information is considered in selecting a compound to go forward to the more regulatory defined activities, where the costs escalate rapidly and thus the cost of failure of a compound becomes very significant. Typical for these types of activities is their exploratory character. This means that the tests do not necessarily comply with regulatory expectations of Good Laboratory Practice documentation. Dedicated testing for regulatory compliance is generally conducted only on the selected clinical candidate.

The newer technologies (e.g. genomics, proteomics) also offer the possibility of developing specific screens for those compounds possessing undesirable toxicity (e.g. the ability to induce oxidative damage, mitochondrial toxicity, endocrine disruption, interference with cell cycle kinases), which can be used to filter out possible toxic compounds at an early stage. Molecular biology is also providing opportunities (e.g. antisense probes, knockout mice) for exploring the receptors chosen as drug targets and discovering at an early stage if changes in such targets result in toxicological liabilities.[27]

3.1.3 Risk–benefit

The regulatory toxicology programme (which supports clinical trials and registration of compounds) runs in parallel with the clinical programme. Single-dose studies in healthy volunteers (phase I studies) require less toxicological support than multiple doses in patients with disease characteristics. There are four phases of the clinical programme (Box 3.1). As the programme progresses through the various phases several things change:

1. The treated population changes from healthy volunteers in phase I to patients specific to the diseased target population in phase II. This is true with a few exceptions, such as in oncology. Here, end stage tumour patients will often be treated with compounds that possess intrinsic toxicities to explore a balance between toxicity and efficacious doses.

2. The duration of exposure to the drug can increase from a single dose in phase I to prolonged repeated dosing for drugs being developed for chronic therapy.

BOX 3.1 Phases of the clinical programme

Phase I
Initial studies in humans to determine tolerance and the safe dosage range and to give an indication to metabolic handling. These studies are usually undertaken with healthy volunteers but may be extended to include patients. Humans exposed: 30–50

Phase II
Early controlled trials in a limited number of patients under closely monitored conditions to show efficacy and short-term safety. These studies will typically also include studies for drug-drug interaction. Humans exposed: 250–500

Phase III
Extended large-scale trials to obtain additional evidence of efficacy and safety, and definition of adverse effects. Humans exposed: several hundred to several thousand

Phase IV
Postmarketing surveillance occurs after the clinical trials programme is complete. It is used to collect adverse event data from a large patient population. Humans exposed: 10,000+

Adapted from Scales, 1990.[28]

---

3. Men are usually the volunteers in phase I and women enter the programme typically in phase II (unless a female-specific medicine is being developed or there is an indication that there may be important gender-specific effects).

4. The monitoring of volunteers/patients becomes less strict throughout the programme. A volunteer in phase I will stay in a clinic and be very closely monitored for any signs of toxicity, whereas a patient in a phase III trial may only be required to return to their physician periodically.

5. The strict control on administration of a drug often changes as it switches from the investigating physician to the patient. Thus, in phase I the drug is administered by the physician whereas in phase III a patient may be sent home with a pack of tablets and instructed to take two a day.

6. The number of people exposed gradually increases.

The hazard to the population therefore increases throughout the trial process as more people are given greater cumulative amounts of the drug in a less controlled and monitored manner. However, with each additional patient treated the clinical experience with the drug is also increasing, providing a greater safety data base in the most relevant species (i.e. humans).

The risk to the individual should therefore decrease as the clinical programme progresses. However, as the numbers of individuals in early stages of clinical trials is low and the numbers of animals studied in toxicology studies are limited, more extensive clinical exposure in later stages of clinical trials may reveal evidence for more, but seldom occurring, potentially problematic types of toxicity. Even more importantly, evidence for such toxicities may not emerge until after marketing authorisation has been granted and even more patients have been treated. In general, this phenomenon is referred to as 'idiosyncratic' toxicity.

It should be noted that the reliance on animal toxicity data changes throughout clinical development. The safety or comfort factor before initial dosing in humans is based largely on general toxicity in animals (i.e. single- or repeated-dose studies), plus safety pharmacology studies measuring pharmacologically mediated adverse effects on vital systems (i.e. respiratory, cardiovascular and central nervous systems) and genetic toxicity studies. Human safety data rapidly reduce the reliance on information based on general toxicity studies in animals. This is not the case, however, for the teratogenic or oncogenic potential of the drug, which will be based on preclinical data for many years even after the drug is marketed.

Box 3.2 shows the toxicity package typically generated before a phase I trial. These trials are usually conducted in males, and thus do not require formal reproductive toxicity studies. In the USA, women can be included in early trials without any animal reproductive toxicity if special precautions are taken to ensure that pregnancy does not occur. An histopathological assessment of the effects of the test compound on the male reproductive tract is made in the repeat-dose toxicity tests.

In a human volunteer study there is obviously no benefit to the individual except perhaps a small financial gain. There is, of course, risk but this is minimised by the small amounts of drug that are administered and the careful monitoring of the volunteer for any adverse signs caused by the drug. Later in the programme, when treating patients who are suffering from a disease, there is a possible, but unproven, benefit that they may be cured or symptoms may be alleviated. Obviously, for incurable, life-threatening or debilitating conditions such as AIDS, some cancers and severe rheumatoid arthritis, a much higher level of risk (i.e. possible toxicity) is acceptable than for other less serious conditions. This is why some cancer chemotherapy, as well as being highly toxic to dividing cells, may in itself be carcinogenic. But any risk for

---

> **BOX 3.2** Basic package of data for phase I trials
>
> 1. *Safety pharmacology* – indication of adverse pharmacologically mediated actions on central nervous, cardiovascular and respiratory systems
> 2. *Pharmacokinetics* – preliminary studies on absorption, distribution, metabolism and excretion
> 3. *Acute toxicity information* – two species either assessed directly or by inference from data of the highest tolerable doses in range finding studies. Usually an evaluation of the maximum repeatable dose (MRD) and possibly local irritancy
> 4. *Repeat-dose toxicity* – rodent and non-rodent species are required. The duration of the test depends on the duration of clinical exposure but many companies conduct two 14-day studies before going into humans. Studies should be performed using the proposed clinical route and at least one species should be a pharmacologically responsive species that expresses the target pathway of the investigational drug
> 5. *Reproductive toxicology* – usually embryo/fetal development studies in two species are required in Europe and Japan if women of child-bearing potential are included. Not required in the USA for some early trials
> 6. *Mutagenicity* – tests for mutagenicity and chromosome damage

---

induction of secondary cancers from the treatment can be tolerated mainly because of the relatively short life expectancies of cancer patients. The various safety studies, from those that are necessary to evaluate the risk of exposing the first human to those required by regulatory authorities in order to market a medicine, are essential elements of a fundamental ICH guideline. This guideline, *Guidance on Non-clinical Safety Studies for the Conduct of Human Clinical Trials and Marketing Authorization for Pharmaceuticals* ('ICH M3', with M as an abbreviation of 'multidisciplinary'), is one of the most important ICH guidelines in that it gives guidance to industry about the expectations of the regulatory agencies on the extent and duration of non-clinical safety studies to cover the various stages of clinical trials.

3.1.4 Good Laboratory Practice

It is important to ensure the quality and reliability of safety studies. This is normally assured by following Good Laboratory Practice regulations.[29] Any deviation from this must be justified.

3.2 Preclinical safety pharmacology

3.2.1 Introduction

Once a compound, or a small series of compounds, has been identified as a potential development candidate, preclinical safety pharmacology studies are considered. It has been estimated that about 75% of acute adverse drug reactions (ADRs) in humans can potentially be predicted by primary, secondary and safety pharmacology studies.[30] Such studies are single-dose studies in animals to determine whether the chosen candidates have (as opposed to frank toxicological) side effects that affect pivotal organ systems in an acute manner and hence would preclude or limit their initial evaluation in humans and hence also impact on their therapeutic use. Because these studies give an indication of potential safety margins after acute doses, it is generally the C_{max} and not the total exposure that is driving the safety margin considerations. Safety pharmacology studies measure the pharmacodynamic actions of drug candidates on vital cardiovascular, respiratory and central nervous systems. There may be concerns that would extend such studies to other systems (e.g. kidney, gastrointestinal tract). The outcome of safety pharmacology studies will generally influence the setting of a safe starting dose for first human volunteer studies, and will give an idea about maximum tolerated doses and what kind of side effects to expect in the first single or repeat-dose human trials for tolerability. In case of severe concerns regarding human pivotal organ system function, studies in humans may nevertheless begin but an online monitoring of human exposure may be warranted including setting a ceiling for human dose/exposure.

3.2.2 Regulatory guidelines

An ICH guideline was agreed in November 2000. This guideline replaces any previous guidance for safety pharmacology studies to register pharmaceuticals in the USA, EU and Japan. This guideline was complemented by a specific guideline on non-clinical studies for delayed ventricular repolarization (QT prolongation) as of 2005.

When deciding on the specific tests to perform on a new chemical entity, the following factors should be considered:

1. Mechanism of action, as adverse effects can be associated with desired effects (e.g. anti-arrhythmic agents in some circumstances can be pro-arrhythmic).
2. Class-specific effects [e.g. disturbances of normal electrocardiogram (ECG) associated with many antipsychotics].

3. Ligand binding or enzyme assay data may suggest a potential for adverse events.

3.2.3 General considerations

When selecting the relevant test models, factors to consider include the pharmacodynamic responses of the model (e.g. changes in blood pressure), pharmacokinetic profile (e.g. differences in adsorption, distribution, metabolism and elimination), species, strain, sex and age of the experimental animals, the susceptibility, sensitivity and reproducibility of the test system, and available background data on the substance. *In vitro* systems, including isolated organs and tissues, cell cultures, cellular fragments, subcellular organelles, receptors, ion channels, can also provide valuable information. These can identify potential problems and also help to define mechanisms of effects seen *in vivo*.

In vivo studies are preferably carried out using unrestrained, not anaesthetised animals. Animals can be fitted with transmitters that allow data to be collected by telemetry. As for all animal studies, avoidance or minimisation of pain and discomfort is an important consideration. Information from the toxicological battery of studies, if they have been adequately designed to address safety pharmacology endpoints, can result in reduction or elimination of separate safety pharmacology studies.

3.2.4 Experimental design

3.2.4.1 Controls

Appropriate controls should be used [e.g. test systems exposed to the vehicle in which the test compound has been dissolved or suspended (negative control)]. The new ICH guideline also suggests that in some cases a compound known to have an adverse effect in a specific test system (positive control) should be used.

3.2.4.2 Route

In general, the expected clinical route of administration should be used when feasible. Regardless of route, exposure to the parent compound and its major metabolites should be similar or greater than that observed in humans. Because safety pharmacology studies are carried out before human studies are initiated, this may have to be inferred from information derived from *in vitro* studies; for example, with human hepatocytes and/or from information from similar compounds that have been used in humans. In some cases, early low-dose human studies may show that significant metabolites are formed in humans but were not formed in the animals used in safety pharmacology studies. In these circumstances, further studies will be needed in animals using isolated or chemically synthesised human metabolites.

3.2.4.3 Dose levels *in vivo*

It is necessary to define the dose–response relationship of any adverse effects observed. The onset and duration of effects should be measured. Because there are differences in sensitivity between species, the doses chosen need to exceed those expected to be used therapeutically. The ICH guideline states that the highest dose tested should be one that produces moderate adverse effects (e.g. dose-limiting pharmacodynamic effects or other toxicities). Such effects should not be so severe that they confound the interpretation of the results being sought. In this context, safety pharmacology studies are normally not conducted to similarly high dose levels as standard toxicity studies. Dose–effect relationships may not follow usual patterns of increase with dose. Instead, saturation on receptors may produce bell-shaped dose–effect relationships, which should not be missed when extrapolating animal data for human safe dosing regimes. Safety pharmacology studies are generally performed by administration of single doses rather than repeated dosing but repeat-dose approaches can be helpful in cases in which an acute effect is expected to attenuate over time. For first human trials this can be very helpful information (e.g. an activation of the autonomic nervous system can be a primary reaction towards treatment but may disappear with repeated treatment).

3.2.4.4 Dose levels *in vitro*

As for *in vivo* studies, it is necessary to establish a concentration–effect relationship. The upper limit of concentrations tested may be influenced by physicochemical properties of the test substance and other factors such as cytotoxicity. In such *in vitro* studies, it is generally desired to obtain a sufficient margin between the concentrations of a test item that produces a desired interaction with the pharmacological target versus the concentrations that can impact on targets relevant for pivotal organ system function.

3.2.5 Safety pharmacology core battery

The preliminary focus of safety pharmacology studies is to measure the effects of the test substance on the cardiovascular, respiratory and central nervous systems.

3.2.5.1 Central nervous system

The ICH guideline lists assessment of the effects of the test compound on motor activity, behavioural changes, coordination and sensory/motor reflex responses. A so-called functional observation battery[31] or Irwin's battery[32] will cover these parameters. Effects on body temperature should also be measured.

3.2.5.2 Cardiovascular system

The ICH guideline lists the assessment of effects on blood pressure, heart rate and ECG. *In vivo*, *in vitro* and/or *ex vivo* evaluations, including methods for electrical repolarisation and conductance abnormalities, should also be considered. These abnormalities can be associated with risks for fatal ventricular arrhythmias [e.g. torsade de pointes (TdP)].

In recent years, pro-arrhythmic properties of some non-cardiovascular drugs received particular regulatory and pharmaceutical industry attention because it was recognized that the highest frequency of drug withdrawals from the market was attributable to a single adverse drug reaction (i.e. fatal ventricular tachyarrhythmias of the TdP type).[33,34] Per definition, the underlying cause for the development of TdP is a delayed cardiac repolarization which can be determined as the prolongation of the QT-interval on the surface ECG.[35] Most if not all of the non-anti-arrhythmic agents associated with the liability to induce TdP prolong the QT-interval with the same mechanism, namely block of the potassium current conducted by the channel encoded by the human ether-a-go-go related gene (hERG).[36] In reaction to accumulating issues in clinical trials and post-marketing events in this area, in 1997 a regulatory 'points to consider' document was issued by the European Committee for Proprietary Medical Products (CPMP, now called the CHMP). This document describes the use of *in vitro* and *ex vivo* test systems for measuring disturbances in electrophysiology.

In 2005, an ICH guideline has been issued entitled *ICH S7B, Note for Guidance on Safety Pharmacology Studies for assessing the Potential for Delayed Ventricular Repolarization (QT Interval Prolongation) by Human Pharmaceuticals*. The core study required by the draft guidelines is an *in vivo* study in telemetered non-rodents to measure ECG changes in the presence of the test compound. This draft guideline also discusses the use of tests for changes in electrophysiology. For example, the guideline discusses the use of hERG potassium (IKr rectifier channel) models. These models use isolated cells (e.g. Chinese hamster ovary cells or human HEK293 cells) that contain cloned hERG genes.[37]

3.2.5.3 Respiratory system
The ICH guideline mentions measurements of airway resistance, airway compliance, tidal volume and blood gases.

3.2.5.4 Supplementary safety pharmacology studies
The core battery of studies should be carried out before a substance is administered to humans for the first time. Any follow-up or supplementary safety pharmacology studies should be carried out if there is a cause for concern raised from the toxicological battery of tests and/or from studies in humans.

Novel centrally acting drugs may need to be tested for abuse potential (see also section 3.8.4.5). Primate self-administration tests may be used preclinically to assess abuse potential. However, it should be borne in mind that regulatory authorities such as the US FDA give more weight to negative evidence of abuse potential from clinical assessment (e.g. in experienced drug abusers) than to negative evidence from animal studies.

Investigation of potential adverse interactions with drugs likely to be co-prescribed with the test drug may also be required. A generalised approach, such as the determination of effects on hepatic drug metabolising enzymes, may be sufficient but in most cases a number of drug-specific interaction studies will also be required.

The effects of the drug on the duration of loss of the righting reflex (sleeping time) in mice pretreated with pentobarbital can be used as a broad screen for detecting effects on hepatic drug metabolism. At the relatively high dose used in this test, pentobarbital is a substrate for a large range of hepatic enzymes. Although sedative actions of drugs can increase sleeping time, unlike hepatic enzyme inhibitors, sedative drugs also potentiate loss of righting reflex induced by barbitone, which is excreted unchanged.

3.3 Single-dose studies

Historically, acute toxicity information has been obtained from single-dose toxicity studies in two mammalian species using both the clinical and a parenteral route of administration. Such studies were generally required to evaluate effects that may result from acute exposure to the maximum non-lethal dose and predict effects of over-dosage in humans. However, according to recent developments in the area of the pivotal ICH guideline that describes the studies needed to cover human clinical trials (the ICH M3 guideline), such information can be obtained from appropriately conducted dose escalation studies or short-duration dose ranging studies that define a maximum tolerated dose in the general toxicity test species. It is also proposed that equally appropriate studies include those that achieve large exposure multiples [e.g. 50-fold the clinical C_{max} or area under the curve (AUC) at the intended human dose], achieve saturation of exposure or use the maximum feasible dose. In all cases, a limit dose of 2000 mg/kg/day in rodents and 1000 mg/kg/day in non-rodents is considered appropriate for acute, subchronic and chronic toxicity studies. When this acute toxicity information is available from any study, separate single-dose studies are not recommended.

3.3.1 Study design
3.3.1.1 Preliminary studies
Groups of four animals (two of each sex) are given a single dose of the test material. For oral dosing studies, animals are not deprived of food overnight before dosing. Groups are treated sequentially, the dosage for each stage being based on the response of the previous group, until the highest dose that does not cause deaths [maximum non-lethal dose (MNLD)] is determined. Animals killed for humane reasons are considered as drug-induced deaths. Animals are observed for 7 days, during which time clinical observations and body weights are recorded. At termination, animals undergo a full macroscopic examination and any unusual abnormalities are examined microscopically.

3.3.1.2 Definitive studies
Groups of 20 animals (10 of each sex) are dosed at the MNLD determined in the preliminary study. Control animals are included only when an unusual vehicle is present in the test formulation or if target organ toxicity is anticipated. Five animals of each sex are observed for 48 h and are then killed for autopsy to allow evaluation of early pathological changes. The remaining five animals of each sex are observed for 14 days before autopsy to evaluate any delayed toxicity that may occur and to assess recovery from early onset changes. Clinical observations and body weight measurements are made during the observation period. At termination, full macroscopic examination and microscopic examination of limited tissues (usually heart, lungs, liver, kidneys, spleen and any tissues related to route of administration tissues) is performed. Blood levels of the drug are not usually determined, as often an assay is still to be developed.

Systemic exposure can be approximated, however, using a scaling model (see section 3.8.5).

Only limited interpretation of the results of single-dose studies is possible. The MNLD can be determined and target organs can be identified. Frequently, death can occur as a result of the exaggerated pharmacological action of the compound and often no target organ toxicity is seen in drug-induced deaths. However, such studies give an indication of what may happen with massive acute over-dosage in the clinic.

3.4 Repeat-dose studies

The duration of repeat-dose animal studies to support both clinical trials and marketing applications is given in Tables 3.1 and 3.2, which are taken from the revised 'ICH M3(R)' guideline on the timing of *Non-Clinical Safety Studies for the Conduct of Human Clinical Trials for Pharmaceuticals*, as of June 2009.

Repeat-dose toxicity studies should be performed in a rodent, typically the rat, and a non-rodent of which at least one species should be responsive to the target pathway on which the investigational drug acts on. The longer the duration of human exposure the longer must be the duration of the toxicity studies. The ICH guideline builds on the general principle that for clinical trials of up to 6 months, the clinical duration can equal the duration of the toxicity studies in all regions. For longer clinical trials, generally those in phase III, a maximum duration of 6 months in rodents and, in general, 9 months in non-rodents is applicable. Filing for registration needs support with study durations as per Table 3.2. For example, application for registration of an antibiotic, which is not used in humans for longer than 4 weeks, needs to be supported by 3-month toxicity study in rodents and non-rodents.

The doses for the definitive repeat-dose studies are usually based on preliminary dose escalating studies. The design of such studies varies between companies. Spurling and Carey[38] have published a study design that allows the maximum amount of both toxicological and kinetic data to be obtained by using a minimum number of animals. The highly predictive nature of these maximum repeatable dose (MRD)

Table 3.1 Duration of repeated-dose toxicity studies to support the conduct of clinical trials in all regions

Maximum duration of clinical trial	Minimum duration of repeated-dose toxicity studies to support clinical trials	
	Rodents	Non-rodents
Up to 2 weeks	2 weeks[a]	2 weeks[a]
Between 2 weeks and 6 months	Same as clinical trial[b]	Same as clinical trial[b]
>6 months	6 months[b,c]	9 months[b,c,d]

[a] In the United States, as an alternative to 2 week studies, extended single-dose toxicity studies can support single-dose human trials. Clinical studies of less than 14 days can be supported with toxicity studies of the same duration as the proposed clinical study.

[b] In some circumstances clinical trials of longer duration than 3 months can be initiated provided the data are available from a 3-month rodent and a 3-month non-rodent study, and that complete data from the chronic rodent and non-rodent study are made available, consistent with local clinical trial regulatory procedures, before extending dosing beyond 3 months in the clinical trial.

For serious or life-threatening indications or on a case-by-case basis, this extension can be based on complete chronic rodent data and in-life and necropsy data for the non-rodent study. Complete histopathology data from the non-rodent should be available within an additional 3 months.

[c] There can be cases where a pediatric population is the primary population, and existing animal studies have identified potential developmental concerns for target organs (toxicology or pharmacology). In these cases long-term toxicity testing starting in juvenile animals can be appropriate.

[d] In the EU, studies of 6 month duration in non-rodents are considered acceptable. However, where studies with a longer duration have been conducted, it is not appropriate to conduct an additional stuey of 6 months.

The following are examples where non-rodent studies of up to 6 month duration can also be appropriate for Japan and the United States: i) When immunogenicity or intolerance confound conduct of longer term studies. ii) Repeated short-term drug exposure even if clinical trial duration exceeds 6 months, such as intermittent treatment of migraine, erectile dysfunction, or herpes simplex. iii) Drugs administered on a chronic basis to reduce the risk of recurrence of cancer. iv) Drugs for indications for which life expectancy is short.

Table 3.2 Duration of repeated-dose toxicity studies to support marketing in all regions

Duration of indicated treatment	Rodent	Non-rodent
Up to 2 weeks	1 month	1 month
>2 weeks to 1 month	3 months	3 months
>1 month to 3 months	6 months	6 months
>3 months	6 months[c]	9 months[c,d]

For footnotes c, and d see Table 3.1.

studies in assessing the outcome of longer duration studies has been established.[39]

Toxicity studies usually follow the sequence: MRD, 2 weeks or 1 month, 3 or 6 months, and 9 months. The choice of duration usually depends on the length of clinical trial to be supported. It should be noted that the ICH guideline for duration of non-rodent species (see footnote to Table 3.1) allows the chronic non-rodent study to be limited to 9 months and nowadays seldom requires a 12-month study (e.g. if a paediatric population is treated). In Europe only, a 6-month non-rodent study is acceptable to support chronic human therapy. It is evident that sometimes chronic toxicity studies can get on the critical path for continuation of clinical trials. Hence, an option is provided to extend a clinical trial to more than 3 months of treatment for serious or life-threatening indications, or on a case-by-case basis, if the non-rodent chronic toxicity study has not been finished. In such cases, in-life and necropsy data from the chronic non-rodent animal study must be provided and the full histopathology data must be available within and additional 3 months. The route of administration should be similar to that employed clinically.

In the early drug development context, it is worthwhile to make reference to considerations of an exploratory clinical strategy, which enables to administer one or several low doses of a pharmaceutical candidate to human volunteers under rather strict conditions. These conditions do not enable dose escalation in human volunteers to the normally explored levels of (in)tolerability in phase I. The EU and the US FDA ('Exploratory IND Studies' as of January 2006) have issued guidelines for such approaches and the new ICH M3(R) guideline also contains various options for an exploratory initial clinical evaluation. The approaches offered to the pharmaceutical industry are characterized by an abbreviated preclinical safety testing program mostly regarding length and dose levels of animal studies to support these exploratory human volunteer studies.

3.4.1 The maximum repeatable dose study

An MRD will be carried out for each species by each route of administration to be used in subsequent repeat-dose toxicity studies. It is usual to conduct an escalating-dose MRD study, in which increasingly larger dosages are administered to the same group of animals every 3–4 days until significant toxicity occurs. The highest dose may then be given for a short period of time in a repeat fashion. However, if local irritancy or target organ toxicity is likely to limit the dose, or if tolerance to repeated dosing is anticipated, a fixed-dose MRD study is more useful. The aims of both types of study are to determine a profile of toxic effects, including target organ toxicity, and to evaluate pharmacokinetic parameters [i.e. to determine evidence of absorption by measuring the time to reach (T_{max}) the maximum plasma concentration (C_{max}) and to provide an indication of exposure by the area under the plasma time–concentration curve (AUC), the plasma elimination half-life ($T^{1}/_2$) and the minimum plasma concentration (C_{min}) after single and repeat doses]. The pharmacokinetic determinations obviously depend on a suitable assay for the drug being available. While in a MRD study in rodents, animals are usually sacrificed at the end of the study and a full histopathological evaluation of organs is carried out, this is not necessarily performed in non-rodents. Hence, non-rodents (dogs, monkeys) may be used for further studies on other compounds after a suitable washout period.

3.4.2 Definitive repeat-dose toxicity studies

The aims of these studies are to further characterise any target organ toxicity identified in earlier studies, to determine any new target organs not seen in earlier studies and to check whether the pharmacokinetics determined in earlier studies are changed and whether dose or exposure levels without evidence for adverse effects are declining over time. Following the dosing period, a number of animals are often retained but undosed to allow for observation of recovery from

Table 3.3 Study design for definitive repeat-dose studies – number of animals of each sex per group

| Group no. | 1 | 2 | 3 | 4 | Total number of |
Group name	Control	Low	Intermediate	High	animals
			1 month toxicity study		
Rat	12(8)	12	12	12(8)	128
Dog/monkey	3(2)	3	3	3(2)	32
			3 month toxicity study		
Rat	16(8)	16	16	16(8)	160
Dog/monkey	3 or 4(2)	3 or 4	3 or 4	3 or 4(2)	32–40
			6 month toxicity study		
Rat	20(12)	20	20	20(12)	208
Dog/monkey	4(2)	4	4	4(2)	40
			9 or 12 month toxicity study		
Dog/monkey	4(2)	4	4	4(2)	40

Figures in brackets are animals retained after cessation of dosing for observation of recovery.

any toxic changes. This recovery period is usually 1 week for 14-day and 1-month studies, and 2 weeks for studies of 3 months or more. However, depending on the turnover or development characteristics of the affected target organs, extended recovery periods may be necessary, especially in chronic toxicity studies. Information on recovery from induced organ changes is needed for safety guidance for humans. The study design is outlined in Table 3.3.

Animals are usually dosed once daily during the dosing period. This may be increased to twice or three times a day to mimic human dosing or to create a kinetic profile in animals similar to that seen or predicted in humans. The low dosage is a small multiple of the estimated clinical dose (usually less than fivefold), based whenever possible on predicted or actual comparative kinetic data. The high dosage may be the MRD, the maximum non-irritant or minimally irritant dose, the maximum practicable/feasible dose (based on the physicochemical properties of the dose, but usually not less than ~100 times the intended clinical dose) or the dose yielding a C_{max} or AUC at least ~100 times that in humans after a clinical dose or the dose at which these parameters become clearly non-linear. Interestingly, the new draft of the ICH M3 guideline suggests that a 50-fold overage in exposure in top dose relative to the desired human efficacious exposure is sufficient. The intermediate dose is usually the geometric mean of the low and high dosages. If tolerance to repeat dosing is shown in the preliminary studies or reduction of exposure by metabolism is observed, an initial period of dose increments may be advisable but should not normally exceed 1 week. In the absence of any human data the

selection of doses in first animal repeat-dose toxicity studies based on likely human exposure often remains a challenge.

3.4.2.1 Study interpretation

The type of observations include those made in MRDs (i.e. clinical observations, body weight, pulse rate in dogs, haematology, clinical chemistry, urine analysis, plasma drug concentration, macroscopic and microscopic post-mortem examination) as well as ophthalmoscopy, electrocardiography (in dogs), organ weights and, in some laboratories, hearing tests. Although some types of toxicity may be obvious, more subtle changes may be difficult to separate from normal variation. Selection of suitable control groups for comparison with drug-treated animals is therefore vital, as is adequate pre-dose evaluation of various measurements.

Control animals usually receive a quantity of vehicle equal to the highest administered to the test groups. When the test material influences pH or toxicity of the dosing solution and these properties are pertinent to the route of administration, the quantities of excipients administered to control animals may have to differ from those administered to the test animals; in such cases it may be more important for test and control solutions to have the same physicochemical properties. Similarly, it may be necessary to administer qualitatively different excipients to the controls in order to keep the physical properties of test and control materials the same (e.g. in an intravenous study, if simple aqueous solutions of the test material are isotonic, the controls should receive physiological saline) and if the test material is administered without a vehicle, the controls are given water or are sham-treated. When the likely effects of a vehicle are unknown, two control groups, vehicle and negative (water, saline or sham-treated), should be included in the study. Statistical comparisons should initially be made against the vehicle control group.

Based on comparisons with an appropriate control group, abnormalities identified during the course of a study may require additional investigations to be undertaken to determine, if practicable, the significance, extent or mechanism of toxicity.

Statistical analysis is essential in order to gain an overview of the very extensive data collected during such studies and to highlight any underlying trends. This analysis also aids in determining the non-toxic effect level required by regulatory authorities.

Finally, any effects present at the end of the dosing period may be investigated during the following recovery period in which a proportion of the animals showing effects are retained undosed while recovery is monitored. Recovery periods of 2 weeks or 1 month are typical. These may not be sufficient to demonstrate complete recovery. However, signs of reversibility should be taken into account when making a risk assessment.

3.5 Carcinogenicity studies

Lifetime bioassays are conducted in animals to detect whether a compound can cause neoplastic changes. Neoplasms are caused by a tissue undergoing growth that is not under the normal control mechanisms of the body. Such growths are often referred to as tumours, but this is an imprecise term which can be applied to any abnormal swelling. If the neoplasm closely resembles its tissue of origin and the growth is slow and does not spread to other tissues it is a benign neoplasm. Neoplasms that grow quickly and invade other tissues and shed cells into blood or lymph vessels which lodge and grow at sites distant from the original neoplasm are termed malignant.

Lifetime bioassays are often referred to as carcinogenicity or oncogenicity studies. A carcinoma is a malignant neoplasm of epithelial cell origin (e.g. adrenal adenocarcinoma); its benign counterpart is referred to as an adrenal adenoma. Malignant neoplasms that arise from connective tissues are termed sarcomas (e.g. fibrosarcoma). The benign counterpart of the malignant fibrosarcoma is a fibroma. Carcinogenicity studies imply to the purist that such studies are designed to detect carcinomas. Oncogeni-

city refers to any neoplasm, benign or malignant, of either epithelial or connective tissue origin. Because the ICH guideline use the term 'carcinogencity' for such studies, this is also used in this chapter.

Carcinogencity studies therefore examine the ability of a material to produce neoplastic changes in a tissue or tissues. Short-term genotoxicity studies provide a good indicator of carcinogenic potential as most carcinogenic agents of concern cause damage to DNA or chromosomes. Normally, long-term lifetime animal studies are required to demonstrate the realisation of that potential and also to detect agents that cause neoplasms by an epigenetic (i.e. non-genotoxic) mechanism. Such epigenetic agents can act by a variety of mechanisms, including immunosuppression, chronic tissue injury, repeated receptor activation and by disturbing hormone homeostasis and thereby increasing cell turnover, which increases the chance of developing a neoplasm.

Because of their size and duration and the corresponding costs involved, carcinogenicity studies are usually conducted towards the end of the development of a pharmaceutical when clinical efficacy has been established and the majority of the toxicity studies have been completed. This means that such studies are normally not completed before an application for a marketing authorisation is made (i.e. at the end of phase III clinical trials). However, it is reasonable to investigate the carcinogenic potential of a pharmaceutical candidate earlier in the development phase under specific circumstances. Guidelines on the Quality, Safety and Efficacy of Medicinal Products for Human Use. Hence, in Europe (*EU Guidelines on the Quality, Safety and Efficacy of Medicinal Products for Human Use* 1989) for example, carcinogenicity studies will usually be required as part of the development of a pharmaceutical preparation in the following circumstances:

1. Where the substance would be used continuously for long periods (i.e. more than 6 months) or have a frequent intermittent use as may be expected in the treatment of chronic illness.

2. Where a substance has a chemical structure that suggests oncogenic potential.

3. Where a substance causes concern as a result of some specific aspects of its biological action (e.g. a therapeutic class of which several members have produced positive oncogenic results), its pattern of toxicity or long-term retention (of drug or metabolites) detected in previous studies the findings in genotoxicity studies.

It is a general rule that for pharmaceuticals developed to treat certain serious diseases, for adults or paediatric patients, carcinogenicity testing, if recommended, can be concluded post-approval.

There is a continuing debate as to whether inbred or outbred strains of rodents should be used. In theory, inbred strains are preferable because a more accurate knowledge of background tumour incidence is available. However, it may be that a particular inbred strain may metabolise the test material in a certain way or have a genetic resistance to the development of a specific tumour type. Usually, outbred strains of rat or hamster are used, but occasionally inbred mice strains are included. An F1 hybrid mouse strain is frequently employed. The most important factor is to have a sound knowledge of the background incidence of tumours in the species or strain selected. This information complements the concurrent control data and provides information on the susceptibility of the strain to rare tumour types. Modifying factors such as diet and cage density must be kept as constant as possible to enable correct interpretation of the results.[40,41]

The 'ICH S1A' guideline, *Testing for Carcinogenicity of Pharmaceuticals*, allows for a one-species carcinogenicity study plus alternative *in vivo* tests such as rat initiator-promoter models, transgenic mouse assays (i.e. p53 +/− knockout mice: Tg.AC mice which carry an activated v-Ha-*ras* oncogene; *ras* H2 mice carrying a human c-Ha-*ras* oncogene and XPA mice which have lost a crucial DNA nucleotide excision repair gene) and neonatal rodent tests. The premise with these alternative carcinogenicity assays is that the animals are predisposed to develop tumours without a lengthy latent period [i.e. induced tumours can appear in 6–9 months (transgenic models) rather than up to the 2 years of the conventional assays]. In addition, animal group sizes are lower than for conventional studies, although at least one agency suggests that in addition to the transgenic animal groups, groups of wild-type animals should also be included in such studies to determine if tumours occur preferentially in the transgenic model.[42] These alternative carcinogenicity studies have been undergoing evaluation for a number of years,[43] but it will be some time before they gain full regulatory acceptance internationally. There have been instances where genotoxicity assessments are equivocal, when regulatory authorities have requested data from a specific transgenic model to aid risk assessment and/or to progress in clinical trials. In the USA, the FDA have requested some companies in these circumstances to provide data from an *in vitro* Syrian hamster embryo (SHE) transformation assay. In this assay pluripotent cells

are grown in culture. It is surmised that if a compound has tumorigenic potential it can induce these cells to lose the contact inhibition of normal cells such that they pile up on top of one another to form a flared colony or 'transformant'.[44] The use of this assay is controversial as scoring of transformants can be subjective, there is no unequivocal marker of transformation and the molecular mechanism of transformation is unknown.[45] If a compound is positive in this assay and a company wishes to progress with development, they have been required to provide data from the P53 transgenic model, which is known to be sensitive to some genotoxic carcinogens. If such an assay is negative, companies have been allowed to proceed with development of the compound in question. If a relevant test compound has been found to be negative in the SHE assay, then development has been allowed without a P53 assay. The use of alternative carcinogenicity studies has reduced the number of traditional 2-year studies for pharmaceuticals by one-quarter.[46] Jacobs[46] also notes that many of the mechanisms of carcinogenicity appear non-genotoxic and may require prolonged treatment to be expressed. Thus, there appears to be a continued need for 2-year carcinogenicity studies in rodents for pharmaceuticals.

The rat will usually be the species of choice for the standard carcinogenicity study because there is greater confidence in its predictivity for human carcinogenicity than the mouse or hamster. The species chosen should be the most appropriate based on considerations such as pharmacology, repeated-dose toxicity, metabolism and toxicokinetics.

3.5.1 Route of administration

In general, the route of administration should be similar to the one intended to be used clinically. Oral administration is the most widely used route of exposure, with the test material mixed in the diet, given in the drinking water or administered by gavage. Each route has advantages and disadvantages.

Dietary and water administration rely on the administered mixture being palatable and stable in the formulation. Accurate administration is not possible, particularly if animals are multiply caged, and cross-contamination, especially from diet mixtures, may be a problem. However, the methods are relatively easy to use, with minimum resource being required, and more or less continual exposure to the material is guaranteed.

Administration by gavage ensures that each animal receives the correct dose but the method is labour intensive and, depending on the kinetics involved, periods of 'drug holiday' may occur during the treatment period.

The other main route used for pharmaceutical preparations is inhalation using a 'head only' exposure system. Parenteral administration, although technically possible, is usually avoided because of the local irritant effects that can occur with repeated injection, particularly by the subcutaneous route. Topical administration is an option for materials intended for administration to the skin.

3.5.2 Dose selection

There has been, and continues to be, considerable debate about the selection of the high dose level for carcinogenicity studies. European and Japanese regulatory guidelines have tended to accept the use of an arbitrary upper limit set at a multiple of 100 times the administered therapeutic dose. In the USA, the selection has been made on the basis of the MTD, a level that causes a moderate decrease in weight gain (not exceeding 10%). Literature has been produced regarding dose selection procedures.[47] The ICH has issued a revised guideline, *Dose Selection for Carcinogenicity Studies of Pharmaceuticals* ('ICH S1R' Guideline as of 2007). In this document, the following six criteria are given for selection of the high dose for carcinogenicity studies of therapeutics:

1. The maximum tolerated dose;
2. A 25-fold AUC ratio (rodent : human);
3. Dose-limiting pharmacodynamic effects;
4. Saturation of absorption;
5. A maximum feasible dose; and
6. A limit dose.

On the limit dose, the guideline text reads as follows: 'In determining the high dose for carcinogenicity studies using the approaches outlined in this guideline it is appropriate to limit this dose to 1500 mg/kg/day. This limit dose applies where the maximum recommended human dose does not exceed 500 mg/day.' On the AUC criterion, it is estimated that 15% of drugs will be caught by the AUC criteria. The MTD, or equivalent, is determined on the basis of the results from a 90-day study, as well as palatability studies if the material is to be administered in the diet or drinking water.

The use of other pharmacodynamic, pharmacokinetic or toxicity-based endpoints in study design should be considered based on scientific rationale and individual merits. In all cases, appropriate dose ranging studies should be conducted. All relevant information should be considered for dose and species/strain selection for the carcinogenicity study. This information should include knowledge of human use, exposure patterns and metabolism. The availability of multiple criteria for dose selection will provide greater flexibility in optimizing the design of carcinogenicity studies for therapeutic agents.

3.5.3 Group sizes

Typically, group sizes of 50 animals per sex are used at each of three dose levels. A double-sized control group is commonly used, often split as two equal-sized groups. This is because concurrent control information is the most important factor in the statistical analysis needed to confirm the presence of an oncogenic effect; splitting the control group gives information on naturally occurring variation in tumour incidence.

Additional animals will be required to provide pharmacokinetic information, especially in mouse studies where blood sampling sufficient for analysis usually requires the animal to be killed.

3.5.4 Conduct of study

Meticulous record-keeping systems are essential to cope with the immense amount of data generated in a carcinogenicity study. Palpations to detect the onset of tumours and follow their duration are an essential part of the study conduct and are carried out with increasing frequency as the study progresses. Regular clinical observations are required to ensure that sick animals are identified, monitored and killed before they die naturally, thus preventing loss of important information through autolysis or cannibalism. A study losing more than 10% of animals through these causes is of questionable validity.

3.5.5 Duration of study

Carcinogenicity studies are usually carried out in rats for 24 months and in mice for 18 months. Although such durations meet guidelines issued by the Office for Economic Co-operation and Development, some authorities believe that these studies should be lifespan studies and would, therefore, expect to see a mortality of at least 50%. The US FDA statisticians impose a further requirement on such studies that for adequate analysis at least 25 animals per sex, per group should survive to the end of the study. In addition, in order to prevent a carcinogenic effect being masked by toxicity, not more than 50% of the intercurrent deaths in any group should be from causes other than tumour formation.

Each sex can be terminated independently when survival is reduced to 50%. In order to meet all the restrictions outlined above, and because the longevity of the Sprague Dawley rat, particularly in laboratories in the USA, is decreasing, many companies start with 60 or 70 animals per sex, per group.

3.5.6 Autopsy and microscopic examination

The importance of undertaking a careful detailed autopsy on each animal cannot be over-emphasised. Organs should be sectioned in a standard manner. The pathologist should adopt a consistent nomenclature and a peer review of the slides has become an accepted part of Good Laboratory Practice.

3.5.7 Evaluation of results

The incidence of neoplasms is compared between the test and control groups for statistical significance and to detect whether there is a trend (i.e. increasing incidence with higher doses). Such a comparison is made by tissue, so that all the neoplasms in the liver, for example, are compared between groups. Also, the total number of animals with single and multiple tumours is compared to see if there is a non-specific increase in tumour burden.

As well as comparing simple incidences, the time when the tumours were detected is taken into account. This is because a compound might not change the overall incidence of a particular type of tumour but it could cause it to develop in much younger animals and cause them to die earlier.

The most important comparison is with concurrent control groups. However, there are occasions when it is necessary to use historical data (i.e. information from control animals of the same strain on other studies). This is more relevant if the studies were conducted in the same laboratory under similar conditions and at the same time. The incidence of a particular neoplasm is often different between laboratories and may change with time. Historical data are most useful to get an idea of the variation in the background range of frequency and also to ascertain that rare tumour types can occur spontaneously.

Statistically, carcinogenicity studies have a low sensitivity because of the small numbers of animals that are used.[48] However, complex statistical analysis, which should include a judgement on whether the tumour was the cause of death, duration to death and trend analysis, can reveal valuable information about the risk to humans of taking the product therapeutically.

3.6 Reproductive toxicology

The assessment of a new pharmaceutical product for effects on reproduction must take into account that mammalian reproduction is a complex cyclical process involving a number of stages, each complicated in themselves. The stages include: gametogenesis, fertilisation, implantation, embryogenesis and fetal growth, parturition, postnatal adaption, development and ageing.

These phases differ in duration depending on the species being considered.

3.6.1 Aims of studies

The two areas of the reproductive process that animal studies focus on are general reproductive effects and developmental effects.

3.6.1.1 General reproductive effects

Studies for general reproductive effects examine the possibility that agents may affect fertility, male or female, by specific pharmacological or biochemical means or by toxicity to a number of cell types, including gametes and their supporting cells. Some agents may alter the delicate hormone balance required for the mammalian reproductive process to maintain its cyclical progress. Others, often potent pharmacological agents, may result in loss of reproductive drive (e.g. loss of libido, sexual dysfunction).

Other agents (e.g. cytotoxic drugs) target reproductive organs because of their ability to affect rapidly dividing cells, and to possibly induce damage to the genetic material.

Studies examining reproductive effects in animals are invariably lengthy and initially 'catch all'. An effect of reduced pregnancy rates in treated females having mated with treated males may be the result of a number of factors that would have to be examined methodically.

3.6.1.2 Developmental effects

The second and more emotive area of examination is developmental effects, where agents may induce abnormalities in the developing offspring. The difficulties in designing studies to detect these types of agents, commonly referred to as teratogens, are that interspecies response is often variable and the abnormalities induced invariably also occur spontaneously. Another confounding factor is that some abnormalities (e.g. cardiovascular and behavioural defects) may only manifest themselves postnatally because of an increase in size or functional abnormalities of the offspring.

3.6.2 Types of studies

Before the ICH guidelines (see below), reproductive toxicity studies were divided into three segments which were designed as follows.

1. *Segment I: Fertility and general reproductive performance study*

This is an overall screening study, covering the entire reproductive cycle of one generation, including the reproductive ability of the offspring of that generation. The test substance is only administered directly to the first (parental) generation and the test animal is usually the rat.

Females are dosed 14 days before mating (NB. there are 5 days between ovulations) and through to lactation. Males were previously dosed 70 days before mating (NB. the spermatogenic cycle is 50 days). However, recent studies in Japan have shown that almost all effects occur late in the cycle. Thus, dosing for 14 days before mating is deemed acceptable.[49]

2. *Segment II: Teratogenicity study*

This concentrates on the most sensitive part of gestation, from the time of implantation until major organogenesis is complete. This is the period during which a test substance is most likely to cause malformation of the embryo. Exposure of the mother to the test substance is usually confined to this period. Conventionally, the study is conducted in the rat and rabbit. Rabbits are intolerant to antibiotics and the mouse is an acceptable alternative in most cases.

3. *Segment III: Perinatal and postnatal study*

This concentrates on the late part of gestation, not covered by the teratogenicity study, on parturition and on the period of lactation. The study can be particularly useful in detecting subtle effects on the brain, which continues physical and functional development during the fetal and postnatal period, after dosing has ceased in the teratogenicity study. The test animal is usually the rat.

There were major differences in the protocol designs for rodent studies between Japanese and European studies. These were resolved by the ICH process which in 1993 published a guideline entitled *Detection of Toxicity to Reproduction for Medicinal Products*.

The ICH guideline's 'preferred option' is a three-study design as follows.

1. *Fertility and early embryonic development (rat)*

Provided no deleterious effects have been revealed by testicular histopathology assessment and testes weight measurements (ICH guideline, *Toxicity to Male Fertility:*

An Addendum to the ICH Tripartite Guideline on Detection of Toxicity to Reproduction for Medicinal Products, as amended in November 2001) in a 1-month repeat-dose study, a premating treatment interval of 2 weeks for both sexes can be used. The treatment period requires justification. Dosing should continue through mating and at least through implantation in the females.

If the short premating dosing interval is used, then the *in vivo* part of the study would take approximately 9 weeks compared with 32–35 weeks for a standard Segment I study.

2. *Embryo-fetal development (rat and rabbit)*

This is a standard Segment II teratogenicity study.

3. *Prenatal and postnatal development, including maternal function (rat)*

Females are exposed to the test substance from implantation to the end of lactation. F1 pups should be evaluated for postnatal development including fertility. The duration of the *in vivo* phase of this study would be approximately 20 weeks if F1 pregnant females are killed for caesarean section examination, 22–24 weeks if allowed to litter.

As an alternative to the 'preferred option', the ICH guideline allows flexibility in the choice of study designs, as long as the combination of studies chosen covers the complete reproductive cycle. This allows the toxicologist to design the reproductive toxicology package so that it is relevant to the compound class under test.

In addition to the above studies, a number of studies examining the pharmacokinetics of the test material need to be conducted to show whether the drug crosses the placenta, whether it is excreted in milk and whether pregnancy affects absorption, distribution, metabolism or excretion.

3.6.3 Timing of studies

Reproductive toxicity tests are not required to support phase I clinical studies in men. Detailed histological evaluations of the male reproductive organs should be performed in the repeated-dose toxicity studies. Male fertility studies in the rodent, however, would be expected to support phase III studies.

Inclusion of women of child-bearing potential (WOCBP) into clinical trials generally requires the completion of reproductive toxicity and genotoxicity studies. However, where appropriate, preliminary reproduction toxicity data are available from two species (essentially studies with a limited number of animals covering the organogenesis period), and where adequate birth control methods are used, inclusion of

WOCBP (up to 150) receiving investigational treatment for a relatively short duration (up to 3 months) can occur prior to completion of definitive reproduction toxicity testing. For shorter clinical studies (e.g. over 2 weeks) and under defined circumstances, WOCBP may be included under intensive control of pregnancy risk without reproductive toxicity study information.

The complete reproductive toxicity package, including the rodent perinatal and postnatal studies, must be submitted with the marketing application.

3.6.4 Juvenile toxicity studies

It is unusual for paediatric trials to be conducted before there is considerable experience in adults, which is obviously more relevant for assessment of risk to children than are studies in juvenile rats.

Juvenile toxicity studies are recommended by both the Japanese and US regulatory agencies before inclusion of children in clinical trials. The studies are usually conducted in the offspring of untreated female rats (although juvenile dog studies have been requested for specific compounds), by giving test material directly to the pups. Dosing usually does not commence until 4 days post-partum, because of technical difficulties, and is continued for 6 weeks. The survival and development of the offspring is monitored and full clinical chemistry, haematological and urine analyses are carried out. At autopsy all major organs and tissues are retained and examined microscopically.

The European agencies recently communicated the expectations for juvenile toxicity studies in a guideline (CHMP, London, 24 January 2008, Doc. Ref. EMEA/CHMP/SWP/169215/2005). In general, the need for and timing of juvenile animals in support of undertaking clinical studies should be justified. If such studies are considered necessary, they should preferably be available before the initiation of clinical studies in paediatric populations. Pharmacokinetic data from humans and animals (including juvenile animals if available) should also be evaluated before the proposed paediatric clinical trial(s).

Key elements in the design of any juvenile animal studies are the following:
1. Reproductive system: development up to adulthood;
2. Pulmonary system: development up to 2 years old;
3. Immune system: development up to 12 years old;
4. Renal system: development up to 1 year of age;
5. Skeletal system: development up to adulthood; and

6. Organs and/or systems involved in absorption and metabolism of drugs: development of biotransformation enzymes up to adolescence.

With this knowledge, the appropriate juvenile studies in animals can be designed if needed. The differences in development of the various organ systems in the usually available animal species such as rats, dogs and monkeys on the one hand and humans on the other hand should be taken into account when deciding over animal age at the start, the duration and the end of treatment.

3.6.5 Evaluation and interpretation of data

The following points should be considered when evaluating the data from reproductive toxicity studies.

3.6.5.1 Antifertility effects in the male

The male rat has a large reserve of spermatozoa and it is difficult to detect antifertility effects by using pregnancy as an endpoint. This is because the ejaculate in rats contains over 1000-fold the number of sperm that will produce maximum fertility. In man the multiple is only 2–4 times and some studies have suggested that in certain Western populations, average human sperm counts appear to have declined over the past 50 years.[50] The rat's testes are also relatively about 40 times the size of man's. If antifertility effects are observed, it can be helpful to measure various sperm parameters (seminology) to help characterise effects.

3.6.5.2 Antifertility effects in females

These would be apparent on examination of the following parameters:
• Number of females failing to become pregnant (any likely contribution of the male to this effect should be eliminated by mating treated females with untreated males);
• Disruption of the oestrous cycle;
• Increased incidence of pre-implantation loss (number of corpora lutea – number of implants *in utero*); and
• Increased incidence of post-implantation loss (number of implants *in utero* – number of live fetuses).

3.6.5.3 Teratogenesis

Evaluation of the data should consider whether there are any fetal abnormalities that have not been observed previously or only occur rarely and whether there is a significant increase in defects that occur spontaneously, especially without any significant maternal toxicity.

3.6.5.4 Postnatal effects

Parturition is a particularly stressful period for both mother and offspring. Delays or protraction of the process may have significant effects on data collected postnatally.

Parameters to consider are the following:
• Perinatal survival of both dam and offspring;
• Postnatal survival of offspring may be influenced by either underlying abnormalities (e.g. of the cardiovascular system) or as a result of poor lactation in the dam;
• The function of vital senses should be evaluated in the offspring (e.g. sight, hearing, balance); and
• Behavioural effects in the offspring can be evaluated by tests for locomotion, habituation, learning and memory.

3.7 Genotoxicity testing

Genotoxicity refers to potentially harmful effects on genetic material (DNA) which may occur directly through the induction of permanent transmissible changes (mutations) in the amount or structure of the DNA within cells. Such damage to DNA can occur at three levels:

1. *Gene (point) mutations* are changes in nucleotide sequence at one or a few coding segments (base pairs) within a gene. They can occur by base substitution (i.e. where one base in the DNA is replaced by another) or by frameshift mutations (i.e. where there is addition or deletion of one or more bases, thus altering the sequence of bases in the DNA, which constitutes the reading frame).

2. *Chromosomal mutations* are recognised as morphological alterations in the gross structure of chromosomes (i.e. they are structural aberrations which can be detected microscopically). Compounds that cause chromosome damage are called clastogens.

3. *Genomic mutations* are changes in the number of chromosomes in a genome, and are also called numerical aberrations. Loss or gain of chromosomes during cell division is called aneuploidy, and chemicals which cause this are called aneugens. It is possible to generate cells containing multiples of the whole chromosome set – these are polyploid cells. Both aneuploidy and polyploidy can result from damage to the mitotic spindle.

Many chemicals possess mutagenic properties, which presents a potential hazard to future generations because mutations in germ cells of sexually reproducing organisms may be transmitted to the offspring. Furthermore, the relationship between mutational changes in DNA and carcinogenesis is strongly supported by the available evidence originating from research into the molecular biology of cancer, and the existence of cancer genes (oncogenes) and tumour suppressor genes. Consequently, the use of short-term genotoxicity tests as pre-screens for carcinogen detection has gained significant importance in drug development. Accumulation of mutagenic events is also associated with atherosclerosis, ageing processes, etc. Thus, there is a necessity to identify and limit the spread of chemicals with mutagenic properties in the environment, and therefore any new therapeutic substance, including new excipients, where a wide exposure can be anticipated, are screened for genotoxicity using testing procedures that detect both gene and chromosome damage, *in vitro* (e.g. using bacterial assays and mammalian cells in culture) and *in vivo* (using rodents).

In the pharmaceutical industry it is usual to carry out genotoxicity screening at an early stage in the drug development programme. This is particularly so with regard to the use of *in vitro* assays. If problems concerning potential genotoxicity can be identified early, using bacterial genotoxicity tests for example, it may be possible to design a useful drug that is devoid of genotoxic properties by the consideration of structure–activity relationships. The *in vitro* tests require small amounts of compound and generate results quickly, making them particularly useful for such studies.

The existing two ICH guidelines for genotoxicity of pharmaceuticals are undergoing a maintenance process and a revised single new guideline ('ICH S2R1') has been released to final consultation in 2008 and is awaiting approval. This revised guideline updates the basic genotoxicity test battery requirements for new chemical entities, the interpretation of test results as well as the need and conditions for follow-up testing in case of questionable results or if a quantitative risk assessment is required.

The general features of a standard test battery for genotoxicity are as follows:

1. Assessment of mutagenicity in a bacterial reverse mutation test. This test has been shown to detect relevant genetic changes and the majority of genotoxic rodent and human carcinogens.

2. Genotoxicity should also be evaluated in mammalian cells *in vitro* and/or *in vivo*.

From these general features, the following options emerge:

Option 1
1. A test for gene mutation in bacteria.

2. A cytogenetic test for chromosomal damage (the *in vitro* metaphase chromosome aberration test or *in vitro* micronucleus test), or an *in vitro* mouse lymphoma *tk* gene mutation assay.

3. An *in vivo* test for genotoxicity, generally a test for chromosomal damage using rodent haematopoietic cells, either for micronuclei or for chromosomal aberrations in metaphase cells.

Option 2

1. A test for gene mutation in bacteria.

2. An *in vivo* assessment of genotoxicity with two tissues, usually an assay for micronuclei using rodent hematopoietic cells and a second *in vivo* assay.

Under both standard battery options, the *in vivo* genotoxicity assays can often be integrated into repeat-dose toxicity studies when the doses are sufficient. Under Option 2, if dose/exposure is not appropriate, an acute *in vivo* study (incorporating two genotoxicity assays in one study where possible) should be performed to optimize dose selection based on exposure/toxicity and, or Option 1, including an *in vitro* mammalian cell assay, should be followed. Compounds from well-characterized classes where genotoxicity is expected may required modification of the test battery to characterize these appropriately in the tests/protocols known to respond to them. Compounds that are toxic to bacteria should still be tested in bacterial reverse mutation tests because mutagenicity can occur at lower, less toxic concentrations. Compounds bearing structural alerts for genotoxic activity are usually detectable in the standard test battery because the majority of 'structural alerts' are defined in relation to bacterial mutagenicity. Compounds for which data on toxicokinetics or pharmacokinetics indicate that they are not systemically absorbed and therefore not available to the target tissues.

Additional testing may include tests for DNA adducts (e.g. the ^{32}P-postlabelling assay[51]), DNA strand breakage (e.g. the so-called COMET assay[52]) or assays measuring unscheduled DNA synthesis (UDS), mutation of transgenes *in vivo* in models such as the Muta-mouse and the Big Blue mouse and rat,[53] or simply the inclusion of both types of *in vitro* mammalian cell assay. Products of biotechnology (e.g. cytokines, monoclonal antibodies) do not normally need to be screened for genotoxicity, unless impurities/contaminants or organic linker molecules cause concern (seen 'ICH S6', *Safety for Biotechnological Products*). However, there is some concern for growth factors that may induce high levels of proliferation in specific tissues, thus increasing the chance of spontaneous mutation in oncogenes and tumour suppressor genes.

Before any human studies, it is common to complete the test battery of genotoxicity tests. However, single-dose clinical trials may begin with having only the information from testing for induction of gene mutations *in vitro* at hand.

For chemical intermediates it is also necessary to carry out bacterial genotoxicity tests for Health and Safety at Work labelling and classification purposes. Additional *in vitro* and *in vivo* assays of the type described for drugs are triggered as the tonnage manufactured per annum increases. The classification and labelling of intermediates in relation to their genotoxicity is important in ensuring that their safe manufacture, storage, transport, use and disposal can be accomplished.

Reactive chemicals are used to manufacture drugs and a proportion of these are genotoxic. The regulatory recommendations on how to test for and assess risk of genotoxic impurities are dealt with in section 3.8.4.3.

3.7.1 Study design

Full study design details for the established regulatory tests for genotoxicity are given in the UK Environmental Mutagen Society (UKEMS) volume on *Basic Mutagenicity Tests*[54] and the relevant Organisation for Economic Cooperation and Development (OECD) guidelines on such tests. OECD testing guidelines are updated periodically and are available from the OECD in Paris, France.

3.7.1.1 Bacterial tests for gene mutation

The most widely used *in vitro* assay is the reverse mutation assay for gene mutation using strains of *Salmonella typhimurium* and *Escherichia coli* which are capable of detecting a wide variety of mutations. This assay measures reversion from histidine dependence to histidine independence for the *Salmonella* strains and tryptophan dependence to independence for the *E. coli* strains and is carried out in both the presence and absence of an exogenous metabolic activation system (usually the post-mitochondrial fraction from the livers of rats treated with cytochrome P450 enzyme-inducing agents). In the test, bacteria are exposed to a range of concentrations of chemical and plated on to minimal agar medium. After a suitable period of incubation at 37°C, the number of revertant colonies is counted and compared with the number of spontaneous revertants obtained in an untreated/solvent control culture.

3.7.1.2 Assays for chromosomal aberrations

The simplest and most sensitive assays for detecting clastogenic (i.e. chromosomal breaking) effects involve the use of mammalian cells. Cultures of established cell lines (e.g. Chinese hamster ovary) as well as primary cell cultures (e.g. human lymphocyte) may be used. After exposure to a range of chemical concentrations in the presence and absence of an appropriate metabolic activation system, the cell cultures are treated with a spindle inhibitor (e.g. vinblastine) to accumulate cells in a metaphase-like stage of mitosis. Cells are harvested at appropriate times and chromosome preparations are made, stained with DNA-specific dye and the metaphase cells are analysed under the microscope for chromosome abnormalities.

3.7.1.3 *In vitro* micronucleus test

Similarly to the assays for chromosomal aberrations, cell cultures are exposed to the test substances both with and without metabolic activation. After exposure to a test substance, cell cultures are grown for a period sufficient to allow chromosome damage as a result of chromosome breakage or effect on spindle formation and incorrect distribution of chromosomes into the daughter cells to lead to the formation of micronuclei in interphase cells.[55] Harvested and stained interphase cells are then analysed microscopically for the presence of micronuclei. Micronuclei should only be scored in those cells that complete nuclear division following exposure to the test chemical.[56] When human lymphocytes are used, the most convenient stage to score micronuclei in this cell system is the binucleate interphase stage. For this purpose, cells are trapped at this stage with the inhibitor of actin polymerisation, cytochalasin B. Cells that have progressed to this stage must have completed one cell division, otherwise they would contain only one nucleus. As micronuclei appear not only as a consequence of chromosome breakage but also if chromosome distribution is affected, the test can be used to investigate the potential of a compound to induce aneuploidy (e.g. via interaction with the spindle apparatus).

3.7.1.4 Mammalian cell tests for gene mutation

A variety of mammalian cell culture systems can be used to detect mutations induced by chemical substances. The L5178Y mouse lymphoma line, measuring mutation at the thymidine kinase (TK) locus, is preferred. TK is an important enzyme involved in DNA synthesis. Cells are exposed to the test substance at various concentrations, in the presence and absence of a metabolic activation system, for a suitable period of time, and then subcultured to assess cytotoxicity and to allow phenotypic expression prior to mutant selection. Cells deficient in TK because

of a forward mutation are resistant to the cytotoxic effects of pyrimidine analogues (antimetabolites) such as trifluorothymidine (TFT). This is because the antimetabolites cannot be incorporated into cellular nucleotides and kill the cell through inhibition of cellular metabolism. After treatment, cells are grown in medium containing TFT; mutant cells can proliferate in the presence of TFT, whereas normal cells containing TK are killed. This allows the detection of an increase in mutant cells after chemical treatment. Analysis of mutant colonies from this assay has shown that they can arise from a variety of genetic changes, including point mutation, large and small chromosomal deletions and recombination.

3.7.1.5 Detection of chromosome damage in rodent bone marrow using the micronucleus test

The micronucleus test is a short-term mammalian *in vivo* assay for the detection of chromosomal damage or damage to the mitotic apparatus by chemicals. The basis of this assay is an increase in micronuclei in the polychromatic erythrocytes present within the bone marrow of treated animals when compared with the controls. The micronuclei, known to pathologists as Howell–Jolly bodies, are formed from chromosomal fragments or whole chromosomes lagging in mitosis. When erythroblasts develop into erythrocytes, the main nucleus is expelled while the micronucleus may be retained within the cytoplasm, and is readily visualised. Animals are exposed to the test substance, usually a single dose, and 24 h and 48 h after treatment they are killed, the bone marrow is extracted and smear preparations are made. After suitable staining, the polychromatic erythrocytes are analysed under the microscope for micronucleus frequency. Following the ICH guideline on genotoxicity, it is sufficient to use only male rats or mice for these tests, as long as no obvious difference in toxicity has been detected between the sexes.

3.7.1.6 Unscheduled DNA synthesis – *ex vivo* assay in rodent liver

This assay is normally carried out only if positive effects have been obtained in earlier *in vitro* tests. The UDS test measures the DNA repair synthesis that occurs after excision and removal of a stretch of DNA containing the region of damage, induced in hepatocytes of animals treated with the test chemicals. UDS is measured by the uptake of radioactively labelled nucleotide, usually tritium-labelled thymidine, into the DNA of the damaged hepatocytes. Animals, usually male rats, are treated with the test chemical, and groups are killed 2–4 h or 12–14 h after treatment. Suspensions of viable hepatocytes are prepared by liver perfusion, and these are cultured in the presence of tritium-labelled thymidine. The incorporation of radiolabel within the DNA is determined autoradiographically. The measurement of DNA damage serves as a surrogate for genetic alterations *in vivo*.

The ICH guideline requires that there must be proof of exposure of the target tissues to the test compound (and its metabolites) to validate the chosen *in vivo* assays. It is known that the type of DNA repair, which is measured in the UDS test, mainly relates to point mutations and not large-scale chromosome damage. Yet, it is mainly the larger scale chromosome damage observed *in vitro* in mammalian cells for pharmaceutical candidate compounds, which requires an *in vivo* approach for better risk assessment. In this context, the UDS test may not have sufficient sensitivity.

3.7.1.7 Comet assay for DNA damage in rodent tissues *in vivo*

The Comet assay, also referred to as the single cell gel electrophoresis (SCG or SCGE) assay, is a rapid, visual and quantitative technique for measuring DNA damage in eukaryote cells, which was introduced by Ostling and Johansson.[57] Under alkaline (pH >13) conditions, the assay can detect single- and double-stranded breaks, incomplete repair sites and alkali labile sites (and also possibly both DNA-protein and DNA-DNA cross-links) in virtually any eukaryotic cell population that can be obtained as a single cell suspension[58] and this test can be attached to a standard rodent toxicity study. Following electrophoresis, broken DNA migrates from the cell nuclei into the gel on coated slides, leaving the image of a 'comet'. Comets form as the broken ends of the negatively charged DNA molecule become free to migrate in the electric field towards the anode. Two principles in the formation of the comet are as follow:

1. DNA migration is a function of both size and the number of broken ends of the DNA; and
2. Tail length increases with damage initially and then reaches a maximum that is dependent on the electrophoretic conditions, not the size of fragments.

In recent years, the *in vivo* Comet assay has become increasingly used for regulatory purposes and acceptance of the test method by regulatory agencies is growing.[52,59] Because many pharmaceutical candidate compounds are associated with findings on chromosomal damage *in vitro*, it is thought that the Comet assay is a suitable *in vivo* follow-up test for cell types other than the highly proliferating bone marrow cells.

3.7.2 Germ cell tests

Because there is no good evidence that mutagens induce mutations exclusively in germ cells, it is not considered necessary to conduct germ cell studies as part of the screening package. Such testing is only carried out if detailed risk assessment data are required (e.g. with anticancer drugs). The newer generation of *in vivo* tests using transgenic animals, and also the Comet assay, has facilitated the study of genetic changes in germ cells and there is a resurgence of interest in this area.

3.7.3 Study interpretation

Guidance on the evaluation of genotoxicity data is given in the revised ICH genotoxicity guideline. Overall, a comprehensive weight of evidence approach is suggested when judging evidence for genotoxicity that comes from single tests or test batteries. Comparative trials have shown that each genotoxicity test can generate both false negative and false positive results in relation to predicting rodent carcinogenicity. Experimental conditions such as the limited capacity of *in vitro* metabolic activation systems can lead to false negative results in *in vitro* tests. Culture conditions (e.g. changes of pH, high osmolality) can lead to false positive results.[60] Further, threshold mechanisms for genotoxic activity become increasingly acknowledged.[61] The test battery approach is designed to reduce the risk of false negative results, while a positive result in any one *in vitro* assay does not necessarily mean that the test compound poses a genotoxic and/or carcinogenic hazard to humans.[62]

For a compound that induces a biologically relevant positive result in one or more *in vitro* tests, an *in vivo* test, in addition to *in vivo* cytogenetic assay, using a tissue other than the bone marrow or peripheral blood, can provide further useful information. The target cells exposed *in vivo* and possibly the genetic endpoint measured *in vitro* guide the choice of this additional *in vivo* test. *In vivo* gene mutation assays using endogenous genes or transgenes in a variety of tissues in the rat and mouse are at various stages of development and have been used to help risk assessments, but there are still concerns regarding the lack of sensitivity of the current assays.

If *in vivo* and *in vitro* test results do not agree, then the differences should be considered and explained, possibly following further studies on *in vitro/in vivo* metabolism[63] and compound class information. If the results of the *in vitro* mammalian cell assay are positive and there is not sufficient weight of evidence or mechanistic information to rule out relevant genotoxic potential, two *in vivo* tests are required, with appropriate endpoints and in appropriate tissues (usually two different tissues), and with an emphasis on obtaining sufficient exposure in the *in vivo* models. Negative results in appropriate *in vivo* assays, with adequate justification for the endpoints measured, and demonstration of exposure will be usually sufficient to demonstrate absence of genotoxic activity.[60]

Additional genotoxicity testing in appropriate models may be conducted for compounds that were negative in the standard test battery but which have shown increases in tumours in carcinogenicity bioassay(s) with insufficient evidence to establish a non-genotoxic mechanism. To help understand the mode of action, additional testing can include modified conditions for metabolic activation in *in vitro* tests or can include *in vivo* tests measuring genetic damage in target organs of tumour induction, such as DNA strand break assays (e.g. Comet or alkaline elution assays), liver UDS test, DNA covalent binding (e.g. by ^{32}P-postlabelling), mutation induction in transgenes, or molecular characterization of genetic changes in tumour-related genes.[64]

3.8 Irritation and sensitisation testing

Topical drug preparations are applied for days or even weeks, cosmetics for a lifetime and skin contact is probably the most common form of exposure to industrial chemicals. Therefore, a knowledge of the cutaneous toxicity is important for an overall hazard assessment. Cutaneous toxicity or localised skin injury can be considered as a primary event, because the compound could be irritant or corrosive, or as a secondary immunologically mediated event causing a delayed hypersensitivity response.

The data obtained from irritation and sensitisation testing can be used for hazard assessment, thereby enabling safe handling precautions to be recommended, and as a basis for classification and labelling. Such studies also have to be performed to meet obligations of regulatory authorities for the clinical trials and marketing of drugs.

3.8.1 Irritancy
3.8.1.1 Skin
Primary irritant-contact dermatitis results from direct cytotoxicity produced on first contact. The cellular injury is characterised by two macroscopically visible events: a reddening of the skin (erythema) and accumulation of fluid (oedema). By observing or measuring these changes one can estimate the extent of skin damage that has occurred. The most widely used single-exposure irritancy test is based on the Draize rabbit test.[65]

In this test, three rabbits are used to assess the irritancy potential following a single 4-h semi-occluded application, to intact rabbit skin, of 0.5 mL or 0.5 g of test material. The skin is observed 30–69 min and approximately 24, 48 and 72 h after patch removal. If irritation is persistent additional observations can be carried out on days 7 and 14. Scores for erythema and oedema at the 24-h and 48-h readings are added together for the three rabbits (12 values) and divided by 6 to give the primary irritation index (PII). This index is used to classify the material from non-irritant (0), mild irritant (>0 to 2), moderate irritant (>2 to >5) to severe irritant (>5).

There is good progress in developing alternative *in vitro* assays for some aspects of irritant potential.[66]

3.8.1.2 Eye
Toxic responses in the eye can result from direct topical ocular exposure of drugs from direct installation into the eye and also from dermal products which patients may accidentally get into their eyes. Until recently the Draize rabbit eye test[65] using three rabbits had served as the major protocol to assess the irritancy potential of topically applied substances.

In the Draize test, a single dose of 0.1 mL or 0.1 g is introduced into the conjunctival sac of the right eye, the left eye acting as a control. The reactions of the conjunctivae, iris and cornea are scored for irritancy at approximately 1, 3, 8, 24, 48 and 72 h and again at 7 days after dosing. Test materials shown to be severe skin irritants or that are below pH 2 or above pH 11 are not tested but are assumed to be eye irritants.

The use of the Draize tests has been receiving attention for a number of years because of animal welfare considerations. Consequently, the modifications of the existing protocol and the development of alternative methods have been extensively examined by the cosmetic and chemical industry to reduce animal usage and the occurrence of severe reactions. One modification of this model uses reduced volumes of 0.01 mL and 0.01 g, which reduces severe reactions but does not compromise the predictive value of the test.

Several *in vitro* methods, including the hen's egg chorioallantoic membrane test (HET-CAM), the bovine cornea opacity and permeability assay (BCOP) and the isolated rabbit eye (IRE) test, have gained regulatory acceptance in Europe for the classification of severe eye irritants.[66] Many companies are using such techniques successfully to reduce *in vivo* testing during development.[67]

3.8.2 Immunotoxicology

3.8.2.1 Sensitisation

The interaction of a chemical (hapten) with epidermal proteins (carrier) can result in a hapten–carrier complex capable of activating skin-associated lymphoid tissue (sensitisation) and dissemination of antigen-specific T lymphocytes (induction). Subsequent encounter with the same or cross-reactive chemicals can result in the elicitation of a characteristic inflammatory skin reaction. The clinical condition is referred to as allergic contact dermatitis and is characterised by erythema, oedema, vesiculation and pruritus. Allergic contact sensitisation is therefore classed as a cell-mediated immunological response to chemicals that contact and penetrate the skin.

There are a number of models for detecting allergic contact dermatitis in guinea pigs. The maximisation test developed by Magnussun and Kligman[68] is the most widely used and employs both an intradermal and topical sensitisation phase, together with the non-specific stimulation of the immune system by the intradermal injection of Freund's complete adjuvant.

Approximately 54 animals are used in the test and the sensitisation response is classified by the percentage of animals showing a stronger response than that seen in the control group. The net response is classified from 0% for a non-sensitiser, up to 8% for a weak sensitiser and over 80% for an extreme sensitiser.

A negative result in this type of test indicates that the potential to sensitise is extremely low and that human exposure is unlikely to be attended by a significant incidence of sensitisation. Because the test can be over-predictive, some toxicologists recommend that a non-adjuvant test such as the Buehler test[69] should be used if a positive is obtained, to give a more realistic determination of the prevalence of human sensitisation. It should be remembered that contact sensitisation is a persistent condition; thus, once sensitised to a chemical, an individual is at risk of dermatitis whenever exposed to the same or antigenically cross-reactive chemical (e.g. nickel in jewellery).

A CHMP guideline, *Non-clinical Local Tolerance Testing of Medicinal Products*, refers to the murine local lymph node assay as a method for the assessment of the induction phase of skin sensitisation. This method measures the ability of compounds to induce proliferate responses in skin-draining lymph nodes. This method uses fewer animals than alternative *in vivo* methods and reduces the trauma to which animals

are potentially subjected.[70] If combined with phenotyping by flow cytometry, the system may also qualify for a semi-quantitative assessment of hypersentivity or allergic contact dermatitis.[71]

3.8.2.2 Immunosuppression

Suppression and enhancement of immune functions are general concerns associated with human risk assessment of pharmaceuticals. An impaired immune response may be associated with a number or risks, among them an impairment of the ability to battle infections or to control tumour growth at early stages. The safety concerns about enhanced immune functions are less well characterised. An ICH S8 guideline on immunotoxicity studies in for human pharmaceuticals has been communicated in 2005. This guideline supersedes earlier guidelines existing in Europe. According to this ICH guideline, immunosuppression or enhancement can be associated with two distinct groups:

1. Drugs intended to modulate immune function for therapeutic purposes (e.g. to prevent organ transplant rejection) where adverse immunosuppression can be considered exaggerated pharmacodynamics.

2. Drugs not intended to affect immune function but cause immunotoxicity as a result, for instance, of necrosis or apoptosis of immune cells or interaction with cellular receptors shared by both target tissues and non-target immune system cells.

For the assessment of effects of pharmaceuticals on immune function parameters, the following endpoints are of importance:

1. Hematological changes such as leucocytopenia/leucocytosis, granulocytopenia/granulocytosis or lymphopenia/lymphocytosis;

2. Alterations in immune system organ weights and/or histology (e.g. changes in thymus, spleen, lymph nodes and/or bone marrow);

3. Changes in serum globulins that occur without a plausible explanation, such as effects on the liver or kidney, can be an indication that there are changes in serum immunoglobulins;

4. Increased incidence of infections; and

5. Increased occurrence of tumours can be viewed as a sign of immunosuppression in the absence of other plausible causes such as genotoxicity, hormonal effects or liver enzyme induction.

An appropriate strategy is to look for changes in these parameters primarily in the standard rodent and non-rodent repeat-dose toxicity studies. Because of differences in the immune system, in particular with respect to lymphocyte subtypes, between rodents, non-rodents and humans, relevance assessment of findings for human risk needs specific attention. Hence, depending on the nature of changes in the parameters in standard toxicity studies, additional specific studies on immune function parameters may be needed, such as a T-cell dependent antibody response (TDAR).

3.8.2.3 Immunogenicity

The number of biological/biotechnology-derived proteins used as therapeutic agents is steadily increasing. These products may induce an unwanted immune response in treated patients, which can be influenced by various factors, including patient- or disease-related and product-related factors. In this context, recent experience with TGN1412, a CD28 antibody introduced into normal healthy human volunteers by Tegenero in March 2006[1] triggered fundamental learning for the industry. TGN1412 at a dose of 0.1 mg/kg triggered a cytokine storm in all treated human volunteers in a phase I study at Northwick Park Hospital in the UK in 2006 (http://www.mhra.gov.uk/NewsCentre/Pressreleases/CON2025434), which came as a surprise for the company, the clinical trial unit and the regulatory authority that approved the trial. This case has constituted major concerns about the appropriateness of regulations for starts of human trials. In hindsight, the initial dose setting based on animal data has been reconsidered with the available data and conclusions have been provided that are indicative of too high a starting dose.[72,73] Subsequently, the case has triggered dedicated regulatory actions around the world of which the CHMP guideline, *Strategies to Identify and Mitigate Risks for First in Human Clinical Trials with Investigational Medicinal Products* (CHMP, London, 19 July 2007, Doc. Ref.EMEA/CHMP/SWP/294648/2007), has to be mentioned in particular.

With a focus on immunological reactions and the TGN1412 case, the guideline implies that animal studies with highly species-specific medicinal products may not reproduce the intended pharmacological effect in humans, give rise to misinterpretation of pharmacokinetic and pharmacodynamic results, and not identify relevant toxic effects. For example, the following modes of action might require special attention:

1. A mode of action that involves a target that is connected to multiple signalling pathways (target with pleiotropic effects), for example, leading to various physiological effects, or targets that are ubiquitously expressed, as often seen in the immune system.

2. A biological cascade or cytokine release including those leading to an amplification of an effect that might not be sufficiently controlled by a physiologic feedback mechanism (e.g. in the immune system or blood coagulation system). CD3 or CD28 (super-) agonists might serve as an example.

For further reasoning related to starting dose calculations for first human trials, see section 3.8.5.

3.8.3 Special routes

Ideally, toxicology studies should mimic, as near as possible, human exposure. Thus, both the route of administration and the exposure should, where possible, be similar to that in humans. The classic route of administration to humans is oral and thus most toxicology studies are conducted by the oral route. However, parenteral routes may be used either to mimic the clinical route or to ensure exposure. The administration of some medicines is directly on to highly differentiated surfaces such as the alveolar surface of the lungs or the skin. It is therefore important to assess the topical irritancy, absorption and subsequent systemic toxicity following such applications. It should be remembered that some compounds (e.g. chlorinated hydrocarbons) may be more toxic when given by the inhalation route than when given orally, or may directly affect the respiratory tract (e.g. formaldehyde vapour). For any such studies, it must be taken into account that excipients that ensure stability of the test compound and help delivery of the test item to the site and will assist in absorption and distribution, may have a considerable impact on the toxicity readout especially by parenteral routes of administration.

Specialised studies may be conducted at any time during the development phase. If a special route is selected as the primary route of administration then this work will be used throughout. Special routes used to supplement the main toxicology programme will usually be conducted before administration or exposure of humans to the test material by the route equivalent to the special route. The duration of dosing recommended for the special routes in different species is presented in Table 3.4. Inhalation studies of 1–3 months' duration should be performed to assess possible local effects on respiratory tissue and also to gain pharmacokinetic data. If carcinogenicity studies have been conducted by the oral route and another clinical route is to be used in humans, the need to repeat such studies should be assessed critically. Carcinogenic potential is related to the concentration of the carcinogen at its site of action. Thus, if the oral

Table 3.4 Maximum duration of dosing by special routes recommended for different species

Route of exposure	Maximum dosing period (months)				
	Mouse	Rat	Dog	Marmoset	Rabbit
Intramuscular	Single	1	1	1	1
Inhalation	Life	Life	12	–	Life
Intratracheal	Single	Single	–	–	1
Intranasal	–	1	6	–	–
Topical	Life	Life	12	12	–
Intrarectal	–	–	1	–	1
Intra-arterial	–	–	–	–	Single[a]

Life, life time; Single, single dose only; – inappropriate or no experience.
[a] Required by some regulatory authorities (e.g. Austria) for injectable products.

route results in adequate exposure of the lung, there should be no need to perform additional inhalation carcinogenicity studies.

These studies generally follow the guidelines for conventional studies (e.g. a control and three test groups receiving differing dosages). The designs are typically as follow.

3.8.3.1 Intramuscular
Varying concentrations of test material are injected into the muscle, using a constant dose volume to a maximum of 1 mL.

3.8.3.2 Inhalation
This can be subdivided into three routes.
1. *Intratracheal* – small quanties, usually less than 1 mL, of varying concentrations of solutions or varying quantities of powder are placed or blown into the trachea of an anaesthetised animal using a cannula placed intratracheally.
2. *Intranasal* – small quantities, usually <50 μL, of varying concentrations of solution or suspension of test material are placed into the nasal cavity by introduction through the external nares.
3. *Pulmonary* – animals are placed in an exposure chamber, either whole body or snout only, or individually exposed via mask systems (dogs, primates and rabbits) and allowed to inhale an aerosol of known concentrations generated from a powder, solution, suspension or a vapour of the test material for periods of up to 23 h/day for durations approaching the animal's natural lifespan.

Typically, exposure periods are 1 h/day 7 days/week using snout-only systems for pharmaceutical products, or 6 h/day 5 days/week using whole-body exposure systems for industrial chemicals.

Aerosols must be respirable (i.e. have a mean aerodynamic diameter of less than 5 μm) to ensure that a reasonable proportion will penetrate the respiratory tract defence systems of the nasal passages and the mucociliary clearance mechanisms.

3.8.3.3 Topical
Test or control material is applied either on to or under an occlusive dressing to the abraded or unabraded shaved skin of animals. Wound healing can be assessed by applying large (e.g. 1 g/L kg) topical doses of test material to an epithelial wound (e.g. an incision) and monitoring wound healing over a period of 14 days.

3.8.3.4 Intrarectal
This is usually performed only in dogs. Different dosages are administered on standard sized suppositories (e.g. size 2 mL).

3.8.3.5 Intra-arterial
This is usually performed only in rabbits. A single injection is made into the central artery of an ear. The contralateral ear artery is given the control material. This is to assess the effects if a subcutaneous or intravenous injection is accidentally injected into an artery, as drugs are rarely given by this route.

3.8.4 Specialty areas
In recent years, regulatory agencies have communicated their expectations about non-clinical studies for human safety assessment of pharmaceutical candidate compounds in a number of specialty areas, which were dealt with in a case-by-case approach so far but now see more strict regulatory expectations.

3.8.4.1 Excipients

Excipients are major components of a drug product in that they are key factors for stability and bioavailability of drugs. As such, a drug substance that is prone to decay by oxidative decomposition can be stabilized by addition of antioxidants. Further, highly lipophilic compounds may not be orally bioavailable without the help of emulsifying and surfactant excipients. A drug product such as a tablet or capsule is often composed of various excipients, the human dose of which can exceed that of the drug substance by far. Experience tells that severe human toxicity can be related to excipients such as sensitization reactions towards intravenous injection of polyethoxylated castor oils (Cremophor), which are non-ionic surfactants. As such, established excipients are normally expected to be well characterised with regard to human safety. Any new excipient has to be treated like a new drug substance including all non-clinical safety testing. A FDA guideline, *Nonclinical Studies for the Safety Evaluation of Pharmaceutical Excipients*, published in 2005 gives the US FDA perspective on this topic. Apart from excipients that are used in the final drug product for the market, there are also excipients that are exclusively used in animal experiments in order to provide a fluid formulation of the drug substance that is applicable to laboratory animals. There may be toxicity associated with these excipients with different animal species being more or less sensitive. The dog has been described to be particularly sensitive to develop anaphylactic reactions in response to preparations containing Cremophor EL or Tween 80 (polysorbate 80).[74] It is therefore indispensable to take potential excipient-related toxicities into account for the selection of appropriate animal species for toxicity testing as well as for the overall safety assessment of a new drug candidate especially if the excipient causing toxicity in animals is not present in the final drug product for human use.

3.8.4.2 Metabolites in safety testing

The appropriate reflection of human metabolites in animal safety testing has always been a challenge. The spectrum of metabolites in animal safety studies and humans may differ considerably and there are many known cases of metabolite-related toxicities for an otherwise non-toxic parent compound. A famous example is the liver toxicity of the reactive metabolite N-acetyl-p-benzo-quinone imine (NAPQI) of acetaminophen, which appears in relevant liver damaging quantities, if the main route of metabolism of acetaminophen, glutathione conjugation, is exceed by

depletion of glutathione pools at high (over)doses. Consequently, the absence of potentially toxic human metabolites in animal safety tests is a concern. Regarding expectations on how animal testing should mirror human metabolism, it is clear that major qualitative differences (i.e. the absence of a certain human pathway in animals) triggers the expectation for synthesis, formulation and testing of such metabolites in animals, possibly even including lifetime carcinogenicity studies. However, major debates in the area have been on which quantitative differences between species should trigger additional animal testing and what constitutes a relevant or major human metabolite in quantitative terms.[75] A decisive study, from which human metabolism and metabolite information can be inferred, is the human ADME study with radiolabelled drug.[76] Depending on information from *in vitro* studies with microsomal preparations or hepatocytes, such studies may be allocated earlier or later during clinical development of a candidate compound. The US FDA guideline, *Safety Testing of Drug Metabolites*, now specifies the regulatory expectations on quantity of human metabolites that can raise safety concerns to 'those formed at greater than 10 percent of parent drug systemic exposure at steady state'. The term systemic exposure refers normally to the AUC. If such metabolites are not present in animal species or in disproportionate amounts, further safety testing and assessment is expected. In practice, the stipulation on '10 percent of the parent' may constitute issues in cases of, for example, low bioavailability of the parent. Under such circumstances, strict obedience to the guideline may lead to additional animal safety testing of metabolites. Smith and Obach[77] argue in favour of using an absolute abundance cut-off instead of using a percentage relative to the parent. Many of the examples on toxicity of human metabolites that trigger concerns relate to liver toxicity, which is discussed in the next section.

3.8.4.3 Liver toxicity

Hepatotoxicity is one of the main failure reasons for clinical candidate compounds in animal toxicity studies. Despite of the prudent and stringent assessment of animal data, it is also one of the major reasons for failure in late stage clinical trials and after marketing.[9,78] Many cases of drug-induced liver toxicity have been demonstrated in humans through covalent binding of protein by reactive metabolites.[9] Measurement of covalent binding to liver microsomal proteins in the presence and the absence of nicotine adenine dinucleotide phosphate (NADPH), as well as the use of trapping agents such as glutathione or cyanide ions to provide structural information on reactive intermediates, have been used routinely to screen drug candidates. Avoidance of pathways that form reactive intermediates early in drug design may be an option to reduce such unwanted toxicities.[79] Frank liver toxicity in form of hepatic necrosis, hepatic steatosis with an early indication of effects based on clinical chemistry data can normally be delineated from animal studies. However, more subtle effects or aspects of liver toxicity that are mainly related to rare cases of potentially fatal human liver toxicity, which often involve immunological reactions, are very hard to tackle in animal studies. One reason is the low incidence of these events in humans, often associated with co-factors (alcohol, food, infections, co-medications), which cannot be assessed with low animal numbers in toxicity studies. The regulatory landscape on this topic is going in two different directions.

The US FDA has issued a draft guidance, *Drug-induced Liver Injury: Premarketing Clinical Evaluation* (US FDA, 2007). Based on the considerations that non-clinical studies have limited possibilities for an enhanced safety assessment, the guidance focuses on an enhanced readout from clinical trials. Because verification of causation is often a critical issue, the guideline addresses rechallenge of patients as follows: 'Generally, rechallenge of subjects with significant (>5xULN) aminotransferase (AT) elevations should not be attempted. If such subjects are rechallenged, they should be followed closely. Rechallenge can be considered if the subject has shown important benefit from the drug and other options are not available or if substantial accumulated data with the test drug do not show potential for severe injury.'

Contrary to the US FDA, the EU authorities follow the idea of a step-wise approach in detecting hepatotoxicity signals from animal studies and conducting mechanistic studies to assess the clinical relevance of non-clinical hepatotoxicity in their draft, *Non-clinical Guideline on Drug Induced Hepatotoxicity* (CHMP, London, 24 January 2008, Doc. Ref. EMEA/CHMP/SWP/150115/2006). The main emphasis of this guideline is to 'optimise the use of data obtained in standard non-clinical studies'.

The following key elements of the step-wise approach are taken form the draft guideline:
1. The identification of compound-related effects in clinical pathology parameters in relevant species and determination of the magnitude of that effect through the comparison of individual animal and group mean data with concurrent controls. Historical control data

can be used to place the magnitude of the changes in perspective but are not the sole determinant of whether or not a change is compound related.
2. For non-rodent studies, attention should be focused on the comparison of individual animal data prior to the treatment and at different experimental time points rather than using the group mean data for such comparisons. Despite the fact that hepatotoxicity findings may not be statistically significant because of the low number of non-rodents used in non-clinical studies, *relevant* hepatotoxicity signals observed in non-rodent studies should be thoroughly investigated.
3. The use of data obtained from mechanistic *in vitro* and/or *in vivo* models.

While both guideline approaches may improve signal detection, it is unclear whether this heightened scrutiny will eliminate compounds similar to those that have posed the concerns in the past. There is also the concern that this goes at the expense of dropping even more potentially valuable new therapeutics during development without having explored all chances for a really improved understanding of human risk for drug-induced liver injury.[80] As the liver is a highly tolerant organ and as such signals are very often detected in animal and human studies, only full immunological understanding is likely to improve the case.

3.8.4.4 Genotoxic impurities
In recent years, the testing and control of pharmaceuticals for the presence of genotoxic impurities have been under regulatory scrutiny. Because of their dedicated use – in many cases chronic use – in humans, pharmaceuticals are expected to be of high purity with little batch-to-batch variability allowed. This focus is justified compared to chemicals of other use areas, for which exposure may be dedicated but limited (e.g. cosmetics), more of an accidental type (e.g. household chemicals), or low and chronic under workplace or use conditions (e.g. pesticides, industrial chemicals).

The relevant 'ICH Q' (with 'Q' for Quality) guidelines concerning the qualification of impurities in commercial manufacture are Q3A(R) and Q3B(R) which focus on impurities in drug substances and drug products, respectively, while Q3C recommends limits for residual solvents in the drug product [ICHQ3A(R), 2002; ICHQ3B(R), 2003; ICHQ3C, 1997]. The guidance given in these regulatory documents is considered to be applicable at the time of registration of a new pharmaceutical entity. The first two guidelines describe threshold levels above which impurities are required to be reported, identified and qualified either in toxicological investigations or in the clinic. The threshold levels vary according to the maximum daily dose of a drug. For drug substance, the identification thresholds are within the range of 500–1000 p.p.m. (i.e. 0.05 and 0.1%). While in general very high purity of more than 98% is attained for pharmaceuticals, the presence of impurities even at low levels of 0.1% or lower may cause unwanted effects or may be of concern for chronic intake. This is of particular importance when the drug is taken at a high daily dose. Hence, the ICH guidelines Q3A(R) and Q3B(R) take precaution for this case and state that although identification of impurities is not generally necessary at levels less than or equal to the identification threshold, 'analytical procedures should be developed for those potential impurities that are expected to be unusually potent, producing toxic or pharmacological effects at a level not more than (≤) the identification threshold'. Thus, in the case of impurities where a potential safety concern for genotoxicity exists, the guidelines imply that the routine identification threshold is not considered to be applicable.

Because genotoxic compounds are usually considered as potentially carcinogenic with a linear dose–response relationship, genotoxic impurities are said to be considered separately from the existing ICH guidelines and limits of acceptability have to be set. As there was no general guidance on how to do this, this has led to considerable differences between regulatory authorities. To reduce the differences in judgement on genotoxic impurities between EU Member States, the CHMP decided to ask the Safety Working Party (SWP) to develop a guideline on genotoxic impurities. This guideline was released after much discussion in June 2006. The central idea in this draft guideline is the concept of the Threshold of Toxicological Concern (TTC). A TTC value of 1.5 µg/day intake of a genotoxic impurity is derived from a large database of animal carcinogenicity studies. It is estimated that the lifetime intake of any genotoxic impurity, with a few exceptions of highly potent genotoxic carcinogens,

below this TTC is associated with an acceptable lifetime cancer risk of <10^{-5}. The use of this TTC approach is proposed as a pragmatic solution for the situation where a genotoxic impurity cannot be avoided and where no compound-specific information is available on the carcinogenic potential of the impurity.

While the generic TTC of 1.5 µg/day is based on a risk delineation from animal data for human lifetime use, it is acknowledged that most pharmaceuticals are not given over lifetime. In addition, the investigation of pharmaceutical candidates compounds in clinical trials will generally involve fewer subjects and treatment for shorter durations than marketing authorization. Based on the knowledge that human tumour risk from exposure to genotoxic carcinogens is not only a function of dose, but also a function of duration of exposure,[81] a so-called 'staged' TTC concept was proposed.[82] According to this concept, generic TTC values can be calculated for durations of exposure that occur typically during clinical trials for pharmaceutical candidate development (Table 3.5). In addition to the back-calculation of lifetime risk data to shorter durations, two additional considerations were taken into account when Müller et al.[82] proposed these values:

1. If clinical use of a pharmaceutical extents beyond a duration of 12 months, a chronic lifetime exposure cannot be excluded; and
2. In the clinical trial stage, the benefits of a pharmaceutical candidate are not fully established.

Hence, the generic TTC value of 1.5 µg/day is proposed for any intake duration of more than 12 months and all staged TTC values for shorter duration of exposure are calculated using an acceptable risk of <10^{-6} instead of <10^{-5}.

In 2008, the CHMP has communicated its regulatory position for the EU on staged TTC values for genotoxic impurities in pharmaceuticals (CHMP, London, 26 June 2008, Doc. Ref. EMEA/CHMP/SWP/431994/2007). These values are given in Table 3.6. Compared with the proposal of a staged TTC according to Müller et al.,[82] these values incorporate a dose rate correction factor of 2 to account for deviations

Table 3.5 Generic staged Threshold of Toxicological Concern (TTC) values for genotoxic impurities during the clinical trial stage for pharmaceutical candidate compounds[82]

	Duration of exposure				
	≤1 month	>1–3 months	>3–6 months	>6–12 months	>12 months
Allowable daily intake (µg/person/day)	120	40	20	10	1.5

Table 3.6 Generic staged Threshold of Toxicological Concern (TTC) values for genotoxic impurities during the clinical trial stage for pharmaceutical candidate compounds proposed by the Committee on Human Medicinal Products (CHMP) in the EU

	Duration of exposure					
	Single dose	≤1 month	≤3 months	≤6 months	≤12 months	>12 months
Allowable daily intake (μg/person/day)	120	60	20	10	5	1.5

from the linear extrapolation model and hence are more conservative. In the meantime, also the US Food and Drug Administration has issued a draft guidance on this topic, which represents a somewhat less conservative approach compared to table 3.6 and hence is not displayed here. Regulatory guidance will certainly further evolve as a globally harmonized approach is certainly needed.

3.8.4.5 Dependence potential

Drugs acting can produce dependence symptoms, in particular the ones acting on the central nervous system. Reinforcing properties and physical withdrawal phenomena are well-known aspects of dependence potential. However, other aspects of withdrawal which are less clear by plain clinical observation, as exemplified by selective serotonin re-uptake inhibitors (SSRIs), also need to be evaluated. In this context, the CHMP has issued the *Guideline on the Non-Clinical Investigation of the Dependence Potential of Medicinal Products* (CHMP, EMEA/CHMP/SWP/94227/2004, 23 March 2006). In this guideline, a tiered approach to the issue by non-clinical studies is proposed. Tier 1 consists of receptorbinding studies, which are usually part of early development of CNS active substances. *In vivo*, confirmation of the binding and functional properties observed *in vitro* can be obtained. Initial investigations could make use of neuropharmacological models such as microdialysis (e.g. dopamine release in nucleus accumbens), neurotransmitter turnover, head twitch, antinociception and locomotor activity. These studies are normally completed prior to first clinical trials. Tier 2 includes:

1. Behavioural models, in which multiple endpoints should be examined such as motor function, cognitive function and appetitively motivated behaviour.[83] The different endpoints should be monitored before, during and after treatment.
2. Studies on withdrawal symptoms once the active substance is withdrawn.
3. Studies on reinforcing properties of active substances in which the self-administration paradigm

is most widely used and may be seen as an approach with great face validity. Such studies may be carried out alongside already running clinical investigations.

3.8.5 Scaling from animals to humans

One of the most difficult tasks in preclinical testing is the scaling from animal data to humans, especially for first-in-human studies. Because various kinds of toxicities are observed for most test items, some kind of safety or exposure margin assessment is expected to result from animal experiments to judge hazard and risk in humans. This will have to be based on measurements of exposure in the toxicity studies compared to the likely human exposure. For any new therapeutic principle, one of the hardest things is to predict likely human therapeutic exposure based on results of *in vivo* pharmacology studies in animals. For prediction of human exposure, a good starting point is usually an assessment of bioavailability in animals by the specific intended route relative to the generally high or absolute bioavailability by the intravenous route. Hence, absorption and systemic toxicity observed using special routes should be compared with the more usual intravenous or oral routes of administration to identify and assess the relevance of any significant differences observed. Plasma levels will obviously depend on the amount of drug absorbed. Higher systemic (i.e. circulating) levels of drug may help explain the differences in toxicity between routes. Corticosteroids are more toxic on the basis of administered dose when given by the inhalation compared with the oral route. It is the ratio of the AUC for the plasma concentration–time curve in the animal to that in humans that constitutes the key element in predicting human toxicity. The art of mechanism-based pharmacokinetic-pharmacodynamic (PK-PD) modelling in drug research has considerably improved over the past few years[84] to the extent that modelling of exposure for first human trials based on animal data became more reliable including those for drugs with, for example, high lipophilicity.[85]

If pharmacokinetic data are not available or not fully trustworthy (e.g. if animal data vary in terms of toxicities associated with exposure and an apparent reason is not obvious), an approximation can be given using a scaling factor that converts body weight to surface area. It was found by Freireich et al.[86] that toxicity of anticancer drugs between species equated to surface area. Using a scaling factor of $X^{0.66}$, where X is the body weight, converts milligram of drug per kilogram of body weight to milligram of drug to metre square of body surface. The US FDA has communicated a draft guideline on estimating the maximum safe starting dose in initial clinical trials for therapeutics in adult healthy volunteers which uses these factors (US FDA, 2005). Table 1 in this FDA guideline indicates factors to convert animal doses into a human equivalent dose (HED). As an example, a mg/kg dose used in the rat needs to be multiplied by 6 to obtain a HED in terms of mg/m^2. For estimation of a safe human starting dose, additional safety factors (e.g. the generic factor of 10) may be used.

On biologicals, the recent Tegenero case[1] suggests that a high level of caution regarding the starting dose and reversibility of side effects has to be applied when highly pharmacologically active principles are about to be tested in humans and for principles for which large pharmacological differences between animals and humans are expected. In this context, McLean[72] has reassessed the appropriate starting dose for the monoclonal antibody TGN1412, a CD28 receptor binding protein, which leads to a massive cytokine release in humans after a single dose. Further, the long half-life of such antibodies implies usually a slow reversibility of side effects.

3.9 Animal numbers, costs and ethics

Toxicity studies are costly in terms of both animals and resources, as indicated in Table 3.7. For a product developed for chronic oral therapy, approximately 4000 rats, 1300 mice, 100 rabbits, 50 guinea pigs and 160 dogs (or a comparable number of monkeys), a total of nearly 6000 animals, is used. If the fetuses and offspring from the reproductive toxicity studies are included, the total doubles. However, the number of animals used in toxicity testing in the pharmaceutical industry compared with the total used is surprisingly low. We recently estimated this to be less than 7.5%. Pharmacological screening for drugs uses by far the greater proportion of animals.

The financial costs are also considerable and have increased significantly over time. To complete the toxicology programme, an inhalation product would cost over £6,000,000 and with the most expeditious planning would take 5 years to complete.

Is all this testing necessary? Retrospective studies show that the detection of clinically relevant toxicities by preclinical animal studies is high and useful, although it is by no means 100%.[3] Fortunately, there has been no repetition on of the scale of the thalidomide catastrophe of the 1960s; however, the recent case of severe immunological reactions towards the first human dose of TGN1412, a CD28 antibody,[1] has renewed discussion on the types of studies required to enter human trials. This has led the European regulatory authorities to quickly generate a specific guidance for strategies to identify and mitigate risks for first-in-human clinical trials with investigational medicinal products.

Most toxicologists agree that if one considers the list of studies required for regulatory approval, there is much room for rationalisation and cutting down on the full range of studies required, without compromising patient safety. There has been a tendency for regulatory authorities to increase the requirements for additional tests on largely theoretical grounds, where there is little or no clinical information to show that current methods do not describe the relevant toxicities adequately. Statistically, carcinogenicity studies are very insensitive and as knowledge increases, it is becoming possible to argue that the large majority of genotoxic carcinogens are detectable by genotoxicity assays and non-genotoxic carcinogens by changes detected in repeat-dose toxicity studies (e.g. hormonal imbalances, tissue specific cell proliferation).[87] It is hoped that the ICH process will continue to be a useful platform not only for a harmonisation of requirements, but also for a complete rationalisation of the toxicity testing programme. Minimization of animal use is an established goal of the ICH guideline process. It has been estimated that the number of animals used in toxicology for registration of a 'standard' compound can be reduced by 50% (pre- and post-ICH).[88,89]

In the future it is possible that the need for animal studies will be further minimised by the use of low and ultra-low dose studies in humans, where refinements in measuring such low doses[90] and the ability to measure and interpret toxicologically relevant changes by use of the 'omic' technologies will increase over time.

Table 3.7 Toxicity studies – approximate cost, test material requirement and reporting times

Study type	Species	No. of animals[a]	Cost[b] (£ thousands)	Test material Factor Q[c]	Report[d] (weeks after study start)
1 month toxicity	Rat	160	70	0.5	20
	Dog	32	120	4	20
	Monkey	32	350	3	20
3 months toxicity	Rat	160	160	1.8	26
	Dog	40	140	15	29
	Monkey	32	450	12	29
6 months toxicity	Rat	192	250	3.7	45
	Dog	40	190	30	45
	Monkey	40	650	25	45
9 (or 12 months toxicity)	Dog	40	400 (600)	60	58 (71)
	Monkey	40	850 (1000)	55	58 (71)
ICH reproductive toxicity study	Rat	200 (1770)	50	1.13	32
Organogenesis	Rabbit	88 (440)	60	1.37	34
Peri-postnatal	Rat	60 (1500)	100	0.35	30
3 months dose range finding study (for cancer study)	Mouse	90	120	0.1	29
Oncogenicity (gavage)	Mouse (80 weeks)	Up to 1000	1000	5.4	150
	Rat (2 years)	600	1000	33.7	150
Genetic toxicology					
Microbial			4	6	3
Mouse lymphoma			18	10	8
Human lymphocyte			18	10	12
Micronucleus	Rat	60	10	24	12

ICH, International Conference on Harmonization of Technical Requirements for Registration of Pharmaceuticals for Human Use.

The figures are for study designs that meet worldwide regulatory requirements for pharmaceuticals. Variations that may be encountered are given in footnotes.

[a] Animal numbers in parentheses are numbers of fetuses/offspring produced.

[b] Costs are approximate (as of 2008) and assume oral (gavage) administration and include costs of assay to confirm dose concentration, bioassay of pharmacokinetic samples and extra groups for assessment of reversibility. Significant variations for the same study design will be found between different contractors (± 20%), different study designs (± 25%) and different routes of administration (intravenous + 25%, inhalation by snout only + 50–100%).

[c] The total quantity of test material required for the study, in grams, is given by the formula Q × sum of the dose levels in mg. Example: a 6-month dog study with dose levels of 100, 200 and 400 mg/kg requires 23.8 kg test material: i.e. $34 \times (100 + 200 + 400)$ g.

Q takes into account, where appropriate, the inclusion in the study design of sufficient animals to study recovery and pharmacokinetics, the projected mean body weight of the animals over the study and a 20% contingency for unexpected losses, etc.

[d] Times given are for a draft report prior to Quality Assurance Unit (QAU) audit, from start of the *in vivo* phase of the study, including a recovery period. It is possible to reduce these times by one-third if given adequate priority.

Acknowledgements

David Scales and David Tweats wrote the earlier editions of this chapter and their insight and knowledge are gratefully acknowledged.

References

All regulatory Guidelines referred to in this chapter can be accessed via the internet addresses of the respective regulatory agency and via the ICH or OECD websites:
EU CHMP guidelines: http://www.emea.europa.eu/
ICH guidelines: http://www.ich.org
Japan MHLW guidelines: http://www.mhlw.go.jp/english/
OECD guidelines: http://www.oecd.org/dataoecd/9/11/
33663321.pdf
US FDA guidelines: http://www.fda.gov/cder/

1 Tegenero TGN1412. Investigators Brochure and Protocol for TGN1412. http://www.mhra.gov.uk, 2006.

2 Zbinden G. Predictive value of animal studies in toxicology. CMR Annual Lecture, 1987.

3 Olson H, Betton G, Robinson D et al. Concordance of the toxicity of pharmaceuticals in humans and in animals. *Reg Toxicol Pharmacol* 2000;**32**:36–67.

4 Pennie WD. Use of cDNA microarrays to probe and understand the toxicological consequences of altered gene expression. *Toxicol Lett* 2000;**112**:473–7.

5 Steiner S, Wiltzman FW. Proteomics: applications and opportunities in preclinical drug development. *Electrophoresis* 2000;**21**:2099–104.

6 Robertson DG, Reily MD, Sigler RE et al. Metabonomics: evaluation of nuclear magnetic resonance (NMR) and pattern recognition technology for rapid *in vivo* screening of liver and kidney toxicants. *Toxicol Sci* 2000;**57**:326–37.

7 Jacobs A. An FDA perspective on the non-clinical use of the X-Omics technologies and the safety of new drugs: the vision of the FDA. *Toxicol Lett* 2009;**186**:32–5.

8 Fenichel RR, Malik M, Antzelevitch C et al. Drug-induced torsades de pointes and implications for drug development. *J Cardiovasc Electrophysiol* 2004;**15**:475–95.

9 Walgren JL, Mitchell MD, Thompson DC. Role of metabolism in drug-induced idiosyncratic hepatotoxicity. *Crit Rev Toxicol* 2005;**35**:325–41.

10 Russell WMS, Burch RL. *The Principles of Humane Experimental Technique*. London: Methuen, 1959.

11 Lynch A, Connelly J. Drug discovery and development: the toxicologist's view – non-clinical safety assessment. In: Wilkins MR, ed. *Experimental Therapeutics*. London: Martin Dunitz, 2003;25–50.

12 Goodsaid F, Frueh FW. Implementing the US FDA guidance on pharmacogenomic data submissions. *Environ Mol Mutagen* 2007;**48**:354–8.

13 Leighton JK, Brown P, Ellis A et al. Workgroup Report: Review of genomics data based on experience with mock submissions – view of the CDER Pharmacology Toxicology Nonclinical Pharmacogenomics Subcommittee. *Environ Health Perspect* 2006;**114**:573–8.

14 Microarray Gene Expression Data (MGED) Society, 2004. MGED Reporting Structure for Biological Investigations (RSBI). Tiered Checklist: A proposed framework structure for reporting biological investigations. http://www.mged.org/Workgroups/rsbi/RSBI-TIRS-Proposal_1_.doc.

15 Tugwood JD, Hollins LE, Cockerill MJ. Genomics and the search for novel biomarkers in toxicology. *Biomarkers* 2003;**8**:79–92.

16 Lühe A, Suter L, Ruepp S et al. Toxicogenomics in the pharmaceutical industry: hollow promises or real benefit? *Mutat Res* 2005;**575**:102–15.

17 Bandara LR, Kennedy S. Toxicoproteomics: a new preclinical tool. *Drug Discov Today* 2002;**7**:411–8.

18 Stapels MD, Barofsky DF. Complementary use of MALDI and ESI for the HPLC-MS/MS analysis of DNA-binding proteins. *Anal Chem* 2004;**76**:5421–30.

19 Dare TO, Davies HA, Turton JA et al. Application of surface-enhanced laser desorption/ionization technology to the detection and identification of urinary parvalbumin-alpha: a biomarker of compound-induced skeletal muscle toxicity in the rat. *Electrophoresis* 2002;**23**:3241–51.

20 Kung LA, Snyder M. Proteome chips for whole-organism assays. *Nat Rev Mol Cell Biol* 2006;**7**:617–22.

21 Hassan S, Ferrario C, Mamo A et al. Tissue microarrays: emerging standard for biomarker validation. *Curr Opin Biotechnol* 2008;**19**:19–25.

22 Nicholson JK, Connelly J, Lindon JC, Holmes E. Metabonomics: a platform for studying drug toxicity and gene function. *Nat Rev Drug Discov* 2002;**1**:153–61.

23 Clarke CJ, Haselden JN. Metabolic profiling as a tool for understanding mechanisms of toxicity. *Toxicol Pathol* 2008;**36**:140–7.

24 Connor SC, Wu W, Sweatman BC et al. Effects of feeding and body weight loss on the 1H-NMR-based urine metabolic profiles of male Wistar Han rats: implications for biomarker discovery. *Biomarkers* 2004;**9**:156–79.

25 Tong W, Harris S, Cao X et al. Development of public toxicogenomics software for microarray data management and analysis. *Mutat Res* 2004;**549**:241–53.

26 Mulrane L, Rexhepaj E, Smart V et al. Creation of a digital slide and tissue microarray resource from a multi-institutional predictive toxicology study in the rat: an initial report from the PredTox group. *Exp Toxicol Pathol* 2008;**60**:235–45.

27 Treinen KA, Louden C, Dennis M-J. Developmental toxicity and toxicokinetics of two endothelin receptor antagonists in rats and rabbits. *Teratology* 1999;**59**:51–9.

28 Scales MDC. An introduction to regulatory toxicology for human medicines. *BIRA J* 1990;**9**:17–21.

29 GLP. *Guide to the UK GLP Regulations 1999*. London SW8 5NQ: Department of Health, UK Good Laboratory

Practice monitoring Authority, MHRA Publications, 2000.

30 Redfern WS, Wakefield ID, Prior H et al. Safety pharmacology: a progressive approach. *Fund Clin Pharmacol* 2002;**16**:161–73.

31 Ross JF, Mattson JL, Fix AS. Expanded clinical observations in toxicity studies: historical perspectives and contemporary issues. *Regul Toxicol Pharmacol* 1998;**28**: 17–26.

32 Irwin S. Comprehensive observational assessment. *Psychopharmacologia (Berl.)* 1968;**13**:222–57.

33 Crumb W, Cavero I. QT interval prolongation by noncardiovascular drugs: issues and solutions for novel drug development. *Pharm Sci Technol Today* 1999;**2**:270–80.

34 Shah RR. Drugs, QT interval prolongation and ICH E14: the need to get it right. *Drug Saf* 2005;**28**:115–25.

35 Dessertenne F. La tachycardie ventriculaire à deux foyers opposés variable. *Arch Mal Coeur Vaiss* 1996;**59**:263–72.

36 Recanatini M, Poluzzi E, Masetti M et al. QT prolongation through hERG K⁺ channel blockade: current knowledge and strategies for the early prediction during drug development. *Med Res Rev* 2005;**25**:133–66.

37 Witchel HJ, Milnes JT, Mitcheson JS, Nancox JC. Troubleshooting problems with *in vitro* screening of drugs for QT interval prolongation using HERG K⁺ channels expressed in mammalian cell lines and Xenopus oocytes. *J Pharmacol Toxicol Methods* 2002;**48**:65–80.

38 Spurling NW, Carey PF. Dose selection for toxicity studies: a protocol for determining the maximum repeatable dose. *Human Exp Toxicol* 1992;**11**:449–58.

39 Scales MDC. Relevance of preclinical testing to risk assessment. *BIRA J* 1990;**9**:11–4.

40 Roe FJC. Food and cancer. *J Human Nutr* 1979;**33**:405–15.

41 Peraino C, Fry RDM, Staffeldt E. Enhancement of spontaneous hepatic tumourigenesis in C3H mice by dietary phenobarbital. *J Natl Cancer Inst* 1973;**51**:1349.

42 CPMP/SWP/2592/04 Rev1. Conclusions and recommendations on the use of genetically modified animal models for carcinogenicity assessment. 2004.

43 MacDonald J, French JE, Gerson RJ et al. The utility of genetically modified mouse assays for identifying human carcinogens: a basic understanding and path forward. *Toxicol Sci* 2004;**77**:188–94.

44 Custer L, Gibson DP, Aardema MJ, Le Boeuf RA. A refined protocol for conducting the low pH 6.7. Syrian hamster embryo (SHE) cell transformation assay. *Mutat Res* 2000;**455**:129–39.

45 Farmer P. Committee on Mutagenicity of Chemicals in Food, Consumer Products and the Environment ILSI/HESI research programme on alternative cancer models: results of Syrian hamster embryo cell transformation assay. International Life Sciences Institute/Health and Environmental Science Institute. *Toxicol Pathol* 2002;**30**: 536–8.

46 Jacobs A. Prediction of 2-year carcinogenicity study results for pharmaceutical products: how are we doing? *Toxicol Sci* 2005;**88**:18–23.

47 Robens JF, Piegorsch WW, Schveler RL. Methods in testing for carcinogenicity. In: Wallace Hayes A, ed. *Principles and Methods of Toxicology*. New York: Raven Press, 1989;79–107.

48 Peto R, Pike M, Day N et al. Guidelines for simple sensitive significance tests for carcinogenic effects in long-term animal experiments. *International Agency for Research on Cancer Monograph* 1980;**Suppl 2**:311–426.

49 Sakai T, Takahashi M, Mitsumori K et al. Collaborative work to evaluate toxicity on male reproductive organs by 2-week repeated dose toxicity studies in rats: overview of the studies. *J Toxicol Sci* 2000;**25**:1–21.

50 WHO. Report and Recommendations of a WHO International Workshop. Impact of the environment on reproductive health. *Dan Med Bull* 1990;**38**:425–6.

51 Reddy MV, Randerath K. Nuclease P1-mediated enhancement of sensitivity of ³²P-postlabelling test for structurally diverse DNA adducts. *Carcinogenesis* 1986;**1**:1543–51.

52 Brendler-Schwaab SY, Hartmann A, Pfuhler S, Speit G. The *in vivo* comet assay: use and status in genotoxicity testing. *Mutagenesis* 2005;**20**:245–54.

53 Thybaud V, Dean S, Nohmi T et al. *In vivo* transgenic mutation assays. *Mutat Res* 2003;**540**:141–51.

54 Kirkland DJ, ed. *Basic Mutagenicity Tests*. Cambridge: Cambridge University Press, 1990.

55 Kirsch-Volders M, Sofuni T, Aardema M et al. Report from the *in vitro* micronucleus assay working group. *Mutat Res* 2003;**540**:153–63.

56 Corvi R, Albertini S, Hartung T et al. ECVAM retrospective validation of the *in vitro* micronucleus test (MNT). *Mutagenesis* 2008;**23**:271–83.

57 Ostling O, Johanson KJ. Microelectrophoretic study of radiation-induced DNA damages in individual mammalian cells. *Biochem Biophys Res Commun* 1984;**123**: 291–8.

58 Singh NP, McCoy MT, Tice RR, Schneider EL. A simple technique for quantitation of low levels of DNA damage in individual cells. *Exp Cell Res* 1988;**175**:184–91.

59 Hartmann A, Agurell E, Beevers C et al. Recommendations for conducting the *in vivo* alkaline Comet assay. *Mutagenesis* 2003;**18**:45–51.

60 Thybaud V, Aardema M, Clements J et al. Strategy for genotoxicity testing: hazard identification and risk assessment in relation to *in vitro* testing. *Mutat Res* 2007;**627**:41–58.

61 Müller L, Kasper P. Human biological relevance and the use of threshold arguments in regulatory genotoxicity assessment: experience with pharmaceuticals. *Mutat Res* 2000;**464**:9–34.

62 Kirkland DJ, Pfuhler S, Tweats D et al. How to reduce false positive results when undertaking *in vitro* genotoxicity testing and thus avoid unnecessary follow-up animal tests: report of the ECVAM workshop. *Mutat Res* 2007;**628**:31–55.

63 Ku WW, Bigger A, Brambilla G et al. Strategy for genotoxicity testing: metabolic considerations. *Mutat Res* 2007;**627**:59–77.

64 Kasper P, Uno Y, Mauthe R et al. Follow-up testing of rodent carcinogens not positive in the standard genotoxicity testing battery: IWGT workgroup report. *Mutat Res* 2007;**627**:106–16.

65 Draize JH, Woodward G, Calvery HO. Methods for the study of irritation and toxicity of substances applied to the skin and mucous membranes. *J Pharmacol Exp Ther* 1944;**83**:337–90.

66 Liebsch M, Spielmann H. Currently available *in vitro* methods used in regulatory toxicology. *Toxicol Lett* 2002;**127**:127–34.

67 Curren RD, Harbell JW. Ocular safety: a silent (*in vitro*) success story. *Altern Lab Anim* 2002;**2**(Suppl. 1):69–74.

68 Magnussun B, Kligman AM. The identification of contact allergens by animal assay: the guinea pig maximisation test. *J Invest Dermatol* 1969;**52**:268–76.

69 Buehler EV. Delayed contact hypersensitivity in the guinea pig. *Arch Dermatol* 1965;**91**:171–5.

70 Kimber I. Skin sensitisation: immunological mechanisms and novel approaches to predictive testing. In: Balls M, Van Zeller A-M, Halder M, eds. *Proceedings of the Third World Congress on Alternatives and Animal Use in the Life Sciences. Progress in the Reduction, Refinement and Replacement of Animal Experimentation.* Amsterdam: Elsevier, 2000;613–21.

71 ICCVAM Murine local lymph node assay. 2008. http://iccvam.niehs.nih.gov/methods/immunotox/immunotox.htm

72 McLean AEM. A calculation of the starting dose for human exposure to a monoclonal antibody TGN1412. *Toxicology* 2007;**231**:102–3.

73 Schneider CK, Kalinke U, Löwer J. TGN1412: a regulator's perspective. *Nat Biotechnol* 2006;**24**:493–6.

74 Lorenz W, Reimann HJ, Schmal A et al. Histamine release in dogs by Cremophor E1 and its derivatives: oxethylated oleic acid is the most effective constituent. *Agents Actions* 1977;**7**:63–7.

75 Baillie TA, Cayen MN, Fouda H et al. Drug metabolites in safety testing. *Toxicol Appl Pharmacol* 2002;**182**:188–96.

76 Smith DA, Obach RS. Metabolites and safety: what are the concerns and how should we address them. *Chem Res Toxicol* 2006;**19**:1570–9.

77 Smith D, Obach RS. Seeing through the MIST: abundance versus percentage – commentary on metabolites in safety testing. *Drug Metab Dispos* 2005;**33**:1409–17.

78 Navarro VJ, Senior JR. Drug-related hepatotoxicity. *N Engl J Med* 2006;**354**:731–9.

79 Doss GA, Baillie TA. Addressing metabolic activation as an integral component of drug design. *Drug Metab Rev* 2006;**38**:641–9.

80 Hughes B. Industry concern over EU hepatotoxicity guidance. *Nat Rev* 2008;**7**:719.

81 Bos PMJ, Baars B, Marcel TM, van Raaij TM. Risk assessment of peak exposure to genotoxic carcinogens. *Toxicol Lett* 2004;**151**:43–50.

82 Müller L, Mauthe RJ, Riley CM et al. A rationale for determination, testing and control of genotoxic impurities in pharmaceuticals. *Regul Toxicol Pharmacol* 2006;**44**:198–211.

83 Balster RL, Bigelow GE. Guidelines and methodological reviews concerning drug abuse liability assessment. *Drug Alcchol Depend* 2003;**70**(Suppl. 1):S13–40.

84 Danhof M, de Lange ECM, Della Pasqua OE et al. Mechanism-based pharmacokinetic-pharmacodynamic (PK-PD) modeling in translational drug research. *Trends Pharmacol Sci* 2008;**29**:186–91.

85 Tang H, Hussain A, Leal M et al. Interspecies prediction of human drug clearance base on scaling data from one or two animal species. *Drug Metab Dispos* 2007;**35**:1886–93.

86 Freireich EJ, Gehan EA, Rail DP et al. Quantitative comparison of toxicity of anticancer agents in mouse, rat, hamster, dog, monkey, and man. *Cancer Chemother Rep* 1966;**50**:219–43.

87 Monro AM, MacDonald JS. Evaluation of the carcinogenic potential of pharmaceuticals: opportunities arising from the International Conference on Harmonisation. *Drug Saf* 1998;**18**:309–19.

88 Tweats DJ. A review of the reduction and refinement of regulatory studies for pharmaceuticals. In: Balls M, Van Zeller A-M, Halder M, eds. *Proceedings of the Third World Congress on Alternatives and Animal Use in the Life Sciences. Progress in the Reduction, Refinement and Replacement of Animal Experimentation.* Amsterdam: Elsevier, 2000;783–91.

89 Lumley CE, Van Cauteren H. Harmonisation of international toxicity testing guidelines for pharmaceuticals: contribution to refinement and reduction in animal uses. *Eur Biomed Res Assoc Bull* 1997;**Nov**:4–9.

90 Lappin G, Garner RC. Big physics, small doses: the use of AMS and PET in human microdosing of development drugs. *Nat Rev Drug Discov* 2003;**2**:233–40.

4 Exploratory development

John Posner

Independent Consultant in Pharmaceutical Medicine, John Posner Consulting, Beckenham, Kent, UK

4.1 Introduction

4.1.1 Definitions

'Exploratory development' (ED) can be defined as 'the first part of clinical drug development in which tolerability, pharmacokinetics and pharmacodynamic activity are defined in humans and in which an early indication of therapeutic efficacy is often obtained'. It begins with preparation for the first study in humans (FIH) and, if all goes well, ends with 'proof of concept'.

The term 'proof of concept' (PoC) is the demonstration that predefined requirements have been met in a clinical trial for the drug to be considered a candidate for full development (FD) in which there will be commitment to doing everything required to gain a product licence. The term 'proof of principle' is often but not always used as synonymous with PoC. These are particularly useful terms when applied to a drug thought to act by a novel mechanism of action. For example, a drug may be the first known inhibitor of a particular enzyme or antagonist at a certain receptor and the PoC will be a demonstration that such inhibition results in a desired pharmacodynamic or clinical endpoint. The terms are perhaps less appropriate when the mechanism of action of the drug class to which the drug belongs is well established. In such cases, the critical success factors relating to the specific drug are often referred to as 'drugability' by which one means the pharmacokinetic profile and resultant dosing schedule or the therapeutic index compared with that of a competitor marketed product. Demonstration of such properties may be critical success factors for the drug but cannot really be considered PoC.

Clinical drug development involves trials with investigational medicinal products (IMPs) but the definition of an IMP includes placebos and marketed products used as controls.[1] In ED we are really focusing on 'new molecular entities' (NMEs), which can be defined simply as 'unlicensed new chemical or biological entities whose therapeutic potential is under investigation'. New chemical entities (NCEs) are small molecules typically of molecular weight ranging 250–500 Da. By contrast, new biological entities (NBEs), often just called 'biologicals', may range from small peptides to proteins of many kilodaltons.

The term 'phase I' is applicable to the FIH in healthy volunteers to determine the safety and tolerability, pharmacodynamic effects and the pharmacokinetics of an NME. However, early evaluation of drugs used in oncology, many biologicals, anaesthetics and others is often performed in patients in whom efficacy may also be demonstrated. The term 'phase I' is also often used to describe such studies. Conversely, human pharmacology studies in healthy volunteer studies are performed throughout the drug development process. For example, studies of drug interactions and pharmacokinetics of new formulations are frequently conducted at a late stage of drug development and studies to support new indications and other line extensions may be performed years after the first licence is granted. Thus, the term 'phase I' has a variety of meanings and is ambiguous.

'Phase II' refers to studies in patients with the target disease to determine safety and preliminary evidence of efficacy. However, what matters is whether proof of concept has been established and with what degree of certainty and in what range of doses. Phase I and at least part of phase II are encompassed by ED but these terms do not capture the exploratory nature of early drug development. They also suggest that the process is linear, whereas in practice the phases of

The Textbook of Pharmaceutical Medicine. Edited by John P. Griffin. © 2009, ISBN: 978-1-4051-8035-1.

drug development are often not well demarcated and different activities run concurrently. For these reasons, I shall not use these terms in this chapter.

4.1.2 Objectives of exploratory development

The overall aim of ED is to reject those NMEs that will not make useful medicines as early as possible and to select NMEs appropriate for full development with the intention of proceeding to 'marketing authorisation application' (MAA) in Europe and 'new drug application' in the USA. Therefore in ED we evaluate a compound critically to establish whether or not it has a certain desired profile.

By contrast, in FD there should be sufficient knowledge about the compound to merit the commitment of enormous resources required to conduct:
• Adequately powered, controlled clinical trials of efficacy and safety;
• Scale-up manufacture of raw material and formulated product;
• Chronic toxicology and carcinogenicity studies;
• Human pharmacology/pharmacokinetic studies;
• Additional clinical studies to address specific issues; and
• Pharmacovigilance and regulatory activities needed for registration.

This approach to drug development has been referred to as 'learn–confirm' in which the effort is invested to learn as much as possible about the NME during ED to make a decision whether to proceed to FD or reject the compound. If the decision is made to continue, the studies should confirm the earlier findings and there should be few nasty surprises in FD. However, it should be recognised that there is never enough information to make 'risk-free' decisions, particularly when working with a novel mechanism of action, and uncommon and rare adverse reactions, which may be critically important, are unlikely to be detected during the course of ED because of the small number of subjects exposed at this stage of development.

Exploratory development begins with the identification of 'critical success factors' for the particular NME. Starting with the first administration to humans, a small number of well-designed and conducted human pharmacology studies should go a long way to describing the profile of the drug and whether it meets the requirements of the previously identified critical success factors.

As early as possible we should try to establish the range of drug doses that produce the desired effect and the relationships between dose, plasma concentration and the magnitude of desired and undesired effects. If

> **BOX 4.1** Objectives of studies in exploratory development
>
> • To identify the relationship between dose and plasma (or other) concentrations – pharmacokinetics
> • To define the shape and location of the dose–concentration–response curves for both desired and undesired effects – preliminary assessment of benefit : risk
> • On the basis of these curves, to identify the range of dosage and concentrations producing maximum benefit with fewest undesirable effects.

successful, much time and resource can be saved later in development because it should be possible to enter clinical trials with the clinically effective dose range.[2,3] The ratio of doses producing a particular undesired effect to that of the desired effect can be determined to provide a preliminary assessment of the therapeutic index. The incidence and clinical significance of adverse events can only be interpreted with reference to the doses, plasma concentrations and their variability and both magnitude and variability of desired effects. The objectives of these exploratory studies are summarised in Box 4.1.

The 'target product profile' of a NME should describe the features that we desire in order for it to be a success with respect to its medical and commercial value. However, from the point of view of exploratory drug development, we need to be more demanding by defining a minimum acceptable profile (MAP), concentrating particularly on the critical success factors. Then, by comparing the actual profile, as revealed by ED, with the MAP, decisions can be made about the future of a project (i.e. whether it is worth taking from ED into FD). The intention is that the findings in ED will predict the benefit : risk ratio that will be established in FD. It is not sufficient to define the MAP simply in terms of 'the drug works and seems to be safe'. The acceptable benefit : risk ratio will depend greatly on the seriousness of the target disease and the availability of other treatments. For an agent that works by a novel mechanism of action and could be the first in class for treatment of a life-threatening disease, the MAP will be quite different from that of a 'me too' for a troublesome but non-serious condition. For the former, demonstration of clinical benefit despite unpleasant and possibly serious adverse effects might be acceptable, whereas for the latter, success might perhaps depend on demonstration of a single advantageous property of the compound over

Table 4.1 Outcomes of exploratory development

Outcome	Likely decision
Meets MAP	Progress the drug into full development
Does not have the desired effect and does not meet MAP	Terminate the project
Has desired effect but does not meet MAP	Bring forward back-up compounds. May be suitable to use as probe in humans to evaluate basis for drug action or to develop methodology to be applied to back-up compounds

MAP, minimum acceptable profile.

its competitors, such as greater oral bioavailability or a longer duration of action with few if any adverse effects, none of which must be clinically significant.

4.1.3 Outcomes of exploratory development

In general terms, there are three possible outcomes of ED, as summarised in Table 4.1. To summarise, while there is always considerable uncertainty in ED and no decision will be infallible, the risk of selecting the wrong compounds for development can be minimised by identifying critical success factors and a MAP that will provide the basis for go/no-go decisions.

4.2 Planning exploratory development

4.2.1 The need for a regulatory strategy

If the purpose of ED is to generate data on which to base decisions about future development, the strategy for future registration of the drug needs to be well defined. It may seem premature to be discussing regulatory matters before the drug has been administered to humans, but the plan for ED may look quite different depending on the 'target product profile'. Even if the design of the first one or two studies might not be affected, the data these studies generate will certainly be critical in deciding whether to continue or stop development, or change direction. For example, a molecule that has been shown to have both anticonvulsant and antinociceptive activity in animal models might be developed as an anti-epileptic, an analgesic or both. The plan for ED will look quite different for these indications, and the MAP of pharmacokinetics and tolerability will probably differ substantially. Similarly, a molecule that is active in animal models of diabetes and obesity might be developed for either indication, or both. Again, the ED plan of studies and desired or acceptable outcomes will depend on the

chosen indication. The strategy may seem relatively straightforward for an antibiotic with a long half-life in animals that would, if translated to humans, give it a clinically meaningful advantage over the competitors. However, even this needs careful definition of the MAP in terms of pharmacokinetics, spectrum of bacterial sensitivity, target diseases, tolerability and safety profiles by different routes of administration. There also has to be a clear understanding of the likely development times needed to achieve registration for different indications by different routes of administration and the impact on the drug's market potential.

4.2.2 Devising the plan

When starting to devise the plan, it is useful to consider a series of questions, shown in Box 4.2. The timeline should be as short as possible and it may be possible to conduct some studies in parallel or at

---

BOX 4.2 Questions to ask when devising the exploratory development plan

- What is the company's strategic goal for this new molecular entity (NME)?
- With a clear understanding of this goal, what is the minimum acceptable profile?
- Which features of this profile are known to be critical to the future of this NME?
- What findings would result in us stopping development?
- What information will expedite and optimise design of clinical trials in full development?
- What is the minimum number of studies required to address these issues?
- How long will it take to carry out the studies and reach a decision milestone?
- What is the most appropriate population for each study? – healthy volunteers or patients and consider age, sex, race, other genetic factors

least with a stagger rather than sequentially; however, this must not be at the expense of the safety of the study subjects. Often there is no choice but to wait for the results of one study before starting the next. On the other hand, predefining the core data required for decision-making and making arrangements for rapid quality control and database-lock can substantially reduce the delays between studies.

The ED plan should lead to one or more decision milestones at which an agreed body of information will be provided in a defined time. The plan may consist of as few as one or two studies in healthy volunteers, to be completed within 6–9 months, or it may involve a complex series of studies in healthy volunteers and patients, which might take 2 or 3 years. Whatever is appropriate, the information available at the decision milestones should enable the company to compare the actual profile with the previously agreed MAP. The company will then be in a position to make a well-founded decision on whether to continue development with a much reduced risk of failure or whether to stop and concentrate precious resources elsewhere.

The first study commonly involves single ascending doses and the second study might involve repeated administration but the specific study objectives must be tailored to the strategic goals and provide clear information that will define the profile. For example, if it is critical that the absorption of an anti-arrhythmic drug is not affected by prior ingestion of food, the effect of food on the bioavailability of the drug should be an objective that can be easily evaluated in the FIH. Or, if an antimigraine drug must be effective in doses that are devoid of sedative activity, tests of sedation, as well as spontaneous adverse event reporting, should be included in the first and subsequent studies. To take an example mentioned above (see section 4.2.1), the patient population, objectives and endpoints of the first study in patients for a drug targeted at diabetes will be quite different from those for a drug targeted at obesity, even if some of the patients may have both conditions. An outline for a generic ED plan is provided in Box 4.3. The documentation required to support the project plan is listed in Box 4.4.

4.2.3 Presentation of the plan

The ED plan is perhaps best composed of two parts:
1. A brief summary of the project presented under the headings suggested in Box 4.3.
2. A more detailed document providing the essential justification, scientific data and commercial information required to support the project, shown in Box 4.4.

BOX 4.3 Outline of an exploratory development project plan

- Therapeutic indication and rationale for development
- Mechanism of action
- Minimal acceptable profile
- Critical features of the profile for go/no-go decisions
- Information that will be generated in exploratory development (ED) for milestone decisions
- List of proposed studies, with a brief outline of each
- Formulations and pharmaceutical material requirements
- Timeline, with critical path to milestone decisions

BOX 4.4 Documentation to support the project plan

- *Medical rationale for development* – medical need, therapeutic target, current therapies available and their deficiencies
- *Scientific rationale* – mechanism of action, novelty, selectivity, potency, etc.
- *Chemistry and pharmacy* – synthetic route, physicochemical properties including stereochemistry, proposed formulation and route(s) of administration
- *Safety* – secondary pharmacology, toxicology
- *Pharmacokinetics and metabolism* – absorption, distribution, metabolism and excretion (ADME), including potential for interactions, polymorphisms of drug-metabolising enzymes and exposures in humans predicted from interspecies allometric scaling
- *Pharmacodynamics* – predicted effective concentrations in humans
- Time to registration with decision milestones
- Discussion of critical features of the minimal acceptable profile for go/no-go decisions
- Patent status
- *Commercial assessment* – competition, present and potential future size of market

---

An overview of the project plan, with timeline and delineated critical path, may be conveniently presented as a Gantt chart. A decision tree is another visual aid that can serve to clarify the critical information required for each milestone decision.

Although the ED plan should be carefully thought out and well defined, it must be recognised that it is not written in tablets of stone. The very scientific nature of ED means that there will be new, often unexpected, findings. Results of one or two doses administered to humans may show that some assumptions were wrong and that the plan must be changed accordingly. For example, if a drug or one of its major metabolites is found to have a much longer half-life than predicted by preclinical studies, this is likely to affect not only the design of present and future studies but also the acceptable tolerability and safety profile and perhaps the commercial potential of the drug, either favourably or adversely. The plan may have to be revised to take these considerations into account. Planning is therefore essential, but execution of the plan needs to be flexible and the plan may have to be modified considerably, even if the overall goals remain unchanged.

4.3 Requirements for administration of an NME to humans

4.3.1 Evidence of primary pharmacodynamic activity

Pharmacodynamics can be defined as 'the action of a drug on molecular or cellular targets or on the whole organism'. The decision to proceed with development of a compound should only be made after thorough characterisation of its pharmacodynamics in terms of dose–concentration–response relationships *in vitro* and *in vivo* in animals. The commitment to take a compound into humans should not be taken lightly because considerable resources are required to meet the demands of the safe and ethical administration of a NME to humans. No pharmaceutical company can afford to waste precious resources on projects that have little chance of success. By contrast, the cost of thorough preclinical evaluation of the mode of action and pharmacodynamic effects of a substance in relation to its desired therapeutic target is small. This is the scientific basis for all rational drug development today and is the information required for the design of the first human pharmacology studies. However, it does not preclude the possibility of serendipitous discoveries, which have played such an important part in drug discovery in the past.

4.3.2 Secondary pharmacodynamic activity and safety pharmacology

Characterisation of the activity of primary interest must be accompanied by an equally thorough evaluation of the pharmacology of the compound at other receptors and in other body systems. Secondary pharmacodynamic activity refers to the pharmacology of a substance not related to its desired therapeutic target.[4] Such studies may reveal desired or undesired properties. Thus, on the one hand, an NME may be found to have the desired effect at sites or in systems other

---

BOX 4.5 Typical safety pharmacology package for a new chemical entities (NCE)

- Receptor ligand and ion channel binding, enzyme assays, etc.
- *Respiratory function* – respiratory rate, tidal and minute volume
- *Cardiovascular system* – *in vitro* systems for potential to prolong electrocardiographic QT interval including ion channel tail current recorded from cells stably transfected with human ether-a-go-go-related gene (hERG) cDNA, recordings of action potentials from isolated dog Purkinje fibres and electrocardiographic recordings from guinea pig atria as well as from *in vivo* studies in rats and dogs; effects on heart rate, blood pressure, cardiac contractility and ECG including anaesthetised and conscious (reflexes intact) animals
- *Central nervous system* – behavioural activity, sensory/motor responses and body temperature
- *Gastrointestinal tract* – bowel transit times
- Additional studies related to findings in the above and to mechanism of action or target patient population for clinical trials

---

than the one first considered. On the other hand, non-selectivity may imply that doses producing the desired therapeutic effect are likely to be accompanied by adverse effects. In short, robust quantitative *in vitro* and *in vivo* non-clinical data are required to avoid wasted effort and, more seriously, potentially dangerous adverse effects in humans during clinical development.

The package of safety pharmacology studies will generally include *in vivo* investigation of effects on all the major systems with parenteral administration of high single/cumulative doses of the compound and any major active metabolites to rodent and non-rodent species. These studies are at least as important as the formal acute toxicity studies for the initial selection of dosage in humans. A typical safety pharmacology package for an NCE is shown in Box 4.5. Such a safety package is not appropriate for biotechnology products.[5] A much reduced package may also be required for substances to be applied topically, which do, however, require specific studies of local irritancy, phototoxicity and photosensitivity.

4.3.3 Pharmacokinetics and drug metabolism

The physical properties and pharmacokinetic profile, with data on absorption, distribution, metabolism and excretion (ADME) in animals, form an essential part of the drug selection process because the desired pharmacokinetic profile should be defined *ab initio*.[6] For example, if it is decided that a potential new antihypertensive drug is to have a half-life in humans of at least 15 h to permit once-daily administration, there really is no point in developing a compound that has a maximum half-life of 45 min in larger mammals. A potential anti-arrhythmic, which is likely to have a low therapeutic index, requires consistent bioavailability; therefore, a compound that undergoes extensive first-pass metabolism or is poorly and inconsistently absorbed in animals is unlikely to be worth developing as an oral therapy to be taken over long periods.

The pharmacokinetics of a drug in rodents, dogs and primates are certainly of some predictive value to humans, although there can often be surprises. If there is good agreement between species, it is likely that humans will handle the drug in a similar fashion. Conversely, if the major clearance mechanism, metabolic or renal elimination of unchanged drug or metabolite profile differ greatly between species, it is far more difficult to predict the pharmacokinetics in humans. Reliable predictions about metabolic clearance in humans can often be made using cloned human metabolic enzymes, human hepatocytes, microsomes or, if available, whole-liver slices.

The potential value of an NME that is metabolised primarily by an enzyme exhibiting polymorphism in the general population, such as CYP2D6, needs to be carefully considered. Potent enzyme induction is another serious disadvantage which should be investigated in animals, and inhibition of cloned cytochrome P450 isozymes should be tested as part of a routine screen, because drug interactions with concomitant medications may be critical to the value of a new therapy.

When a compound undergoes metabolism, the pharmacokinetics of major metabolites, particularly those that have pharmacological activity or are responsible for toxicities, should be examined. A long half-life of a metabolite may result in accumulation long after the concentration of the parent molecule has reached steady state. Much of the evaluation of the pharmacokinetics and the rates and routes of metabolism will be studied in animals using radio-labelled drug, but should be supported by 'cold' assays.

4.3.4 Toxicology

This topic is covered comprehensively in Chapter 3 and the discussion here will be confined to a few salient points.

Physicians and other clinical scientists responsible for ED are unlikely to be expert in toxicology but they must be familiar with the preclinical safety requirements for human studies in general[7] and with the detailed toxicology of the NME under consideration. The final responsibility for the decision whether and how to conduct the FIH lies with the physician. Toxicity findings that give cause for concern should always be discussed with the toxicologist even if they are considered to be unrelated to the drug. Explanation may suffice but if reassurance is inadequate, additional studies may be needed or it might be necessary to limit exposure in humans until further information becomes available.

It should be appreciated that the objective of the toxicologist is to identify target organ toxicity, whereas that of the clinical pharmacologist is to minimise risk and avoid significant toxic effects. Thus, the clinical pharmacologist needs to know:

1. The organs in which toxicity was demonstrated and any abnormalities in laboratory tests.
2. The maximum no observed (non-toxic) effect dose level (NOEL).
3. The maximum no observed adverse (toxic) effect dose level (NOAEL).
4. The toxicokinetics, in particular the peak concentrations (C_{max}) and exposure [area under the plasma concentration–time curve (AUC)] to parent drug and any major metabolites at the NOAEL and at higher (toxic) doses in the animal species tested.

This information may affect selection criteria for the study population and choice of tests additional to routine safety monitoring. It will certainly contribute to selection of the starting dose, range of doses, maximum exposure and dose increments to be studied. Pharmacokinetics in humans may be quite different from those in animal species but the relationship between plasma concentrations and effects frequently holds across species so that plasma and, if possible, tissue concentrations are generally more important than dose. Acute toxicity may be attributable to pharmacological effects which are related to the C_{max} while chronic toxicity often unrelated to the primary pharmacology is more likely to be related to exposure (AUC) over time. For compounds with very extensive plasma protein binding, allowance may be required for differences in the extent of binding in different species compared with that in human plasma.

While the importance of plasma concentrations rather than dose cannot be over-emphasised, an important exception to this occurs in the case of hepatotoxicity resulting from exposure of the liver to portal rather than systemic blood drug concentrations. In this case, the oral dose administered to the animals is more relevant than the systemic plasma concentrations, which reflect the extent of first-pass metabolism as well as absorption and distribution.

Before administration of an NME to humans, a mutagenicity test in bacterial cells (Ames test), with and without metabolic activation, and tests for chromosomal aberrations in mammalian cells should be negative.[8] Any positive or equivocal results will require additional tests to be performed before proceeding to humans. Studies of embryo-fetal toxicity should be performed before administration of an NME to women of reproductive potential. Studies of fertility, early embryonic development and prenatal and postnatal development are not required at this stage of development; neither are carcinogenicity studies.

An additional consideration is the safety assessment of agents that will be used for challenge stimuli in the evaluation of pharmacodynamics. In some cases there is a long history of uneventful clinical use of tests (e.g. bronchial challenge with histamine and methacholine). If used in a similar manner, there may be no need to consider performing safety studies in animals prior to their application in ED. On the other hand, the use of agents that are much less well established and that have an unproven safety record must raise the question of whether appropriate toxicology and pharmacological safety assessments should be performed in animals.

4.3.5 Drug substance and pharmaceutical formulations

The size and quality of the batch of bulk chemical or biological material that will be formulated for the FIH are critical to the expeditious transfer from animals to humans. Required details of the drug substance are shown in Box 4.6. Wherever possible, the same batch that has been used for toxicology should be used for the human studies. This avoids difficulties in attributing toxicity findings to different impurities or different proportions of the same impurities which are frequently encountered in early batches. Although the batch size may be limited, the amount of material required for the initial human studies is generally small compared with that used for toxicology.

It is always difficult to provide the pharmacist with sufficient information to facilitate manufacture of an optimal formulation. The dose range of interest is not known, and careful consideration should be given to selection of unit doses that will provide the greatest

flexibility. Good communication is essential and adequate lead time must be allowed. Compounds with poor absorption are difficult to formulate and may take considerable time and resources. Repeated *in vitro* and *in vivo* testing in animals may be required before a satisfactory formulation is found.

All formulations for administration to humans must be prepared in compliance with Good Manufacturing Practice (GMP) and the certificates of analysis must be provided. The European Clinical Trials Directive[1] requires that details of the formulations be provided to, and approved by, regulatory authorities and a 'qualified person' at the investigator site(s). In principle, the Directive has been in force throughout the EU since May 2004 although it has been implemented at various times in different member states. The Directive applies to healthy volunteer as well as patient studies. The requirements for pharmaceutical products for administration to humans are summarised in Box 4.6.

The need for placebos generally from the first human study onwards typically involves manufacture of dummy capsules or tablets, and if oral solutions or

---

BOX 4.6 Pharmaceutical requirements for administration to humans

Drug substance
- Chemical structure
- Physical properties: e.g. appearance, solubilities, pH, pKa
- Details of the synthetic route
- Manufacturing process and controls
- Elucidation of structure
- Batch analysis
- Analytical procedures
- Stability data

Formulation
- Description and composition
- Manufacturing process and controls
- Control of excipients
- Analytical methods
- Proof of structure
- Purity, proportions of impurities, identity of major impurities
- Stability of formulated as well as raw material
- Certificate of analysis giving date of manufacture, batch number, weight of material and range, dissolution characteristics, appearance, excipients, expiry data and assurance of compliance with Good Manufacturing Practice
- Compatibility of injections with intravenous fluids and with plastics

suspensions are to be used, these must be matched as closely as possible for taste, colour and appearance.

Consideration must also be given to agents that are intended to be used for challenge stimuli. Some may be available commercially for use in humans, others may not and considerable work may have to be done to obtain raw material of sufficient purity and stability, followed by development and manufacture of an appropriate formulation.

4.4 Preparation for the first administration to humans

4.4.1 Transfer from preclinical to clinical

The establishment of good working relationships between the preclinical scientists (e.g. chemists, immunologists, pharmacologists, toxicologists, drug metabolism) and the clinical scientists responsible for ED is of enormous value. This is sometimes hard to achieve when the different groups are separated geographically or an NME is licensed from another organisation. However, it should be recognised that at this stage, the preclinical scientists generally have far more knowledge about the compound and of the related science and their contribution to the ED plan can be extremely valuable. On the other hand, the clinical pharmacologist has an important part to play in assessing the preclinical data. Consideration of the ED plan may reveal that studies additional to those planned may be required. Review of the toxicity, safety pharmacology and metabolism data acquired to date may raise concerns and indicate that further work is necessary.

Close cooperation before the first administration to humans is likely to lead to a smooth transfer of the compound and the rapid movement of a compound out of preclinical trials into humans. This lead time can be used to devise the ED plan, design the first studies and, when appropriate, to select and develop methodologies that will contribute to the drug's evaluation in humans. This may include validation of pharmacodynamic measures to be used in the clinical pharmacology unit, assessment of the possible contribution of imaging techniques and development of bioanalytical methods. Not infrequently, assays that were perfectly adequate to support preclinical work are insufficiently sensitive, specific or accurate to quantify the comparatively low concentrations of parent drug and major metabolites in humans. At the very least, assays require validation in human matrices.

4.4.2 Preparation of the clinical investigator's brochure

The rate-limiting step, which usually defines when an NME can be transferred to clinical, is the subacute (usually 28 day) toxicology. While reports of these studies are being written, preparation of the key documents required for the FIH can begin. Once the toxicology reports are available, and are supportive of proceeding to humans, the documentation can be completed. In addition to the protocol (see section 4.4.3), and information for volunteers with consent form, the investigator's brochure (IB) needs to be prepared. It is usual for each of the preclinical disciplines to contribute sections to this document, but the clinical scientists need to ensure that the document is appropriate for a clinical readership. The outline content and format of the IB is provided in a guideline of the International Conference on Harmonisation (ICH) published by the European Medicines Agency.[9]

It should always be remembered that the IB is not a promotional document aimed at presenting the NME in its best light; on the contrary, it is intended to inform investigators and ethics committees about every aspect of the drug, to enable them to make wise judgements in the interest of study subjects, be they healthy volunteers or patients. The IB is necessarily a summary, but less than full disclosure of important information about the drug, whatever the source, is not acceptable and all documents should be referenced and made available on request.

The first edition of this important document will contain no clinical information, but the next edition should be produced immediately after completion of the FIH, with a summary of the findings. The principal investigator must become fully familiar with the IB when the protocol is being developed and, once finalised, the IB should be submitted to the relevant independent ethics committee (IEC) and competent (regulatory) authority as providing the scientific background in support of the protocol.

4.4.3 Aspects of the first protocol and ethics review

A protocol for the first and other early studies with an NME in humans is similar to those for later studies in healthy volunteers and patients but has some particular features that are worth special consideration. The protocol should be written to satisfy not only the needs of regulatory authorities and personnel who will be involved in conduct of the study, but also to facilitate the work of the IEC, which bears considerable responsibility in such cases. The nature of the scientific material contained in the protocol is often complex, highly specialised and quite unlike most protocols for clinical trials handled by such committees.

The emphasis is essentially on safety rather than ethics, although, a study that does not minimise risk and is of dubious scientific quality is also unethical. As well as a summary of the preclinical information, some comment and interpretation about its significance should be provided. The choice of starting dose and increments for dose escalation should be justified. The number of subjects and amount of data that will form the basis for a decision to escalate should be clearly stated, as should the criteria for stopping the escalation – the stopping rules.

The clinical procedures that will be undertaken and intended doses may need to be revised after review of the first results. The protocol should therefore be written with some flexibility so that, for example, within a defined dose range, adjustments of dose can be made. Similarly, while the minimum interval between doses should be explicit, there should be an option to increase the proposed interval if the half-life is longer than expected. There should be some flexibility in timing of blood samples and urine collections, which may need to be changed in light of pharmacokinetic and pharmacodynamic data generated during the study, although the maximum number of samples and total blood volume to be sampled should be unchanged. On the other hand, this flexibility, which is necessary for the smooth conduct of an FIH, must not be taken to imply that ill-defined or vague objectives and procedures are acceptable and the IEC cannot and should not be expected to give carte blanche. Therefore, the basis for decisions and alternatives should be detailed carefully.

When the IEC meets to review the protocol, it is advisable for a senior toxicologist and the principal investigator to be available to answer questions if required. Of course, members of the committee may have access to any other company documents, such as toxicology reports, if they desire. More detail about the design of such studies is provided in section 4.7.

Pharmaceutical companies frequently establish a committee of senior management to authorise the first study of an NME in humans, the review and approval generally being a prerequisite for submission to the external IEC. However, as stated in section 4.3.4, the clinician responsible for the FIH must be personally satisfied that the preclinical data, relating to efficacy and safety, justify administration to humans. A useful test is for the physician and other responsible personnel to ask themselves: 'Would I be prepared to volunteer for this study and would I be happy for a loved-one to do so?'

4.4.4 Request for clinical trial authorisation

The application for a clinical trial authorisation (CTA) for the first administration of an NME to humans comprises the same elements as all other CTAs but there will be no clinical data. The regulatory authority known as the competent authority (CA) of the EU member state requires receipt of confirmation of the European Clinical Trials Database (EudraCT) number, a covering letter, a completed application form, the protocol with all current amendments, the IB and a full Investigational Medicinal Product Dossier (IMPD) (see below). If the study is to be conducted in more than one member state, a list of CAs should be included. If the opinion of the IEC is available, it should be provided.

The IMPD should summarise the quality, manufacture and control of the IMP including chemical (drug substance), pharmaceutical (drug product) and biological data, derived from tests carried out to current standards of GMP, and the non-clinical pharmacology, pharmacokinetics and toxicology conducted to the standards of Good Laboratory Practice (GLP). Assessors and reviewers prefer data presented as tables with a brief discussion of the most important results and any conclusions. The application should draw attention to and justify any deviations from the standards described in available guidelines. There should be sufficient detail in the summaries and tables for assessors to reach their own conclusions about the potential toxicity of the IMP and the safety of its use in the proposed study. The IMPD should include a section in which the data are integrated to provide an assessment of overall risk. Potential hazards should be identified and the safety margins based on the preclinical information and estimated exposure in humans over the proposed dose range should be presented with measures that will be taken to monitor safety.

The suggested headings and arrangement of the document may be found in *The Rules Governing Medicinal Products in the European Union Volume 2, Notice to Applicants Volume 2B*, which can be accessed at the Commission website (www.pharmacos.eudra. org). Information is also available at the European Medicines Agency website (www.emea.eu.int).

4.5 Studies in healthy volunteers

4.5.1 What is a healthy (non-patient) volunteer?

In a report of the Royal College of Physicians on studies in healthy volunteers,[10] a healthy volunteer is described as 'an individual who is not known to suffer any significant illness relevant to the proposed study, who should be within the ordinary range of body measurements such as weight, and whose mental state is such that he is able to understand and give valid consent to the study'. In the Association of the British Pharmaceutical Industry (ABPI) guidelines for medical experiments in non-patient human volunteers,[11] it is stressed that the individual cannot be expected to derive therapeutic benefit from the proposed study. While these descriptions are correct, I would suggest that words such as 'relevant to the proposed study' are too ambiguous and the definition should state unequivocally that a healthy volunteer must indeed be in good health. Perhaps a more satisfactory definition of a healthy or 'non-patient' volunteer (the word 'human' is superfluous) is as follows: 'An individual who is in good general health, not having any mental or physical disorder requiring regular or frequent medication and who is able to give valid informed consent to participation in a study.' Thus, a healthy young man taking an antibiotic for acne does not qualify but a woman taking an oral contraceptive does (unless specifically excluded by the protocol). Similarly, a migraine or hayfever patient who takes daily prophylactic medication is excluded but one who takes medication only at the time of infrequent acute attacks is acceptable, in principle. Obviously, individuals will not be able to participate if suffering from an acute attack or if they have taken medication within a period defined in the protocol.

Even with this somewhat stricter definition, there is room for discretion. A sportsman who takes an occasional puff of a bronchodilator for exercise-induced asthma but is otherwise asymptomatic may be considered eligible by some. Individuals who have undergone surgery for a congenital condition and are in excellent health may or may not be suitable. The decision to include a subject with a 'normal variant' electrocardiogram (ECG) can sometimes be difficult and may merit an expert opinion. An asymptomatic patient with a hip prosthesis who is taking no medication may be acceptable whereas an equally healthy individual with a prosthetic heart valve should be excluded from a study involving a cannula because of the risk, however remote, of endocarditis. Clearly,

whatever definition of a healthy volunteer is used, sensible clinical judgement is still required.

The use of healthy volunteers has revealed findings that are generally thought to be pathological but in fact are not associated with any adverse prognosis. For example, short runs of non-sustained ventricular tachycardia were found in 2% of healthy individuals with normal hearts on 24-h ambulatory ECG monitoring.[12] Microscopic haematuria is also a common finding. Epileptiform activity on electroencephalography (EEG) is found in subjects with no history of epilepsy. In addition, laboratory values will frequently fall outside the 'normal' range for the laboratory, simply on the grounds of statistical probability which is dependent on the criteria used to define the normal range.

Although not of direct relevance to screening, it should also be recognised that some of the procedures to which a volunteer may be subjected can affect test results. Perhaps, the most important example of such findings is the rise in transaminases that occurs in some subjects resident in a clinical pharmacology unit for a week or more, possibly because of dietary factors. The importance of a placebo group to help distinguish between effects resulting from active drug and procedural-related abnormalities cannot be over-emphasised.

Healthy volunteers can be of either sex, although early studies are mostly confined to men because results of reproductive toxicity are generally not available at the time. Companies are not usually prepared to incur the cost of a reproductive toxicology package before there is some confidence that the compound is a reasonable candidate for development. In the absence of such data, medicolegal and ethical considerations relating to the risk of causing embryo-fetal damage have deterred companies from including women in FIH. Men are also frequently favoured for later studies because of concerns over the inability to detect very early pregnancy and the possibility that the menstrual cycle or oral contraceptives may affect drug metabolism. Concerns that the results from studies conducted mainly in men may not be representative of both sexes are rarely justified because, unlike in the rat, there are few important sex-related differences in drug metabolism in humans.

For legal reasons, the lower age limit for volunteers is generally 18 years. The first studies with a new candidate drug are usually conducted in young healthy male volunteers with an upper age limit of 35–40 years. The lower age limit for the elderly is usually 65 years but when specifically addressing tolerability, pharmacokinetics and pharmacodynamics in the elderly, a representative population should certainly include many subjects in their seventies and eighties.[13]

4.5.2 Healthy volunteers or patients?

The decision to use healthy volunteers, a particular patient population or a combination of the two should be based on ethical, safety, scientific and practical grounds. While risk must be minimised for all studies in humans, there is clearly a difference in the ratio between benefit and risk for a healthy volunteer and a patient who has severe, perhaps life-threatening disease. Therefore, it has long been accepted that some drugs are too toxic or produce effects that would be unacceptable in healthy volunteers. These include cytotoxic agents, neuromuscular blocking drugs and anaesthetics.

Less well established is the appropriate population for study of biologicals such as monoclonal antibodies, growth factors and interleukins. These may target the immune system, exhibit agonist activity on targets within a biological amplification cascade, result in activation of signalling pathways and affect multiple systems. Ethics committees and regulatory authorities as well as physicians may hold different views about the most appropriate choice of population for a particular NBE. While recognising that many monoclonal antibodies have proven to be innocuous, my own view is conservative and to consider administration to healthy volunteers only for vaccines. The half-life of immunoglobulins is approximately 2 weeks, which implies that exposure will continue for at least 8–10 weeks. Furthermore, many of these agents will change the immune system in both predicted and unpredicted ways in the long term. This is in marked contradistinction to small molecules, which are generally present and whose effects last for a few hours or days at most. An important additional consideration for many biologicals that target specific cell populations expressing a particular epitope, is that more information of relevance to efficacy and indeed pharmacokinetics may be obtained in the patient population.

On the other hand, physicians responsible for patient care are, rightly, conservative about exposing their patients to unknown risks. Thus, asthmatics, who have hyperactive airways, are far more likely to develop serious impairment of respiratory function because of bronchoconstriction from an inhaled material, drug or vehicle than are healthy volunteers. An elderly patient with an acute stroke is far more susceptible to the sedative effects of an NME than is

a young healthy subject. Furthermore, the appropriate dose range to be studied can frequently be established in healthy subjects using biomarkers (see section 4.6.3) so that exposure of patients to excessively high (or low) doses can be avoided. Of course, this does not imply that less caution is required when dosing healthy volunteers; it simply recognises that the risks may be considerably less in this population.

In addition to the greater risk in patients, results of studies in patients are frequently confounded by the effects of disease, concomitant medication, age and other variables. By contrast, healthy subjects are much more homogeneous and subjects are studied under standardised conditions. It is sometimes argued that healthy volunteers are not representative of the patient population and therefore that the studies are of less relevance. This argument fails to take the study objectives into account; some questions about a drug are much more easily answered by deliberately excluding sources of variation.

In addition to the scientific benefit to be gained from studies in healthy volunteers, there are a number of practical advantages.

• Healthy volunteers can generally be recruited much more rapidly than patients.

• Healthy volunteers are generally willing and able to make themselves available on scheduled study days so that groups of subjects can be studied together, thereby expediting the study and enabling efficient use of staff and laboratories.

• Human pharmacology studies are frequently very intensive, with a tight schedule of complex measurements, often requiring training and a high degree of cooperation from subjects. Young healthy volunteers are more suited to this type of study than most patients.

In summary, studies in healthy volunteers are an integral part of the development of most drugs because they are capable of rapidly providing a large amount of data that are not confounded by other variables and that can thereby expedite the subsequent evaluation of the drug in patients. However, the choice of population should be considered carefully for every NME on a case-by-case basis and the absence of benefit to a healthy subject and the possibility of long-term risk to the well-being of healthy individuals will often mean that studies in patients are more appropriate.

4.5.3 Source of healthy volunteers

The majority of healthy volunteer studies are conducted by contract research organisations (CROs), which recruit subjects from the general public by advertising and word of mouth. The composition of the volunteer database depends to some extent on the location, some being comprised mainly of students or the local residential population, others, particularly in large cities, having a preponderance of backpackers and temporary workers. The source of volunteers does have implications for safety, motivation and withdrawal rates. The more itinerant volunteers may not be available for follow-up and little may be known about their medical background. While the 'professional volunteer' is wholly inappropriate, volunteers who understand what is involved and are well motivated and who have long-term medical screening records is highly desirable. For more details of volunteer recruitment see section 4.5.5.

4.5.4 Facilities and staff

The minimum standards for the facilities in which clinical pharmacology studies should be conducted are described in the ABPI guidelines.[11] Clearly, the same standards should apply to all organisations involved in conducting studies. In the UK, the Medicines and Healthcare products Regulatory Agency (MHRA) has instituted inspection of facilities and a system of accreditation is now in place.

Provision of adequate competent medical staff is essential for the safe and ethical conduct of studies in humans. Decisions about whether a volunteer fulfils the entry criteria or should be withdrawn from a study, how to respond to an unexpected adverse event and when to discontinue a study can prove challenging to the most experienced physician. Similarly, research nurses need many organisational and technical skills over and above those that they acquired during their basic clinical nursing training. Scientific staff must be competent in the techniques that will provide the essential data. All must be properly briefed about what will be required of them during the course of a study, and must be fully familiar with local standard operating procedures (SOPs) and working in compliance with Good Clinical Practice (GCP).

Non-clinical as well as clinical staff involved in conducting studies in humans should be trained in basic life support with regular updates, preferably every 6 months, and medical staff should also receive training in advanced life support. Training records should be kept for each member of staff and practice emergency call sessions should be run frequently. Staff development is a subject beyond the scope of this text but it is worth emphasising the value of offering training for clinical research nurses in the medical and

scientific aspects of their work, as well as expecting them to learn on the job under supervision. Motivation and performance will be greatly enhanced by staff who understand something of the science behind the compound being tested and the medical as well as commercial rationale for its development.

4.5.5 Volunteer recruitment procedures

Procedures for recruitment of volunteers vary slightly between organisations conducting healthy volunteer studies, but the checklist of procedures provided in Box 4.7 is generic.

Detailed written information, which generally constitutes part of the consent form, should not be provided to potential volunteers until ethics committee approval has been obtained. A checklist of the items that should be covered in the volunteer information is given in Box 4.8. Most importantly, the information should be provided in clear non-technical language.[14] A balance must be struck between provision of adequate information and an excessively long and detailed document, which may provide some legal protection for the investigator but is too long and complex to be comprehensible to the average lay person.

A copy of the study schedule and an oral explanation should complement the written information. Volunteers should be given every opportunity to ask questions and to obtain additional information. They should be encouraged to contact the study physician about any symptoms, however trivial, that occur between study occasions, particularly if they wish to take medication, such as analgesics, decongestants or antihistamines. A cooling-off period of at least 24 h should be allowed after provision of information to allow the volunteer to consider and have the opportunity to discuss with their partner, family or friends.

BOX 4.7 Volunteer recruitment procedures

- Provide brief information about study to potential volunteers
- Arrange to meet potential volunteers
- At meeting, provide written and oral information
- Check volunteer's understanding, giving ample opportunity for questions
- Check volunteer's interest in volunteering
- Allow at least 24 h for volunteer to consider
- Obtain witnessed written consent
- Obtain consent to write to his or her doctor
- Medical screen
- Check that the volunteer fulfils all entry criteria; review screening tests

BOX 4.8 Information for volunteers

- The rationale and objectives of the study, with some background information
- Information about the drug in animals and humans, including possible adverse effects
- Dosages to be employed, comparison with dosage in animals and previous exposure in humans, route of administration
- If appropriate, information about comparator drugs that may be used, including possible adverse effects
- What will be required of the volunteer (e.g. number of study days and nights, insertion of cannulae, urine collections, follow-up blood samples)
- Possible adverse effects of procedures
- Restrictions of, for example, food, caffeine, alcohol, smoking, driving or operating machinery, contraception
- Requirements for medical screening, including urine tests for pregnancy and drugs of abuse
- Arrangements for transport
- The right to withdraw at any time without prejudice
- The right to obtain more information
- Confidentiality of records, with access limited to study personnel and auditors
- The right to no-fault compensation
- Approval of the protocol by an ethics committee
- The honorarium that will be paid
- How to contact the physician or nurse out of hours

Therefore, it may be inappropriate for consent and medical screening to follow immediately after an information session.

If volunteers are required to give specimens for genotyping for drug metabolising enzymes or for proteins that might be involved in pharmacodynamic responses, a separate consent form should be provided for this purpose. If it is intended that a DNA sample be stored for future analysis, consent should be requested and it should be made clear that all data will be held in a format that will make it impossible to link the data to an identifiable individual. Subjects should be free to refuse or withdraw consent independent of their consent to participation in the study. In the event of a withdrawal, any samples taken should be destroyed.

The size of the honorarium should reflect the amount of inconvenience that the study causes to the participant, and not the perceived risk. It is best decided by relatively disinterested parties, such as a medical director in consultation with a senior research nurse. The sum must be submitted for IEC approval with the protocol and is non-negotiable.

The chance of a mishap occurring in a volunteer study is increased when little or nothing is known about the subject. It should be a precondition of acceptance of a volunteer into a study that he or she is registered with a general practitioner (GP) and that permission is given to contact the GP to inform them of the study and to seek confirmation that their patient is suitable to participate.[15] The information that can be obtained can help to ensure that the volunteer is in good health; therefore every attempt should be made to contact GPs including those of volunteers living abroad. Although communication about a patient between physicians is always confidential, a GP may recommend that their patient does not participate without giving a specific reason; there is no obligation to do so and their opinion should be respected.

Another concern is that a volunteer may fail to disclose that they have recently participated in another trial or may even be currently doing so. To deal with this problem, efforts have been made on a voluntary basis to establish national databases that can cross-check volunteer participation. Of course, the value of such databases is dependent on the number of CROs, academic units and pharmaceutical companies who participate. In the UK, a database called TOPS (The Overvolunteering Prevention System) is now well established. It is of proven benefit in preventing accidental or deliberate over-volunteering.[16] Similar arrangements are in place in some other European countries.

A list of procedures comprising a medical screen is given in Box 4.9. Particular studies may require additional procedures, such as lung function tests, coagulation studies, exercise or 24-h ECG or a psychiatric interview.

BOX 4.9 Medical screens

- Medical history
- Physical examination
- ECG, with report on intervals as well as rhythm and morphology
- Full blood count and plasma biochemistry
- Immunology for hepatitis B and C and HIV
- Urinalysis
- Screen for drugs of abuse
- Pregnancy tests for women of reproductive potential
- Other tests as appropriate (e.g. tests of coagulation, respiratory function, cognition)

4.5.6 Good Clinical Practice

The requirements of GCP, as described in the ICH guidelines,[17] are presented in Chapter 7 and will not be discussed further here. However, it is emphasised that the standards required of large clinical trials in patients apply equally to small clinical pharmacological studies in healthy subjects. Studies should be conducted in accordance with SOPS. Many SOPs will resemble those pertaining to later phase clinical trials, but some will be specific to healthy volunteer studies. Details of procedures not covered by SOPs should be specified in the protocol. Studies must be monitored by the sponsor or a representative; the monitor should not be one of the investigators so that monitoring visits and assessments can maintain objectivity.

4.5.7 Adverse reactions in volunteer studies

There are no accurate data that provide a comprehensive picture of the extent of healthy volunteer studies and hence of the incidence of adverse reactions. However, surveys and clinical series have been published from time to time. In 1984, the ABPI requested information from its member companies on their activities in this area.[18] Of the 43 companies that responded, 28 conducted in-house studies and all but two commissioned external work. In the in-house studies, there were 18,671 subject exposures to drugs. There were no deaths or life-threatening suspected reactions. The incidence of serious suspected reactions that might have been attributable to drug was 0.27 per 1000 subject exposures. Of the 8733 subject exposures in external studies, there was one death on which the inquest reported an open verdict and no life-threatening suspected reactions. The incidence of suspected serious reactions was 0.91 per 1000 subject exposures.

In another survey conducted by the clinical section of the British Pharmacological Society over a 1-year period from 1986 to 1987, 8163 healthy volunteers received drugs for research purposes.[19] Potentially life-threatening adverse effects were reported in 0.04% and moderately severe adverse effects in 0.55%, with no lasting sequelae. The three severe reactions were skin irritation and rash requiring hospitalisation, anaphylactic shock after an oral vaccine, and perforation of a duodenal ulcer after multiple-dose non-steroidal anti-inflammatory drug; all made a complete recovery. The results were similar to those reported in the earlier ABPI survey and the authors concluded that the risk involved in these studies is very small and that most of the moderately severe reactions are of the predictable kind, generally being attributable to the known pharmacological activity of the drug.

In a much larger survey of 93,399 subjects participating in non-therapeutic research in the USA,[20] 37 subjects were reported to be temporarily disabled and one to be permanently disabled. The latter was from a stroke occurring 3 days after investigation, and its attributability is unknown.

In a report of two 5-year periods in a single centre in France, the incidence of adverse events in 1015 healthy volunteers was 13.7% in subjects receiving active drug and 7.9% in those receiving placebo.[21] Headache, diarrhoea and dyspepsia occurred in more than 10 per 1000. Three per cent of adverse events were rated severe but there were no deaths or life-threatening events. Some events, such as vasovagal attacks, were related to procedures rather than treatment.

Thus, over a period of several decades involving the administration of thousands of NMEs to humans, the incidence of serious adverse events in such studies was very low. However, in March 2006, a study conducted in the UK involving the first administration to humans of a novel recombinant humanised monoclonal antibody resulted in a 'cytokine storm' in all six volunteers who received the first dose of the drug. The immediate effects and the subsequent multiorgan failure were life-threatening in two subjects and were very serious in the remaining four. Fortunately, the study unit was within a hospital and the volunteers were transferred to the intensive care unit. All the volunteers survived although not without permanent injury in at least one case. There are a number of lessons to be learned from this disastrous event, some of which are discussed in section 4.8.4. At this point, it will suffice to point out that although the probability of a life-threatening adverse reaction in volunteers is historically very small indeed, the risk is ever-present and everything possible must be done to minimise it.

4.5.8 Insurance and compensation

These topics are covered at some length in the Report of the Royal College of Physicians[10] and the much more recent ABPI guidelines.[11] Essentially, the company must undertake to pay compensation to any volunteer who has suffered bodily injury as the result of participating in a study, without proof of negligence or evidence that a test drug or procedure failed to fulfil a reasonable expectation of safety. This contractual agreement should be stated in the consent form that the volunteer signs. Ethics committees should ensure that arrangements for such 'no-fault' compensation are in place. Regarding personal insurance, companies will not normally exclude cover for accidents occurring as the result of research, but volunteers are advised to seek clarification on this from their insurers, particularly when taking out a new policy.

4.6 Study objectives in first-in-human studies

The first and subsequent studies of an NME in humans should aim to obtain dose–concentration–response relationships for desired and undesired effects. These objectives may be summarised as follows. To investigate over a range of doses:

- Tolerability and safety;
- Pharmacokinetics; and
- Pharmacodynamic activity.

4.6.1 Tolerability and safety

The word 'tolerability' is perhaps a little clumsy but it describes accurately what is assessed, namely how well the drug is tolerated by those to whom it is administered. This last qualification is necessary because there are many instances in which a drug is better tolerated or less well tolerated by young healthy volunteers than by patients. For example, anxiolytics and first generation antidepressants are usually far better tolerated by patients with depression than by healthy volunteers. However, healthy volunteer studies generally provide useful information about tolerability even if it may underestimate the dose at which central effects will become evident in patients. Many adverse reactions will be directly related to the known pharmacological activity of the drug and are therefore predictable.

The investigation of tolerability must cover a number of doses thought to be in the range required for therapeutic benefit. The relevance of these data can only be interpreted when they are related to plasma concentrations and, if appropriate, measurements of pharmacodynamic activity. Adverse reactions occurring at 10 times the therapeutic dose may not pose a problem; conversely, the absence of adverse reactions at one-tenth the therapeutic dose is of little relevance and, if misinterpreted, may give unfounded confidence. This may seem obvious but has important implications for study design which are frequently ignored (see section 4.7).

'Tolerability' should not be confused with the term 'tolerance', which describes the diminution in effects of a drug on prolonged exposure. Tolerance may be caused by increased clearance because of autoinduction of enzymes responsible for the drug's metabolism, such as occurs with some antiepileptic drugs (e.g. carbamazepine). Tolerance may also result from

altered pharmacodynamics, which is common with drugs acting on the CNS.

'Tolerability' should also be distinguished from 'safety'. A drug that causes mild sedation may be safe except to individuals undertaking certain activities that are affected adversely by sedation such as driving a car. On the other hand, a drug may be tolerated well in the short to medium term but may cause elevation of liver transaminases as a result of hepatotoxicity. Similarly, a drug may be tolerated extremely well by healthy volunteers and by the vast majority of patients but may cause prolongation of the ECG QT interval, which poses a significant risk of cardiac arrhythmias in susceptible patients. A preliminary assessment of safety may be obtained in exploratory repeat-dose studies in healthy volunteers and patients but it should be recognised that the chances of detecting an uncommon serious adverse event are remote because of the relatively small number of subjects exposed.

4.6.2 Pharmacokinetics

An explanation of the underlying concepts of pharmacokinetics is to be found in Chapter 5. The pharmacokinetic information that can be obtained from the FIH is dependent on the route of administration. When a drug is given intravenously, its bioavailability is 100%, and the true values of pharmacokinetic parameters clearance and apparent volume of distribution can be obtained in addition to the plasma elimination half-life. Over a range of doses it can be established whether exposure, measured as the AUC, increases in proportion to the dose and hence whether the kinetic parameters are independent of dose (Figure 4.1). When a drug is administered orally, the half-life can still be determined, but the values obtained for apparent volume of distribution and clearance will usually differ from those after intravenous dosing, partly because they will be uncorrected for bioavailability, which is usually unknown. However, if the maximum concentration (C_{max}) and AUC increase proportionally with dose, and the half-life is constant, it can usually be assumed that clearance is independent of dose. If, on the other hand, the AUC does not increase in proportion to the dose, this could be the result of a change in bioavailability, clearance or both.

In addition to the pharmacokinetics of a drug, the FIH can provide important information about its metabolites. If assay methodology has been developed, metabolites in plasma can be detected and the AUC and half-lives determined. Further information can be obtained from assaying urine for drug and

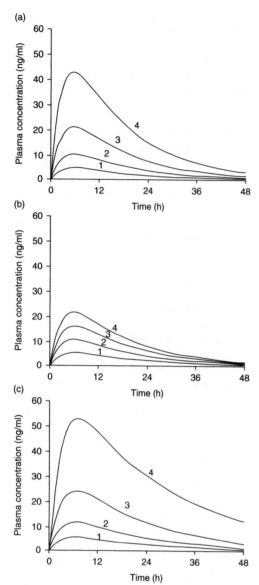

Figure 4.1 Plasma concentration profiles after doubling doses showing: (a) proportional increase with dose; (b) less than proportional increase with dose; (c) greater than proportional increase with dose.

metabolites. Renal clearance can be calculated over time intervals and the ratio of renal : systemic clearance calculated so that the relative importance of renal and metabolic clearance can be assessed. The relative proportions of parent compound and identifiable metabolites will give an important, albeit incomplete, picture of how the drug is excreted in urine. The total amount of parent compound and metabolites measured in urine will give a minimum value for bioavailability of the drug. Early administration by both intravenous and oral routes can be extremely useful to ascertain the bioavailability and, if low, whether this is because of poor absorption or extensive first-pass metabolism.

It is a great mistake to think that the information obtained from such a study is mainly the concern of pharmacokineticists. The data are essential for making rational decisions about the future development of a compound. At the simplest level, a half-life that is so short that the drug would have to be administered five or six times a day in order to maintain therapeutic benefit may be a good enough reason to discontinue development. A drug that has to be administered in very large doses to achieve adequate plasma concentrations, or fails to reach them at all because of poor absorption, is obviously unattractive. Large variability in bioavailability because of inconsistent absorption or extensive first-pass metabolism might constitute another reason for stopping development, particularly for a drug predicted to have a low therapeutic index. Saturation of clearance mechanisms which, at the very least, will make dosing complicated, could result in unacceptable toxicity. The presence of a large number of metabolites may be undesirable, particularly if not all of them were present in the animal species used for toxicology so that additional toxicity studies might be required to support further work in humans. The presence of a major metabolite with pharmacological activity and a half-life much longer than the parent drug may be a useful way of extending the duration of action but its predicted accumulation on repeat dosing may pose a serious safety concern.

At the end of the FIH, the pharmacokinetic profile should be compared with that desired for the compound. If reality compares unfavourably with the ideal, the unpleasant decision to discontinue development may have to be taken. Even if single-dose pharmacokinetics are acceptable, a further assessment will need to be made after repeat-dose administration of the drug, because this may reveal plasma concentrations that do not match the predictions from single doses. For example, saturation of elimination resulting in higher than predicted steady-state concentrations, with associated toxicity, may make dosing too difficult for practical purposes. Conversely, autoinduction of metabolic enzymes, with resultant increased clearance, may occur, making it necessary to increase the dose over a period of weeks and also rendering the drug susceptible to interactions with other drugs.

Another consideration may be the accumulation of a metabolite that has a much longer half-life than that of the parent compound and which was perhaps undetectable after single doses. Some common reasons for stopping development on the basis of pharmacokinetic data are given in Box 4.10.

However, none of the reasons given for stopping development is applicable to all drugs. Thus, a short plasma half-life may be perfectly acceptable when the effect of the drug persists long after the drug has gone (e.g. the effect of aspirin on platelet cyclo-oxygenase) or when only brief exposure is needed to obtain therapeutic benefit (e.g. penicillin for pneumococcal pneumonia). Saturation of metabolism at high doses may be irrelevant if much lower doses are required for therapeutic benefit. Low bioavailability may not constitute a problem if the therapeutic index is high (e.g. propranolol for hypertension) or the dosage can be readily adjusted to meet the needs of the individual patient (e.g. oral morphine for chronic pain). The presence of multiple metabolites does not necessarily contraindicate proceeding; many useful lipophilic drugs undergo extensive metabolism. A persistent active metabolite may actually convert a drug that would have been unattractive into a very useful one; that, after all, is the principle of prodrugs. The point is that rational decisions can only be made if the information is actively sought and then matched against the desired profile.

Pharmacokinetics may also form the basis of a decision on the choice of compound from a series for development. It is not uncommon for a company to take three or four compounds of a series as far as the FIH and to choose for development the compound that is most attractive from the pharmacokinetic point of view. Similarly, the development of achiral compounds rather than racemic mixtures is generally preferred and it may be necessary to establish whether stereoselective metabolism occurs in humans and, if so, which enantiomer has the more desirable profile.

With the advent of extremely sensitive bioanalytical techniques such as accelerator mass spectrometry, it is now possible to make such selections of candidate compounds based on microdosing at a very early stage of evaluation. Evidence of drug distribution to target tissues (e.g. in the skin) may also be achieved by such sensitive assays and support further development of a particular compound.

From the pharmacokinetics of single doses it is possible to simulate the expected accumulation and concentrations on reaching steady state that will occur on repeat dosing. However, it cannot be assumed that these predictions will hold, and repeat dosing studies in ED should generally include a comparison of pharmacokinetic profiles after the first dose and then at steady state. An increase in clearance because of autoinduction will result in lower C_{max} and AUC and a shorter half-life than predicted. However, this may only become apparent after dosing for 10–14 days. Conversely, saturation of metabolic enzymes at steady state may result in higher than predicted plasma drug concentrations. Accumulation of metabolites that were only present in low, perhaps undetectable, concentrations after single doses may be observed after repeat dosing.

4.6.3 Pharmacodynamics

The third major objective of ED studies in humans is to evaluate pharmacodynamic effects that may serve as biomarkers. A 'biomarker' is 'a characteristic that is objectively measured and evaluated as an indicator of a normal physiological process, pathogenic process or pharmacological response to a therapeutic intervention'. Biomarkers may be mechanistic (e.g. increased expression of a protein, phosphorylation of an enzyme, occupation of a receptor) or they may be functional (e.g. cardiac output, forced expiratory volume, cognitive performance). They may be measures of efficacy (e.g. blood pressure, cholesterol, CD4 counts) or of toxicity (e.g. liver function tests, proteinuria, QT_c).

When a biomarker is not merely a measure of pharmacodynamic effect but is intended to substitute for a clinical endpoint, it is called a 'surrogate endpoint'. The implication is that extensive study of the biomarker has generated sufficient confidence that linkage to a clinical endpoint has been established. A 'clinical endpoint' is defined as 'a characteristic or variable that measures how a patient feels, functions

Table 4.2 Examples of biomarkers of established utility in healthy volunteers

Activity	Biomarker	Drug class/activity
Enzyme activity *ex vivo*	Serum ACE + renin, A-I, A-II	ACE inhibitor
	Platelet MAO_B	Antiparkinsonian
	Neutrophil LO or urinary isoprostanes	Anti-inflammatory LO inhibitors
	Blood factor Xa	Anticoagulant
Physiological response without challenge	Psychomotor tests, for example, reaction time, tracking tasks, saccadic eye movements, body sway, EEG	Sedatives
	Tests of cognition	Cognitive enhancer
	Spirometry, flow-volume loops, plethysmography	Bronchodilators
	Vasodilatation by venous occlusion plethysmography, laser Doppler	Vasodilators
	Acid secretion by gastric pH electrode	Gastric antisecretory drugs
	Gastrointestinal transit time by hydrogen breath test and radio-opaque markers	Gastrointestinal motility agents
Antagonism of response to challenge *in vivo* or *ex vivo*	Skin wheal and flare to i.d. histamine	H_1 antagonist
	Bronchoconstriction to inhaled histamine	
	Bronchoconstriction to inhaled leukotrienes	Leukotriene antagonist
	Late asthmatic response to inhaled antigen	Steroids, other anti-inflammatories
	Nasal airways resistance and cytology to inhaled antigen	Antiallergics
	Cytokine, stress hormone and vascular response to intravenous endotoxin	Immune modulators for shock and inflammation
	Vasoconstriction to A-II	A-II antagonist
	Exercise-induced increase in heart rate	β-blocker
	Blood pressure response to tyramine	MAO_A inhibitor
	Ex vivo platelet aggregation	IIb/IIIa antagonists, NSAIDs
	Impairment of cognition to scopolamine	Cognitive enhancer
	Pain response to cold water	Opioid analgesic
	Gastric acid secretion to pentagastrin	H_2 antagonists, proton pump inhibitors
Immune response	Antibody response	Vaccine
	T-cell responsiveness	Immunosuppressant

ACE, angiotensin-converting enzyme; A-I, A-II, angiotensin I, II; H, histamine; i.d., intradermal; LO, lipoxygenase; MAO, monoamine oxidase; NSAID, non-steroidal anti-inflammatory drug.

or survives'. When the validity of a surrogate endpoint is widely accepted, it may very occasionally replace a clinical endpoint for registration purposes. Table 4.2 lists examples of established biomarkers that may be employed to assess the pharmacological properties of drugs in healthy volunteers.

As mentioned in the introduction to this chapter, decisions in ED will often depend on the dose–response curves for desired and undesired effects, and hence predictions about benefit : risk. It may be just as important to assess undesired as well as desired effects. For example, the decision to develop a new histamine H_1 antagonist will depend on assessments of the dose–response curves for sedation and effect on the QT interval of the ECG, as well as demonstration of the dose–response for antagonism of weals and flares to intradermal histamine, or histamine bronchial challenge.

Whenever possible, investigation of pharmacodynamics should be combined with pharmacokinetic measurements to understand the relationship between concentration and effect. Such relationships can be handled very simply or with sophisticated pharmacokinetic–pharmacodynamic (PK-PD) modelling.

Some of the most exciting advances in biomarker development are in the area of imaging. Here, we are not referring to the important contribution imaging makes to assessment of efficacy in late-phase clinical trials. The contribution that ultrasound scanning, positron emission tomography (PET), single positron emission computed tomography (SPECT) and magnetic resonance imaging (MRI) can make to decision-making early in clinical development is becoming increasingly recognised. For example, measurement of receptor occupancy using specific PET ligands to visualise cerebral receptors and enzymes (e.g. opioid, $5\text{-}HT_{1A}$, $5\text{-}HT_2$, dopamine D_2, muscarinic, nicotinic MAO_B) can frequently provide a rapid and relatively simple means of selecting one or more doses for inclusion in clinical trials. This is of enormous value for trials of treatment of diseases in which group sizes can be extremely large, such as stroke and dementia. It also can set an upper limit to the dose of a drug, above which no additional efficacy is likely and adverse effects are more likely.

The limitations of the use of biomarkers in healthy volunteers must be recognised. For example, although there have been attempts to simulate migraine headache in volunteers, to date none of these models can be considered adequate to serve as a surrogate endpoint. Patients with migraine are not difficult to recruit and are usually healthy apart from their migraine. In this case, it may be more appropriate to establish tolerability and pharmacokinetics in healthy volunteers and then to select a maximum well-tolerated dose with which to perform a small PoC clinical trial in patients. This will need to be followed by larger trials to establish the dose–response relationship.

The value of biomarkers to establish the dose–response and concentration–response curves at the earliest stage of drug development cannot be over-estimated. However, it should be recognised that the utility of any biomarker depends at least in part on the expertise of the experimentalists. Long before the study takes place a decision will need to be made about where the study will be placed and who precisely will perform the measurements. Whether assaying the concentrations of a hormone, performing respiratory function tests or measuring receptor occupancy with a PET ligand, adequate time must be allowed to assess the quality of data produced by a potential investigator or laboratory, whether in-house or in collaboration with an academic centre or CRO. Choice of an investigator must also take into account logistic concerns, such as availability of suitable subjects, capability of staff and access to particular equipment. All developmental methodology work must take place before its application to assessment of an NME so that results are sufficiently reliable to provide the basis for decisions about the NME.

Even if a technique is well established and the methodology has been used many times by the chosen investigator, it is usually worth including an active comparator in such studies. First and foremost, this acts as a verum – it is a concurrent control that verifies that the technique is capable of producing a positive result in that study, thereby avoiding the false negative conclusion. In addition, it will provide a measure with which the magnitude, duration and quality of responses obtained with the NME can be compared (i.e. a bioassay). The main exception to the use of an active comparator is the FIH in which formal statistical comparisons are rarely appropriate and the emphasis is on safety. Aspects of the design of the FIH are now discussed.

4.7 Design of the first-in-human study

The first study of an NME in humans will inevitably involve an escalating-dose design, usually with single doses, although in oncology, repeat dosing is often more appropriate for ethical reasons. The choice of starting dose, increments, range and interval between occasions, number of subjects and use of placebo all need to be considered. Paramount is the safety of the subjects.

4.7.1 Choice of dose range

Factors that must be taken into account in selecting the dose range to be studied are listed in Box 4.11. An excellent guidance document which considers all the factors that must be taken into account when considering the starting dose is available from the European Agency for the Evaluation of Medicinal Products (EMEA).[22]

BOX 4.11 Factors to be considered in selecting dose range for study in humans

- The range of doses and plasma concentrations that exhibited pharmacodynamic effects in animals, the nature of the effects, and the slope of the dose–response curve
- Maximum concentration (C_{max}) and exposure (AUC) in toxicity studies at NOAEL using the most sensitive species, based on the concentrations of drug unbound to plasma proteins (for which substantial corrections may be necessary if plasma protein binding in one or more species is above 95%)
- The nature and severity of toxicity seen in animals – some findings are of more serious consequence than others
- The comparative disposition in different species and predicted exposure in humans, with particular attention to the presence of active metabolites with long half-lives
- The range of doses and number of increments likely to be required in humans

Knowledge of the concentration–response relationship and the nature of both the pharmacodynamic responses and toxicity in animals are the only sound basis for deciding on the starting dose and dosage increments to be used in humans. This information needs to be interpreted and applied using common sense and caution; unthinking application of formulae is not appropriate. A guidance document issued by the US Food and Drug Administration (FDA) bases estimation of a maximum safe starting dose on the NOAEL in animal toxicity studies and subsequent application of algorithms for calculation of human equivalent doses based on body surface area.[23] This approach may be suitable for establishing the maximum safe starting dose but this is rarely the dose one wishes to use at the start of a dose escalation as it takes no account of pharmacological effects of interest, which may occur at doses many orders of magnitude lower than the NOAEL. It also ignores plasma concentration data in tests considered to be of relevance to the putative therapeutic range. There can be no certainty in estimation of the starting dose because the pharmacokinetics in humans are unknown. Nevertheless, prediction from allometric scaling and careful application of all PK-PD information from animal studies, including the steepness of the dose–response curve and the estimated therapeutic window, should all be used to justify a starting dose that is predicted to be below that which will produce any biological effect. For biologicals, this dose has recently been called the minimum anticipated biological effect level (MABEL)[22,24] but the approach should be no different for NCEs.

4.7.2 Magnitude of dose increments

It is quite usual to escalate the doses by doubling or trebling, which is consistent with the linear relationship between logarithm of the dose and response. However, if the slope of the dose–response curve is steep, such increments may be excessive, and for some drugs the relationship between dose (rather than log dose) and response is linear. Sometimes it is preferred to start with a very low dose, examine the pharmacokinetics and then increase the dose four- to fivefold if appropriate. Once into the expected therapeutic range, increments should not generally be greater than doubling. Even when all this has been considered, the doses scheduled are only tentative and they may well need to be modified in the light of the first experience in humans.

4.7.3 Should we dose to toxicity?

The choice of the top dose in a dose-escalating study may be difficult. The view is often expressed that dosing should continue to 'toxicity' (i.e. the dose should be escalated until intolerable adverse effects are experienced by one or more volunteers). Although an adequate definition is lacking, this suggests that the maximum tolerated dose (MTD) will be one increment below that toxic dose. There are certainly some drugs for which the therapeutic index is expected to be low and the putative therapeutic dose will be close to that which can just be tolerated. However, deliberate production of serious adverse events is never acceptable in healthy volunteers and usually unacceptable in patients (an exception to the latter being haematological toxicity with cytotoxics). Therefore, for most ED studies of drugs with a low therapeutic index, it is of much greater relevance to determine a dose that produces some mild non-serious effects. The term minimum intolerated dose (MID)[25] has been applied to patients, and although the dose may be different, the term can equally be applied to healthy subjects. Examples of effects that determine the MID may be sedation, flushing, headache, loose stools or a small change in heart rate or blood pressure. Of no less importance is the dose below the MID, which may be defined as the maximum well-tolerated dose (MWTD). The MWTD is frequently used as the top dose in subsequent ED dose range finding studies in healthy volunteers and patients.

The 'dosing to toxicity' approach was adopted because investigators did not take the trouble to measure pharmacodynamic effects or even follow plasma drug concentrations during the course of a study. Many drugs have a reasonably high therapeutic index and for these it should be perfectly possible to stop the escalation based on a predefined pharmacodynamic endpoint, such as maximum inhibition of a target enzyme. Similarly, the dose of an NME that is devoid of pharmacological effects with a high therapeutic index (e.g. many antibiotics) can usually be escalated to a particular plasma concentration that is in excess of that predicted to be of therapeutic benefit from *in vitro* and perhaps *in vivo* animal studies.

4.7.4 Number of doses for individual subjects

A widely practised approach to the dosing of subjects participating in an FIH is to administer a dose to individual subjects just once, with a new cohort of subjects recruited for each dose level. This has the advantage of simplicity with avoidance of drop-outs, unblinding and carry-over. However, it is an extremely uneconomic use of volunteers involving recruitment of large numbers of potential subjects and screening of many more. It also precludes intra-individual comparisons of data and tends to lead to highly variable data.

The alternative approach, which has been widely practised in Europe for many years, is to administer several doses to an individual on separate occasions, which may be called a multiple single-dose design. If the number of dose increments is expected to be no greater than four, the study can often be conducted with a single group of volunteers. If the estimated number of dose levels is 6–8, two cohorts may be dosed consecutively or on alternate occasions. Such a design enables the relationship between dose and any adverse events to be studied within an individual and a set of pharmacokinetic and dynamic data to be obtained for each individual over a range of doses. Because intra-individual variation is generally much less than interindividual variation; it permits comparisons of pharmacokinetic parameters at each dose to establish whether the pharmacokinetic parameters are independent of dose. With respect to pharmacodynamics, it is often possible to plot a dose–concentration–response for each individual.

If the half-life of a drug or of a metabolite is more than about 24 h, the multiple single-dose design with alternating cohorts can be used with the first cohort receiving dose levels 1, 3 and 5 (or placebo) and the second cohort dose levels 2, 4 and 6. This allows individual subjects to be dosed with a longer interval between doses, say 2 weeks, with dose escalation in the alternate cohort on the intervening weeks. However, drugs (or metabolites) with very long half-lives are best studied using a new cohort of volunteers for each dose.

Situations may arise when the dose range that has to be studied is very wide and the number of increments required to cover the range is large. It may then be advisable to use successive cohorts of volunteers so that the first cohort might receive dose levels 1–4, the second dose levels 4–7 and so on. Note that each cohort is introduced at the top dose level received by the preceding cohort, the overlap being necessary to avoid exposure of a naive subject to what might be a high dose. Whichever design is preferred, the interval between dose escalations should be determined on grounds of safety, not convenience or availability of subjects. For drugs with half-lives of 2 or 3 h it may theoretically be possible to escalate the dose very frequently and thereby conclude the study quickly. However, analytical laboratories can rarely support a turnaround time of less than a week and there is a limit to how quickly data can be collated and reviewed. Failure to obtain, scrutinise and evaluate all the data puts volunteers at unnecessary risk (see section 4.8), as does inadequate time for follow-up safety assessments of subjects. For drugs or metabolites with long half-lives, clinical assessment and blood sampling for pharmacokinetics and clinical pathology may have to continue for many days or weeks before it is prudent to escalate dose, whether in the same or different individuals.

4.7.5 Use of placebo

In general, FIH should be placebo-controlled. In a dose-escalating design, it is obviously not possible to randomise or balance the order of doses, and there may be insufficient power to subject pharmacodynamic endpoints to statistical analysis. However, the advantages of a placebo group outweigh the disadvantages. It is not uncommon for a large number of trivial symptoms to be reported by volunteers and it may only be possible to interpret the significance of these when the incidence in the placebo and treated groups is compared. Substantial changes in vital signs, such as heart rate and blood pressure, occur in the course of a day, and a placebo is invaluable in distinguishing drug-induced effects from others. Similarly, it is not uncommon for some external factor such as an influenza epidemic, food poisoning or caffeine withdrawal to

Table 4.3 Parallel-study design with two alternating cohorts of eight subjects and a 6 : 2 randomisation to active drug (A) or placebo (P) – each subject receives either A on four occasions or P on four occasions

Subject	1	2	3	4	5	6	7	8	9	10	11	12	13	14	15	16
Dose 1	P	A	A	A	A	A	P	A								
Dose 2									A	P	A	P	A	A	A	A
Dose 3	P	A	A	A	A	A	P	A								
Dose 4									A	P	A	P	A	A	A	A
Dose 5	P	A	A	A	A	A	P	A								
Dose 6									A	P	A	P	A	A	A	A
Dose 7	P	A	A	A	A	A	P	A								
Dose 8									A	P	A	P	A	A	A	A

Table 4.4 Crossover study design with two alternating cohorts of eight subjects and a 6 : 2 restricted randomisation to active drug (A) or placebo (P) – each subject receives A on three occasions and P on one occasion

Subject	1	2	3	4	5	6	7	8	9	10	11	12	13	14	15	16
Dose 1	P	A	A	P	A	A	A	A								
Dose 2									A	P	A	A	A	A	P	A
Dose 3	A	P	A	A	A	P	A	A								
Dose 4									A	A	P	A	P	A	A	A
Dose 5	A	A	P	A	P	A	A	P								
Dose 6									P	A	A	A	A	P	A	A
Dose 7	A	A	A	A	A	A	P	A								
Dose 8									A	A	A	P	A	A	A	P

affect a study. Frequently, minor elevation of liver transaminases or lymphocytosis occurs as the result of intercurrent viral infections. Liver transaminases also tend to rise with prolonged periods of incarceration in a study unit, probably because of diet, lack of exercise or other lifestyle factors. A placebo group can be invaluable in deciding whether the problem is likely to be drug-related.

4.7.6 Blinding

As far as possible, the study should be conducted under double-blind conditions. Sometimes, pharmacological effects – desired or undesired – tend to unblind the study, but even in these circumstances the identity of treatment will be unknown to subjects and observers at the time of dosing and before onset of effects, thereby minimising bias. Specified personnel, such as the pharmacist, bioanalyst and pharmacokineticist, may need to know the treatment allocation code but this should not compromise the blinding of all other study personnel.

4.7.7 Parallel groups or crossover

If subjects are to receive more than one dose level of active drug in the multiple single-dose study design,

there are a number of ways in which subjects can be allocated to active drug (A) or placebo (P) but essentially they fall into two approaches:
1. Subjects are randomised to receive either A or P throughout the study (i.e. parallel groups).
2. Subjects are randomised to receive A or P on different occasions in a crossover design.

Tables 4.3 and 4.4 show examples of parallel and crossover designs, with two alternating cohorts of eight subjects randomised to A or P in a dose-escalating design involving eight dose levels.

The advantages of a parallel group design can be summarised as follows:
1. The design is simple and robust.
2. No doses are omitted so the full dose–response and linearity of pharmacokinetics can be established within individuals.

The disadvantages of a parallel group design can be summarised as follows:
1. It can be very difficult to maintain the blind throughout the study because as soon as pharmacodynamic effects are observed both subjects and investigators will know whether an individual has been allocated to the active or placebo group for the remainder of the study.

2. Subjects cannot serve as their own placebo controls for intrasubject comparisons of pharmacodynamic effects, including adverse events.

3. Variability in intersubject data may confound meaningful comparisons unless cohorts are large.

4. Only a proportion of subjects participating in the study receive active drug.

The advantages of a crossover design are as follows:

1. Maximum information is obtained from a comparatively small number of subjects.

2. Randomisation to A or P is different on every study day, therefore it is comparatively easy to maintain the blind throughout the study.

3. Intrasubject variability in pharmacodynamics is generally much less than intersubject variability, allowing meaningful comparisons with placebo.

The disadvantages of a crossover design are as follows:

1. Individual subjects skip a dose level when they receive placebo so that no pharmacokinetic data are available for this subject/occasion and the subject is exposed to a large dose increment on the next occasion.

2. The dose escalation may stop before all subjects have received placebo so that the crossover is incomplete.

4.7.8 Size of cohorts

The number of subjects per cohort needed for the initial study depends on several factors. If a well-established pharmacodynamic measurement is to be used as an endpoint, it should be possible to calculate the number required to demonstrate significant differences from placebo by means of a power calculation based on variances in a previous study using this technique. However, analysis of the study is often limited to descriptive statistics such as mean and standard deviation, or even just recording the number of reports of a particular symptom, so that a formal power calculation is often inappropriate. There must be a balance between the minimum number on which it is reasonable to base decisions about dose escalation and the number of individuals it is reasonable to expose to an NME for the first time. To take the extremes, it is unwise to make decisions about tolerability and pharmacokinetics based on data from one or two subjects, although there are advocates of such a minimalist approach. Conversely, it is not justifiable to administer a single dose level to, say, 50 subjects at this early stage of ED. There is no simple answer to this, but in general the number lies between 6 and 20 subjects.

4.8 Minimising risk

4.8.1 Minimal risk

The principle governing all studies in humans is that of 'minimal risk', so that a healthy volunteer leaves a study in as good health as when he or she entered it. The Royal College of Physicians has stated that, 'A risk greater than minimal is not acceptable in a healthy volunteer study'.[10] A healthy volunteer stands to gain nothing directly from a new medication and the risk should therefore be negligible but it can never be reduced to zero. One must never be deluded into believing that an NME is going to be 'safe'. If all the toxicity studies are reassuring and the molecule belongs to a well-known class that has an exemplary safety record, the NME must still be treated with the greatest respect. Some of the ways in which risk can be minimised are mentioned below.

4.8.2 Practical aspects of study design and conduct

A comprehensive knowledge of the preclinical information about a compound is an essential requirement for the safe conduct of the FIH. Toxicology, metabolism, pharmacokinetics and pharmacodynamics are all important, despite their limited predictive power for humans. As explained above (see section 4.7.1), selection of the starting dose is dependent on all these preclinical findings but many other aspects of the study design must also take the preclinical findings into account. For example, in deciding the interval between dosing subjects, the pharmacokinetics in animals and the time course of pharmacodynamic effects (desired and undesired) must be considered carefully. If a drug to be administered orally is expected to exert its maximum effects at the time of peak plasma concentrations after rapid absorption, it may be reasonable to dose subjects at 30- or 60-min intervals. On the other hand, if the effects are not directly related to plasma concentrations and/or are expected to occur many hours after dosing, the interval may need to be 24 h or more. If subjects are dosed with an interval that is too short, drug-related adverse reactions would be likely to occur at the same time in several or all the subjects. This could be very difficult to manage and puts subjects at unnecessary risk. Indeed, it may be wise to stop the study after the first significant adverse reaction has been seen and reconsider the dose or whether to proceed at all.

It is wise to study two or three lead volunteers on the first day at a new dose level with one of the subjects receiving placebo before the remaining subjects receive the same dose on another day. It is also often sensible to limit the number of subjects studied on one day to 6 or perhaps 8, at least two of whom will receive placebo.

The route of administration is also a key factor. It is a common misconception that the intravenous route is of higher risk than the oral route. The advantages of the intravenous route are that the infusion can be administered slowly over an hour or several hours and the rate of administration can be reduced if necessary. Should significant adverse events appear while the infusion is in progress, it can be discontinued altogether before the full dose has been administered. Administration of a bolus or rapid infusion is never justified for a first administration to humans. For orally administered drugs, there is no chance to alter anything once the dose has been swallowed.

The most carefully designed study and the most ethical protocol do not guarantee safety. A study that is not prepared and executed properly is likely to put volunteers at unnecessary risk. There must be sufficient staff to cover all practical aspects of the study. At least one nurse and a doctor should be present for dosing and for a specified period afterwards, usually at least a few hours. All staff should be thoroughly briefed by the investigator, the case report forms checked against the schedule, and every member of staff should know precisely what he or she will be doing during the course of a study day. The detailed schedule for each study day must also be optimal. An antidote to the NME, if available, should be present on the unit with staff fully briefed what treatment will be administered, should the need arise, however remote the possibility.

4.8.3 Interim reviews

Interim reviews of the data are an essential requirement to minimise risk during dose-escalation studies. After each study day, or certainly after a predefined number of volunteers have received the next dose increment, the investigator, nurses, study physicians and medical and other representatives of the sponsor should meet (face-to-face or by video/teleconference) to review the data. A decision to stop, modify or continue dose escalation should be made jointly between the principal investigator at the CRO and the sponsor's physician. Such reviews should be conducted with maintenance of the double-blind and steps should be taken to avoid inadvertent unblinding, such as by coding of subject numbers. The data that should be reviewed are listed in Box 4.12.

> **BOX 4.12** Interim review of data
>
> - Overall progress: number of subjects, doses, etc.
> - Adverse events: type, severity, duration, action taken, outcome, likelihood of attributability to study drug
> - Vital signs, ECGs, other procedures for safety monitoring
> - Pharmacodynamic measures
> - Plasma concentrations, pharmacokinetics, any difficulties with assay methodology
> - Laboratory data: blood and urine tests
> - Procedures: any difficulties, compliance

It should be noted that pharmacokinetic data are included, which places a strain on the bioanalysts and laboratory facilities. However, with proper planning and adequate development time, preliminary but reasonably reliable data can usually be obtained within 2 or 3 days of receiving samples. Knowledge of maximum concentrations, dose proportionality of AUC and half-lives of the parent molecule and major metabolites greatly adds to making rational decisions about adverse events, times for sampling and measurements, the appropriate next dosage increment and the interval that should be allowed between study occasions.

Adverse events should be tabulated for easy inspection but the case report form should be available and all laboratory data such as blood counts, renal function and liver function tests should be inspected closely. The absence of obvious adverse events does not mean that all is well, and careful scrutiny of data by an experienced physician can often spot problems before they become troublesome. Not infrequently, one or more volunteers become unwell during the course of a study, usually because of intercurrent viral infections, and decisions about postponement of study days, subject withdrawal and follow-up can be made during these meetings. Data that are missing because of non-attendance of volunteers, for whatever reason, may lead to a delay in the study, with postponement of dose escalation until they have caught up.

The review requires that all the data be collated for presentation, which is a useful discipline. An opportunity is also provided for practical problems to be discussed and acted upon. All decisions should be documented and it is good practice for the sponsor to confirm the main outcome decision in writing to the CRO. Any significant modifications to the protocol will have to be put before the IEC before proceeding and substantial amendments required review by the competent authority. The volunteers also need to be updated about any changes to the schedule and adverse events as the study unfolds. As always, a volunteer must be free to withdraw from a study at any stage.

The decision to halt a dose escalation is not always straightforward. There may have been adverse events that are not serious but that are disliked by the volunteers. While decisions about safety must always be in the hands of the physicians, the investigator must listen carefully to the volunteers and nurses. When hitherto sensible and well-motivated volunteers begin to adopt a negative attitude to a study for whatever reason, it is usually time to stop.

4.8.4 Higher risk new molecular entities

In Section 4.5.7 mention was made of the life-threatening adverse reactions to the first dose of a new biological entity known as TGN1412 that occurred in a study conducted in the UK in 2006. It is not appropriate to discuss the details of this case here but some important aspects relating to management of risk are pertinent. TGN1412 was a recombinant IgG4 monoclonal antibody, which acted as an agonist binding to CD28 present on T cells. The T-cell stimulation bypassed the normal requirement for co-stimulation by T-cell receptor triggering. It was intended for reconstitution of T cells in diseases such as chronic lymphoctytic leukaemia and autoimmune diseases such as rheumatoid arthritis.

Following the event, the UK Department of Health established an inquiry which was conducted by an Expert Scientific Group (ESG). In their final report, the ESG enumerated a number of properties that confer higher risk.[24] The advent of biologicals and novel engineered molecular structures leads to many more factors contributing to risk than in the past. Some of these are listed in Box 4.13.

While any of these factors may confer higher than normal risk, there is no simple formula for assessment of risk. Indeed, the ESG emphasised that considerations with respect to trial design and safety should be on a case-by-case basis. It must never be forgotten that any drug can be dangerous if administered in excessive doses.

4.9 Subsequent studies in healthy volunteers

The limitations of the FIH should be recognised. Even if the study has achieved all its objectives in terms of

---

BOX 4.13 Some factors that contribute to higher than normal risk

- Mechanism of action may be poorly understood
- Species specificity may make non-clinical tests of safety and efficacy of questionable relevance to humans because of absence of on-target effects
- Dose calculations based on biological activity in non-clinical species may be erroneous because of absence of on-target effects
- Actions on the immune system may be difficult to predict
- Amplification, cascades and multiple signalling pathways may result in multiple steep dose–response curves
- Quality of the product used in human studies may be different from that used in non-clinical testing

---

tolerability, pharmacokinetics and pharmacodynamic endpoints, the data will only be of a preliminary nature. It is then necessary to re-examine the provisional plan of exploratory studies and reconsider priorities and data, which require early verification in carefully designed, controlled studies. The objectives of these studies should be driven by the critical questions in the ED plan. A few points about the design of commonly required studies are made in the next paragraphs.

4.9.1 Effect of food ingestion

An assessment of the effect of food on the pharmacokinetics of a drug can generally be examined in a single-dose two-arm randomised crossover design study, which may be included in the same protocol as the dose-escalating study. Preliminary information can also be obtained by including a 'fed' occasion at one dose level in the dose escalation. These studies will be insufficient for registration purposes, which require an adequately powered study performed with the final formulation, but the information should be sufficient to indicate whether there is need for restrictions on dosing with respect to meals in repeat-dose studies in healthy volunteers and patient clinical trials.

4.9.2 Multiple doses

Frequently, information on tolerability, safety and pharmacokinetics of multiple doses for up to about 14 days is the highest priority. A placebo-controlled parallel-groups dose-escalating design is generally appropriate, with each cohort receiving a single dose level or placebo for the defined duration. Typically, such a study would involve three or four dose levels, selected on the basis of results of the first study. If three dose levels were chosen to be studied, cohorts of 12 subjects might be randomised 9 : 3 A : P so that at the end of the study nine subjects will have received each dose level and nine will have received placebo. If biomarkers are to be employed to assess the relationships between dose, concentration and response, consideration should be given to use of a positive control as well.

Plasma pharmacokinetic profiles should generally be obtained with the first dose and at the end of the dosing period, when steady state has been achieved (i.e. when input rate of drug is equal to the elimination). Blood should be also be sampled immediately before dosing at selected times during the dosing period to obtain trough concentrations. The pharmacokinetics at steady state can then be compared with those after single doses within each subject. So-called 'time-dependent kinetics' in which the single-dose data do not accurately predict the kinetics at steady state may result from a number of causes. For example, autoinduction, when the drug induces its own metabolism, will result in clearance increasing with time. Conversely, if metabolism becomes saturated at high concentrations, the steady state concentrations may be higher than predicted from the pharmaco-kinetic parameters obtained after single doses.

Many drugs active on the CNS will be subject to pharmacodynamic tolerance (i.e. effects will diminish on repeat dosing despite maintenance of plasma concentrations). If development of tolerance is considered likely, consideration should be given to designing dose-escalation steps within each cohort with pharmacokinetic and pharmacodynamic assessments at some of these interim steps. Usually, it is the central effects of drugs acting primarily on the CNS that limit the dose that can be administered to healthy volunteers rather than any target organ pathological changes. The MWTD generally is lower than that which may subsequently be defined in patients.

With drugs acting primarily on other systems, the limit to dose escalation may also be determined by the incidence or severity of adverse events, but for drugs that are well tolerated, the dose may be limited in accordance with plasma concentrations and total exposure defined by the NOAEL in the most sensitive toxicity species. Indeed, the NOAELs and the nature of target organ toxicity are far more relevant for limiting the dose in multiple-dose than single-dose studies.

4.9.3 Pharmacodynamics

The use of pharmacodynamic biomarkers is discussed in section 4.6.3. While it may be extremely valuable to include such measures in the FIH, the data that can be obtained in a dose-escalating study are necessarily limited. The first study will usually suggest the dose range of interest and the magnitude and time course of effects but these will need to be characterised more fully. For example, it may be crucially important to know whether a drug causes sedation and, if so, over what dose range. There may be some evidence from the first study that subjects felt drowsy or light-headed at the upper end of the dose range studied. It will then be necessary to perform a study specifically to investigate this using a battery of psychopharmacological and cognitive tests.

Study of single-dose pharmacodynamics of desired or adverse effects in healthy volunteers is best performed using double-blind crossover designs, typically with three or four dose levels, placebo and active controls, randomised and balanced for order according to Latin squares. For studies in patients, multiple-limb crossover designs are less appropriate but crossover studies with single doses of A versus P are certainly feasible and, of course, parallel groups, single or repeat dosing are commonly employed designs.

4.9.4 Studies in the elderly

For a drug that will be used commonly in the elderly, it is important to obtain early information about tolerability and pharmacokinetics in this age group. Because glomerular filtration rate declines with age, exposure to drug is likely to be greatly increased in the elderly if the drug is eliminated primarily by the kidney. In the case of a high extraction drug, impairment of cardiac output in the elderly is likely to increase exposure because of reduced first-pass metabolism. Single- and multiple-dose studies in healthy elderly volunteers can provide extremely valuable information prior to exposure of patients in this age group, who are a vulnerable group and in whom many factors may confound results.

4.9.5 Drug interactions

If a drug is to be tested in patients who will inevitably be receiving other medications with which the NME is likely to interact, it may be important to design interaction studies in healthy volunteers early in ED. This is not simply a matter of whether dosage adjustment may be required. For example, the demonstrated ability of an NME to inhibit metabolism and thereby double the concentrations of a standard therapy which will almost always be given concomitantly, may lead to a decision to stop development altogether. At the very least, it will have implications for the recruitment of subjects in subsequent clinical trials.

The design of such studies will usually involve repeat dosing of one or both drugs to achieve steady-state concentrations. Potential interactions with drugs used commonly by the elderly, such as digoxin, antihypertensives and warfarin, need not be studied in the elderly but some of these studies may need to be performed before exposing patients in clinical trials. Data from *in vitro* and *in vivo* studies in animals and preclinical characterisation of metabolism and other aspects of pharmacokinetics are crucially important in selecting appropriate interaction studies to be performed early in clinical development.[26]

4.9.6 Radiolabelled studies

A mass-balance study to gain a comprehensive understanding of the metabolic fate of drug-related material requires administration of radiolabelled material to humans. Such studies generally involve administration of single doses, with subsequent collection of excreta as well as blood sampling until virtually all drug has been eliminated. The clinical phase of such studies is generally not complex, but preparation for the study, with synthesis of the radioactive molecule and development of 'cold' assays of metabolites as well as parent molecule, may take many months. Such studies also require submission of applications with detailed dosage and radioactive exposure calculations for authorisation by external bodies such as the Administration of Radioactive Substances Advisory Committee (ARSAC) in the UK (www.advisorybodies.doh.gov.uk/ARSAC/).

The timing of the study during the course of development is often a subject of much debate. The information gained may be critical but there is an understandable reluctance to commit to all the preparatory work before it is clear that the NME will be going all the way to MAA. Fortunately, microdose radiolabel studies are now possible to establish the metabolic fate of molecules very early in development (see section 4.6.2).

4.10 Exploratory studies in patients

The ED plan will enumerate which studies are to be performed in healthy volunteers and which in patients. While the first studies progress, the information generated needs to be constantly evaluated and the decision to proceed to patients should be driven by the data and how well the studies have actually achieved their objectives. The first consideration, as always, will be safety. Information that can be obtained more safely in healthy subjects, which may subsequently reduce risk to patients, should prompt a debate on whether it is wise to progress according to plan or whether an additional study should be performed in healthy subjects. Another option that may be considered is to proceed with the planned study in patients but to admit them to hospital or a clinical investigation unit for all or part of the dosing period. However, this might not be feasible because suitable facilities and staff are not available or because the anticipated rate of patient recruitment might be considered unacceptably slow.

Perhaps the most frequent problem at this stage of ED is that the dose range of interest has not been adequately defined. If this can be achieved only in the target patient population there is no point in carrying out more studies in healthy subjects. If, on the other hand, an additional study using established valid biomarkers in healthy subjects would clarify the dose range of interest, thereby avoiding under- or over-dosing and reducing the number of dose levels that need to be examined in the patient population, this option should be considered. While competition demands that drug development should proceed at a fast pace, time is often wasted in development because of a failure to maximise the information that can be obtained in ED – the learn–confirm paradigm. A delay of a few months to obtain critical data in ED may save a year or two of development time later on.

However, the mechanistic demonstration of a drug's effects must, before too long, lead to the proof of concept of efficacy in patients with the target disease. Such studies typically involve 50–200 patients, administration of two or more active doses, placebo and reference treatment controls. Endpoints may be clinical or biomarkers or a combination of these. While the random allocation to different parallel treatment groups of fixed size is traditional, there is a growing appreciation of the use of adaptive designs and more exploratory statistical approaches.

The use of biomarkers and surrogate endpoints in patients is well established in virtually all therapeutic areas. After all, blood pressure has been used as a surrogate for cardiovascular risk for many decades. Some other examples are given in Table 4.5.

An important qualification must be made. While a biomarker may be of proven value in establishing whether a drug has the desired effect in patients or

Table 4.5 Examples of biomarkers of established utility in early drug evaluation in patients

Clinical endpoint	Biomarker	Drug class
Risk of cardiovascular events	LDL : HDL serum cholesterol	Statins
Complications of diabetes	FBG, HbA$_{1C}$, insulin sensitivity	Some oral antidiabetic agents
Relapse rate and disability in MS	Demyelination plaques on MRI scan	Various agents for MS
Frequency of epileptic fits	EEG photostimulation	Antiepileptics
Progression to AIDS	Serum viral mRNA	Anti-HIV drugs
Fracture rate in osteoporosis	Bone mineral density	Bisphosphonates, HRT, etc.
Progression of prostatic carcinoma	Serum PSA and testosterone	GnRH analogues

EEG, electroencephalography; FBG, fasting blood glucose; GnRH, gonadotrophin releasing hormone; HbA$_{1C}$, glycosylated haemoglobin A$_{1C}$; HDL, high-density lipoprotein; HRT, hormone replacement therapy; LDL, low-density lipoprotein; MRI, magnetic resonance imaging; MS, multiple sclerosis; PSA, prostate specific antigen.

healthy volunteers and for evaluation of the dose–response relationship, it may not be a surrogate for the clinical endpoint.[27] Thus, suppression of testosterone after an initial rise will give an almost immediate endpoint for the effect of gonadotrophin releasing hormone analogues in prostate cancer but the relationship breaks down later in the disease. Measures of blood glucose control are vital for establishing dose–response in early studies of new oral agents for type 2 diabetes but they are not surrogates for the complications of the disease, despite the proven relationship between glycaemic control and complications. Furthermore, the benefit of some long-acting insulins appears to be the reduction in nocturnal hypoglycaemia with no effect on the traditional measures of glycaemia. Bone mineral density is inversely related to fracture rates in osteoporosis and is an endpoint for efficacy but for regulatory purposes vertebral fracture rates constitute the primary outcome variable. An important exception is mRNA viral load in HIV-positive patients, which is accepted by regulatory authorities as a surrogate for a delay in progression to AIDS and survival.[28] Such a conservative approach may sometimes seem to place unnecessary demands on the pharmaceutical industry but there is precedent. Suppression of ventricular extrasystoles seemed at one time to be an obvious marker of efficacy of type Ic anti-arrhythmic agents. The complete failure of this outcome to serve as a surrogate to predict the incidence of sudden death in patients with heart disease justifies the extremely cautious position of regulatory authorities in accepting surrogate endpoints for registration purposes.[29]

An interesting aspect of the use of biomarkers as surrogates is exemplified by the statins, which lower serum low-density lipoprotein cholesterol. It has recently been shown that their contribution to improved prognosis in patients with cardiovascular disease is not entirely a result of lowering of cholesterol and may be related to anti-inflammatory activity. Thus, the apparently obvious surrogate turns out to be an inadequate biomarker for predicting outcome.

Of course, it is not always necessary to rely on biomarkers for rapid evaluation of dose–response relationships in ED. Thus, efficacy of new drugs is readily demonstrated in terms of the clinical endpoint for diseases, such as migraine, inflammatory pain, asthma, psoriasis, glaucoma and many others.

4.11 Outcomes of ED

As discussed in the introduction to this chapter, results of ED are intended to give a clear indication that the drug is a serious candidate for FD to product licence, or that it is not viable and development should be stopped forthwith. Sometimes it takes a little longer before the picture becomes clear but the aim should be to make a go/no-go decision at the earliest opportunity.

Overall, results of ED should impact on both the project itself and on the research programme from which additional compounds are actively being sought. Some common reasons for discontinuing a project and their possible impact on the research programme are shown in Table 4.6.

Table 4.6 Discontinuation of a project and impact on basic research

Findings leading to project termination	Impact on research
Poor tolerability at effective concentrations	If due to specific compound, need back-up
	If a class effect, stop programme
Unsatisfactory pharmacokinetics or metabolism	May be possible to design a better molecule
Low potency	May be possible to design a more potent molecule
Low or absent efficacy	If principle disproved, stop programme

A more successful outcome of ED will usually commit the company to proceed to full develoment. If ED has achieved its objectives it should be possible to make use of the PK-PD information obtained to optimise the design of subsequent pivotal clinical trials. In particular, it should be possible to use dosage regimens that are rational and justifiable on scientific as well as commercial grounds. Active research programmes should proceed with the search for follow-up compounds.

References

1 Directive 2001/20/EC Article 2(d) of the European Parliament and of the Council of 4 April 2001 on the approximation of the laws, regulations and administrative provisions of the member states relating to the implementation of good clinical practice in the conduct of clinical trials on medicinal products for human use. Eur-Lex. *Official Journal of the European Communities* 2001, L121 Vol. 44:34–44. http://europa.eu.int/eur-lex/.

2 European Agency for the Evaluation of Medicinal Products. *ICH Tripartite Guideline. Dose–Response Information to Support Drug Registration.* London: EMEA, 1994.

3 Schmidt R. Dose-finding studies in clinical drug development. *Eur J Clin Pharmacol* 1988;**34**:15–9.

4 European Agency for the Evaluation of Medicinal Products. *ICH Topic S7 Safety Pharmacology Studies for Human Pharmaceuticals CPMP/ICH/539/00.* London: EMEA, 2000.

5 European Agency for the Evaluation of Medicinal Products. *ICH Topic S6 Safety Studies for Biotechnological Products CPMP/ICH/302/95.* London: EMEA, 1995.

6 Center for Drug Evaluation and Research, US Food and Drug Administration. *Guidance for Industry, Drug Metabolism/Drug Interaction Studies in the Drug Development Process: Studies In Vitro.* Rockville, MD: FDA, 1997.

7 European Agency for the Evaluation of Medicinal Products. *ICH Topic M3 Non-Clinical Safety Studies for the Conduct of Human Clinical Trials for Pharmaceuticals CPMP/ICH/286/95.* London: EMEA, 1995.

8 European Agency for the Evaluation of Medicinal Products. *ICH Topic S2B Genotoxicity: A Standard Battery for Genotoxocity Testing of Pharmaceuticals CPMP/ICH/174/95.* London: EMEA, 1995.

9 European Agency for the Evaluation of Medicinal Products. *ICH Topic E6, 1996, Guideline for Good Clinical Practice, Section 7.3. Content of the Investigator's Brochure.* London: EMEA, 1996.

10 Royal College of Physicians. Research on healthy volunteers. *J R Coll Physicians Lond* 1986;**20**:243–57.

11 Association of the British Pharmaceutical Industry. *Guidelines for Phase I Clinical Trials.* ABPI, 2007.

12 Stinson JC, Pears JS, Williams AJ et al. Use of 24 h ambulatory ECG recordings in the assessment of new chemical entities in healthy volunteers. *Br J Clin Pharmacol* 1995;**39**:651–6.

13 Lacey JH, Mitchell-Heggs P, Montgomery D et al. Guidelines for medical experiments on non-patient human volunteers over the age of 65 years. *J Pharm Med* 1991;**1**:281–8.

14 Jackson D, Richardson RG. Essential information to be given to volunteers and recorded in a protocol. *J Pharm Med* 1991;**2**:99–103.

15 Watson N, Wyld PJ. The importance of general practitioner information in selection of volunteers for clinical trials. *Br J Clin Pharmacol* 1992;**33**:197–9.

16 Boyce M, Nenthwich H, Melbourne W et al. TOPS: the overvolunteering prevention system. *Br J Clin Pharmacol* 2003;**55**:418P–9P.

17 European Agency for the Evaluation of Medicinal Products. *ICH Topic E6 Guideline for Good Clinical Practice CPMP/ICH/135195.* London: EMEA, 1995.

18 Royle JM, Snell ES. Medical research on normal volunteers. *Br J Clin Pharmacol* 1986;**21**:548–9.

19 Orme M, Harry J, Routledge P et al. Healthy volunteer studies in Great Britain: the results of a survey into 12 months activity in this field. *Br J Clin Pharmacol* 1989;**27**:125–33.

20 Carden PV, Dommel FW, Trumble RR. Subjects in nontherapeutic research. Survey of United States Department of Health, Education and Welfare. *N Engl J Med* 1976;**295**:650–4.

21 Sibille M, Deigat N, Janin A et al. Adverse events in Phase I studies: a report in 1015 healthy volunteers. *Eur J Clin Pharmacol* 1998;**54**:13–20.

22 Committee for Medicinal Products for Human use (CHMP). Guideline on strategies to identify and mitigate risks for first-inhuman clinical trials with investigational medicinal products. EMEA/CHMP/SWP/28367/07.

23 Guidance for Industry. Estimating the maximum safe starting dose in initial clinical trials for therapeutics in adult healthy volunteers. US Department of Health and Human Services, FDA, Center for Drug Evaluation and Research (CDER) Pharmacology and Toxicology, July 2005.

24 Expert scientific group on Phase one clinical trials. Final report 30 November 2006. Publ. TSO (The Stationery Office).

25 Cutler NR, Sramek J, Greenblatt DJ et al. Defining the maximum tolerated dose: investigator, academic, industry and regulatory perspectives. *J Clin Pharmacol* 1997;**37**:767–83.

26 Committee for Proprietary Medicinal Products. *Note for Guidance on the Investigation of Drug Interactions EPMP/EWP/560/95.* London: CPMP, 1995.

27 Rolan P. The contribution of clinical pharmacology surrogates and models to drug development: a critical appraisal. *Br J Clin Pharmacol* 1997;**44**:219–25.

28 Deyton L. Importance of surrogate markers in evaluation of antiviral therapy for HIV infection. *JAMA* 1996;**276**: 159–60.

29 Echt DS, Liebson PR, Mitchell B et al. Mortality and morbidity of patients receiving encainide, flecainide or placebo: the Cardiac Arrhythmia Suppression Trial. *N Engl J Med* 1991;**324**:781–8.

5 Clinical pharmacokinetics

Paul Rolan[1] and Valèria Molnár[2]

[1] University of Adelaide, Adelaide, Australia
[2] Clinical Pharmacology Consulting Ltd, Beaumont, Australia

5.1 Introduction

The term 'pharmacokinetics' refers to the time course of the passage of a drug and its metabolites through the body. It can be thought of as 'what the body does to the drug' in contrast to pharmacodynamics, which can be thought of as 'what the drug does to the body' (Figure 5.1). The processes involved are absorption, distribution, metabolism and excretion, and are defined in Box 5.1. Together, these processes have an important role in determining the duration and magnitude of both the desired and undesired pharmacodynamic effects of drugs.

It is not usually possible to measure the concentration of a drug at its site(s) of action. Plasma, which can be conveniently sampled, is generally used instead, but drug concentrations may be determined in other bodily fluids such as saliva and cerebrospinal fluid, as well as the excreta, urine and faeces. There is often a relationship between plasma concentration and response, although this may sometimes be complex. Therefore, estimation of plasma concentrations, and how they are altered by the many factors that can

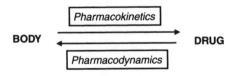

- the study of the time course of a drug's passage through body fluids and tissues
- 'what the body does to the drug'

Figure 5.1 Pharmacokinetics – definition.

The Textbook of Pharmaceutical Medicine. Edited by John P. Griffin. © 2009, ISBN: 978-1-4051-8035-1.

> **BOX 5.1** The pharmacokinetic processes
>
> *Absorption* – the process of getting drug into the body (not necessarily the systemic circulation)
> *Distribution* – the processes of distribution into and out of the tissues
> *Metabolism* – the processes that change the drug to another molecule
> *Excretion* – the processes that remove drug from the body
>
> Collectively, these processes are referred to as ADME

affect drug handling, may be used to make predictions about dosage in the otherwise healthy individual and in the presence of organ failure or concomitant medications.

A growing appreciation of the predictive value of pharmacokinetics, together with a change in the attitude of regulatory authorities to the whole question of dosage, has led to increased importance of the clinical pharmacokinetics regulatory submission. It is no longer acceptable to register a dosage regimen based on a single empirically derived dose of proven efficacy and safety. Drug developers are now rightly required to demonstrate, wherever possible, that the optimum dose and frequency of dosing have been selected to give the greatest benefit for the least risk of adverse reactions. Regulatory authorities also require pharmacokinetic information to support clinical data in order to make recommendations on how dosage should be modified for particular patient populations. The clinical significance of altered pharmacokinetics, and hence the requirement for dosage adjustment, will, to some extent, depend on the therapeutic index of the drug. Thus, while a clinical pharmacokinetics package forms a mandatory part of every regulatory submission for a systemically administered drug, a more comprehensive package will be generally required for drugs of low therapeutic index.

Although, like statistics, the details of pharmacokinetic analysis are best left to the experts, a pharmaceutical physician who is familiar with the basic concepts of how pharmacokinetic information contributes to a dossier will be able to interact more effectively with company colleagues and regulatory authority staff. It is the aim of this chapter to provide such a preliminary grounding.

5.2 Basic concepts

The reader is referred to one of several texts giving detailed accounts of clinical pharmacokinetics.[1] However, an understanding of the basic concepts is essential in order to appreciate how pharmacokinetic data can provide insight into the physiological processes that determine the time course of a drug in the body, and implications this has for the toxicity and therapeutic efficacy of drugs, particularly new active substances in development.

5.2.1 Overview of the fate of administered drug

A drug can be administered directly into the vascular compartment or by an alternative route such as orally. It can usually be assumed that the entire dose administered by the intravenous route reaches the systemic circulation. After oral administration, only a proportion may reach the systemic circulation because of incomplete absorption or because absorbed drug may be metabolised in the mucosa of the gastrointestinal tract or liver, a process known as first-pass metabolism. Once in the systemic circulation, drug is transferred from the circulation to tissues and back again; this is called distribution. Rates and extent of distribution to different tissues may depend on blood perfusion, diffusion, active transport and binding to plasma and tissue proteins. Also, once the drug is in the plasma, it can start to be removed, either by changing it to another molecule (metabolism) or by removal from the plasma in unchanged form (excretion) most frequently into urine, but sometimes bile or, more rarely, breath. Collectively, metabolism and excretion are known as elimination.

5.2.2 Plasma concentration–time curve

The effects of the processes listed above on the time course of the plasma concentration with time is as follows. Initially, as absorption starts, the plasma drug concentration will rise. As soon as there is some drug in the plasma, distribution and elimination will start. Absorption will start to slow down as there is less drug to be absorbed. Eventually, the rate of drug going into the plasma from absorption will be equalled by the rate of drug leaving the plasma by distribution and elimination, so temporarily a plateau of maximum concentration is reached. Absorption continues to slow (as by now most of the drug has been absorbed) and the plasma concentration will continue to fall because of ongoing distribution and elimination. Often, elimination is slower than distribution, resulting in an initial fast fall, caused mainly by distribution and then a slower fall largely as a result of elimination.

Most physicians will be familiar with the basic shape of a plasma concentration–time curve following oral or intravenous administration, and are likely to be familiar with, or at least readily understand, the simple terms that relate to this shape. Such terms – maximum plasma concentration (C_{max}), time to maximum plasma concentration (t_{max}), area under the plasma concentration–time curve (AUC) and half-life ($t_{1/2}$) – are illustrated in Figure 5.2.

5.2.3 Descriptive versus conceptual parameters

These simple descriptive terms can be used for any concentration–time profile, and do not require any conceptual understanding of how the drug is handled by the body. Although these descriptive terms are useful in designing a dosage regimen (see below), there is no way of understanding why two drugs dosed at the same nominal dose could have very differing values of C_{max} and half-life. To understand why the values are as they are, it is necessary to use a new set of parameters, which assist in the conceptual understanding of how the drug is handled by the body. The three most important parameters in this conceptual group are illustrated in Figure 5.3. These parameters are clearance (CL), bioavailability (F) and volume of distribution (V), and are discussed in turn below.

5.2.3.1 Clearance

Clearance is a measure of the body's ability to eliminate the drug substance from the plasma or blood by either metabolism or excretion. The main organs of clearance are the liver and the kidneys, although other organs can take part as well (e.g. gut, lung, peripheral tissues). Clearance is an important parameter because it is the property of a drug that determines the maintenance dosing rate needed to maintain a desired

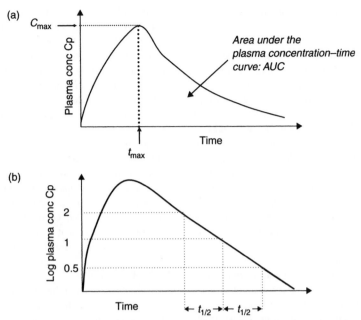

Figure 5.2 Descriptive pharmacokinetic parameters: (a) plasma concentration–time plot; (b) semi-logarithmic plot.

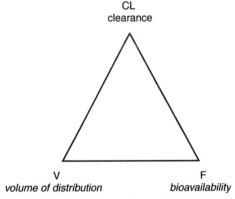

Figure 5.3 The triad of primary pharmacokinetic parameters.

BOX 5.2 Clearance – definitions and concepts

- Defined as 'rate of drug elimination divided by the plasma concentration'
- Equivalent to 'the volume of plasma completely cleared of drug per unit of time'
- Sum of metabolism and excretion
- Has units of flow (mL/min), which can be corrected for body weight (mL/min/kg)
- Total clearance is the sum of all organ clearances:
  $$CL_{total} = CL_{renal} + CL_{hepatic} + CL \ldots$$
  CL = dose/AUC for intravenous drug
  CL = bioavailable dose/AUC for all routes
  $$CL = F \times dose/AUC$$
- Note that there is *no* half-life term

plasma concentration. Clearance can be defined in several ways but the two most useful definitions are listed in Box 5.2.

When clearance is otherwise unspecified, the term 'clearance' is used to mean 'total clearance', which is the sum of the individual organ clearances (e.g. hepatic clearance, renal clearance). Measuring or estimating individual organ clearances can be used to predict changes in drug handling under different physiological circumstances (see below). Given that one of the definitions of clearance is 'the volume of plasma

completely cleared of drug in unit time', it can be readily seen that this is equal to the total plasma flow (or blood flow if the measurements have been carried out in blood) multiplied by the proportion of drug removed by the organ during the passage. This latter proportion defines the concept of 'extraction ratio' of an organ. If there is a high (>70%) extraction ratio across an organ, increasing the blood flow is likely to increase clearance. Conversely, when the extraction ratio is low (<30%), changes in blood flow are unlikely to change clearance because the eliminating capacity is not limited by the amount of drug being supplied.

5.2.3.1.1 Clearance units and range for values

As indicated in the definition, clearance has units of flow (e.g. mL/min or L/h); it can also be corrected for body weight, body surface area or age. For drugs that undergo negligible renal elimination and are very stable metabolically, clearance values can be <1 mL/min. The maximum values for organ clearance approach total organ plasma or blood flow. Hence, the maximum limit for hepatic clearance is approximately 1500 mL/min. Higher values for clearance would suggest that more than one organ is responsible for clearance or that the drug is metabolised in the plasma. For example, diamorphine has a systemic clearance of approximately 3000 mL/min because it is deacetylated in the plasma.

The kidney is a special case because, unlike with other organs, we can measure the amount of drug eliminated by that organ, in this case by measuring the amount of unchanged drug in urine. For all small molecules, the unbound drug in plasma is readily filtered at the glomerulus where the normal glomerular filtration rate (GFR) is approximately 120 mL/min. Hence, if the renal clearance of a drug is much higher than the GFR, we can conclude that active tubular secretion must exist as a renal excretion pathway. This is important because, unlike filtration, which is a passive process, competition for tubular secretion, and hence the potential for clinically relevant drug interactions, can occur. Conversely, if the renal clearance is substantially lower than the filtered free drug clearance, we can conclude that tubular reabsorption must be occurring. This raises the possibility of renal clearance being dependent on urinary flow rate or pH.

In addition to metabolism, the liver is also able to secrete unchanged drug into the bile, sometimes against a high concentration gradient. An example of a drug that is almost exclusively eliminated by biliary secretion is the antimalarial drug atovaquone.

Whether a drug is eliminated largely unchanged in urine or primarily metabolised is a function of its physicochemical properties and its suitability as a substrate for metabolising enzymes. As a broad generalisation, hydrophilic (water-loving) drugs will be excreted in unchanged form in the urine and lipophilic (fat-loving) drugs will be primarily metabolised. The metabolites may subsequently be excreted via the kidneys.

For most drugs, clearance is a constant and thus independent of dose. This would mean that, for

example, when you double the dose, the plasma concentration is doubled (Figure 5.4a) but clearance is the same. However, for some drugs, clearance may change with dose. This usually occurs when a drug is eliminated primarily by metabolism (and this is a saturable process) and the mass dose of the drug is high. For example, alcohol is a drug that is consumed in gram doses where the rate of metabolism is saturated after a small intake. A more clinically relevant example is phenytoin, where metabolism is saturated within the therapeutic dosage range (Figure 5.4b). Terms used to describe this include 'non-linear kinetics' and this results in disproportionately high increases in plasma concentration when the dose is increased. Under such circumstances, clearance is concentration-dependent and thus will have to be stated for each dose separately, as the value will differ.

5.2.3.2 Bioavailability

Bioavailability is the other important conceptual pharmacokinetic parameter, in addition to clearance. The key concepts are summarised in Box 5.3. Bioavailability is defined as 'the proportion of an administered dose that reaches the systemic circulation'. It has no units and is usually expressed as a percentage. Values range from 0 to 100%, and will be 100% or 'complete' for an intravenously administered drug. After oral administration, only a proportion of the drug may reach the systemic circulation because of incomplete absorption or because absorbed drug may be metabolised in the gut wall or liver (first-pass metabolism). For orally administered drugs, bioavailability will be the product of the fraction of the dose absorbed into the body and the fraction of the dose that escapes gut and hepatic first-pass metabolism. For example, if a drug is 50% absorbed but the subsequent passage through the liver (i.e. first-pass metabolism) removes 75% of the absorbed

---

BOX 5.3 Bioavailability – definition and concepts

- The proportion of an administered dose that reaches the *systemic circulation*
- No units – often as expressed as a percentage
- Ranges from 0 to 100%
- Is affected by absorption and first-pass metabolism
- The proportion of an absorbed dose that escapes metabolism before it reaches the systemic circulation (1 – hepatic extraction ratio); therefore high (hepatic) clearance drugs will have low bioavailability
- Usually calculated as AUC_{oral}/AUC_{iv} for the same dose

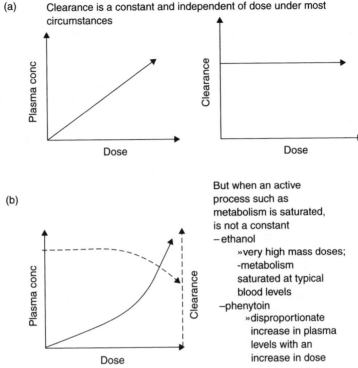

Figure 5.4 (a) Clearance is a constant; saturation of metabolism. (b) Factors affecting a dosage regimen. After Rowland and Tozer (1995),[1] with permission.

drug, the bioavailability is $0.5 \times (1 - 0.75) = 12.5\%$. Examples of drugs with low bioavailability because of high first-pass metabolism include propranolol, verapamil and morphine.

As with clearance, the physicochemical properties of a drug can determine its absorption and hence have an effect on bioavailability. Hydrophilic drugs may dissolve well in the gut lumen and hence cause few formulation problems, but cross cell membranes poorly and hence may be poorly absorbed, although there are some mechanisms of absorption of hydrophilic drugs between cells. In contrast, lipophilic drugs may dissolve poorly and hence cause formulation problems, but they may be well absorbed. These opposing constraints mean that very hydrophilic or very lipophilic drugs are often poorly bioavailable, and intermediate values are often sought by drug discovery to retain good bioavailability.

5.2.3.3 Volume of distribution

Volume of distribution is the third parameter to complete the triad of primary pharmacokinetic parameters. The key concepts are summarised in Box 5.4.

BOX 5.4 Volume of distribution – definition and concepts

- Defined as the amount of drug in the body divided by the plasma concentration
- Has units of volume (L) or can be corrected for body weight (L/kg)
- Minimum value is the plasma volume – large molecules that are confined to the plasma, and drugs that are highly protein bound
- Maximum value is much larger than body volume: means that drug must be concentrated in tissue(s) means that drug probably crosses membranes drug is often lipophilic
- Usually calculated as terminal elimination slope × clearance
- Least useful of the three primary pharmacokinetic parameters

---

Volume of distribution is defined as a proportionality constant relating the total amount of drug in the body to the plasma concentration. Overall, volume of distribution is a complicated concept and can be one of the most difficult to understand. It is also not a single parameter, as the volumes of distribution can vary depending on when it is calculated following the dose. For example, it can be readily understood that shortly after an intravenous bolus, the volume of distribution may be quite small because the drug is still largely in the plasma compartment. However, once steady state has been reached, the volume of distribution may be larger. In the terminal elimination phase, when tissues are loaded with drug and the plasma concentrations are being reduced by clearance, the volume can be even larger again.

It is rare for the volume of distribution to represent a real volume. It can occur – the smallest possible distribution volumes will occur for drugs that are largely physically confined to the plasma compartment (e.g. large highly protein-bound drugs), such as some intravenous contrast agents. However, there is no upper limit to volume of distribution and it can be very much larger than body volume. Under such circumstances one can conclude that the drug must be highly concentrated in at least one tissue. This may have important implications for therapeutic potential or for toxicity. For example, a lipophilic drug is likely to penetrate and be concentrated in the CNS, which may be desired or undesired.

The units of volume of distribution are those of volume (i.e. L) and can be adjusted for, for example, body weight. The two main uses of volume of distribution are in the calculation of loading doses for rapid onset of drug effect, and in understanding changes in half-life (see below).

5.2.3.4 Calculation of primary parameters

It is important to understand that the primary parameters clearance and volume of distribution can only be calculated following intravenous administration of drug. This is because it is necessary to know the amount of drug that has reached the systemic circulation for these calculations. This is not known for a non-intravenous dose, unless one makes an estimate of bioavailability (e.g. from urinary recovery of unchanged drug). Given the usefulness of knowing these primary parameters in being able to make physiological predictions about the drug, this is one reason why some regulatory authorities insist on having this information, which requires intravenous administration of the drug, even when there are no plans to administer the drug therapeutically intravenously. Calculation of bioavailability requires a comparison of the area under the plasma concentration–time curves following a non-intravenous and an intravenous dose, after correction for dose size. Without know-

---

> **BOX 5.5** Half-life – definition and concepts
>
> - Time taken for plasma concentration to fall by 50%
> - Determined by *both* volume of distribution *and* clearance
> - $t_{1/2} = 0.7\ V/CL$
> - Used in calculation of dosing regimens – the frequency of dosing is adjusted to keep the fluctuation of concentration between doses within acceptable limits
> - Steady state is reached after 4–5 half-lives
> - Time to reach 50% of steady state is one half-life ($t_{1/2}$)

ing the bioavailability, only 'apparent' clearance and volume of distribution can be calculated and the ability to make predictions from these values is very limited.

5.2.3.5 Half-life

Physicians may be surprised to see that mention of half-life has been dealt with so late in this chapter, as it is likely to be the pharmacokinetic term most familiar to them. The key concepts are summarised in Box 5.5. Half-life is not a primary pharmacokinetic parameter but is one of the descriptive terms. Although many physicians will readily accept that changes in clearance will alter half-life, what is not quite so obvious is that half-life is equally determined by volume of distribution and in fact there is an equation relating these three terms:

$$t_{1/2} = 0.7\ V/CL$$

Thus, if we are comparing half-life values between two groups of patients, or in an individual before and after a potentially interacting drug, we cannot automatically assume that a prolonging of the half-life is the result of a reduction in clearance. This may well be the case, but is also possible that there are differences in volume of distribution. Furthermore, if drug has a long half-life it cannot be assumed to have a low clearance. For example, digoxin has a half-life of over a day but this is the result of a large volume of distribution because the drug is concentrated in tissues. In fact, its clearance is relatively high, and this is why measures to increase clearance (such as haemodialysis) are ineffective in removing a significant amount of drug from the body in cases of overdose, unless additional measures are taken to reduce volume of distribution (e.g. digoxin antibodies).

The plasma elimination half-life can be determined from a semi-logarithmic plot of the plasma concentration–time plot (Figure 5.2b), following an intravenous dose, as the time taken for the plasma concentration to fall by 50%. The elimination half-life of some drugs is very short (seconds or minutes) whereas for others it may be very long (weeks).

The half-life determines the time it will take to achieve steady state and is useful for determining a dosing regimen. However, it does not give any clue to the processes involved in handling of the drug, so that knowledge of the half-life alone cannot be used to make predictions about factors that are likely to affect the rate of elimination.

5.2.4 Predictions from pharmacokinetic parameters

Earlier we stressed the utility of being able to make predictions from knowledge of the primary pharmacokinetic parameters, and some examples have been given. A further example is as follows. Imagine we have undertaken a first-in-human study where the drug has been given intravenously. Negligible amounts of unchanged drug were recovered in the urine, and the total plasma clearance was calculated to be 750 mL/min. Based on *in vitro* data it is likely that the drug is metabolised. It is reasonable to assume that the total plasma clearance is likely to be largely brought about by hepatic clearance and hence we have a hepatic extraction ratio of about 50% (750/1500 mL/min). Already we can assume that the drug will have oral bioavailability no higher than 50% (because first-pass metabolism is likely to be about

50%) and that changes in hepatic blood flow and/or metabolising capacity will affect steady-state plasma concentrations. This is without having yet given an oral dose of the drug.

5.2.5 Use of pharmacokinetic information to design dosage regimens

An understanding of the pharmacokinetic properties of a drug is one of the major sources of information used in designing a dosing regimen:

• The volume of distribution can be used to determine the size of the dose required to reach a desired target plasma concentration with the first dose: 'loading dose'.
• Clearance will determine the maintenance dosing rate to maintain an average plasma concentration.
• The half-life (i.e. both volume of distribution and clearance) will guide the choice of a dosing interval such that the fluctuations in plasma concentration are kept within acceptable limits.

However, there are other major factors in determining the dosing regimen, such as the nature of the concentration–response relationship for both efficacy and toxicity and commercial/compliance factors. There are additional reasons why caution should be applied in assuming an efficacy–time profile from a given plasma concentration–time profile. Some reasons why the time course of drug concentration and effect may differ are given in Table 5.1.

Table 5.1 Factors that may affect the relationship between drug concentration and effect

	Effect	Examples
Pharmacokinetic factors	Long time for tissue uptake	Plasma digoxin only correlates with effect >6 h after dose
	Drug trapped in tissues	Omeprazole, salmeterol: drug disappears from plasma but effect is long-lasting
	Active metabolite(s)	Terfenadine: delay in onset of effect because it is mediated by a metabolite
Pharmacodynamic factors	Pharmacological tolerance	Benzodiazepines
	Threshold effects	Anticonvulsants
	Steepness of concentration–effect curve	LAAM – opioid for management of dependence – short duration of effect with high steepness
	Effect takes time to develop through a chain of effects, 'cascade effect'	Time course of onset of action of antidepressants and warfarin
	Irreversible effect	Selegiline (irreversible MAO_B inhibitor): short plasma half-life but effects last a week
Dosing factors	Drug concentration may be supramaximal due to high dose	Frusemide and penicillin, the effect is at its maximum throughout the dosing interval

LAAM, ; MAO, monoamine oxidase;

Furthermore, it should not be assumed that a constant plasma concentration is desirable. For example, aminoglycoside antibiotics are safer and more effective for systemic Gram-negative infection in immunocompetent individuals when given once daily rather than three times daily for the same total daily dose, despite a plasma half-life of less than 2 h. Secondly, although traditionally pharmaceutical companies have tried to have the 'one dose for all' approach for dose selection, this may be increasingly hard to maintain with the increasing amount of genetic and related information on an individual's capacity to handle and respond to a drug.

5.3 Bioavailability and bioequivalence

Bioavailability and bioequivalence are related terms but they can be confused. Bioavailability as defined in section 5.2.3.2 is also known as absolute bioavailability and is simply the fraction of the administered dose that reaches the systemic circulation; it is therefore defined only in terms of the *extent* of drug absorption. However, in the Committee for Proprietary Medicinal Products (CPMP) guideline for the investigation of bioavailability and bioequivalence,[2] bioavailability is defined as the 'the rate and extent to which the active substance of therapeutic moiety is absorbed from a pharmaceutical form and becomes available at the site of action'. The reason that bioavailability has been defined in this way is because *rate*, as well as extent, is important when comparing bioavailability of two pharmaceutical forms of an active substance to determine whether they are bioequivalent. Bioequivalence and comparative bioavailability are discussed below but the absolute bioavailability is described first.

5.3.1 Bioavailability

It would seem that that when developing a drug that is intended purely for oral administration there would be no need to administer the drug intravenously. However, the primary pharmacokinetic parameters cannot be determined without giving the drug intravenously. As drug regulators find these parameters helpful, they like to see this information.

It can be assumed that the bioavailability of an intravenous dose is 100% and a calculation of oral bioavailability can therefore be obtained by comparison of the AUCs after oral and intravenous administration, after correction for the exact dose:

$$F = \frac{AUC_{oral}}{AUC_{iv}} \times \frac{Dose_{iv}}{Dose_{oral}}$$

The AUCs can be obtained by administration of intravenous and oral formulations in a crossover study. The size of the intravenous dose should be reduced compared with the oral dose in proportion to the expected bioavailability so that the AUCs will be similar. This avoids assumptions about linear kinetics and maximises safety, because high plasma concentrations by the intravenous route are avoided. Similarly, it is appropriate to infuse the intravenous drug over a period comparable with the time to maximum concentration (t_{max}) after oral administration in order to avoid transient high peaks.

There may not be any intention to develop an intravenous formulation for therapeutic use but it will usually be a necessary to produce one for the purposes of the study. For prodrugs (i.e. where the main pharmacological activity comes from a metabolite), the appropriate intravenous comparator is the active metabolite. However, there are some drugs that cannot be administered by the intravenous route, either because it would not be safe or because it is not technically feasible to develop a suitable formulation. If there is a very high recovery of unchanged drug in urine, it may be possible to obtain a reasonable estimate of absolute bioavailability from oral administration. However, metabolites in urine cannot be assumed to derive from drug that was bioavailable because they may have been formed in the gut by the action of intestinal bacteria, for example, and subsequently absorbed and excreted in urine. An alternative to intravenous administration is a reference oral solution; if this is not feasible, an oral suspension of standardised fine particles size may be the best option. Clearly, these do not enable calculation of absolute bioavailability but might indicate whether the test formulation has less than optimal bioavailability. For a drug that exhibits high intra-individual as well as interindividual variability of clearance, or which has time-dependent kinetics, it may be useful to give the intravenous and oral formulations simultaneously. Drug administered by one route will need to be labelled with either a radioactive or stable isotope so drugs administered by the two routes can be distinguished.

5.3.2 Bioequivalence

Two medicinal products containing the same active ingredients are therapeutically interchangeable if they produce the same clinical effect. However, assessment of clinical response would require a clinical trial for every new formulation, which is simply not feasible or justifiable. It is reasonable to assume that the effects of drug molecules, once they have reached the systemic circulation, should be independent of the formulation from which they came. Therefore, two products containing the same active ingredient can be regarded as bioequivalent if they produce the same plasma concentration–time profiles. This enables manufacturers to market a new formulation of a licensed products on the basis of bioequivalence rather than a full clinical package. Similarly, a generic formulation can be licensed with the only clinical study being a bioequivalence study. It should be recognised that pharmacokinetic bioequivalence may not be a perfect surrogate for therapeutic equivalence because adverse reactions may differ because of biological effects of excipients. Furthermore, equivalent plasma concentrations may not imply indistinguishable clinical effects in the case of topical agents acting locally on the skin, lung, eye or within the gut lumen.

In contrast to the measurement of absolute bioavailability, for which only the extent of absorption is important, establishment of bioequivalence requires demonstration that the rates of absorption are also indistinguishable. This can be clinically important; for example, a capsule formulation of phenytoin produced higher and earlier peak plasma concentrations, which were associated with a higher incidence of adverse reactions although the extent of absorption was similar to the standard formulation.[3] Fortunately, a comparison of plasma AUCs is universally accepted as a valid means of comparing the extent of absorption, although there is little agreement as to the best measure of the rate. Because peak concentration (C_{max}) is obviously of great importance for many drugs, it is generally taken as the second important kinetic parameter for tests of comparative bioavailability or bioequivalence. Nevertheless, as C_{max} occurs at the time after drug administration (t_{max}) when the rate of entry of drug into the plasma equals the rate of its removal, therefore t_{max} is determined by the rate of distribution and elimination as well as the rate of absorption. t_{max} is also dependent on discrete sample times, in contrast to a continuous variable such as concentration, and it therefore has less statistical power to reflect a real change in absorption rate.

Testing of bioequivalence is an area where drug regulatory authorities have produced extremely detailed and specific guidelines, not only on the design and conduct of the study, but also on statistical analysis, sample analysis and drug sample retention. One reason for this is that manufacturers of generic medicines can obtain registration of a generic version of a drug of proven clinical safety and efficacy on the basis of a single bioequivalence study, without the need to perform clinical trials of safety or efficacy. Commercial pressures are clearly great and there have been a number of examples of misconduct, and a scandal involving gross fraud. The result is that the guidelines are extremely strict, and for products of high therapeutic index and excellent safety records they seem excessive. However, there is little room for flexibility, and adherence to the guidelines is strongly recommended. Recently, the US Food and Drug Administration (FDA) has proposed a classification of drug bioavailability which stratifies the need for a human study, depending on the physicochemical characteristics of the compound and its bioavailability. This has reduced the need for bioequivalence studies of minor changes in formulation of well-absorbed drugs with the granting of a 'biowaiver'.[4] A reasonable approach to the problem is suggested as series of questions, provided in Table 5.2.

Protein drugs also represent a special case. Unlike small molecules, two protein drugs with the same chemical formula (i.e. amino acid sequence) might have subtle changes in folding or sites of glycosylation which might affect function. Hence, regulatory authorities do not in general accept pharmacokinetic bioequivalence to licence 'generic' biopharmaceuticals. For such products, the concept of 'essential similarity' is proposed, which includes some relevant measure of drug effect, in addition to pharmacokinetics as well as extensive product characterisation. For example, there may be a complex relation with excipients which are not thought to be therapeutically active. An excellent review of this subject has been published.[5] Hence, in this complex area, expert advice will be required when reformulating a protein drug and ideally the formulation should be optimized before the first human study so that all development continues with the one formulation.

It should be remembered that the role of regulatory authorities is to protect the public. For entirely justifiable reasons, they will apply very strict criteria to products with a low therapeutic index, non-linear kinetics or unfavourable physical properties. Digoxin, phenyotin and primidone provide notable examples of drugs where bioinequivalence issues have led to clinical problems.

Table 5.2 Factors to be considered when deciding whether a new formulation requires a study to establish bioequivalence

Factors to be considered	Suggests study is required
Difference from reference	Substantial
Bioavailability	Low
Therapeutic index	Low
Kinetics	Non-linear
Dispersal/dissolution properties	Poor
Relationship to another drug	Other drug has known poor bioavailability or bioequivalence problems
Likely attitude of a regulatory authority in a commercially important territory	Authority has shown little flexibility in the past
Importance of drug to your portfolio	Commercially important drug

5.4 Drug interactions

5.4.1 Selection of studies

It is reasonable that data should be required to demonstrate whether the response of patients to a new active substance is likely to change or be changed by concomitant medication. However, there is clearly a huge number of potential drug combinations and some rational selection is required. To assist with the selection of drug combinations for which data are required, at least the following seven questions should be asked.

1. *What are the ADME characteristics of the drug?*

For drugs that are metabolised, there are a number of enzyme inhibitors and inducers which may potentially affect the same pathway. Selection of a drug interactions study at the level of hepatic metabolism is becoming much more rational with the identification of a variety of isozymes of hepatic cytochrome P450 and the association of specific drug metabolising processors with each isozyme (see section 5.4.3). Similarly, a drug that is mainly excreted in the urine, with a renal clearance much greater than GFR, is likely to be actively secreted by the renal tubule. If the drug is an organic acid, probenecid is likely to reduce its elimination; if it is basic, its renal clearance may be reduced by cimetidine.

2. *Does the drug belong to a class of compounds known to interact with many other drugs?*

For example, drugs containing an imidazole ring (e.g. cimetidine and many antifungal agents) inhibit many reactions mediated by cytochrome P450. Therefore, a new compound of this chemical class is likely to

behave similarly, and evaluation of its potential interactions will be required.

3. *What is the therapeutic index of the drug?*

If the drug has a low therapeutic index, interactions are much more likely to have clinical consequences, so a variety of kinetic studies will be needed.

4. *Is the drug likely to be co-prescribed with a drug of narrow therapeutic index?*

For example, a drug for angina, cardiac failure or an anti-arrhythmic agent is likely to be co-prescribed with warfarin. If there is any evidence of enzyme induction or inhibition, a clinical study with warfarin may be required.

5. *What are the chances of the drug being co-prescribed with a wide range of medicines?*

A drug that is to be given to young adults in single doses (e.g. for migraine) is far less likely to cause many clinically significant interactions than one that is intended for long-term administration, particularly in an elderly population who often receive several concomitant medications.

6. *Pharmacodynamics*

Although this chapter concentrates on clinical pharmacokinetics, it would be wrong to omit mention of pharmacodynamic interactions in a section on drug interactions. It is difficult to generalise, but drugs with marked pharmacological effects, particularly on the cardiovascular system and CNS, are potentially subject to clinically important pharmacodynamic interactions.

7. *Does the drug share a common mechanism of absorption or disposition with another likely co-prescribed drug?*

Two drugs that are intended to be co-administered

might compete for active absorption or a common route of elimination.

5.4.2 Study design

There are several factors to take into account in the design of drug interaction studies.[6] Single-dose studies have been criticised but may be useful to exclude major effects. If an interaction is detected with single doses, it may be necessary to conduct a study at steady state, mimicking the dosage used in clinical practice to determine the true clinical consequences of interaction.

Whenever possible, interaction studies should not only be pharmacokinetic but should also include pharmacodynamic measurements in order to assess the likely clinical effect of an observed pharmacokinetic interaction. Furthermore, if possible the design should go some way to explaining the mechanism of interaction. For example, measurement of a metabolite in plasma or urine may help to distinguish changes in elimination from changes in absorption as the reason for the change in AUC of the parent drug.

There are certain special cases which can seem difficult. For example, chronic full dosing of warfarin to volunteers has safety concerns, and the concentrations following a single standard dose can be regarded as subtherapeutic. To address this, a design using a single large dose of warfarin has been shown to be reliable in detecting or excluding clinically significant interactions with warfarin.[7]

5.4.3 Enzyme induction and inhibition

Drugs that cause induction or inhibition of enzymes may affect the metabolism of concomitantly administered drugs, as well as of hormones and other endogenous substances. For this reason, such properties are considered undesirable and sometimes they might constitute sufficient reason to discontinue drug development. At the very least, studies will be required to assess the magnitude of effect of likely interactions. Metabolic and toxicity studies in animals will usually provide the basis for suspicion, and studies in human liver slices, cultured hepatocytes and microsomal preparations can be extremely valuable in establishing metabolic pathways and the likelihood of enzyme induction or inhibition in humans. There have been some important developments in this field in recent years and it is now possible to identify:
• Which cytochrome P450(s) is/are responsible for the metabolism of the test compound; and
• Which cytochrome P450(s) is/are inhibited by relevant multiples of the therapeutic concentrations of the test compound.

These data will help predict other drugs that may affect the handling of the test drug and alternatively, concomitant medication for which the handling, and hence clinical response, may be altered by administration of the test drug. There is an increasingly extensive library of known inhibitors, inducers and substrates for each isozyme. This information can be used to predict which groups of drugs are unlikely to interact with the test drug, which can be justification for not performing unnecessary studies. Unfortunately, extrapolation from the *in vitro* data is not perfect and hence *in vivo* data may be required with a likely concomitant medication of narrow therapeutic index.[8]

Once the *in vitro* screen has been performed, it is an increasingly common practice to use well-validated markers of each individual cytochrome P450 in order to make generalisations about the presence or lack of interactions of a certain group of compounds. Several reference probe compounds can even be given simultaneously using the 'cocktail' approach so that, for example, the presence of absence of an effect of the test compound on several cytochrome P450s can be studied conveniently in a single human study. This can be a powerful tool and can be very cost-effective.[9]

One potentially serious consequence of enzyme induction relates to the oral contraceptive pill (OCP), which may be rendered ineffective by induction of its metabolism. The effect of a period of drug administration on circulating concentrations of the appropriate oestrogen and progestogens over the course of menstrual cycles may be examined in women taking the OCP, with additional non-hormonal precautions taken to avoid unwanted pregnancy.

Another approach is to investigate whether the drug causes autoinduction – whether its own clearance is increased by a period of drug administration compared with that after a single dose. This has implications for starting and maintenance dosage of the drug, as well as potentially for other drugs.

Environmental factors that may affect drug handling include changes in the diet (barbecued meat causes enzyme induction; grapefruit juice and some other fruit juices can inhibit cytochrome P450 3A4); the herbal St John's wort causes significant enzyme induction; smoking (induction), and alcohol (acutely causes inhibition; chronically causes induction) and these must be avoided for a period before the study and until its completion. The duration of dosing with the test drug also needs some consideration. While enzyme inhibition may occur after a single dose, it may take 7–10 days for enzyme induction to be fully develop as the new protein synthesis occurs.

5.4.4 Protein binding

Although at one time, displacement from plasma protein binding sites was thought to be an important cause of clinically significant drug interactions, it is now recognised that it is only likely at most to produce a temporary increase in drug effect in most drugs. It is only for a very few drugs that alterations in protein binding may be clinically important, and only following intravenous administration. For clinically significant drug interactions that have been attributed to displacement of plasma protein binding, alternative mechanisms, such as inhibition of metabolism, have been found to be responsible (e.g. warfarin–phenylbutazone and tolbutamide–sulphonamide interactions). If the drug is highly protein bound, screening *in vitro* for protein binding displacement may help guide a search for suitable probe drugs to assess the clinical effect. However, displacement *in vitro* does not necessarily mean a clinically significant interaction *in vivo*. This subject and the implications for drug development have been reviewed elsewhere.[10]

5.5 The elderly

The elderly, who for the purposes of drug regulation are generally defined as over 64 years of age, are a disproportionately large group of consumers of medicines. In the industrialised world the proportion of the elderly in the population is increasing and will continue to do so for at least the next quarter of a century. Many drugs in development, such as those for ischaemic and degenerative diseases, are targeted almost exclusively at the elderly. It therefore becomes much more than a 'box-checking exercise' to evaluate both the dynamics and kinetics of new active substances in this population.

Age-related differences in pharmacokinetics between the elderly and young are primarily caused by:
• Diminished renal function;
• Altered proportions of body fat and water;
• Reduced cardiac output;
• Some degree of altered hepatic metabolism;
• Disease;
• General debility; or
• Concomitant medication.

For a drug that is to be developed for a disease that occurs mainly in the elderly, it is often advisable to evaluate tolerability and pharmacokinetics in healthy elderly volunteers before clinical trials in the patient population. Dosage may need to be reduced and par-

ticular care taken when the kidney is the major organ of elimination, which should be established in the healthy young before administration to the elderly. It should be remembered that the GFR in the healthy elderly with normal plasma creatinine and urea is generally much lower than that in the young. One reason why 'healthy elderly' studies have attracted heavy criticism is that the carefully selected, well-preserved subjects with normal ECGs, laboratory results and physical examinations do not really resemble the frail heterogeneous elderly population that they are meant to represent. This might result in a poor appreciation of the range of pharmacokinetic alterations in the elderly patient group.[11] It has been suggested in an FDA guideline[12] that the 'population approach' can be adopted to obtain information about pharmacokinetics in the elderly. Although this approach has a certain appeal, it also has serious drawbacks. This subject is discussed in section 5.10.

5.6 Renal impairment

As the kidney is one of the major organs of drug elimination, renal impairment is likely to affect the kinetics of many drugs. Although a wide range of processes (filtration, tubular secretion, and active and passive tubular reabsorption) underlie renal drug handling, the overall renal clearance of drugs generally declines in parallel with GFR or creatinine clearance ('the intact nephron hypothesis'). However, the extent to which this affects total clearance depends on the proportion of renal clearance to total clearance. Pharmacokinetic studies in patients with renal impairment might therefore seem to be redundant for drugs that are cleared predominantly by non-renal processes, but experience has shown that studies may still be needed. For example, if a highly metabolised compound has a renally cleared metabolite with pharmacological activity, metabolite accumulation will occur if standard doses are given. Clinically significant effects resulting from an accumulation of an active metabolite from a highly metabolised drug include:
• Seizures produced by the accumulation of norpethidine after administration of pethidine;
• Toxicity from thiocyanate accumulation following administration of nitroprusside;
• Rash and allergy from accumulation of oxipurinol following administration of allopurinol; and
• Narcosis from morphine 6-glucuronide after administration of morphine.

Even when the major metabolite is inactive, clinically important pharmacokinetic changes for metabolised drugs may occur in patients with renal failure. The non-steroidal anti-inflammatory drugs that derive from propionic acid (e.g. ibuprofen, naproxen, ketoprofen, indoprofen and benoxaprofen) are metabolised to ester glucuronides in the liver. These are inactive and are normally rapidly eliminated by the kidney. However, when renal function is impaired, elimination of the glucuronide is delayed and plasma esterases convert the metabolite back into the parent compound, producing accumulation of the parent drug ('the futile cycle'). In the light of these examples, it is reasonable that if the drug is to be prescribed to patients with renal impairment, an appropriate study should be performed even for drugs that are highly metabolised.

A single-dose study is usually conducted before patients with chronic renal failure are included in clinical trials. The dose employed can be similar to that used for studies in subjects with normal renal function because C_{max} is unlikely to be increased greatly. The study of pharmacokinetics and tolerability at steady state may then be necessary, for which a lower dosage should be used if clearance was shown to be reduced in the initial study. When it is expected that renal disease will have only a modest effect on drug handling, it may be sufficient to compare the pharmacokinetics in a group of patients with advanced renal disease with those in healthy controls. However, when the kidney is the main organ of elimination, it would usually be necessary to examine the changes in kinetics in several groups of patients graded with respect to renal function. The effect of dialysis in patients with end stage renal disease should also be investigated.

5.7 Liver disease

As with renal impairment, a study in patients with liver disease is required to avoid a contraindication in this patient population. Unlike renal disease, there is no single clinical variable that can be used to predict reliably the extent of change of hepatic drug clearance of a given compound. However, the most widely used is the Child–Pugh classification,[13] which is based on several clinical and laboratory variables and has been useful in producing dosing information. In general, drug handling is more likely to be affected in advanced decompensated cirrhosis than when the disease is well compensated. Reactions mediated by mixed function oxidases (phase 1) are thought to be affected earlier in the disease and to a greater extent than are large capacity conjugation (phase 2) reactions. Alcohol further complicates the metabolic picture because it has a significant enzyme-inducing effect when taken chronically but when present in high concentrations it may acutely inhibit oxidative capacity.

In addition to changes in clearance, drug distribution may be altered in liver disease by the resulting low plasma protein concentrations and ascites. Intrahepatic and extrahepatic cholestasis are also likely to affect biliary transport of more drugs and studies in patients with these conditions may need to be considered for some drugs. Bioavailability may be increased by portal–systemic shunting allowing absorbed drug to escape first-pass metabolism. Pharmacodynamic changes that are not related directly to alterations in pharmacokinetics also occur in liver disease (e.g. increased sensitivity to anticoagulants).

When designing a pharmacokinetic study in patients with liver disease, it is important to keep the target population for the disease indication in mind. Patients with severe liver disease are ill, and may not be likely to take medications for relatively minor illnesses. This is in contrast to patients with advanced renal failure, who may be otherwise relatively well. Given that the hepatic drug handling for a highly metabolised drug may be disturbed by advanced liver disease in a highly unpredictable manner (unlike in renal disease), it may be prudent to limit a study with the test drug to patients with relatively mild and compensated cirrhosis rather than decompensated cirrhosis, where marked changes and perhaps adverse clinical consequences could be expected. This restricted approach might be appropriate for a non-life-threatening indication (e.g. migraine) but for the treatment of Gram-negative sepsis it would be essential to study the kinetics and tolerability in advanced liver disease.

5.8 Disposition, rates and routes of elimination of radiolabelled drug

In the development of most new active substances, it is required to investigate the disposition of the compound and its metabolite(s) and their rates and routes of elimination. This is generally carried out with radiolabelled compound, usually [14]C. In the UK, approval of the Administration of Radioactive Substances Advisory Committee (ARSAC) is required for administration of radiolabelled compound to humans. The purpose of the submission is to demonstrate that the dose of absorbed radiation is minimised by administration of the lowest dose that is consistent with meeting the objectives of the study. In general, the estimated absorbed radiation dose should be less than 500 μSv, but higher amounts are permissible if they can be justified. The estimate is based on tissue distribution of radioactivity in animals and the pharmacokinetics in animals and humans.

In addition to ARSAC approval, the protocol must also be approved by ethics committees in the normal manner for studies in humans. The study should be conducted in between four and eight consenting subjects, in facilities where any spills of radiolabelled materials can be contained and monitored. Normally, subjects will be required to provide blood samples and to collect all excreta for a period determined by the known or estimated half-lives of the parent compound and metabolite. With cooperative subjects, recoveries of radioactivity should be close to 100%. Samples will be assayed for radioactivity and by standard chromatographic methods, and every attempt should be made to identify major metabolites which may be revealed by radiochromatographic profiling.

The study should provide unique information on the plasma–concentration profiles of parent drug and metabolite. The rates and extended excretion in urine, faeces and if appropriate, expired air can be defined.

Given the increasing public concern over radioactivity, it is becoming increasingly difficult to recruit adequate numbers of subjects to such studies. A new approach to undertaking these studies has recently become available. In conventional studies, drug-related material is detected by measuring the disintegration of ^{14}C. Accelerator mass spectrometry, in contrast, can count individual atoms of ^{14}C and this can enable measurements of ^{14}C concentrations even when the dose is reduced by a thousand-fold or more compared with conventional studies. Such low doses may not require ARSAC approval or specific measures for dispensing of study drugs.[14]

5.9 Pharmacokinetic–pharmacodynamic modelling

There is usually a relationship between drug concentration and the effect. Although the relationship might be simple, sometimes it is not obvious and may be complex. For example, as we are usually assaying plasma, time delay for drug to reach the active site might obscure the underlying relationship between effect and the concentration at the active site (which we usually cannot measure). Similar complications arise with the impact of active metabolites or the development of tolerance. However, data analytical tools, generally collectively referred to as 'pharmacokinetic–pharmacodynamic (PK-PD) modelling' can be used to extract the underlying relationship[15,16]. If such a relationship is found, this is potentially very powerful as it enables extrapolation of the effect (which is often hard to measure) from plasma concentration (which is usually easier to measure). Dosing recommendation for special patient groups (e.g. children, those with organ impairment) may be based on such models. PK-PD analysis has been used to support the licensing of a dose which was not one of the doses tested in pivotal studies but an intermediate dose. The FDA has also stated that a 'well-characterised' PK-PD relationship might be the supporting evidence of efficacy additional to one clinical trial proposed under the Modernisation Act.

5.10 Population analysis

The usual way to examine the effect of a clinical variable (e.g. age, disease, concomitant medication) on the pharmacokinetics of a drug is to perform a small controlled study in which the experimental and control groups are homogeneous and closely matched and differ only in the variable of interest. This classic scientific method is well accepted by the scientific and regulatory communities and enables examination of a variable in a small group of subjects before including patients with that variable in a large clinical trial. However, there are some deficiencies with this approach. Perhaps the most important is that the small sample may not be truly representative of the population intended (see section 5.5 on the elderly). A summary of some of the advantages and difficulties of the traditional approach is given in Table 5.3.

An alternative method for searching for factors affecting variability in pharmacokinetics is the 'population approach'. This refers to a technique in which estimates of individual pharmacokinetic parameters are made from subjects from a potentially large population in which the PK and/or PD characteristics and PK-PD relationship of a drug are investigated in a population of subjects, and the factors associated with between- and within-subject variability are sought. Such factors could include gender, age, race, smoking status, body weight, concomitant medications,

Table 5.3 Advantages and difficulties of detailed pharmacokinetic studies in small groups of subjects – the traditional approach

Advantages	Difficulties
Well accepted	Not usually useful for 'screening'
Provides rich and high quality data	Frequent sampling is very difficult in patients in large clinical trials or in children
Causation between factor and altered pharmacokinetics to be established (e.g. in interaction studies)	Relationship between altered pharmacokinetics and clinical response cannot be examined directly
Early results from specific studies enable expansion of patient population in phase III studies; not usually difficult to perform	Study sample usually does not represent the target population
Relatively straightforward and simple data analysis	Small sample may fail to elicit extremes of altered kinetics

genetics, abnormal liver function tests. It is also possible to examine whether altered pharmacokinetics are associated with altered efficacy or safety (i.e. making a population PK-PD model). Although this form of analysis can be performed within a single (usually large) trial, it is also particularly helpful to include the data from subjects in all trials, including small data-rich phase I and II studies with the large but less data-rich phase III studies. Such an analysis may be a powerful tool with which to justify an overall dosing regimen or a dosing recommendation for special patient groups, and is favoured by the FDA for this purpose.[17]

In order to appreciate the difference in approach, it is necessary to describe how pharmacokinetic analysis is traditionally performed. In a typical conventional pharmacokinetic study, a large number of samples is taken from a limited number of subjects and pharmacokinetic parameters are calculated for each individual, with estimation of errors associated with these calculations. Average values of each parameter can then be calculated for the group.

By contrast, in the population approach, the raw data set that is analysed consists of concentration–time points (and other necessary data such as demographic information) taken from a large number (up to hundreds to thousands) of patients. Only a few data points (perhaps 1–4) may have been obtained from patients in phase II and/or phase III trials. Even with these few samples, it is possible to estimate the individual pharmacokinetic characteristics of each subject and hence a measure of the mean parameters and their variability can be assessed. If an effect on pharmacokinetics is found, its consequence may be examined by looking for altered efficacy or safety which may not be possible in a traditional volunteer study.

This might lead to demonstration of a therapeutic concentration range.

When planning to incorporate a population PK or PK-PD analysis some extra resource is required (e.g. to collect, transport and assay large number of samples – may be thousands), in studies where, traditionally, pharmacokinetic sampling had not been carried out in the past (e.g. phase III trials). For a meaningful analysis to be performed, the patient needs to be asked when the last dose (and perhaps one or two preceding ones) were taken in relation to the sample and this is to be recorded in the Clinical Report Form (CRF). How much dosing information is needed is governed by the pharmacokinetic characteristics of the drug. From a technical point of view, large databases need powerful computers and user-friendly software to avoid very time-consuming data analysis and to allow for the inclusion of phase III data in the analysis. Even if these matters are resolved, the lack of people with the necessary expertise, both at pharmaceutical companies and regulatory agencies, may be limiting.

As with any technique there are some difficulties. The demonstration of a statistical association does not necessarily imply causation. If a clinical variable is associated with altered pharmacokinetics, it might be necessary to perform a specific study to confirm or refute this as it could be a chance finding. The approach may not be appropriate to safely explore clinical variables that are likely to have a major effect on pharmacokinetics. For example, for a renally cleared drug which is likely to require a reduced dose in patients with renal failure, it may be necessary, for safety reasons, to perform a careful traditional pharmacokinetic study to determine the appropriate dosing regimen before these patients can be included

Table 5.4 Advantages and cautions/difficulties of the population approach

Advantages	Cautions/difficulties
Allows gathering of data in target population	Not widely understood and appreciated methodology
Can be used for screening for the effect of a large number of variables to identify factors important for variability and thus dosing	Can demonstrate correlation but not causation
Provides a tool to predict (e.g. different dosing regimens) and the PK of an individual from clinical/demographic data	Logistically challenging with large number of plasma samples, exact sample times and dosing history required
Possible to establish relationship between concentration, clinical response and adverse reactions using a large patient population	If this is to be obtained from the last phase III trial, it may require late changes to the dossier or become rate-limiting in submission
Limited sampling per patient makes the technique particularly appealing for studies in vulnerable patient groups (e.g. the elderly and children)	Technically difficult; complex software; limited number experienced operators

PK, pharmacokinetics.

in the main phase III trials. The FDA has suggested that the population method is a suitable method with which to explore the changes in pharmacokinetics in the elderly, but because age is often associated with altered pharmacokinetics, it is often necessary, again for safety reasons, to explore this before including elderly patients in the main efficacy studies using a standard dose. However, the results of a population analysis may eliminate the need for several smaller studies by answering questions relating to, for example, impact of age, concomitant medication or gender on the drug's pharmacokinetics, or pharmacodynamics.

The decision to utilize a population approach should preferably be made early in the development of a drug to allow for the maximization of its benefits. Preferably, data should be pooled starting with the early studies in healthy volunteers and new data should be added to the database, data analysis carried out and the previous results challenged. By doing so, the knowledge of the drug will accumulate throughout its development, which will aid the developmental process by supporting the design of future studies and allowing timely scientific and strategic decision-making based on all available information. The results of a population pharmacokinetic analysis may not be available until several months after the end of the main phase III trials programme. This is likely to be around the time of the regulatory submission, and it is very late to find out about important clinical variables that affect handling of the drug. A way around this is to use only part of the patient population from the

phase III trial(s) and to carry out the data analysis while the clinical programme is still ongoing. In this case, careful consideration has to be placed on the issue of blinding and dispersion of results prior to finalisation of phase III trial.

The population approach has found widespread application throughout all phases of drug development, and is generally perceived as beneficial for the development and approval of drugs.[18–23] With the accumulation of experience in this field, increased understanding and appreciation by drug developers, and combined with feedback from regulators it may be expected that population analysis will be used increasingly in the future. At present the most appealing way forward appears to be a judicious mix of the traditional approach combined with population analysis in an interactive fashion, as data accumulate throughout the drug development process. A summary of some of the advantages and difficulties of the population approach is given in Table 5.4.

5.11 The rest of the typical clinical pharmacokinetics package

Box 5.6 lists the elements of a typical clinical pharmacokinetics package for a systemically acting drug. Not all will be required for every submission, but omissions do need to be justified. Topically administered drugs with local action, and sustained-release drugs, are special cases that require a specialised approach.

BOX 5.6 The clinical pharmacokinetics regulatory submission

1. Single-dose pharmacokinetics including relationship between dose and plasma concentration, absorption rate, total, metabolic and renal clearance, volume of distribution, elimination rate constant and half-life
2. Multiple-dose pharmacokinetics
3. Dose proportionately
4. Absolute bioavailability by a given route
5. Bioequivalence of any particular formulation compared with standard formulation used in clinical trials
6. Identification and pharmacokinetics of major metabolites, often using radiolabelled drug
7. Interactions with other drugs likely to be administered concomitantly, including enzyme induction and inhibition
8. Pharmacokinetics in specific populations to demonstrate the effect of age and disease on kinetics (e.g. young, elderly, patients with renal failure, liver disease, cardiac failure)
9. Effect of gender on pharmacokinetics
10. Effect of food on drug absorption
11. The relationship between pharmacokinetics and pharmacodynamic effects

BOX 5.7 The ideal drug in terms of pharmacokinetics

- Intermediate lipophilicity/good hydrophilicity → good absorption
- Small (molecular weight <300) → good absorption
- Low clearance → good bioavailability and long half-life if this is important in the clinical situation
- Cleared by both renal and hepatic mechanisms so reduced capacity of one pathway (e.g. as a result of disease or drugs) will not lead to dramatic accumulation
- Not an inducer or inhibitor of cytochrome P450 enzyme → low drug interaction liability

5.12 The ideal drug from the point of view of pharmacokinetics

There are many examples of drugs that are successful in the marketplace but which have less than optimal pharmacokinetics. However, when a compound that has desirable pharmacokinetic characteristics is selected for clinical development, this can lead to a smoother clinical development programme, fewer regulatory concerns, a more straightforward datasheet and, ultimately, better clinical utility. In today's competitive marketplace such characteristics may be key determinants of commercial success. A summary of some desirable pharmacokinetic characteristics, along with the reasons for those characteristics, is given in Box 5.7.

5.13 Role of pharmacokinetic properties in determining a dosage regimen

Determining the optimal dosing regimen for a new drug can be very difficult. However, considerable commercial superiority can be obtained by one drug over another by thoughtful selection of the dosing regimen, even if the two drugs have comparable pharmacokinetic and pharmacodynamic properties. Because pharmacokinetic properties of the drug determine the time course of plasma concentration, it is obvious that this information will have some role in determining a dosing regimen. However, there are many other important types of information that are also relevant in determining a dosing regimen, and excessive reliance on pharmacokinetic properties alone can result in a suboptimal dosing regimen. There is not space here for a full discussion of all of the factors that go into designing a dosing regimen, but a diagrammatic representation of the factors and their categories is presented in Figure 5.4(b).

5.14 Conclusions

To summarise, pharmacokinetics describes the absorption, distribution, metabolism and excretion of a drug by the body. Plasma concentration profiles, and in particular half-life, are important factors to consider in designing a dosage regimen. Calculation of primary pharmacokinetic parameters such as clearance and volume of distribution can provide insight into the physiological processes affecting plasma concentrations and enable some predictions to be made about the effects of age, disease and concomitant medication of these concentrations. The clinical pharmacokinetic regulatory package can therefore be assembled in a rational manner, providing sound support for the clinical trials regulatory submission. Increasingly, a global model of linking pharmacokinetics to pharmacodynamics is a source of competitive advantage, allowing more rational dose selection, especially for special patient groups, and assisting regulatory review.

References

1 Rowland M, Tozer TN. *Clinical Pharmacokinetics: Concepts and Applications, 3rd edn.* Philadelphia: Lea and Febiger, 1995.

2 CPMP. *Note for Guidance on the Investigation of Bioavailability and Bioequivalence.* London: CPMP, 2000.

3 Neovonen PJ. Bioavailability of phenytoin: clinical pharmacokinetic and therapeutic implications. *Clin Pharmacokinet* 1979;22:247–53.

4 Food and Drug Adminstration (FDA). *Guidance for Industry. Waiver of In Vivo Bioavailability and Bioequivalence Studies for Immediate-release Solid Dosage Forms Based on a Biopharmaceutics Classification System.* Rockville, MD: FDA, 2000.

5 Schellekens H. Bioequivalence and the immunogenicity of biopharmaceuticals. *Nat Rev Drug Discov* 2002:1:457–62.

6 FDA Guidance for Industry. *In Vivo Metabolism/ Drug Interaction Studies: Study Design, Data Analysis and Recommendations for Dosing and Labelling.* Rockville, MD: FDA, 1999.

7 Toon S, Hopkins KJ, Garstang FM, Rowland M. Comparative effects of ranitidine and cimetidine on the pharmacokinetics and pharmacodynamics of warfarin. *Eur J Clin Pharmacol* 1987;32:165–72.

8 Tucker GT, Houston BJ, Huang S-M. Optimising drug development: strategies to assess drug metabolism/transporter interaction potential: towards a consensus. *Clin Pharmacol Ther* 2001;70:103–14.

9 Frye RF, Matzke GR, Adedoyin A et al. Validation of the five-drug 'Pittsburg Cocktail' approach for assessment of selective regulation of drug-metabolising enzymes. *Eur J Clin Pharmacol* 1977;62:365–76.

10 Rolan PE. Plasma protein binding displacement interactions: why are they still regarded as clinically important? *Br J Clin Pharmacol* 1994;37:125–8.

11 Lacey JH, Mitchell-Heggs P, Montgomery D et al. Guidelines for medical experiments on non-patient human volunteers over the age of 65 years. *J Pharm Med* 1991;1:281–8.

12 Food and Drug Administration (FDA). *Guidance for Industry. Study of Drugs Likely to be Used in the Elderly.* Rockville, MD: FDA, 1989.

13 Food and Drug Administration (FDA). *Guidance for Industry. Pharmacokinetics in Patients with Impaired Hepatic Function: Study Design, Data Analysis and Impact on Dosing and Labelling.* Rockville, MD: FDA, 1999.

14 www.xceleron.co.uk.

15 Colburn WA. Combined pharmacokinetic/pharmacodynamic (PK/PD) modelling. *J Clin Pharmacol* 1988;28:769–71.

16 Sheiner LB, Stanski DR, Vozeh S et al. Simultaneous modelling of pharmacokinetics and pharmacodynamics: applications, to d-tubocurarine. *Clin Pharmacol Ther* 1979;25:358–71.

17 Food and Drug Administration (FDA). *Guidance for Industry. Population Pharmacokinetics.* Rockville, MD: FDA, 1999.

18 Steimer JL, Vozeh S, Racine-Poon A et al. The population approach: rationale, methods and applications in clinical pharmacology and drug development. In: Welling PE, Balant LP, eds. *Handbook of Experimental Pharmacology.* 1994;110,405–51.

19 Samara E, Granneman R. Role of population pharmacokinetics in drug development: a pharmaceutical perspective. *Clin Pharmacokinet* 1997;4:294–312.

20 Tett SE, Holford NHG, McLachlan AJ. Population pharmacokinetics and pharmacodynamics: an underutilized resource. *Drug Inf J* 1998;32:693–710.

21 Reigner B, William P, Patel I et al. An evaluation of the integration of pharmacokinetic and pharmacodynamics principles in clinical drug development: experience within Hoffman La Roche. *Clin Pharmacokinet* 33:142–52.

22 Minto C, Schnider T. Expanding clinical applications of population pharmacodynamic modeling. *Br J Clin Pharmacol* 1998;46:321–33.

23 Sheiner LB, Steimer J-L. Pharmacokinetic/pharmacodynamic modeling in drug development. *Annu Rev Pharmacol Toxicol* 2000;40:67–95.

6 Purpose and design of clinical trials

Steve Warrington

Hammersmith Medicines Research Ltd, London, UK

6.1 Introduction

6.1.1 History of the controlled clinical trial

We will probably never know for certain who carried out the first controlled clinical trial but, according to the written history of the western world, it was James Lind, a ship's surgeon in the British Navy. In 1753, he published his account of a trial of six potential remedies for scurvy.[1] He allocated two scorbutic sailors to each treatment: cider, sulphuric acid, vinegar, seawater, nutmeg paste with barley water, or citrus fruit (two oranges and one lemon), once daily. Even though the citrus fruit ran out after only 6 days, both recipients were nearly cured. Of the other treatments, only cider had any useful effect. The trial was open, had no placebo arm, used a mere 12 patients and cost almost nothing; yet it led eventually to profound and permanent changes in clinical practice and in the health of countless people.

About 50 years later came what might well be the first placebo-controlled double-blind clinical trial. In 1796, Dr Elisha Perkins, a Connecticut (US) physician, received the first medical patent to be issued under the Constitution of the United States, for a device known as Perkins Patent Tractors. The tractors comprised two 7.5-cm pointed metal rods made of steel and brass. Perkins claimed that they contained rare alloys and were efficacious in treating inflammation, rheumatism and pain in the head and the face, when passed over the affected part for about 20 min.[2] The international success of the devices was such that in 1799 a retired UK physician, John Haygarth, was moved to write: 'the Tractors have obtained such a high reputation at Bath, even amongst persons of

rank and understanding, as to require the particular attention of physicians. Let their merit be impartially investigated, in order to support their fame, if it be well-founded, or to correct the public opinion, if merely formed upon delusion . . . Prepare a pair of false, exactly to resemble the true Tractors. Let the secret be kept inviolable, not only from the patient but also from any other person. Let the efficacy of both be impartially tried.' Haygarth persuaded two physicians to undertake the trial, which was carried out on five rheumatic patients in hospitals in Bath and Bristol, UK. The result seemed clear-cut: the tractors did not work. However, even though the trial was placebo-controlled and blinded, it involved only five patients and it was not randomised – all five patients had the placebo tractors one day before they had the 'genuine' ones. Moreover, the result cannot have been statistically significant, as there were only five patients. Perhaps Perkins Patent Tractors deserve a retrial!

Medicines were not subjected to systematic trial until the 20th century, even though powerful and effective preparations had by then been in use for millennia. For example, opium came into use at least 5000 years ago; quinine treatment of malaria began in the 1600s; and the use of digitalis in heart disease was first described in 1785.

The design of the first large-scale randomised controlled clinical trials leaned heavily on agricultural experiments carried out by Fisher in the 1930s, in which randomisation had been used to reduce bias attributable to the observer or to confounding factors such as differences in soil, moisture, sun and wind. That work led others, including the distinguished statistician Sir Austin Bradford Hill, to adopt similar experimental designs in clinical trials.[3] The first large-scale randomised controlled clinical trial is generally reckoned to be the UK Medical Research Council's comparison of streptomycin + bed rest with bed rest

The Textbook of Pharmaceutical Medicine. Edited by John P. Griffin. © 2009, ISBN: 978-1-4051-8035-1.

alone, in the treatment of pulmonary tuberculosis.[4] That trial began recruiting patients in 1947, and the results were published in 1948. It remains a landmark in the development of clinical trial methodology, because of its inclusion of a 'best existing treatment' control group, its scrupulously careful organisation and its use of sealed randomisation envelopes.[5] Previous trials had used 'alternate-patient' or 'coin-tossing' methods of allocating treatments to patients, both of which were susceptible to investigator bias.

6.1.2 Phases of drug development in humans

Clinical drug development is conventionally divided into four phases. The results from each phase determine the design of the next.

1. *Phase I – is it bioavailable? Is it tolerated? Does it do anything that might be therapeutically useful?*

Clinical pharmacology in small numbers (tens) of healthy non-patient (or patient) volunteers to assess tolerability, safety, pharmacokinetics and pharmacodynamics – if a biomarker or surrogate endpoint is available.

2. *Phase II – does it seem to work?*

Phase IIa – clinical pharmacology in patients with the target disease (small numbers: 10–200) to assess pharmacodynamics, pharmacokinetics and dose–response (or concentration–response) relationships.

Phase IIb – larger trials in several hundred patients to formally assess the dose–response relationship and increase understanding of efficacy, safety and tolerability.

3. *Phase III – how well does it work?*

Formal randomised controlled therapeutic trials (in hundreds or thousands of patients) to test efficacy and safety of two or more dose levels, and to compare new drug with existing ones; usually an international programme.

4. *Phase IV – look how well it works*

Post-licensing studies in the target population, with wide entry criteria, to broaden experience in clinical practice; objectives are typically surveillance for safety, or further comparisons with other therapy. The results are more likely to be used for marketing purposes than in support of applications to regulatory authorities.

Trials may be further classified according to their purpose.[6] Table 6.1 shows such a system, which reflects the construction of a regulatory application. Note the inclusion of pharmaco-economic studies, which entail assessments of quality of life and health care cost; these are now almost essential for a successful application, and are valuable in negotiating pricing and reimbursement schemes.

Clinical trials are required for five purposes:

1. To move a drug through a development programme;
2. To gain marketing authorization;
3. To guide treatment of individual patients;
4. To investigate a specific property of the drug, such as incidence of an adverse event; and
5. To select one drug rather than another for addition to a therapeutic formulary and inform a health policy.

The randomised controlled trial (RCT) aims to demonstrate that an observed effect is not the result of chance. However, no-one should be convinced by the results of a single comparative clinical trial, even though it be scrupulously designed, conducted and analysed. In any case, regulatory authorities invariably require more than one RCT (see Chapters 17, 18 and 21–26).

6.1.3 Controlled trials versus observational studies

RCTs are an essential part of drug development, but they do not tell us everything we need to know about the use of a medicine. The RCT is an experiment in which the medical management of the patients almost always differs substantially from routine clinical practice. First, the randomisation process, not the doctor, determines which treatment the patient receives; secondly, the entry criteria lead to the exclusion of patients who might well be given the drug if it were licensed rather than experimental.

Once the drug is marketed, it is important to try to identify how patients respond to it in routine medical practice. To achieve that, it is essential to observe the clinical use of the drug without disturbing or influencing the behaviour of prescribers and patients. RCTs are useless for that purpose: the correct tool is the observational study, which in pharmaceutical medicine offers surveillance of a medicine's actual (rather than recommended) usage, its clinical efficacy and, in particular, its safety in normal use. The observational study is an important pharmaco-epidemiological tool, and may be prospective (prescription event monitoring and cohort studies) as well as retrospective (see Chapter 16).

6.1.4 Global trials

The enormous cost of research and development of a drug can be recovered only if a global market can be accessed, so there is a strong incentive to carry out global trials. Such multicentre trials can use a large pool of suitable investigators, sites and patients, so can accrue completed patients very quickly. That

Table 6.1 A classification of clinical trials by type and purpose. From ICH[6]

Phase	Type of trial	Purpose of trial	Examples
I	Human pharmacology	Assess tolerability	Dose tolerability trials
		Define PK and PD	Single and multiple dose PK and/or PD trials – some in special patient groups
		Explore drug metabolism and drug interactions	Drug–drug interaction trials
		Estimate activity	
II	Therapeutic exploratory	Explore use for the targeted indication	Earliest trials of short duration in narrowly defined, subject populations, using biomarkers or surrogate endpoints
		Estimate dosage for subsequent trials	Dose–response exploration trials
		Provide basis for confirmatory trial design, endpoints and methods	
III	Therapeutic confirmatory	Demonstrate/confirm efficacy	Large, controlled trials to establish efficacy
		Establish safety profile	Randomised parallel dose–response trials
		Provide an adequate basis for assessing the benefit: risk relationship to support licensing	Clinical safety trials
		Establish dose–response relationship	Trials of mortality/morbidity outcomes
			Large simple trials
			Comparative trials
IV	Therapeutic use	Refine understanding of benefit–risk relationship in general or special populations and/or environments	Comparative effectiveness trials
		Identify less common adverse reactions	Studies of mortality/morbidity outcomes
		Refine dosing recommendations	Trials of additional endpoints
			Large simple trials
			Pharmaco-economic studies

PD, pharmacodynamics; PK, pharmacokinetics.

means that a definitive result can be achieved rapidly, or that the size of the trial can be increased to yield enough statistical power to show small differences between treatments. Multinational trials that generate data acceptable in all major territories have been facilitated by the International Conference on Harmonisation (ICH) of Technical Requirements for the Registration of Pharmaceuticals for Human Use.[7]

Multicentre trials are not without drawbacks. They are very expensive, yet it is unlikely that all trial procedures will be carried out in the same way in all centres. Medical practice varies between countries.

Similarly, patients vary in their reporting of adverse events, and doctors vary in their recording of them. Multiple centres introduce another source of variation in the results, so a multicentre trial has lower statistical power than a single-centre trial of the same sample size.

6.2 Pharmacogenetics

The design of a clinical trial – particularly its size and entry criteria – should take account of the likely variability in response to a drug. That response depends not only upon factors such as the patient's age, sex, ethnicity, the severity of target disease, presence of other disease and other medication, but also upon the patient's genetic make-up.

Pharmacogenetics is the study of the genetic differences between individuals in clinical response to a particular drug. Pharmacogenomics is a broader term, and means the 'application of genomic technology in drug development and therapy'. Pharmacogenetics is not a new science, but it is only recently that genomic technology has permitted the identification of polymorphisms in genes linked to drug effects and then to phenotypic responses.[8,9] This has led to the concept of 'the right medicine for the right trial subject'.

Pharmacogenetics has been introduced into some phase I–III clinical trials, particularly those that focus on drug disposition, pharmacodynamics and adverse drug reactions.[10,11] Advances have been made in understanding the pharmacogenetics of drug metabolic enzymes (cytochrome P450), and a comprehensive listing of genetic polymorphisms of potential clinical relevance has been compiled. In future, trial designs may also need to take account of genetic polymorphisms other than in cytochrome P450 enzymes. For example, lack of a functional protein (enzyme or transporter) might affect drug response; subjects may not be able to activate a prodrug or to metabolise a drug efficiently.

However, the current evidence for the clinical importance of genetically determined variability is not impressive; it is important to read the original literature with a critical eye.[12] At present, pharmacogenetics alone can rarely account for intersubject variation in pharmacokinetics. That is disappointing, but perhaps not surprising. The pharmacokinetic consequences of variation in an enzyme that shows genetic polymorphism depend on, for example:
• Whether the enzyme mediates metabolism of the parent drug, primary metabolite or both;
• The overall contribution of the enzyme to clearance of the drug;
• The capacity of alternative pathways of metabolism and elimination; and
• The potency of active metabolites.

Even if significant pharmacokinetic differences do arise from the polymorphisms, they may have no important effects. Alterations in pharmacodynamics (and clinical efficacy) depend upon the operating region of the concentration–response relationship; the therapeutic index; whether kinetic variability is outweighed by variability in sensitivity or number of receptors; or in the turnover of the natural receptor ligand.

Pharmacogenetics has advanced our understanding of pharmacodynamics less than our understanding of pharmacokinetics. Variability in pharmacodynamics is inherently greater than in pharmacokinetics. Whether pharmacokinetic–pharmacodynamic variability translates into clinically relevant differences in drug response depends on other factors such as compliance, doctor and/or patient perception of efficacy and side effects. To date, there are few solid examples, shown in replicated well-controlled trials, of associations between genotype and pharmacodynamic responses to a drug.[13]

Classification of pharmacogenetics into types I and II has helped the understanding of the genetic contribution to variation in drug response:
• *Type I pharmacogenetics* relates to genotypic variants in pharmacological receptors and other processes that contribute to a disease or syndrome; hence, unrecognised or undiagnosed disease heterogeneity contributes to differences in drug response.
• *Type II pharmacogenetics* represents genotypic variation that is not related to the pathogenesis of the disease but nevertheless influences the response to a drug.

Both type I and II pharmacogenetics may contribute to a variable extent, and this may help to explain variable responses to a drug in multifactorial disease such as essential hypertension or asthma. In spite of the rather modest impact of pharmacogenetics to date, the influence of pharmacogenetics on trial design is likely to increase in future.

6.3 Trials in special groups

Special groups include children, the elderly, patients with renal or hepatic impairment and some ethnic groups. Women of child-bearing age may also be a special group in trials of drugs other than those – such as the oral contraceptive pill – that are specifically designed for them. Data generated from one ethnic group may not be accepted by the regulatory authority in a country of a different ethnic composition.

6.3.1 Paediatrics
The scientific basis of the development and clinical usage of drugs in children, with some notable exceptions, lags sadly behind that in adults. The reasons include lack of commercial incentive, practical and

ethical difficulties in trial conduct, and a historical perspective that children are 'small adults'. There are two important consequences. First, there is a lag phase before medicines used in adults become available for use in children (e.g. treatments for asthma). Secondly, many drugs prescribed for children are used either 'off label' or are licensed for another indication in children.

In Europe, the ICH E11 guideline,[14] based on the existing EU Committee for Proprietary Medicinal Products (CPMP) guideline,[15] has been adopted. In the USA, in 1997, the Food and Drug Adminstration (FDA) introduced 'stick and carrot' legislation, whereby market exclusivity for an extra 6 months is granted for the whole product range after the sponsor has completed an agreed clinical trial programme in a paediatric population. The FDA also has stipulated under the Pediatric Rule (1998)[2] that a development plan for a new or marketed product must include a paediatric programme, unless the FDA specifically waives or defers trials.

There is clearly a huge difference between a newborn infant and a teenager. For the purposes of development of paediatric medicines, it is usual to divide 'children' into five categories according to age and development:

1. Preterm newborn infants;
2. Term newborn infants (0–27 days);
3. Infants and toddlers (28 days to 23 months);
4. Children (2–11 years); and
5. Adolescents (12–16 or 12–18 years, depending on the region).

While trials may not be required in all age bands, and some bands might be too wide in certain diseases, this categorisation is a useful and practical framework to use in formulating a clinical development programme.

The guidelines on development of paediatric medicines advise that the need for a paediatric component must be considered on the basis of the seriousness of the indication and the lack of satisfactory alternative therapy. It recognises three main categories:
1. Medicines for diseases that mainly or exclusively affect children. A full development programme, with the possible exception of initial safety and tolerability, is required at an early stage.
2. Medicines for serious or life-threatening diseases occurring in both adults and children, where there are currently no, or limited, therapeutic options. The paediatric component should be started early after initial proof of safety and of concept has been generated in adults, and the paediatric trials should form part of the marketing application.

3. Medicines intended for other diseases. Trials in children are less urgent, and are started only when results of adult phase II/III trials are reassuring. However, companies should have a clear plan, and should give reasons for timing.

The types of trials to be carried out demand a flexible approach, and depend on the seriousness of the disease, on the availability of other treatments and on pharmacokinetics at different ages. For example, if the disease process and efficacy endpoints are similar in adults and children, then extrapolation from adult efficacy data, together with pharmacokinetic and safety trials in the appropriate paediatric age range, could form the basis of a successful application. Likewise, it may be possible to extrapolate efficacy from older to younger paediatric groups, such that only pharmacokinetic and safety trials are needed in younger children. However, when there is no known correspondence between efficacy and blood levels, the regulatory authority will expect clinical or pharmacological effect trials to be carried out in the relevant age groups. For novel indications, or where the disease course and therapeutic outcome are likely to be different in adults and children, clinical efficacy trials are needed.

Other important considerations in trials of children are:
1. An appropriate formulation that is palatable.
2. Volume of blood to be taken for pharmacokinetics.
3. The need for long-term follow-up in trials, post-marketing surveillance and safety assessment of marketed medicines to determine effects of the drug on physical function and development, such as bone maturation, growth and sexual development.

6.3.2 Ethnic factors in clinical trial development

The influence of ethnic factors on drug response in clinical trials is important in two contexts. First, the regulatory application should contain data generated from subjects whose ethnic mix is similar to that in the population where the medicine will be used. Secondly, an applicant may wish that data generated in one country with one ethnic predominance should be used to gain marketing approval in another country where the ethnicity of the population is different.

The ethnic factors that may affect drug response can be classified as intrinsic or extrinsic. Intrinsic factors are either genetically determined, such as polymorphisms of drug metabolism and genetic diseases that could influence response, or physiological and pathological, such as age, major organ dysfunction and diseases peculiar to a geographical region. Some intrinsic factors that affect kinetics and dynamics, such as height, weight, body surface area and receptor sensitivity, may be influenced by both mechanisms.

Extrinsic (environmental) factors include climate, culture (educational status, socioeconomic factors), medical practice (especially the use of other medicines) and differences in regulatory practice, endpoints and methodology (especially for subjective endpoints, such as rating scales).

Factors such as smoking, food habits and alcohol intake influence drug responses, probably by both intrinsic and extrinsic mechanisms.

The influence of ethnicity on efficacy has not been studied extensively. The notion of ethnic differences is supported by anecdote, but such differences probably contribute little to the variability in drug response, compared with differences within an unselected population drawn from a single ethnic group. However, it is prudent to ensure that at least the major ethnic groups in whom the drug is to be used are represented in a clinical development programme.

Some properties of a medicine that might make it sensitive to ethnic factors include non-linear pharmacokinetics; a steep dose–response curve for efficacy and/or safety, a narrow therapeutic dose range; significant metabolism through a single pathway that is subject to polymorphism; low bioavailability; and the likelihood of multiple (and varying) co-medication.

A regulatory authority may accept, for registration purpose, data predominantly generated in a 'foreign' ethnic group. However, bridging trials may be required in the locally dominant ethnic group to determine if differences exist.[7] The need for bridging trials depends on whether the medicine is 'ethnically sensitive' or 'insensitive' on the basis of the criteria discussed above. For example, if the drug is metabolised via a route that shows no genetic polymorphism, has a high therapeutic index, a shallow dose–response curve and there are universally agreed endpoints to determine efficacy and safety, then bridging trials may not be needed.

When the fate of a major development programme rests on 'foreign' data, it is wise to discuss their acceptability with the appropriate regulatory authorities at an early stage, and to be guided by ICH topic E5.[7]

6.3.3 The elderly

Most new drugs will be used in elderly patients, and many diseases (e.g. Alzheimer's) are strongly age-related. Clinical trials of the efficacy and safety of medicines in the elderly must take account of the following:

1. Will the drug be used mainly or entirely in the elderly?
2. How might age affect the pharmacokinetics and pharmacodynamics (tolerability and efficacy) of the drug?
3. To what extent can results be extrapolated from younger people?
4. To what extent are the effects of age separable from those of deterioration in specific organ function (especially kidney and liver)?
5. Can the important questions about development and clinical use of the drug in the elderly be answered by a 'population screen' approach, or will specific trials be needed in the elderly?

Definition of 'elderly' is arbitrary, and chronological age does not always correspond with actual physiological or pathological state. As the people of industrialised countries grow older, experience of the drug, either in pre-registration or surveillance studies, in the frail and very elderly will become increasingly important. ICH guidelines on trials in geriatric patients[16] adopt 65 years as the cut-off point, but recognise that older age ranges should also be studied. They point out that it is important 'not to unnecessarily exclude trial subjects with concomitant illnesses'. That is all very well, but including subjects with concomitant illnesses can create ethical difficulties; and phase II and III protocols often have restrictive entry criteria to maximise the chance of a positive result.

Trial endpoints must be given particular consideration in the elderly. For example, health questionnaires that include practical outcomes, such as the ability to walk further or rise unaided from a chair, may be more appropriate than measures of surrogate dynamic effects. Conversely, declining intellectual function and attention span may make questionnaires and rating scales inappropriate. Correlation between changes in rating scale and clinical outcome is problematic in the elderly. Also, the duration of phase III comparative efficacy trials needs careful consideration. Another issue is whether to conduct phase I safety and tolerability trials only in elderly subjects if the drug is specifically for use in that age group.

6.3.4 Patients with impaired hepatic or renal function

The proposed indications for the candidate drug, together with knowledge of its pharmacokinetics and metabolism in healthy volunteers, will show whether specific trials in patients with impaired hepatic or renal function will be needed for the Marketing Approval Application and New Drug Application.

Relevant guidelines are available on the FDA website,[17] but it is always advisable to discuss proposals with the relevant regulatory authorities. The topic is considered in more detail in Chapter 5.

6.4 Clinical trial design

6.4.1 Selection of response variables
6.4.1.1 Efficacy endpoints
Efficacy endpoints are chosen according to the objectives of the trial. They may be the therapeutic effect itself (e.g. eradication of infection, healing of peptic ulcer), a factor related to the therapeutic effect or some surrogate effect.

There is a substantial literature on surrogate endpoints.[18,19] The characteristics of an 'ideal' surrogate endpoint in phase I–IV trials depend on whether the emphasis is on the efficacy or the safety evaluation of the potential medicine. An ideal surrogate efficacy endpoint is:
• At an early stage in the biological process that leads to therapeutic benefit;
• Easy to record and measure;
• Reproducible on different occasions and with different investigators;
• Cheap;
• Of acceptable sensitivity and specificity;
• Non-invasive;
• Applicable across a wide range of patients; and
• Highly predictive of a therapeutic or clinical endpoint.
The last point (i.e. a high validity) can be confirmed only in phase III or IV trials, when enough subjects have achieved a therapeutic response that can be correlated with the change in surrogate marker. Thus, surrogate markers, in this context, are most valuable for selecting second-in-class or follow-up drugs, when validity has already been tested with the first compound. This is an important point that is often glossed over in debates with regulatory authorities as to whether a surrogate endpoint is an indication in its own right.

In the evaluation of pharmaceutical products, commonly used surrogate efficacy endpoints include:
1. Pharmacokinetics, when there is an *in vitro* measure of drug effect, such as minimum inhibitory concentration of an antimicrobial against a bacterial culture.
2. An *ex vivo* measure of drug action, such as inhibition of ADP-induced platelet aggregation by a fibrinogen receptor antagonist.

3. An *in vivo* marker of the pharmacological effect of the drug (e.g. hypoglycaemic HbA_1c response to an antidiabetic agent); change in concentration of a 'serum marker of disease' such as C-reactive protein with antirheumatoid agents.
4. The *in vivo* antagonism by the potential drug of an exogenous agonist [e.g. inhibition of 'weal and flare' response to intradermal serotonin by 5-hydroxytryptamine $(5-HT)_3$ antagonists; inhibition by a leukotriene LTD_4 antagonist of bronchoconstriction induced by inhaled LTD_4].
5. The investigational appearance of tissues or organs (e.g. endoscopy findings of a peptic ulcer); the radiological appearance of joint erosions.

Surrogate endpoint data can yield:
1. 'Proof' of physiological–pharmacological effect;
2. Determination of dose–response relationship before phase III trials;
3. Confidence, from phase I and IIa trials, that the drug is worth testing further;
4. Help in choosing among several compounds in the same biological or chemical class, for progression to phase II;
5. Comparative effect or safety data for two drugs with a similar mechanism of action; and
6. Enough data to register a drug for an indication.

Surrogate endpoints are a nearly constant feature of 'proof of principle' or 'proof of concept' trials. Sponsors try to use 'small scale', short-term trials as the basis for a go/no-go decision on the future of the development programme. The aim is to control the increasing cost of clinical development – most novel substances that enter phase I never reach the marketplace.

6.4.1.2 Safety endpoints
Adverse effects of drugs are broadly of two kinds: those related to the known pharmacological effects of the drug, and those that are unpredictable. Known pharmacological effects require specific tests to detect and quantify them, and the tests should be performed at time points appropriate to the pharmacodynamics and pharmacokinetics of the drug. Such tests may be especially important in vulnerable subject groups, such as the elderly or those with renal or hepatic disease, or during long-term trials when drug or metabolite accumulation might occur. It may be possible to measure surrogates markers of toxicity, such as prolonged QT interval for the life-threatening arrhythmia 'torsade de pointes'. The characteristics of safety surrogates are similar to those of efficacy surrogates as described in the previous section.

Unpredictable adverse events are detected in five main ways:

1. Haematological and biochemical screening tests. These tests generate a large volume of data that often includes adverse results that are not caused by the drug.

2. Measurement of vital signs (blood pressure, pulse rate, respiratory rate).

3. Serial 12-lead electrocardiograms (ECGs), mainly looking for QT prolongation.

4. Non-directed physical examination – which also ensures that the doctor is brought into close contact with the patient.

5. Non-directed questioning about adverse events, using an open question such as 'How has the medicine suited you?'

6.4.1.3 Subsidiary assessments

Highest priority must be given to the assessment and recording of primary endpoints, as they determine the outcome of the trial. Moreover, the power calculation for sample size is based on the most important primary endpoint.

Subsidiary assessments should be kept to the minimum compatible with the safety of the subject: the temptation to add secondary endpoints should be resisted, unless they usefully enhance the trial. The protocol must state clearly whether the secondary endpoints are to be statistically evaluated (in which case power statements will need to be given) or are simply descriptive.

In long-term trials, extra visits may be scheduled, at which critical trial data are not recorded but the subject is assessed for general well-being and tolerability of trial medication. Such visits help to maintain good relationships between the doctor and patient, and may encourage compliance with treatment.

6.4.2 Patient population in trials and in clinical practice

For some drugs, the target patient population is clear at the start of the clinical development programme: for example, a 'me-too' lipid-lowering drug, or a novel delivery system for insulin. That certainly is not the case for drugs that interfere with one or more steps in a complex biochemical or immunological process, such as anti-tumour necrosis factor agents. Furthermore, serendipity may come into play during the course of the trial programme, as was the case with the phosphodiesterase-4 inhibitors; sildenafil was originally designed for the treatment of heart failure, but was licensed and is now widely used for treatment of male erectile disorders.

The usual pattern in the development of a drug is to move from highly selected and well-defined subject groups to an ever broader and less selected population, up to and beyond the granting of a marketing authorisation.

6.4.2.1 Eligibility criteria

The population for a clinical trial is selected on the basis of inclusion and exclusion criteria, which together constitute the entry, or eligibility, criteria. Entry criteria are of two kinds: general and specific. General criteria include age, sex, race, weight, previous medical history, previous and concurrent medication and function of major organs such as liver, kidney and heart. Specific criteria are of two kinds: endpoint-related and trial population-related.

Endpoint-related criteria specify acceptable values of variables that are to be used as endpoints. For example, in a trial of an antihypertensive drug, the acceptable range of systolic and diastolic blood pressure would be stated, as would the position of the subject, the apparatus to be used and the required stability over a specified number of visits. Trial population-related criteria apply to trials of drugs in special groups, such as patients with renal or hepatic impairment.

6.4.3 Choice of trial design

Box 6.1 lists different aspects of trial design.

6.4.3.1 Pilot trials

A 'pilot' is a type of trial, not a design feature. A pilot trial is usually open (unblinded) and small in scale, but can follow any design (e.g. double-blind, parallel or crossover). Performing a pilot trial implies uncertainty about the safety (e.g. narrow therapeutic ratio) or efficacy of the medicine, or about testing it in a particular context or indication. Pilot trials usually examine feasibility, so that resources are not wasted

---

BOX 6.1 Aspects of clinical trial design. Groupings do not necessarily imply strict alternatives or mutual exclusion

- Pilot/pivotal
- Open/blind
- Controlled/uncontrolled
- Placebo/active comparator
- Parallel/crossover/matched pairs
- Dose–response/final dose/dose escalation
- Dose titration (response)
- Concentration–response

by using an endpoint that is not appropriate or sensitive.

Pilot trials do not imply 'quick and dirty' research, or a sloppy approach. They demand as much careful thought as do pivotal trials. They are usually carried out early in drug development, but can be useful at any stage. A pilot trial may be converted into a definitive trial; that possibility should be discussed with a statistician at the design stage.

6.4.3.2 Pivotal trials

The term 'pivotal trial' (as with a 'pilot trial') does not imply a particular design, but rather the use to which the results will be put. A pivotal trial should yield convincing evidence of efficacy, and should allow important decisions to be made about the medicine – such as the dosage schedule. Because of its importance, the trial will be subjected to comprehensive quality control and and quality assessment, and will attract close scrutiny by sponsors and regulators.

Pivotal trials typically form phase III, but can occur at any phase in a drug development programme. In regulatory terms, pivotal trials are those that the sponsor hopes will persuade the regulatory authority of the efficacy and safety of the drug.

6.4.3.3 'Blindness' to treatment

The term 'blind' refers to ignorance of the identity of the trial treatment. The aim of 'blinding' is to minimise bias in trial execution, and sometimes also in the interpretation of results. Blinding is achieved by disguising the identity of the trial medication. The simplest method is to use formulations that look identical, which is usually simple with tablets or capsules, but is more difficult for oral solutions that look and taste different.

Blinding can be achieved for non-identical treatments by the use of the 'double-dummy' technique, whereby each active agent has a matched placebo and trial subjects in each limb of the trial take two sets of tablets: one active and one placebo. The double-dummy technique can be used successfully to compare treatments given by different routes (e.g. oral and intravenous). Even such exotic dose forms as suppositories, eye drops, skin patches or inhalers can be tested in a double-blind fashion.

There are various levels of blinding:
• In an 'open' or 'open label' (a term used by US investigators) trial, all concerned with the trial are aware of the identity of the trial medicine.
• In a 'single-blind' trial, the subject is unaware of the identity of the trial medicine, but the investigator

knows what it is. Rarely, the subject is aware but the investigator in unaware.
• In a 'double-blind' trial, neither subject and investigator, nor anyone else at the trial site, is aware of the identity of the treatment.
• In a 'treble-blind', or 'totally blind' trial, no-one is aware of the treatment allocation – not even the pathologist, statistician, efficacy review committee, or even the experts who review objective endpoints.

The double-blind design is the most commonly used. It yields reliable data, but is not too complex. 'Treble-blindness' sounds impressive, but it increases complexity and cost, and usually incurs time penalties. The protocol author must use common sense: for example, when a drug and placebo are to be given intravenously, and product must be made up freshly for each administration, must the pharmacist be 'blind' to the identity of the material? In multicentre trials in which mortality or morbidity is the endpoint, it is usual to have a blinded 'efficacy endpoint' committee but an unblinded 'safety review' committee.

Open or open-label trials are always liable to be criticised. It is a golden rule of clinical research that, whenever possible, trials must be double-blind. But there are circumstances when an open design must be used (Box 6.2). The protocol must include rules governing the unblinding of the trial. Usually, unblinding is scheduled to be carried out just after the trial database is 'frozen' or 'locked'.

BOX 6.2 When an open clinical trial design may be used

1. Phase I pharmacokinetic trials
2. Phase I dose-ranging trials in patients, as opposed to volunteers (e.g. in severely or terminally ill subjects)
3. Uncontrolled non-comparative trials
4. Phase II or III long-term continuation trials, particularly those following on a short-term double-blind efficacy trial, in order to increase subject exposure
5. If a double-blind design would be unethical
6. Compassionate plea protocols – by definition, these must be open, and have the advantage to the subject of allowing early access to a potentially valuable medicine
7. Treatment Investigational New Dry (IND) (or non-US regulatory authority equivalent) – as in 6, the investigator takes the responsibility for the trial
8. Some large multicentre post-marketing surveillance trials comparing the newly marketed drug with standard therapy

Premature 'breaking of the blind' is a serious matter, as it can spoil part or the whole of the trial. A medically serious adverse event is the usual reason for premature unblinding. When that happens, it is rarely necessary to unblind the treatment allocation of subjects other than the affected one(s), which is why the treatment code must be held in individual sealed envelopes for each subject. The investigator has the inviolable right to unblind, but should always try to discuss the matter with the sponsor first.

6.4.3.4 Controlled trial

A controlled trial is one that includes a comparator treatment, and/or 'population', as a control. An uncontrolled trial does not include a comparator treatment or population group, so is often described as a non-comparative trial.

Control groups are included in a clinical trial so that the medicine under test can be compared with a contemporary reference treatment. If there is no control group, then the effect of the drug can be compared only with baseline or historical data which is so unreliable that the results have little or no credibility. However, it may well be helpful to include baseline values in the analysis of data from both the drug-treated and the comparator group. The types of control groups used in clinical trials include:

- Concurrent placebo;
- Concurrent active medication;
- No treatment; or
- Concurrent use of usual or standardised care.

The control group must be as similar as possible to the group receiving the medicine under investigation. Whenever possible, a prospective control group must be used, rather than historical data: historical controls are notoriously unreliable and hence of little value. The choice of control depends on:

1. Phase of the drug development programme;
2. Primary objective of the trial;
3. Likely response to placebo;
4. Ethical acceptability of using placebo in serious conditions, such as epilepsy;
5. Availability and appropriateness of an active comparator; and
6. Length of the trial.

The main purpose of a placebo control group is to allow discrimination of the effects of the test treatment from the natural progression of the disease, or from observer or subject bias, or other extraneous factors. For further discussion on control groups and placebo in clinical trials, see Temple and Ellenburg.[20]

6.4.3.5 Placebo

A placebo is an inert preparation (or a sham procedure) that is used in double-blind trials to prevent bias in the selection of trial subjects, and to minimise bias in the assessment of treatment effects. A placebo treatment helps to distinguish the pharmacodynamic effects of a drug from the psychological effects of the act of medication and the circumstances surrounding it, such as increased interest on the part of the doctor, more frequent hospital visits and emotional support. Placebo also helps to distinguish drug effects from spontaneous fluctuations in disease state. The value of the placebo-controlled trial in the early evaluation of a new potential medicine cannot be over-emphasised. It is particularly valuable under the following circumstances:

1. No standard medical treatment exists;
2. Standard medical treatment exists, but has never been shown to be effective;
3. The drug under trial has a novel mechanism of action and/or a new route of administration;
4. The standard treatment is inappropriate as comparator (e.g. different route of administration);
5. The response can only be measured only subjectively; or
6. A large placebo response is known to occur in the condition to be treated.

However, a placebo treatment is not always appropriate or possible:

1. It is unethical to withdraw an effective treatment in serious conditions such as epilepsy and tuberculosis.
2. No suitable placebo is available.
3. It may be too cumbersome to use placebo if the trial aims to compare, for example, an intravenous with an oral formulation.
4. Previous trials have convincingly defined the placebo response rate, and the trial is designed to test dose–response relationships.
5. The trial compares the new treatment against a positive control.
6. A very long treatment period is essential, there has been a good response to a previous treatment or the identity of the active treatment is obvious because of its adverse effects.

Although some of those arguments against the use of a placebo involve questions of ethics, a placebo-controlled trial is always preferable to the continued use of treatments of unproven value. Some old remedies that are widely used have never been subjected to a placebo-controlled trial, and the development of a new medicine may create a unique opportunity to include them in a comparison with placebo.

Some disease states or trial conditions are associated with a large placebo response, so a placebo treatment is essential in a comparative trial. Such factors include long treatment periods; previous treatments and response to them; characteristics of the trial subjects (e.g. social class, educational level and personality type); influence of medical staff, environment and supervision during the trial; appearance and taste of trial drugs; and presence (or absence) of unwanted pharmacological effects. Some conditions may permit only a short period of placebo treatment (e.g. 2–6 weeks in chronic heart failure) but thereafter an active comparator must be introduced, whether routinely or 'as needed'.

6.4.3.6 Comparator medicines

Active comparators are included as a 'benchmark' or 'gold standard' against which the new drug is to be compared. The choice of comparator depends on the following:

1. Does the trial aim to test pharmacological or therapeutic effect?
2. Is it possible to 'blind' the trial?
3. Is the active comparator the standard treatment that many eligible patients will already be taking, and will it be feasible to then randomise them to a standardised dose?
4. Will one active comparator serve for all countries in which the drug will be marketed?

In practice, in phase II or III, the positive control or comparator is usually the medicine that is most widely prescribed, in a dose that seems optimal, on the basis of clinical experience. In some disease states, the standard treatment may comprise several drugs with different mechanisms of action. For example, for patients who have survived an acute myocardial infarction, the treatment regimen may include aspirin, an angiotensin-converting enzyme inhibitor, a lipid-lowering drug and a fibrinogen receptor antagonist. The potential new medicine will thus need to be tested in combination with those drugs rather than as a single agent. The comparator would then be the standard combination. It is usually both feasible and ethical to compare the new medicine with placebo, each combined with the standard regimen of drugs.

Trials comparing a new medicine with existing treatments have three possible aims: to show superiority, equivalence or non-inferiority of the new medicine. Statistical and regulatory guidelines are available for each type of trial.[21–26]

6.4.3.6.1 Superiority trials Superiority trials provide convincing evidence of efficacy – but a placebo-controlled trial is even better, because it could be argued that an active comparator might actually worsen the condition under study. Superiority trials are chosen when it is ethically unjustifiable to use a placebo. The trial design must have the same key features (e.g. the 95% confidence interval of the observed treatment difference should be entirely to the right of the point of equivalence; Figure 6.1). That is hard to achieve, unless the new medicine is truly much superior to the existing: a huge sample size is needed to show reliably a small difference. For that reason, superiority trials carry a high risk of failure, and so are not popular, in spite of the marketing advantage that might accrue from a successful outcome.

6.4.3.6.2 Equivalence There are two main categories of equivalence trial: bioequivalence and clinical equivalence. Bioequivalence is easy to test: certain pharmacokinetic variables (C_{max}, AUC) of a new formulation must fall within specific (and regulated) margins of the standard formulation (see Chapter 5). Clinical equivalence is much harder to show, but is of

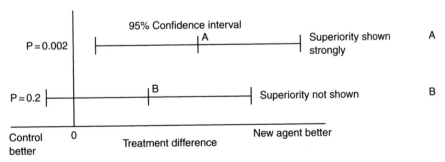

Figure 6.1 Relationship between significance tests and confidence intervals for the comparison between a new treatment and control. The treatment differences A and B are in favour of the new treatment, but superiority is shown only in A. In B, the outcome might meet criteria for equivalence, or non-inferiority, as defined in the protocol.

interest when the standard therapy is of some benefit but the newer treatment is easier to use, has fewer side effects or is cheaper. The trial protocol must clearly state that its objective is to demonstrate clinical equivalence, and the equivalence margins must be defined and justified. A positive outcome is achieved only if the entire confidence interval of the main trial endpoint lies within the limits defined in the protocol.

6.4.3.6.3 Non-inferiority trials
These are much more common than clinical equivalence trials in phase III of drug development. In a non-inferiority trial, the objective is to show that a new treatment is not less effective than an existing treatment whose efficacy has been proven. It might be more effective or equivalent but, using the confidence interval approach, the only interest is in a possible difference in one direction. Design of such trials must include the key features described for superiority trials, and definition of purpose and clinical equivalence as for clinical equivalence trials. A positive outcome depends on demonstrating that the lower margin of the confidence interval of the main study endpoint lies above the lower limit of clinical equivalence, as defined in the protocol.

6.4.3.7 Parallel or crossover design
Most clinical trials in phase III of drug development use two groups of trial subjects. In a parallel design, patients are randomly allocated to one of the two treatments, and never receive the other. In a crossover design, each patient receives both treatments, allocated in randomised order, 'crossing over' at a halfway point.

In a parallel design, the response of one group of subjects is compared with that of the other. The crossover design allows comparison of the effects of the treatments in the entire trial population. So, in a parallel design, the comparisons are between subjects; in a crossover design, the comparisons are within subjects.

The advantages and disadvantages of crossover and parallel-group designs are summarised in Table 6.2. In practice, crossover designs are often preferred in the early phases of drug development, particularly for the first dose-ranging trials – but only in very stable disease states. Parallel designs are almost always needed for the definitive dose-ranging trials and for therapeutic efficacy trials.

The critical weakness of crossover designs is their susceptibility to carry-over effects (i.e. the effect of the first treatment has not worn off before the start of the second treatment). Statistical analysis can detect carry-over effects, but it is then too late to modify the trial design. Crossover designs are susceptible also to period effects (i.e. the order in which the treatments are given affects the response to each treatment). Randomisation – a random but balanced allocation of subjects to treatment sequences – ensures that all treatment sequences are equally represented, but period effects may still reduce the power of the trial.

6.4.3.8 Single-centre trials
Single-centre trials are usual in the early stages of the drug development. Most phase I trials are single-centre, and are carried out in healthy volunteers in a specialist clinical pharmacology unit. Such units have the

Table 6.2 Comparison of crossover and parallel designs in clinical trials

	Parallel	Crossover
Robust to trial violations (e.g. missed visits, missing data)	Yes	No
Variability of data	High, because treatment effects are compared *between* subjects	Low, because treatment effects are compared *within* subject
Subject numbers	Large	Small
Disease state	Stability desirable	Stability essential: baseline at each crossover point must be similar
Carry-over effect	No	Yes
Period effect	No	Yes
Treatment effects must develop within treatment period	Not essential	Yes

expertise and equipment to do the intensive monitoring required.[27] Early phase II trials may be small enough to be performed in a single centre, but most require several centres simply because it would take a single centre too long to recruit and study enough patients.

Using a single centre minimises the variability in the patient population that may arise from differences in social, ethnic or environmental factors. Using a single centre also minimises (or may even eliminate) interobserver variation: such variation can influence patient selection as well as the assessment of outcome measures. Because variability in outcome measures is minimised, a single-centre study almost always has higher statistical power than a multicentre one of the same size.

Although the results from a single centre may not be so reliably generalised to a much wider population, that does not usually matter in the early stages of development of the drug. The later studies, in phase II and III, remedy that deficiency by including patients drawn from a much wider population.

6.4.3.9 Multicentre trials

Most trials in phase II, and almost all trials in phase III, are carried out in multiple centres, because a single centres cannot recruit patients fast enough: phase III studies typically require hundreds of patients in order to achieve enough statistical power to detect a difference between active treatment and placebo. Even larger numbers are needed to show superiority over an existing effective treatment, or to show non-inferiority of the new medicine (see Chapter 8 for discussion of statistical power).

Although multicentre trials are usually essential to the generation of evidence of efficacy within a reasonable time, they carry substantial penalties in terms of both cost and quality, as follows:

1. Different centres may interpret the protocol – and other instructions – differently.
2. Patient populations vary among centres, especially ones in different countries.
3. Diagnostic and treatment practices (both for target disease and for incidental illnesses) vary among centres.
4. Measuring procedures and equipment vary among centres.
5. Clinical laboratory results vary (sometimes sharply) among centres. Using a central laboratory avoids that problem, but creates risks and logistical difficulties in the shipment of samples.
6. High administrative and financial overheads for coordination, set-up and monitoring, and for shipment of samples and Clinical Report Form.

7. Adverse event recording is near-impossible to standardise among centres: recording rates vary, and attribution of causality is certain to vary among investigators.

This is a daunting list. However, multicentre trials cannot be avoided, so the sponsor must do everything possible to mitigate their disadvantages. The protocol must be detailed and specific enough to minimise intercentre variation in patient selection, methods of measurement and recording of adverse events. It is usual to specify a central laboratory, and to centralise the processes of coding of adverse events, data management and statistical analysis. Procedures for setting up and monitoring the study must be immaculate.

In spite of the important drawbacks of multicentre trials, the pharmaceutical industry now has long experience of the design, management and reporting of multicentre studies to a high standard – high enough to allow their successful use in applications to market new medicines.

6.4.3.10 Dose selection

In clinical practice, the optimal dose is the smallest that yields the desired therapeutic response. However, the optimal dose differs among patients because of variation in body size, drug metabolism and excretion, race, age, state of disease and so forth. In drug development, it is not possible to investigate more than a few dose levels – often only one or two – for the registration of a given indication. It is only after extensive clinical experience, and further clinical trials, that the optimal dose is defined. The optimal dose often proves to be lower than that studied in phase III, as was the case with atenolol and captopril, for example.

6.4.3.10.1 Dose–response relationships, potency and efficacy An understanding of the dose–response relationship is enormously helpful in both drug development and therapeutic practice. The relationship between the concentration of a drug at its site of action and the intensity of the pharmacological effect is best shown by a concentration–response curve (Figure 6.2), in which (by convention) the intensity of the response is plotted against the logarithm of the concentration. It is possible to construct such concentration–response curves using *in vitro* experiments but, in the intact human, the serum or plasma concentration is used as an indicator of drug concentration at the receptor. If circulating concentrations are not available, then the dose of the drug is used instead. The typical dose–response curve is sigmoid (S-shaped) as in Figure 6.2. The 'plateau' at the top of

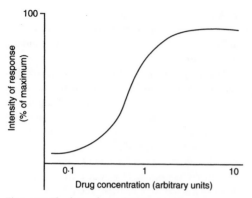

Figure 6.2 The shape of most dose–response (or concentration–response) curves is sigmoid – the increase in response eventually flattens off despite increasing concentrations.

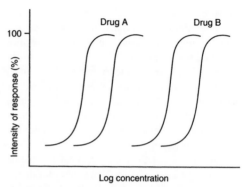

Figure 6.3 Dose–response curves for two drugs, A and B; B is less potent than A. The curves under A and B represent theorised positions of efficacy and toxicity relations. The distance between the individual pairs represents the therapeutic index.

the curve has two possible explanations. First, there is a limit to the response of all biological systems (e.g. heart rate, blood pressure, urine flow, neuronal firing rate, enzyme activity or neurotransmitter release) cannot be increased beyond a certain point. Secondly, a drug may be incapable of maximal activation of its receptor, even when it occupies 100% of the receptors; such a drug is termed a partial agonist.

The position of the curve describes the potency of the drug. Potency is the overall relationship between a quantity of drug and its effect.[28,29] In Figure 6.3, a low dose of drug A has an effect similar to a high concentration of drug B so A is more potent than B. The higher potency of A is obvious at a glance because its dose–response curve is well to the left of the curve for B. However, A is not more powerful (or efficacious) than B, because B is capable of producing the same clinical effect as does A, if it is given in high enough doses.

If one drug is less powerful than another, this is shown by the dose–response curve reaching a plateau at a lower level than that of the more powerful drug. For example, thiazide diuretics are less powerful than 'loop' diuretics: the dose–response curve for a thiazide diuretic plateaus at a lower effect level than that for 'loop' diuretics, and increasing the dose produces no additional diuretic effect.

The term 'potency' is often used wrongly – it is often confused with power or efficacy. The actual weight of a drug that has to be administered has no clinical significance, unless it is high: a large weight of drug is more likely to interact with other drugs, by competing for enzymatic metabolism or protein binding, for example.

Antagonists

An antagonist shifts the respective agonist's dose–response curve to the right – a higher dose of agonist is needed to yield the same effect.

A *competitive antagonist* competes for the same receptor as the agonist, and causes a parallel shift of the dose–response curve: the slope and plateau level remain unchanged, but the whole curve is moved to the right.

A *non-competitive antagonist* acts at a site different from the agonist, and the effect on the dose–response curve is unpredictable. It will certainly shift to the right, but the slope and plateau level are both likely to change. So, the potential maximum response to agonist may be reduced, whereas the effect of a competitive agonist can be fully reversed by increasing the dose of agonist.

A *partial agonist* occupies receptors without fully activating them, so behaves like an antagonist in that it shifts the dose–response curve to the right. However, because it partially activates the receptors, the starting point of the dose–response curve will be higher before any agonist is given. Translated into clinical practice, this means that partial agonists increase receptor activity when stimulation by the natural agonist is at a low level, but decrease it when activation by natural agonist is at a high level. For example, pindolol is a partial agonist at β-adrenoceptors: it slightly increases heart rate at rest, but reduces it during exercise.

Efficacy

Efficacy has both pharmacological and therapeutic definitions. Pharmacological efficacy refers to the strength of response induced by an agonist occupying

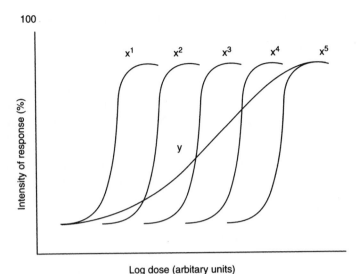

Figure 6.4 X^1–X^5 are individual dose–response curves; Y is the average dose–response curve for the population. Note that X curves cannot be predicted from Y.

a receptor. It describes how agonists vary in the response they produce, even when they occupy the same number of receptors.

Therapeutic efficacy, or effectiveness, is the ability of a drug to produce a useful effect, and refers to the drug's maximum effect. Thus, if drug A produces a greater therapeutic effect than drug B, regardless of how much of drug B is given, then drug A has the higher therapeutic efficacy.

Therapeutic index

A drug may have several dose–response curves: one for the main therapeutic effect, and one for each type of toxicity. The shape and position of the dose–toxicity curve, in relation to the dose–response curve for the desired effect, shows the relative toxicity or therapeutic index of the drug. The interval between the curves is the ratio between is the maximum tolerated dose and the minimum effective dose.

In humans, it is never possible to define the efficacy and toxicity curves well enough to calculate an accurate numerical therapeutic index. Nevertheless, Figure 6.3 illustrates the concept, which usefully illustrates the relativity between safety and efficacy. Drugs with steep dose–response curves for efficacy are difficult to develop and to use in patients, because small changes in dose can have dramatic clinical effects. A steep dose–toxicity curve is also a problem, unless the curve is far to the right of the dose–response curve (i.e. the therapeutic index is high).

The shape and position of the dose–response curve of any drug will vary among patients, as a result of factors that may include age, sex, disease states and pharmacogenetics. Figure 6.4 shows hypothetical dose–response curves for five individual patients. Curve 'y' shows the hypothetical dose–response relationship for the complete population of patients. Notice that its slope differs from that of the individual patients, because of the contribution that each patient makes to it. It is curve 'y' (not the individual patient's curve) that determines what is the correct dose for both clinical trials and therapeutic use.

6.4.3.10.2 Dose titration and concentration–response designs In a dose titration trial, the subjects are studied while taking a predetermined dose, which is increased incrementally until the desired therapeutic effect is achieved. Interpretation of such trials is complicated by the difficulty in distinguishing between the effect of the dose increase and the increased duration of exposure – continued treatment at a lower dose might have achieved the same effect.

Dose titration trials of antihypertensives have been criticised by the FDA, because such trials tend to lead to higher doses being recommended for clinical use. However, Sheiner et al.[30,31] have revived interest in dose titration, by proposing methods of taking account of the potential for period effects and period–dose interactions. They suggested the inclusion of a randomly assigned placebo arm for the duration of the trial, with the subsequent analysis using parametric subject-specific dose–response models. Using such complex dose–response models, they showed (in a simulation) that dose titration designs could perform better overall than a fixed-dose parallel-group design, and only slightly worse than a crossover design.

In a concentration–response design, subjects receive either a fixed dose (or dose range) of a medicine and their plasma concentrations are determined, usually at steady state. Alternatively, various doses of a medicine are titrated until a predefined plasma concentration is achieved. In both designs, plasma concentrations are plotted against clinical response, in order to determine if a relationship exists. These designs are suitable for only a few types of drug, such as short-acting intravenous anaesthetic agents. Their wider use is limited by the difficulty in extrapolating from plasma concentrations to effective oral dose.

Whatever their merits, none of these designs has found a regular place in the drug development process.

6.4.3.10.3 Dose: size and schedule   Dose selection for exploratory trials is discussed in Chapter 4.

Choosing the dose for phase II studies

Phase I studies usually define well the pharmacokinetics of the new medicine. However, if there is not a good biomarker of the medicine's potential therapeutic efficacy, the correct doses to study in phase II will remain a matter of informed guesswork. Most commonly, the doses chosen for phase II are ones that the phase I pharmacokinetic data suggest will yield plasma concentrations in a range that was efficacious in animal models of the target disease. Of course, allowance has to be made for interspecies differences (e.g. in protein binding).

Frequency of dosing may be decided on the basis of pharmacokinetic data, but it is often possible to give medicines less often than the pharmacokinetic parameters suggest. This is partly because pharmacological effects are generally proportional to log concentration of drug, not to the concentration itself: so, halving the concentration does not halve the effect of the drug. Other mechanisms for the unexpectedly long persistence of a drug's effect include long-lasting changes downstream from the drug receptor (e.g. changes in intracellular effector mechanisms); persistence of drug in an extravascular compartment, such as brain tissue; or a drug effect that takes time to reverse, such as volume depletion by a diuretic. In the design of the first phase II trials, there is a strong prejudice against giving the test medicine more often than twice daily, because of the perceived marketing disadvantage of thrice (or more frequent) dosing. Taking all these factors into account, it is usual to give medicines either once or twice daily in phase II studies.

Choosing the dose for phase III studies

If all goes well, the phase II trials will give a strong indication (but not proof) of the medicine's efficacy. However, phase II usually includes too few patients to achieve a high level of confidence that the drug is effective. The result is that the dose in phase III often has to be decided on the basis of inadequate evidence. Because it would be disastrous to give too low a dose and thus conclude falsely that the drug was ineffective, there is an understandable tendency to give larger rather than smaller doses in phase III. This has led in the past to drugs being marketed at a higher dose than necessary, because even large phase III studies have a limited capacity to distinguish an effective dose from placebo.

6.4.3.11 Trial subject compliance, tolerability and acceptability

Poor patient compliance (fashionably known as 'adherence' or 'concordance') with the treatment regimen can ruin a clinical trial, as can failure to comply with other requirements of the protocol.

Compliance with treatment can arise from poor acceptability (bad taste, pills too large or awkward in shape), complicated regimen or poor tolerability. These issues must be addressed in subsequent clinical trials. Even so, compliance will never be 100% in a phase II or III trial – human beings are intrinsically unreliable, forgetful, or both. The following measures may help to improve compliance:

1. Giving medicines under supervision – either in a research unit or in the patient's home (by a clinical trials assistant).

2. Questioning the patient about compliance, and emphasising its importance at frequent intervals.

3. Informing the patient that the trial includes taking blood and/or urine samples to measure the medicine or its metabolites.

4. Doing a 'pill count', either in the clinic or as a 'spot check' in the patient's home. It is usual to do pill counts at clinic visits, but it is easy for the patient to cheat by throwing away pills or, worse, by taking too many just before the clinic visit.

5. Using an electronic counter in the cap of a specially designed medicine bottle: the counter records the date and time of each opening of the container. The counters add to the cost of the trial, and there is no guarantee that the patient has actually taken the medicine. It is not generally suitable for very large trials.

6. Having the patient collect their trial medication from a pharmacist separate from the investigator. The pharmacist keeps a record of the number of units

dispensed and returned. This system might improve compliance, because patients seem reluctant to cheat a 'third party' dispensing the drugs.

If patients' compliance falls below a threshold level (which should be determined at the outset), a decision must be taken as to whether their data should be excluded from the analysis. As a general rule, non-compliant patients should be excluded from the analysis of phase II ('explanatory') trials, but not from phase III or IV trials, which are sometimes termed 'pragmatic'.

The logic of this policy is that phase II trials are designed to test if the drug works if the patient actually takes it; phase II trials do not attempt to show that it is a good policy to treat a general patient population with the medicine. Patients' data are usually included up to the point at which they stop treatment, but the policy 'last observation carried forward' is not applied in the statistical analysis. Of course, all safety data from all subjects are included in the analysis.

Non-compliant patients are included in the analysis of phase III trials because the objective of such trials is to test the medicine under conditions similar to routine clinical use. So, the analysis is performed on an 'intention to treat' principle, and the 'last observation carried forward' policy is applied to replace missing values. Gross non-compliance may justify the exclusion of individual patients. The rules governing the inclusion or exclusion of data from non-compliant subjects must be determined during the protocol design phase, with the aim of forestalling any accusation of bias.

6.4.4 Bias

Bias is the introduction a systematic error that distorts the data and may lead to a false positive or false negative outcome. Bias is distinct from random error, which occurs by chance. Random error may lead to a false negative result, but is very unlikely to cause a false positive (for further discussion see Chapter 8).

Bias may occur in the selection of subjects for the trial, in allocating the treatments, in measuring the critical endpoints, and in recording safety and tolerability data. Bias may be introduced consciously or unconsciously by sponsor, investigator or trial subject. Many of the features of trial design mentioned in this chapter were developed to minimise the pernicious effects of bias.

Prospective double-blind controlled trial designs incorporating stratification of subjects and randomisation of treatments, rather than retrospective observational, cohort, case-controlled or uncontrolled designs,

will at least minimise the risk of bias. A statistician must be consulted during the protocol design stage, as many biases have a statistical basis that may not be obvious to the untrained investigator.

Bias in execution of trial manoeuvres can be reduced or avoided by choosing objective rather than subjective assessments wherever possible, and by using, for example, standardised questions about adverse events. Digit preference, usually for 0 or 5 as the last digit of each number, is well recognised in the recording of numerical data such as blood pressure; it can be minimised by using automated devices that display the result in digital rather that analogue format.

In spite of randomisation, bias in subject selection may still occur. Randomisation prevents weighted allocation to one treatment regimen rather than another, but it does not prevent selection of the wrong kind of subject in the first place – which will subsequently affect the degree to which the data can be extrapolated. For example, an investigator may have preconceived ideas about the safety of a drug, or about its effectiveness in a particular subset of subjects who nonetheless meet the entry criteria. Even if randomisation is double-blind, this may lead to selection bias caused by the investigator rejecting eligible patients.

6.4.5 Sample size

Statistical aspects of sample size are considered in Chapter 8. Some implications are considered here. 'Sample size' refers to the number of subjects who must finish a trial, not to the number who must enter it. It depends on:

1. The size of the expected treatment effect on the primary efficacy endpoint.
2. The variability the primary endpoints (i.e. the standard deviation of the treatment mean).
3. The 'power', or desired probability of detecting the treatment difference with a defined significance level. In most controlled trials, a power of 80% or 90% (0.8–0.9) is often chosen, although higher power is sometimes specified.

The general rule is that the smaller the difference to be detected, and the greater the variability in the primary endpoint, the larger the sample size must be. Figure 6.5 gives an example of power curves, or statistical nomogram,[29] that show how sample size is related to size of effect, variability of effect, and power. An undersized sample can lead to type I or II errors:

1. Type I error finds a difference between treatments when, in reality, none exists. It is most likely to occur when multiple comparisons are made (see Chapter 8).

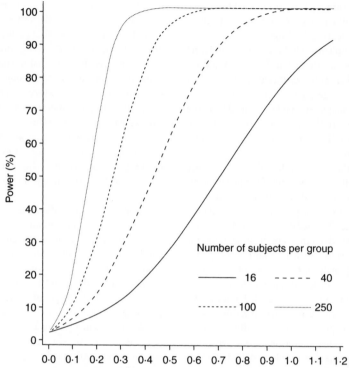

Figure 6.5 Power curves show the number of subjects needed to achieve given levels of power in a trial. The curves are constructed for 16, 40, 100 and 250 subjects per group in a two-limb comparative trial. The graphs show: (i) how many subjects must be studied, given the desired power of the trial and the expected difference between the two treatments; (ii) the power of a trial, given the number of subjects and the expected difference; and (iii) the difference that can be detected between two groups of subjects of a given size, with varying degrees of power.

2. Type II error fails to find a difference between treatments when, in reality, they differ, to an important extent. It is a serious problem in clinical trials, because sample size is so often limited by clinical resources and availability of patients.

The aim of any clinical trial is to have low risk of type I and II errors, and hence enough power to detect a difference between treatments, if it exists. Of the three factors in determining sample size, the power (probability of detecting a true difference) is arbitrarily chosen. The magnitude of the drug's effect is estimated from previous experience with drugs of the same or similar action, and the variability of the primary endpoint is derived from the literature. If the drug is a novel substance in a new class, the sample size in the early phase of development is chosen on an arbitrary basis.

Clinical trials that aim to show a difference between two effective drugs must be very large; for example, trials to detect improvement in mortality after myocardial infarction or coronary artery bypass surgery involve tens of thousands of trial subjects. Such trials are major undertakings for the sponsor, and require commitment at the highest management level. Large trials are also needed if there is a high placebo response rate. While the literature may help in determining the placebo response rate, it often turns out to be quite different in a new trial.

It is tempting to maximise experience of a new drug by giving placebo to as few subjects as possible, using an unequal randomisation technique. For example, a ratio of 1 : 2, or 1 : 3 may be chosen in a large clinical trial. However, it is important to obtain statistical advice before using unequal randomisation – not all statisticians favour it.

6.4.6 Statistical analysis of clinical trials

Statistical analysis is covered in Chapter 8. Here, we offer some general guidelines on the statistical analysis of clinical trials.

6.4.6.1 Statistical analysis plan

Most trials in phase III need input from a statistician. At the draft protocol stage, statisticians can advise on the design strategy, avoidance of bias and the sample size. Statisticians can also advise on how the primary endpoints should be analysed, what factors should be included in the statistical model and how the results should be expressed. However, it is for the physician, not the statistician, to decide what size of effect it is important to detect, with what degree of statistical significance (usually at the 5% or 1% level) and with what power (usually at least 80% chance of detecting the chosen effect).

The statistical analysis plan (SAP) should be written before the trial starts and must be in place before the data are unblinded. It specifies all the statistical analyses and presentations that will be performed. The SAP should state how the baseline (point of randomisation) values of primary endpoints will be analysed. Common potential problems must be addressed; for example, differences in baseline values between treatment groups are a potential threat to the success of the study, and their analysis must be specified in advance. Also, it is important to minimise the use of multiple comparisons, which tend to arise when endpoints are measured at multiple timepoints. Repeated measures, ANOVA and ANCOVA, are often appropriate methods of analysis in such circumstances.

Criteria for accepting data from patients who violate the entry criteria, or who have incomplete data, should be defined before the trial starts and certainly before the final analysis begins. If an interim analysis is essential, its timing, purpose and possible consequences must be included in the SAP, together with any necessary adjustments to the final statistical analysis. Some regulatory authorities have their own statistical criteria that must be observed (e.g. for bioequivalence trials).[21]

6.4.6.2 Statistical and clinical significance

The statistical significance of a trial defines how often a difference of the observed size could occur by chance alone if there were, in reality, no difference between the treatments. The most widely accepted level of probability in therapeutic trials is 5%, which indicates that, if the 'no-difference' or null hypothesis were true, a difference as large as the observed one would occur only five times if the experiment were repeated 100 times. This is evidence that the null hypothesis is likely (but not certain) to be untrue; so, there is probably a real difference between the treatments.

Any level of significance can be set for a given test; for example, at the 1% level, the chance of the null hypothesis being true is only 1 in 100, so a negative result would occur only once if the experiment were repeated 100 times. However, statistical significance must not be confused with clinical significance. Small p-values are of no consequence at all, unless they relate to a difference large enough to benefit patients with the target disease. For that reason, confidence intervals (see next section) are now given greater prominence than p-values.

6.4.6.2.1 Confidence intervals Suppose that a trial shows that a drug reduces systolic blood pressure ($p < 0.0001$). That is statistically highly significant, but clinically meaningless. Doctors are interested not in p-values but in the estimated size of the drug's effect and in what confidence they can have in the estimate.

Confidence intervals are expressed as a range within which it can be 95% (or other chosen percentage) certain that the true value lies. The range may be broad, indicating uncertainty, or narrow, indicating a high level of confidence. The mean difference between treatments, and the confidence interval of that difference, are thus extremely useful in the interpretation of small trials: they show not only the size of the drug's effect, but also the degree of uncertainty related to it.

If the mean difference between treatments is substantial but its confidence interval is wide, a real difference might well be missed because the sample size is too small (Figure 6.6).[32] On the other hand, if the mean difference between treatments is trivial but the confidence interval of the mean difference is very narrow and does not encompass zero, the treatment effect is statistically significant but (probably) clinically unimportant.

6.4.7 Drawing conclusions from efficacy data

Four simple calculations enable the non-statistician to answer the question 'How much better would my chances be if I took this new medicine than if I did not take it?'[19]: the relative risk reduction; the absolute risk reduction; the number needed to treat; and the odds ratio (Box 6.3).

6.5 Conclusions

The controlled clinical trial is invaluable. It has been developed and refined so that it offers reliable answers

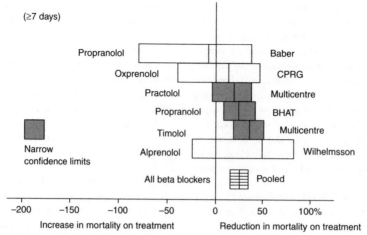

Figure 6.6 Effect of beta-blockers on post-infarction mortality. Difference in mortality is expressed as percentage of control rate in six controlled trials of beta-blockers (95% confidence intervals based on odds ratio). Narrow confidence intervals are associated with the largest trials, which are the major contributors to the pooled result.

BOX 6.3 Summarising benefit

Group	Outcome event		
	Yes	No	Total
Control group	a	b	a+b
Experimental group	c	d	c+d

Control event rate (CER) = risk of outcome event in control group:

$$CER = \frac{a}{a+b}$$

Experimental event rate (EER) = risk of outcome event in experimental group:

$$EER = \frac{c}{c+d}$$

Absolute risk reduction (ARR) = CER − EER

Relative risk reduction (RRR) = $\dfrac{CER - EER}{CER}$

Number needed to treat (NNT) = $\dfrac{1}{ARR} = \dfrac{1}{CER - EER}$

Odds ratio is the ratio of the odds of the outcome event occurring in the experimental group relative to the odds of that event occurring in the control group. So:

$$\text{Odds ratio} = \frac{EER/1 - EER}{CER/1 - CER}$$

More simply, odds ratio $= \dfrac{c/d}{a/b} = \dfrac{b \times c}{a \times d}$

---

to most questions but, like all tools, it is sometimes misused. The discipline of pharmaceutical medicine has adopted the RCT because new medicines must be proven to be therapeutically effective and safe before they are licensed for prescription. Much therapeutic research is now sponsored by pharmaceutical companies, and their staff contribute greatly to the design, conduct, analysis and reporting of clinical trials. Pharmaceutical medicine has embraced the clinical trial, and has developed it into the fundamental tool of drug evaluation.

References

1 Lind J. A treatise of the scurvy. In three parts. Containing an inquiry into the nature, causes and cure, of that disease. Together with a critical and chronological view of what has been published on the subject. Edinburgh: printed by Sands, Murray and Cochran for A Kincaid and A Donaldson, 1753;viii.

2 Booth CC. John Haygarth FRS (1740–1827). The James Lind Library www.jameslindlibrary.org 2002. Accessed 26 August 2008

3 Armitage P. Bradford Hill and the randomised controlled trial. *Pharm Med* 1992;6:23–7.

4 Medical Research Council. Streptomycin treatment of pulmonary tuberculosis. *BMJ* 1948;2:769–782.

5 Yoshioka A. Use of randomisation in the Medical Research Council's clinical trial of streptomycin in pulmonary tuberculosis in the 1940s. *BMJ* 1998;317: 1220–1223.

6 International Conference on Harmonisation of Technical Requirements of Pharmaceuticals for Human Use (ICH). *Topic ES Note for Guidance on General Considerations for Clinical Trials, CPMP/ICH/291/95.* London: European Medicines Agency, 1997.

7 International Conference on Harmonisation of Technical Requirements of Pharmaceuticals for Human Use (ICH). *Topic E5 Note for Guidance on Ethnic Factors in the Acceptability of Foreign Clinical Data, CPMP/ICH/289/95.* London: European Medicines Agency, 1998.

8 Roses AD. Pharmacogenetics and future drug development and delivery. *Lancet* 2000;**355**:1358–61.

9 Wolf CR, Smith G, Smith RL. Pharmacogenetics. *BMJ* 2000;**320**:987–90.

10 Pharmacogenetics Working Party Report. *Int J Pharm Med* 2001;**15**:59–100.

11 Meyer UA. Pharmacogenetics and adverse drug reactions. *Lancet* 2000;**356**:1667–71.

12 Dickins M, Tucker G. Drug disposition: to phenotype or genotype. *Int J Pharm Med* 2001;**15**:70–3.

13 Lindpaintner K, Foot E, Curlfield M et al. Pharmacogenetics: focus on pharmacodynamics. *Int J Pharm Med* 2001;**15**:74–82.

14 International Conference on Harmonisation of Technical Requirements of Pharmaceuticals for Human Use (ICH). *Topic E11 Note for Guidance on Clinical Investigation of Medicinal Products in the Paediatric Population, CPMP/ICH/2711/99.* London: European Medicines Agency, 2001.

15 Committee for Proprietary Medicinal Products. *Note for Guidance on Clinical Investigation of Medicinal Products in Children, CPMP/EWP/462/95.* London: European Medicines Agency, 1997.

16 International Conference on Harmonisation of Technical Requirements of Pharmaceuticals for Human Use (ICH). *Topic E7 Note for Guidance on Studies to Support of Special Populations: Geriatrics, CPMP/ICH/379/95.* London: European Medicines Agency, 1994.

17 Pharmacokinetics in patients with impaired hepatic function; pharmacokinetics in patients with impaired renal function. http://www.fda.gov/cber/gdlns/imphep.htm (hepatic); and http://www.fda.gov/cber/gdlns/renal.pdf (renal); accessed December 2008.

18 Rolan P. The contribution of clinical pharmacology surrogates and models to drug development: a clinical appraisal. *Br J Clin Pharmacol* 1997;**44**:219–25.

19 Greenhalgh T. *How to Read a Paper: The Basis of Evidence-based Medicine.* London: BMJ Publishing, 1997;93–5.

20 Temple R, Ellenburg SS. Placebo-controlled trials and active-control trials in the evaluation of new treatments. *Ann Intern Med* 2000;**133**:455–63.

21 Committee for Medicinal Products for Human Use (CHMP). *Guideline on the Investigation of Bioequivalence, CPMP/EWP/QWP/1401/98 Rev 1.* London: European Medicines Agency, 2008 (Draft).

22 International Conference on Harmonisation of Technical Requirements of Pharmaceuticals for Human Use (ICH). *Topic E10 Note for Guidance on Choice of Control Group in Clinical Trials, CPMP/ICH/364/96.* London: European Medicines Agency, 2001.

23 Jones B, Jarvis P, Lewis JA et al. Trial to assess equivalence: the importance of rigorous methods. *BMJ* 1996;**313**:36–9.

24 Lewis JA. Switching between superiority and non-inferiority. *Br J Clin Pharmacol* 2001;**52**:223–80.

25 Senn SJ. Cross-over, sequential and dose-finding studies. In: Senn S, ed. *Statistical Issues in Drug Development.* Chichester: John Wiley, 1997;237–9;257–64;275–7.

26 International Conference on Harmonisation of Technical Requirements of Pharmaceuticals for Human Use (ICH). *Topic E9 Note for Guidance on Statistical Considerations in the Design of Clinical Trials, CPMP/ICH/363/96.* London: European Medicines Agency, 1998.

27 Resuscitation Council (UK). *CPR Standards for Clinical Practice and Training in Hospitals.* London: Resuscitation Council, 2008. Accessed at http://www.resus.org.uk/pages/standard.pdf December 2008.

28 Baber NS. What does the investigator need to know about the drug? In: Cohen A, Posner J, eds. *A Guide to Clinical Drug Research, 2nd edn.* London: Kluwer Academic, 2000;17–37.

29 Bowman WC, Rand M. *Textbook of Pharmacology, 2nd edn.* Oxford: Blackwell Scientific, 1980.

30 Sheiner LD, Hoshimoto Y, Beal SL. A simulation study comparing design for dose-ranging. *Stat Med* 1991;**10**:303–21.

31 Sheiner LD, Beal SL, Sambol NC. Study designs for dose ranging. *Clin Pharmacol Ther* 1989;**46**:63–77.

32 Lewis JA, Ellis SH. A statistical appraisal of post-infarction in beta-blocker trials. *BMJ* 1982;**31**–7.

Further reading

Friedman LM, Furberg CD, DeMets DL. *Fundamentals of Clinical Trials, 3rd edn.* New York: Springer-Verlag, 2006.

Laurence D, Bennett P, Brown M. *Clinical Pharmacology, 8th edn.* Sidcup, UK: Churchill Livingstone, 1997.

Rang HP, Dale MM, Ritter JM. *Pharmacology, 6th edn.* Sidcup, UK: Churchill Livingstone, 2007.

Senn S. *Statistical Issues in Drug Development.* Chichester, UK: John Wiley, 1997.

Spilker B. *Guide to Clinical Trials.* New York: Raven Press, 1991.

Useful internet addresses

British Pharmacopoeia. www.pharmacopoeia.org.uk

Centers for Disease Control. www.cdc.gov

Central Office for Research Ethics Committees (COREC). www.corec.org.uk

Drug Information Association. www.diahome.org

European Drug Regulatory Affairs. www.eudra.org

European National Medicines Authorities. www.heads.medagencies.org

Food and Drug Administration (FDA). www.fda.gov

Food and Drug Law Institute (FDLI). www.fdli.org

International Conference on Harmonisation (ICH). www.ifpma.org/ichl.html

Medicines and Healthcare products Regulatory Agency (MHRA). www.mhra.gov.uk

National Institutes of Health. www.nih.gov

National Library of Medicine. www.nim.nih.gov

Pharmaceutical Research Manufacturers Association. www.phrma.org

Regulatory Affairs Professional Society (RAPS). www.raps.org

US Pharmacopeia. www.usp.org

World Health Organization (WHO). www.who.ch

7 Conduct of clinical trials: Good Clinical Practice

Kate L.R. Darwin

Hammersmith Medicines Research Ltd, London, UK

7.1 Introduction

This chapter is written primarily as a guide to running trials of new chemical entities during drug development. The principles described are relevant to all other trials, such as those comparing two or more licensed treatments, and those conducted in academic institutions without any support from the pharmaceutical industry. There will be some differences of detail in those other circumstances.

7.2 Good Clinical Practice

The procedures for assuring quality of clinical trials have evolved over the past 30 years, culminating in several published guidelines and regulations. There are four key Good Clinical Practice (GCP) documents:
1. GCP guideline of the International Conference on Harmonisation (ICH) of Technical Requirements for the Registration of Pharmaceuticals for Human Use;[1,2]
2. Code of Federal Regulations (21 CFR) of the USA;[3,4]
3. EU Clinical Trials Directive (2001/20/EC);[5]
4. EU GCP Directive (2005/28/EC).[6]
All of those documents have their origin in the Declaration of Helsinki.[7]

The US Food and Drug Administration (FDA) Code of Federal Regulations provides information on the requirements for registration of new drugs in the USA. Most potential new drugs will be marketed in the USA in order to reap a financial return. Apart from a few minor differences, the FDA has adopted the ICH GCP guideline.[3,4] The ICH GCP guideline

remains the most comprehensive GCP standard in Europe, although the EU Clinical Trials Directive and the EU GCP Directive impose requirements additional to those in ICH GCP. In today's global climate, the pharmaceutical physician should work to ICH GCP, in the context of local regulations.

7.2.1 Declaration of Helsinki

The Declaration of Helsinki[7] originated from a set of guidelines for medical experiments called the Nuremberg Code, which was a consequence of atrocities committed in the name of medical science during the Second World War. Since 1964, the general assemblies of the World Medical Association (WMA) have made recommendations to guide physicians in clinical research involving human subjects. Although not legally binding, the Declaration forms the foundation of all other significant international documents on the ethical conduct of biomedical research.

The Declaration of Helsinki covers all the important ethical considerations, such as the involvement of a qualified physician in any clinical trial, putting the well-being of the trial subject before science and society, the use of scientific principles in the design of the trial and the need for informed consent and a review by an ethics committee: in fact, all areas covered by ICH GCP.

The WMA reviews the Declaration of Helsinki every 4 years. The 2000 version contained significant changes from previous versions; in particular, changes that aimed to avoid exploitation of developing countries. The changes included a requirement that subjects have access to the best treatment identified by the trial after the trial has finished; a recommendation that local participants in a trial should be able to benefit from the trial results; and a requirement for greater transparency about economic incentives. In addition, the Declaration stated that placebo controls

The Textbook of Pharmaceutical Medicine. Edited by John P. Griffin. © 2009, ISBN: 978-1-4051-8035-1.

should be avoided, in favour of comparator controls – a requirement that was later watered down in an interim revision to the Declaration.

Controversy over the changes in the 2000 version led to publication of an EU Clinical Trials Directive (in 2001) that referred to the 1996 revision of the Declaration, rather than the 2000 version. As a result, clinical trial protocols in Europe refer to the 1996 version. Furthermore, in 2004, the FDA published regulations requiring foreign studies to be performed in accordance with ethical principles stated in the 1989 revision of the Declaration, and, in 2008, the FDA replaced that requirement with one that the studies be carried out in accordance with GCP. Nevertheless, continual review of the Declaration of Helsinki ensures continued debate of the ethical issues surrounding clinical trials. This is particularly important as pharmaceutical companies turn their attention to advanced therapies, such as gene therapy and gene transfer, which raise new ethical problems.

7.2.2 ICH GCP

In the 1950s, several events led to greater control and harmonisation of drug development. In the USA, a terrible mistake in the formulation of a children's syrup in the 1930s forced the US government to create a product authorisation system under the FDA. The thalidomide tragedy in Europe alerted many regulatory authorities to the dangers as well as the benefits of new synthetic drugs. Safety considerations, in addition to efficacy, became paramount in new drug treatments. With the public expectation that new drugs be both safe and effective came an escalation of the cost of research, and an ever-increasing health care bill for governments.

Global harmonisation was felt to be an acceptable solution, reducing costs by avoiding unnecessary duplication of clinical trials in humans and by minimising the use of animal testing. Hence, in 1990, drug regulatory authorities of the EU, Japan and the USA got together with representatives from the pharmaceutical industry to try to reach a consensus on the safety, quality and efficacy requirements for authorisation new medicinal products. This was the beginning of the ICH.

In 1996, the ICH approved the final draft of GCP, and recommended it for adoption by the regulatory authorities of the EU, Japan and USA. ICH GCP is based on 13 principles (Box 7.1).

Before ICH GCP, there were many guidelines from various regions and countries relating to the conduct of clinical trials. With the advent of ICH GCP, the

---

BOX 7.1 The principles of ICH GCP

1. Clinical trials should be conducted in accordance with the ethical principles that have their origin in the Declaration of Helsinki, and that are consistent with GCP and the applicable regulatory requirement(s)
2. Before a trial is initiated, foreseeable risks and inconveniences should be weighed against the anticipated benefit for the individual trial subject and society. A trial should be initiated and continued only if the anticipated benefits justify the risks
3. The rights, safety and well-being of the trial subjects are the most important considerations and should prevail over interests of science and society
4. The available non clinical and clinical information on an investigational product should be adequate to support the proposed clinical trial
5. Clinical trials should be scientifically sound, and described in a clear detailed protocol
6. A trial should be conducted in compliance with the protocol that has received prior institutional review board (IRB)/independent ethics committee (IEC) approval/favourable opinion
7. The medical care given to, and medical decisions made on behalf of, subjects should always be the responsibility of a qualified physician or, when appropriate, of a qualified dentist
8. Each individual involved in conducting a trial should be qualified by education, training and experience to do his or her respective task(s)
9. Freely given informed consent should be obtained from every subject prior to clinical trial participation
10. All clinical trial information should be recorded, handled, and stored in a way that allows its accurate reporting, interpretation and verification
11. The confidentiality of records that could identify subjects should be protected, respecting the privacy and confidentiality rules in accordance with the applicable regulatory requirement(s)
12. Investigational products should be manufactured, handled and stored in accordance with applicable Good Manufacturing Practice (GMP). They should be used in accordance with the approved protocol
13. Systems with procedures that assure the quality of every aspect of the trial should be implemented

---

conduct of clinical trials globally has become more uniform. Many countries have modified the format of ICH GCP to the local conditions but, in general, the principles of ICH GCP have been observed.

7.2.3 EU Clinical Trials Directive (2001/20/EC) and EU GCP Directive (2005/28/EC)

In 2001, the European Parliament published the EU Clinical Trials Directive,[1] which governs clinical trials of investigational medicinal products (IMPs) undertaken in the EU. Each European country had to implement the Directive by 1 May 2004. In 2005, the European Parliament published the EU GCP Directive, laying down the principles and detailed guidelines for GCP in clinical trials of IMPs in Europe. The GCP Directive complemented the Clinical Trials Directive, and European countries had to implement it by 29 January 2006.

Before the EU Clinical Trials Directive, European countries varied in the legal requirements and procedures for conducting clinical trials, some countries adopting more vigorous ethical and scientific methods than others. For example, the GCP inspectorate in the UK had to be 'invited' to conduct most inspections, because there was no legal basis for normal routine inspections. The EU Clinical Trials Directive was designed to simplify and harmonise the administrative provisions governing trials and applies to both commercial and non-commercial trials of IMPs, including healthy volunteer (phase I) trials. Only non-interventional trials are excluded from the scope of the Directive. In non-interventional trials, the diagnosis, monitoring and treatment of the subject falls within current practice, and prescription of the medicine is separate from the decision to include the subject in the trial. The Directive does not apply to clinical trials of products that are not IMPs, such as diagnostic agents or agents used to elicit a physiological response (e.g. immunogens). Such trials must be performed in accordance with ICH GCP but do not need to comply with the Directive.

The EU Clinical Trials Directive covers:
• Protection of trial subjects (including risk–benefit assessment of the trial, insurance and indemnity to cover the liability of the sponsor and investigator, and informed consent);
• Clinical trials in children and adults who are unable to give consent;
• Establishment of ethics committees and of inspectorates to verify GCP standards;
• Approval of a clinical trial by the national regulatory authority and by a single ethics committee, within 60 days of receipt of a valid application;
• Conduct of trials (including arrangements for approval of amendments to the protocol);
• Arrangements for suspension of trials by regulatory authorities;
• Creation of a European database to allow regulatory authorities in member states to share information;
• Application of Good Manufacturing Practice (GMP) to IMPs, including requirements for manufacturers and importers of IMP to be licensed, for each batch of IMP to be signed off by a Qualified Person, and for labelling;
• Pharmacovigilance standards; and
• Special considerations for gene therapy trials and xenogenic cell therapy.

7.3 Preparation of documentation for the clinical trial

7.3.1 Trial master files

A huge number of documents are generated during a clinical trial. Those documents are kept in the sponsor's and investigator's trial master files. Section 8 of GCP lists the essential documents which must be filed in the trial master file. Some documents must be filed before the trial starts; others will be added during or after the trial. Many documents will be present in the trial master file of both the sponsor and the investigator, but some documents (such as monitoring visit reports) will be present only in the sponsor's file, and others (such as the screening log, which lists subjects' names) will be present only in the file of the investigator. Separate files will contain financial and budget-related documents.

It is essential that each version of each key document involved in the control and conduct of the trial (e.g. the protocol, information and consent form, IMP dossier and investigator's brochure) be properly identified. A version number, date and page number (in 'page x of y' format) must appear on each page of the document. Systems must be in place to control the versions of documents, such that it is clear which version has been approved by the regulatory authority and/or the ethics committee, and which version is currently in use. Superseded documents must be withdrawn from use. In the case of information and consent forms, it must be possible to verify that trial subjects have signed the correct approved version.

7.3.1.1 The protocol

The protocol is key to the control of a clinical trial. It describes the rationale, objectives, design, methods, statistical considerations and organisation of the trial. ICH GCP[1] section 6 specifies the information that should be included in the protocol (Box 7.2).

BOX 7.2 The main contents of the protocol (ICH GCP section 6)[1]

The following elements should be present:

General information
- Trial title, identifying code, version and date
- Name and address of sponsor
- Name, title, address and telephone number(s) of the: sponsor's medical expert, monitor, investigator(s), clinical laboratory and other medical or technical institutions involved in the trial

Signature page
Signed by:
- Sponsor
- Statistician responsible for the statistical plan
- Investigator

Summary
- Introduction
- Objectives
- Trial population
- Treatments
- Trial design
- Criteria for assessment

Contents page

Background information
- Name and description of the IMP(s)
- Summary of relevant nonclinical and clinical studies
- Known and potential risks and benefits
- Description of and rationale for the route of administration, dose and regimen
- Statement that the trial will be performed in compliance with the protocol, GCP and applicable regulatory requirement(s)
- Description of the trial population

Trial design
- Objectives and purpose of the trial
- Primary and secondary endpoints
- Type of trial (e.g. double-blind, placebo-controlled, parallel design)
- Schematic diagram of trial design
- Follow-up period
- Measures taken to avoid bias, such as randomisation and blinding
- Description of trial treatment(s)
- Duration of treatment and participation
- Stopping rules
- IMP accountability procedures
- Procedures for maintaining and breaking randomisation codes
- Identification of source data

BOX 7.2 continued

Selection and withdrawal of subjects
- Inclusion and exclusion criteria
- Withdrawal criteria

Treatment of subjects
- Trial treatment(s): dose form, packaging, labelling, dose, regimen
- Concomitant and rescue medication
- Compliance

Assessment of efficacy
- Efficacy variables
- Timing and methods of assessment of efficacy

Assessment of safety
- Safety variables
- Timing and methods of assessment of safety
- Procedures for handling and reporting adverse events and serious adverse events
- Follow-up of adverse events

Statistics
- Statistical methods
- Definition of analysis populations and criteria for inclusion in analyses
- Timing of any planned interim analysis
- Justification for the sample size
- Level of significance
- Criteria for termination of the trial
- Procedure for missing, unused and spurious data
- Reporting procedures for deviations from the statistical plan

Quality control and quality assurance
- Monitoring
- Statement confirming direct access to source data and documents
- Quality control procedures
- Audit

Ethics and regulatory aspects
- Trial approval
- Notification of the general practitioner
- Consent

Data handling and record keeping
- Data management
- Archiving

Financing and insurance (if not in a separate agreement)

Publication policy

References

7.3.1.2 Approach to construction of the protocol

Most pharmaceutical companies have their own format for a protocol. Independent investigators will adopt their own or their institution's format. Typically, the protocol will be generated from a standard template, designed to comply with regulatory requirements and company policy. Certain sections may be 'copied and pasted' from a previous protocol, but care needs to be taken to avoid information specific to the previous trial suddenly appearing in the text of the new protocol. It is advisable to avoid repetition of information in multiple sections, because inconsistencies may be introduced as the draft protocol develops into the definitive trial design.

Many individuals may be involved in preparing the protocol. In a pharmaceutical company, it is usually left to a project manager to coordinate the contributions, which should include those of the pharmaceutical physician and the statistician. Input from the principal investigator at an early stage in the development of the protocol is essential. He or she can contribute on practicalities (e.g. selection of subjects, feasibility of design), ethical issues and primary endpoints. The protocols for independent trials may be prepared by the investigator but the advice of an experienced statistician familiar with clinical trials should be sought. Whether the protocol is for a commercially sponsored or an independent trial, vigorous proof reading and review should take place. Reputable pharmaceutical companies have protocol review boards with representatives from quality assurance (QA), and data management as well as the pharmaceutical physician and statistician. A respected and disinterested colleague should review the protocols for independent trials.

The following questions must be answered before the final version of the protocol is ready.

1. Does the protocol contain all the information required by ICH GCP? In particular, consider the following:

• Is there a clear description of what source data will be recoded directly into the case report form (CRF) and what will be recorded in the medical records? As a minimum, the trial code, date of consent, date of enrolment, visit dates, administration of IMP and concomitant medication, adverse events and key efficacy variables should be in the medical records. The protocol must state that monitors, auditors and inspectors from regulatory authorities will have access to source data and documents.

• Are there clear instructions for reporting adverse events and serious adverse events (SAEs)? The investigator must be obliged to report SAEs to the sponsor within specified time limits, and 24-h contact details must be given. It should be clear that these 'rules' also apply to SAEs that occur in subjects who have finished the trial. In a blinded trial, there should be clear instructions on when and by whom the code for a particular subject should be unblinded in an emergency.

• Does the protocol clearly state that the trial cannot begin without approval of the regulatory authority and the ethics committee? It should describe when and how informed consent should be obtained.

2. Is the protocol flexible enough to allow the sponsor and investigator to respond appropriately to emerging trial results, and thereby minimise the need for future amendments? This is especially important in early trials. In a first-in-human trial of single escalating doses, the protocol should specify the planned doses to be tested, but allow those doses to be adjusted on the basis of emerging trial data. Without flexibility, any change to the planned doses would constitute a protocol amendment which might cause a substantial delay to the trial. Also consider whether it is appropriate to allow limited flexibility in entry criteria, dose regimen, washout periods, and timing and number of assessments.

3. Does the protocol make sense? Someone other than a physician should read the protocol. In the case where there are many investigator sites, the individuals reading the protocol may be tired and overworked. Also, laypersons in the ethics committee will need to understand the document.

4. Is the document professionally presented and internally consistent? There should be no spelling mistakes, and the table of contents and cross references to section numbers and the reference list should be correct.

The final draft should be signed off by a senior representative of the medical department sponsoring the clinical trial, the statistician involved in the preparation of the protocol and, perhaps, a medical advisor specialising in the indication or procedure. These signatories take professional responsibility for the content of the protocol. In addition, each individual investigator involved in the clinical trial will sign the protocol, thereby agreeing to comply with it.

After approval of the protocol by the ethics committee and the regulatory authority, any changes must be documented. If the changes are substantial, they should be documented in a formal numbered protocol amendment, and signed off by the same people who signed the original protocol. The EU Clinical

Trials Directive requires that substantial protocol amendments be approved by the regulatory authority and the ethics committee before implementation, unless the changes are urgent safety measures to protect the trial subjects (see section 0). The FDA has similar requirements for changes to the protocol that are not logistical or administrative.

7.3.1.3 The informed consent form

The information and consent form (ICF) consists of two documents: the information sheet and the consent form. They should be considered as a pair of documents, not separate entities. The ICF should contain core information that applies to trials in general; that information may need modification to comply with local regulations. The ICF should also contain trial-specific information; for example, an explanation of the purpose of the trial, entry criteria, anticipated risks and benefits, and trial procedures.

The sponsor must ensure that the ICF contains all the information listed in section 4.8.10 of ICH GCP[1] and any additional information required to meet local regulations. For example, the detailed guidance to the EU Clinical Trials Directive on applications to the ethics committee[1] requires details of conflicts of interest, and the subject's right, on withdrawal from the trial, to request destruction of identifiable stored samples. In addition, most countries have specific requirements for their ICF. For example, in the UK, reference should be made to the Association of the British Pharmaceutical Industry (ABPI) guidelines on compensation of clinical trial subjects.[9,10] In other countries (e.g. Ireland), the trial subject is allowed a specific length of time to decide whether to enter the trial. It is essential that local requirements be checked when a country-specific ICF is prepared. The information in the protocol, investigator's brochure and ICF, particularly that on possible adverse events, must be consistent.

In Europe, personal data are subject to strict regulation (Directive 95/46/EC).[1] The ICF must tell subjects who will see their personal data and explain how their confidentiality will be protected. Subjects should also be told that they have the right to check that the data relating to them are correct. If data from a European clinical trial are to be sent outside of Europe, subjects should be told that the trial results may be sent to countries where laws about keeping information are less strict than in Europe.

The ICF must be written in language that can be understood by the average trial subject.[1,4,12,13] Simple words must be used instead of complex ones; for example, 'stop' instead of 'discontinue', 'avoid' instead of 'abstain' and 'cause' instead of 'induce'. Most trial subjects will not understand technical jargon such as 'placebo' and 'erythema', so alternatives (such as 'dummy medicine' and 'redness') must be used. Volumes should be described in familiar terms such as 'teaspoons' rather than 'millilitres'. Ethics committees often request changes to the ICF, because of local conditions, customs, or interpretation of words, or because the committee considers the language to be too technical. In making any modifications to an ICF, ensure that the changes do not result in removal of information required by ICH GCP and local regulations. The sponsor must ensure that the ICF is read and signed by trial subjects only after it has been approved by the relevant IEC.

If the ICF is to be translated into another language, then someone fluent in that language should carry out the translation. Expensive translation agencies often provide a grammatically correct translation but in archaic language. The translator should provide a translation certificate stating what was translated (including the version number and date of the document) and when, and the translator's name, status and appropriate qualifications. The translator should state that the translation was carried out to his or her best ability, and the statement should be signed and dated. A different person should then translate the translated ICF back into the original language. The latter document will confirm that nothing was left out of the original translation.

7.3.1.3.1 Obtaining informed consent Each subject must give written informed consent before he or she participates in the clinical trial. The patient should be given sufficient time to read the information sheet, and to discuss any concerns with the investigator, personal physician, partner, family or friend, before giving consent and entering the trial (see section 6.2.3). No trial-specific procedure (e.g. blood sampling or radiological examination) should be carried out to decide the suitability of a potential subject until that subject has given written consent. In addition, no drug or placebo should be administered to the subject before written consent is given, unless it is part of ongoing treatment of the subject for a previously established diagnosis. In some clinical trials there is a 'wash out' period when the subject is not allowed to take his or her routine medication; again, this must not begin until the subject has given written consent.

In some situations, data may have been acquired from routine medical procedures before consent was given: it may be inappropriate and unethical to repeat the procedure (e.g. radiological examination) after the subject has entered the trial. In those situations, the protocol and ICF should explain what pre-existing data can be used after consent has been obtained.

Phase I units may have a separate protocol for screening tests to establish the volunteer's suitability as a potential subject (sometimes called 'panel screening'). This protocol and the informed consent procedures must have the approval of an ethics committee. Before a volunteer screened in this way enters a specific trial, the consent process must be repeated with the trial-specific ICF.

In trials of adults who are mentally or physically unable to give proper consent, and in trials of children, special arrangements must be made. Trials in which the subjects cannot provide informed consent will become more frequent as more difficult indications (e.g. trauma, stroke or dementia), and very young children, become the focus of clinical trials. The pharmaceutical physician should ensure that established mechanisms for consent are followed with agreement of the ethics committee and in compliance with ICH GCP chapter 4.8,[1] FDA Title 21 CFR Part 50 sections 24–27[1] and the EU Clinical Trials Directive Articles 4 and 5.[5] Further guidance for UK researchers is given in the standard operating procedures issued by the National Research Ethics Service (NRES).[14]

7.3.1.4 Investigator's brochure

The investigator's brochure contains detailed information on the background of the IMP, and should facilitate a better understanding of the rationale for the trial and the key features of the protocol. The potential investigator should review the investigator's brochure before agreeing to participate in the trial. The brochure, together with any published papers, should give the investigator sufficient information to decide if the proposed trial is justified, and allow him or her to answer any questions from trial personnel and the ethics committee.

ICH GCP[1] specifies the minimum information that should be presented in an investigator's brochure:
• Physical, chemical, pharmaceutical properties and formulation of the IMP;
• Non clinical pharmacology studies;
• Pharmacokinetics and metabolism in animals;
• Toxicology;
• Effects on humans;
• Pharmacokinetics and product metabolism;
• Safety and efficacy;
• Marketing experience; and

• Summary of data and guidance for the investigator, including details of how to recognise and treat a possible overdose or adverse reaction caused by the IMP. Various specialists will contribute to the brochure, including toxicologists, pharmacokineticists and pharmacists. A pharmaceutical physician should review the document carefully.

As more information becomes available, the investigator's brochure should be updated. In any case, it should be updated at least once a year. Anything that might alter the risk–benefit assessment of the IMP, such as a serious finding in a preclinical study, must be communicated in writing to the investigators, and reported promptly to the regulatory authority and ethics committee.

Updates to the investigator's brochure must be distributed to investigators of all ongoing trials. Receipts will be required from the investigator, and old brochures should be recalled and accounted for. The investigator's brochure is a confidential document; the principal investigator is responsible for its security.

7.3.1.5 Investigational medicinal product dossier

In Europe, sponsors must prepare an IMP dossier (IMPD), which contains detailed physical, chemical and pharmaceutical information on the drug substance (the active pharmaceutical ingredient) and the drug product (the final formulation). It includes details of the manufacturing method, analytical tests and methods, storage conditions, packaging and shelf-life of the IMP. In particular, it contains a specification for the IMP: details of the tests that will be performed on each batch, and the acceptance criteria against which the IMP will be released for use in trial subjects. It also contains information on the preclinical and clinical studies of the IMP, or cross-refers to that information in the investigator's brochure.

The IMPD forms part of the application for regulatory approval of a trial. It allows the regulators to assess the quality of the IMP. The investigator will not normally need to see the IMPD. However, if the investigator site is to do any manufacturing work on the IMP (such as dispensing individual subjects' doses from bulk supplies), the investigator should have access to the IMPD.

7.3.1.6 Case report form

The case report form (CRF) is the document in which the trial data are recorded. The CRF must capture all the information specified by the protocol: data that confirm the suitability of the subject, and all the trial results, through to follow-up. Some of the trial results will not be recorded in the subject's medical records, so the CRF will be the only source of the data. However, much information will be transcribed from original documents (e.g. radiological report, medical correspondence, laboratory results and original medical records).

Each page of the CRF should include an investigator-specific identifier, subject number, protocol code and time point (e.g. visit or day). The CRF must be designed such that it is clear and unambiguous, contains sufficient space for data to be entered and is arranged in a logical order: consider, for example, whether it is more appropriate to record data in chronological order of procedures, or to have sections, separated by labelled section dividers, for different variables (such as vital signs, pharmacodynamic endpoints). For categorical data (such as ethnic origin or tests with a 'positive' or 'negative' result), tick boxes should be provided. It should be clear to how many decimal places numerical data should be recorded. CRFs should be appropriate to the situations in which they are to be used. For example, in an endoscopy study, the site of lesions and other features could be recorded on a diagram. Manipulation of data in the CRF by trial site personnel should be kept to an absolute minimum: calculations (such as change from baseline) are more likely to be done correctly by computer programs at the end of the trial than by busy site personnel.

A data manager usually prepares the CRF using a template, which has standard page formats that have been developed, using experience gained in previous trials, to avoid ambiguities and mistakes. Good quality control (QC) procedures must be in place to ensure that the CRF matches the protocol, and that sections of the template that have no relevance to the present trial have been deleted. Design features may be used to avoid errors in, and increase the efficiency of, data entry (e.g. ensuring that 'Yes' tickboxes are always on the left, and 'No' tickboxes are on the right).

The investigator should be required to sign each appropriate section of the CRF (e.g. confirmation of a subject's eligibility to take part in the trial). The investigator should sign the last page of the CRF, to confirm that the data were measured according to the protocol and accurately recorded.

There should be guidance notes to assist the investigor's team in completing the CRF, and a flowchart showing the timing of key trial activities (e.g. blood samples). The CRF will contain objective measures (e.g. blood pressure, heart rate, peak expiratory flow rate) and subjective measures (e.g. assessment of whether side effects might be related to the trial treatment and rating of their severity). Where the investigator is required to make subjective judgements, clear guidance on the criteria to be used must be given in the protocol, to ensure consistency among investigators and sites.

Investigators should be invited to review the CRF and, ideally, it should be 'field tested' by colleagues and investigators before the start of the trial. The trial statistician should review the CRF, to ensure that it will capture the data required for the statistical analysis.

Preparation, QC and review of the CRF takes time. The transfer of the final format to 'no carbon required (NCR)' paper prolongs the process. The printer's proofs should be checked for accuracy before the printing begins. NCR paper should be of high quality whatever the budget for the trial; otherwise, only the top copy will be readable.

7.3.1.7 Source documents

'Source documents' are original records, such as medical records, laboratory reports, subjects' diaries, pharmacy dispensing records, recorded data from automated instruments and radiographs. They contain 'source data'.

The protocol should specify what data will be recorded in the medical records and transcribed into the CRF (data for which the medical records are the source document), and what data will be recorded directly into the CRF (data for which the CRF is the source document). For example, the following data will usually be transcribed from the medical records: date of consent, key baseline medical findings, visit dates, start and finish dates of trial treatment, concurrent medication, adverse events, key efficacy results, and any actions or interventions (such as escape medication). Additional information in the medical records, such as biopsy reports and radiographs, will provide confirmation that the data in the CRF have been recorded correctly. Furthermore, trial data in the subject's medical record may be of use to any future consulting physician responsible for the care of the subject.

Monitors, QA auditors and inspectors need to see all the medical records available to the investigator. It is not acceptable to create copies of data from CRFs or checklists derived from medical records and claim that these are source documents.

7.3.1.8 Storage of medical records

The investigator should know what will happen to the medical records of trial subjects who have participated in clinical trials at his or her institution. The medical authorities or the institution should have guidelines for the retention of records before they are scanned into an electronic form, microfiched or destroyed. Usually, when they are changed into another form, the medical records will be reviewed by administration staff and those items deemed not essential will be removed and destroyed. The investigator should be aware that complete medical records will be required for any future inspection by a regulatory agency. The medical record for each participating subject should be labelled on the front, stating that the record should not be destroyed without consultation with the investigator or before a certain date (for further information on length of storage of documents see section 0). The routine medical record-keeping procedures must be adequate to support running of the clinical trial to GCP standards at each investigator site.

7.3.1.9 Subject diary cards

Some trials employ subject diary cards: source documents that allow the subject to record, on a daily basis, information such as doses of IMP taken at home, concomitant medication, adverse events or an efficacy variable (such as a change in their medical condition). Care should be taken in the preparation of the diary card, so that it is a simple 'user friendly' document. It must not comprise a collection of standard pages from the CRF. It should use layman's language, and give full and clear instructions on how it should be completed. If subjects are required to rate their medical condition or adverse events, the diary card should contain clear guidance on the criteria to use. Clearly, data recorded by subjects at home will be less complete and reliable than those recorded by trial personnel in an inpatient trial. To increase the chances of capturing important information, keep to a minimum the number of data fields.

Diary cards must be approved by an ethics committee, so they must be prepared at an early stage in the trial. The process for transfer of data from diary cards on to CRFs or directly into the trial database should be defined in advance.

7.3.1.10 Alert card

The use of an alert card is not a specific regulatory requirement. However, in many clinical trials, it is appropriate that an alert card be given to subjects, particularly if they are outpatients. In an emergency, the alert card will identify that the subject is in a clinical trial and provide information on the nature of the clinical trial and whom to contact for information.

The alert card should contain the investigator's name and contact details, and a 24-h contact number (the contact should have knowledge of the trial and not just be a hospital duty physician), the protocol code and the indication (perhaps modified to be more acceptable to the subject).

7.3.1.11 Standard operating procedures

Standard operating procedures (SOPs) are detailed written instructions designed to achieve uniformity in the performance of a specific function. Many pharmaceutical companies, hospitals and institutions work to SOPs. SOPs should be written so that they can be of use to new or experienced staff, both for training and for information. Forms, templates and checklists should be referenced in the SOPs, and, where appropriate, flow charts[1] should illustrate the procedures being described. All SOPs should be reviewed and, if required, updated on a regular basis.

Most SOPs will provide guidance that can be applied to any clinical trial; for example, the method for measuring blood pressure, the procedure for storing clinical trial material or procedures for putting contracts in place. However, some SOPs might be trial-specific, to ensure uniformity of procedures in a global multicentre trial (e.g. unblinding procedures). Laboratories involved in the trial should have SOPs defining maintenance, validation and use of their equipment and methods.

In the UK, ethics committees follow the SOPs issued by NRES. These SOPs, which are available from the NRES website, are a useful reference for investigators in the UK. They summarise the regulations governing clinical trials, and explain how investigators should submit applications, and what information investigators and sponsors must report to the ethics committee during and after a trial.

7.4 The IMP and its documents

The time taken to prepare, pack and label medication in accordance with regulatory requirements can delay the start of clinical trials. Not so long ago, the care and attention devoted to the preparation of IMPs was far from stringent. However, the regulators pointed out that it was illogical that IMPs were not subject to the controls that would apply to the formulations of which they are the prototypes.[1] Nowadays, all IMPs used in trials in Europe must be produced according to GMP.[16–18] IMPs used in trials in patients in the USA must be made to GMP. However, in 2008, the FDA made most IMPs for use in phase I trials exempt from

GMP requirements. Instead, the FDA will oversee manufacture of those IMPs through their general statutory GMP authority and through review of applications for approval of phase I trials [investigational new drug (IND) applications].

The EU Clinical Trials Directive requires that every batch of IMP used in a clinical trial in Europe be signed off by a Qualified Person, to confirm that it has been made to GMP, and that it is of suitable quality. Manufacturers and importers of IMP for use in clinical trials in Europe must be licensed. IMPs must be labelled in line with the requirements of Annex 13 to EU GMP.[1]

Manufacture of the IMP should start as early as possible. Foresight is not easy, particularly when a series of related trials using the same IMP is being planned and scheduled to start over perhaps a 2-year period. The scale of and uncertainty in this task are self-evident.

7.4.1 Manufacture

Manufacture of the IMP may be carried out by the pharmaceutical company sponsoring the clinical trial or may be contracted out. The manufacture of clinical trial medication requires a long run-in period, probably 6 months or longer. It is affected by other manufacturing commitments and the stage of development of the formulation. Changes to the formulation during clinical development can cause delays, particularly if different formulations have different dissolution rates, as this may lead to variation in the extent and timing of the clinical response. If such variation is potentially significant, a clinical comparison of the formulations (bioequivalence trial)[1] may be required. If the differences are marked, it could throw doubt on the relevance of the clinical trial(s) already completed.

It is most efficient to make one order for all the medication for a clinical trial programme. However, the size of the order can be immense, equalling the order for start-up stock for the product when it is eventually launched. Its manufacture is therefore a major undertaking. Also, consider that development of the IMP may cease after the results of early trials have been analysed. Furthermore, it is not possible to make one order for the entire programme if the formulation is at an early stage of development or has a short shelf-life.

The manufacturer of the IMP should provide a standard request form for the investigator or sponsor to use when ordering supplies. Well-designed forms help the person completing the form to provide critical information.

7.4.2 Comparators

In addition to manufacturing placebo, the sponsor may need to obtain clinical trial supplies of a marketed comparator from another manufacturer. The precise requirements for blinding (e.g. similar size, colour and no identifying features) can be difficult to meet. Not surprisingly, any approach by the sponsor may be met by the manufacturer with some hesitation, or even obstruction, with unreasonable requests for access to information. It is customary to provide a copy of the protocol, or at the least an outline, with clear indication of the material needed and the timeframe for its supply.

Faced with difficulties in obtaining supplies directly from a rival manufacturer, the sponsor may decide to elect for a 'double-dummy' technique, or to mask the identity of the IMP and the marketed comparator (e.g. by over-encapsulation). In doing the latter, it must be considered that the absorption characteristics of the comparator might be changed, and the bioavailability[1] of the modified and the original formulation should be compared. In the case of over-encapsulation of IMP and comparator in gelatin capsules, simple *in vitro* dissolution studies may be sufficient to demonstrate that the absorption characteristics of the formulation are unlikely to be affected. The results of such studies should be presented in the application for regulatory approval of the trial.

7.4.3 Presentation

The clinical trial material must be suitably packaged for the trial. In early trials, it will usually be appropriate to provide bulk supplies to the investigator, so that the dose can be determined, and dispensed at the site, as the trial progresses. In later trials, optimal pack size will be dictated by the duration of treatment and the intervals between visits. In outpatient trials, excess medication is usually dispensed to the patient, to allow for possible delays in renewing stocks of IMP. Furthermore, a count of the returned medication at each visit will reveal compliance.

The material must be appropriately labelled. IMP that has been packaged for individual subjects in trials in Europe must be labelled in accordance with Annex 13 to GMP,[1] in the local language. The labelling requirements of Annex 13 are summarised as follows:
• Name, address and telephone number of the main contact for information on the IMP, trial and emergency unblinding (sponsor, contract research organisation or investigator);
• Pharmaceutical dosage form, route of administration, quantity of dose units and, in open trials, the name and strength of the IMP;

- Batch number;
- Trial code;
- Subject number and visit number;
- Name of the investigator;
- Directions for use (reference may be made to a leaflet or other explanatory document);
- 'For clinical trial use only' or similar wording;
- Storage conditions;
- Expiry date; and
- 'Keep out of reach of children', unless the IMP will not be taken home by subjects.

Procedures must be in place, and monitored, to ensure that each subject receives the correct treatment allocation. The dosing instructions must be clear. In a blind trial, it is advisable to establish any differences between the test drug and the comparators in smell, appearance, consistency to touch and taste: many blind trials have been unblinded by differences in such basic characteristics.

7.4.4 Shipping and importation

The transfer of IMP to the investigator site requires forward planning. If the site is abroad, knowledge of the local import/export rules is essential. Importation documents will be needed, customs dues must be paid or waived, and certification may be required to confirm that use of the IMP has been approved. Special arrangements may need to be made in advance to ensure that the IMP is stored under suitable conditions while it clears customs.

The principal investigator may be the direct recipient of IMP at the point of importation. Alternatively, local company staff may sign for and collect the IMP. Local company staff will be able to provide the documentation necessary for accreditation and clearance of the IMP, and to advise on procedures and potential causes of delay.

Each shipment should be accompanied by a document listing the contents of the shipment. Particular attention should be given to the dates when the IMP was dispatched from the supplier and when it arrived at the investigator site. A long interval implies that the IMP may have been stored in an unsuitable area on the way to the site (e.g. on a tropical airport runway in high summer). The investigator should acknowledge in writing receipt of each shipment.

7.4.5 Control and documentation of IMP

The investigator site must check, acknowledge and record each batch of IMP. All IMP received, used and returned or destroyed must be accounted for. Any relaxation of drug accountability, as is seen sometimes in multicentre trials of many thousand subjects,

---

BOX 7.3 Documents present in master files concerning the investigational medicinal products (IMPs)

- IMP dossier (for clinical trials in Europe)[a]
- Instructions for handling IMP (may be in protocol or IMP dossier)
- Technical agreement to cover any manufacturing work carried out at the investigator site (if applicable)
- Certificate of analysis
- Certificates of conformity with pharmacopoeial standards (e.g. for excipients or packaging materials)[a]
- Certificates of Good Manufacturing Practice (GMP) compliance or, in Europe, Qualified Person (QP) release certificate for each batch of IMP, confirming compliance with GMP and the IMP specification given in the application for regulatory approval
- Shipping records
- Import licence (if appropriate)
- Sample IMP label and (if appropriate) translation certificate[a]
- Records of manufacturing carried out at the investigator site (e.g. dissolution and dilution of IMP, repackaging and relabelling of IMP)
- Accountability records, with batch number and expiry date, showing receipt, storage location, use, return to pharmacy, and destruction or return to sponsor of each dose unit of IMP
- Dosing records
- Certificate of destruction of IMP (if destroyed at site)
- Emergency code-break procedures (usually a sealed envelope for each subject)
- Investigator's confirmation of receipt of code-break documents[a]
- Code-break documents returned to supplier at end of trial (in sealed containers)[a]
- Master randomisation list in sealed envelope (if trial still blind)[a]

[a] Usually present only in sponsor office

---

can cause problems in monitoring the correct formulations and doses given to the subjects. The significance of the results in such a trial may then be called into question. Records of accountability and manufacture of IMP are kept, with other supporting documents (Box 7.3), in the trial master files.

The IMP should be stored in a secure facility, free from pests and vermin. The environment where the IMP is kept should be controlled and monitored for temperature and humidity. Records must show where the IMP was stored throughout the trial.

In most investigator sites, the pharmacy will play an important part in the storage and accountability of the trial material. In some countries (e.g. France), the local regulations insist that a pharmacist supervises the storage and ensures the traceability of the IMP. Occasionally, there is no pharmacy at the site, or the investigator makes independent arrangements with the sponsor.

Procedures at the investigator site must ensure that each subject gets the correct medication and that the IMP has not expired. Monitors should check that the amount of IMP leaving the pharmacy on any given date matches that administered to subjects. The investigator, pharmacist or their staff, and the monitor, must check any returned IMP. The number of capsules or tablets in the returned containers must be recorded and must be consistent with the information in the CRFs and the dispensing records.

In Europe, repackaging and relabelling of IMP are classed as manufacturing, and must be carried out in a licensed unit, in accordance with GMP, and checked by a Qualified Person. There is an exemption in the UK for repackaging and relabelling of IMP in a hospital or health centre by a physician, pharmacist or person being supervised by a pharmacist if the IMP is to be used in an investigator site that is a hospital or health centre. Typically, in early trials, the IMP may need to be repackaged and relabelled from bulk supplies, or a primitive formulation may need to be reconstituted and diluted. Many early trials are performed by contract research organisations (CROs). They are not hospitals or health centres, so they must have a licence if they are to do any manufacturing work on an IMP. Manufacturing work needs to be covered by a contract called a technical agreement. Additional licences are required if investigator sites import or store controlled drugs, which may be used as IMPs or as part of trial procedures (e.g. subjects may be sedated with midazolam before endoscopy).

In early trials of an IMP, the expiry date may be extended as more stability data become available. The labelling should always meet the local GMP regulations. In Europe, an additional label, showing the batch number of the IMP and the new expiry date, should be attached to the container such that it does not obscure the batch number on the original label. This should be carried out at a licensed site but, where justified, can be performed or supervised by a pharmacist or by an appropriately trained monitor. The process must be carried out in line with the principles of GMP, checked by a second person, covered by a contract and fully documented.

At the end of the trial, the IMP should be destroyed or returned to the supplier. Destruction of IMP must be witnessed and recorded on a signed certificate. Return of IMP to the supplier should likewise be recorded.

7.4.5.1 Emergency unblinding

Emergency code-break information is usually provided in sealed envelopes, 'advent' sheets or sealed label covers on the IMP containers which, when opened, will indicate which treatment the subject has been administered in a blind trial. Their purpose is to provide the information the investigator needs for treating a subject in an emergency.

Normally, the investigator should ask the sponsor to unblind the subject if necessary, thus improving the chances of maintaining the blinding of the whole trial. There must be adequate arrangements for emergency unblinding outside normal working hours.

The sealed codes should be provided with the IMP, and a blinded trial should not start until the sealed codes are available at the investigator site. Investigators must be informed that they must not unblind their own trial subjects, out of curiosity, when the trial has been completed at their site. All sealed (and unsealed) codes should be checked and returned to the supplier at the end of the trial.

7.5 Running the clinical trial

7.5.1 Before the start of the trial

7.5.1.1 Selection of investigators

The selection of investigators is critical to the success of a clinical trial. The principal investigator should have previous experience of clinical trials and qualifications that reflect experience in the relevant indication. Exceptions can be made when an IMP is being investigated in general practice. In this situation, not every practitioner will be trained to undertake clinical trials or have special knowledge of the disease being treated. The sponsors should overcome any deficiencies by providing training and good monitoring. However, many of the most relevant criteria of sufficient and suitable staff support, facilities and trial subject population will be determined in the so-called pre-trial visit (see section 0).

The pharmaceutical physician may be an investigator or part of a sponsor organisation selecting investigators for a trial.

7.5.1.1.1 Considerations before becoming an investigator The investigator must decide whether it is feasible for a clinical trial to be carried out in his or her facilities. The most important considerations are availability of time and resources. In particular, the investigator should consider whether other interests (e.g. other clinical trials in the same patient population) might interfere with his or her participation in the trial. The investigator should seek information about the sponsor: does the sponsor provide adequate monitoring and support, and user-friendly protocols and CRFs? The potential investigator should examine his or her motivation for doing the clinical trial. It is often financial, perhaps to provide additional funds for new equipment or staff, but it may be scientific curiosity, the desire to improve patient treatment or to improve the investigator's professional status by publication.

7.5.1.1.2 Considerations by the sponsor in selecting suitable investigators

There are various ways to select good investigators but none is foolproof. Investigators found to be satisfactory in previous trials may be selected. However, circumstances change, supporting staff leave, enthusiasm wanes or other trials demand attention. The best investigator in a previous trial may fail in the next trial.

There will often be a need for one or two opinion leaders to be involved in the trial. They may have helped in the design of the trial, and will contribute to any future publications. Their influence among their peers may help later to promote the use of the product. They may wish to actively participate in the trial, although most of the clinical trial work at their site will be delegated to a more junior physician. It should never be assumed that a physician with high professional standing in his or her field will necessarily be a good investigator.

Sometimes, pharmaceutical companies have previous experience of working with suitable investigators in a particular therapeutic area. The opinion leaders themselves may know individuals suitable as investigators. Young investigators with some clinical trial experience may have suitable patients, and the ability and patience to cope with the considerable amount of paperwork required in most clinical trials.

There are now several commercial organisations that can provide a list of 'suitable' investigators for a particular indication. Any assumption that the individuals are in fact suitable should be based on an independent assessment. For phase I trials in the UK, the ABPI guidelines[1] give guidance on the education and experience expected of principal investigators.

7.5.1.2 Pre-trial visit

Experienced sponsor staff should visit the investigator site before a clinical trial starts, even if the investigator has been involved in previous trials. Most pharmaceutical companies have checklists and SOPs dictating the requirements of an investigator site. Sponsor staff should inspect the clinical, pharmacy, storage and administration facilities, and speak to key site staff. The sponsor should check: SOPs; staff levels and competence; workload of the site; maintenance and calibration of equipment; and available resources. Questions should always be asked about the site staff's understanding of GCP, in particular, the importance of informed consent and ethical approval, and of the importance of maintenance of confidentiality of the sponsor's documents.

Finally, the sponsor will need to explore the protocol with the investigator, which may be still in draft form. The investigator must know what will be required of him or her and the site staff, and must be asked whether the procedures in the protocol are acceptable to him or her. When the protocol is finalised, the investigator will need to follow the protocol exactly.

7.5.1.3 Preparing for the trial

At the time of the pre-trial visit, and certainly before any subjects are recruited, many other activities will need to take place. The medical management must select the laboratories to be used, and organise QA auditors to audit IMP manufacturers and distributors, investigator sites and suppliers of software for the clinical trial [e.g. electronic diaries or interactive voice response technology (IVRT)]. Team cooperation at the sponsor site is essential for the future success of the trial.

Only in very exceptional circumstances do the qualifications and experience of the pharmaceutical physician warrant their involvement in these exercises. He or she should understand that these activities need to be undertaken and the contribution that each activity will make to the trial. However, the pharmaceutical physician will be involved if part of the clinical work is to be delegated to a CRO or a site management organisation (SMO), or they are part of a strategic team planning the clinical trial.

7.5.1.4 Contract research organisations and site management organisations

There is a growing reliance by sponsors on contracting out part or all of the work of the clinical trial to a subcontractor. The reasons are many, but commonly reflect limited staff resources, pressures of time and inability to identify and organise investigators, especially into a collaborative group (for instance, general practitioners in one locality). In independent trials by investigators, additional expertise may be needed in areas such as regulatory affairs, statistical analysis or data management. Subcontractors offer different services, ranging from large CROs capable of conducting an international clinical trial with minimal contribution from the sponsor; CROs specialising in the conduct of early phase trials; specialised groups for data management, regulatory affairs, monitoring and auditing; to a single consultant for statistical analysis or medical writing.

A recent development has been the emergence of SMOs, which manage investigator sites. Many delays in clinical development occur in the setting up and initiation of trials at investigator sites. These delays result from obtaining ethics committee approval, subject recruitment or the training of staff. Individual SMOs should be able to identify investigators capable of conducting the trial who have access to a large number of suitable subjects and are familiar with GCP and the local regulations. In addition, they can save the sponsor time by providing a single contact for contract and budget negotiations. Several varieties of SMO exist, some specialising in particular indications – perhaps attached to an institution focused on that indication, some providing support for independent investigators and some being totally independent business enterprises.

The pharmaceutical physician should be involved in the selection of CROs and SMOs. He or she is often best qualified to judge the professional competency of the physicians involved in any contractual work. There needs to be a clear understanding as to who will provide medical advice to the investigator and to the non-physicians in the clinical trial teams, who will be responsible for the assessment of the medical significance of adverse events, SAEs and safety issues in general, and who will do any medical coding. The responsibility for custody of the clinical data should be clearly defined at each stage from initial recording to final analysis. It is essential to document the roles and responsibilities of the sponsor, the contracted organisation and the investigators, who will always have ultimate responsibility for the safety and care of their trial subjects.

7.5.2 Technical considerations

Before a clinical trial starts, the sponsor must consider the use of technical aids such as IVRT, remote data entry, electronic diaries and electronic tracking systems which provide status and monitoring reports. All these systems utilise computer systems that must be validated. Double and McKendry[1] described validation as the process that documents that a computer

system reproducibly performs the functions it was designed to do. In other words, validation ensures that the system is 'fit for purpose'. The document *Guidance for Industry – Computerised Systems used in Clinical Trials*, published by the FDA in 1999,[1] and *Good Automated Manufacturing Practice Guidance* (GAMP5)[22] give recommendations of what is required (see also section 0).

7.5.2.1 Interactive voice response technology

The use of IVRT[23] can improve efficiency at the investigator site. Investigators and their staff interact with the system by pressing keys on their touchtone telephone in response to a recorded voice request. In a typical example, when a new subject is recruited to a clinical trial, the subject randomisation number is allocated in return for demographic information, such as subject initials, eligibility criteria, age, sex and weight. In addition, IVRT can be used to track clinical trial material and ensure that the correct treatment is provided to each subject. Patient packs of IMP will be prepared in sub-batches containing all possible treatments in the ratio specified by the protocol: sub-batches of two, for trials with two treatments and a 1 : 1 treatment allocation ratio; sub-batches of three, for trials with two treatments and a 2 : 1 treatment ratio. This ensures that the ratio of subjects at a site receiving each treatment is as defined in the protocol.

7.5.2.2 Electronic data capture and remote data entry

Electronic data capture is the process by which data are entered directly into a computer database (called an electronic CRF, or eCRF), rather than onto a paper CRF, at the investigator site. Remote data entry is the process by which data are entered at the investigator site from the paper CRF into an electronic database, which is available to sponsor staff to review. The design of the computer database mirrors that of the paper CRF.

Electronic data entry systems provide screen prompts and automatic checks. These remind the investigator to complete missing responses, and can immediately flag values of potential clinical concern, inconsistencies and invalid entries. It may be possible to automatically download some data, such as laboratory data, thus avoiding the need for data entry. Each user is identified by a specific username and password, so that entries and changes to data can be traced.

Using web-based eCRFs and databases, monitors can review the data from the sponsor's office, and notify the investigator of any corrections required. As the sponsor has access to the data in real time, the most up-to-date results can inform decisions on the conduct of the trial, such as changes to the dosing regimen in early phase trials.

If an eCRF is used, it is essential to have a back-up paper CRF, for use in case of disaster, such as power failure. Security of any web-based system must be ensured (e.g. by use of encryption).

7.5.2.3 Electronic subject diaries

Paper subject diaries are notorious for being illegible, incomplete and inaccurate. Electronic diaries are small portable devices that can present text and graphics to the subject. They allow the subject to record and store responses, which can be automatically time-stamped. The data can then be downloaded directly into the clinical trial database. The main drawbacks include the need for training the subject in use of the diary, possible variations in local time settings and the logistics of distribution, maintenance and recovery of the diaries.

7.5.2.4 Clinical laboratories

Traditionally, the local hospital pathology department provided laboratory safety data for clinical trials. Increasingly, sponsors are using central laboratories to which some or all the laboratory samples from a multicentre trial are sent. Central laboratories ensure that standard methods and reference ranges are used, which reduces variation among investigator sites. In addition, all the laboratory results can be transferred electronically to the main database, thus avoiding the opportunity for errors in the transcription of data from the laboratory report into the CRF and then into a database.

However, there are drawbacks as well as advantages. Clinical trials for certain intensive care indications (e.g. trauma and acute myocardial infarction) will require frequent monitoring of certain laboratory parameters, and the rapid turnaround of results, by a local laboratory, is essential. Some laboratory variables, such as coagulation variables, must be measured quickly, before degradation occurs. That may not be possible if the central laboratory is a different part of the country or even in another continent. Some investigators may request laboratory data on the same sample from two sources – local and central. This may be due to poor training, but may reflect the investigator's mistrust of data from an unfamiliar and perhaps foreign central laboratory. The protocol must clearly specify which results will be used in any safety analysis. The regulatory authorities will not accept an arbitrary selection based on favourable or unfavourable results that may bias any future safety analysis.

A good central laboratory will provide adequate packaging and arrange the delivery of samples by courier. The International Air Transport Association (IATA) regulations for the transport of biological samples across national borders need to be observed. Most blood samples will fall into risk group II (moderate individual risk, limited community risk). Further information can be obtained from the IATA website (www.iata.org). Staff responsible for the packaging of the samples for dispatch will require appropriate recognised training.

7.5.2.5 Training of the investigator and site staff

The competence of the investigator and the site staff is, overall, the responsibility of the institution or employing authority, and the immediate responsibility of the investigator. The sponsor cannot train the site team in the medical, scientific or technical aspects of trial procedures, or the care of the subjects. However, the sponsor must provide training to ensure that the staff understand the basic requirements of the trial and any specific trial-related procedures. All staff involved in a clinical trial must have had documented training in GCP and in the key elements of the specific clinical trial.

7.5.2.6 Investigator meetings

Investigator meetings contribute to the smooth running of the trial. To the pharmaceutical physician they are an important opportunity to meet investigators, obtain expert advice on trial design and learn about potential problems before they occur.

Investigator meetings can be single-centre or multicentre meetings, and may have global representation. Meetings should be attended by the investigators, their staff and key individuals from the sponsor. There should always be an investigator meeting, called an initiation meeting, before the clinical trial begins at a particular site. At that meeting, the sponsor must discuss with the investigator and site staff trial-specific procedures, including procedures for recording data in the CRF. Other investigator meetings may take place during a trial to update investigator site staff and train new investigators to the trial. They should normally include sections relating to GCP and safety aspects, IMP accountability and administration, recording of data, and review of the protocol. Such meetings are opportunities to ensure uniformity of procedures and to resolve any misunderstandings.

7.5.2.7 Ethics committee application

The investigator is usually responsible for making the ethics application. Since the implementation of the EU Directive in 2004, ethics committees in the UK have followed common SOPs under direction of NRES [previously called the Central Office for Research Ethics Committees (COREC)]. The application process is briefly summarised below.

An application for a clinical trial of an IMP must be submitted to an appropriate committee, called the main committee. The chief investigator – the investigator with overall responsibility for the trial – makes the application to the main committee. Each principal investigator – the investigator with responsibility for the trial at a site – makes an application locally (to an ethics committee or NHS care organisation) for review of site-specific issues. In a single-centre trial, the chief investigator is also the principal investigator; likewise, the chief investigator might be the principal investigator at one of the sites in a multicentre trial.

The sponsor should provide assistance to the chief investigator, to enable him or her to meet the deadline for submission. In particular, the sponsor must provide: supporting documents, such as evidence of insurance; and information that the chief investigator needs to complete the NRES application form, such as details of subcontractors to be used in the trial, and duration of storage of samples taken during the trial. The sponsor must also review promptly drafts of the ICF and any diary cards, to ensure that they are finalised before the deadline. The sponsor's pharmaceutical physician will usually be responsible for ensuring that the description of the risks of the IMP and trial procedures given in the ICF is accurate.

The chief investigator is invited to attend the ethics committee meeting to answer questions about the application. There are four possible outcomes of the ethical review:

1. Approval, with or without conditions that must be satisfied before the trial can start;
2. Provisional approval, with details of what further information is required to secure approval;
3. Rejection; or
4. Referral, pending advice from an expert.

The chief investigator is notified in writing of the decision within 10 working days of the meeting. In the case of provisional approval or deferral, the ethics committee will give a final decision within 60 days of receipt of the initial application (but note that the 60-day clock stops ticking while the committee waits for any further information from the investigator).

A full description of the process, and the forms, are available on-line from NRES.[1]

After the investigator has obtained ethics approval, he or she can begin recruiting subjects for the trial, but the trial cannot start until it also has the approval of the regulatory authority. Procedures in other EU countries differ, but throughout Europe, ethics committees are required to give a single opinion on each trial within 60 days. Further details are in the detailed guidance to the EU Clinical Trials Directive on the application format and documentation to be submitted in an application for an Ethics Committee opinion on the clinical trial on medicinal products for human use.[1]

In the USA, the investigator applies for IRB approval. Multicentre trials may be reviewed separately by each site's IRB, or by one central IRB, or the responsibilities for review may be shared between a central IRB and local IRBs (e.g. the central IRB may be primarily responsible for the review, but local IRBs might review the ICFs for local concerns).[1]

7.5.2.8 Regulatory approval

Clinical trials must be approved by the appropriate government agency before they start. The EU Clinical Trials Directive[1] has almost standardised the process of regulatory approval within Europe. In each EU country, the regulatory authority has 60 days to consider an application for clinical trial authorisation (CTA).

Before submitting an application for a CTA, the sponsor obtains a EudraCT trial number on-line, and then completes the on-line application form. The sponsor sends the application form to the relevant competent authority, with supporting documents. In the UK, those supporting documents include: email confirmation of the EudraCT number, protocol, investigator's brochure, IMP dossier, the IMP label and the manufacturer's licence. The supporting documents required differ from country to country. Full details are in the detailed guidance to the EU Clinical Trials Directive on application for a clinical trial authorisation, notification of substantial amendments and declaration of the end of a trial.[25]

In the UK, the Medicines and Healthcare products Regulatory Agency (MHRA) initially has 30 days to respond to the application. There are two possible outcomes of the review:

1. Approval with or without conditions; or
2. Notification of grounds for non-acceptance.

If the application is not accepted, the sponsor may respond to the grounds for non-acceptance within

14 days, and the MHRA will give a final decision within 60 days of receipt of the original application.

In the USA, an IND application is made to the FDA using Forms 1571 and 1572, the latter giving details of the investigators, facilities, and IEC(s).[1]

7.5.2.9 Additional approval

Depending on the nature of the trial, additional approval may be needed before the trial can start. For example, in the UK:
• Trials involving administration of radioactive substances need approval of the Administration of Radioactive Substances Advisory Committee (ARSAC);
• Trials of investigational medicinal products for gene therapy may need approval of the Gene Therapy Advisory Committee or a specialised ethics committee;
• Investigator sites in the NHS need management (research governance) approval from the investigator's NHS care organisation.

7.5.2.10 Budgets and contracts

Responsibilities must be clearly defined in a contract.[1] The contract and, in particular, arrangements for compensation of subjects in the event of a trial-related injury, should be in place before the trial begins. However, a letter of intent may allow the trial to start before the final budget has been agreed, provided that a signed general agreement is in place obliging the sponsor and investigator to comply with ICH GCP and local regulations, and setting out arrangements for compensation of trial subjects and indemnification of the investigator.

There should be a clear understanding of the costs and expenses that the site's institution or hospital will absorb and what the sponsor will pay for either directly or indirectly. It is helpful to try to separate the cost of materials and equipment hire from the cost of the services provided by staff. In some cases, the investigator's institution will demand a 'handling charge' for handling the contract and dealing with the invoices. This may cover some or all the salaries of the site staff, the use of the facilities and equipment, and disposable supplies. Many pharmaceutical companies now utilise a contracts manager to manage trial costs. In all financial matters concerning clinical trials, all costs and expenses must be clearly recorded.

The means and timing of payments must be documented in the contract. Agreement should be reached on contractual arrangements for premature trial termination and payments to be made when data from a trial subject are not evaluable; for example, because the subject withdraws from the trial, or the investiga-

tor deviates from the protocol. The contract with the investigator's institution must cover all subcontracted duties, including those that will be subcontracted by the investigator (e.g. laboratory tests or use of the pharmacy).

In addition to the undertakings relating to the particular trial, standard provisions should be included either in the contract, in the protocol, or in both. These include statements on indemnity, compensation of subjects, confidentiality and publication, and agreement to audits and inspections. The investigators' responsibilities under ICH GCP guidelines, related guidelines (such as the ABPI guidelines),[9,10] and local regulations should be identified.

7.5.2.11 Financial disclosure

Globally, there is concern that biased results could be produced from trials conducted by investigators who own shares in or receive other financial benefits from the sponsor. The Declaration of Helsinki[7] requires that 'sources of funding, institutional affiliations and conflicts of interest should be declared' in any publication and the protocol. All trials conducted on products that are likely to be part of a submission to the FDA require the sponsor to make a disclosure of financial holdings of the investigators that participate in all trials. Any significant payments (US$25,000) that could influence the outcome of the trial, proprietary interest in the product under trial or significant equity interests (excess of US$50,000) need to be declared by the investigator.[1]

Most future products will need to benefit from the potential sales of the US market. So, before commencing a trial, the investigator should make a financial disclosure. Even when there is a considerable financial interest in the success of the product, the financial disclosure will not necessarily rule out the investigator's role in the trial totally. Most inspectorates are more interested in what is not declared than what is. Ethics committees may also require financial benefits and conflicts of interest to be declared.

7.5.3 During the trial

7.5.3.1 Subject recruitment

In the past, the recruitment of patients has been highly dependent on the activities of the investigator and the patients who were attending his or her clinic. Recommendation of a patient by the treating physician is still the preferred method for recruiting trial subjects. However, increasingly, advertisements are being used – on notice boards in clinics, in the local press and on television, radio and the internet.

CROs that specialise in healthy volunteer trials have databases of volunteers who have expressed an interest in participating in clinical trials. CRO staff can search the database for suitable volunteers, and contact them with details of the trial. However, advertising is often still necessary to meet recruitment targets.

There are guidelines and regulations[1] to observe before embarking on an advertising campaign for a clinical trial. Before the advertisement is placed, an ethics committee must approve it, whether it be a newspaper advertisement or a video or audio message. The information presented should be limited to that required by prospective subjects to determine their interest and eligibility. The following may be included – the name and address of the investigator, the purpose of the research, a summary of the entry criteria, a description of any benefits to the subject, the time or other commitment required, the location of the research and the person to contact for information.

Advertisements should not be coercive. No claims should be made, either explicitly or implicitly, that the drug or device is safe or effective for the indication. Terms such as 'new drug', 'new medication' or 'new treatment' should not be used without an explanation that the treatment is experimental. Advertisements should not promise 'free medical treatment' when the intention is only to say that subjects will not be charged for taking part in the trial. The key aspect is that patients should not enter clinical trials purely because they cannot afford to obtain medical treatment for their illness. Advertisements may state that subjects will be paid, but should not emphasize the payment (e.g. by using bold type).

7.5.3.2 Collection of the data

The expertise of the sponsor's pharmaceutical physician will be used to support the clinical trial team in four main areas during a clinical trial:

1. *Monitoring.* The physician must understand the function of the monitor, and provide support. In particular, he or she may have to give medical advice when the suitability of a potential subject is considered.
2. *Safety.* The physician must review, understand the importance of, and respond appropriately to adverse events, particularly SAEs. He or she must be aware of new safety information, such as new toxicological data, and interpret that information in the context of the trial.
3. *Data interpretation.* The physician must interpret the significance of test results, such as laboratory data, in relation to the IMP.

4. *Coding.* The physician may be required to give support to the data manager who codes medical terms (such as adverse events) before the data are analysed.

7.5.3.3 Monitoring visits

One of the advantages of working with a large institution or pharmaceutical company is that there should be systems in place to monitor the trial properly. Investigators conducting independent trials should be aware that a trial nurse or another physician does not replace the role of the independent monitor.

The clinical trial monitor acts as a QC supervisor, usually covering several sites in the same trial, and so ensuring uniformity in the recording of trial data. The clinical trial monitor checks that the information in the CRF is complete, accurate and legible. He or she must do source data verification (i.e. check the data in the CRF against individual subject's medical records and other supporting documents). Omissions such as concomitant drug treatment or development of a concurrent illness must be corrected. In addition, protocol deviations (such as missing visits) and details of subjects who do not complete the trial (including the reason) must be recorded. The monitor must ensure that each subject gave written informed consent before they underwent any trial specific procedure. The monitor will also help site staff to interpret the protocol, and relay procedural instructions.

After each visit to the site, the monitor records in a visit report any errors in the CRF and omissions from the trial master file. Each error is recorded, and recurring errors are highlighted. Efforts to produce high-quality (or 'clean') CRFs will be rewarded later when preparing the clinical trial database for analysis, as any corrections made after the CRF has left the site must be signed off by the investigator.

Monitoring reports also summarise the status of each subject recruited at the site. In some pharmaceutical companies, the information is recorded on an electronic tracking system, which provides rapid updates on the progress at each investigator site. These updates, together with those from other investigator sites, allow rapid assessment of the progress and status of the whole trial.

The clinical trial monitor is a temporary member of the site team, and should make scheduled visits to the site. The investigator and the site staff should allocate sufficient time to answer the monitor's questions and correct errors in the CRF. The monitor will need space to work and access to all the necessary documents, including medical records.

The role of the monitor is to verify that the rights of human subjects are protected; the trial data are accurate, complete and verifiable from source documents; and the trial is conducted in accordance with GCP, the protocol and regulatory requirements. The investigator and the site staff have primary responsibility for these aspects of clinical research. However, the regulatory inspectorates have, on numerous occasions, observed failures in consent and ethical approval procedures, and in data recording, when there has been no, or inadequate, monitoring.

7.5.3.4 Use of the independent data-monitoring committee

The pharmaceutical physician may be asked to serve on an independent data-monitoring committee (IDMC). It is an independent committee, comprising mainly physicians, that may be established to assess, at intervals, the progress of clinical trials with respect to the safety data and critical efficacy endpoints. The members of the committee may recommend the continuation, modification or stopping of a clinical trial. When working on a 'blind' trial, any unblinded members must take great care not to unblind the other members. Another use for an IDMC is to provide an independent pool of experts to evaluate a particular measure of efficacy in a multicentre trial, such as the size of a growth in a radiograph. This provides some degree of uniformity when many different physicians and specialists at individual sites are measuring many radiographs.

7.5.3.5 Adverse events and reactions

ICH GCP defines adverse reactions and adverse events as follows:

• *Adverse drug reaction.* 'In the pre-approval clinical experience with a new medicinal product or its new usages, particularly as the therapeutic dose(s) may not be established: all noxious and unintended responses to a medicinal product related to any dose should be considered adverse drug reactions. The phrase responses to a medicinal product means that a causal relationship between a medicinal product and an adverse event is at least a reasonable possibility, i.e. the relationship cannot be ruled out.

Regarding marketed medicinal products: a response to a drug which is noxious and unintended and which occurs at doses normally used in man for prophylaxis, diagnosis, or therapy of diseases or for modification of physiological function (see the ICH *Guideline for Clinical Safety Data Management: Definitions and Standards for Expedited Reporting*).'

• *Adverse event.* 'Any untoward medical occurrence in a patient or clinical investigation subject administered a pharmaceutical product and which does not necessarily have a causal relationship with this treatment. An adverse event (AE) can therefore be any unfavourable and unintended sign (including an abnormal laboratory finding), symptom, or disease temporally associated with the use of a medicinal (investigational) product, whether or not related to the medicinal (investigational) product.'

Note that the FDA uses the term 'adverse experience' rather than 'adverse event'. In a clinical trial, an adverse event is an adverse outcome that occurs while a subject is taking an IMP, but is not necessarily attributable to it. For an adverse event to be classed as an adverse reaction, there must be at least a reasonable probability that the event was caused by the IMP. In clinical trials, it is not always possible to ascribe causality.

7.5.3.5.1 Types of adverse drug reaction There are several classifications of adverse reactions, but the most commonly employed define two principal kinds (A and B) and three subordinate classes (C, D and E):[1]

1. *Type A* (augmented) reactions are brought about by the pharmacological effect of the drug, often in exaggerated form. They are dose-related and predictable, and they can occur in anyone.
2. *Type B* (bizarre) reactions occur only in some people and are not part of the known pharmacology of the drug. They are not dose-related, and are the result of unusual interaction of the trial subject with the drug. These effects may be predictable where the mechanism is known (e.g. genetic polymorphism associated with hepatic metabolising enzymes), or they may be unpredictable (e.g. caused by immunological processes).
3. *Type C* (continuous) reactions are a result of long-term use of the drug (e.g. analgesic nephropathy or peripheral neuropathy with reverse transcriptase inhibitors).
4. *Type D* (delayed) reactions are teratogenic or carcinogenic responses.
5. *Type E* (end-of-use) reactions occur with rebound withdrawal phenomena.

Recently, a Type F has been added: unexpected failure of therapy.

In phase I and II trials, type A reactions are by far the most frequent. Type B are rare, which is fortunate, as some can be serious or even fatal. Table 7.1 shows the number of subjects that need to be studied to give

Table 7.1 Number of patients that need to be studied to give a good chance of detecting adverse events

Expected incidence of adverse reaction	Required number of patients for event		
	1 event	2 events	3 events
1 in 100	300	480	650
1 in 200	600	960	1300
1 in 1100	3000	4800	6500
1 in 2000	6000	9600	13,000
1 in 10,000	30,000	48,000	65,000

Source: Council for the International Organisations for Medical Science. *Safety Requirements for the First Use of New Drugs and Diagnostic Agents in Man.* Geneva: CIOMS (WHO), 1983.

a good chance (95%) of detecting an adverse event when there is no background incidence. The problem is many orders of magnitude worse if the adverse reaction closely resembles spontaneous disease that has a background incidence in the trial population.

7.5.3.6 Reporting adverse events and establishing causality

Sponsors will have their own set of SOPs governing reporting of adverse events. The following account is generally applicable to most situations.

Adverse events can be described as serious or non-serious. ICH GCP[1,30] classifies an event as an SAE if it:
- is fatal;
- is life-threatening;
- results in persistent or significant disability or incapacity;
- requires or prolongs hospitalisation; or
- is associated with a congenital abnormality or birth defect.

The term 'life-threatening' in the definition of an SAE refers to an event or reaction in which the subject was at risk of death at the time of the event; it does not refer to an event or reaction that hypothetically might have caused death had it been more severe.

In addition, in accordance with the ICH *Guideline on Clinical Safety Data Management: Definitions and Standards of Expedited Reporting*,[1] events or reactions that are not immediately life-threatening or may not result in death or hospitalisation, but might jeopardise the subject or require intervention to prevent one of the other outcomes listed in the definition of an SAE, should usually be considered serious.

An 'unexpected' adverse event or reaction is one, the nature or severity of which is not consistent with the applicable product information (e.g. invest-igator's brochure for an unapproved IMP or package insert/summary of product characteristics for an approved product).

A suspected serious adverse reaction (SSAR) is an adverse event that is suspected to be an adverse reaction (i.e. related to the IMP), and is serious. A suspected unexpected serious adverse reaction (SUSAR) is a SSAR that is unexpected.

The investigator must notify the sponsor as soon as he or she becomes aware of an SAE in a trial subject. Where applicable, the ethics committee and regulatory authorities should also be informed either by the sponsor or by the investigator (see section 0). The reporting of SAEs, whether considered alarming or not, should have priority over most other activities in a clinical trial.

Establishing a cause–effect relationship between an adverse event and a drug is a serious and difficult problem. Karch and Lasagna[1] proposed degrees of certainty for attributing an adverse event to a drug, as shown in Box 7.4. With this kind of classification in mind, how can a sponsor (or anyone else interested) assess whether an adverse event is associated with a particular medicine? Broadly, there are two approaches: global introspection and use of algorithms. Both rely on the application of logic to the set of circumstances presented. Global introspection is most frequently used and involves one or more experts considering the factors associated with the medicine and the institution. The main factors to consider are as follows:

1. Previous experience with the medicine and background incidence of reaction in this disease group.
2. The trial subject's medical history (e.g. age; hepatic or renal impairment; previous exposure to the medicine; and presence of other disease).

> **BOX 7.4** Karch and Lasagna's[32] proposed degrees of certainty for attributing an adverse event to a drug
>
> - *Definite.* Time sequence from taking drug is reasonable. Event corresponds to what is known about the drug. Event ceases on stopping drug. Event returns on restarting drug.
> - *Probable.* Time sequence reasonable. Corresponds to what is known of the drug. Ceases on stopping drug. Not reasonably explained by subject's disease.
> - *Possible.* Time sequence reasonable. Does not correspond to what is known of the drug. Could not be reasonably explained by the subject's disease.
> - *Conditional.* Time sequence reasonable. Does correspond to what is known of the drug. Could not be reasonably explained by the subject's disease.
> - *Doubtful.* Event not meeting the above criteria.

3. The characteristics of the adverse event (e.g. timing of event, plasma concentration of parent drug and metabolites, laboratory tests).

4. Effects of rechallenge, dechallenge and response to treatment.

5. Alternative explanations of adverse event (e.g. other therapies).

The risk of rechallenge has to be very carefully considered. Its use will depend on the severity of the reaction, availability of a specific antidote, ease and speed of reversing the effect and the subject's willingness to be exposed for a second time. Rechallenge was once fairly common in phase I trials when an exaggerated response (type A reaction) occurred and a smaller dose could be used for the rechallenge. However, since the introduction of GCP and the increase in regulation of clinical trials in Europe, rechallenge has become rare. To rechallenge a volunteer, approval of an amendment to the protocol and ICF would normally be needed; by the time the amendment were approved (if it were approved), the volunteer's enthusiasm to take another dose of IMP would no doubt have waned.

7.5.3.7 Determining clinical significance of an adverse event

If an adverse event has been causally linked to the use of the IMP, the sponsor, usually in conjunction with the investigator, will need to decide on the clinical relevance of the event and the action that needs to be taken. The issue is important to:

- The individual subject;
- The other subjects in the trial;
- Those about to receive the drug in other trials; and
- The overall future of the drug.

The clinical significance (in both the narrow and wider context) of the adverse event will be determined by considering the following factors:

- What is the nature of the event?
- Will it reverse spontaneously and completely?
- What specific therapy is available?
- Are particular groups of subjects at risk and should clinical use be restricted?
- Are there any clinical or investigational factors that could predict who may develop the adverse event?
- What is the risk–benefit ratio?
- Is the drug a novel medicine for an otherwise poorly treated and severe disease?
- Are alternative medicines toxic?

These deliberations may result in several outcomes. Clinical development may continue as planned, but additional vigilance, with more frequent monitoring and special tests, may be introduced into protocols. The dose may be reduced, or certain 'at-risk' subjects may be excluded from further trials. The drug may proceed to registration, but the authorities may stipulate that a post-marketing surveillance study be conducted. Alternatively, the drug may be withdrawn from further clinical development.

7.5.3.8 Pharmacovigilance in clinical trials

The sponsor must keep the regulatory authority and ethics committee informed of developments that affect subject safety. Rules on what should be reported to the regulatory authorities vary among countries.

In Europe, SUSARs must be reported within 15 calendar days; SUSARs that are fatal or life-threatening must be reported within 7 calendar days, and a follow-up report must be provided within a further 8 calendar days. The minimum information that should be included in an initial report is identity of the IMP; subject identifier; SUSAR; source of the report; trial identifier (e.g. EudraCT number); and mandatory administrative information, including a unique case identifier (refer to the ICH E2B guideline).[1] Reports should be unblinded, so the sponsor is usually responsible for reporting SUSARs to the regulatory authority.

In the USA, sponsors must report unexpected serious adverse events in an expedited fashion; the timelines match those in Europe. Rules for reporting to ethics committees are still more variable. In the UK, only SUSARs that have occurred in the UK need be reported to the ethics committee in an expedited fashion; the ethics committee is informed of SUSARs that occur outside the UK in 6-monthly safety reports from the sponsor.

Other information requires expedited reporting to the regulatory authority and ethics committee in Europe if it materially alters the current risk–benefit assessment of the IMP, or warrants changes in the way the IMP is administered or the overall conduct of the trial. Some examples are:
• A clinically important increase in the incidence of, or qualitative change in, an expected serious adverse reaction;
• A SUSAR that occurs after the clinical trial has finished;
• Significant findings and recommendations of the Data Monitoring Committee;
• A major new safety finding from a completed animal study (e.g. carcinogenicity);
• An SAE that could be associated with the trial procedures and that could modify the conduct of the trial; or
• Any anticipated early termination or temporary halt, for safety reasons, of a trial of the same IMP in another country.
In the USA, the FDA must be notified within 15 calendar days of any findings from animal tests that suggest a significant risk for trial subjects (e.g. carcinogenicity).

Sponsors of trials in Europe and the USA must send the regulatory authorities and the ethics committee annual safety reports on the IMP. Currently, there is no such requirement in Japan. However, work is ongoing to harmonise the requirements for annual safety reports in the three ICH regions.

7.5.3.8.1 Council for International Organization of Medical Science
The Council for International Organization of Medical Science (CIOMS) provides various forms, such as the form normally used to report SAEs and SUSARs (CIOMS I), but also many other types of forms (e.g. CIOMS II for the international reporting of periodic drug-safety update reports). The council is active as a medium for international discussion on safety and bioethics (see Chapter 15).

7.5.3.9 Laboratory safety data
In general, the interpretation of laboratory safety data is undertaken for the following reasons:
1. To identify abnormal values or changes in an individual subject. Delta check 'flags' on individual laboratory reports indicate variables that have changed by more than a predetermined amount from baseline. They could indicate change in the subject's condition or an error in sample collection or analysis.

2. To identify trends in the data, even if the individual or mean values lie entirely within the 'normal' reference ranges.
3. To identify predictable or unpredictable laboratory abnormalities, which may need particular attention in further trials.
4. To identify groups who are potentially at high risk.
5. To establish a 'denominator' for any problems that may occur in this or subsequent trials.

The pharmaceutical physician may be called upon at various stages of the trial to interpret laboratory data (e.g. to determine eligibility of a subject; identify risk factors; monitor the progress of the disease or treatment; detect adverse reactions; and determine appropriate doses for certain 'at-risk' subject groups, such as those with renal impairment).

7.5.3.9.1 Abnormal findings and sources of error
Laboratory values are interpretable only if the tests are reliable and the reference ranges are known. To ensure reliability, each laboratory test should be validated to confirm that it is accurate (it gives the correct result) and precise (there is acceptable assay-to-assay variability in the results). Clinical laboratories should run standard QC samples alongside test samples, and should participate in external QA schemes.

Reference ranges are usually based on the 95% confidence interval of a variable measured in a sample of healthy individuals. Thus, they usually encompass the mean value and two standard deviations on either side of the mean. However, 5% of people who are free of disease will fall outside this range, with 2.5% above and 2.5% below. The sponsor should know the source of subjects who provide the normal range. Most laboratories periodically update their ranges of reference values to reflect the population they serve.

A subject with one or more safety values outside the normal range may have responded adversely to the drug, but other causes should be considered: concurrent and intermittent illness; concurrent medication; alcohol or drug abuse; and progress of the disease. The careful follow-up of the subject with repeated laboratory tests during and after treatment will usually help to resolve whether the observations are attributable to the drug.

In groups of subjects, some changes in laboratory values which remain within the normal range are more difficult to interpret. Seeking similar trends in other clinical trials may help the pharmaceutical physician to decide whether the abnormal findings should be attributed to the IMP. A fairly common finding of this kind is a transient rise in liver transaminases or creatine kinase, but usually a careful history and follow-up investigations will determine whether the enzyme changes are, for example, due to an acute viral infection or an exposure to the IMP. In phase I trials, increases in liver enzymes, unrelated to the IMP, are common.[1] The reason for the changes is not clear, but the imbalance resulting from reduced physical activity and high carbohydrate intake (especially sucrose) is thought to be a factor.[1]

Laboratory safety data can be erroneous, and this must always be considered when abnormalities are reported. There are numerous sources of error, which may be related to the trial subject (e.g. self-medication, diet, strenuous exercise); collection, storage and transport of the sample; the analytical technique (e.g. high variability, inappropriate reference ranges, interfering substance in the sample); or to administrative errors (e.g. transcription errors). Some of the sources of error are listed in Table 7.2. When there is doubt about the validity of the test, it should be repeated, if necessary, at a different laboratory.

7.5.3.9.2 Action taken in response to abnormal findings
Individual trial subjects may have to be withdrawn from the trial if abnormalities in laboratory safety data are confirmed and considered serious. Trends in laboratory findings in certain groups (e.g. the elderly) or in all trial subjects may necessitate additional investigations in subsequent clinical trials (e.g.

measurement of hepatic transaminases). Further clinical trials will provide information on how well the IMP is tolerated and whether the benefits revealed by laboratory safety and efficacy data outweigh the overall risk.

7.5.3.10 Amendments
Even if the trial protocol is flexible, it may be necessary to amend it, or other key trial documents, during the trial. In Europe, an amendment to a clinical trial authorisation is an amendment to:
- The terms of the request for clinical trial authorisation from the regulatory authority or approval from the ethics committee;
- The protocol; or
- Any other particulars or documents submitted with the applications to the regulatory authority or the ethics committee.

The detailed guidance to the EU Clinical Trials Directive on application for a clinical trial authorisation, notification of substantial amendments and declaration of the end of a trial[1] requires that *substantial* amendments be approved by the regulatory authority and/or the ethics committee, unless the changes are urgent safety measures to protect the trial subjects. The regulatory authority and the ethics committee must be notified as soon as possible of amendments that have been implemented to eliminate an immediate hazard, and have not been given prior approval.

Table 7.2 Sources of error in laboratory values

Reason for error	Possible result
Delayed or slow separation of blood	Increase in plasma potassium, phosphate, total acid phosphatase, lactate dehydrogenase, hydroxybutyrate dehydrogenase or aspartate aminotransferase
Haemolysis of blood during venesection,	Increased potassium and possibly lactate dehydrogenase and aspartate aminotransferase
Prolonged venous stasis	Increased thyroxine, total protein, lipids or subfractions
Infusion in same arm as sampling	Increased electrolyte or glucose levels, dilution of all other variables
Thawed samples	Loss of plasma enzyme activities
Inaccurately timed urine collection	Erratic clearance data
Palpation of bladder and prostate catheterisation	Rise in tartrate-labile acid phosphate and PSA
Glucose not in fluoride bottle	Low glucose (after 4 h)
Incorrect container for blood	EDTA or oxalate cause low calcium with high potassium or sodium
Underfilled coagulation tubes	Prolonged prothombin time and activated partial prothrombin time

EDTA, edetic acid ethylenediaminetetra-acetate; PSA, prostate-specific antigen.

Table 7.3   Approval required for changes to trial

Type of change	Approval required
Change to information submitted to the regulatory authority only (e.g. amendment to IMP dossier reflecting extension to shelf-life of IMP)	Regulatory authority only
Change to information submitted to the ethics committee only (e.g. amendment to information and consent form reflecting change in arrangements for payment of trial subjects)	Ethics committee only
Change to information submitted to the regulatory authority and the ethics committee (e.g. protocol amendment changing the dosing regimen)	Regulatory authority and ethics committee
Restarting a trial after a temporary halt	Regulatory authority and ethics committee

The detailed guidance[1] further defines a substantial amendment as an amendment that is likely to affect *to a significant degree*:

1. Safety or physical or mental integrity of the subjects of the trial;
2. Scientific value of the trial;
3. Conduct or management of the trial; or
4. Quality or safety of any investigational medicinal product used in the trial.

The EU Clinical Trials Directive sets a time limit of 35 days for review a substantial amendment. The sponsor is responsible for deciding whether a non-urgent amendment is substantial, and deciding whether to request approval from the ethics committee and/or the regulatory authority (Table 7.3). The regulatory authority must be notified of any substantial amendment submitted to the ethics committee only, and vice versa. Non-substantial amendments need not be notified to the regulatory authority or the ethics committee, but they must be documented.

In the USA, amendments that significantly affect the safety of trial subjects or, for phase II and III trials, that significantly affect the scope or scientific quality of the trial, need approval of the FDA and the ethics committee. In Europe and the USA, investigators can implement without prior approval urgent amendments to protect subjects from an immediate hazard, but the regulatory authority and the ethics committee must be informed promptly.

7.5.3.11 Reporting requirements during the trial

During the trial, the sponsor must ensure that the required reports are made to the ethics committee and the regulatory authority. Regulatory authorities in Europe must receive:

1. Pharmacovigilance reports (see section 0); and
2. Notification of:

- Urgent, substantial amendments;
- Any temporary halt to the trial; and
- The end of the trial.

In addition, the UK MHRA requires that sponsors report serious breaches of GCP or the protocol (see section 0).

In the UK, the following must be reported to the ethics committee:

1. Investigator's annual reports of the progress of the trial, if the trial lasts for more than a year;
2. Pharmacovigilance reports (see section 0);
3. Reports of any serious breaches of GCP or the protocol (see section 0);
4. Updates to the investigator's brochure (but only if there is a change to the risk–benefit assessment of the trial); and
5. Notification of:

- Absence of the principal investigator for more than 4 weeks;
- Urgent, substantial amendments;
- Any temporary halt to the trial; and
- The end of the trial.

7.5.4 Data management

The workload in assembling clinical trial data for analysis is dictated by the quantity and the quality of the data. If the quality is poor, the process is extended by remedial steps going all the way back to the investigator site. Therefore, all the preceding efforts to bring high-quality data from investigators are amply justified by the resources and time saved during the data management process.

Two essential features of modern data management are a validated computer system and trained specialist staff. Data management is a recognised discipline, with professional associations and university courses. Any temptation to avoid the use of trained staff, and instead rely on secretaries, investigator site monitors or nurses, could prolong the process and may endanger the integrity of the results.

7.5.4.1 Computer systems in clinical trials

Computerised systems are essential for handling the large quantity of data, and for future interrogation. Non-validated computer systems are unacceptable. The FDA documents *Computerised Systems Used in Clinical Trials*[1] and 21 CFR part 11 Regulations[36] should be followed when processing clinical data in any computer system, and when using electronic signatures, even if the results will never be used in any US regulatory application.

Because the use of computer systems in data management is so important, it is appropriate to have a basic understanding of what is required to validate a computer system. In simple terms, the validated computer system is developed, implemented, operated and maintained in a controlled manner, from the design stage to its decommissioning. Each stage must be fully documented.

The software developer should follow written functional specifications for the system, and keep evidence that appropriate tests were carried out on the software. It is usually appropriate for the software user's QA staff to audit the software developer.

The user must document their requirements for the system (the user requirements), and document in a validation plan the strategy for testing the system against the user requirements, including acceptance criteria, assumptions, exclusions and responsibilities. The user of the system, not an IT specialist, should test the system. Each test, including the expected results and the actual results must be documented and then summarised in a validation report. The formal acceptance of the system for use must also be recorded. Evidence of staff training must be kept, and SOPs must be written, governing use of the system.

Installation of the system must be documented, and any changes to the system must be controlled. Revalidation should be carried out if necessary, and updated user manuals, SOPs and training records must be filed. Computer systems that handle clinical trial data should be secure, backed up and have a date- and time-stamped audit trail which independently records changes to data such that the previously recorded information is not obscured.

7.5.4.2 The process

The system shown in Figure 7.1 reflects the process undertaken in many data management groups.

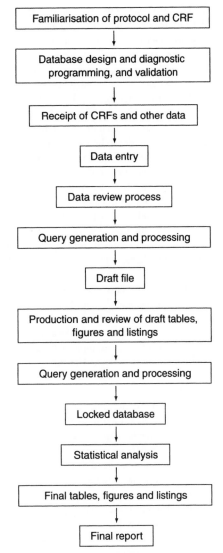

Figure 7.1 Data management process.

Although the order of some of the stages, such as data entry and query generation, may vary, as in the case of electronic data capture at the investigator site, the activities will be similar for all data management. The clinical data may arrive in various forms: CRFs by fax, post or courier – sometimes a few pages at a time; central laboratory data by email or on portable media; and ECG and Holter data by courier or post. It is therefore essential that proper tracking systems are in place.

The CRF will be a major determinant of the database design, so it is essential that the data manager review the CRF before the start of the trial. The data manager may need to liaise with programming and statistical specialists to decide the structure of the database.

The requirement for interim analyses may impact on the data management processes, and is of major significance if a trial is blinded. That is because separate staff will be needed for the interim analysis if the regular staff are to remain blinded for the final analysis.

Other considerations include the coding of the data and the dictionaries to be used, when and how SAE and adverse event data will be incorporated into the database, and the electronic checks to be run on the data during and after data entry. If data entry is carried out in several centres (for instance, different countries), the standards must be identical. A centrally based validation group will monitor that these standards are being maintained and will identify early any persistent problems, so that these can be avoided everywhere.

Once all the queries have been resolved, and the data have undergone final QC checks, the database is 'locked'. Only by a controlled and fully documented process should the database be unlocked to allow changes to be made. For example, late SAEs may necessitate additions to the locked database.

7.5.4.3 Coding

Coding ensures reproducibility and standardisation of data. It also allows advanced medical terminology to be used and facilitates searching and manipulation of data. Many large data management groups have professionals who concentrate solely on coding, ensuring that the coding is standardised.

The pharmaceutical physician will have a role in ensuring that the coding has been carried out correctly. Specific clinical data could be lost or misrepresented because a particular disease or adverse event is coded too generally. Conversely, a term could be coded in a way that fails to describe the disease or event because it is too specific. This can cause problems when the clinical trial report is written and when safety data are being interpreted. Translation can be a source of problems during the coding process; it is important that the translation of medical information be done by a trained translator.

The Medical Dictionary for Regulatory Activities (MedDRA)[1] has been adopted by ICH as the standard medical terminology for regulatory communication.

7.5.4.4 Audit and data trails

A fundamental principle of GCP is that the data recorded in the CRF or in any of the accompanying documents (e.g. diary cards) cannot be changed without the written agreement of the investigator. The data manager notes omissions and errors identified during the data management process, and generates lists of data queries, which must be resolved and signed off by the investigator before the database can be updated. The data manager must track all queries, and only when all the queries have been resolved can the data be considered 'clean'. Many individuals, including senior pharmaceutical physicians, have wanted to alter data on CRFs because 'they know the data are wrong'. However, an unauthorised change to any data supplied by the investigator is unacceptable. The only exception is an uncontroversial change (such as correction of a typographical error) that is covered by written data entry conventions agreed in advance.

Data management systems keep an audit trail: an electronic record of all the changes that have been made, by whom and when. At inspections, regulators may ask to see the audit trail, to trace changes to the data. Any changes must be justified and agreed by all concerned.

Another important series of steps is extraction of data to create listings, tables and graphs. A 'data trail' should be established, showing the source of the data used in analyses. The manner in which analysis sets were constructed (i.e. rules applied, identifiers of data sets) should be recorded, so that the analyses can be reproduced later, for instance when more data from other trials are available. The statistician's analysis is valid only if it truly reflects the original CRF data. Understandably, the statisticians' confidence in the data presented to them is of paramount concern and their questioning of data should be regarded as legitimate.

7.5.4.5 Statistical analysis

A qualified statistician must be consulted about the design of the trial and the planned statistical analysis. The statistician should, ideally, have experience of clinical trials and be a chartered statistician or equivalent.

A summary of the analysis plan will be included in the protocol but, usually, it is described in more detail in a separate signed statistical analysis plan. The plan should describe the criteria for excluding subjects from the analysis, the statistical methods to be used, and general principles, such as the significance level and how missing data will be dealt with. In a blinded trial, the plan must be finalised and signed before the randomisation code is broken. Unblinding of the trial must not take place until all the subjects at all the investigator sites have completed the trial and the database has been checked and locked. In an open trial, the plan must be signed before the analysis of the data begins. It may be necessary to revise the plan as a result of a protocol amendment. Such changes should be documented in an amendment to the statistical analysis plan.

It is essential that the statistical analysis described at the beginning of the trial be used at the end of the trial. If there are deviations from the planned analysis, the reasons must be documented in the trial report. Frequently, the results of the planned analysis are not as expected. It may be tempting to modify the analyses or datasets in an attempt to produce the desired results. However, the original planned analysis must be presented in the report, and any additional analyses that were unplanned must be described as unplanned in the report.

The ICH has produced a number of guidance documents on statistical considerations in clinical trials.[38-40]

7.5.4.6 Data integrity

The institution, pharmaceutical company or independent investigator carries considerable responsibility as custodian of trial data and is potentially exposed to charges of bias, of suppression or even of alteration of data. Data may be modified in order to correct errors, but all changes must be tracked. Documented QC and quality assurance steps must be part of the process (see section 7.7).

7.5.4.7 The end of the trial

The closing down of the trial at the site after the last visit of the last subject, and resolution of the data queries in the CRF, is an important part of the clinical trial. Archiving of documents, both at the site and at the sponsor, needs to be peformed as soon as possible after the end of the clinical phase of the trial. The effort required to do this well is very much less than that which would be required if deficiencies were identified later – particularly if that occurred during a regulatory authority inspection.

The investigator may wish to archive the site's documents, or may wish the sponsor to supply archiving space. In the latter case, the documents should be sealed so that there is no opportunity for anyone but the investigator to see them. All the documents at the sponsor's office, whether paper or electronic, should also be archived.

The length of time required to archive the documents is at least 2 years after the last approval of the marketing application or any contemplated marketing application, or at least 2 years after the formal discontinuation of clinical development (ICH GCP 5.5.11).[1] These requirements make long-term planning for archiving difficult because usually one does not know what the status of the IMP will be in 6 months' time, and certainly not in 2 or 3 years. Typically, sponsors and investigators should plan to archive documents for at least 15 years.

At the end of the trial, the clinical trial monitor should make a close-out visit to each investigator site, and do the following:
- Ensure that arrangements have been made to archive: the documents in the investigator's master file, the investigator's copies of the completed CRFs, and any trial-related records in the pharmacy.
- Advise the investigator to try to prevent the medical records of the trial subjects from being deleted or lost.
- Check that all randomisation codes have been returned from blind trials without being opened except in a recorded emergency.
- Do a final accountability check of any remaining IMP, and arrange for the IMP to be destroyed or sent back to the supplier.
- Ensure that the end of the trial has been notified to the regulatory authority and the ethics committee, as applicable.

7.5.4.8 Regulatory inspections and QA audits

The EU Clinical Trials Directive (2001/20/EC)[1] has reinforced the need for European agencies, as well as those of the USA and Japan, to inspect clinical trials. Sponsors, mindful of the implications of failed inspections, routinely audit investigator sites to try to ensure that standards meet the regulatory requirements and ICH GCP.

In Europe, regulators do routine inspections of holders of trial authorisations, and organisations to which trial-related duties have been subcontracted, including investigator sites. Sponsors and investigators are notified of routine inspections in advance. Before a routine inspection, the inspector will normally request written information about the site (e.g. a list of SOPs, a list of ongoing trials, copies of key SOPs, and an overview of the facilities). During the inspection, the inspectors will review in detail the documents in the trial master file, source documents, pharmacy records, SOPs and the site's facilities. The inspectors will request documents, and the organisation must be prepared to provide them promptly during the inspection. The inspectors will also interview site staff. At the end of the inspection, the inspectors will give feedback at a close-out meeting. After the inspection, the inspector will send the organisation a written report of the findings and recommendations. The organisation must respond to the report in writing until all the queries have been resolved to the satisfaction of the regulatory authority. Further information can be obtained from FDA guidance manuals[41,42] and the MHRA website.

In a similar manner, sponsors will audit investigator sites. The job of the auditor is to question the conduct of the trial and the integrity of the data. Investigators may be annoyed that their conduct is questioned, particularly as auditors are usually not physicians, but both investigators and auditors must understand that each has a job to do, and be tolerant. The regulators may also do inspections without notice, or at very short notice, usually as a result of a report of suspected violation of the regulations.

In the UK, the MHRA may inspect phase I research sites under a voluntary accreditation scheme. The scheme was introduced following a recommendation by the Expert Scientific Group (ESG) that was formed to review phase I clinical trials after six healthy volunteers in the TGN1412 trial were admitted to intensive care, in March 2006, after they had been given an IMP (a superagonist anti-CD28 monoclonal antibody).[1] Phase I sites can apply for standard or supplementary accreditation. Units with supplementary accreditation are considered suitable to do first-in-human trials of 'higher risk' IMPs, such as those that act via a species-specific mechanism, for which animal data are a poor predictor of likely effects in humans.

7.6 Preparation of the clinical report

7.6.1 General considerations

ICH GCP requires that a report of the trial be written. This ensures that the results are documented and interpreted, even if only one trial subject is involved (ICH GCP 5.22).[1] This is another safeguard, along with ethical approval and informed consent, against unapproved and poor quality experimentation on humans. It also facilitates the use of the new knowledge gained during the clinical trial to influence decisions on therapy or the development of the IMP. For the manufacturer, the results of clinical trials determine what claims can be made about the efficacy, safety and quality of a new medicine when applying for a marketing licence and when persuading doctors to use the medicine. Whether the report is of a small academic investigation or part of the research for a

future commercial product, its preparation justifies care and attention.

Reports of clinical trials should be prepared in line with ICH Guideline E3.[42,44,45] Clinical trial reports are accompanied by extensive listings and tables of data, so that the regulators can run an independent analysis.

In Europe, a copy of the summary of the clinical trial report must be submitted to the ethics committee and the regulatory authority within 1 year of the end of the trial. Whereas extensive data packages are submitted to regulators, only limited data are published in journals. Publication of trial results as early as possible should be encouraged, with a view to prevent unnecessary trials and improve subject safety. However, owing to factors such as lack of time, commercial sensitivity and unwillingness of journals to publish negative results, the majority of clinical trials remain unpublished.[1]

7.7 Quality management

The final principle of ICH GCP states: 'systems with procedures that assure the quality of every aspect of the trial should be implemented' (ICH GCP 2.13).[1] The word 'quality' is often misunderstood, although freely used when referring to processes and documentation in clinical trials. It should mean that a standard of excellence has been reached in: the care of the subjects' physical and mental well-being; protection of the subjects' rights; compliance with the protocol and with scientific, ethical and regulatory standards; and the integrity of the data. Quality is the responsibility of every person who works on a clinical trial.

Regulatory authorities require that trials supporting a licensing application for a new medicine be carried out in accordance with GCP, and the quality principles inherent in the guideline. Sponsors should ensure that everyone working on a clinical trial follows a quality system, with SOPs to ensure that each task is performed in a controlled and uniform way. ICH GCP has not always been fully applied to other biomedical research, such as some independent trials on marketed products initiated by clinicians without support from the manufacturer. The training that clinicians, scientists and technicians receive from company-based staff before and during a sponsored clinical trial can considerably enhance the quality of the trial.

In some pharmaceutical companies and institutions, the principles of total quality management (TQM),[46] philosophies associated with European Foundation for Quality Management (EFQM)[1] or ISO 9001[1] have been adopted. Sweeney[49] has provided details of how the original versions of ISO 9000 standards could be applied to clinical trials. However, all these quality systems can provide only a limited foundation. Independent reviewers, auditors from QA groups and inspectors from regulatory agencies must reinforce the quality systems.

7.7.1 QC and QA

Many scientists confuse the terms QC and QA. In clinical trials, there is a very real difference. QC comprises the operational techniques and activities undertaken by all participants to verify that the quality requirements of the clinical trial have been fulfilled, whereas QA verifies that the QC has satisfied these requirements. In other words, QC includes checks: that the data recorded are consistent with source documents; that the subjects are given the correct dose; that accountability records can be reconciled with the IMP remaining in pharmacy; that equipment is calibrated and suitable for use; and that the relevant SOPs and the protocol are followed. QA includes the establishment of SOPs that oblige staff to follow uniform practice, and checks by independent individuals that QC is in place and is effective.

7.7.1.1 Quality control

Quality control must be employed at all stages of a clinical trial. The clinician has been perceived as reluctant to introduce QC in clinical research, perhaps because of a fear of finding mistakes that reflect on clinical professionalism, a lack of time or – in some unfortunate cases – arrogance that nothing could be wrong. This has resulted in the drug industry recruiting non-medical scientists to independently monitor the activities occurring at the investigator site.

If the investigator and site staff do not scrupulously follow the protocol, this could alter the outcome of the trial. The site must have the right subject, with the right disease, and administer the right treatment at the correct dose at the right time. The investigator must make the correct observations, at the right time, and make a complete and accurate record of the results. All this must be checked. Furthermore, the investigator must use calibrated equipment, and reproducible and – in some cases – validated, methods. Methods for making objective measurements (e.g. blood pressure, peak expiratory flow, gastric emptying times, skin thickness, reaction times) can be defined, sometimes calibrated, and the reproducibility of repeated measurements validated. Subjective endpoints may be validated (e.g. anxiety or depression rating scales and questionnaires). Criteria for subjective judgments by clinical staff must be clearly defined in advance. The training of staff in consistent use of subjective endpoints is essential before the trial starts.

7.7.1.2 Role of the clinical trial nurse or coordinator

Many investigator sites employ part- or full-time nurses to support clinical trials. Nurses should never be considered to be an extravagance because, without them, the burden of administration and QC is solely on the investigator. The clinical trial nurse can help the investigator in many ways, but two of the most important are ensuring that the data in the CRF are consistent with information in source documents, and liaising with the sponsor's monitor.

7.7.1.3 Quality assurance

All clinical trials should be subjected to QA, either by an in-house department or by external consultants. QA is defined as 'all those planned and systematic actions that are established to ensure that the trial is performed and the data generated, documented (recorded), and reported in compliance with GCP and the applicable regulatory requirements(s)' (ICH GCP 1.46).[1]

QA staff should be independent from those who work on or manage the clinical trial. Their independence facilitates the reporting of deficiencies without bias. QA conduct audits of clinical trials, to establish whether QC has taken place, whether SOPs are being followed, and whether the quality systems in place will provide clinical data to GCP standards. The word 'audit' should be reserved for QA activities. If a regulatory authority conducts an audit, it is usually called an 'inspection'.

QA has many other functions, including review of new protocols, and audits of the facilities and systems of investigators and non clinical contractors, such as laboratories, software developers, contract archives or data managers. For example, to ensure that the high-quality clinical data that have so laboriously been obtained are accurately reflected in the trial report, QA should audit data management, statistics and reporting groups.[1] They should also audit the final clinical trial report. Robust QC procedures should be in place, but quality of data can be affected if suitable QC staff are unavailable or because of pressure to meet timelines. The regulatory agencies will expect all functions in the clinical trial that are subcontracted to meet the requirements of GCP.

Often, the QA department will provide a supporting function in the preparation and revision of SOPs and in the training of staff involved in clinical trials.

7.7.2 Fraud/misconduct

The FDA defines fraud as the deliberate reporting of false or misleading data or the withholding of reportable data. Although the agency has used the word 'fraud', in the USA the word usually implies injury or damage to victims and therefore the word 'misconduct' is preferred. Fraud in clinical research may be a rare phenomenon[1] but no one really knows how many cases are undetected or not reported. In the UK, a pharmaceutical company reporting an investigator for fraud may experience a backlash from the local professional and lay community before the full facts become known. The motives of a fraudulent investigator may be financial gain or professional promotion, trying to produce results either too quickly or too precisely. In some cases, work overload or mental illness provide a backdrop to the crime.

Fraudulent investigators may add data where the original are missing, possibly not wanting to admit that they forgot to obtain or record them, or that they lost them (e.g. broken blood sample tube). Serious cases involve falsification of data for trial subjects who do not exist, or creation of ethical approval and consent documents at the site.[51–53]

Certain quality management measures already outlined, and summarised in Table 7.4, will reduce the opportunities for fraud. Fraud should be contained with regular monitoring, an active QA unit and an increasing role for inspectors from the regulatory agencies. Statisticians should routinely scrutinise demographic differences in the subjects recruited at one centre compared with other centres, clustering of laboratory data, and variations in data to establish both the scientific significance of the results and also whether the data of a particular site need investigation for fraud.[1]

Sponsors must have an SOP describing what to do when fraud is suspected. Where possible, additional evidence should be obtained, usually by a competent QA auditor. In the meantime, only the minimum key individuals should be made aware of the problem until sufficient evidence has been obtained to establish the truth. The appropriate authorities such as the national drug industry organisation and the regulatory authorities should be informed if fraud has taken place. In the UK, the sponsor is obliged to report serious breaches of the protocol or GCP (such as fraud or misconduct) to the regulatory authorities and the ethics committee within 7 days. Sometimes, other sponsors will have reported additional evidence that fraud is taking place at a particular site. The site must be closed if trial subjects are still being recruited, and a full explanation provided to the authorities. Any clinical data collected will need to be reviewed and a decision made as to whether any of the data can be included in the analysis. To a pharmaceutical

Table 7.4 Methods of detecting fraud

Method	Comment
Check whether the original source data match those that are recorded and reported	Importance of sufficient source documents (e.g. medical records, radiographs and laboratory results)
Do the data fit the chronological order of events?	Do visit dates match collection dates of samples? Is there any evidence that data were recorded or corrections were made out of chronological order?
Check reasons for missing records	Missing records should be explained, file notes or correspondence should confirm explanation
Can you read the deleted entries? Are all the records perfect, without any corrections?	No whiteout; erasures can be read; 'perfect' results on paper without wear and tear should be checked
Establish who is recording the data	Is the investigator signing off the CRF? Are appropriate staff carrying out trial procedures? Do signatures match those on the investigator's signature log? Consent forms should contain more than one handwriting style
Do the data look real?	There should be some variability in the data, and erratic data points. Check variation with other sites using biostatistics
Is the site meeting expectations or does it appear 'too efficient' to have achieved all the work?	Can all the work be carried out in the timeframe allowed with the facilities and equipment available?

physician, fraud is never an easy situation. It usually involves a professional colleague and there is always the worry that the established facts have been misinterpreted. However, a fraudulent individual cannot be tolerated in modern clinical research.

Fraud is not limited to the investigator and his or her staff. Staff of pharmaceutical companies and institutions may alter CRFs, modify data sets, alter tables, suppress reported side effects or bias written reports. The detection of such activities, inside or outside an institution, by investigators or company staff relies on others in the same team recognising that something is suspicious. Double-checking of data by colleagues and authentication of those data is the best deterrent to misconduct.

7.8 Conclusions

Increased regulation of clinical trials in the last few years, particularly in Europe, has led to greater bureaucracy. However, the application of GCP and GMP to all trials, including non-commercial ones, should result in greater protection of subjects and data of a higher quality. The challenge for sponsors and investigators is to keep up-to-date with the ever changing regulatory requirements, and to interpret those requirements in the best interests of trial subjects without impeding research.

There is no evidence that the investment in manpower and other resources necessary to execute clinical programmes will decrease, and the use of specialist contract organisations in all areas – trial monitoring, data handling, report writing and consultancy – is likely to continue. As companies strive harder for shorter surer paths to regulatory approval, the well-conceived, well-executed and correctly interpreted clinical trial will continue to be pivotal.

References

1 International Conference on Harmonisation (ICH) of Technical Requirements of Pharmaceuticals for Human Use. *Topic E6(R1) Note for Guidance on Good Clinical Practice: Consolidated Guideline, CPMP/ICH/135/95.* London: European Medicines Agency, 1996.

2 European Agency for the Evaluation of Medicinal Products. *Explanatory Note and Comments to the ICH Harmonised Tripartite Guideline E6: Note for Guidance on Good Clinical Practice, CPMP/768/97.* London: European Agency for the Evaluation of Medicinal Products, 1997.

3 Food and Drug Administration (FDA). International conference on harmonisation, good clinical practice: consolidated guidelines. *Fed Regist* 1997;**62**:25692–709.

4 Food and Drug Administration (FDA) *Protection of Human Subjects Code of Federal Regulations, Title 21, Part 50–55.* Washington: US Government Printing Office, 1997.

5 European Parliament. Directive 2001/20/EC of the European parliament and of the council of 4 April 2001 on the approximation of the laws, regulations and administrative provisions of the member states relating to the implementation of Good Clinical Practice in the conduct of clinical trials on medicinal products for human use. *Official J Eur Commun* 2001;**L121**:34–44.

6 European Parliament. Commission Directive 2005/28/EC of 8 April 2005 laying down principles and detailed guidelines for Good Clinical Practice as regards investigational medicinal products for human use, as well as the requirements for authorisation of the manufacturing or importation of such products. *Official J Eur Commun* 2005;**L91**:13–19.

7 World Medical Association (WMA). Declaration of Helsinki, 59th WMA General Assembly, Seoul, October 2008.

8 European Commission. Detailed guidance on the application format and documentation to be submitted in an application for an Ethics Committee opinion on the clinical trial on medicinal products for human use. February 2006. *ENTR/CT 2*, Revision 1.

9 Association of the British Pharmaceutical Industry. *Clinical Trial Compensation Guidelines, 418/94/6600M.* London: ABPI, 1994.

10 Association of the British Pharmaceutical Industry. *Guidelines for Phase 1 Clinical Trials, 4th edn.* 1 July 2007.

11 European Parliament. Directive 95/46/EC of the European Parliament and of the Council of 24 October 1995 on the protection of individuals with regard to the processing of personal data and on the free movement of such data. *Official J Eur Commun* 1995;**L281**:31–50.

12 Hochhauser M. The informed consent form: document development and evaluation. *Drug Inf J* 2000;**34**:1309–17.

13 National Research Ethics Service. *Information Sheets and Consent Forms: Guidance for Researchers and Reviewers.* Version 3, 2 May 2007.

14 National Research Ethics Service. *Standard Operating Procedures for Research Ethics Committees.* Version 4.0. April 2009.

15 Doclo RJ. Improving SOP writing with process mapping. *Appl Clin Trials* 2000;**9**:62–70.

16 European Commission. Volume 4. Good manufacturing practices. Annex 13. *Manufacture of Investigational Medicinal Products.* July 2003. F2/BL D(2003). Revision 1.

17 European Commission. The rules governing medicinal products in the European Union. Volume 4. *Good Manufacturing Practice (GMP) Guidelines.* Luxembourg: Commission Office for Official Publications of the EC, 1992.

18 Food and Drug Administration (FDA). *Current Good Manufacturing Practice in Manufacturing, Processing, Packaging or Holding of Drugs; General. Code of Federal Regulations 210, 211*. Washington DC: National Archives and Records Administration, 1997.

19 European Medicines Agency, Committee for Proprietary Medicinal Products. *Note for Guideline on the Investigation of Bioequivalence, CPMP/EWP/QWP/1401/98. Rev 1*. London, July 2008 (Draft).

20 Double ME, McKendry M. *Computer Validation Compliance*. Buffalo Grove, IL: Interpharm, 1994.

21 Food and Drug Administration (FDA). *Guidance for Industry: Computerised Systems Used in Clinical Trials*. Rockville, MD: Division of Compliance Policy, 1999.

22 International Society for Pharmaceutical Engineering (ISPE). Good Automated Manufacturing Practice (GAMP). *GAMP 5: A Risk-based Approach to Compliant GxP Computerized Systems*. January 2008.

23 O'Shea K. Interactive voice response technology. *Appl Clin Trials* 1998;7:30–4.

24 Food and Drug Administration (FDA). *Guidance for Industry: Using a Centralized IRB Review Process in Multicenter Clinical Trials*. March 2006.

25 European Commission. Detailed guidance for the request for authorisation of a clinical trial on a medicinal product for human use to the competent authorities, notification of substantial amendments and declaration of the end of the trial. October 2005. *ENTR/F2/BL D(2003)/CT 1.* Revision 2.

26 Food and Drug Administration (FDA). *Investigational New Drug Application. 21 Code of Federal Regulations Part 312.* Washington DC: National Archives and Records Administration, 1998.

27 Tarantowski R. Writing a clinical trial budget. *Appl Clin Trials* 1996;5:26–40.

28 Food and Drug Administration (FDA). Financial disclosure by clinical investigators. Title 21 Code of Federal Regulations Parts 54, 312, 314, 320, 330, 601, 807. *Fed Regist* 1998;63:5233–54.

29 Food and Drug Administration (FDA). Recruiting study subjects. In: *Guidance for Institutional Review Boards and Clinical Investigators Section in Information Sheets*. Rockville, MD: Office of the Associated Commissioner for Health Affairs, 1998 (update).

30 Edwards RI, Aronson JK. Adverse drug reactions: definitions, diagnosis and management. *Lancet* 2000;356: 1255–9.

31 International Conference on Harmonisation (ICH) of Technical Requirements of Pharmaceuticals for Human Use. *Topic 2A Note for Guidance on Clinical Safety Data Management: Definitions and Standards for Expedited Reporting, CPMP/ICH/377/95*. London: European Medicines Agency, 1995.

32 Karch FE, Lasagna MD. Adverse drug reaction. *JAMA* 1975;234:1236–41.

33 International Conference on Harmonisation (ICH) of Technical Requirements of Pharmaceuticals for Human Use. *Draft Consensus Guideline: Revision of the E2B(R2) ICH Guideline (previously coded E2B(M)) on Clinical Safety Data Management Data Elements for Transmission of Individual Case Safety Reports*. 2003.

34 Rosenzweig P, Miget N, Brohier S. Transaminase elevation on placebo during phase I trials: prevalence and significance. *Br J Clin Pharmacol* 1999;48:19–23.

35 Purkins L, Love ER, Eve MD, Wooldridge CL, Cowan C, Smart TS et al. The influence of diet upon liver function tests and serum lipids in healthy male volunteers resident in a Phase I unit. *Br J Clin Pharmacol* 2004;57: 199–208.

36 Food and Drug Administration (FDA). Code of Federal Regulations Title 21, Part 11, electronic records and electronic signatures. *Fed Regist* 1997;62:13 430–66.

37 Medical Dictionary for Regulatory Activities (MedDRA). http://www.meddramsso.com/MSSOWeb/index.htm

38 International Conference on Harmonisation (ICH) of Technical Requirements of Pharmaceuticals for Human Use. *Topic E10 Note for Guidance on Choice of Control Group in Clinical Trials, CPMP/ICH/364/96*. London: European Medicines Agency, 2001.

39 International Conference on Harmonisation (ICH) of Technical Requirements of Pharmaceuticals for Human Use. *Topic E9 Note for Guidance on Statistical Considerations in the Design of Clinical Trials, CPMP/ICH/363/96*. London: European Medicines Agency, 1998.

40 International Conference on Harmonisation (ICH) of Technical Requirements of Pharmaceuticals for Human Use. *Topic E4 Note for Guidance on Dose Response Information to Support Drug Registration, CPMP/ICH/378/95*. London: European Medicines Agency, 1994.

41 Food and Drug Administration (FDA). *Compliance Program Guidance Manual (7348.811) Clinical Investigators*. Rockville, MD: Division of Compliance Policy, 1999.

42 Food and Drug Administration (FDA). *Compliance Program Guidance Manual (7348.810) Sponsors, Contract Research Organisations and Monitors*. Rockville, MD: Division of Compliance Policy, 1999.

43 Expert Scientific Group on Phase One Clinical Trials. *Final Report*. The Stationery Office, UK: 30 November 2006.

44 International Conference on Harmonisation (ICH) of Technical Requirements of Pharmaceuticals for Human Use. *Topic E3 Note for Guidance on Structure and Content of Clinical Study Reports, CPMP/ICH/137/95*. London: European Medicines Agency, 1996.

45 International Conference on Harmonisation (ICH) of Technical Requirements of Pharmaceuticals for Human Use. *Topic M4 Common Technical Document for the Registration of Pharmaceuticals for Human Use – Organisation CTD, CPMP/ICH/2887/99*. London: European Medicines Agency, 2004.

46 Feigenbaum AV. *Total Quality Control*. New York: McGraw-Hill, 1951.

47 European Foundation for Quality Management. The Excellence Model. Brussels: European Foundation for

Quality Management. Available at: http://www.efgm.org.html.

48 International Organization for Standardization. *ISO 9001: 2008. Quality Management Systems – Requirements.* Bsi (British Standards), 30 Nov 2008.

49 Sweeney F. Merging GCP and ISO 9000 requirements: a source of synergy in quality management of clinical research. *Drug Inf J* 1994;**28**:1097–104.

50 Campbell H, Sweatman J. Quality assurance and clinical data management. In: Rondel RK, Varley SA, Webb CF, eds. *Clinical Data Management, 2nd edn.* Chichester, UK: John Wiley, 2000;123–41.

51 Buyse M, George SL, Evans S et al. The role of biostatistics in the prevention, detection and treatment of fraud in clinical trials. *Stat Med* 1999;**18**:3435–51.

52 Mackintosh DR, Zepp VJ. Detection of negligence, fraud and other bad faith efforts during field auditing of clinical trial sites. *Drug Inf J* 1996;**30**:645–53.

53 Lock S, ed. *Fraud and Misconduct in Medical Research, 2nd edn.* London: BMJ Publishing, 1996.

Further reading

Friedman LM, Furberg CD, DeMets DL. *Fundamentals of Clinical Trials, 3rd edn.* New York: Springer-Verlag, 1998.

Senn S. *Statistical Issues in Drug Development.* Chichester, UK: John Wiley, 1997.

Spilker B. *Guide to Clinical Trials.* New York: Raven Press, 1991.

Useful internet addresses

British Pharmacopoeia. www.pharmacopoeia.org.uk

Centers for Disease Control and Prevention. www.cdc.gov

Drug Information Association. www.diahome.org

European Drug Regulatory Affairs. ec.europa.eu/enterprise/pharmaceuticals/eudralex/eudralex_en.htms

European National Medicines Authorities. www.heads.medagencies.org

Food and Drug Administration (FDA). www.fda.gov

Food and Drug Law Institute (FDLI). www.fdli.org

International Conference on Harmonisation (ICH). www.ifpma.org/ichl.htmi

Medicines and Healthcare Products Regulatory Agency (MHRA). www.mhra.gov.uk

National Institutes of Health. www.nih.gov

National Research Ethics Service (NRES). www.nres.npsa.nhs.uk

Pharmaceutical Research Manufacturers Association. www.phrma.org

Regulatory Affairs Professional Society (RAPS). www.raps.org

US Pharmacopeia. www.usp.org

World Health Organization (WHO). www.who.ch

8 Medical statistics

Andrew P. Grieve

Formerly at Pfizer Global Research and Development Sandwich, UK

8.1 Introduction

The rapid accrual of biomedical information has led to considerable interest both in the notion of evidence-based medicine and also in the history of the use of quantitative evidence in medicine. Tröhler[1] has shown that the origins of a quantitative approach to medicine can be traced back to the 18th century in Britain. It was a movement begun by physicians who believed that there was a need to move to an empirical approach to medicine and away from the systemic pathophysiological approach of antiquity.

Today, statistics is a necessary and important link in the interdisciplinary chain of drug discovery and development. There is no part of the drug development process where statistics does not have a place: from screening chemicals for activity in drug discovery, through all phases of clinical development, through pharmaceutical development and manufacturing, to the forecasting of the potential sales of a new drug. In all of these contexts statisticians and statistics are involved in helping scientists understand the size of effects relative to considerable variability, whether it is biological variability, in the animal or human case, or seasonal variability when it comes to forecasting sales of an antihistamine. In this chapter, we concentrate on the application of statistics to clinical research.

8.2 Probability

The basis of all statistical inference is probability and in order to understand ideas such as confidence inter-

vals and significance tests, a basic understanding of probability is necessary.

8.2.1 What is probability?

What does it mean to say 'The probability of heads is half when a coin is tossed?' It simply means that if we were to toss a coin very many times, heads would occur approximately half of the time. If we were to toss the coin 1000 times we would expect to get about 500 heads – not exactly 500 heads, but about 500 heads. Of course, if we were to toss the coin only twice, there is no guarantee that heads will occur only once. If we were to toss the coin four times, there is no guarantee that heads will occur twice. So what can we say about the distribution of likely outcomes in this latter case? How likely is it that we might get three heads and a single tail? We can determine how likely different outcomes are by enumeration. Table 8.1 gives the possible outcomes from tossing a coin four times.

Allowing for the order of the occurrences of heads and tails, we can readily determine the probability

Table 8.1 Enumeration of the results of tossing a coin four times

	Number of heads				
	0	1	2	3	4
	TTTT	TTTH	TTHH	THHH	HHHH
		TTHT	THTH	HTHH	
		THTT	THHT	HHTH	
		HTTT	HTTH	HHHT	
			HTHT		
			HHTT		
Total (16)	1	4	6	4	1

The Textbook of Pharmaceutical Medicine. Edited by John P. Griffin. © 2009, ISBN: 978-1-4051-8035-1.

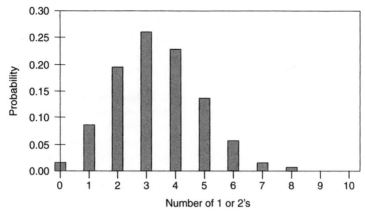

Figure 8.1 Distribution of the number of one's or two's out of 10.

of given outcomes. For example, the probability of getting three heads and one tail can be seen to be $^4/_{16} = 0.25$.

As a second example, the chance of getting a one or two from throwing a fair die is $^1/_3$. What is the likely outcome if the fair die is tossed 10 times? Enumeration could again be used to determine the probability of zero, one, two, etc., occurrences of one or two. As a result of the process the distribution of outcomes is shown in Figure 8.1 from which it is determined that the most likely outcome is three out of 10 with a probability of just over one-quarter; the probability of getting zero occurrences is approximately one in 60; there is a very small probability of getting eight or more occurrences.

The distribution illustrated in Figure 8.1 is an example of what is called a sampling distribution and it will be important when we come to consider statistical tests.

8.2.2 Inductive probability

The sampling distribution determined in the previous section is an example of a deductive use of probability. Given that the probability of an occurrence of a one or two is known, we were able to deduce the probability of the outcomes that could arise if the die was tossed 10 times. In medical research, however, we do not know what the true probability (response probability) is. Ours is the reverse problem, we observe a response rate, for example, 23 out of 80 patients respond positively to a given treatment, and want to infer what the true population response rate is. The requirement is to be able to make inductive probability statements.

To illustrate, consider the following information about asymptomatic women participating in breast screening given by Gigerenzer.[2]
1. The probability of any woman having breast cancer is 0.8% (less than one in 100);
2. If a woman has breast cancer, the probability of a positive mammogram is 90%;
3. If a woman does not have breast cancer, the probability of a positive mammogram is 7%.

Suppose that a woman has a positive mammogram. What is the probability that she in fact has breast cancer? To solve this problem statisticians use Bayes' theorem, a theorem in conditional probability introduced by the non-conformist minister Reverend Thomas Bayes in 1763.[3] Gigerenzer explains how Bayes' theorem works by converting the problem into 'natural frequencies'.

If there are 100,000 asymptomatic patients in the population, then 800 will have breast cancer (0.8%; 1). Of these, 720 (90%; 2) will have a positive mammogram. The remaining 99,200 women do not have breast cancer, but 6944 (7%; 3) will nevertheless have a positive mammogram. Therefore, in total 7664 women will have a positive mammogram, of which 720 would in reality have breast cancer. Thus, the probability that a woman with a positive mammogram has breast cancer is 720/7644 = 9.4%.

While the use of Bayes' theorem in this context is not generally controversial, its use more generally in medical and clinical research has not always been positively received.[4] It is not the scope of the present chapter to illustrate the use of Bayesian statistics in a more general context and interested readers should read the excellent introduction to the use of Bayesian methods in health care evaluation provided by Spiegelhalter et al.[5]

8.3 Scales of measurement and clinical endpoints

When you can measure what you are speaking about, and express it in numbers, you know something about it; but when you cannot measure it, when you cannot express it in numbers, your knowledge is of a meagre and unsatisfactory kind: it may be the beginning of knowledge, but you have scarcely, in your thoughts, advanced to the stage of science.[6]

The movement towards quantification in medicine required the development of measures of clinical effect. When assessing the effectiveness of his approach to removing bladder stones, the lithotomist William Cheselden measured the impact on mortality by determining the proportion of patients who died.[1] Similarly, when measuring the pain relief of a treatment for migraine headache we need to define and measure pain. In whatever circumstances we are researching – heart disease, depression, etc. – we have to measure the severity and extent of the disease. From a statistical perspective, what is important is the scale of measurement. Statisticians generally recognise three types of scale: qualitative, ordinal and quantitative.

8.3.1 Qualitative data

The simplest form of qualitative data is binary data in which there are only two possible values (e.g. death/survival, or success/failure), each of which needs to be defined within a specified time interval, has pain relief been achieved within 2 h of treatment, success – or not, failure. This form of data is extremely common in medical research and yet it ignores the possibility of gradation, success may not be total but only partial and yet not be total failure. These considerations lead naturally to the concept of ordered categorical or ordinal data.

As its name implies, the defining property of ordinal data is that there is a natural ranking in the outcome. For example, the pain associated with migraine headache is often measured on a 4-point ordinal scale: absent, mild, moderate or severe; wherein the pain being absent is better than experiencing a mild pain, is better than experiencing a moderate pain, is better than experiencing a severe pain. Often the categories are assigned a numerical value: 0 = absent, 1 = mild, 2 = moderate and 3 = severe,

but care needs to be taken in the interpretation of such numbers because they do not comprise a true numerical scale. Thus, the difference between absent and mild is not necessarily equivalent to the difference between mild and moderate.

8.3.2 Quantitative data

There are two main types of quantitative data: discrete and continuous. Discrete quantitative data usually come about by the counting of numbers of events. Examples of this form of data are the number of asthma attacks, the numbers of rescue tablets taken or the number of relapse events. There are two types of continuous quantitative data defined by whether there is a true zero point of the scale or not. If there is such a zero point the scale is a ratio scale, otherwise it is an interval scale. Examples of the former are height, weight or volume, while a typical example of the latter is temperature in which the origin is essentially arbitrary – 0°F is not equivalent to 0°C. In practice, this distinction has no impact on the statistical analysis of data and the same techniques are applied to data from both ratio and interval scales.

8.3.3 Measurement and endpoints

It is important when choosing a particular measurement scale to answer a number of questions. Is the choice that is made of clinical relevance? How is the endpoint to be measured? Can we measure the clinical endpoint directly, or must we choose an indirect approach? Is the choice that is made sensitive enough to measure real treatment effects? Having collected the information how are we to analyse it? Some of these issues are illustrated in the following sections.

8.3.3.1 Responder rates

Increasingly, clinical researchers ask questions such as: what proportion of patients responds to treatment A? Do a greater proportion of patients respond to active treatment rather than placebo? In these circumstances, the endpoints tend not to be directly measured but are derived from other measurements. For example, suppose we are interested in measuring the reduction in blood pressure following treatment, in particular the primary interest is in determining the proportion of patients who experience a reduction of at least 15 mmHg – defining such improvement as being a response. Figure 8.2 shows data from 100 patients with the responder cut-point also being displayed. We can determine from the distribution

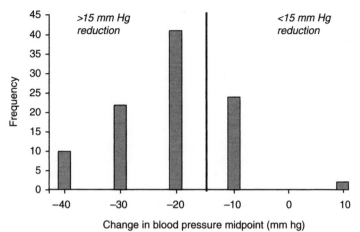

Figure 8.2 Distribution of change in blood pressure (mmHg).

that 73% of patients are classified as responders. Alternatively, we can fit a mathematical distribution to the data and estimate the rate from properties of the distribution. From the data in Figure 8.2 we can estimate the arithmetic mean of the data as well as the standard deviation (defined in sections 8.4.1.1 and 8.4.1.2) giving values of 26.8 and 10 mmHg. If the data can be assumed to follow a normal distribution then we can estimate that 76% of the distribution will lie below −15 mmHg.

The first point to be made is that if we can use a mathematical distribution to estimate the responder rate, it is more efficient than to count the number of observations meeting the condition. Such efficiency gains mean that using the distribution we will need fewer patients to estimate the rate to the same degree of accuracy. Senn[7] reports that the former approach can give rise to sample sizes 40% higher than using the original measurements. Intuitively, this is reasonable because the use of a cut-point essentially says that we can distinguish between a reduction of 14.9 and 15.1 mmHg, whereas in reality those two measurements are essentially equivalent in terms of the information they provide about the benefit of a treatment. Secondly, the choice of the cut-point is itself arbitrary. Why should a reduction of 15 mmHg be any more important than any other? In his article, Senn strongly criticises this approach. However, it is widely used and does have its own supporters.[8]

8.3.3.2 Biomarkers and surrogate endpoints

In clinical trials intended to provide sufficient evid-

ence for marketing approval of drugs, what is most important is to collect unequivocal evidence of a positive risk–benefit profile relative to an active comparator or placebo. For diseases that are life-threatening or those associated with severe morbidity, it is preferable that the primary endpoint is of clinical relevance, examples being mortality, a measurement of the patient's quality of life, such as relief of disease-related symptoms, improvement in ability to carry out normal activities or reduced hospitalization time. Unfortunately, such trials may need to be very large; consequently, they tend to have a long duration, and can be extremely costly.

In such circumstances there is an inevitable desire to find alternative surrogate endpoints that allow the length and size of clinical trials to be considerably reduced.[9] A common approach has been to utilise endpoints that are correlated with the outcome of primary interest. Minimally, all that this may require is that patients who experience some benefit on the surrogate tend to experience benefit on the clinically meaningful endpoint. While such an approach may be useful to demonstrate biological activity, in general it is not sufficient to make a reliable demonstration that a treatment will also positively impact the true clinical endpoint. As Fleming and DeMets[10] note, 'a correlate does not a surrogate make'. What is required is that the effect of treatment on the biomarker correlates well with that on the final endpoint, so that a valid surrogate endpoint allows correct inference to be drawn regarding the effect of an intervention on the true clinical endpoint of interest.

Many statistical approaches have been proposed to ensure the validity of surrogates. The seminal work of Prentice[11] which focused on hypothesis testing has been followed by estimation-based methods such as Buyse and Molenberghs,[12–15] which aim to quantify the degree of validity of a surrogate.

There are many examples of biomarkers, which have been used as surrogates[10] in prominent clinical trials that have been subsequently found to be inadequate, illustrating the difficulty in identifying a surrogate endpoint. One notable scenario is that of a biomarker that responds to therapy and is highly predictive of survival, but does not predict the effect of treatment on survival. The use of $CD4^+$ counts in HIV trials is an example of such a biomarker.[16,17]

Temple[18] has argued that there may be problems in correctly assessing the risk–benefit profile of a drug on the basis of findings on a surrogate. This may be the case, if the relationship between the biomarker and the clinical endpoint is coincidental or corelated by a third factor. Furthermore, favourable or unfavourable drug effects may remain undetected by the surrogate.[19]

Finally, there are time issues associated with biomarkers and surrogates. Biomarkers may be better predictors of short-term treatment effects than long-term effects[20] and therefore we need to be specific about the timing of outcome assessment when evaluating a biomarker. A distinction is drawn by Hughes et al.[21] between a concurrent surrogate, measured during the same time period as the clinical endpoint and an intermediate surrogate, which explains the effect of treatment on a clinical endpoint at some future time point.

8.3.3.3 Rating scales

In section 8.3.1 we introduced the idea of a simple ordinal rating scale such as the four-point scale for a migraine headache: absent, mild, moderate, severe. Another simple approach to measurement is the so-called visual analogue scale (VAS). The VAS is simply a line – normally 100 mm long – the ends of which are associated with descriptions of opposite extremes of the disease. For example, in the treatment of depression the descriptions might be: 'Couldn't be feeling better' and 'Couldn't be more depressed'. The patient marks on the line where his or her current experience of depression falls.

The advantage of this approach over a simple ordinal scale is that it has the characteristics of a continuous scale, and hence more sensitive methods can be used and potentially at least will result in smaller

sizes. However, there are questions that are often raised concerning this approach:

• Can patients understand what they are supposed to do?
• If patients rate themselves on a VAS scale on two occasions when their disease is stable, will they provide similar results?
• Do patients use the scale in a similar way?[22]

All the evidence available in the literature suggests that in general these concerns should not preclude the use of VAS scales in clinical studies.

In some diseases, a simple ordinal scale or a VAS scale cannot describe the full spectrum of the disease. There are many examples of this including depression and erectile dysfunction. Measurement in such circumstances involves the use of multiple ordinal rating scales, often termed items. A patient is scored on each item and the summation of the scores on the individual items represents an overall assessment of the severity of the patient's disease status at the time of measurement. Considerable amounts of work have to be carried out to ensure the validity of these complex scales, including investigations of their reproducibility and sensitivity to measuring treatment effects. It may also be important in international trials to assess to what extent there is cross-cultural uniformity in the use and understanding of the scales. Complex statistical techniques such as principal components analysis and factor analysis are used as part of this process and one of the issues that need to be addressed is whether the individual items should be given equal weighting.

The use of these multiple rating scales is an attempt to develop a simple representation of what may be an extremely complex construct. Part of the statistical developments of these scales will be to identify so-called subdomains of the disease (e.g. physical, emotional and sexual). The identification of these subdomains will require close collaboration between the statistician and the clinical researcher in the interpretation of the results.

8.4 Basic statistical principles

There are two principal forms of statistics: descriptive and inferential. The purpose of descriptive statistics is to give a description of the data that have been collected, whether from a clinical trial, epidemiological investigation or survey. Inferential statistics is aimed at making probability-based statements about hypotheses, parameters of populations, etc.

8.4.1 Descriptive statistics

A major part of descriptive statistics is the use of graphical methods to represent data. It is not the scope of this chapter to cover graphical methods; however, it is good statistical practice to produce a visual summary of data. In the following sections we concentrate on summary statistics that describe important aspects of data.

8.4.1.1 Measures of location and central tendency

The idea behind measures of location and central tendency is contained within the notion of the average. There are predominantly three summary statistics that are commonly used for describing this aspect of a set of data: the arithmetic mean – normally shortened to the mean, the mode and the median.

1. The mean of a set of values is determined by dividing the sum of the values by the number of values. It is mostly utilised for quantitative data, but if applied to binary that has been coded 0 or 1, the mean is the proportion or rate with the given characteristic.

2. The median is the typical value. It is the midpoint of the values when arranged in ascending order and has 50% of the values above it and 50% below it. The median can be used for both quantitative and ordinal data. If there are an even number of values and therefore strictly no middle value, the average of the two middle values is taken.

3. The mode is the most commonly occurring value and can be used for qualitative, ordinal as well as quantitative data.

The data listed below and displayed in Figure 8.3 are random measurements of blood glucose (mmol/L) taken from 40 first year medical students.[23]

2.2	2.9	3.3 3.3 3.3
3.4 3.4 3.4	3.6 3.6 3.6	3.7 3.7
	3.6	
3.8 3.8 3.8	3.9	4.0 4.0 4.0
4.1 4.1 4.1	4.2	4.3
4.4 4.4 4.4	4.5	4.6
4.7 4.7 4.7	4.8	4.9 4.9
5.0	5.1	6.0

The arithmetic mean is:

$$\frac{2.2 + 2.9 + \cdots + 5.1 + 6.0}{40} = \frac{162.2}{40}$$

$$= 4.055 \text{ mmol/L}$$

As there are 40 values the median is determined by the average of the 20th and 21st values. Because these are both 4.0, the median is 4.0 mmol/L. The value 3.6 mmol/L occurs four times, more than any other, so 3.6 mmol/L is the modal value. The three summary statistics are displayed in Figure 8.3. Clearly, for this data the mean and median are similar, and this is true for any distribution of values that is symmetric, which is the case here. The mode is somewhat removed from both the mean and median. In fact, the mode is not often used as a summary of data because it records only the most frequent value, and this may be far from the centre of the distribution. A second difficulty with the mode is that there can be more than one mode in a sample. For example, had one of the values 3.6 been instead 3.5, there would have been eight distinct modal values: 3.3, 3.4, 3.6, 3.8, 4.0, 4.1, 4.4 and 4.7 mmol/L.

The median does not use the actual numerical values; rather it uses their relative magnitudes. The

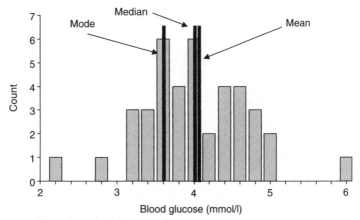

Figure 8.3 Distribution of blood glucose levels from 40 students.

median remains unaffected by extreme values far out into the tails of the distribution. For example, had the value 6.0 mmol/L been 16.0 mmol/L, the median value would have remained unchanged at 4.0 mmol/L.

The mean uses the most information from the sample, relying as it does on the actual numerical values. It is the most commonly used measure of location and therefore can be misused. For example, we have noted that it is inappropriate to use it for ordered categorical data such as: 0 = absent, 1 = mild, 2 = moderate, 3 = severe, because in taking an average the implicit assumption is being made that a change from absent to mild is identical to a change from moderate to severe. The arithmetic mean is also sensitive to discrepant values. For a sample in which the value 6.0 mmol/L is replaced by 16.0 mmol/L, the mean changes from 4.055 mmol/L to 4.305 mmol/L. For this reason, the mean should not be used when data are asymmetric.

Figure 8.4 shows serum triglyceride level in cord blood from 282 babies.[23] Clearly, these data are not symmetric. The arithmetic mean is 0.506 units, while the median is 0.460 units. Bland[23] has shown that the logarithms of the data are remarkably symmetrical and, under such conditions, a more appropriate measure of location is the geometric mean, which can be calculated in two steps. First, the data are log-transformed and the arithmetic mean of the log-transformed data is calculated. Second, the arithmetic mean is back transformed using an exponential function to give the geometric mean. For the triglyceride data, the arithmetic mean of the log-transformed data is −0.761, and the corresponding geometric mean is 0.467 units, which is considerably closer to the median.

A final measure of location is the harmonic mean. This is rarely used explicitly although again it may be implicitly used. For example, when considering the analysis of heart rate data, many statisticians would recommend that the reciprocal of the heart rate be analysed rather than the heart rate itself. Again, this has to do with an attempt to make the distribution of the transformed variable be more symmetric. The resulting variable is the duration of a heartbeat. If the arithmetic mean of the durations is determined and the reciprocal of this value taken, the resulting summary is the harmonic mean of the original heart rate data.

8.4.1.2 Measures of variability

In the previous section, we covered different summary measures for the location of a set of data. Measures of location on their own are not sufficient to characterise data. We also need to be able to measure the variability in data, a measure that indicates to what extent individual measurements differ from one another.

The simplest such measure is the range measuring the interval between the smallest and largest values in the sample. Although simple, it has the disadvantage that it tends to increase with sample size, because in larger samples we are increasingly likely to see extreme values. For the blood glucose data the range is 6.0 − 2.2 = 3.8 mmol/L.

A second simple measure of variability is the interquartile range which is the interval between the upper and lower quartiles. The upper quartile of a set of data is that value that is less than 25% of the data and greater than 75%; similarly, the lower quartile is the value that is greater than 25% of the data and less than

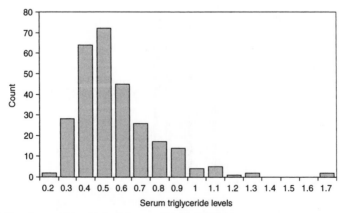

Figure 8.4 Distribution of serum triglyceride levels from cord blood of 282 babies.

75%. For the blood glucose data the lower quartile is 3.6 mmol/L and the upper quartile 4.55 mmol/L, giving an interquartile range of 0.95 mmol/L.

Like the median, neither of these ranges accounts for the numerical values of all the data, only their relative magnitudes. The standard deviation, which is the square root of the variance, accounts for the individual magnitudes and is a measure of the average squared-deviation of individual values from the sample mean. If the individual values are denoted by y_i, $i = 1, \ldots, n$ and the sample mean by $\bar{y}$, then the sample variance is:

$$\frac{\sum_{i=11}^{n}(y_i - \bar{y})^2}{n}$$

from which the standard deviation is directly

$$s = \sqrt{\frac{\sum_{i=11}^{n}(y_i - \bar{y})^2}{n}}$$

It is usual to replace the n in the denominator by $(n-1)$ so that the resulting estimate of the population value is unbiased. For the blood glucose data the variance is 0.488 and the standard deviation 0.698.

The measures we have considered have been to do with the sample and while this may be of interest in its own right, more often we will be interested in understanding the variability not of the sample, but of a statistic based on the sample. In order to think about the variability of a statistic we need to consider again the sampling distribution of a statistic in just the way we did in section 2.1.

To illustrate the point we can conduct a sampling experiment. Suppose that the 40 blood glucose measurements in Figure 8.3 comprised the total population of values. A sampling experiment can be carried out by randomly selecting values from the original 40, calculating their mean and repeating the process for a given number of times. Concretely, we took 40 random samples of size 10 from the population of blood glucose values. This gives us 40 sample means that are not equal to one another, so like the original measurements they show random variability. There are a very large number of ways of choosing 10 values from 40, and the 40 that have been chosen are a random sample from the so-called sampling distribution of the mean.

In Figure 8.5 we display both the population histogram as well as the histogram of sample means, and clearly these distributions differ. Because the 40 values are themselves a random sample from a distribution, we can determine certain characteristics of the distribution, for example, the sample mean and standard deviation. The mean of the means is 4.102 mmol/L and the standard deviation is 0.177 mmol/L. The original population mean was 4.055 mmol/L so that the mean of the sampling distribution is reasonably close to it. In contrast, the standard deviation of the population was 0.698 mmol/L and that is considerably larger than the standard deviation from the sampling distribution. This result mirrors intuition

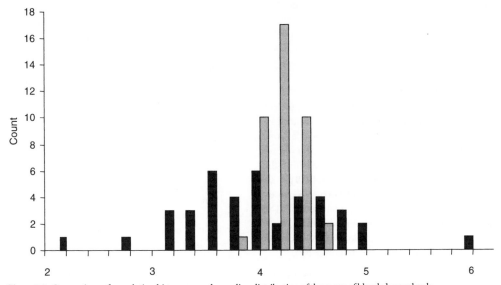

Figure 8.5 Comparison of population histogram and sampling distribution of the mean of blood glucose levels.

because we would expect sampling means to be less variable than the individual population values. The standard deviation of this sampling distribution is known as the standard error of the mean. For the original 40 blood glucose level values the standard of the mean is $0.698/\sqrt{40} = 0.110$.

This example shows that the standard deviation of the sampling distribution is less than that of the population. In fact, this reduction in the variability is related to the sample size used to calculate the sample means. For example, if we repeat the sampling experiment, but this time based on 15 rather than 10 random samples, the resulting standard deviation of the sampling is 0.159, and on 25 random samples it is 0.081. The precise relationship between the population standard deviation or and the standard error of the mean is:

$$\text{s.e.(mean)} = \frac{\sigma}{\sqrt{n}}$$

The difference between these two concepts, the population standard deviation and the standard error of the mean, is important and we will return to it when considering confidence intervals.

8.4.2 Inferential statistics

Historically, the role of statistics in biomedical research has been largely to test hypotheses. More recently, there has been a move to supplant hypothesis tests from their dominant position by confidence intervals. This move has been endorsed by the International Committee of Medical Journal Editors and climaxed with the publication, under the auspices of the British Medical Journal, of *Statistics with Confidence*.[24] Hypothesis tests and *p*-values continue to be, and will continue to be of importance; this review of medical statistics covers all three.

8.4.2.1 Confidence intervals

The estimation of a parameter alone is not sufficient since a single estimate tells us nothing about how accurate the estimate is. The main purpose of confidence intervals is to indicate the precision, or imprecision, of the estimated statistic as representing the population values. The confidence interval will give us a range of values within which we can have a chosen confidence of it containing the population value. The degree of confidence usually presented is 95%.

When estimating a population mean, the 95% confidence interval is approximately given by

$\bar{y} \pm 1.96 \times s/\sqrt{n}$ (sample mean $\pm$ 1.96 $\times$ standard error of the mean)

Applying this to the blood glucose level data for which we know that the sample mean is 4.055 mmol/L and the standard error is 0.110 mmol/L, the 95% confidence limits are approximately $4.055 \pm 1.96 \times 0.110$ = 3.84–4.13 mmol/L.

One question that is often asked of statisticians is: in what sense can we be 95% confident that the population mean lies within the limits 3.84 and 4.13? To answer the question we can again conduct a sampling experiment as follows. Suppose that the 40 blood glucose measurements in Figure 8.3 comprised the total population of values. For random sample of size 10 from the populations of blood glucose values determine the sample mean, standard error and the corresponding 95% confidence interval. Repeat the process 100 times. The results of such an experiment are shown in Figure 8.6.

In this figure, each individual confidence interval has been drawn as a vertical straight line joining the lower and upper limits. The horizontal line is positioned at the value 4.055 mmol/L – the population mean. This gives us 40 sample means that are not equal to one another, so they on their own – like the original measurement – show random variability. There a very large number of ways of choosing 10 values from 40, and the 40 that have been chosen are a random sample from the so-called sampling distribution of the mean. Clearly, most of the 100 intervals include the population mean value. In fact, 95 of the 100 include the population value, while five of them, indicated by the dashed lines, do not. This demonstrates the basis of confidence in a confidence interval. It is a confidence based on the idea that if we repeat sampling from a population a large number of times and each time determine the confidence interval, then in 95% of the cases the interval will include the population value and in 5% of cases it will not.

From the formula for a confidence interval, its width is determined by three parameters: the sample size, population variability and the degree of confidence. Plainly, if the sample size is increased then we have seen the standard error will be reduced and hence the width of the interval will also be reduced. If we can reduce the variability of the characteristic being studied then we can again reduce the standard error and hence reduce the width. The reduction of variability is not always simple because part of variability is natural biological variability. However, there is also a component of variability that is dependent on the measurement process. For example, when measuring blood pressure we can attempt to reduce variability by: consistently measuring the blood

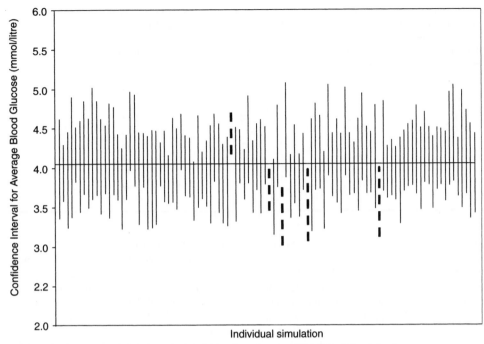

Figure 8.6 Confidence intervals from 100 samples of size 10 from the population of blood glucose levels.

pressure while sitting after a period of rest; taking the measurement at the same time of day; ensure the measurement is taken by the same nurse or doctor; make use of an automatic sphygmomanometer. Finally, by increasing the degree of confidence – say to 99% from 95% – the width of the interval will be increased.

8.4.2.2 Hypothesis tests, tests of significance and p-values

So far we have concentrated on estimation and confidence intervals. Often, however, researchers will be interested in testing specific hypotheses. The vehicle that is used to test hypotheses is generally the significance test. We will illustrate the concepts behind significance tests using the data in Table 8.2.

The data in Table 8.2 are taken from a study reported by Hindle et al.,[25] the purpose of which was to determine whether a new dry powder inhaler (DISK) was equivalent to a traditional metered-dose inhaler (MDI) in its ability to deliver doses of a bronchodilator to the lungs of volunteers. The data are the percentages of an inhaled dose of salbutamol recovered in a urine sample taken 30 min post-inhalation for each method of delivery in nine volunteers. A measure of treatment effect is the difference in percentages within volunteers, shown in the fourth

column. Of these differences seven are negative and two are positive (fifth column) and the question we need to answer is how likely is it that if there is no difference between the inhalers, we would see this degree of imbalance between negatives and positives?

The significance test requires us to specify:

1. A null hypothesis to be tested – defining that there is no difference between the treatments.
2. The null hypothesis is tested against an alternative hypothesis – which defines how the treatments may differ. This will be important when considering sample sizing and power in section 8.5.8. This difference can be in either direction, giving rise to one-sided and two-sided tests.
3. A test statistic – a measure of how much the data depart from the null hypothesis.

If there were truly no difference between the inhalers then we would expect that any individual difference is as likely to be negative as it is to be positive. In other words, in these circumstances the probability of a negative is $1/2$. The null hypothesis then will be:

$$\text{Probability}(MDI > DISK)$$
$$= \text{Probability}(MDI < DISK) = 0.5$$

This is precisely the situation considered in section 8.2.1 where we considered the distribution of heads

Table 8.2 30-min post-inhalation urinary salbutamol excretion (% inhaled dose) in nine subjects following inhalation of 4 × 100 mg salbutamol using a metered-dose inhaler (MDI) and a dry powder inhaler (DISK)

Volunteer	MDI	DISK	Difference	+/−
1	0.70	0.85	−0.15	−
2	0.26	0.80	−0.54	−
3	1.18	0.92	0.26	+
4	1.32	3.45	−2.13	−
5	0.37	3.85	−3.48	−
6	2.18	4.96	−2.78	−
7	2.62	2.11	0.51	+
8	0.85	1.97	−1.12	−
9	1.27	2.47	−1.20	−
Mean	1.19	2.38	−1.18	

and tails from the toss of a coin 10 times. As there, we can determine the sampling distribution of the number of negatives as shown in Figure 8.7. From Figure 8.7 we can see that the probability of achieving exactly seven negatives out of nine is approximately 0.07. This probability is not the p-value. The p-value is the probability that a value of the test statistic as large, or larger than that seen in the study would occur by chance if there were no difference in the treatments. For this example, the p-value is the probability of observing either seven, eight or nine negatives out of nine and this is approximately 0.09. This is a one-sided p-value. If we are interested in alternatives in both directions, we have to consider values as far from the expected number in the other direction. The

expected number of negatives is 4.5 and it is clear from Figure 8.7 that the distribution is symmetric about this value and therefore in the other direction we will be interested in zero, one or two negatives out of nine and this has the same probability, 0.09. The two-sided p-value is the sum of theses two values giving a value of 0.18.

How is the p-value to be interpreted? On one level, it can be interpreted as a measure of how likely it is that pure random variation would give the magnitude of differences seen in the study. If the p-value is small then it can be argued that, all other things being equal, it is unlikely that the differences could be due to chance variation alone. Standardly, a value of 0.05 is often used as a cut-point to determine whether the

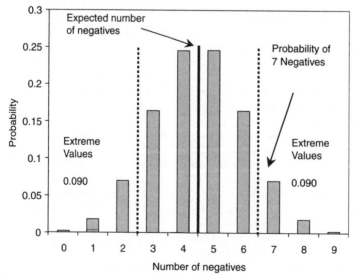

Figure 8.7 Distribution of the number of negatives out of nine given the null hypothesis is true.

p-value is small or not. If the *p*-value is smaller than 0.05 then we could 'reject the null hypothesis', or state the treatments are statistically different. If we strictly follow this rule, then if we were to carry out 100 studies in circumstances in which there was no true difference between the treatments then we would expect, by chance, five times out of these 100 to conclude that the null hypothesis was false. Making a decision to reject a true null hypothesis is termed an error of the first kind, and the probability of such an error under the null hypothesis is called the type I error, significance level or false positive rate.

The test of significance that we used as an illustration utilised only the sign of the differences – whether it was negative or positive. Generally, the actual differences are used. If we think about the differences themselves then if there were no difference between the treatments we would expect the average difference to be zero. This defines the null hypothesis. The sample mean of the differences divided by its standard error is the test statistic and a large value of this statistic would indicate that there is likely to be a difference between the treatments.

The data in Table 8.2 give a sample mean difference of −1.181 percentage units with a standard error of 0.459 giving a test statistic of −1.181/0.459 = −2.573. This should be compared to a so-called Student's *t*-distribution which tells us that – given a suitable tabulation of values – the *p*-value for a difference as large or larger than the average difference seen here is 0.0165 for a one-sided test or 0.0330 for a two-sided test.

8.5 Issues in design

The medical statistician's role in regard to the investigation should be that of obstetrician, rather than morbid anatomist, for it is unfair to expect him or her to extract scientific knowledge by performing a kind of mathematical post-mortem upon the numerical remains of a badly planned study.[26]

Many of the important statistical aspects of clinical trials design are dealt with in detail in Chapter 6 of this volume (S. Warrington) and so here only specific statistical aspects are discussed. The prospect facing us before we conduct a clinical trial is that:

1. We want to collect data concerning the efficacy and safety of a new treatment regime.

2. We want to test hypotheses concerning the drug that are of interest to us.

3. We want to convince the regulators as to the results.

4. We want to convince the prescribers as to the value of the drug.

An important aspect of achieving this is that in the protocol we say what we are going to do; in the statistical analysis plan, developed before the data are collected, we implement what we said we were going to do and carry it through to the statistical analysis itself; finally, in the study report we verify that we did what we said we were going to do. Many of the problems associated with the running of clinical trials would be minimised if clinical researchers followed this simple recipe. This is no more than Good Clinical Practice,[27] or thought of in another way it is similar to Total Quality Management, which recognises that it is preferable to build quality into a product than to try and correct its output. Critical to much of this is a careful understanding of the aims and objectives of the clinical trial.

8.5.1 Study aims and objectives

A key figure in the development of clinical trials methodology in the 20th century was Sir Austin Bradford Hill. In his *Principles of Medical Statistics*,[28] which first appeared as a series of articles in *The Lancet* and was subsequently published as a book, he described the clinical trial as being 'a carefully, and ethically, designed experiment with the aim of answering some precisely framed question'. It is notable that this definition talks of a question, not questions. To illustrate he describes an early trial of streptomycin in which the object was 'to measure the effect of the drug on respiratory tuberculosis'. He points out is that this objective is too vague. Questions that need to be answered are:

• Which aspects of the illness are important?

(a) the minimal lesions on acquisition;

(b) the advanced progressive disease with poor prognosis;

(c) the chronic, relatively inactive state.

• Because speed of recovery depends on age, we need to specify more closely the age groups to be included.

Greater precision is required in the objectives. We need to have:

• A defined population;

• Defined endpoints;

• Relatively few questions to be answered.

As Hill pointed out: 'it would of course be possible deliberately to incorporate more and different groups (of patients) in a trial, but to start out without thought and with all and sundry included, with the hope that the results can somehow be sorted out statistically in the end is to court disaster'. In essence, simplicity is to be admired.

The need for clarity in the objectives of a study is also addressed in drug regulations. Here are four examples:

1. Is a difference sought or is equivalence the objective? The International Conference of Harmonisation (ICH E9)[29] makes it clear that 'it is vital that the protocol of a trial, designed to demonstrate equivalence or non-inferiority contains a clear statement that this is its explicit intention' (ICH E9, Section 3.3.2). In the past if a trial failed to show that a new treatment gave benefit compared to a standard, it was commonplace to claim that the new treatment was therefore as effective as the standard. Such an argument is no longer acceptable as will be discussed in section 8.5.6.

2. Is there a specific subgroup of patients of extra interest? In this case ICH E9 states, 'any claim of treatment efficacy (or lack thereof) or safety based solely on exploratory subgroup analyses are unlikely to be acceptable' (ICH E9, Section 5.7).

3. Is one specific treatment comparison important? 'any aspects of multiplicity . . . should be identified in the protocol; adjustment should always be considered . . . an explanation of why adjustment is not thought necessary should be set out in the analysis plan.' (ICH E9, Section 5.6)

4. Is one variable more important than others? 'Redefinition of the primary variable after unblinding will almost always be unacceptable, since the biases this introduces are difficult to assess' (ICH E9, Section 2.2.2).

The issue covered in the second and third examples relate to elevating the type I error as we carry out more and more individual tests. There are three circumstances in which this may occur:

1. *Multiple comparisons* – in which comparisons are made amongst more than two treatments;
2. *Multiple endpoints* – in which two treatments are compared with many endpoints;
3. *Multiple looks at the data* – examples of which are interim analyses and subgroups.

To illustrate the problem in subgroups, suppose we separately compare treatments in both males and females. Then we have the following possibilities:

		Females	
		Type I error (α)	No type I error $(1-\alpha)$
Males	Type I error (α)	α^2	$\alpha(1-\alpha)$
	No type I error $(1-\alpha)$	$\alpha(1-\alpha)$	$(1-\alpha)^2$

Table 8.3 Impact of multiple subgroup testing on the overall probability of at least one type I error

Number of subgroups	Probability of at least one type I error
2	0.0975
3	0.1426
4	0.1855
5	0.2262
6	0.2649
7	0.3017
8	0.3366
9	0.3598
10	0.4013

From which we can determine the probability of at least one type I error as:

$$\alpha^2 + \alpha(1-\alpha) + \alpha(1-\alpha) = 2\alpha - \alpha^2$$
$$= \alpha(2-\alpha) > \alpha$$

If we are using a standard 5% type I error then this probability $= 0.05(2 - 0.05) = 0.0975$ which is almost twice the prespecified value. As the number of subgroups is increased, this probability grows as is shown in Table 8.3 and this provides the caution that ICH E9 expresses about subgroup analyses.

To illustrate how the type I error may be elevated by using interim analysis we conduct a sampling experiment. The data below are 50 values of the Ritchie Index, a measurement of joint stiffness in patients with rheumatoid arthritis taken from a study reported by Barnes et al.[30] The values were obtained during the study run in a pre-treatment phase.

14	9	8	9	1	20	3	3	2	4
2	3	6	1	2	11	16	24	16	21
19	22	33	12	12	12	19	10	33	2
19	40	1	20	1	2	4	7	9	4
9	6	14	8	27	10	27	7	24	21

The mean of these data is 12.18 units and the standard deviation is 9.69 units. Let us suppose that we wish to test the null hypothesis that the population mean is 12.18, in other words the null hypothesis is true. Suppose also that we can conduct the study in one of the two ways. In the first, we take a random sample of 20 subjects from the population and test the hypothesis at the 5% level at the end of the trial. In the second, we plan to take a maximum of 20 patients from the population, but allow ourselves the option of testing after 10 patients, again at the 5% level, and if the result

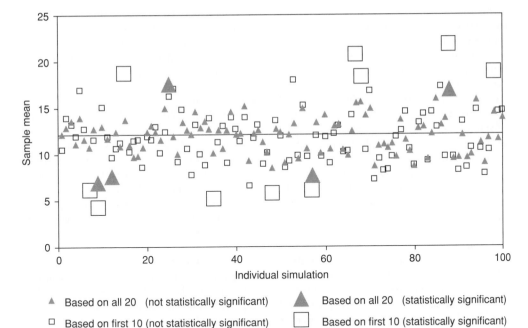

Figure 8.8 Results of a simulation experiment comparing a design with analyses after 10 and 20 patients, and a design with a single analysis after 20 patients.

were significant stopping the trial, otherwise continuing to the end at which point a second 5% level test would be conducted. The sampling experiment consists as before of randomly sampling from the population under each design and then repeating the process a large number of times, in this case 100 times.

The results of the simulation are shown in Figure 8.8. In this figure, we see that in the first design in which there is one analysis after 20 patients, there are five cases where we would falsely declare a significant result and this is consistent with a 5% level of significance. On the other hand, if we were to test at the interim, and if not significant continue to the end, we find that there are in total 12 cases where we would falsely conclude significance. In other words, by repeating the test the false positive rate is increased. In 1969 Armitage et al.[31] investigated issues associated with multiple tests of accumulating data. Their work led directly to the development of group sequential designs and the use of stopping rules initially by Pocock in 1977,[32] O'Brien-Fleming in 1979[33] and the α-spending function of Lan and DeMets in 1983.[34]

There are two potential solutions to this problem. First, we can pre-specify a single test (group) on the primary endpoint at a single point in time, much in line with Hill's views. Or, we can attempt a statistical

solution based on adjusting the type I error for the individual tests.

The group sequential tests are such a statistical solution to the repeated testing case. For multiple subgroups, we can use the so-called Bonferonni[35] correction. In the case of two subgroups this requires us to test each individual subgroup at a type I error of 0.0253 leading to a probability of making at least one type I error of 0.05 as required.

8.5.2 Explanatory/pragmatic trials

As we have seen in many ways, good research is characterised by studies that address a well-defined question. There are essentially two types of questions to be answered: explanatory and pragmatic, a distinction originally drawn by Schwartz et al.[36] Explanatory studies focus on mechanisms looking for a potential benefit by adhering to laboratory conditions, and can be thought of as proof of concept studies. They tend to be scientific in nature, concentrating on furthering scientific knowledge. Pragmatic studies, on the other hand, assess whether such potential can be realised in a more realistic setting, first in phase III confirmatory trials and then ultimately in phase IV or post-marketing trials. They are more likely to be 'technological' in nature with the aim of providing clinically relevant recommendations for treating patients. The distinction between these two types of trials is crucial because it has direct influence on the designs, conduct, analysis and interpretation of the results of the studies. Many studies attempt to answer both type of questions simultaneously but care should be taken in recognising and acknowledging this: 'The protocol should make a clear distinction between the aspects of a trial which will be used for confirmatory proof and the aspects which will provide the basis for explanatory analysis' (ICH E9 Section 2.1.3).

To illustrate how explanatory and pragmatic trials differ from one another we look in turn at subjects, treatments and delivery, outcome measures, conduct and analysis.

8.5.2.1 Subjects

Subjects in an explanatory study are more likely to be high-risk patients in whom a high response can be anticipated, for example, because of a good history of treatment compliance. The population of patients will tend to be relatively homogeneous, controlled by tight inclusion/exclusion criteria and hence the sample size will tend to be relatively small. In contrast, pragmatic studies are more likely to have a much wider inclusion criteria, to ensure representation from the target population. As a consequence, the patients will tend to be more heterogeneous leading to larger sample sizes.

8.5.2.2 Treatment and delivery

In explanatory studies, there is a tendency to compare a new treatment with placebo and to rigidly adhere to single doses of the new treatment in anticipation of maximising treatment compliance. On the other hand, pragmatic studies are more likely to compare the new treatment with the best available alternative and to use a more flexible attitude to dosing, for example, including the possibility of individual dose titration. The delivery of treatment is likely to mimic real-life usage.

8.5.2.3 Outcome measures

In explanatory trials, endpoints are likely to be objective, possibly surrogate, and may be chosen to maximise the sensitivity to detect treatment differences. In contrast, endpoints in pragmatic trials will tend to be more patient-centred including, for example, survival and quality of life.

8.5.2.4 Conduct

The conduct of explanatory trials will include close monitoring of the study in an attempt to ensure strict adherence to the protocol. There is likely to be exhaustive recording of data. In contrast, the conduct of pragmatic trials will tend to mirror real life. There will be attempts to minimise data recording, but there is likely to be exhaustive follow-up of all patients.

8.5.2.5 Analysis

In explanatory trials, we are likely to exclude both protocol violators and treatment non-compliers. The objective behind these exclusions is to increase the efficiency. However, the exclusions may give rise to bias and hence to compromise the results if too many patients are excluded. Such an analysis population is termed as completers, or per protocol, population. In pragmatic trials, we generally include all patients using the intention to treat (ITT) principle.

8.5.2.6 Intention to treat

The purpose of utilising an ITT analysis population is to minimise the bias that can occur by excluding patients who do not complete a trial. The late Professor Ken McRae illustrated the concept using the following simple example.

A physician believes that fell-running is the best treatment following a myocardial infarction. He decides to test this by sending patients to run up Ben Nevis. Of the 25 patients who complete the course (of treatment), all 25 survived for at least 10 years. However, before concluding that fell-running is the best treatment, we should not forget the 25 who refused to the treatment, the 25 who were lost on Ben Nevis and the 25 who die while running.

There are many different definitions of an ITT population tailored to specific diseases or trial designs. Amongst these are the following:
• All randomised patients (in the groups to which they were randomised);
• All randomised patients (correctly allocated);
• All randomised patients with at least one dose of study drug; and
• All randomised patients with at least one dose of study drug and at least one observation of the efficacy variable after baseline.
Whichever definition is to be used it must be defined in the protocol.

One issue that is important to determine is how missing data will be handled in an ITT analysis. ITT was largely developed in clinical trials in which the major endpoints were events, mortality, infarctions, etc. In such studies it is possible to follow-up on patients who withdraw from treatment and determine whether the event has occurred or not and indeed in such trials every effort should be made to do this. For other types of data (e.g. a pain scale) other approaches are necessary.

Very often, a last-observation-carried-forward analysis is carried out in which the last available observation in any patient is used.

8.5.3 Choice of endpoint

It was noted in section 8.3.3 that in choosing the primary endpoint to be used in a study there are a number of questions that need to be considered:

• Which aspects of the disease are we interested in measuring?
• Of the potential endpoints:
(a) Are they clinically meaningful?
(b) Are they relevant to patients?
(c) How is each measured? Can they be measured directly?
(d) Are they sensitive to treatment?
• How do we analyse what we have measured?

To illustrate how there can be a strong link between the endpoint of the method of analysis we consider the case of binary data in the next section.

8.5.3.1 Defining the endpoint for binary data

The data in Table 8.4 have been extracted from an investigation reported by Miranda-Filho et al.[37] who compared the treatment of tetanus by the intrathecal route with the standard intramuscular route. The primary endpoints of the study were disease progression and death and we concentrate here on the former.

Any inferences about the difference between the effects of the two treatments that may be made upon such data are the observed rates, or proportions of deteriorations by the intrathecal route. In this example, amongst those treated by the intrathecal route $22/58 = 0.379$ of patients deteriorated, and the corresponding control rate is $37/60 = 0.617$. The observed

rates are estimates of the population incidence rates, π_t for the test treatment and π_C for the controls. Any representation of differences between the treatments will be based upon these population rates and the estimated measure of the treatment effect will be reported with an associated 95% confidence interval and/or p-value.

Typically, statisticians use one of the three approaches to represent treatment differences for such data: absolute rate reduction (ARR), relative risk (RR) and the odds ratio (OR). In the first approach we look at the difference between rates $\delta = \pi_C - \pi_t$. For this tetanus data, the estimated ARR is $0.617 - 0.379 = 0.238$, indicating that the intrathecal route reduces the rate of deterioration by approximately 24%. The 95% confidence interval associated with this estimate is 0.0621–0.4127 and because the interval does not contain zero the p-value is less than 0.05.

In the case of RR, we look at the ratio of the rates: $\phi = \pi_C/\pi_t$. For the tetanus data, the estimated RR is $0.617/0.379 = 1.63$; in other words, the risk of becoming infected with typhoid among controls is approximately twice that among those inoculated. The 95% confidence interval for the estimated RR is 1.35–2.03, and again because the interval excludes the null value, in this case one, the p-value is less than 0.05.

Finally, the OR is defined as: $\theta = \pi_C(1 - \pi_t)/[\pi_t(1 - \pi_C)]$. For the tetanus data the estimated OR is $0.617 \times 0.621/(0.383 \times 0.379) = 2.63$ and its associated 95% confidence interval is 1.25–5.53 once again indicating a p-value of less than 0.05.

In Table 8.5, we compare the response rates for the two primary endpoints – disease deterioration and mortality for the Hindle et al. study.[25] What is interesting is that for the mortality endpoint ARR shows less deviation from the null than in the case of disease deterioration, while the converse holds for the RR. This is often regarded as a major defect of the RR as a measure of treatment effect, in that it does not

Table 8.4 Incidence of deterioration and death in patients treated for tetanus by the intrathecal and intramuscular routes

	Treatment	Deteriorated	Stable/improved	Total
Disease deterioration	Intrathecal	22	36	58
	Intramuscular	37	23	60

	Treatment	Died	Survived	Total
Mortality	Intrathecal	4	54	58
	Intramuscular	10	50	60

Table 8.5 Incidence of deterioration and death in patients treated for tetanus by the intrathecal and intramuscular routes

Endpoint	Rates		Summary measures	
	Intrathecal	Intramuscular	ARR	RR
Disease deterioration	0.617	0.379	0.238	1.626
Mortality	0.161	0.063	0.092	2.339

ARR, absolute rate reduction; RR, relative risk.

take account of baseline, or control risk. In fact, there are examples in which the converse is true, increased ARR but reduced RR. The choice between the measures cannot, or should not be based upon such differences but upon the relevance of absolute or relative effects.

There is considerable evidence that the form in which data is reported has an impact on the understanding of the results, and on the decisions which are taken on the basis of the data.[38–47] For example, Misselbrook and Armstrong[44] report the results of an investigation in which hypertensive and matched non-hypertensive patients were offered treatment for chronic mild hypertension. They were provided information of the positive impact of the offered treatment on the likelihood of their developing a future stroke. The information was presented in different formats, including RR and ARR. When the information of the benefit of treatment was given in the form of RR, 92% of patients responded that they would accept treatment. In contrast, when the same information was presented in the form of ARR, only 75% patients reported that they would accept treatment. The confusion is not restricted to patients. Forrow et al.[41] report the results of a study in which physicians reported they were more likely to treat both hypertension and hypercholesterolaemia when data were presented in the form of RR rather than ARR.

Laupacis et al.[48] introduced the number needed to treat (NNT) into the medical literature as an easily understood and useful measure of treatment effect for clinical trials in which the main outcome variable is binary. It has been argued that the NNT is more easily understood by practising physicians than more statistically based measures. Mathematically, the definition of the NNT is extremely simple as it is just the reciprocal of the ARR:

$$NNT = \frac{1}{ARR} = \frac{1}{\pi_C - \pi_t}$$

Conventionally, this is interpreted as meaning that if NNT patients are treated with each treatment, one additional patient will benefit from being treated with the new treatment compared to the control. Applying this definition to the mortality data from the Hindle et al. study[25] gives an NNT of $1/(0.161 - 0.063) = 10.83$. Conventionally, this is interpreted as meaning that approximately 11 patients need to be treated intrathecally to save one life.

Since its inception the NNT has been widely used, not only to report the results of individual clinical trials, but more particularly in the evidence-based medicine world to report the results of systematic reviews, or meta-analyses (see section 8.6). Its use by the evidence-based medicine fraternity has led to the NNT being incorporated into a number of treatment guidelines. Three of four recent clinical practice guidelines issued by the Australian and New Zealand College of Psychiatrists used the NNT in summarising results.[49–51] Despite its popularity with clinicians, not all statisticians have been as supportive.[52,53]

8.5.4 Prevention of bias

As pointed out in ICH E9, 'the most important design techniques for avoiding bias in clinical trials are blinding and randomisation, and these should be a normal feature of most controlled clinical trials intended to be included in a marketing application'. The avoidance of bias is absolutely crucial if the interpretation of the results of a clinical trial is to be valid. We noted in section 8.4.2.2 that the logic of significance test is that 'all other things being equal' a small p-value would allow us to conclude that there was a significant difference between the treatments. The meaning of the phrase 'all other things being equal' is that the only differences between the patients in the treatment groups are the treatments that the patients receive. Randomisation and blinding provide us with the means to ensure this.

8.5.4.1 Randomisation

Why do we randomise? Randomisation is a procedure based on a chance allocation of subjects to treatments. Its purpose is to produce groups of patients comparable, or balanced, with respect to factors that may influence outcome apart from the treatments themselves, thus allowing us to make a strong causal connection between the treatments and their different outcomes. What is important here is to realise that randomisation protects us not only against imbalance with respect to important known prognostic factors but also against imbalance with respect to the unknown, possibly unmeasured factors. While many people would argue that the justly famous Medical Research Council study of streptomycin for the treatment of tuberculosis[54] was the first trial to use randomisation, this is not the case.[55,56] Indeed, the notion of balance was known to be important in the 18th century.[1]

A second reason for randomisation is that from a statistical perspective it ensures the validity of the standards approaches to statistical inference, t-tests, analysis of variance (ANOVA), etc.

8.5.4.1.1 Unrestricted randomisation The simplest form of randomisation is unrestricted randomisation. Suppose we need to randomise 12 patients to two treatments, A and B, and that we have access to a table of random numbers (e.g. Table A in Campbell and Machin).[57] Choosing randomly the 21st row and fourth block, the next 12 random numbers in this table are 316427816281. If even numbers are assigned to A and odd numbers to B, then the randomisation which is generated is: BBAAABABAAAB giving seven A's and five B's. Although unrestricted randomisation is simple in principle, it does not guarantee that there are equal number of patients per treatment group, as here.

8.5.4.1.2 Blocked randomisation If using blocked randomisation, we ensure balance between treatments within a block of patients. Suppose, for example, we again wish to randomise the two treatments, A and B, to 12 patients in blocks of size four. Then within each block of four patients, treatments are randomly allocated to patients to ensure that two patients receive both A and B. For example:

Block		
2	1	3
AABB	ABBA	BABA

The advantages of blocked randomisation are that it protects against time effects, by which it is meant that if the characteristics of the patients entered into the study change, blocking protects against lack of balance. Secondly, in multicentre trials it reduces the risk of serious imbalance with respect to the numbers of patients allocated to each treatment. The disadvantages are that the last treatments allocated in each block may become known if there is the possibility of functional unblinding through known properties of the treatments. Secondly, it is practically implemented with only a small number of stratification factors (see section 8.5.4.1.3). The first disadvantage can be mitigated by making the block size long enough to avoid predictability or having block length (e.g. four, six or eight) and, secondly, by making investigators blind to block length.

8.5.4.1.3 Multicentre studies and stratified randomisation In multicentre trials it is usual to use a separate randomisation procedure within each centre to ensure that there is balance – or at least near balance within each centre. In such circumstances ICH E9 (see section 2.3.2) recommends that the randomisation be performed centrally, with several blocks allocated to each centre. This procedure is a simple form of stratified randomisation.

A second important use of stratified randomisation is in those cases where it is known that a particular set of variables are, or are believed to be, important prognostically. It is desirable in such cases to ensure balanced allocation within each combination of the levels of these prognostic variables that can lead to enhanced efficiency in comparing treatments. As a simple illustration, suppose that gender and age are important, and that the strata for the latter are defined by: <40, 40–59, >60 years. Within each combination of the strata, a separate randomisation list, perhaps based on blocks, is prepared to give:

Strata		Blocks		
Sex	Age	1	2	3
F	<40	AABB	BABA	ABBA
F	40–59	BARB	AABB	BBAA
F	>60	BBAA	AABB	AABB
M	<40	ABBA	BABA	BBAA
M	40–59	BABA	BABA	AABB
M	>60	ABBA	BAAB	ABAB

Table 8.6 Balance of four prognostic factors in a hypothetical trial after 50 patients have been randomised

Factor	Level	No. on each treatment	
		A	B
Disease severity	Moderate	30	31
	Severe	20	19
Age	<55 years	18	17
	≥55 years	32	33
Length of illness	<10 years	21	22
	≥10 years	29	28
Centre	1	19	21
	2	8	7
	3	23	22

The advantages of stratified randomisation are to:
1. Minimise the chance of accidental bias with respect to important factors;
2. Increase the precision with which the treatments are compared and the power (see section 8.5.7) to detect treatment differences;
3. Make the trial results more convincing by being able to demonstrate the balance with respect to the important factors.

As far as disadvantages go, the need for central randomisation may slow the process of randomisation for an individual patient, although computer systems make this less of an issue than was previously the case. Secondly, there is always a danger that misclassification of patients to strata can occur and this is only found out later, leading to a danger of increased imbalance. Thirdly, while there are improvements to precision and power, the gains are limited. Finally, while stratified randomisation can reduce bias and imbalance, there is a school of thought that suggests that post-stratification, for example, analysis of covariance (ANCOVA) can reduce bias.

8.5.4.1.4 Dynamic randomisation – minimisation

When there are a large number of prognostic variables to account for, it may be practically difficult to implement a fully stratified randomisation scheme. The reason being that with a large number of factors there are even more individual stratum combinations and therefore there will be very few patients in many of the combinations. In such circumstances, the method of dynamic allocation, or minimisation, has been recommended.

Minimisation is based on the idea of biasing the treatment allocation so as to minimise the total imbalance between treatments according to some criterion. To illustrate, consider the case shown in Table 8.6. This shows the current balance of individual prognostic factors in a hypothetical study with three prognostic factors run in three centres. So far 50 patients have been randomised to each treatment. Suppose that the next patient has following characteristics:

Disease severity	moderate
Age	<55 years
Length of illness	>10 years
Centre	2

For each treatment, we add together the numbers corresponding to the characteristics of the next patient to give:

Treatment A: $30 + 18 + 29 + 8 = 85$
Treatment B: $31 + 17 + 28 + 7 = 83$.

Minimisation then favours B because this has the smallest total. There are two ways of favouring B. One is to bias the allocation probability in favour of B; for example, B has an 80% chance of being chosen, and A a 20% chance. The other approach – deterministic minimisation, allocates B with 100% chance.

The main advantages of minimisation are that it achieves good balance on prognostic factors and thereby increases efficiency. However, it has been criticised – particularly deterministic minimisation – for not guaranteeing the underlying randomness assumed by the statistical methods used to analyse the data. A second disadvantage is that because minimisation is a dynamic process it uses information on subjects already entered to allocate to future patients. Because these patients may be in other centres the process is usually carried out by a centralised system using the internet, fax or telephone.

8.5.4.1.5 Ethical issues and randomisation There are ethical issues with randomisation. There are two types of ethics that are associated with human medical research: individual and collective ethics.[58,59] Individual ethics recognises the primacy of the individual and is aimed at doing what is best for the subjects in the current trial. In contrast, collective ethics is aimed at doing what is best for all future patients who will benefit from the results of the current trial. Clearly, there is a tension between these two principles which is recognised in the Declaration of Helsinki, which comes down on the side of the individual: 'Concern for the interests of the subject must always prevail over the interest of science and society.'[60]

Many have argued that concerns for the individual intuitively lead to the use of adaptive designs in which randomisation is biased towards the more successful treatment or treatments. One type of adaptive design is the randomised-play-the-winner (RPW) design. Such designs are often described in terms of the following urn model. At the start of the trial, an urn contains a balls, each of two colours, white and red, representing the two treatments, A and B, respectively. When a patient requires treatment, a ball is selected at random from the urn and subsequently replaced. If it is white then the patient is allocated to A, if red to B. When the response of a previously allocated patient becomes available, the content of the urn is updated in the following way. If the patient was located to treatment t, either A or B, and responded positively, β balls of colour t and γ balls of colour s (the complement of t) are added to the urn. On the other hand, if the patient was located to treatment t, and responded negatively β balls of colour s and γ balls of colour t are added to the urn. In time, the urn will contain a higher proportion of the more successful treatment.

Despite their ethical appeal, RPW designs have rarely been used in medical research in general, or drug development in particular. This may be because of the negative impact of a study reported by Bartlett et al.[61] This trial in newborn babies with severe respiratory failure compared extracorporeal membrane oxygenation (ECMO) with a standard ventilator. The endpoint was survival and given that it was anticipated there would be a major benefit of ECMO, it was decided to run it as an RPW (1,1,1). It resulted in the following sequence of allocation and data (S: success, F: failure):

Patient number												
Treatment	1	2	3	4	5	6	7	8	9	10	11	12
ECMO	S		S	S	S	S	S	S	S	S		S
Standard		F										

The study was stopped after the result from the 12th patient was known because the statistical analysis showed that there was significant evidence favouring ECMO. These results generated controversy, first about the appropriate statistical analysis of such data, and secondly about the wisdom of definitely concluding benefit in favour of ECMO when only one patient was treated with the standard. This latter issue could have been addressed either by increasing the number of balls in the urn initially, for example, by using an RPW (10,1,1), which would have slowed down the imbalance in favour of ECMO, or by using a randomised block of say 10 patients before an urn model was used and in which the initial ratio of coloured balls is determined by the results of the randomised block.

However, there is a counter argument. In the ECMO trial, after the result of the ninth patient became known, the RPW design requires that the patients be randomised to ECMO compared to the standard ventilator in the ratio 9 : 1. Clayton[62] argues that if the one treatment is so much superior to the other that 90% of patients are allocated to it, it is unethical to withhold it from the remaining 10%. If we accept that argument, is it also true if the ratio is 8 : 1 or 7 : 1? How much information is sufficient to make us, ethically, refuse to randomise patients? Such questions are not simple.

8.5.4.2 Blinding
The primary purpose of blinding is to minimise any conscious, or unconscious, bias in the conduct of a clinical trial. Such biases may arise through allocation, through assessment of treatment effects by physician, the attitude of the patient knowing that they are receiving a particular treatment, decisions made by the physician as to the cause of adverse events, withdrawal of treatment, etc. All of these may be influenced by knowledge of the treatment. The purpose of blinding is to prevent the identification of treatments until such time as there is no longer a possibility of bias.

There are generally three levels of blindness:
1. *Double-blind* – in which neither the patient nor any clinical staff involved in the management and assessment of the patient are aware of the treatment.

2. *Single-blind* – in which the patient alone is unaware of the treatment.

3. *Open-label* – in which both the patient and physician are open to the treatment.

In these trials, it is often sensible to have the assessment of the patient handled by a physician who is blinded, even if the treating physician and the patient are open.

There is an ethical imperative, despite blinding, to protect the patient from harm. Therefore, it is most important that a system is developed to allow the blind to be broken in some circumstances (e.g. when a patient suffers a serious adverse reaction). The study protocol should describe those conditions under which the blind may be broken and the system itself should allow the breaking of the blind in a single patient, rather than the whole study.

8.5.5 Control groups

Often statisticians are asked to consider the use of control data other than those arising from contemporaneous randomised controls and, more often than not, they reply that such use is inappropriate. What are the alternatives that need to be considered and why are they not appropriate?

8.5.5.1 Concurrent non-randomised controls

A trial is conducted in which a physician decides to allocate some patients to a new treatment, and other patients he or she treats with what until now has been his or her first choice of treatment. The physician monitors the changes in all the patients over time and at a predetermined time compares the results from the two groups of patients. A difference is found. In order to be confident that the observed difference is real, the physician needs to assume that the patients in the two groups are essentially identical in respect to all important factors that are important to the disease and its prognosis. Unfortunately, without randomisation we cannot be sure that such an assumption is valid. As we noted in section 8.5.4.1, the strength of randomisation is that it protects against biases, unconscious or conscious.

8.5.5.2 The patient as their own control

There are two circumstances in which patients act as their own control: crossover designs and pre-test/post-test designs.

8.5.5.2.1 Crossover designs

The essential feature of a crossover design is that each patient receives at least two of the treatments under consideration. In the simplest two-period two-treatment crossover, with treatments A and B, patients are allocated to one of the treatment sequence AB. As is often the case, the most succinct statement of advantages and disadvantages of crossover design is to be found in Hill.[28]

In some instances it may be better to design the trial so that each patient provides his or her own control – by having various treatments in turn. This is known as a 'crossover' trial. By such means we may sometimes make the comparison more sensitive because we have eliminated the variability that must exist between patients treated at the same stage of the disease in question (so far as can be judged). We have done so, however, at the expense of introducing as a factor the variability within patients from one time to another, i.e. we may be giving the patient treatment A and treatment B at different stages of the disease.[28]

The primary advantage of such a design is that the patient being his or her own control increases the precision of the treatment comparisons because they are made within patients rather than between patients. This has important ethical and economic consequences. Ethical, in that we would want to minimise the number of patients who receive the less efficacious treatments; economic, because the use of fewer patients will reduce the costs. Such advantages might suggest that crossover designs should be the design of choice if not for three disadvantages.

1. Crossover designs, because they last approximately twice as long as parallel group designs, may be more prone to patient withdrawal.

2. They are only applicable in stable chronic diseases where patients would be expected to return to their pre-treatment severity after a short period without treatment.

3. Most importantly, if the effect of treatment is not confined to the period in which it is applied – so-called carryover – or if the treatment effect differs from period to period, estimates of treatment effects may be biased.

This latter disadvantage led the crossover design to be described as 'not the design of choice in clinical trials, where unequivocal evidence of treatment effects is required'. Over the last 25 years, many statisticians have been more positive about the place of the crossover design in clinical research.[64,65]

Of course, the control in a crossover design is not contemporaneous because it occurs within different treatment periods. Nonetheless, such trials are randomised and the effect of differential period effects can be allowed for in the analysis and does not give rise to bias in treatment estimates.

8.5.5.2.2 Pre-test/post-test designs In a pre-test/post-test design, each individual subject is measured on two occasions separated by the same treatment and the difference between the two measurements, appropriately averaged across subjects, is an estimate of the effect of treatment. In order for this to be a valid measure of the treatment intervention, we need two assumptions. First, there is no change in the experimental conditions, an example would be that in estimating a treatment for hayfever the pollen count remains constant over the period of the experiment. Secondly, there is no natural progression of the disease over time, an example would be the treatment of a common cold which might be expected to improve within 4 or 5 days without treatment.

This second assumption is equivalent to an assumption that there is no 'regression-to-the-mean'.[66] Regression-to-the-mean is a phenomenon originally reported in 1885 by Galton[67] who showed that the children of tall parents tend to be shorter than their parents, and conversely children of shorter parents tend to be taller than their parents. This is of importance in the context of clinical research because patients are chosen to participate in a clinical trial because they have in some sense extreme values. As an example, high blood pressure is a surrogate for coronary artery disease and patients entered into a study to reduce blood pressure will have high values, in expectation that it can be lowered.

Changes seen after treatment may not be brought about by the treatment alone because untreated patients will generally improve because of regression-to-the-mean. There is therefore a need to disentangle the treatment effect from regression-to-the-mean. In order to this we need concurrent randomised controls.

8.5.5.2.3 Historical controls Because many clinical trials are conducted in the same diseases, with the same control treatments, there is an obvious desire to make the most use of this potentially valuable information. Can we compare the results of a new treatment in a group of patients with a group of control patients extracted from a historical database? For example, suppose we are testing a new treatment for migraine headache and 60% of patients improve in the first 2 h post-treatment, compared with 30% in a group of historical control patients treated who had been treated with the current 'gold standard'. Are we able to conclude that the new treatment is preferable to the 'gold standard'?

In order to be able to sustain this conclusion we need to assure ourselves that the groups are essentially similar in every respect but treatment. They need to be similar with respect to their demographic profiles; similar with respect to disease severities; there should have been no changes to the way patients are treated – no new standard method for handling patients apart from a pharmacological intervention. To assure all of these is difficult because we can only investigate characteristics that are measured. As we have already remarked, randomisation protects against lack of balance with respect to all characteristics, measured or not.

8.5.6 Active control groups

In active control trials, there is a natural tendency to believe that if we show no statistical difference between a new treatment and active control then we are justified in concluding that the treatments are equivalent. To illustrate consider the data below taken from a report of 1904 by Pearson[68] on prevention of typhoid by inoculation.

Treatment	Infected	Not infected	Total
Inoculated (I)	7 (25.0%)	21	28
Not inoculated (NI)	3 (23.1%)	10	13

A test of the null hypothesis that the rates of infection are equal – $H_0 \times \pi_I/\pi_{NI} = 1$ gives a p-value of 0.894 using a chi-squared test. There is therefore no statistical evidence of a difference between the treatments and one is unable to reject the null hypothesis. However, the contrary statement is not true that therefore the treatments are the same. As Altman and Bland[69] succinctly put it, 'absence of evidence is not evidence of absence'. The individual estimated infection rates are $\pi_I = 0.250$ and $\pi_{NI} = 0.231$ that gives an estimated RR of 0.250/0.231 = 1.083 with an associated 95% confidence interval of 0.332–3.532. In other words, inoculation can potentially reduce the infection by a factor of three or increase it by a factor of three, with the implication that we are not justified in claiming that the treatments are equivalent.

Consider a second example. A surgeon devises a new method of carrying out a surgical procedure and pilots the technique in 10 patients of whom none develop a postoperative infection. Can the surgeon claim therefore that the new technique is safe? The answer again is no because in this case the upper end of the 95% confidence for the true infection rate is 0–26% so that infection rate could be as high as one in four. (Hanley and Lippman-Hand[70] developed a simple approximation for the 95% confidence for cases in which the observed data are of the form 0 out of n. They show that approximately the interval is $0-3/n$ %. This is known as the rule of three.) In order that we can claim equivalence of treatments, specially designed studies need to be conducted.

8.5.6.1 Equivalence and non-inferiority studies

What was missing in the previous section was a definition of what is meant by equivalence. Because it is unlikely that two treatments will have exactly the same effect, we will need to consider how big a difference between the treatments would 'force' us to choose one in preference to the other. In the typhoid example there was a difference in rates of 1.9% and we may well believe that such a small difference would justify us in claiming that the treatment effects were the same. But had the difference been 5% would we still have thought them to be the same? Or 10? There will be a difference, say 8%, for which we are no longer prepared to accept the equivalence of the treatments. This is the so-called equivalence boundary. If we want then to have a high degree of confidence that two treatments are equivalent it is logical to require that an appropriately chosen confidence interval (say 95%) for the treatment differences should have its extremes within the boundaries of equivalence.

In Figure 8.9 we illustrate various cases that can arise from studies intended to show equivalence and the relationship between significance in the traditional sense and clinical significance as determined by the confidence interval and the boundaries of equivalence. In case A, the 95% confidence interval includes both the null hypothesis of no difference and is within the boundaries of equivalence and from both a stat-

istical and clinical perspective there is no evidence of a difference between the treatments. In case B, in contrast, the confidence interval is still within the boundaries, but does include the null hypothesis, so from a statistical perspective there is a difference between the treatments but it is not clinically relevant. Case C shows both statistical and clinical significance, as the confidence interval lies outside the equivalence boundaries and therefore cannot include the null hypothesis. In the final case, D, the confidence interval includes the null hypothesis but its extremities lie outside the boundaries of equivalence, so that statistically there is no difference but clinically the result is equivocal.

If in Figure 8.9 a positive difference between treatments were indicative of a benefit for the test treatment then case C would indicate significant superiority of the new treatment. In such circumstances, we would not wish to conclude that only the treatments were not equivalent. In such circumstances, we can use a single boundary and such studies are called non-inferiority studies in which the objective is to show that the new treatment is no more than a small amount worse than the standard. The conduct of the inference remains similar: if the confidence interval is to the right of the non-inferiority boundary, we can conclude that the new treatment is non-inferior to the standard.

There are a number of issues in using such studies to achieve marketing authorisation. First, there needs to be a justification of the boundaries. How can we be sure that the choice of S is appropriate? Secondly, has an appropriate choice comparator been made? Is the dose of the comparator appropriate? Is the

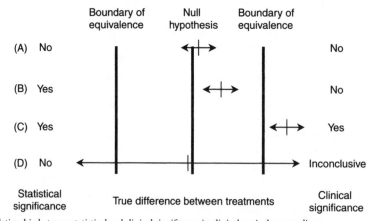

Figure 8.9 Relationship between statistical and clinical significance in clinical equivalence studies.

Table 8.7 Pre-treatment and post-operation maximum rate of urea synthesis (MRUS) values in a randomised trial of spleno-renal shunts

Control operation		New operation	
Pre-treatment	Post-treatment	Pre-treatment	Post-treatment
34	16	51	48
40	36	35	55
34	16	66	60
36	18	40	35
38	32	39	36
32	14	46	43
44	20	52	46
50	43	42	54
60	45		
63	67		
50	36		
42	34		
43	32		

population of patients appropriate? Thirdly, while for superiority trials it is generally accepted that the appropriate analysis population is an ITT population, it has been argued that for equivalence and non-inferiority studies that the as per protocol population also has a role. Finally, we need to be sure that an equivalence or non-inferiority study is capable of showing a difference between treatments, should one exist. This is termed assay sensitivity. The difficulty here is that in superiority trials the achievement of statistical significance is by definition proof of capability while in equivalence or non-inferiority studies there is no equivalence proof of capability from within the study itself. Many of these issues are discussed in ICH E10[71] and Jones et al.[72]

8.5.7 Choice of analysis

The appropriate choice of analysis depends on many of the issues that we have already considered. For example:

1. The study objective – is it to show that the treatments are different or that they are different by no more than a small amount (see section 8.5.6.1)?
2. The scale of measurement – quantitative compared with qualitative (see section 8.3).
3. The endpoint itself (see section 8.5.3.1).

In studies in which there are important prognostic factors, accounting for them as part of the analysis can be important in increasing the precision with which treatment effects can be estimated. Such analyses

generally involve the use of an analysis of covariance (ANCOVA) type of approach.

To illustrate ANCOVA we consider the data in Table 8.7 taken from a study reported by Rikkers et al.[73] which compared the effect of two types of splenorenal shunts in the treatment of cirrhotic patients. The primary measurement was the maximum rate of urea synthesis (MRUS) measured both pre- and post-treatment. The basic question here is: how do we interpret treatment effects in the light of potential differences in baseline severity? One simple approach is to take the difference between pre- and post-treatment measurements and to analyse these. Statistically, it is more appropriate to use ANCOVA, a technique that provides a mathematical adjustment of the treatment to allow for baseline imbalance in severity.

Figure 8.10 illustrates how ANCOVA works for the MRUS data. In this figure, we have plotted the post-treatment MRUS values against the pre-treatment values with the treatment groups being separately identified. A linear regression line is determined for each treatment group, assuming that there is a common slope. Then, for any value of the pre-treatment the vertical separation of these two lines is an estimate of the treatment differences in post-treatment values adjusted for a common baseline value. For these data the pre-treatment adjusted estimate of the treatment difference is -12.8 with an associated 95% confidence interval (-21.1 to -4.5). Had the treatments been

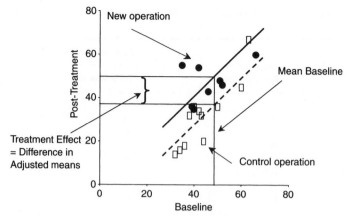

Figure 8.10 Illustration of analysis of co-variance using data from Rikkers et al.[73]

compared without this adjustment, the treatment difference would have been estimated as −15.7 with associated confidence interval (−28.0 to −3.3). This latter interval is almost 50% larger than the adjusted interval, indicating that ANCOVA has resulted in a more precise treatment estimate.

8.5.8 Sample size and power calculations

In section 8.4.2.2 we encountered the concept of the type I error which was defined as rejecting the null hypothesis when it is true. When considering how to sample size a study we need to consider a second type of error – the type II error. The relationship between this second error and the null hypothesis is illustrated below.

		H_0 True	H_0 False
Decision	Accept H_0	✓	Type II error
	Reject H_0	Type II error	✓

We see that in contrast to the type I error, the type II error is defined as occurring when accepting the null hypothesis if it is false. The power of a test is defined to be the probability of detecting a true difference and is equal to 1 − probability (type II error). The type II error and power depend upon the type I error, the sample size, the clinically relevant difference (CRD) that we are interested in detecting and the expected variability. Where do these values come from?

1. Type I error – this is preset and usually takes the value of either 0.05 or 0.01;

2. The CRD, as its name implies, needs to be relevant; an example might be a drop in 15 mmHg in diastolic blood pressure;

3. An estimate of the population variability may be obtained from a pilot study, a literature meta-analysis (see section 8.6) or phase I/II studies.

In most cases we will be interested in determining the sample size for a given type II error, which is typically fixed at values of 0.1 or 0.2. Many sample size determinations take the form:

$$n = \frac{2\sigma^2}{CRD^2} \times f(\alpha, \beta)$$

where n is the number of patients in each group, σ is the population variability, CRD is as above, α is the type I error, β is the type II error and $f(\alpha, \beta)$ is a function that depends upon the cumulative normal distribution function and takes the form:

		β			
		0.05	0.1	0.2	0.5
α	0.1	10.8	8.6	6.2	2.7
	0.05	13.0	10.5	7.9	3.8
	0.02	15.8	13.0	10.0	5.4
	0.01	17.8	14.9	11.7	6.6

What is clear form this formula and the tabulated values of $f(\alpha, \beta)$ are that:

1. Sample size will increase if the type I and II errors, α and β, are stricter in the sense that they are smaller.

2. If σ is large, sample size will be large; this is related to the relationship between sample size and a reduced standard error (see section 8.4.1.2).

3. If the clinically relevant difference is large, the sample size will be small.

To illustrate the use of the formula suppose we are designing a trial to compare treatments for the reduction of blood pressure. We determine that a clinically relevant difference is 5 mmHg and that the between-patient standard deviation α is 10 mmHg. A type I error is set at 0.05 and the type II error at 0.20. Then the required sample size, per group, is:

$$n = \frac{2 \times 10^2}{5^2} \times 7.9 = 63.2 \sim 64$$

There are a number of ways to sample size a trial. The scientific approach is:
• To specify what we are interested in detecting – the CRD;
• Determine the likely variability – σ;
• Decide what probabilities of type I and II error we can tolerate;
• Determine the sample size;
and this is the approach illustrated above. The resource planning approach is:
• To specify the likely budget and thence the sample size;
• Determine the likely variability – σ;
• Decide what probabilities of type I and II error we can tolerate; and
• Determine the minimum difference that is detectable.
The argument against this approach is that this minimum difference may be clinically unrealistic and hence the true power will be much less than specified and this can be regarded as unethical, because patients are being exposed to a new therapy when there is little likelihood of a successful outcome. There is evidence that many studies are underpowered at the planning stage. Freiman et al.[74] investigated 71 'negative' taken principally from the *New England Journal of Medicine*, *The Lancet* and the *Journal of the American Medical Association*. They restricted their attention to studies with a binary outcome and for which there was a clear statement of lack of statistical significance. For 67/71 (94%) of the studies, they determined that there was >10% type II error of missing a 25% therapeutic improvement; in 50/71 (70%) there was >10% type II error of missing a 50% therapeutic improvement.

There are of course practical considerations in clinical research. We may find patient recruitment difficult in single-centre studies and this is one of the major drivers to multicentre and multinational trials. Alternatively, we may need to relax the inclusion/exclusion criteria or lengthen the recruitment period. Unfortunately, while each of these may indeed increase the supply of patients, they may also lead to increased variability that in turn will require more patients. A second issue is the size of the CRD which, if it is too small, will require a large number of patients. In such circumstances we may need to consider the use of surrogate endpoints (see section 8.3.3.2). Finally, the standard deviation may be large and this can have a considerable impact on the sample size – for example, a doubling of the standard deviation leads to a four times increase in the sample size. The issues concerning components of variability in section 8.4.2.1 are relevant here. It is generally the case that when more complex statistical analysis strategies and designs are under consideration, standard sample size calculations are inadequate to cover them. In such circumstances simulation is often used to determine the type I and II errors of the proposed studies for a given sample size.

8.6 Meta-analysis and summaries

Meta-analysis is the practice of using statistical methods to combine and quantify the outcomes of a series of studies in a single pooled analysis. The ideas of meta-analysis are not new. One of the first recognisable meta-analyses is by Pearson[68] in a paper in 1904 in which he provided an overview of the results of inoculating British soldiers against typhoid. In the 1930s the idea of combining results from independent experiments arose both in physics[75] and in agricultural research.[76,77] In contrast, the term itself did not appear until 1976 when Glass first coined it.[78] In all of these contexts a meta-analysis or, as it is sometimes also termed, an overview, can be seen to be a retrospective analysis of studies that have already been conducted.

In simple terms, meta-analysis is the practice of using statistical methods to combine and quantify the outcomes of a series of studies in a single pooled analysis. What is crucial in this definition is the emphasis on the use of statistical methods. In most biomedical research, the scientific review has a lengthy history and is still widely used. However, in so far that it does not utilise statistical methods for pooling results, and tends to summarise more in qualitative rather than quantitative terms, it cannot be regarded as meta-analysis.

Many of the published meta-analyses in clinical research have been as a result of the extraction of summary data from published sources (e.g. death rates in the treatment of patients after a myocardial infarction). For such studies, much of the research interest has centred on issues surrounding the appropriateness of the statistical techniques and on the methods that should be used to reduce the almost inevitable bias associated with meta-analyses. In the case of the former, the issues relate to the use of fixed effect or random effect models and whether the treatment effect may be assumed to be homogenous across studies. For the latter, one needs to consider problems associated with publication bias, selection bias, size bias and the premature termination of studies because of a positive result in an interim analysis.

More recently, there has been evidence that the results from meta-analyses are not always confirmed by very large randomised studies and it has been argued that meta-analyses based on individual patient data provide a much more reliable method of combining data from similar studies. In particular, basing meta-analysis on individual data is the best method for looking at subgroups of patients and for incorporating prognostics variables and other important co-variates. In the context of drug development, such individual data are almost always available and this leads to the possibility of a planned series of trials that can be subjected to a meta-analysis of the raw data.

8.6.1 Uses of meta-analysis and their strengths and weaknesses

It is useful to make a distinction between the exploratory and confirmatory uses of meta-analyses.

8.6.1.1 Exploratory use of meta-analysis

There are a number of uses to which meta-analyses can be put in an exploratory mode.

First, they can be used to generate hypotheses. Because of their nature when data are extracted from the literature across diverse study protocols meta-analyses can be extremely useful in generating hypotheses, particularly concerning subgroups of patients. In this sense their use mirrors one potential objective of a population pharmacokinetic study that may be to determine interesting co-variates, which influence drug absorption and elimination. Secondly, they can generate data that can subsequently be used to help plan new studies. When designing new studies we need to have some idea, not only of the level of effect that we may see in the study, but also some idea of the likely variability. Meta-analyses can be an invaluable source of such data. Thirdly, they can be used to judge the consistency of results across different settings. Fourthly, they can be used to appropriately present result from a series of studies. Finally, they can help in increasing the precision of treatment estimates; this

can be important in its own right or again in the context of study planning.

8.6.1.2 Confirmatory use of meta-analysis

It might be hoped that a meta-analysis of small studies could in some way replace the registration requirement of two individual positive pivotal phase III studies supporting a drug's registration. It seems that this is unlikely to be satisfactory in the classic sense of a meta-analysis in which data are extracted from the literature. However, it is possible to envisage circumstances in which a planned meta-analysis as part of drug development program could be acceptable. For example, suppose that the treatment of recurrence of a condition within a fixed time period is a secondary endpoint in a drug development program and that recurrence occurs in, say, only a small proportion of patients. Studies sized for the primary endpoint would be too small for the secondary endpoint but a planned meta-analysis over a number of similar studies would be feasible. A second use might be in terms of supporting a claim based upon one or two studies.

8.6.1.3 Weaknesses of meta-analysis

There are two major types of weakness associated with meta-analysis: bias and heterogeneity. When planning a clinical trial every effort is made to minimise the impact of bias on the results. For example, clinicians and patients are kept unaware of the treatment being used for each individual patient, so-called double-blind studies, and patients are randomly allocated to a treatment. However, in meta-analysis there is the potential for the reintroduction of bias as an issue. For example, there is a tendency that only positive studies are published and that negative studies remain unpublished. This so-called publication bias can lead to an overestimation of the true effect of a drug if it remains unknown. There are graphical techniques (e.g. the 'funnel plot') that endeavour to identify when publication bias is occurring.[79] A similar problem is selection bias which can occur if not all published trials are used in the meta-analysis. Both of these biases should be addressed in the planning phase of the meta-analysis, before data have been collected. In studies in which interim analyses are performed, biased treatment estimates may arise if the study is terminated early and account needs to be taken of this in combining this information with other studies. These bias issues are unlikely to be as important in a drug development program because the sponsor will be able to exercise a far greater degree of control than in a classic meta-analysis.

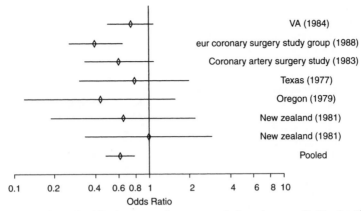

Figure 8.11 Meta-analysis of mortality following coronary bypass surgery in the study reported by Yusuf et al.[80]

8.6.1.4 An example of a meta-analysis

Coronary artery bypass surgery has been used for more than 30 years to treat ischaemic heart disease, but the evidence for its efficacy to reduce mortality in individual studies has been varied. Some studies have questioned whether bypass surgery, while undoubtedly improving quality of life, has any impact on increasing life expectancy. A meta-analysis reported in *The Lancet* in 1994[80] combined the evidence from seven trials comparing bypass surgery with medical treatment. It estimated that 5 years after treatment the mortality rate in bypass patients was 10.2%, while in the medically treated group the corresponding rate was 15.8%. The advantage was maintained at 7 and 10 years after treatment.

Figure 8.11 illustrates the result of the meta-analysis using the OR as an endpoint. Values of the OR less than one indicate a reduction of mortality in favour of bypass surgery, greater than one in favour of medical therapy. What is clear here is that while only one of the seven studies showed any significant evidence of benefit for surgery, all but one of them showed an excess mortality in the medical treatment group. The pooled estimate of the OR clearly shows a benefit in favour of bypass surgery.

References

1 Tröhler U. *To Improve the Evidence of Medicine: the 18th Century Origins of a Critical Approach.* Edinburgh: Royal College of Physicians of Edinburgh, 2000.

2 Gigerenzer G. *Reckoning with Risk: Learning to Live with Uncertainty.* London: Allan Lane, Penguin Press, 2002.

3 Bayes T. An essay towards solving a problem in the doctrine of chances. *Philos Trans R Soc* 1763;53:370–418.

4 Feinstein AR. Clinical biostatistics. XXXIX. The haze of Bayes, the aerial palaces of decision analysis, and the computerized Ouija board. *Clin Pharmacol Ther* 1977;21: 482–96.

5 Spiegelhalter DJ, Abrams KR, Myles JP. *Bayesian Approaches to Clinical Trials and Health-Care Evaluation.* Chichester: John Wiley and Sons, 2003.

6 Thomson W (Lord Kelvin). Lecture to the Institution of Civil Engineers (3 May 1883). In: *Popular Lectures and Addresses, Vol. 1.* London & New York: Macmillan and Co., 1891;80.

7 Senn S. Disappointing dichotomies. *Pharm Stat* 2003;2: 239–40.

8 Lewis JA. In defence of the dichotomy. *Pharm Stat* 2004;3:77–9.

9 Biomarker Definitions Working Group. Biomarkers and surrogate endpoints: preferred definitions and conceptual framework. *Clin Pharmacol Ther* 2001;69:89–95.

10 Fleming TR, DeMets DL. Surrogate endpoints in clinical trials: are we being misled? *Ann Intern Med* 1996;125: 605–13.

11 Prentice RL. Surrogate endpoints in clinical trials: definition and operational criteria. *Stat Med* 1989;8:431–40.

12 Buyse M, Molenberghs G, Burzykowski T et al. Statistical validation of surrogate endpoints: problems and proposals. *Drug Inf J* 2000;34:447–54.

13 Buyse M, Molenberghs G. Criteria for the validation of surrogate endpoints in randomized experiments. *Biometrics* 1998;54:1014–29.

14 Buyse M, Molenberghs G, Burzykowski T et al. The validation of surrogate endpoints in metaanalyses of randomized experiments. *Biostatistics* 2000;1:49–67.

15 Molenberghs G, Geys H, Buyse M. Evaluation of surrogate endpoints in randomized experiments with mixed discrete and continuous outcomes. *Stat Med* 2001;20: 3023–38.

16 Tsiatis AA, DeGruttola V, Wulfsohn MS. Modeling the relationship of survival to longitudinal data measured

with error: applications to survival and CD4 counts in patients with AIDS. *J Am Stat Assoc* 1995;**90**:27–37.

17 Ellenberg SS. Surrogate markers in AIDS and cancer trials: discussion. *Stat Med* 1994;**13**:1437–40.

18 Temple RJ. A regulatory authority's opinion about surrogate endpoints. In: Nimmo WS, Tucker GT, eds. *Clinical Measurement in Drug Evaluation*. New York: Wiley,1995;1–22.

19 Lesko LJ, Atkinson AJJ. Use of biomarkers and surrogate endpoints in drug development and regulatory decision making: criteria, validation, strategies. *Annu Rev Pharmacol Toxicol* 2001;**41**:347–66.

20 Albert JM, Ioannidis JPA, Reichelderfer P et al. Statistical issues for HIV surrogate endpoints: point/counterpoint. *Stat Med* 1998;**17**:2435–62.

21 Hughes MD, DeGruttola V, Welles SL. Evaluating surrogate markers. *J Acquir Immune Defic Syndr Hum Retrovirol* 1995;**10**:S1–S8.

22 Grieve AP. Do statisticians count? A personal view. *Pharm Stat* 2002;**1**:35–43.

23 Bland M. *An Introduction to Medical Statistics*. Oxford: Oxford University Press, 1987.

24 Altman DG, Machin D, Bryant TN, Gardner MJ, eds. *Statistics with Confidence, 2nd edn*. London: BMJ Books, 2000.

25 Hindle M, Newton DAG, Chrystyn H. Dry powder inhalers are bioequivalent to metered-dose inhalers. *Chest* 1995;**107**:629–33.

26 Green FHK, Principle Medical Officer, Medical Research Council. *Lancet* 1954;**ii**:1084–1091.

27 International Conference of Harmonisation. E6: Guideline for Good Clinical Practice, 1996. http://www.emea.eu.int/pdfs/human/ich/013595en.pdf [Accessed January 2005.]

28 Hill AB. *Principles of Medical Statistics, 11th edn*. Edinburgh: Livingstone, 1984.

29 International Conference of Harmonisation. E9: Statistical Principles for Clinical Trials, 1998. http://www.emea.eu.int/pdfs/human/ich/036396en.pdf [Accessed January 2005.]

30 Barnes CG, Berry H, Carter ME et al. Diclofenac sodium (Volarol®) and indomethacin: a multicentre comparative study in rheumatoid arthritis and osteoarthritis. *Rheumatol Rehabil* 1979;Supplement **2**:135–46.

31 Armitage P, McPherson CK, Rowe BC. Repeated significance tests on accumulating data. *J R Stat Soc [Ser A]* 1969;**132**:235–44.

32 Pocock SJ. Group sequential methods in the design and analysis of clinical trials. *Biometrika* 1977;**64**:191–99.

33 O'Brien PC, Fleming TR. A multiple testing procedure for clinical trials. *Biometrics* 1979;**35**:549–56.

34 Lan KKG, DeMets DL. Discrete sequential boundaries for clinical trials. *Biometrika* 1983;**70**:659–63.

35 Perneger TV. What's wrong with the Bonferonni adjustments. *BMJ* 1998;**316**:1236–8.

36 Schwartz D, Flamant R, Lellouch J. *Clinical Trials* (translated by Healy MJR). London: Academic Press, 1980.

37 Miranda-Filho D, Ximese R, Barone A et al. Randomised controlled trial of tetanus treatment with antitetanus immunoglobulin by the intrathecal or intramuscular route. *BMJ* 2004;**328**:615–8.

38 Bobbio M, Demichelis B, Giustetto G. Completeness of reporting trial results: effect on physicians' willingness to prescribe. *Lancet* 1994;**343**:1209–121.

39 Bucher HC, Weinbacher M, Gyr K. Influence of method of reporting study results on decision of physicians to prescribe drugs to lower cholesterol concentration. *BMJ* 1994;**309**:761–4.

40 Fahey T, Griffiths S, Peters TJ. Evidence based purchasing: understanding results of clinical trials and systematic reviews. *BMJ* 1995;**311**:1056–9.

41 Forrow L, Taylor W, Arnold RM. Absolutely relative: how research results are summarized can effect treatment decisions. *Am J Med* 1992;**92**:121–4.

42 Hoffrage U, Lindsay S, Hertwig R et al. Communicating statistical information. *Science* 2000;**290**:2261–2.

43 Malenka DJ, Baron JA, Johansen S et al. The framing effect of relative and absolute risk. *J Gen Intern Med* 1993;**8**:543–8.

44 Misselbrook D, Armstrong D. Patients' responses to risk information about the benefits of treating hypertension. *Br J Gen Hypertens* 2001;**51**:276–9.

45 Moriarty PM. Using both 'relative risk reduction' and 'number needed to treat' in evaluating primary and secondary clinical trials of lipid reduction. *Am J Cardiol* 2001;**87**:1206–8.

46 Naylor CD, Chen E, Strauss B. Measured enthusiasm: does the method of reporting trial results alter perceptions of therapeutic effectiveness. *Ann Intern Med* 1992;**117**:916–21.

47 Sheridan SL, Pignone M. Numeracy and the medical student's ability to interpret data. *Eff Clin Pract* 2002;**5**:35–40.

48 Laupacis A, Sackett DL, Roberts RS. An assessment of clinically useful measures of the consequence of treatment. *N Engl J Med* 1988;**318**:1728–33.

49 Royal Australian and New Zealand College of Psychiatrists. Australian and New Zealand clinical practice guidelines for the treatment of panic disorder and agoraphobia. *Aust N Z J Psychiatry* 2003;**37**:641–56.

50 Royal Australian and New Zealand College of Psychiatrists. Australian and New Zealand clinical practice guidelines for the treatment of depression. *Aust N Z J Psychiatry* 2004;**38**:389–407.

51 Royal Australian and New Zealand College of Psychiatrists. Australian and New Zealand clinical practice guidelines for the treatment of schizophrenia and related disorders. *Aust N Z J Psychiatry* 2005;**39**:1–30.

52 Hutton JA. Number needed to treat: properties and problems (with discussion). *J R Stat Soc [Ser A]* 2000;**163**:403–19.

53 Grieve AP. The number needed to treat: a useful measure or a case of the emperor's new clothes. *Pharm Stat* 2003;**2**:87–102.

54 Medical Research Council Streptomycin in Tuberculosis Trials Committee. Streptomycin treatment for pulmonary tuberculosis. *BMJ* 1948;**ii**:769–82.

55 Chalmers I. Why transition from alternation to randomisation in clinical trials was made. *BMJ* 1999;**319**:1372.

56 Chalmers I. Comparing like with like: some historical milestones in the evolution of methods to create unbiased comparison groups in therapeutic experiments. *Int J Epidemiol* 2001;**30**:1158–64.

57 Campbell MJ, Machin D. *Medical Statistics: A Commonplace Approach*. London: Wiley & Sons, 1993.

58 Palmer CR, Rosenberger WF. Ethics and practice: alternative designs for phase III randomised clinical trials. *Control Clin Trials* 1999;**20**:172–86.

59 Palmer CR. Ethics, data-dependent designs, and the strategy of clinical trials: time to start learning-as-we-go? *Stat Methods Med Res* 2002;**11**:381–402.

60 World Medical Association. *52nd Assembly, Declaration of Helsinki: Ethical Principles for Medical Research Involving Human Subjects*. Edinburgh: World Medical Association, 2000.

61 Bartlett RH, Roloff DW Cornell RG et al. Extracorporeal circulation in neonatal respiratory failure: a prospective randomised trial. *Paediatrics* 1985;**76**:479–87.

62 Clayton DG. Ethically optimised designs. *Br J Clin Pharmacol* 1982;**13**:469–480.

63 Food and Drug Administration. A report on the two-period crossover design and its applicability in trials of clinical effectiveness. Minutes of the Biometric and Epidemiology Methodology Advisory Committee (BEMAC) Meeting, 1977.

64 Senn SJ. *Crossover Trials in Clinical Research*. London: Wiley,1983.

65 Jones B, Kenward MG. *Design and Analysis of Cross-Over Trials*. London: Chapman-Hall, 1989.

66 Bland M, Altman DG. Regression towards the mean. *BMJ* 1994;**308**:1499.

67 Galton F. Regression towards mediocrity in hereditary stature. *J Anthropol Inst* 1885;**15**:246–63.

68 Pearson K. Report of certain enteric fever inoculation statistics. *BMJ* 1904;**3**:1243–46.

69 Altman DG, Bland JM. Absence of evidence is not evidence of absence. *BMJ* 1995;**311**:485.

70 Hanley JA, Lippman-Hand A. If nothing goes wrong is everything all right? Interpreting zero numerators. *JAMA* 1983;**249**:1743–45.

71 International Conference of Harmonisation. E10: Choice of Control Group and Related Issues in Clinical Trials. http://www.emea.eu.int/pdfs/human/ich/036496en.pdf [Accessed January 2005.]

72 Jones B, Jarvis P, Lewis JA et al. Trials to assess equivalence: the importance of rigorous methods. *BMJ* 1996; **313**:36–9.

73 Rikkers LF, Rudman D, Galambos JT et al. A randomized, controlled trial of the distal splenoral shunt. *Ann Surg* 1978;**188**:271–82.

74 Freiman JA, Chalmers TC, Smith HJ et al. The importance of beta, the type II error and sample size in the design and interpretation of the randomized control trial. Survey of 71 'negative' trials. *N Engl J Med* 1978;**299**:690–4.

75 Birge RT. The calculation of errors by the method of least squares. *Phys Rev* 1932;**40**:207–27.

76 Cochran WG. Problems arising in the analysis of a series of similar experiments. *J R Stat Soc* 1937;**4** (Supplement):102–18.

77 Yates F, Cochran WG. The analysis of groups of experiments. *J Agric Sci* 1936;**28**:556–80.

78 Glass GV. Primary, secondary and meta-analysis. *Educ Res* 1976;**5**:3–8,

79 Light RJ, Pillemer DB. *Summing Up: The Science of Reviewing Research*. Cambridge, MA: Harvard University Press, 1984.

80 Yusuf S, Zucker D, Peduzzi P et al. Effect of coronary artery bypass graft surgery on survival: overview of 10 year results from randomised trials by the Coronary Artery Bypass Graft Trialists Collaboration. *Lancet* 1994;**344**:563–70.

9 Development of medicines: full development

Peter D. Stonier

Amdipharm plc, Basildon, Essex, UK

9.1 Introduction

Full drug development involves management of the whole project from early proof of concept to post-launch activities. The very large financial and human resource costs associated with scale-up of a development project from early phase work through to phase III and launch in major markets require that the risks associated with the investment are managed appropriately.

Nevertheless, rapid progress through phase III development will allow a longer effective patent life, which will increase the commercial return on a new medicine, and in recent years this factor alone has been a major driver for large pharmaceutical companies to project manage their product portfolios more efficiently.

The changing nature of the pharmaceutical industry, with increasing numbers of small companies whose survival depends on rapid registration and successful marketing of one drug candidate, means that additional risks such as intellectual property rights, shareholder return, contractual and legal relationships are part of the risk associated with the investment. Management of business risk, which is outside the scope of this chapter, has been identified as a significant problem for small companies.[1]

9.2 Background

Total drug development costs are huge and continue to increase over time. In 2003, development costs of 68 randomly selected new drugs were US$403 million each (year 2000 dollars).[2] Capitalising out-of-pocket

costs to the point of marketing approval at a real discount rate of 11% yields a total pre-approval cost estimate of US$802 million for each new medicine (year 2000 dollars) and the costs have increased at an annual rate of 7.4% above general price inflation.[2] The majority of drug development costs are in phase III development: these include not only the clinical trial programme itself, but significant associated regulatory and manufacturing scale-up costs.

The long-forecasted consolidation in the pharmaceutical industry happened in the 1990s, and has paused in the mid-2000s. The impact of this consolidation was demonstrated by an increase in product failures and increased trial cancellations in 1999 and 2000. However, during 2001, phase III activity increased again, albeit by a small 1.8% increase (to 385 projects) compared with 2000, and this activity has continued to increase to 404 projects in 2004, 423 in 2006 and 540 projects in 2008. Pharmaprojects in mid-2006[3] was reporting on 1633 companies researching 7406 drugs currently in active research and development (R&D) in 218 therapy areas. The number of companies in R&D continues to rise so that in 2008 there were 1967, almost double the 998 figure recorded in 1998.[4] The number of drugs in active R&D also continues to rise, with 7737 in 2007 and 9217 in 2008. Nevertheless, the pharmaceutical industry is concentrated amongst the major companies, with the top 25 companies originating >20% of all drugs in development and each showing a pipeline expansion in 2008 over 2007. In 2006, over 23% of all drugs in development were in the anticancer field.

9.2.1 Senior management perspective

Taking into account all marketing and development failures, cost calculations demonstrate that companies must develop more 'blockbuster' products with annual sales over US$1 billion if they are to maintain historical

The Textbook of Pharmaceutical Medicine. Edited by John P. Griffin. © 2009, ISBN: 978-1-4051-8035-1.

rates of returns to shareholders, or they must significantly cut development costs. Thus, the focus of management is increasingly on the high costs of phase III programmes, and there is a need to reduce risks and costs in phase III by:

• Aggressive portfolio management in early phases of development;
• Life cycle management, including risk management; or
• Continued spend on local trials after submission to fill gaps in the development programme such as paediatric or geriatric subjects in phase IIIb and IV.

Clearly, there is a limit to how much the research costs can increase and companies are beginning to think in new ways about how to manage their R&D costs. There is an increase in the number of alliances and partnerships with academic groups, small biotechnology companies and health care providers who, it is hoped, will provide the entrepreneurial drug development skills that large pharmaceutical companies are currently unable to generate internally. Networks, modelled on successes such as cancer,[5] and involvement of patient groups will continue to increase in importance.

The biotechnology explosion has also finally arrived. Globally, the total number of companies working on pharmaceutical R&D continues to rise and in May 2004, 656 companies were working on only one or two compounds.[4] The number of companies with one product in development, which is a useful proxy for biotechnology-driven or emerging pharmaceutical companies, has increased each year from 212 in 1998 to 373 in 2001 and 656 in 2004. Moreover, the top 25 pharmaceutical companies have a significant proportion of R&D drugs in development which are licensed in, typically from smaller pharmaceutical companies or research laboratories.[4]

Ranked by total numbers of drugs in R&D in 2008, the top five companies are GlaxoSmithKline (254 drugs in development), Pfizer (213), Merck & Co (211), Sanofi-Aventis (211) and AstraZeneca (184). Of the 254 R&D drugs that GlaxoSmithKline has in development, 167 (66%) are their own drugs; Pfizer has 162 (76%); Merck & Co 148 (70%); Sanofi-Aventis 151 (72%); and AstraZeneca 137 (74%).[4]

This changing picture of full drug development means that the largest pharmaceutical companies are now having to be adept at intellectual property protection, legal and contractual development and co-marketing agreements, as well as accelerated drug development. The single-product companies must also be skilled at managing their cash flow, relationships with their shareholders and the marketplace in which they need to thrive.

Recovery of costs by successful marketing of products is essential in order to maximise shareholder return. As R&D costs continue to increase by 8–11% per annum, and sales turnover increases by 5–7% per annum, R&D takes up an increasing proportion of the pharmaceutical budget and, for the largest pharmaceutical companies, is about 17% of turnover.

The International Conference on Harmonisation (ICH), the EU Clinical Trials Directive (2001/20/EC) and the Good Clinical Practice Directive (2005/28/EC) provide a more unified standard for clinical trials and also facilitate mutual acceptance by the regulatory authorities in Europe, Japan and the USA. Development of the guidelines and, in the European Union, the Directives has allowed companies to streamline their drug development programmes by mandating a more uniform approach through the European Union. Consequently, the approach is probably better driven from head office rather than at a country or company subsidiary level, especially as regulatory convergence develops within Europe.

9.3 Taking products into later development phase

9.3.1 Clinical perspective

This chapter focuses on the clinical development of new medicines. This is an area where companies can plan and control much more of their activity. As more drug development projects are terminated at phase II, companies have to be careful that the phase II studies are particularly well designed to avoid the likelihood of a type II error. This means that the studies do not miss a significant clinical difference or advantage for the product. Clarity of thought and detailed design considerations for phase II studies are increasingly important in drug development. The use of external advisory boards can be especially helpful, and it can be useful to include drug development and regulatory specialists on advisory boards together with the more traditional academic staff members.

If the area of endeavour is crowded there will be significant competition for patient recruitment to clinical trials. Currently, these therapy areas include diabetes, oncology and cardiovascular medicine, and it may become necessary to seek patients outside Western Europe and the USA. Investigator fees are rising and competition for patients is helping to increase fees in these geographical areas and also in some areas of Central and Eastern Europe. However, even significant investigator fees may not be sufficient to encourage recruitment if there is little investigator excitement about the product. Investigators are keen to work on innovative products and may well seek increased fees to support other academic work if the product is not particularly exciting for them.

The likely effectiveness of the product, derived from the preclinical and early clinical work, will determine study design, complexity and size. It is a mistake to try to answer too many questions in a single study, despite the apparent commercial attractiveness of such a strategy. A study over-burdened by many secondary objectives is more likely to fail when the design is implemented in many centres worldwide. What seems a good idea at head office can often be hard to implement in the clinic. Statistical advice is vital, and statisticians offer excellent opinions about the utility of complex study designs.

The expected adverse event profile will also determine the study design. A drug for which the prescription is to be initiated in a tertiary referral clinic by leading experts in the field, such as many oncological compounds, will have a different safety profile than a product which will be widely used across many different specialties in primary and secondary care. Characterisation of the risk–benefit profile is an important consideration in study design.

Consideration needs to be given to suitable clinical endpoints. It can be tempting, because of cost and speed of development, to use surrogate endpoints in a pivotal study. A surrogate endpoint is defined as an endpoint that is intended to relate to a clinically important outcome but does not, in itself, measure clinical benefit. A surrogate endpoint should be used as a primary endpoint when appropriate; for example, when the surrogate endpoint is reasonably likely to, or is well known to, predict clinical outcome. However, great care needs to be taken in basing a pivotal and full development programme on the use of surrogate endpoints. Typically, these endpoints are used in early development and discussion with the regulatory authorities is advised before using such endpoints in a full development programme. The use of surrogate markers is discussed in the *ICH Guideline E8: General Considerations for Clinical Trials*. The Guideline makes the point that these markers are most often useful in exploratory therapeutic trials in well-defined narrow patient groups.

9.3.2 Regulatory perspective

The regulatory authorities are increasingly welcoming informal as well as formal discussions about drug development programmes. There are differences in approach between the European Medicines Agency (EMEA) and the US Food and Drug Administration (FDA) and it is wise to take regulatory advice before contacting the agencies. The FDA tends to require a formalistic approach to the development programme. This can have strengths in that the programme direction is clear, but it can be rather limiting in terms of defining a mandatory series of trials and a particular development strategy. Nevertheless, it can be particularly useful if the development programme is likely to be in a new area of medicine or unusual in any way.

The National Institute for Health and Clinical Excellence (NICE) was set up in 1999 as a Special Health Authority for England and Wales. Its role is to provide patients, health professionals and the public with authoritative, robust and reliable guidance/guidelines on current 'best practice'. The guidance covers individual health technologies following appraisal, and guidelines are developed relating to the clinical management of specific conditions. In practice, the pharmaceutical industry has tended to see NICE as an additional 'fourth' hurdle after the Medicines and Healthcare Products Regulatory Agency (MHRA) or EMEA has approved the quality, safety and efficacy of a new product. Consideration has to be given in any development programme to applications to NICE and other bodies throughout the world, and companies may need to consider special and additional studies to meet any objections these bodies may have in allowing a product to be satisfactorily commercialised.

The Common Technical Document (CTD) (ICH M4)[6] is now a requirement. The CTD is the agreed common format for the preparation of a well-structured application to the regulatory authorities and has had an impact on all organisations as database integration and electronic submissions become more common.

The ICH has had an important role in establishing guidelines for drug development. Although these are only guidelines and not legal documents, companies would have to justify deviations from the guidelines in any application for approval. The World Health Organization (WHO) has recently stated that it expects the ICH guidelines to be adopted in non-ICH countries eventually. Based on ICH, the European Union has recently developed a new system (Directive 2001/20/EC) of clinical trial regulation, transposed into national law in each Member State. This will have the effect of making failure to comply with the 'GCP Directive', for example, a criminal offence.

The EU Clinical Trials Directive (2001/20/EC) and associated guidelines and Directives, such as the Good Clinical Practice Directive (2005/28/EC), should allow regulatory convergence over time in Europe. The guidelines provide benefits for clinical trial subjects: they are protected during studies, and they can be confident that the studies are based on good science. The Trials Directive is associated with a large number of Guidance and other Directives. These include the following Guidance: Competent Authority Submission, Ethics Submission, EU Clinical Trials Database, EU Suspected Unexpected Serious Adverse Reactions (SUSARs) database, Adverse Reaction Reporting, Revised Annex 13, Qualification of Inspectors for GMP Inspection, and two Directives: 2003/94/EC (The 'GMP Directive') and 2005/28/EC (The 'GCP Directive'). All the key principles applying to the new system are mentioned in 2001/20/EC. These include: Legal Representation, Compliance with GCP, Obligations to Regulatory Authorities, Obligations to Ethics Committees, Compliance with CMP, EU Database of Clinical Trials, Pharmacovigilance, and GMP and GCP Inspections.

As always, increased regulation has resulted in increased costs, offset slightly by an increase in standardisation of procedures across regions of the world. There are new databases to master, including the European Clinical Trials Database (EudraCT), and a new pharmacovigilance database for SUSARs; responsibility for both of these lies with the EMEA. In time, these new relationships with competent authorities, ethics committees, EudraCT and SUSAR databases and the need for legal representation will become easier and more routine. The value of regulatory convergence will then become more apparent.

9.3.3 Commercial perspective

Apart from the traditional costs associated with commercial development, the costs of selling and marketing the product will require evaluation. Decisions have to be made about whether the product will be sold by the company's own sales force or licensed to partners in some markets. Such discussions are beyond the scope of this chapter.

The company franchise in a particular area of therapeutic endeavour may be enhanced or compromised by active patient groups. There is increasing pressure to place more development and clinical trial information in the public domain. For example, in the UK, the pharmaceutical industry trade association, the Association of the British Pharmaceutical Industry (ABPI), has agreed to develop a register of phase III trials conducted in the UK, 3 months after drug approval in a major market – which might not be the UK. Patients will therefore be in a position to seek entry into trials and may demand this from their physicians.

The development of AZT (Retrovir, zidovudine) by Wellcome (now GlaxoSmithKline) is an interesting example of patient power. Patient groups obtained copies of early phase drug development protocols and some subjects demanded to be placed into these clinical trials for HIV/AIDS. The scrutiny of the protocols by patient groups resulted in improvements in clinical trial designs and the political pressure exerted by these groups ensured that the drug regulatory process became more politicised. This resulted in more rapid approval of drugs by some regulatory authorities and also pushed forward discussions about surrogate markers. It is probable that AZT did not fully meet the established principles of safety and efficacy when it was approved, and further development was required after approval. Whether this approach was beneficial to the entire community of AIDS patients remains debatable.

Other patient groups, in areas as diverse as osteoporosis research, dementia and oncology, have learnt from the AIDS patient groups the power of politics in medicine, and these groups will have an increasing impact on drug development. Some of this impact will be positive but some is likely to be negative and may encourage a too rapid assessment of drug efficacy and safety by the authorities. Indeed, there is evidence of increased product withdrawal by the FDA. Eleven products have been withdrawn between 1997 and mid-2001, compared with eight product withdrawals in the previous 10 years. Whether this is a result of more rapid early development, a more rapid assessment process or simply a result of bad luck is open to conjecture. However, it is clear that a product withdrawal in either late-phase development or early post-marketing can have a devastating effect on a company's share price as a result of the expected decrease in revenue and the potential for poor public relations. Within a day of announcing the withdrawal of rofecoxib (Vioxx), more than £14 billion was wiped from Merck's stockmarket value, equivalent to one-quarter of its worth, and the share price plunged to an 8-year low.[7]

The market potential of a drug or device is clearly critical in determining the desirability of proceeding into later phase development. An increasing number of programmes are stopped at phase II because it is not economical for the company to develop these products. DiMasi[8] in 2001 estimated that, compared with the 1981–86 period, where 29.8% of products were terminated because of economic reasons, between 1987 and 1992 the number of terminations was 33.8% and that this upward trend has continued.

Likely shifts in demographic factors and prescribing mean that drugs for the elderly, such as therapies for Alzheimer's disease or osteoporosis, are increasingly attractive as targets for drug development. Oncological drugs and drugs for chronic diseases also continue to be important for companies' financial health.

The political environment continues to be important. All governments want to constrain health care costs, and an easy target is prescription drug costs. This is not necessarily the most sensible target, as improving health service management may have as important an effect on the national purse. Nonetheless, there is a continuing downwards pressure on health care prescribing.

9.3.4 Exit strategy

Most pharmaceutical companies cannot market products by themselves in all countries of the world. This may be because there is no subsidiary in the relevant country, or because the sales forces' other commitments mean that this drug cannot be adequately marketed in one particular market. For whatever reason, all development programmes must consider an exit strategy for the product in each market. Are there to be co-licensing, co-marketing or other agreements? Is the drug to be licensed out in other markets? Such discussion is beyond the scope of this chapter, but involves important considerations for any full drug development programme.

9.4 Preparing the plan

9.4.1 Structure of the plan

The candidate drug has passed the early development hurdles. In particular, the early preclinical toxicology and commercial environments are suitable. Care must be taken regarding any intellectual property concerns, and that preliminary drug supply and manufacturing forecasts look favourable. Early evaluation and planning will take about 12 months to execute, being a complex process with many interactions and requiring the integration of many different processes. Typically, and best practice for the development of such a plan, this requires a relatively senior project manager or development scientist to take primary

responsibility and ownership of the project. The 'owner' must have the authority to obtain the necessary information from different departments within the organisation and from external suppliers.

The plan will eventually prescribe a likely filing date for a Marketing Authorisation Application (MAA) (product licence). This date is vital and when the plan becomes public information, any slippage in the date is likely to impact on the share price of the company. Accordingly, senior members of the company must be confident that the date can be met. There will always be pressure to bring the date forward but this has a cost in resources, and risks damaging credibility with investors if the accelerated timelines cannot be met.

Thus, a sequential plan is safe, cost effective in terms of resources and manageable by most organisations. Unfortunately, such a plan has a cost in terms of unacceptable delays to shareholders. In the early 1990s there was a vogue for massively parallel plans which ran many activities simultaneously in order to address and bring forward 'stop-go' decisions and filing dates. Stop-go decisions were made aggressively and the plans were continually examined to review ways to bring the filing date forward. Such plans are now less common. The principal reason cited by organisations is that such plans throw many of the company resources onto a single product. If the product fails in late-stage development, other candidate compounds will have been neglected. Such plans therefore are a significant gamble for even well-resourced and capitalised organisations. If they fail, a gap appears in a company's product pipeline, with serious consequences for the well-being of the organisation.

Quite how the plan is reviewed depends on the organisation, the therapeutic class and regulatory priority rating. Large organisations will review on a 12-monthly cycle the overall shape of the drug development portfolio for, say, the next 10 years, the near-term portfolio and resource requirements, say over 3 years, and closely review the detailed plan for the next 12 months. This allows the company to define the next 12 months in terms of budget and resource, and the next 3 and 10 years in some detail to establish if there are likely to be gaps in the portfolio 10 years hence that can be filled by in-licensing of compounds. Such a strategic review is vital for the successful integration of new compounds into the company. Furthermore, such a review allows integration of a registration package which will be acceptable to most major markets into a single dossier. This avoids fragmentation of the clinical development programme.

Duplication of activities is minimised and the major pivotal phase III studies and analysis are performed only once and integrated. Knowledge of the compound and likely questions from the regulatory authorities from the major markets can be centralised. This saves time and resources.

Smaller companies and venture capital funded organisations are likely to be focused on a single compound, its analogues, metabolites and differing formulations. Without the luxury of a 10-year strategic development plan, such organisations are naturally tightly focused on the success of their product. Within these companies, pressure to bring the filing date forward can be intense and if the date is missed this can have serious consequences for the market capitalisation of the company.

9.4.2 Therapeutic targets

Clinical success rates and attrition rates by phase of clinical trial for new drugs are important indicators of how effectively companies are utilising drug development resources. The proficiency with which this is carried out reflects a complex set of regulatory, economic and company-specific factors. Success rates differ by therapeutic class, and typically vary from about 28% success rate for an anti-infective compound to 12% for respiratory drugs.[9] It is mandatory to ensure that the therapeutic target is appropriate and commercially attractive, and to define the required product performance to ensure successful marketing. These activities demand close cooperation between discovery, development and marketing departments before embarking on a full development plan. In the treatment of herpes zoster infection, for example, there is a precedent using the speed of crusting of the vesicular lesions as a marker for the efficacy of drug treatment, with significantly more rapid crusting, associated with the active agent, permitting registration. This is hardly of major relevance to the clinical situation as a beneficial effect on the disappearance of vesicles is of minor consequence to the patient who has a painful condition. The important clinical question is the effect of treatment on pain acutely, and in the longer term in the prevention of post-herpetic neuralgia. This creates an interesting dilemma. Should the primary clinical endpoint be crusting of lesions, given that this approach will undoubtedly result in more rapid execution of studies and therefore faster registration, or should it address the real medical issue (i.e. pain), an area where the clinical evaluation of the efficacy of treatment will be more complex? The responsible clinical decision is to measure

both endpoints, but the implications for marketing must be understood.

The use of the different therapeutic targets, and the implication for the organisation, surrounds competitive advantage. What may be a minor clinical advantage for a new compound can sometimes be converted into a significant commercial lever that will facilitate marketing. Many companies use the draft Summary of Product Characteristics (SmPC) to establish needs and wants, allowing a useful dialogue between the drug development and marketing groups.

Draft labelling and a draft SmPC are produced at the beginning of the development process and these embody the features that the marketing group regards as minimal to ensure commercial success ('needs'). These needs must be tempered by input from medical and development to ensure that the requirements are realistic. The draft would also include features that are perceived to have significant advantages over competitor agents ('wants') and those that would provide useful talking points ('nice to have').

It is always tempting to design a minimalist programme of studies (i.e. the minimum required to obtain registration for a given indication), but this approach may not even address the 'needs', particularly in an area where there is relative satisfaction with available therapy and therefore intense competitor activity. For example, the development of a non-steroidal anti-inflammatory drug may include studies in relatively small numbers of patients, aiming to demonstrate less gastrointestinal blood loss than that associated with an established comparator. In such a competitive area this is likely to be insufficient without demonstrating that this translates into real clinical benefit compared with the comparator (e.g. reducing the incidence of major gastrointestinal blood loss requiring transfusion). A large-scale clinical study such as this may not therefore be required for registration but would be required for launch in order to demonstrate to clinicians the place of a new agent in a crowded therapeutic area.

During this process it is necessary to establish that the marketing 'wants' are indeed achievable. For example, there may be a need for an adequate therapy for delayed nausea and vomiting associated with chemotherapy. Clinicians may state that this is a clinical need. Depending on the current therapies and the early profile of the candidate drug, a good estimation of the drug's likely effectiveness in the indication can be made. However, if there are already therapies in later development or in the marketplace that partially address the clinical need, it might require significant therapeutic endeavour, usually through late phase III and phase IV clinical trials, to establish the product in the marketplace. It is therefore important to identify the place of an individual drug in the therapeutic armamentarium.

The prescriber will base a decision on a consideration of the relative risk–benefit, whereas the regulator will consider the drug entirely on its own merits and will tend to assess the efficacy, safety and quality of a drug in its own right. A relative judgement is straightforward in an area of high unmet medical need, when there is simply a consideration of whether it is better to have the disease treated or untreated, but much more difficult and subtle in an area where drug treatment is already available. The complexity of the decision tends to increase with an increasing number of treatment options and under these circumstances the prescriber will be more inclined to consider the options for the individual patient. For example, when treating hypertension in a middle-aged man the first choice may be a beta-blocker. The choice of which beta-blocker may depend on whether the particular drug has been shown to have any primary or secondary role in preventing myocardial infarction, on its effect on cholesterol, its propensity to affect adversely the peripheral vasculature, whether it limits exercise tolerance or has undesirable effects in a patient with asthma. It is therefore important to mirror this thought process when considering the market support programme and also to take account of preclinical data that may point to establishing clinical differentiation from a competitor. Studies examining such endpoints are always attractive to marketing departments.

The use of surrogate markers is always attractive. They allow drug development timelines to be shortened and may allow particular marketing angles to be pursued (e.g. a cholesterol-lowering effect in a cardiovascular agent). Regulators are increasingly likely to question the use of surrogate markers for large-scale pivotal phase III studies. Typically, at least one clinical endpoint trial is necessary. Such a trial is large and costly and it may take a considerable time to enrol and follow-up subjects in the study. The large cardiovascular intervention and survival studies are examples of such studies.

Regulators may require specific studies to address specific questions (e.g. use of the drug in the elderly, in children or other at-risk populations). Design of these studies needs detailed consideration: the subjects might be difficult to recruit, and comparative or placebo studies may be complex, potentially unethical

or unduly expensive in terms of time and resources. Drug development expertise, as well as good support from the biostatistical and biometrics groups, is vital. The ICH guidelines can be particularly helpful when conducting clinical trials in special populations. However, sometimes the guidelines are ambiguous at best.

9.4.3 Safety

About 20% of new drugs will fail because of safety concerns.[9] Nevertheless, with a clinical development programme involving an average of about 4500 patients (see below), the potential prescriber of a new drug is faced with the absence of a large amount of safety data. The safety profile of a drug will develop over time as adverse reactions occur spontaneously in a normal clinical setting. While there is no substitute for spontaneous reporting in the identification of rare side-effects, it is important to consider whether useful safety information can be generated soon after launch.

In this context, a decision on whether post-marketing surveillance studies should be built into the development programme must be taken. Such an observational study may signal the occurrence of adverse events or, alternatively, it may signal and quantify the frequency of adverse events. At this point in the life cycle of a new medicine, post-marketing surveillance is likely to involve cohort observational studies of 10–20,000 patients. The value of these studies is likely to be threefold:

1. To generate safety data during use of a drug in routine clinical practice, to enable a comparison to be made of the safety profile in an uncontrolled population and the controlled clinical trial population;

2. To provide safety data in a defined group incompletely covered in the registration package (e.g. the elderly); and

3. To enlarge the 'formal' safety database and thereby act as an insurance policy to address problems occurring at a later stage in a drug's evolution.

The possibility for such studies will depend on the disease, disease frequency and whether the prescribing setting is in primary or secondary care. The value of these studies is likely to be greatest if data are generated as soon as possible after launch, and plans for implementation must occur well in advance of submission of the regulatory dossier. Such studies might also be a condition of registration.

Post-marketing (phase IV) studies also generate safety data, but qualitatively these are likely to be similar to those collected during the pre-registration phase. In Western Europe, larger phase IV studies that have the evaluation of clinical safety as a primary objective have been embraced by the Post-Authorisation Safety Assessment (PASS) or Safety Assessment of Marketed Medicines (SAMM) guidelines, which have superseded previous guidelines on post-marketing surveillance and which are incorporated into the EMEA pharmaco-vigilance guidelines.

In recent years, there has been a growth in the field of mega-studies, usually clinical outcome studies involving 5000–25,000 patients, with a simple primary endpoint such as mortality and a number of secondary morbidity endpoints. The potential for studies of this magnitude to throw up less frequent side-effects than those seen in the pre-registration programme is clear.

9.5 The detailed clinical development plan

In this section we consider the requirements for the clinical programme leading to global registration, as well as other studies which will form part of the overall programme. Scheduling is covered elsewhere in this volume, but it must be emphasised that each activity in the clinical study programme has to be identified and an appropriate order determined. A realistic estimate of timing can thus be made and, when the sequence and timing of events has been determined, the critical path can be established. This is the chain of essential events that must be accomplished to achieve a particular goal; clearly, a change to one of these events has a fundamental effect on development time.

As with any plan, well-defined milestones and checkpoints must be incorporated and subsequent activity should not proceed until these have been achieved. The plan must always be sufficiently detailed to identify supporting activities such as toxicological studies that must be completed to allow development to continue without interruption. Many of these activities can, and should, run in parallel.

9.5.1 Number of patients

Although there are no fixed rules on devising the phase III programme, the more subjects admitted the better in terms of a safety evaluation, but it must be kept in mind that ethical considerations demand that only sufficient patients to meet the scientific criteria of study endpoints should be randomised. For example, for a disease-modifying drug for rheumatoid arthritis,

approval has been granted on a database of up to approximately 6000 subjects; however, a novel immuno-suppressant agent has been granted an approval with fewer than 2000 subjects. Based on their experience, Blake and Ratcliffe[10] suggested that approximately 3000 patients per indication is average for a New Drug Application (NDA) in 1991. The Tufts Institute in 2001 suggested that about 4500 subjects is average for an NDA.[11] These two numbers are consistent with an annual compound increase in numbers of about 7%. Others have suggested that about 100 patient-years experience is satisfactory for some established drugs for well-understood disease areas, such as new formulations of insulin. Much also depends on the additional supportive data that can be included in the application.

The number of subjects is likely to vary depending on the degree of unmet medical need and the seriousness of the disease indication. It is likely that a drug shown to be effective in treating stroke, a condition with a high mortality and morbidity where no effective treatment is available, will require a database of fewer than 3000 patients. Conversely, an anxiolytic, used to treat a non-life threatening condition where effective treatments already exist, may require a much larger database. However, 4500 patients represent a reasonable working total.

9.5.2 Number of studies

Having established the number of patients to be included in the pre-registration clinical programme, it is important to consider how these will be distributed and hence how many studies are required. This is very variable. The Tufts Institute reported that, for biopharmaceuticals, there were on average only 12 studies and 1014 subjects per NDA compared with 37 studies and 4478 subjects for a conventional pharmaceutical NDA.[11]

Generally speaking, the FDA will require placebo-controlled studies wherever possible to demonstrate efficacy at the dose to be marketed and these are termed pivotal studies. Pivotal studies do not have to be placebo-controlled, and in some areas, such as depression, the ICH guidelines suggest a three-arm study, with both an active comparator and a placebo control. The Declaration of Helsinki, revised in 2000, suggested that in some disease areas, placebo-controlled studies are to be examined very carefully for their ethical content. This includes areas where conventional best therapy is generally acceptable. In this case, great care needs to be taken with the choice of active comparator.

It is widely accepted that two placebo-controlled pivotal studies are necessary, although it is not clear that this is a mandatory regulation in the FDA or EMEA regulations. However, there is a certain insurance in this approach as studies, even of drugs that are effective, can occasionally fail to show a statistically positive result if the treated population somehow deviates from the norm or if the placebo response is unexpectedly increased. In Europe the use of an active comparator in a pivotal study is more common.

Sample sizes for clinical trials are discussed more fully elsewhere in this book and should be established in discussion with a statistician. However, sample sizes should be sufficient to be 90% certain of detecting a statistically significant difference between treatments, based on a set of predetermined primary variables. This means that trials utilising an active control will generally be considerably larger than placebo-controlled studies in order to exclude a type II statistical error (i.e. the failure to demonstrate a difference where one exists). Thus, in areas where a substantial safety database is required (e.g. hypertension), it may be appropriate to have in the programme a preponderance of studies using a positive control.

The increasing use of active comparator studies has meant that more studies are being powered on a 'non-inferiority' basis. It is essential to discuss such designs with statisticians. Other novel designs (e.g. initial open-label therapy followed by a randomised treatment arm following disease exacerbation) are becoming more common. These novel designs must be discussed with a statistician and with the regulatory authorities before expensive mistakes are made.

Conversely, if demonstration of efficacy is more critical than establishing safety (e.g. in Alzheimer's disease), then placebo-controlled studies are appropriate. Although the studies may include fewer patients, the number of studies may be approximately the same as for a hypertension programme.

It is eminently sensible to aim to have the smallest number of studies in the dossier as this makes data management and analysis less complex and therefore less time-consuming. It is inevitable that some studies which are not universally necessary will find their way into the core dossier. In France, for example, pricing is inextricably linked to technical approval and, when granting a price, the authorities make reference to an already available treatment wherever possible. It would therefore be virtually impossible to obtain pricing approval unless a comparative study with a reference drug had been undertaken. As pricing approval is the immediate step after technical approval, the 'pricing study' needs to begin at the same time as the core registration studies, hence it becomes part of the regulatory dossier.

While it is desirable to avoid duplicating activity, there will undoubtedly be some duplication of studies in the clinical programme given the foregoing discussion. It is important nevertheless to ensure that ad hoc studies do not find their way into the plan by default. The importance of studies designed to demonstrate competitive advantage has been mentioned and while data from many of these studies may not find their way into the regulatory dossier, the studies are nevertheless part of the overall clinical programme. Under these circumstances, there is little point in allowing duplication of comparator drugs between studies. For example, there is a considerable variety of drugs for the treatment of depression, ranging from the old tricyclic compounds such as amitriptyline and imipramine to the more recent and less toxic compounds such as the selective monoamine and serotonin reuptake inhibitors. In between there is a host of antidepressant drugs with distinguishing properties; some are sedative, while others have anxiolytic activity. The most widely used drug will also vary from country to country. This situation therefore presents an opportunity to implement an international programme to test the new agent against a variety of competitors in order to tease out differences and provide data that may be required to support registration and that will also be of major use at the time of launch and subsequent marketing in individual countries. Care must be taken at head office that local studies do not jeopardise the overall regulatory and marketing plan, as embodied in the draft SmPC. A study in which the drug dosage is halved for local marketing reasons might have the potential to undermine the whole regulatory package unless there are clear medical reasons for such a study.

Finally, in addition to studies that may be included to address potential regulatory questions, it is important to consider whether 'in-filling' is needed. In an attempt to speed drug development, a high-risk strategy is to take the decision to enter full development as early as possible. This may mean that many elements of the phase IIb programme are not carried out sequentially. One strategy is to carry out formal dose-ranging studies as part of the large-scale phase IIa efficacy and safety programme. 'In-filling' can be used to describe any study that forms part of the essential regulatory package that is not conducted in conventional phase I–III sequence.

9.5.3 Duration of treatment

In Europe, a drug that is likely to be administered long term will require a minimum of 100 patients treated for 1 year to gain approval. This will vary depending on the circumstances. It is likely that a new antihypertensive agent will require significantly more long-term experience than this before a licence is granted, whereas a drug that is effective in treating gastric cancer may require less. It is important to remember that data generated as a result of long-term administration will be required to support registration applications for drugs used to treat recurrent diseases, such as peptic ulcer, as well as chronic diseases such as hypertension.

Most phase III studies in a chronic disease will require 1 year of therapy. Most oncology studies will require 12 months' survival data.

9.5.4 Dose

The FDA demands, at opposite ends of the dose range, a dose that demonstrates efficacy but is associated with side-effects and a dose that is largely ineffective. A range of doses may be studied within these limits, with the aim of identifying a dose that is both effective and tolerable. In Europe, there is greater scope to justify the choice of dose in a particular set of clinical circumstances. Choice of dose should also take account of further development for new indications; for example, an antihypertensive drug may also be effective in treating angina or heart failure but the dose is likely to differ significantly.

9.5.5 Patient categories

It is important to include all age ranges that are of clinical importance. Development of an anti-asthma drug, for example, should include a programme of evaluation in children as well as adults because they will form a significant portion of the database and risk–benefit considerations will be different. Development of an anti-arthritis compound, on the other hand, will be undertaken predominantly in older patients and particularly detailed information on efficacy and safety in the elderly will be required.

This raises the important question of 'what is elderly?' In the average regulatory dossier, the majority of patients are likely to be less than 75 years old, yet population demographics point to the increasing importance of the 'older elderly' – those aged more than 75 years. Abernethy[12] reports, reassuringly, that there is little or no evidence to date to suggest that the toxicity of any drug is unique to the elderly and therefore it follows that the 'older elderly' are probably not a discrete group. It would appear prudent, however, in a clinical situation where a drug is likely to be taken by large numbers of patients in this category for there to be an appropriate evaluation of the risks and benefits. This may not need to form part of the regulatory package but data could be generated by a cohort observational study as part of a post-marketing surveillance programme.

The FDA Modernisation Act of 1997 (FDAMA) included a number of elements that have increased the number of studies being performed in children. This was largely successful at increasing data on paediatric studies in the USA and has been now replaced by the Best Pharmaceuticals for Children Act, 4 January 2002 (Public Law No. 107-109). In September 2004, the European Commission released a proposal for a Regulation on medicines for children.[13] The aim of this Regulation is to ensure that medicines for children are efficacious and safe, and will mean that all development plans will have to consider actively paediatric studies in the future.

9.5.6 Coexisting medical conditions/concomitant drug interactions

It is important to ensure adequate collection of data in patients who have coexisting medical conditions in whom drug elimination may be reduced, particularly those with hepatic or renal impairment, as lower doses are likely to be required in these patients. It is also important to investigate potential drug interactions, both clinically and pharmacologically, particularly for drugs prescribed for conditions that are likely to coexist, and specific clinical pharmacology studies must be built into the programme. For example, it is necessary to determine the effect of a new antihypertensive agent co-prescribed with an angiotensin converting enzyme (ACE) inhibitor, nitrate, calcium-channel blocker, beta-blocker and diuretic, in terms of both drug interactions and potentiation of antihypertensive effect. Interaction via an effect on the cytochrome P450 system must also be investigated should there be any suggestion from preclinical data that this may occur.

9.5.7 Dosage form

Is the dosage form to be used for large-scale development and hence commercialisation the same as that used for earlier phase studies and is the choice underpinned by an appropriate toxicology work-up? It is common for the dosage form to change during the course of the development process. Early studies may be carried out using liquid or capsule preparations because of the ease of formulation. Almost invariably, the marketed formulation will be different and it is important to ensure that inclusion in the regulatory dossier of data obtained using the early formulations can be justified by appropriate bioavailability studies, which may be required as part of the full pre-registration plan. It is highly desirable that the full development programme, which will generate the largest amount of data for the registration file, utilises the formulation to be marketed in order that safety and efficacy data can be amalgamated. Phase III studies should be undertaken with the intended market formulation.

It is important to consider the impact of different formulations. The requirements for an inhaled drug, for example, will be quite different from the requirements for the same drug given orally.

Is the development of two formulations to proceed in parallel or sequentially? The size of the programme may be doubled if a second formulation is aimed at a different target group. However, it may be more cost-effective to carry out a larger programme than to come back at a later date. For example, in the development of a new agent to treat inflammatory bowel disease it may be inappropriate to use an orally active formulation in a patient with disease confined to the distal end of the large bowel. While this situation may account for a relatively small proportion of patients, it is nevertheless desirable to have available a range of formulations suitable for use by all patients. Under these circumstances it would substantially increase the cost of the programme to study these patients at a later date, given that during the screening process to identify patients suitable for inclusion in a trial of oral medication; these patients would be identified and would not be included in the study. The length of time taken to gather data on the major formulation is unlikely to be increased as there is no competition for patients, but gathering data on the secondary formulation represents an increase in workload. The trade-off is therefore an increase in workload versus a more cost-effective and clinically comprehensive programme.

9.5.8 Clinical trial supplies

This is a crucial area and one that should be given maximum attention during the planning process, as the length of time required to ensure adequate clinical trial supplies can never be underestimated. Inadequacy of clinical trial supplies can be a reason for delay in the execution of a clinical development programme. The Clinical Trials Directive (2001/20/EC),

GMP Directive (2003/94/EC) and Annex 13 Guidance allow verification of compliance with Good Manufacturing Practice (GMP) as well as Good Clinical Practice (GCP). Investigational medicinal products (IMPs) have to be manufactured to a standard 'at least equivalent to' EU GMP. This relates to the finished dosage form and not just the active pharmaceutical. Placebo has to be manufactured to GMP as well. GMP codes vary across the world and specific steps must be taken to ensure that EU GMP standards are met. In practice, this relates mostly to drugs manufactured in the USA, as there is no Mutual Recognition Agreement between US and EU GMP. A Qualified Person (QP) release is required for each batch of all IMPs and this might be especially difficult to achieve for active comparator products.

The explanation for delay is likely to be threefold:
1. Insufficient information is provided to colleagues in pharmaceutical development early enough, so that insufficient compound has been synthesised and manufactured according to the relevant GMP standards.
2. Insufficient time is allowed for packaging and distribution. Clinical trials packaging is becoming increasingly complex, particularly when a drug that may be a second-line treatment is being tested. For example, it would be unethical to stop an ACE inhibitor and diuretic in a patient with heart failure, therefore administration of a new drug will be against this backdrop. In order to maintain double-blind conditions, it will be necessary to employ a double-dummy technique and therefore a minimum of four different agents per patient must be packaged: the ACE inhibitor, diuretic, new agent and placebo. The situation can be hugely complex as, for example, the testing of a new antiparkinsonian agent, where packaging of more than a dozen tablets per patient per day may be necessary. Complexity is further increased if the trial is international and dosage instructions have to be supplied in a number of languages. Despite this, drug supplies have to be distributed to a number of different countries, each of which requires different documentation to satisfy local customs regulations. It is hardly surprising that this aspect of the clinical development plan sometimes does not receive the attention it warrants. The use of an interactive voice randomisation system (IVRS) becomes increasingly useful as the study design becomes more complex. IVRS also allows scarce drug supplies to be rapidly dispatched to the appropriate site.
3. Insufficient time is allowed to obtain supplies of comparator drugs. Companies are notoriously bureaucratic, or even obstructive, in dealing with requests

for supplies of active drug and placebo; it therefore pays to start negotiations early. Protocols involving comparator drugs from other companies must be targeted for early drafting, particularly if they are on the critical path, as the approval process is likely to be prolonged. If adequate time is allowed then it is always possible, should there be a refusal to supply active drug and placebo, to extract the active substance from a marketed formulation, reformulate, demonstrate bioequivalence with the approved formulation, and manufacture sufficient supplies for the clinical programme, together with matching placebo. This is clearly much less efficient than negotiating successfully with another company.

9.5.9 Length of the programme

The importance of taking a long-term strategic view when designing the full development programme has already be stressed, but clearly it is impossible to plan in detail studies which may or may not start some years in the future. The most crucial timing in the programme is the point at which the clinical cut-off will occur to permit compilation of the clinical section of the registration dossier. From this point, the timing of submission of the dossier can be predicted and hence the timing of regulatory approval and launch. It is thus important to be able to estimate with some degree of accuracy the length of time necessary to achieve the goal of clinical cut-off and to ensure that the major pivotal studies will be finished at that point. This fact mandates that the pivotal studies should receive high priority in the execution of the plan.

As anyone involved in the conduct of clinical trials knows, it is notoriously difficult to estimate the length of time it will take to recruit patients into a study. Formal inclusion and exclusion criteria can severely restrict the numbers of patients suitable for a trial, even when common conditions are being studied. An additional and common complication is the 'over-optimistic investigator syndrome'.

It is becoming increasingly common to conduct fairly rigorous feasibility studies to determine the likelihood of patient and investigator recruitment in different countries. A complicating factor is competing studies. This is particularly so in areas of great scientific endeavour such as oncology. It is not uncommon for large oncology centres to be running upwards of 50 different studies. Competition for patients can be intense.

In more recent years, in an attempt to overcome these problems, it has become fashionable to include more centres than may be necessary in a study on the basis that some will be successful at recruiting whereas others will not. All, of course, have to be assessed to ensure that they can operate within the principles of GCP. It is important to be realistic in estimating the speed at which recruitment will occur, and even in common disease areas it is often unreasonable to expect centres to recruit at the rate of more than one to two patients per month. Nevertheless, the geographical distribution of clinical research is of major commercial concern because involvement of influential clinicians in the evaluation of a product is vital. It necessarily follows that involvement of influential clinicians in potentially large markets is of prime importance. Studies should therefore be conducted in these areas as first choice. However, that mandates a willingness on behalf of the investigator to participate in pivotal studies and to meet development deadlines which, of course, assumes the existence of an appropriate patient population and facilities for the conduct of the study.

A further factor that will impact the speed at which the clinical programme can proceed is the human resource committed to the programme. There are some activities that will not be affected by manipulation of resource, such as the 'in-life' phase of a 2-year carcinogenicity study. However, reporting time for the study can be reduced if more resource is applied. Various models for predicting resource allocation exist but none is particularly reliable. While trial monitors and data handlers may be a resource dedicated to one programme, physicians and statisticians invariably have a range of commitments and will therefore be called upon to deal with unexpected problems, which cannot be taken into account in the planning process. Blake and Ratcliffe[10] have generated a model describing drug development, running either sequentially or in parallel. For reasons that have already been considered, the former situation generally does not exist because of time constraints, although it makes more efficient use of human resources. Blake and Ratcliffe estimated that for an average NDA of about 3000 patients, with studies proceeding in parallel, it is necessary to recruit around 200 centres. Clearly, for an NDA that requires an average of about 4500 subjects, these numbers should be extrapolated upwards. Blake and Ratcliffe estimated that the programme would require the dedicated tie-in of 25–30 staff, three-quarters of whom would be trial monitors and data processors and the remainder physicians and statisticians. This gives some idea of the level of resource commitment required to discharge a successful programme and some notion of the continued commitment of resource to market support studies.

9.5.10 Data management

In many companies, data collection, handling and analysis constitute a major bottleneck and are a source of irritation to investigators and of frustration to commercial colleagues. The process of data collection begins with the protocol, which must be clear and unambiguous. If it is confusing in English it will be more so in a foreign language. There must be a flow diagram. The practical parts of the protocol (i.e. those in daily use during the running of a trial) should be separate from the remainder and in a form allowing easy reference. If the protocol facilitates the study it will reduce error and hence rework.

The case report form (CRF) should be unambiguous and simple to use. Its completion should minimise the need for text. CRFs should consist of three modules. One module is common for all trials (e.g. laboratory data), one is common for all trials in the clinical programme for a given compound, and one is specific to the study in question. In this way data handlers become familiar with the forms and can therefore manage a larger number with fewer mistakes. A mechanism should be in existence to ensure that the clinician completes the CRF adequately.

Recently, significant efforts have been made in most organisations to reduce the time from last patient out to final report. As always, a balance must be struck between satisfactory resource utilisation and cost. Most companies are now looking at an 8–12 week period from last patient out to final report. The most significant delay is in resolving final data queries at study sites and this depends principally on the clinical research associate monitoring schedules and the availability of study personnel at the study site. It should be the objective of every trial monitor to produce a complete set of clean data within 1–2 weeks of the last patient completing the trial, with the target of closing the database and initiating the analysis and statistical reporting of the primary variables with the minimum of delay. Data are of little value unless they are analysed and reported; indeed, data left in an office may be potentially dangerous.

To simplify the process it is important that a single database is developed for the whole programme. This is particularly relevant to the production of safety data, not only in the interests of efficiency, but also so that any safety issues will be recognised as they arise.

If a particular set of adverse events is suggested by preclinical toxicology then they should be flagged in the database so that the monitors' attention is drawn to them.

9.5.11 Cost

The full clinical development plan will be a major expense, so has to be costed accurately and conducted as economically as possible. The conduct of clinical trials is being increasingly seen by investigators as a business, and grants to investigators are the largest out-of-pocket expense incurred in the clinical development phase. It is estimated that drug development costs about US$403 million per drug, on average, at 2000 prices,[2] but this includes manufacturing and all on-costs, rather than just the drug development programme.

9.5.12 Technology

Although superficially attractive, there has not been the widespread adoption of technology that many have predicted for the past 15 years. The use of electronic data capture (EDC) remains in its infancy. There are many suppliers, and most companies have conducted studies with EDC. However, the difficulties in training investigators and ensuring consistent technological support 24 hours a day, 365 days a year, in many different countries remain formidable. As internet access improves, electronic diaries may become more widely used for some particular types of studies, such as asthma and diabetes, where patients are accustomed to keeping diaries in any event.

Electronic medical records are not yet useful for significant clinical development research.

9.6 Executing the plan

There can be no substitute for excellent planning and this is why a substantial portion of this chapter has been devoted to a consideration of the important elements of the clinical development programme. There needs to be a clear and concise map of activities leading to compilation of the clinical section of the regulatory dossier and beyond. However good the programme is, there will be a successful outcome only if it is executed in an efficient and timely manner. The important factors are:

- Selection of sites;
- Prioritisation of trials;
- Quality control;
- Quality assurance;

- Use of contract research organisations (CROs);
- Training – technical and process;
- Communication; and
- Process improvement.

9.6.1 Selection of sites

Reference to the principles of GCP has been made; only investigational centres whose personnel and facilities are capable of working to GCP should be selected to participate in the programme. The selection of an investigator is a balance between value for money and desirability of having a particular individual working within the programme.

9.6.2 Prioritisation

The importance of identifying pivotal studies and studies on the critical path was discussed in a previous section. It is important that these studies are given the highest priority, both in execution and reporting, and that provision is made to identify early if there are problems recruiting patients so that appropriate remedial action can be taken. The studies of longest duration should be started first.

9.6.3 Quality assurance

While quality assurance of data is rightly demanded by the FDA and EMEA, it increasingly forms an integral part of other aspects in the execution of clinical trials. Investigators must understand that this is part of the process of participating in a study and must expect to be audited and the quality of their data recording to be monitored. Most companies now have a quality assurance function which, for management reasons, reports outside the clinical organisation. This function can also be outsourced.

9.6.4 Quality control

One of the measures of the quality of the pre-registration clinical programme is the total time from the decision to enter full development to the first regulatory approval in a major market. It is also important to monitor quality in other ways. One option is to assess the frequency with which predetermined milestones are achieved. More subtly, quality can be assessed by examining the number of incomplete, inaccurate or indecipherable CRFs that are returned or the number of protocol amendments made that are not based on new information. Milestones may still be achieved when quality is poor (i.e. when there is inefficiency), but this means that they were wrongly established and can be improved if efficiency improves.

9.6.5 Contract research organisations

In a discussion on the allocation of resource and analysis of workload, the decision on whether to engage a CRO for an element of the programme should be taken during the planning stage. It is important to remember that a CRO has to be managed and this can be as much as 5–10% of the company resource which would otherwise be directly involved in carrying out the programme. It is important that the objectives for the CRO are clear and that the scope of the task involved, including cost and milestones, is agreed by both parties before any contractual commitment. It must also be remembered that the CRO has to be audited and quality assured.

CROs are likely to be more efficient, and on occasion can be faster than the company. A balance has to be struck between the outsourcing costs, internal costs (which are often underestimated) and the management requirements and skill sets of the CRO and internal staff.

9.6.6 Training

It is obvious that appropriate technical training should be provided for anyone joining a development programme, and staff already working on the programme should be encouraged to keep abreast of developments in the therapeutic area. Equally important is process training to ensure that the principles of GCP are fully understood and applied, and that internal processes in the form of standard operating procedures (SOPs) are fully documented and understood. The process, and hence the SOPs, will need to satisfy all those customers and providers who will contribute to the development programme and ensure that the many tasks involved will be performed once and once only to avoid waste. The ability of all staff to work to SOPs and therefore work between countries and disciplines with a degree of consistency is paramount in executing a successful programme and this ability should be tested by regular audit. This is a particular advantage in times of stress when personnel may become interchangeable.

9.6.7 Communication

All personnel involved in the programme should have the same level of knowledge of progress and this can only be achieved using a computer-based clinical trials management system, which must be constantly and accurately updated. The central monitors who have an overview of the programme must initiate remedial action should recruitment, especially into pivotal studies, be less than anticipated. Equally, information concerning adverse reactions should be disseminated promptly so that investigators can be kept closely informed and enjoy a uniform level of knowledge. Finally, in order to develop and foster teamwork, regular meetings involving internal and external staff must be arranged so that a two-way exchange of information can occur and problems solved.

9.6.8 Process improvement

The importance of documenting internal processes in the form of SOPs has already been mentioned. Any activity forming part of the development plan is a process. Each SOP should be looked on as a dynamic document and opportunities for improving each process should be sought continually. For example, the time that elapses between the last patient completing a clinical trial and production of the statistical report is an activity very much on the critical path.

This activity or process can be broken down into its smallest components, each of these examined carefully for opportunities to reduce cycle time, and pieced together again, with the objective of producing a significantly quicker time overall. The implications in terms of total development time are huge and yet many companies do not attempt to harness the benefits that process improvements can bring by establishing formal process improvement initiatives.

Acknowledgements

Dai Rowley-Jones and Paul A. Nicholson, who authored this chapter in the Third Edition of this textbook, and Alan G. Davies, co-author to the Fifth Edition, are acknowledged for their leadership and the free use of their material when preparing this chapter.

References

1 Arthur Anderson. *Managing Risk, Building Value. Risk Management in the UK Life Sciences.* London: Arthur Anderson, 2001.

2 DiMasi JA, Hansen RW, Grabowski HG et al. The price of innovation: new estimates of drug development costs. *J Health Econ* 2003;**22**:151–85.

3 Pharmaprojects Annual Review 2006: http://www.pjbpubs.com/pharmaprojects/annual_review.htm. Accessed 17 October 2008.

4 Pharmaprojects Annual Review 2008. http://www.pharmaprojects.com/therapy_analysis/annual-review-0508.htm. Accessed 24 October 2008.

5 Geoff Watts. Negotiating research priorities. *BMJ* 2004;**329**:704.

6 Committee for Proprietary Medicinal Products. *ICH M4. Common Technical Document for the Registration of Pharmaceuticals for Human Use – Organisation CTD.* CPMP/ICH/2887/99. London: CPMP, 1999.

7 Debashis S. Merck withdraws arthritis drug worldwide. *BMJ* 2004;**329**:816.

8 DiMasi JA. Risks in new drug development: approval success rates for investigational drugs. *Clin Pharmacol Ther* 2001;**69**:297–307.

9 DiMasi JA. New drug development in the United States from 1963 to 1999. *Clin Pharmacol Ther* 2001;**69**:286–96.

10 Blake P, Ratcliffe MJ. Can we accelerate drug development? *Drug Inf J* 1991;**25**:13–8.

11 Tufts Center for the Study of Drug Development. *Outlook 2001.* Boston: Tufts Center, 2001.

12 Abernethy DR. Research challenges, new drug development, preclinical and clinical trials in the ageing population. *Drug Saf* 1990;**5**(Suppl 1):71–4.

13 European Commission. *Proposal for a Regulation of the European Parliament and the Council on Medicinal Products for Paediatric Use.* Brussels 29.9.2004.

Part II Medical department issues

10 The medical department

Peter Stonier[1] and David Gillen[2]

[1] Amdipharm plc, Basildon, Essex, UK
[2] Primary Care BU Europe Canada Australia and NZ, Pfizer, Walton Oaks, UK

10.1 Introduction

Medical departments may be large, as in the head-quarters of a multinational company, or small, as in one of its subsidiary operating companies. There are probably as many ways of organising a medical department as there are companies. Although there may be national, cultural and regulatory differences between countries, which further complicate their construction, the influence of the EU, through the introduction of guidelines and directives, is leading to medical departments across Europe operating in similar ways. No matter how they are organised, there are certain responsibilities that all medical departments should accept.

This chapter outlines these areas of responsibility and the key players who are needed to fulfil these. It also describes how, by working in cross-functional teams, the members of the medical department contribute to the process of product development.

10.2 Role of the medical department

The common objective of all pharmaceutical companies is to discover, develop and market safe, efficacious and cost-effective medicines that will bring benefits to patients, health care professionals and consumers, and result in profitable returns to the company. In this process it is important that, at all stages in the life cycle of a pharmaceutical product, the needs and interests of those who will receive these medicines should be paramount. To this end, the major areas of responsibility for the medical department are to:

The Textbook of Pharmaceutical Medicine. Edited by John P. Griffin. © 2009, ISBN: 978-1-4051-8035-1.

• Act as the medical conscience of the company;
• Ensure adherence to relevant legal requirements and guidelines;
• Provide a medical perspective to product development;
• Provide the medical input to the servicing and support of marketed products throughout their life cycle;
• Provide general as well as specialised medical expertise, as required; and
• Act as the company's expert interface with all sectors of the medical profession as well as other external stakeholders (e.g. regulatory authorities, press, health technology assessment bodies).

How these responsibilities are shared among the members of a medical department will become apparent from the descriptions of the various roles in section 10.3. The degree to which the medical department is usually involved in what is traditionally described as the four phases of clinical development will also be outlined.

There exist guidelines and regulations, described elsewhere in this book, to control:
• The conduct of clinical evaluation during the development of a new product;
• The regulatory process which allows the product to be marketed; and
• The way in which the product can be promoted.
Beyond these guidelines, the medical department has the important role of keeping the company aware, at all times, of the needs of patients and of the medical and allied professions. It is therefore important that there should be medical input to a company's strategy by having the head of the medical department (in the UK) usually in the role of medical director, as a member of the senior management team. The development of pharmaceutical medicine into a specialty (see section 10.3.1) has strengthened the role of the

pharmaceutical physician, who is qualified not only to provide medical expertise but also, through the tradition of the Hippocratic oath, to represent the needs and interests of patients. While the pharmaceutical physician remains bound by the requirements of Good Medical Practice, as laid down in the UK by the General Medical Council,[1] recently specific guidance has also been provided in a report produced by the Faculty of Pharmaceutical Medicine.[2]

10.3 Who are the key players in the medical department?

The medical department is usually headed by a senior pharmaceutical physician (the medical director), who is supported by a team consisting of other physicians, graduates and administrative staff. The non-medical graduates are normally pharmacists or life scientists and, in addition to providing informed scientific input, may look after some administrative areas. In some companies they, rather than the physicians, may be responsible for staff management, thus allowing the physicians to concentrate on their advisory roles.

In a modern pharmaceutical company, members of the medical department can expect to have an important role at all stages in a product's life cycle. Working with commercial new product development colleagues from the earliest planning stages, their specialist skills and expertise help the team to drive the development process down the right path from earliest clinical development to product marketing and beyond.

Key players from the medical department are likely to be as follows, although not every company will place all these specialists within the medical department:

- Pharmaceutical physicians;
- Clinical research scientists;
- Statisticians and data managers;
- Medical information scientists;
- Scientific advisers;
- Regulatory executives;
- Drug safety/pharmacovigilance scientists; and
- Pharmacoeconomics advisers.

In whatever way it is organised, the medical department works closely with cross-functional colleagues such as finance, human resources and other departments. Thus, while it is not possible to propose any specific organisational structure for a medical department, the organogram presented in Figure 10.1 reflects the issues that need to be considered when deciding on the preferred organisation within the company.

Let us now consider what each player brings to the process of product development.

10.3.1 The pharmaceutical physician

Currently, there are few specific regulatory and legal requirements for medically qualified approval (e.g. final approval of promotional material).[3] This can now be carried out by a pharmacist for materials more than 1 year old.[3] It is possible for a small organisation to meet these requirements by employing physicians on a part-time advisory basis. In the UK, over 700 physicians are employed full time in the pharmaceutical industry, so it is evident that companies see them having a wider role. Although the legal requirement for medical signatories may be limited, the internal policies of many companies require that certain matters can only be conducted or approved by a registered medical practitioner. For example, standard operating procedures (SOPs) might require a medical signatory on clinical trial protocols and amendments, clinical study reports, clinical investigators' brochures, 'Dear Doctor' letters and 'named patient' supplies of medicines.

It is expected that, before entering the industry, the physician has acquired a good base of medical knowledge and broad clinical experience. However, pharmaceutical physicians are not usually employed for their clinical expertise because although many retain honorary clinical posts – with the consent of their employing companies – this is rarely sufficient for them to remain clinical 'experts' and clinical advice is best sought from current full-time clinicians. On the other hand, it is possible for a pharmaceutical physician to become an internationally recognised expert on clinical research in a particular therapeutic area and, through this clinical contact, to have valuable access to key opinion leaders.

There are certain personal attributes over and above a medical degree and clinical experience that make for a successful pharmaceutical physician. To be valued, the pharmaceutical physician must be able to provide insight into the clinical benefit, and hence the commercial potential, of a compound at any stage in its development. He or she must also have the planning skills to realise that potential, and an ability to communicate at all levels, both inside and outside the company, increasingly needed for 'leadership' qualities as well as technical knowledge. If the medical department is to act as the company's medical conscience (see section 10.2), it will need to have a medically qualified and suitably experienced person on its staff. The physician might take a high-profile

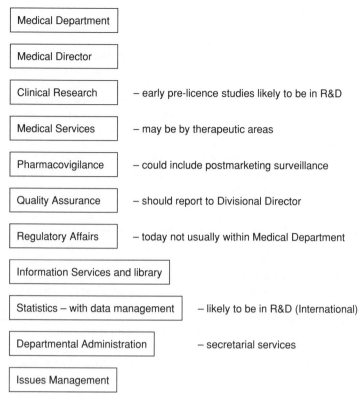

Figure 10.1 Roles within or associated with the company's medical operations.

role in drug withdrawals from the market and in addressing the reputational challenges of the industry; there is an increasingly important role for pharmaceutical physicians as the external face of the company and its interactions with stakeholders in the health care marketplace and other public and governmental bodies. In addition, a good pharmaceutical physician can be a credible ambassador for the company when lecturing to external audiences or dealing with the communication media.

Most physicians in the pharmaceutical industry work in one of three main areas, which correspond to the well-defined phases through which a drug passes in its clinical evaluation:

1. Clinical pharmacology;

2. Clinical research – particularly clinical development; or

3. Medical affairs or medical services.

The ratio of pharmaceutical physicians in each area is approximately 1 : 4 : 8. In some small companies, a physician's responsibilities may extend across more than one of these areas. In larger companies, clinical

pharmacology is likely to be responsibility of the research part of a company, while the medical services function resides within local operating companies.

In recent years, an increasing proportion of early clinical research involving healthy volunteers (phase 1), falling under the responsibility of the clinical pharmacologist, is conducted in clinical research units as part of the contract research sector working with, but outside, the pharmaceutical companies.

Historically, the medical department's involvement in clinical research was in late-stage (phase IIIb and phase IV) studies for local market needs. Nowadays, although pre-licence clinical studies are most likely still driven by the research part of the company, the medical departments of local operating companies will probably coordinate these early international clinical studies in their own countries. As a result, clinical research now tends to be much more integrated, with Good Clinical Practice (GCP) being applied to all phases both pre- and post-licence. Similarly, phase IV or post-marketing studies tend to be international as registration and marketing strategies become pan-European or global in nature. The pharmaceutical physician has an important role in determining the therapy area and product strategy well before product launch, and this requires close liaison with colleagues in research and development.

To be effective, the pharmaceutical physician in the medical department has to recognise both the clinical needs of patients and the commercial needs of the company. Commercial colleagues look for constructive advice on how to fulfil these needs while operating within ethical and legal constraints. Such advice would include providing insight into the decision-making processes of clinical colleagues.

The specialty of pharmaceutical medicine and the concept of the pharmaceutical physician have developed in the last 40 years from the role of 'medical adviser in the pharmaceutical industry'. In the UK this development led, in 1989, to the foundation of the Faculty of Pharmaceutical Medicine within the Royal Colleges of Physicians. From this, Europe-wide recognition of pharmaceutical medicine as a specialty is slowly becoming reality. Legal and regulatory changes are also driving a requirement for specialist registration and accreditation.

The pharmaceutical physician provides a medical direction to marketing strategy and ensures that product literature and promotional material are legal and factually accurate. This is an important contribution to the medical department's role as 'medical conscience' (see section 10.2). Medical input remains necessary to the servicing and support of marketed products throughout their life cycle.

Such support can involve responding to complaints about promotional activities, which may come from other companies or external agencies such as, in the UK, the Prescription Medicines Code of Practice Authority and the Medicine and Healthcare products Regulatory Agency (MHRA; Blue Guide). A medically qualified person should certainly have overall responsibility for clinical drug safety issues (see section 10.3.6). Pharmaceutical physicians are often involved in the training of sales representatives. The medical director is not only a senior pharmaceutical physician, but also a senior manager and needs to be fully conversant with all the issues facing the company and understand all the principles and procedures that govern its operation. Nowadays this will include human resource issues, such as awareness of the laws related to employment. Without this broad understanding, the medical director will not be able to lead the activities of the medical department in a way that is optimal for the organisation while maintaining all the required professional and ethical standards.

10.3.2 The clinical research scientist

The clinical research scientist (CRS) is involved in all aspects of clinical trials from planning and design, through initiation and monitoring, to report-writing and publication. The medical department is likely to be involved in organising late pre-licence or post-licence clinical studies, with volunteer and phase II studies being the responsibility of the research and development part of the company. The primary objective of phase III studies is to contribute to the dossier for marketing authorisation which, once approved, is a watershed in a product's life. This will establish the initial profile of the product. In addition, there is a need to incorporate economic parameters into clinical at an early stage; while these aspects were addressed in late phase IIIb trials, they are now being introduced in phase II studies with the recognition that phase III is too late in the development process. There is also a need to broaden patient populations so that they more accurately reflect the real world. For successful marketing, clinical trials will be needed very shortly after product launch to further define the product profile, any additional claims that can be made about it and the treatment options. In certain therapeutic classes there may also be opportunities to switch some form of the product to a non-prescription classification. The studies needed to obtain the data to satisfy all these requirements will need to be planned, and probably started, before the first marketing authorisation. It is clear therefore that those involved in each set of trials need to collaborate closely.

The organisational structure for clinical research depends on size and whether the department is within headquarters or a local operating company. The transition through the phases of clinical research needs to be smooth and the decision-making process behind the research clear and well communicated. In larger companies the responsibilities of clinical scientists may be divided into therapy areas. Alternatively, monitoring responsibilities may be divided geographically, especially in the case of field-based staff.

Given the uncertainty of clinical research, one major asset of any CRS is flexibility. If this is combined with an aptitude for self-motivation, as well as team working, then the individual should be well qualified for the task.

The introduction of GCP has accelerated the need for quality control and quality assurance, particularly in the field of clinical research. Quality control is carried out by the staff who are responsible for the particular activity, working to SOPs – which cover all the tasks under scrutiny – within an overall quality management system. SOPs not only need to be written, but must also be updated regularly. Quality assurance is the process that seeks to confirm that SOPs have been observed; this is accomplished by the process of auditing. Internal audit departments should be under separate management from the medical department. Regular audits can not only assure external bodies such as regulatory authorities (MHRA/EMEA/FDA) that proper procedures have been followed, but also serve to deter those rare attempts at fraud on the part of clinical investigators.[4]

In most companies it is likely at some time that CRSs within a company will collaborate with counterparts within contract research organisations (CROs). CROs range from small, often specialised, groups, to large multinational companies. The services offered cover virtually every facet of clinical research, as well as of the regulatory process necessary for obtaining a marketing authorisation. CROs provide a flexible resource to cope with peaks of activity without the need to employ additional staff. As well as contracting projects out to them, it is possible to take staff on 'secondment' from a CRO for a set period of time. These arrangements can work very well but there may be some disadvantages. For example, an in-house clinical research team will probably be more familiar with the company's products and, through closer relations with the sales force, have greater commercial awareness. In addition, while clinical investigators may see CRO staff as representing the pharmaceutical company, the company is unlikely to have direct control over their day-to-day activities. Finally, by using a CRO, there is less opportunity to develop professional relationships between clinicians and the company.

Agreements drawn up between companies should include not only financial arrangements, but should also define SOPs and methods of monitoring and auditing. In the UK, the Association of Clinical Research (ACR) was founded in 1988 to help ensure high standards. Its members agree to operate to the standards and practices set out in the ACR code and undergo regular independent inspections to ensure that they do.

10.3.3 The statistician

Although increasingly statisticians are not based within a medical department but in the research and development (R&D) departments of a company, possibly at international rather than affiliate level, their role in clinical development has, in recent years, expanded from the tradition of providing advice on patient numbers and data analysis. Statisticians are likely to have input not just to individual studies but across entire development programmes. By providing general statistical advice they can completely change the design of studies and later provide not only the analysis, but also valuable advice on how to interpret the results and use them appropriately. Such advice may be equally valuable in relation to the results from published studies used in support of promotional claims. It is essential to have a sound statistical rationale behind a clinical research project if it is to stand up to scrutiny by regulatory agencies and ethics committees.

10.3.4 The data manager

Date managers too, are allied to R&D operations of a company rather than the medical department. Data managers need to work closely with the CRS, the statistician and the pharmaceutical physician to design reliable and practical methods of capturing and storing data gathered in clinical trials. Whether these data are recorded on the traditional case record form (CRF) or by means of computer-based technology, such as remote data entry, the data manager must ensure that the method used is investigator-friendly. If it is not, it will lead to erroneous data, which no amount of statistical analysis can repair. Confidentiality and anonymity in pooled data are important and the source of the data must be kept secure.

Time invested by both the data manager and statistician in designing the structure of the database should also reap rewards at the analysis stage. In addition, a good-quality database is essential if the study is to pass the auditing process.

10.3.5 The medical information scientist

Within the medical department there may be two types of information support. There will be medical information scientists, who provide the external 'scientific service', required by Article 13 of Directive 92/28/EEC (on advertising) of the Council of the European Communities. In addition there may be those, sometimes called 'scientific advisers', who provide specialised information support to a product or therapy area within the company. Many medical information scientists are qualified pharmacists.

Requests for information about a company's products come from many sources, both inside and outside the company. Hospital information pharmacists, often on behalf of hospital doctors, are the most frequent source of enquiries, but community pharmacists and individual clinicians may also contact the company. Sometimes, a suspected adverse drug reaction lies behind the enquiry and the medical information scientist should be trained to recognise this. The adverse event report can then be passed to the company's pharmaco-vigilance department in order to initiate documentation, follow-up and appropriate reporting to regulatory authorities. Other sources of enquiries are nursing staff, consumer groups, the media and, increasingly, patients and other members of the public. Companies offer an out-of-hours emergency enquiry service for both product information and emergency enquiries arising from clinical trials.

In the UK, until recently, the provision of information in response to enquiries from members of the public was not allowed, and individuals were referred to their medical practitioner. However, as the provision of information about medicines directly to the public has increased through such innovations as patient pack inserts and greater access to the internet, so a better informed public now demands greater involvement in their own clinical management. This demand is likely to be fuelled further as an increasing number of medicines are reclassified from prescription only (POM) to over-the-counter (P). Consequently, it is now accepted that members of the public can be provided with factual answers to questions about their medicines, which can include copies of a product's summary of product characteristics (SmPC), European public assessment reports and package leaflets, all of which may be published on the internet. The medical information scientist is trained to respect the principle that, like a pharmacist, in providing such information they must not come between a patient and their doctor and, when appropriate, should encourage the enquirer to seek medical advice.

10.3.6 The scientific adviser

In larger companies this role has evolved from the medical information service. The scientific adviser is the product or therapy area expert, who is custodian of all the information related to their specialist field. The scientific adviser is a key member on crossfunctional teams with commercial and medical colleagues and will work with advertising agencies on the creation of a product's promotional platform. In some companies scientific advisers are also key 'customer facing' medical department colleagues.

10.3.7 The regulatory executive

The regulatory department may be part of the medical department, the research function or report directly to the head of the company. Wherever it is placed, the role of regulatory executive is crucial to the success of the company. The regulatory executive defines the pharmaceutical, toxicological and clinical data required to prove the quality, safety profile and efficacy of a product and to obtain a medically and commercially favourable marketing authorisation (product licence), as ultimately reflected in its SmPC. This includes defining the appropriate regulatory strategy to achieve rapid product development and registration. Because this advice will need to be given several years before the submission is made, this requires the regulatory executive to be completely up to date not only with national, European and international regulations and guidelines, but also with their own national regulatory authority's thinking. To this end, strong and effective working relationships need to be built up with regulators. The regulatory executive also needs to keep the company informed of the potential impact of any proposed changes to regulations and, if necessary, provide comment on these to the regulatory authorities via the appropriate trade associations. In the local operating unit much of the regulatory executive's role is to update and maintain company licences, and product information (SmPCs, patient information leaflets and packaging).

It is often not appreciated how much work is required to ensure that the marketing authorisations are kept up to date through being renewed and amended as necessary. Similarly, it may not be realised that a 'simple' variation to a product licence, such as a small change in the amount of excipient, will require the submission of a variation document to the authorities.

Other responsibilities include applications for regulatory approval of clinical trials and ensuring that promotional material for a product is in line with its licence.

10.3.8 The drug safety/pharmacovigilance scientist

Effective handling of all information relating to drug safety is one of the most important responsibilities, if not *the* most important responsibility, of the medical department. The size of a company and the volume of work will dictate whether the responsibility for monitoring drug safety resides with members of staff who have other responsibilities for the various compounds, or with a specialised drug surveillance group.

Every company is required by European law to have a nominated Qualified Person responsible for pharmaco-vigilance (QPPV) (Directive 2001/83/EC Article 8(3)(n)). The QPPV need not be a physician but must have access to one.

The most important task relating to drug safety monitoring is the timely processing of spontaneously reported suspected adverse drug reactions relating to marketed products, as well as adverse events reported in clinical trials of both pre-licensed drugs and marketed products. Timelines for passing such reports to national and international regulatory authorities are closely regulated. The reason for such defined timelines is that if any reports of suspected adverse reactions could lead to changes in the regulatory status of a product, they need to be received as soon as is practicable.

Clearly, those involved in drug safety monitoring need to liase closely with both clinical research and medical information scientists. In addition, those responsible for clinical drug safety must undertake periodic safety update reports at predetermined intervals, in accordance with current International Conference on Harmonisation (ICH) guidelines (ICH E2C). Such routine analyses can identify new safety signals as soon as they become detectable.

Other activities that may fall within the area of post-marketing surveillance require input from, if not handling by, those responsible for clinical drug safety. These may include observational (non-interventional) studies, which may be retrospective or prospective, and other projects specifically designed to investigate a safety issue. In addition, many drug safety units are responsible for ensuring that *all* staff in the company are trained (and logging training) on adverse event reporting guidelines and the recognition of potential safety information and concerns relating to the company's products.

Overall responsibility for clinical safety matters must rest with a senior pharmaceutical physician who will be able to provide appropriate professional opinion and advice.

10.3.9 The pharmaco-economics adviser

It is no longer sufficient to demonstrate that a drug is efficacious and well tolerated, with an acceptable safety profile. Increasingly, in many countries health care decision-makers are mandating what medicines doctors can prescribe. With health care costs rising, it is necessary to provide evidence of effectiveness of the medication and economic measurements of the benefits that a new drug can provide. Such comparisons will need to include not only measurements against competitor drugs, but also against other medical interventions. The science of pharmaco-economics has arisen in response to this challenge and, as a member of the medical department team, the pharmaco-economics adviser, like the statistician, should be involved in the early stages of clinical development planning.

The role of the pharmaco-economist in the pharmaceutical company is therefore increasingly important. These professionals include physicians, pharmacists and economists, who work within or close to the medical department. These professionals are involved with clinical trial development, earlier stage development, and also in the UK work with bodies such as the National Institute for Health and Clinical Excellence (NICE) and the Scottish Medicines Consortium (SMC) on pharmaco-economic submissions on medicines within their licensed indications.

In many ways the Health Technology Assessment (HTA) submission is one of the most important pieces of work for pharmaceutical companies in the UK. With a positive HTA appraisal comes access to medicines by patients in the NHS. Conversely, a negative HTA appraisal from NICE or SMC can have very adverse effect on the availability of a medicine, as NHS funding cannot be guaranteed. The process of HTA appraisal is covered in another chapter; what concerns us here is the role of the medical department in a company. One of the major roles of the medical or scientific adviser in the medical department is to develop the clinical effectiveness part of the HTA appraisal submission. In addition, the company pharmaco-economist may work in a medical department or will work closely with medical colleagues. The process can be very protracted and require further 'working' with other cross-functional colleagues.

10.4 Team working

It is clear from their roles that, to work effectively, members of the medical department need to interact not only with other members of the department but also with colleagues in other departments, such as commercial, legal and communications. An effective medical department is one that fulfils the major responsibilities described in section 10.2 in a creative and constructive way. If successful, commercial colleagues will perceive the medical department as having the role of a facilitator rather than a policeman. Commercial and medical staff can facilitate the work of each other on a daily basis. For example, a sales representative may put a doctor interested in clinical research directly in contact with a company's clinical research manager. Conversely, a doctor who has developed a favourable view of a company from working as a clinical investigator may be more disposed to granting interviews to sales representatives from that company. It is a powerful asset to a company that pharmaceutical physicians have unique channels of access to clinicians that are not afforded to commercial colleagues.

Many companies have found that bringing the different contributors together in cross-functional teams can produce synergistic results. For example, a team responsible for ensuring the successful launch of a newly licensed product might include a product/marketing manager, a pharmaceutical physician, a clinical trial scientist, a scientific adviser, a market researcher, an advertising agency representative, a financial manager and a senior member of the sales team. They may invite other members of the team, such as lawyers and public relations, as required. Similar cross-functional working continues throughout the life cycle of the medicine. The role of the pharmaceutical physician and other medical department colleagues, as part of this team, is to protect and enhance the medicine for which they are responsible. By 'protect' we mean the compliance and safety issues discussed earlier in the chapter, and by 'enhance' we mean producing, interpreting and communicating the clinical trial data that continues throughout a medicine's life. By sharing commonly agreed objectives, the members of the team are encouraged to work together to achieve the same goal. An increasingly important role for senior medical department colleagues is acting as external ambassadors for the company. This means working proactively, or reactively, to issues with the media, as well as representing the company on external NHS/ Department of Health/or industry bodies.

Historically, many pharmaceutical companies have chosen not to talk proactively about R&D innovation for example, but this is changing. As industry becomes more transparent, the need for well-informed credible medical spokesmen or women will increase. It is increasingly important that medical department colleagues are willing and able to engage with external bodies to discuss their medicines. In the past, many companies have relied on external spokesman, and while collaboration between industry and academic medicine will and must continue, the balance must change.

Clinical trial strategy teams bring together clinical research scientists with statisticians, data managers, regulatory executives, pharmaceutical physicians and marketing managers to discuss the clinical data that are needed, and the timescales and costs, to achieve specific commercial objectives.

Another area requiring a pooling of expertise is issues management. Pharmaceutical companies must be geared to respond quickly and appropriately when faced with external issues, which are often medical issues such as drug safety. A core team, whose individual roles are clear, needs to be prepared to deal with such situations. The principal elements of issues management relate to anticipating an issue wherever possible, identifying and documenting the true facts of the case, preparing reasoned arguments and answers to potential questions, and training in facing the press, media and public to debate the issue. The facts of the case and 'question and answer' documents should be prepared. Key members of such a team are therefore the medical director, or a designate, senior managers who are able to quickly implement actions, a legal adviser if appropriate, and a member of the public relations/communications department, who knows how to communicate the team's outputs effectively.

Training for media appearances, and regular 'refreshers', are essential for anyone who might be required to represent the company. Professional guidance enables individuals to make best use of the media in communicating the factual messages relating to a particular issue. Similarly, staff required to give presentations, particularly outside the company, should undertake training in presentation skills if they are to be successful ambassadors of the company. The professionalism of any presenter is thrown into question when they appear to have little enthusiasm for the subject or empathy for the audience and cannot communicate clearly, either verbally or by means of audiovisual aids.

10.5 Conclusions

It is clear that while the medical department can be seen to be a team in itself, its members play on many different teams. A successful medical department is one that contributes to the commercial success of the company while maintaining the highest professional and ethical standards.

Acknowledgement

We are indebted to Dr Darrall Higson, who authored this chapter up to the Fifth Edition, for his leadership and free use of his material when preparing this chapter.

References

1 General Medical Council. *Good Medical Practice.* London: 2006.

2 Ethics and pharmaceutical medicine: the full report of the Ethical Issues Committee of the Faculty of Pharmaceutical Medicine of the Royal Colleges of Physicians of the UK. *Int J Clin Pract* 2006;**60**(2):242–52.

3 Prescription Medicines Code of Practice Authority. *Code of Practice for the Pharmaceutical Industry 2008.* London: PMCPA, 2008.

4 Wells F, Farthing M, eds. *Fraud and Misconduct in Biomedical Research, 4th edn.* London: RSM Press, 2008.

11 Medical marketing

David Galloway and Bensita Bernard

Cytosystems Ltd, Aberdeen, Scotland, UK

11.1 Introduction

The pharmaceutical industry is a business and as such medical marketing has a key role in the development of that business and hence the survival of the company to which the medical practitioner has been exposed. Most physicians, regardless of specialty training, have little or no idea of the complexities nor indeed the excitements which the Pharma business can offer them. In my own case, with a formal training in hospital medicine and a specialty interest in clinical pharmacology, medical marketing was a foreign field in which my sole contacts had been through specialised hospital representatives.

However, there is so much more to medical marketing, requiring specialist knowledge in areas in which most doctors have never been trained such as product competition, market segments, inventory, formulation issues, public relations campaigns, opinion leader development and new techniques in approaching specialist subscribers; all part of the usual armamentaria of our colleagues in the medical marketing department. Such a process from the laboratory to the marketplace and the dispensing of pharmaceutical products may take up to 10–12 years and cost upwards of £800 million.

There is little doubt that these days everyone is much more aware of the power of marketing and the importance of brand and brand image. The complexity of medical marketing is simply one aspect of a business proposition in the pharmaceutical industry. This encompasses the most detailed and demanding of scientific specialties and basic sciences, as well as the translation of these sciences from the laboratory

and animal and early studies in humans to subsequent development of a pharmaceutically approved medical product.

Many of the chapters in this textbook focus on the various aspects of research, development and the licensing of pharmaceuticals. Both physicians and non-medical scientists working in departments other than sales and marketing require some understanding of marketing. Such techniques, even in the last 3 or 4 years, have developed as a consequence of increased communications worldwide between different areas of the company working in different countries across the world, each of which may have different health care needs.

Thus, the requirements of an individual working in a phase I clinical pharmacology unit may be vastly different from the physician working as a medical advisor along with sales and marketing colleagues. A medical advisor for a single product or a number of products, depending on the size of the company, makes demands upon training quite different from the National Health Service (NHS) or country-based health care systems. This chapter focuses on the role of physicians working as medical advisors and the kind of knowledge base that will help them to understand not only the areas in which they work, but also the importance of those areas in relation to the overall development of a new medicine.

Although this chapter is geared towards pharmaceutical products, it is equally important to note that medical input is a valuable source of information in the marketing of diagnostic products, either in the early detection of disease states such as coronary artery disease or cancer, or in the monitoring of such disease states once the diagnosis has been established to determine the nature and rate of disease progression. This chapter is written from a UK perspective so readers in countries outside the UK will need to

The Textbook of Pharmaceutical Medicine. Edited by John P. Griffin. © 2009, ISBN: 978-1-4051-8035-1.

make allowances for this. Some specific points may not be relevant to other countries but, in general, the principles apply to most health care systems.

11.2 Pharmaceutical market

The world pharmaceutical market represents the outcome of successful medical marketing. It continues to grow, although the rate of expansion in the last 3–5 years has varied both by country and by product (Figure 11.1). Indeed, it is of interest that from 1998 to 2007 global pharmaceutical sales have more than doubled. Not surprisingly, with regard to both size and dynamics, the US market is in the lead and, at about 33%, sales in the US market from 2001 to 2004 increased significantly faster than other markets. Overall, the USA represents 43% of the pharmaceutical market worldwide, Europe some 31%, Japan 9% and all other markets approximately 17%. In a more recent appraisal of the development of the largest pharmaceutical markets, the US and Spanish pharmacy market increased by almost 50% during the period 2001–2007. During the same period, both the UK and France exceeded Germany, Japan and Italy in rate of growth worldwide.

The largest group of products on a worldwide basis used to be antibiotics but, more recently, and particularly in the last 5 years, the importance of hypolipidaemic, anti-asthma, antihypertensive and antiplatelet products should not be underestimated. The dismal record of the UK, which spends less on medicines per head than almost any other industrialized country, has continued over the past 5 years. Indeed, the spend on medicines as a percentage of gross domestic product (GDP) in various countries in 2007 indicates that the UK spends 0.85% of GDP on medicines compared with the USA which spends some 2.08% of GDP on medicines (Figure 11.2).

The conservativism which is a key marker of the UK's policy provides an increasing challenge to the medical marketeer as it takes a very long time for UK prescribers to take up a new product. General practitioners (GPs) in the UK, and in some instances the specialist hospital consultant – similarly conservative

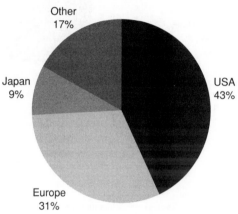

Figure 11.1 Pharmaceutical market worldwide (2003–2007).

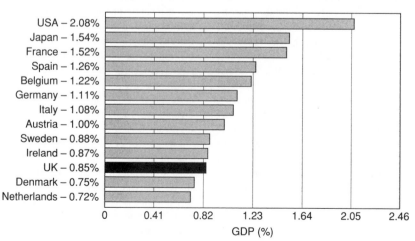

Figure 11.2 Spend on medicines as a percentage of GDP in various countries, 2007.

Table 11.1 Top five leading pharmaceutical corporations UK market share, 2007

Corporation	Nat	Primary care market sales (£m)	Share of primary care market (%)	Hospital sales (£m)	Share of hospital market (%)	Total market sales (£m)	Share of total market (%)
1 Pfizer	USA	955.16	11.2	136.38	4.2	1091.54	9.3
2 GlaxoSmithKline	UK	873.76	10.3	183.16	5.7	1056.92	9.0
3 Sanofi-Aventis	F	587.25	6.9	194.78	6.0	782.03	6.7
4 AstraZeneca	UK	585.21	6.9	82.38	2.5	667.59	5.7
5 Novartis	CH	288.47	3.4	170.46	5.3	458.93	3.9

in their view – may recognise significant advances in therapeutic outcomes only by virtue of effective medical marketing. For most therapeutic classes there is a relatively slow pattern of uptake and the demand for evidence-based medicine to convert earlier established medical prescribing practices to somewhat newer and more definitive or targeted therapy takes both time and marketing effort.

There is little doubt that the pharmaceutical market is both complex and diverse. Differences in therapeutic areas and in the ways in which countries use medicines vary widely across the globe. It is of interest that, unlike most other global industries, the pharmaceutical industry is highly fragmented and the importance of small companies amongst those global giants such as Pfizer, GlaxoSmithKline (GSK) or Sanofi-Aventis should not be underestimated, in that many of those have provided targeted therapeutic advances which in larger companies may not be readily achieved or achievable (Table 11.1).

Pfizer remains the market share leader not only in the UK but globally but, as many practitioners know, has only a limited number of therapeutic areas. Its rival companies GSK, Sanofi-Aventis, AstraZeneca, Novartis, Roche and Wyeth, together with Merck & Co, Lilly and Boehringer Ingelheim compete for market share in the UK and worldwide. It is clear that companies with a knowledge base and expertise in particular areas tend to retain those areas both for investment and for medical marketing. Such activity is commonly referred to as a 'franchise' and the ability of leading companies for such a franchise area is often a key factor in remaining successful by which is meant market share, cash return and shareholder profit. The role of franchises should not be underestimated and will be dealt with later in the chapter.

The sales of genetically manufactured pharmaceuticals, a relatively recent set of products in pharma-

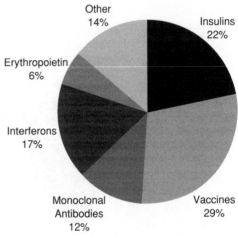

Figure 11.3 Sales of genetically manufactured pharmaceuticals, 2007.

ceutical medicine, is constantly increasing. In 2000, this share of the pharmaceutical market was 7.6%. By 2006 this had risen to 10.9% of market share and the increase over the intervening years from 2003 to 2007 is illustrated in Figure 11.3. Just under half of these sales were recorded for insulins to treat diabetes and interferons used for immune disorders. Other important applications include blood disorders, rheumatic diseases, monoclonal antibodies against cancer, enzymes for metabolic disorders and vaccines.

The growth in sales of genetically manufactured pharmaceuticals has risen from 1.89 billion Euro in 2003 to 2.38 billion Euro in 2006. Thus, it is clear that the pharmaceutical market, despite a recent downturn in worldwide sales as a result of the global financial crisis, continues to expand and respond not only to market opportunities but to patient need.

11.3 Strategic planning

The importance of marketing in the success of any product cannot be underestimated. A marketing plan, just like a clinical research project plan, requires considerable thought and clarity of execution and remains under constant revision and updating, depending on changes in marketing needs and targeted patient opportunities. The sheer cost of research and development (R&D) for new pharmaceuticals demands active cooperation between marketing and clinical development groups and this includes all areas of clinical research activity if the product and the company are to be successful.

In my own experience, it was not unusual for the clinical research group and the marketing team not to interact or even know each other until the product was within 2 years or so of launch. This particular paradigm is no longer viable. Today, the interaction of the medical marketing team occurs at a very early stage in product development and a representative of that team may well be involved in the initial introduction of the product to humans and part of the phase I and II programmes for elaboration of the product and its role as a novel development with a good safety profile and an early effective therapeutic response. Thus, the medical marketing department is now commonly involved with the product from the time of discovery right through the product life cycle from phase I to IV until such time as the patent expires.

Most individuals involved in specialist marketing activity still consider that the first 6 months following the launch of a new product are the most important. The strategy surrounding the launch and its follow-up is designed to maximise the early sales potential of the novel therapy. Relaunch of a product in the first year or two following a failed first launch is possible, but very few products are relaunched with any degree of success.

Strategic planning for the medical marketing team determines the balance between the risks of the product getting into the marketplace and how successful it will be commercially once it gets there. The targets need to be clearly defined, and the area in which the product is to be launched needs to be well documented.

In some ways, the area of greatest potential is also that of greatest risk; this is when a condition for which a biological target has been identified but no proven product has yet been developed. Much more commonly, when developing a compound for a condition where therapeutic agents have been identified and proof of concept studies completed, the product may achieve a smaller market share but the outcome in terms of acceptance may be of value to the company when it is introduced relatively early into the market for that therapeutic field.

The other area of strategic planning, somewhat less favoured by our more aggressive marketing companions, is the development of so-called 'me too' compounds. In this instance the target is well known and the compounds already established, and the new compound being considered offers similar indications, fewer contraindications and possibly a better safety profile. On these particular characteristics, the new compound being considered may offer significant advantages over those already in the market and can be successful although it requires substantial input from the marketing department. In such instances the medical marketeer can highlight improved pharmacokinetics, a greater degree of selectivity in therapeutic areas, improved tolerance or a marketing package that allows, perhaps, once a day as opposed to more frequent administration of the product via an oral formulation.

Internationally, the larger companies may embark on one or all of the above strategies, depending upon the mix and therapeutic areas of the products they have in their portfolios. Such decision-making cannot be taken in isolation and clearly needs the agreement of the both the R&D and the marketing groups. Such relationships are not always easy to achieve and again, experience determines that leadership in both areas is an absolute key to effecting a high profile product launch. The head of R&D and his or her senior associates need to understand the needs of the marketing group and vice versa. Strategic planning involves an early understanding of the limitations as well as the advantages of the R&D process for the product in question and the targeted marketing objectives for the group undertaking the sale of the product in the marketplace. Throughout this process, the head of R&D and the head of marketing must jointly agree that flexibility and alteration in priorities has to be part of the overall strategic plan, more particularly when regulatory claims need to be modified as clinical development progresses. At some point the strategic plan needs to come to fruition and the marketing launch associated with product delivery to the prescribers needs to represent fairly the R&D achievements of its early and subsequent development as well as the overall anticipation of market size by the commercial and business needs of the company.

11.4 Customers

There is little doubt that in this highly competitive marketplace there are a number of key elements that need to be considered when formulating a marketing plan. The strategy and tactics, some of which have been illustrated above, will vary depending on the stage of the product in its life cycle (i.e. the stage at which it is launched, developed, re-invented and extended as a therapeutic product for the treatment of a particular disease or therapeutic area). For example, such a plan would be markedly different for a product not yet launched from one near the end of its patent life and, with the increasing recognition of the importance of patent life and the relevance of generic competition, one of the fundamental elements of any marketing plan must be an understanding of the customer and his or her needs.

Clearly, the aim of marketing is to meet the target customers' needs and wants. It is clear from research both in the pharmaceutical industry and other businesses, that understanding customers' behaviour is never simple. Customers may say one thing and do quite another and this is as true in pharmaceutical marketing as it is in the automotive industry. Doctors, who may indicate their particular therapeutic desire in one disease or another, may say one thing to the representative and yet do quite another. In this respect, the pharmaceutical market is unique in that the end user of the product (i.e. the patient) for the most part leaves the choice of medicine to his or her physician. However, this pattern is changing. Indeed, with the advent of the internet, apart from specialised areas open only to a selective browser audience such as the British Medical Association (BMA), Doctors.net.uk and a variety of other limited specialty websites, the internet provides a non-regulated source of information, factually correct or otherwise, to the patient who has access to electronic data sets and surveys. Such changes produce not only an increasing awareness of the advantages and disadvantages of particular medicines and particular conditions, but also often unregulated insights into new medicines which may be entirely inappropriate for their particular needs.

Thus, the patient is increasingly more involved in the choice of medicines and the approach to their particular disease. This is especially true in the USA where the patient may bear most of the cost of the prescribed drug. In Europe, and in particular in the UK, the cost is partly or largely borne by the patient's insurance or by the State. Such involvement of the patient on a cost basis is less noticeable, although with increasing demands on the social services available in each nation state, personal costs for medicine may increase in the future. It is of interest that, looking at the UK in particular, the overall cost of the NHS is steadily rising but as a percentage of total NHS costs, the medicines bill remains around 10% (10.3% in 2007). This figure has remained remarkably constant despite a growth year by year in the number of prescriptions issued (Table 11.2). Indeed, more than 912 million prescriptions were dispensed in the UK in 2007 at an average cost of £10.37 each. As the Association of the British Pharmaceutical Industry (ABPI) has indicated, this represents remarkable value for money in that medicines often reduce or eliminate the need for more costly treatments in hospital and maintain the concept of ambulatory patient care. In the UK, the industry provides the nation's medicines at an average cost of only 47p per person per day.

The definition of 'the customer' is complex in the pharmaceutical market and it would be reasonable to assume that the physician who prescribes the medicine is the customer. Usually in the UK this would be the GP. Nowadays, however, that prescriber does not operate in a vacuum and is heavily influenced by a number of external factors.[1] As the National Institute for Health and Clinical Excellence (NICE), the Scottish Medicines Consortium (SMC) and the All Wales Medicines Strategy Group (AWMSG) are linked to recommended therapies in England, Scotland and Wales, respectively, prescribing practice outside their remit or recommendation is not readily tolerated by local or regional formularies.

All these different stakeholders in the prescribing process will need to be considered in the company's promotional strategy. All have markedly different agendas that need to be addressed in the marketing plan. The marketing plans are themselves encompassed in the strategic overview of the way in which the medicines are presented to the market. The relative importance of these customers clearly needs to be established and a number of questions which the medical marketeer needs to address include:

• What do we wish to achieve and how do we wish to achieve it?

• What are the customers' needs, bearing in mind the customer may be cost limited?

• What behavioural changes are we expecting either in the prescriber or in the customer?

• How best can we deliver this message and what medium may be the most useful for doing so?

Table 11.2 NHS expenditure per person in the UK

	Total NHS cost (£million)	Total NHS cost per person (£)	All NHS medicines cost (£million)	NHS medicines cost per person (£)	Medicines as a % of total NHS cost
1980	9,456	168	732	13.00	7.7
1985	16,349	290	1550	27.46	9.5
1990	26,169	458	2370	41.50	9.1
1995	40,432	698	4316	74.54	10.7
1996	42,326	729	4657	80.21	11.0
1997	43,921	755	4992	85.76	11.4
1998	46,240	792	5447	93.35	11.8
1999	48,770	833	5988	102.32	12.3
2000	53,429	910	6641	113.07	12.4
2001	58,279	989	7138	121.10	12.2
2002	64,430	1089	7879	133.17	12.2
2003	74,741	1259	8813	148.40	11.8
2004	82,202	1379	9722	163.05	11.8
2005	89,567	1494	10,334	172.40	11.5
2006	98,959	1640	10,373	171.95	10.5
2007	104,678	1725	10,829	178.45	10.3

There is little doubt that hospital specialists still have an important influence in prescribing practice but it is recognised that the majority of patients are treated in general practice so this is where the bulk of prescribing occurs. It is therefore not surprising that the GP remains the main focus for the industry and 'targeting' the GP is often the key element in customer appreciation. Recent changes in the UK health care system, however, have altered some aspects of the relative importance of the GP as a customer. Reforms in the NHS, which have continued almost without cessation in the last decade or so (nine reorganisations in the past 10 years), and the increase of primary health care organisations (PCOs) have altered the GP's role and in particular their prescribing practice. Some GPs are affected more than others by these changes and it is important for any company to be aware of how GPs are reacting to the pressures put upon them by pricing policies. Most districts, areas and regions have some form of local formulary and it is difficult both for the hospital practitioner as well as the GP to prescribe medicines outside that formulary prescription, more especially because these are selected by a group of therapeutic experts within the region and based on national guidelines. Such restrictions may be a result either of cost (i.e. the individual cost of the product such as new anticancer

agents or novel cardiovascular agents), or may have some aspects of therapeutic efficacy unproven by current standards.

Most companies have therefore developed databases that are constantly updated by the sales representatives as they come in contact with customers whether in hospital or in general practice or more commonly now in the local pharmacy. It is absolutely critical that the company builds relationships with all the stakeholders in the prescribing process and keep updating the information on these particular individuals. Such detailed knowledge of what customers are doing and saying is important to the staff at headquarters as they track and evaluate sales and promotional strategies, not only in increasing prescribing practice but also increasing sales returns and therefore cash to the company. It is vital that promotional campaigns are targeted accurately and resources are not wasted.

11.5 Market research and market intelligence

As in any business organisation, we have seen how companies update their intelligence on prescribers and other stakeholders via representatives, both in general practice and in hospital medicine, but this is only one aspect of a wider collection of data on how the market is reacting. Not only is it important to know what prescribers are thinking and doing, but it is also important to track the competition in this and related areas.

Most companies will purchase a range of data sets from a variety of commercial companies who specialise in collecting and collating such data by individual drug and by therapeutic area. Such sources of information are both wide and varied and include panels of GPs and specialists who record what they are prescribing and for what indication, to information from wholesalers and pharmacists. Some companies also sponsor individual market research studies with questionnaires, personal interviews with individual panels of doctors and, more frequently nowadays, focus groups of patients.

There is little doubt that to be successful in the pharmaceutical market it is vital that data on how your product is progressing and what the competition is doing is constantly updated and evaluated. Larger companies are particularly adept at collating such diverse sources of information and keeping track of what might be occurring in alternative fields. They are acutely aware of novel or rival products that impact on the market in their particular therapeutic area and recognise that a new surgical technique, new medical device or new therapy may be introduced that completely alters the way in which the disease is managed. This is even more significant when endorsed by one of the advisory panels in the UK such as NICE or the SMC.

It is clear that one of the most critical times when accurate competitor intelligence is needed is when a company is considering developing a new product or device. With the development time of around 10 years for the former and 5 years for the latter, as much information as possible needs to be gathered about competitor activity before any decision is made to commit to the development of a new product.

It is recognised that in the past such considerations were of less importance. Companies 20 or 30 years ago could look to upwards of 10 years of exclusivity in a therapeutic area before a competitor in the same therapeutic class entered the marketplace. More recently, that gap has reduced and in some cases – depending on development time – may last for only a few months. Additionally, the growth of pharmaceutical R&D in countries where costs of such activities are notably lower, such as India and China, highlights the fact that a competitive entrant may only be months behind this novel introduction.

The requirements for phase I and II programme developments are quite clear. In the majority of countries worldwide, safety of a new therapy as part of the phase I programme needs to be established at a very early stage. Therapeutic efficacy in phase II development relates to a small group of patients with the targeted disease and this will also require early definition. However, when developing a phase III programme for a new drug, this is the area in which accurate competitor intelligence and a detailed knowledge of the drugs used are required and need to be built into the clinical plan. This is the phase in which considerable financial commitments are made by the company on the basis both of safety and efficacy and in which a much broader development programme related to market research and intelligence and the opportunity for market penetration is needed.

In many therapeutic areas there is increasing harmonisation between countries in the use of major drugs, and this is particularly true of the industrialized world including the USA and Canada, the European Union including the UK, and Japan. It is also important to recognise that one particular product may dominate that market, whether through therapeutic efficacy or successful marketing policies. The decision at this point relates to whether, medically speaking, such a competitor product should be included in the phase III programme or whether that should be recognised as a question in the phase IV programme and the wider marketing of the product post-launch. In an ideal world, particularly as related to the market researcher, data should be available for comparing the new product against the leading competitor in the major markets at the time of launch. It is common, however, that financial or time pressures may limit the scope of the phase III programme, and in this case the phase IV study will be needed to fill the gaps.

11.6 Promotion

We are all familiar with the process of promotion, whether to buy the latest soap powder or hair product. It is now commonplace for marketing and marketing activities to be involved early in the development of a compound and much more usually now, in early R&D. One of the earliest elements in a promotional campaign, and this should be established well before launch, is a public relations (PR) programme. Often, this is foreign territory for the medical marketeer and certainly for the medic joining the industry. This is a skilled process and involves close integration between the marketing department of the company, senior management and in-house specialists. The alternative for smaller companies is to bring in specialist promotional personnel with a particular interest in pharmaceutical products. The key here is that once a product is under clinical development then this can be announced to the financial press and financial analysts at a time that is appropriate to the benefit and shareholder value of the company. Companies clearly have obligations to their shareholders and to the financial markets to disclose information that may have an effect on the share price and hence return to the shareholders. Such analysts' briefings therefore have a dual role of informing the financial community about drugs or drug opportunities under development but also raising the company's profile to a wider audience. Novelty is something that all pharmaceutical companies strive for in their promotional activity and, if sufficiently novel, such financial information may well spill over into the general press or television. This PR media campaign early in the development of a compound is valuable in creating awareness of the product and creating demand by physicians but needs careful and thoughtful management. Clinical trial publications and their dissemination not only in the scientific community but also those within the marketing arena will also be part of a PR campaign to increase awareness of the product and its potential benefits both to patient and prescriber.

Often, at the time of launch, symposia will be organised to further increase the exposure of a new therapeutic agent to prescribers. A common approach is to arrange company-sponsored symposia as satellites to regional or international medical meetings at which large numbers of specialists within the target therapeutic area will be invited to attend. It is particularly important, more especially in the last few years, that such symposia are of a high scientific standard if they are to attract the interest of physicians and avoid the criticism, often quite appropriate, of being purely promotional. These symposia are carefully tailored and planned, often to open with a keynote presentation on the current knowledge of the disease under discussion by a noted researcher in the field. The product itself can then be reviewed in relation to current treatment options, showing how the new therapeutic agent fits into the management of the condition and its benefits for patient care. There is much criticism of the industry at present in that keynote speakers must be independent authorities facilitating a lively debate and discussion in the symposium and

involving both the merits and the limitations of the new product together with suggestions for further studies. Even the venue for the meeting should be chosen carefully. It is often perceived that a university or academic facility may be preferable but that a local hotel is more convenient or offers better conference facilities. There is increasing pressure on the industry to ensure that the scientific content of the meeting takes precedence over the facilities and level of hospitality offered to attendees.

The launch date of the product is a critical time for the company and at launch and beyond, plans need to be in place for journal advertising and detailing of the product to doctors by sales representatives. This simply emphasises that the customer base of pharmaceuticals and diagnostics is complex and the needs of individual customers, whether prescriber or patient, clearly differ. For many GPs and specialists, information about the product will be via advertising, representative detailing and mailings, whereas for NHS staff such as those working in Health Authorities or PCOs, the information will need to be more focused both on cost and effectiveness as well as improved service provision. At a practice nurse level, the emphasis will be on educational material and the practical aspects of the product's use. Cost of therapy here will also be an issue as part of general practice and disease awareness and indeed as one other aspect of promotion by the company. Disease awareness programmes may be developed where appropriate to illustrate the value of the new product to that disease entity.

In the UK at least, the main customer remains the physician. GPs gain information about new products from a variety of sources including their peers and hospital colleagues. It is clear that although advertisements in medical journals are an expensive but important element in building awareness among prescribers, they are not usually the basis on which physicians start to prescribe a new compound.

Hospital specialists will readily start to prescribe a new product if they are convinced both of its safety and efficacy, provided it is for use in their own specialty. It is also clear they are much less ready to try a new compound if it is outside their area of expertise. Many examples exist whereby individual specialisms for cardiology, gastroenterology, rheumatology and so on develop their own focus for preferred prescriptions in their own therapeutic area. Those physicians will become powerful influences on their GP colleagues, and then on the local pharmacist and prescribing nurse practioner.

GPs, by the very nature and the variety of their jobs, may initiate new drug therapies in many different therapeutic areas. In general, they will be guided by what the local hospital specialists recommend and by discussion and/or focus groups with their peers. In the past, detailing by company representatives has been a significant factor in influencing prescribing behaviour and the information delivered by the representative is seen to be valuable by both hospital specialists and GPs. However, this is changing and the training of these representatives, skilled as they may be and often with a scientific background, may be seen by an increasing number of specialists as being wholly company-focused and product-based rather than independent messengers of the safety and efficacy of their product. This is a further reflection of the cynicism affecting much of today's society in the ever-widening search for increasing safety, widening therapeutic efficacy and absence of adverse affects for the preferred prescription at a cheaper price.

11.7 Medical information

An important element to consider when discussing the increasing awareness of a product is the use of the company medical information department. It is quite clear that this is not and must not be a promotional element in the marketing sense, but rather the provision of accurate and up-to-date scientific data about the company's products for an interested observer or potential prescriber. This can be valuable in establishing and maintaining not only the company's image but its integrity and honesty in providing a sensible and practical response to an interested request for information. There is little doubt that if a company is known by prescribers to provide an excellent and responsive scientific service, then its image and reputation amongst the prescribing fraternity – let alone the interested patient – will be enhanced. A strong positive company image can only be of assistance to the company's representatives when dealing with customers face to face, more particularly in the light of increasing competition in any one therapeutic area.

Most companies, especially the larger ones, have developed an international computerised system to ensure that the information given out in response to enquiries is both comprehensive and as up-to-date as possible. The data that support the individual statements in the summary of product characteristics (SPCs) are collated and fully referenced and are used to respond to enquiries from prescribers and

pharmacists. It is not uncommon that a question is not easily answered and the response requires a detailed literature search by the medical information department. Such a search often requires considerable expertise and one of the major advantages of pharmaceutical databases is that once validated, usually by headquarters staff, the search – both the question and the answer – are made available to other subsidiaries throughout the world. This avoids duplication of effort, ensures consistency of response across the globe and highlights the need for sharing of information across the company as a whole. Critics of the industry, and there are many of these, quite rightly look for evidence of dual standards between the USA and Europe and less well-developed parts of the world. Linking medical information departments around the world and sharing such information with all parties ensures that the company delivers a consistent message which limits the opportunities for tailoring messages and responses to individual markets.

11.8 Brands

Pharmaceutical drug marketing is in many ways similar to the marketing and branding of other products such as in the automobile industry, the cosmetics industry and a wide range of consumer products. Thus, when a new drug comes to the market it will have a series of properties outlined in the SPC including indications, dosage, form, precautions, frequency of dosing, contraindications and side effect profile. All these features, both individually and collectively, establish the product in the marketplace (i.e. its position), and form the basis of the 'brand'. Like other marketing segments, the creation of a strong brand image is fundamental to advertising and this is as true for pharmaceuticals as it is for other sectors in the marketplace. Marketing is concerned with perception and a successful brand will be perceived by the consumer as having not only unique benefits that meet their needs but specific benefit for them. In this instance, perception is reality and the brand image aims to create a reality relevant to the individual and their needs.

Prescribers form opinions and beliefs about drugs or devices in the same way as they do about consumer products. Shaping their perceptions and the creation of a strong positive brand image is key to differentiating the product from the competition and to financial success in the marketplace. Companies go to great lengths to build the brand image of their products and endeavour to achieve consistency of brand messages on a global basis. In pharmaceuticals, not only is the message of suitability and efficacy a key feature of branding, but the over-riding element of safety is central to new product introduction. Over time in the product's life cycle, new indications and formulations will be developed and introduced to strengthen brand image, to further differentiate the product and to expand the marketplace whereby cash sales mark success and hence promotion of the company and its products.

11.9 Patients

One of the features of prescription medicines in the UK and the European Community is that companies are not allowed to communicate directly with patients, but in the USA and New Zealand direct to consumer (DTC) advertising of prescription medicines by indication is allowed. In the UK, the ABPI Code of Practice has been relaxed a little in this area in recent years and companies can now communicate in a very limited fashion with the general public. Clause 22.1 of the current Code of Practice (ABPI 2008)[2] still prohibits the advertising of prescription-only medicines to the public. However, the promotion of medicines to the public for self-medication purposes is covered by the consumer code of the Proprietary Association of Great Britain (PAGB). In addition, methods of sale of medicines through pharmacies are also covered by the code of ethics for pharmacists and pharmacy technicians of the Royal Pharmaceutical Society of Great Britain. Nonetheless, these limitations are strictly applied and one of the areas in which companies can comment on rival medicines is the extent and nature of public relations activities, particularly advertised in the medical, nursing and allied press, of their product versus rival competitors.

Over the past few years, there have been a number of novel initiatives by companies in the UK to carry out disease awareness programmes whereby patients or potential patients are advised about the need to recognise both symptoms and/or signs in themselves as an early index of potential disease. However, prescription medicines are explicitly not mentioned in this context.

More recently, there has been debate at the European level over relaxing DTC advertising in a limited number of therapeutic areas. Although discussion continues at present, there are no specific plans to allow even limited DTC advertising within the EU. However, one of the areas in which a number of changes have taken place is in over-the-counter (OTC) prescriptions of reduced doses of patent expired products as part of requested self-medication overseen by a pharmacist. This is seen as not only useful but of cash benefit to the manufacturing company once patents have expired on particular products for that indication.

In an earlier Government White Paper (Saving Lives: Our Healthier Nation) published in July 1999,[3] plans were set out for an Expert Patients programme. The concept being that patients, especially those with a chronic illness such as diabetes, chronic obstructive lung disease or hypertension, might be best placed to cope with their disease. The emphasis here is that the former doctor–patient relationship where 'the doctor knows best' is changing and will continue to change. The Government is encouraging patients not only to have a more active role in their disease management but, where appropriate, to initiate physician contact and active intervention based on increasing patient knowledge and awareness.

The concept of the Expert Patient and hence the development of patient focus groups is evolving and companies need to be aware of these changes and the challenges as well as the opportunities that they pose. Patients demand the best, and are not satisfied with second best, as for instance in 'postcode prescribing', and this can only be a valuable asset to companies introducing new therapies.

11.10 Franchises

Earlier in this chapter, we saw that the pharmaceutical market is not one specific market but is composed of a number of highly diverse segments. Some companies dominate specific fields and the ability to build and defend their franchise within a market segment seems to be one of the more important features that single out successful companies from others who are either smaller or less successful in that area. It is perceived that it takes years if not decades to build a franchise and once established in any particular area, companies will do all they can to maintain their position within that therapeutic field. Companies thus develop relationships with their customers, whether hospital specialists, general practitioners, PCOs or even patient focus groups, and through these relationships build a powerful marketing platform. Such relationships also lead to a group of influential local or international opinion leaders, usually physicians or surgeons, who are recognised as pre-eminent in their field. Such individuals will work on the early development trials for a new product and will act as experts at the time of regulatory approval, publish papers on the product and discuss its use and its place in management of the disease in question at global conferences and influential technical and board meetings.

The long-term relationships that form the basis of a franchise activity mean that physicians in a particular field tend to work with a selected group of companies that they both know and trust. Such relationships create a barrier to entry in the given market for a new competitor and although the new entrant may choose to enter it alone and here a large pharmaceutical company will have all the resources to break into a market, a small start-up or biotech company may choose to form an alliance with an established player. Competition in these areas is fierce and small companies often have difficulty in establishing their product where such dominance is widely recognised. Similarly, and to the benefit of smaller companies, large Pharma with an established franchise and facing the expiry of patents may specifically wish to licence in compounds in its field of expertise to maintain its market position. Such strategies may not always be successful and where companies have dominant positions in particular areas, the expiry of the patent and the development of competitive generic products may lead to the disappearance of the franchise in that area and its subsequent influence may evaporate appropriately.

In contradiction to this, as one of the ways in which building and maintaining a franchise in any particular market (e.g. GSK in the asthma market), this is largely achieved by the introduction of new compounds to the market at regular intervals. This may be associated with improved delivery technology. For example, GSK were particularly adept in developing drugs for asthma delivered to the lung via inhaler devices. Thus, investment in delivery technology meant that GSK maintained its market dominance long after the patents on certain products had expired. Device innovation is similarly not easy, although shorter in terms of development pathway. The introduction of a new device delivery system requires all the skills of the marketing department as well as the technical expertise which enables physicians and patients alike to become familiar and comfortable with the new system. Such a mix of product and delivery device has created significant barriers to new entrants into the inhaler market and similar examples can be identified both in the device as well as the diagnostic fields in other areas of pharmaceutical medicine.

11.11 Patent expiry and generics

The key feature for medical marketing is that all members of the team have a very early understanding of the limited life cycle of the pharmaceutical product under development and that once the patent expires, generic competitors rapidly enter the market. There are a number of strategies that companies can adopt to try to extend patent life and these include such well-known phenomena as line extensions, reformulations, combination products or switching to OTC sales. At present, in the USA, and more recently in the European Union, a 6-month extension of exclusivity may be granted if studies are performed demonstrating safety and efficacy in a paediatric population. In the European Union, the problem of off-label use in paediatrics has been well recognised by the Commission and has resulted in the introduction of new legislation in 2006.[4]

There are some instances where it is not possible to reformulate or develop combination products and the response in the marketplace to the loss of a patent can be not only very dramatic, but financially very concerning. In the UK particularly, and also to an increasing extent in the USA, generic competitor entry and penetration of the market can be very swift, particularly those medicines developed substantially more cheaply and often originating from India or elsewhere. In other European countries there tends to be much more brand loyalty and the penetration of the market by generic competitors is on the whole much slower. There are several examples of how rapidly the market in the UK can change following patent loss and where, within a few months, prescription volumes for the branded product had fallen to a fraction of pre-patent loss level. Such an example following patent loss is Innovace (enalapril) where, within a few months, prescription volumes of the branded product had fallen to a fraction of the pre-patent loss level.[5]

11.12 Demonstrating the benefits of medicine

The clinical trial programme of a new compound through phases I–III is well documented and highly regulated and is concerned with the collection of sufficient data to pass the regulatory hurdles regarding both safety and efficacy. In the present climate, however, the possession of a product licence demonstrating efficacy may not be enough to satisfy the market in terms of clinical effectiveness. In many markets, including the UK by way of NICE, and other similar bodies such as the SMC in Scotland and in Wales through the AWMSG, safety and clinical effectiveness must be demonstrated. Such effectiveness must then be balanced against associated costs and net patient benefits.

There is little doubt that publications in a variety of journals and papers demonstrating clinical efficacy as well as safety are important to keep the product in the physician's mind and form the basis of promotional claims. More may be needed, however, if the product is to succeed in the marketplace. In these circumstances, decisions need to be made on whether sufficient data exist for modelling of clinical effectiveness or whether an outcome study over a varying period of time needs to be performed. In some therapeutic areas, such as cardiovascular disease and cancer therapy, it may be possible to add some cost and quality of life questions on to the phase III programme without making the study too complex. Phase III programmes are both extensive in terms of numbers of patients exposed to novel therapy as well as expensive in terms of numbers of patients required by many regulatory agencies. In other therapeutic areas, however, such an approach in phase III may not be feasible. This is particularly true for conditions where the endpoint in phase III is a surrogate for the endpoint of interest to physicians and payers (e.g. in hypercholesterolaemia, diabetes or HIV infection).

Very often, outcome studies looking for a hard clinical endpoint (e.g. death, myocardial infarction or gastrointestinal bleed) are often long, very large and very expensive to perform. Such trials in the industrialized world may dominate the R&D budget over a number of years until the trial is concluded and the results analysed. Currently, the R&D budget expenditure in the UK alone is approaching £4 billion per annum. More recently, the advent of China, India and Eastern Bloc countries, among others, to the range of clinical trial centres with adequate patient numbers at a much reduced cost, have proved attractive to western-based pharmaceutical companies. Where the result of the trial – carefully controlled, well monitored and well documented – is positive, they can transform a product's performance in the marketplace very significantly. Examples of impressive trial outcome figures include a number of trials involving hypertension, hypercholesterolaemia and diabetes mellitus and, in these instances, well-conducted trials involving novel therapies or combination treatments have proved to be potent mediators of change towards increased patient benefit and improved financial

returns for the companies involved. Such studies require a thorough understanding of the background pharmacology of the product, a relevant and close appraisal of its toxicology as well as a reasoned appraisal of its short as well as medium and long-term benefits in the management of disease for a patient population of sufficiently sizable proportions. Thus, in modern terms, effective single drug or drug combination therapy in the reduction of raised levels of blood pressure in 20% of the adult population in the industrialized world is a continuing magnet for drug companies seeking innovative approaches for the control of blood pressure in adults and children. Likewise, the explosion in diabetes mellitus, both type 1 and particularly type 2, illustrating a western lifestyle which seems geared to excess, has stimulated substantial endeavour in the pharmaceutical industry towards medication that not only reduces appetite and hence weight, but also leads to improved glycaemic control in those patients, more especially those with type 2 diabetes mellitus.

11.13 National Institute for Clinical Excellence

The National Institute for Health and Clinical Excellence (NICE) as a special Health Authority was introduced by the Government in 1999, the objectives of which were ostensibly to encourage the faster uptake of effective new medicines, to promote more equitable access to treatments and to improve the use of NHS resources. This seemed a sensible and straightforward initiative by Government and, in one sense, industry welcomed the introduction of NICE. It was well recognised that the UK had one of the slowest uptakes of innovative therapies in Europe despite having amongst the highest rates of cancer and heart disease and the social irritant of 'postcode' prescribing. It is quite clear, however, that in practice, industry's concern is that far from encouraging faster uptake of medicines as the Government had suggested, the reverse has proven to be the case. NICE is sometimes referred to as the fourth hurdle to a successful market launch of any new therapy. The consequence of this as perceived by industry is increased costs for research and investment in marketing and promotion. In some ways this has been the case in that NICE has transformed the UK marketing landscape and now companies need to build the capability to respond to an appraisal of one of its compounds via NICE and related mechanisms. The NICE website (www.nice.org.uk), whereby guidance on the elements and the timing of technology appraisal lies in the public domain, has opened companies to general and competitor scrutiny. There are few changes in the four main elements of a technology appraisal and a summary of the components of these subsections is shown below:

1. Introduction:
(a) Epidemiology;
(b) Development of the technology;
(c) Problem definition.
2. Clinical effectiveness:
(a) Inclusion and exclusion criteria for studies used in the submission;
(b) Comparisons;
(c) Clinical data.
3. Cost effectiveness:
(a) Resource use and costs;
(b) Discounting;
(c) Dealing with uncertainty.
4. Wider implications of the technology for the NHS:
(a) Budget impact;
(b) Service impact;
(c) Consideration of equity.

A large proportion of the technology appraisals so far performed by NICE on pharmaceuticals has been on products recently introduced into the marketplace and this has created difficulties for manufacturers trying to answer the questions posed by the appraisal. For most compounds, as one would expect, at the time of launch it is very unlikely that outcome studies will have been completed to allow accurate cost-effectiveness calculations to be performed. The clear emphasis in phase III studies is on clinical efficacy and safety to satisfy the regulatory requirements of the authorities. In most instances and in such circumstances, it is impossible (and probably unethical) to perform 'pragmatic' studies on the general population until safety and efficacy have satisfactorily been demonstrated in a tightly defined trial population.

The only alternative that is reasonably open to manufacturers faced with a technology appraisal soon after launch, is to base their cost-effectiveness argument on computer modelling or simulation. This is not really satisfactory and does not represent best clinical practice but under the circumstances is probably all that can be reasonably done at present.

NICE is a UK (strictly English) institution, but has provided a model whereby many countries already have or are establishing bodies that are designed for evaluating the clinical effectiveness of new compounds. The comments applicable to the UK on the need for

outcome studies as part of phase III programmes extend both the cash spend and the timing of such programmes beyond anything currently in practice.

There are additional uncertain elements which need to be built into a company's plans for NICE or its equivalent in Scotland (SMC) or in Wales (AWMSG) on how to handle the uncertainty in the marketplace when an appraisal is announced and then performed by NICE or other advisory bodies. Once an appraisal of a compound has been announced and the timetable for the appraisal made public by NICE there is a clear tendency for prescribers and NHS bodies to adopt a 'wait and see' approach to the prescribing of the new medicine regardless of its apparent efficacy. This process, which may take anything up to 2 years on average, is a substantial hurdle to the initiation and use of the product until such time as the appraisal process and its recommendations are considered.

11.14 Conclusions

For many physicians and non-clinical scientists working in industry, more particularly in early clinical development, their involvement with marketing and marketing-related activities will be peripheral to their roles in the company. Nonetheless, for those in medical advisory roles, particularly those involved in strategic planning and medical marketing, this knowledge base will be central to their everyday work. There are a number of key areas that are useful to those in an advisory role within the medical marketing sphere. These include essentially aspects of 'good housekeeping' including a literature search and collection and collating of publications on advantages and disadvantages of current treatments. It is always useful to write a review of the proven and potential benefits of the new product, not only for the education of internal staff and possibly for publication, but also for the further enlightenment of more senior staff who may be further away from the basic science.

In addition, it is useful for those involved to make a list of the likely questions which include aspects of phase I and II activities of the drug, more particularly mechanism of action, safety profile and its use in paediatric and elderly populations, and its benefits or otherwise in pregnancy. Standard answers to these questions (and these are the ones that are frequently asked of physicians in the medical marketing team) will also cover either in depth or in principle those same questions asked by pharmacists, government agency physicians and research workers. This will represent the best currently available scientific and medical opinion which for the company will provide a response that is consistent throughout the world.

Early attention to lecture notes for presentations at national and international symposia as well as for educational purposes within the company are important. These will include presentations of a straightforward and structured nature for the sales representatives.

It is important that the messages given to all sections of the company are clear, consistent and at an appropriate level to satisfy their particular needs whether at the board room, at research symposia or at the grass roots in making an impact on the customer base of the company. Patient information sheets containing the essential information that the patient will want to know is the forerunner to the patient information leaflet. Here it is vital, particularly for the medical advisor of the proposed promotional literature, that the information is consistent with the product licence, obtains legal approval of the proposed literature from the corporate legal department in writing and is relevant to the prescribing perspective of the patient under treatment.

In many ways this is the most difficult area for the medical marketeer to oversee in that if there is any possibility for misinterpretation of any promotional statement then it requires further review. Such examples include a safety assessment or definition of net benefit by the relevant internal consultant. Substantial pressure may be put upon such an individual to release the documentation but when in doubt adequate supporting documentation should be prepared and a formal response made with copies to appropriate colleagues including legal counsel.

Any promotional material that is not in accordance with the marketing authorisation, is inconsistent with labelling approved by the regulatory authority or is misleading, whether deliberate or otherwise, is a criminal offence under the Medicines Act (1968). This carries both financial penalties, which may be substantial, and the potential for a custodial sentence. This is already part of Case Law. Conviction of such an offence usually leads to removal from the Medical Register by the General Medical Council and an end to that individual's medical practice.

Thus, it is readily seen that medical marketing is a balancing act between the commercial aspects of the company and its cashflow and the responsibility of the individual doctor as the voice of practical ethics for the company. However, in the final analysis, it is the responsibility of the medical advisor to the company to ensure that the interests of and benefit to the health of the patient take precedence over all other considerations. This will ensure the proper conduct of the medical advisor and his or her understanding of the Hypocratic oath.

References

1 Young JH. Medical marketing. *Textbook of Pharmaceutical Medicine, 5th edn.* Oxford: Blackwell Publishing, 2006;344.

2 Association of the British Pharmaceutical Industry. *Code of Practice for the Pharmaceutical Industry.* 2008. Available at http://www.abpi.org.uk/publications/pdfs/pmpca_code2008.pdf

3 *Saving Lives: Our Healthier Nation.* Royal College of General Practitioners Summary paper, Cm4386. The Stationery Office, 1999.

4 EU Regulation on Paediatric Medicines, Regulation (EC) No. 1901/2006 and the amending Regulation (EC) No. 1902/2006.

5 Young JH. Medical marketing. *Textbook of Pharmaceutical Medicine, 5th edn.* Oxford: Blackwell Publishing, 2006;350.

12 Information and promotion

Charles de Wet

Boehring Ingelheim Limited, Bracknell, Berkshire, UK

Knowledge is of two kinds. We know a subject ourselves, or we know where we can find information upon it.
Samuel Johnson (1709–84)

12.1 Introduction

The demand for relevant quality information has increased in line with rapidly changing technology and the internet has become the most referenced source of health information. Health care communications have also been expeditiously changing, with the removal of barriers to channels, disciplines and marketing, often under proactive guidance from regulators and authorities. At the same time, there has been much debate about the promotional practice of the pharmaceutical industry, culminating in the UK in the publication in 2005 of the Health Committee report on the *Influence of the Pharmaceutical Industry*.[1] This report urges greater restraint in the promotion of medicines, a sentiment reflected by calls for greater state and federal regulation of statements made by pharmaceutical manufacturers in the USA.[2]

These developments have contributed to issues of information and promotion becoming a key focus for the pharmaceutical physician. On the one hand, there is an obligation to provide accurate factual up-to-date data to enable the appropriate use of medicines; on the other hand, the obligation is to consult and interpret the databases to guide brand teams to develop promotional strategies and materials that will maximise the competitive position in the marketplace, while ensuring that the materials are appropriate, factual, fair and capable of substantiation. Publication

of misleading promotional material is a criminal offence and the Health Select Committee has recommended punishment befitting such a status.

Communication by pharmaceutical companies to physicians, and the provision of information on and promotion of their medicinal products, devices and diagnostic agents, have a unique status in both legal and business terms. Over and above the general legislation and controls on advertising applying to other industries, claims made by pharmaceutical companies about their products are subjected to additional legislation. Because medicines have the potential for harmful as well as beneficial effects and can cause serious problems if not used safely, they cannot be regarded as ordinary general commodities. To ensure high standards, responsibility and the safe use of medicines, there are specific regulations that strictly control the advertising and promotion of medicinal products in the UK. Central to this is that the regulations prohibit advertising of prescription only medicines (POM) to the public.

The control of medicines advertising in the UK is based on a long-established system of self-regulation supported by the statutory role of the Medicines and Healthcare products Regulatory Agency (MHRA) acting on behalf of government health ministers. The Medicines Act 1968[3] and its detailed regulations[4,5] comprehensively control the manufacture, packaging, labelling, distribution and promotion of medicines for both human and animal use, setting out standards of conduct to which pharmaceutical companies should abide. These standards are detailed in the British Code of Advertising Practice,[6] the Code of Practice for Advertising Over-the-Counter (OTC) Medicines, incorporating the Proprietary Association of Great Britain (PAGB) Consumer Code and the PAGB Professional Code,[7] the Independent Television Commission Code of Advertising Standards and Practice,[8] the Radio

The Textbook of Pharmaceutical Medicine. Edited by John P. Griffin. © 2009, ISBN: 978-1-4051-8035-1.

Authority Code of Advertising Standards and Practice and Programme[9] and the Association of the British Pharmaceutical Industry (ABPI) Code of Practice for the Pharmaceutical Industry.[10] The ABPI Code of Practice reflects and extends beyond the relevant UK law and aims to ensure that the promotion of medicines to health professionals and to administrative staff is carried out within a robust framework to support high quality patient care.

12.2 Legislation, controls and codes and their enforcement

12.2.1 Legal controls

Advertising of medicines in the UK is controlled by both statutory measures (with both criminal and civil sanctions) enforced by the MHRA, and self-regulatory measures (through Codes of Practice for the pharmaceutical industry) administered by trade associations. A combination of specific European and national legislation underpins the advertising of medicines alongside the general legislation on advertising which includes medicines.

12.2.1.1 European legislation

Title VIII of European Directive 2001/83/EC ('the Codified Directive')[11] as amended by Directive 2004/27/EC[12] contains the relevant European legislation on advertising.

12.2.1.2 UK legislation

12.2.1.2.1 The Medicines Act 1968 The Medicines Act 1968[3] came into effect on 1 September 1971 and introduced provision to control all matters and activities relating to medicinal products. Part VI of the Act (Promotion of Sales of Medicinal Products) deals specifically with the advertising of medicines; Section 92 defines 'advertisement'. Most provisions, however, have been superseded by subsequent legislation, and recently it has been announced that the Medicines Act 1968 will be reviewed in full over the next few years.

12.2.1.2.2 Medicines Regulations Existing controls on advertising under the Medicines Act 1968[3] have been reinforced by the Advertising and Monitoring Regulations,[4,5] which came into force on 9 August 1994 implementing Title VIII of the European Codified Directive.[11] Together with their subsequent amendments, these two Medicines Regulations constitute the most relevant UK legislation relating to the advertising of medicines. The Medicines (Advertising) Regulations 1994[4] set out the provisions for advertising, including homeopathic medicines and advertising directed at the public and at health professionals. The Advertising Regulations also make provisions for breaches that constitute a criminal offence and specify the penalties for such breaches. The Medicines (Monitoring of Advertising) Regulations 1994[5] specify procedures whereby advertisements considered to be inconsistent with the Advertising Regulations can be acted upon, either by reference to an administrative body established for that purpose or by civil proceedings.

The provisions of Advertising Regulations[4] apply to 'advertisements' for 'relevant medicinal products'. However, not all provisions apply to all advertisements or all relevant medicinal products. Separate sections apply, for example, to advertisements to health professionals, the public and registered homeopathic medicines.

Regulation 2 (2) of the Advertising Regulations,[4] referencing Section 92 of the Medicines Act[3] and underpinned by the definition of 'advertising of medicinal products' of Article 86 of the Codified Directive,[11] defines 'advertisement' as activities 'designed to promote the prescription, supply, sale or consumption of medicinal products'. The definition applied to medicines is not limited to specific media. It covers both written and spoken words intended to encourage prescription or supply of medicines by health professionals and use by the general public, in published journals, magazines and newspapers, photographs, film, broadcast material, video, electronic transmissions and the internet. The Regulations do not include all materials, and reference material, factual informative statements or announcements, trade catalogues and price lists are excluded provided that they do not make a product claim. The product labelling and package leaflet, which complies fully with the requirements of Statutory Instrument (SI) 1994/3144[13] and Title V of European Directive 2001/83/EC,[11] would also fall outside of the definition of 'advertisement'.

Regulation 2 (1) of the Advertising Regulations[4] defines a 'relevant medicinal product' broadly as a substance that either claims to or has the actual function of treating or preventing disease in human beings or animals. The vast majority of medicines are included and, since October 2005, also traditional herbal medicinal (THM) products with a 'traditional herbal registration' under the THM Registration Scheme.[14] Unlicensed herbal medicines and homeopathic medicines covered by product licences of right usually fall outside of the definition.

The Regulations require an advertisement to: comply with the particulars listed in the summary of product characteristics (SPC); encourage rational use by presenting the medicine objectively and without exaggerating its qualities; and not to be misleading.[4] They prohibit the advertising of unlicensed medicines (except provision of relevant factual information on novel medicines or methods of administration to health authorities, trust hospital budget holders and public advisory bodies).[4] Advertising materials for THM products have to include the statement 'Traditional herbal medicinal product for use in . . . exclusively based upon long-standing use as a traditional remedy'. Moreover, in advertising registered homeopathic medicines, information on the product labelling only may be used with no mention of a specific indication.[15]

12.2.1.2.3 Other relevant legislation Consumer advertising generally (excluding medicines) is regulated by the Trade Descriptions Act 1968 and supporting Regulations,[16] in particular, the Control of Misleading Advertisements 1988 (SI 1988/915).[17] The Office of Fair Trading and the Advertising Standards Authority (ASA) administer this legislation on behalf of the Department of Trade and Industry. Broadcast advertising (including medicines) is regulated by the Broadcasting Acts of 1990 and 1996[18] and the more recent Communications Act 2003.[19] The ASA on behalf of the Office of Communications (OFCOM) is responsible for the administration of this legislation. Guidance and specific information on the advertising of medicinal products to health professionals and the general public is published in the MHRA Guidance Note 23 'The Blue Guide'.[20] The ABPI and PAGB Codes of Practice[10] also address the advertising of medicinal products, with provision for areas not included in the Regulations.

12.2.1.3 Advertising, control and enforcement
The advertising of medicines is controlled partly by statutory measures enforced by the MHRA. The key function of the MHRA is to protect public health by promoting the safe use of medicines and ensuring that they are promoted honestly as to their benefits, uses and effects, and in compliance with current legislation. As a licensing authority, the MHRA has a statutory duty on behalf of government ministers to consider all breaches of the Medicines Act and Regulations. To ensure compliance with the legislation, the MHRA conducts a number of activities:
• Checking compliance with the law prior to publication (vetting) in defined circumstances;

• Monitoring of published advertising materials;
• Handling complaints about advertising; and
• Enforcement in relation to materials not compliant with the Regulations.

12.2.1.3.1 Vetting The MHRA has statutory powers under the Monitoring Regulations to require companies to submit advertising material before use for vetting. In implementing recommendations by the Health Select Committee's Report,[1] the MHRA has committed to vet newly licensed products subject to intensive monitoring and all new active substances. Vetting may also be required with product reclassification, such as from POM to P (i.e. from being available on prescription only to being available in a pharmacy without prescription, under the pharmacist's supervision) or where previous advertising for a product has breached the Regulations. Normally, the vetting period is no longer than 6 months.

12.2.1.3.2 Monitoring of published advertising material The MHRA's Advertising Standards Unit routinely scrutinises medical journals, magazines and other types of media, including the internet, for non-compliance with the Advertising Regulations. Marketing authorisation holders are contacted for clarification where there is doubt or the complaints procedure is initiated where there is cause for concern.

12.2.1.3.3 Handling of complaints Promotion or advertising of medicines in both POM and OTC health care sectors is controlled principally through the pharmaceutical industry's self-regulatory codes. However, the MHRA is required to investigate the complaint where a complaint has not been dealt with in a satisfactory manner within a reasonable time frame by the designated self-regulatory body, or where a complaint has been made to the MHRA directly. The MHRA generally investigates all complaints received but may refer to a self-regulatory body where an initial investigation has found no breach of the legislation but a potential breach of an ABPI Code of Practice.[10] At its discretion, and with the agreement of the complainant, other cases may also be referred.

Where a complaint about a broadcast advertisement is received by both the MHRA and the ASA, or by the ASA alone, it is the responsibility of the ASA to investigate the complaint. Accelerated action is taken where there is a serious risk to public health. Generally, the MHRA endeavours to complete an investigation within 30 days. The decision is communicated to the complainant and the advertiser, and the outcome is published on the MHRA's website. The MHRA occasionally issues a statement about a specific case to highlight concerns and provide guidance on good practice; it may also request or compel the issue of a corrective statement by the advertiser.

12.2.1.3.4 Enforcement The Monitoring Regulations[5] set out the statutory powers available to the MHRA. The MHRA can and will resort to formal procedures, such as issuing notices during case investigation, enforcement action or prosecution, if it considers there to be a public health justification. However, in most cases, it is expected that companies will collaborate with the MHRA to resolve potential breaches. The MHRA can serve a 'minded to' notice upon any person responsible for the issue or publication of an advertisement, although such action is usually taken against the marketing authorisation holder. It is also entitled to take an injunction in the courts either as part of its investigation of a complaint or of its own volition. Companies may make written representations to the non-statutory Independent Review Panel (IRP) in defence against a proposed determination of breach. The IRP's view has to be taken into consideration by the MHRA in their assessment. The MHRA's final decision closes the case, subject only to any judicial review of the decision before the courts or any criminal prosecution.

Importantly, any breach of the provisions of the Advertising Regulations, Regulation 23, is a criminal offence that could result in a fine and/or imprisonment for up to 2 years. Similarly, failure to comply with any requirement enforced by a notice served under the Monitoring Regulations is a criminal offence with a similar penalty. Civil sanctions, such as requiring publication of a corrective statement, can also be applied.

12.2.2 Self-regulation

Promotion or advertising for prescription and consumer medicines remains principally controlled through the self-regulatory codes established and operated by the pharmaceutical industry. Specifically, these are the ABPI Code of Practice for the Pharmaceutical Industry[10] and the Code of Practice for Advertising OTC Medicines, incorporating the PAGB Consumer and Professional Codes.[7]

The ABPI Code of Practice[10] has strong support from the industry with all companies employing considerable resources to ensure compliance of their activities. A condition of ABPI membership is to abide by the Code in both the spirit and letter. In addition

to over 75 ABPI member companies that are responsible for the supply of more than 80% of medicines to the National Health Service (NHS), over 60 non-member companies have also given formal agreement to accept the jurisdiction of the Prescriptions Medicines Code of Practice Authority (PMCPA). Complaints made against companies under the Code are regarded as serious both by the companies and the industry as a whole. Sanctions are applied against companies ruled in breach of the Code.

12.2.2.1 ABPI Code of Practice

The year 2008 marked 50 years of self-regulation of the promotion of medicines, with the first Code of Practice, the 'Code for the sales promotion practice for medical specialities' published in October 1958 by the ABPI. Despite this first Code being only two pages long (compared with 60 pages of the edition published in 2008), it took just 12 days for the first complaint to be received. The Code has since been reviewed and updated regularly.

The two most recent updates deserve special mention. The revised Code of January 2006[21] recommended a radical overhaul of how the industry regulated its own marketing and promotion to address some of the concerns of the Health Committee report.[1] The July 2008 Code[10] confirmed the process of ongoing review and improvement in establishing a system of self-regulation that could be seen as robust and effective by the public. It also incorporated the latest revision of the European Federation of Pharmaceutical Industries and Associations (EFPIA) Code of Practice on the Promotion of Medicine (2004),[22] which became effective from January 2000, as well as the EFPIA Code of Practice on Relationships between the Pharmaceutical Industry and Patient Organisation.[23]

While the industry has a legitimate right to promote medicines to health professionals, the ABPI Code of Practice aims to ensure that it is done within a robust framework to support high quality patient care, in a responsible, efficient and professional manner. Indeed, standards for the conduct and training of company staff are defined by the Code. The Code applies to the promotion of medicines to members of the UK health professions and to appropriate administrative staff. Promotion of an OTC medicine to health professionals (if designed to encourage doctors to prescribe the medicine) and advertisements to pharmacists for medicines other than OTC medicines also come within the scope of the Code. Code compliance is not limited to the UK but also applies to promotion at meetings for UK health professionals and administrative staff held outside the UK, and when such individuals attend international meetings outside the UK. Promotional material distributed at an international meeting outside the UK also needs to comply with the local requirements of the regulatory body of the host country.

The Code definition of promotion is broad and encompasses any activity by a pharmaceutical company (or with the company's authority) that promotes the prescription, supply, sale or administration of its medicines. The Code also applies to some areas not related to promotion, including declaration of sponsorship, non-interventional studies, provision of medicines and samples, grants and fees for services, use of consultants and relations with patient organisations. Moreover, joint working with health authorities and trusts and the like, as well as activities designed to enlarge the market in defined therapeutic areas, such as disease awareness campaigns, need to be conducted in ways compatible with the Code.

The Code does not apply to the promotion of OTC medicines to health professionals when the object of the promotion is to encourage their purchase by members of the public. It also excludes replies made in response to individual enquiries or specific communications from health professionals or appropriate administrative staff. Factual accurate informative announcements and references concerning licensed medicines are also excluded, provided they contain no product claims. Such information supplied to national public organisations, such as the National Institute of Clinical Excellence (NICE), the Scottish Medicines Consortium (SMC) or the All Wales Medicines Strategy Group (AWMSG), is also exempt. The SPC, European and UK public assessment reports, labelling on medicines and accompanying package leaflets are also excluded.

In summary, the principal requirements of the Code are that all promotion is in accordance with the product licence and the SPC. It must be accurate, balanced, fair, unambiguous and objective, and based on an up-to-date evaluation of all the evidence. It must not mislead either directly or by implication. All information, claims and complaints must be capable of substantiation, with such substantiation provided promptly on request. Promotion must never be disguised. It must recognise the special value of medicines, the professional standing of the recipients and the principles of good taste. Certain obligatory information (i.e. the prescribing information) must be included in all promotions, with exemptions for abbreviated advertisements and some promotional aids. Requirements are discussed in more detail in section 12.3.

12.2.2.2 Enforcement of the ABPI Code of Practice

The Code requires each company to appoint a senior employee responsible for ensuring that the company is adherent to its provisions. Names of signatories have to be submitted to the MHRA and to the PMCPA. Unless other formal arrangements are made, this person is assumed to be the company's managing director or chief executive or equivalent. Signatories take personal responsibility for the material they authorise and, under the law, may be held accountable. One of the two signatories must be a registered medical practitioner (or, where a product is for dental use only, a registered medical practitioner or dentist) and the other an appropriately qualified person or senior official of the company. Promotional material for products or indications that have been on the UK market for more than 1 year and not part of a new and novel promotional campaign may be certified by a practising UK registered pharmacist working under the direction of a registered medical practitioner.

All promotional material (including arrangements for meetings outside the UK) must be examined. None can be issued until the final form, to which no subsequent amendments can be made, has been accepted by two signatories. It is the belief of these signatories that the material is compliant with the requirements of the Code and relevant advertising regulations, is consistent with the marketing authorisation and the SPC, and is a fair and honest presentation of the facts about the medicine. Materials still in use must be recertified at intervals of no more than 2 years to ensure continued adherence, and copies of certificates and the final form of the material should be preserved for not less than 3 years after their final use.

Similar to the pharmaceutical industry's global agreements to disclose certain clinical trial data, operation of the Code is seen as a demonstration of the industry's commitment to transparency. In 1993, the PMCPA was established to operate the Code for the pharmaceutical industry independent of the ABPI. Comprising a director, a secretary and a deputy secretary, it is responsible for the provision of advice, guidance, conciliation and training on the Code, as well as for the complaints procedure. It is also responsible for scrutinising journal advertising and monitoring meetings on a regular basis.

Complaints submitted under the rulings of the Code are considered firstly by the Code of Practice

Panel (CPP), which consists of the members of the PMCPA, acting with the assistance of independent expert advisers. Rulings are made on the basis that a complainant has to prove their complaint on the balance of probabilities. Both the complainant and the respondent company may appeal to the Code of Practice Appeal Board (CPAB) against the rulings made by the CPP. The CPAB is chaired by an independent, legally qualified chairman and includes representatives of the pharmaceutical industry within the UK and independent members from outside the industry. Details appear in the PMCPA's 'Constitution and Procedure', which are published with the Code.[10]

The CPAB has a dual role, acting over the activities of the CPP and the PMCPA, as an appeal body and as a supervisory body. All complaints received by the PMCPA and all rulings by the CPP are reported to the CPAB, thus ensuring independent scrutiny from outside the pharmaceutical industry of both the PMCPA's and the CPP's activities by the independent chairman and independent members of the CPAB. Where promotional material or activities are ruled in breach of the Code, the company concerned must cease to use the material or cease the activity in question forthwith and provide a written undertaking to that effect. Reports on all cases under the Code are published, naming companies ruled in breach of the Code. These reports receive wide coverage, particularly in the pharmaceutical press and occasionally reaching the lay press.

The CPAB may also require a company ruled in breach of the regulations to take steps to recover items distributed in connection with the promotion of a medicine. A variety of additional sanctions are available to the APBI Board of Management following receipt of a report from the CPAB. The APBI Board of Management can reprimand a company and publish details of that reprimand. It can order the PMCPA to audit company procedures in relation to the Code and, following that audit, impose a requirement on a company to improve its procedures in relation to the Code. The ABPI Board of Management can also require a company to publish a corrective statement and, in extreme cases, suspend or expel members from the ABPI. With regard to a non-member company, the board can remove that company from the list of non-members that have agreed to comply with the Code, and then advise the MHRA that responsibility for that company will no longer be accepted under the Code.

In addition to the ABPI subscription, all members of the ABPI are required to pay an annual Code of Practice levy to assist in funding the PMCPA. Certain administrative charges, payable by both members and non-members of the ABPI, may also be levied by the PMCPA in relation to complaints under the Code. These charges are akin to the costs awarded in civil cases in the courts. Charges are based on the number of matters ruled in a case, which is determined by the PMCPA director. Charges are fixed at two levels, dependent on whether the final case ruling is made by the CPP or, on appeal, by the CPAB. Charges are paid by either the company ruled in breach of the Code or the complainant (where the complainant is a pharmaceutical company) where there is a rule of no breach of the Code. Complainants from outside the industry are not required to pay any charge, regardless of outcome.

Perhaps unsurprisingly, the two largest sources of complaints are health professionals (mainly doctors and pharmacists) and the pharmaceutical companies themselves. However, criticisms of pharmaceutical advertising and/or promotional activities in the public domain, such as in the medical, pharmaceutical or lay press, or on radio or television, are also routinely taken up and dealt with as complaints under the Code. Additionally, the CPP and the CPAB can investigate possible breaches of the Code in promotional material that has been brought before the CPP or CPAB but not raised by the complainant in the case.

Companies are encouraged to attempt to settle inter-company disputes over advertising material without recourse to the formal complaints procedure. Generally, before progressing a formal complaint, the PMCPA would like evidence of inter-company dialogue. Guidelines on proceeding with inter-company dialogue are available on the PMCPA website. Companies may also seek the assistance of a conciliator to reach an agreement on inter-company differences about promotion and can contact the PCMPA director in regard of this. The PMCPA is also willing and able to provide informal guidance and advice on the requirements of the Code and, where appropriate, may seek the views of the CPAB.

12.2.2.3 Complaints under the ABPI Code of Practice and their management

Even for the experienced pharmaceutical physician, it is difficult to anticipate how promotional material will be perceived by its recipients. What may be entirely clear to the 'informed' approver of the material may be entirely unclear to the 'uninformed' or even 'informed' recipient. If the recipient is misled, there is no defence against the material not being misleading. Therefore, it is essential for those who develop, review and approve promotional materials to stand back and think objectively about how a recipient could perceive what is said, written or visualised.

Typically, about half of complaints to the PMCPA relate to Code Clause 7: 'Information, Claims and Comparisons' (Clauses 7.2–7.4, 7.10),[10] which addresses accuracy, balance, fairness, objectivity, lack of ambiguity and full representation of the total and up-to-date evidence. Comparisons must be carefully and appropriately presented, and information, claims and comparisons must be capable of substantiation.

The majority of the remaining complaints received by the PMCPA and the CPAB relate to hospitality, travel and meetings, to the promotion of unlicensed indications (i.e. not specified in the product licence), the conduct of medical representatives and to not maintaining high standards. The highest judgement is on those involved with meetings and hospitality. A complaint in this regard could constitute a breach of Code Clause 2, bringing 'Discredit to, and Reduction of Confidence in, the Industry'. Sponsors and recipients can be guided by asking themselves 'Would you and your company be willing to have these arrangements generally known?' and 'Does the educational content of the meeting outweigh the hospitality offered?' Prejudicing patient safety and/or public health, excessive hospitality, inducements to prescribe, inadequate action leading to a breach of understanding, promotion prior to the grant of a marketing authorisation, conduct of company employees or agents that falls short of competent care, and multiple or cumulative breaches of a similar and serious nature in the same therapeutic area within a short period of time, are all likely to be in breach of Clause 2. Particular censure is reserved for a breach of Clause 2, including public reprimanding, suspension or expulsion from the ABPI, and publishing of brief case details in the medical, pharmaceutical and nursing press.

12.2.2.4 Other codes

The system of self-regulation in the UK is underpinned by the statutory powers of the MHRA and supported by a number of regulatory bodies, the majority of which operate their own Codes of Practice. Second to the ABPI Code of Practice,[10] the pharmaceutical physician will most commonly have to refer to the Code of Practice for Advertising OTC Medicines.[7] The PAGB is the largest trade association and self-regulatory body for the OTC medicines industry. The two PAGB Codes (Consumer Code and Professional Code) are drawn up in consultation with the MHRA, ASA, Committee of Advertising Practice (CAP), OFCOM, Broadcast Advertising Clearance Centre and the Radio Advertising Clearance Centre. The Consumer Code presents standards for the advertising of OTC medicines to the general public and the Professional Code controls advertising directed at persons qualified to prescribe or supply medicines. The PAGB provides training programmes on its Advertising Codes, and its Complaints Committee will consider complaints, which can be referred to its Appeal Board. However, the PAGB does not vet advertising directed at professional or trade audiences.

The ASA is responsible for ensuring that all advertising is honest and respectful. It administers the British Code of Advertising, Sales Promotion and Direct Marketing (the CAP Code).[6] Since November 2004, the ASA also assumed responsibility for radio and television advertisements in a co-regulatory partnership with OFCOM. The Health Food Manufacturers Association, a trade association operating on behalf of the industry, administers a Code of Advertising Practice covering the advertising of specialist health products to the public and to health care professionals.[24] The British Dental Trade Association, the body that represents manufacturers, wholesalers and distributors of products and services to the dental profession, has Code of Practice to ensure the highest quality of dental service.[25] Additionally, a Code governing the promotion of medicines for use in animals is administered by the National Office of Animal Health.[26]

There are also a number of International Codes, with which local codes usually have to be in line and incorporate their provisions. A list for reference only is provided below; the interested reader is referred to the full publications:

• International Federation of Pharmaceutical Manufacturers and Associations' (IFPMA) Code of Pharmaceutical Marketing Practices;[27]

• European Federation of Pharmaceutical Industries and Associations' (EFPIA) Code on the Promotion of Prescription-Only Medicines to, and Interactions with, Health Professionals;[22]

• EFPIA Code of Practice on Relationships between the Pharmaceutical Industry and Patient Organisations;[23]

• World Health Organization's Ethical Criteria for Medicinal Drug Promotion;[28]

• International Pharmaceutical Congress Advisory Association's Code of Conduct.[29]

The detailed provisions provided in the available codes are to ensure that pharmaceutical companies operate in a responsible, ethical and professional manner. Measures should be taken by pharmaceutical companies to ensure that they comply with all applicable codes, laws and regulations. This includes the national code of the host country where activities are planned or carried out outside the UK.

12.3 Marketing, advertising and promotion of prescription medicines

Physicians working for, or under contract to, pharmaceutical companies selling medicinal products including medicines, vaccines, medical or surgical devices and diagnostic agents, will find themselves in an environment very different from their undergraduate teaching, subsequent postgraduate training and clinical or non-clinical practice. With reforms within the NHS, general practitioners and doctors in private practice are mindful of the importance of a businesslike or commercial approach to their practices. This aspect of pharmaceutical medicine may be difficult to comprehend on joining the industry as a medical adviser. Therefore, it is essential that the more experienced company physicians, such as the medical director or medically qualified department heads, provide support, advice and training about these matters to physicians who are new to the medical department.

Sales and marketing departments within a company require service and support from the whole medical department as well as from individual physicians who are usually assigned to provide medical advice on specific products that are currently being promoted. The demand for that service is usually directly related to the need for the commercial success of that product or products in the medical market place. As trained professional advisers, pharmaceutical physicians can encourage and guide the methods used by marketing departments in bringing medicinal products to the attention of the prescribing physician. In providing a professional service, they may assist sales and marketing colleagues in maximising the benefits of the product when prescribed by clinicians for disease management. Once the subtlety of this medico-marketing interface is understood, pharmaceutical physicians come to realise that their ethical or professional instincts are not compromised.

Open dialogue is essential between medical and marketing departments so that areas of potential contention or disagreement are discussed before actions are taken, costs are incurred and complaints are received. Indeed, marketing colleagues usually appreciate good ideas that are medically acceptable in promotional terms and especially so when review of the data allows strong support of claims or advantages for a particular product. Marketing colleagues are best advised to consult the relevant medical adviser early in the process. When both meet with blank paper and a few ideas, discussions usually lead to good promotional material that is ethically acceptable and non-contentious. The task is likely to be more arduous when the product manager prepares a draft, which the medical adviser is then expected to edit to meet the ABPI Code of Practice.[10]

The creation of ethical promotional material is a team exercise, the key players being the product manager, the product physician, the scientific adviser, and a colleague from the regulatory affairs department. A competent review of the data relevant to the claims being made for the product, together with a reading for compliance with the product licence and the Code of Practice,[10] are the minimum needs in the generation of material intended for promotional use. The final document then has to be approved by the company's senior executives, usually the medical director or senior medical colleagues and possibly the marketing director. The managing director is also involved since any breach of the Code of Practice[10] and/or Medicines Act 1968[3] and its Regulations[4,5] will be notified to the senior company executive.

12.3.1 Methods of promotion
12.3.1.1 Verbal promotion
Verbal promotion is carried out by company sales representatives, who visit prescribing doctors at their surgeries or institutions and present information about the company's medicinal products. Representatives must take care to ensure that all aspects of their calls, such as frequency and duration, do not cause the doctor inconvenience, and that certainly no fee should be paid or offered for the interview. Usually with aid of printed or prepared material (see section 12.3.1.2), the representative engages in a dialogue with the doctor regarding the attributes of the product, presenting any advantages and comparative data. The representative will also try to ascertain whether the doctor has patients for whom the medicine might be indicated, such as for those whose disease may be inadequately controlled by their current prescribed medication. In this case, if the physician can be persuaded to try the promoted medicine, and the treatment is at least as successful as the current prescription, then the physician may

consider using the product the next time a patient with the same disease presents. A well-trained and well-informed representative can also discreetly and tactfully educate the doctor, because few doctors know about all medications and/or are able to read all the scientific literature. Equally, should the representative learn any information in relation to the product's safety they must report it back to the company.

The pharmaceutical physician has an important role in the training of representatives, who are required to have full knowledge of the products they promote and maintain a high standard of ethical conduct in the manner in which they promote them. The ABPI requires of member companies that all medical representatives are professionally trained under their Code of Practice. In-house training on the Code is carried out by companies and by the PMCPA in accordance with an approved syllabus drawn up by the ABPI. Representatives must take the appropriate ABPI examination within their first year of joining the company, and are required to pass within 2 years if they wish to continue in that employment. The pharmaceutical physician will generally be required to teach representatives sufficient understanding of the diseases and their treatment, relevant to the company's products. Additionally, their knowledge of product clinical data, and published and unpublished reports and articles, can be applied to teaching representatives about the issues surrounding the product characteristics, which may arise in discussions with prescribing doctors. Importantly, representatives must learn the details of the product licence to avoid being in breach of the Medicines Act, its Regulations, or the Code of Practice. In particular, they must be aware that claims or comparisons which are outside the terms of a product's marketing authorisation or inconsistent with the SPC are unacceptable.

While the personal attributes and knowledge of medical representatives are fundamental in promoting a product successfully, pharmaceutical physicians have an important role in informing, guiding and advising them so that their verbal promotion is appropriate. Content usually varies according to whether the recipient is a general practitioner or a hospital consultant or specialist. General practitioners tend to prefer clear messages about the possible advantages and disadvantages of particular products in conditions that are commonly treated in general practice. Hospital physicians or specialists who are familiar with the literature regarding key medicines in their speciality are likely to want a more sophisticated discussion. Both increasingly wish to know the likely medication costs in relation to the benefits. Pharmaceutical physicians should therefore provide representatives with comprehensive information regarding the company's ethical medicinal products.

12.3.1.2 Written, printed and documentary promotion

Pharmaceutical companies typically employ the help of advertising and marketing, public relations and other specialist agencies to produce company promotional literature, as well as their own marketing professionals. All written, documentary and published promotional items are usually reviewed by the company medical advisers for conformity with the known data, the Code of Practice and relevant advertising regulations. Written and published promotional material must not be made available to prescribing doctors unless it has been certified by two appropriate persons on behalf of the company, one of whom may be the pharmaceutical physician. As the company and responsible medical signatory could be prosecuted for breach of the regulations, the importance of 'getting it right' cannot be underestimated.

Additionally, part of the pharmaceutical physician's role is to ensure that the literary content is appropriate for the promotional purpose. This may be both time-consuming and complex, and companies usually have standard operating procedures (SOPs) that cover the generation and approval of all ethical promotional material. These SOPs should be written by experienced colleagues who know the relevant parts of the Medicines Act and the Code of Practice, in conjunction with those whose actions are governed by these rules to ensure that they 'work'. They should then be approved by those who hold relevant positions of authority within the company, including the medical director. Such SOPs should also have the approval of the marketing and managing directors because procedures and performance are evaluated by the MHRA and the PMCPA.

In terms of promotional materials, written and published items constitute the majority of the pharmaceutical physician's workload because these are generally left with prescribing doctors as sources of information and reminders about the product. Such items vary from lengthy detail aids (presenting the product profile) to abbreviated advertisements, simple 'mailers' (promotional letters) and reminders (small items that can be used in day-to-day practice, such as note pads, pens, coffee mugs and wall charts) to large advertisements that appear in the medical press. For all items, there are both general and specific rules.

Generally, prescribing information must form part of all promotional material (excludes abbreviated advertisements and promotional aids meeting specific requirements); more specifically, abbreviated advertisements are largely restricted to journals and other professional publications intended for health professionals, and must be no larger than 420 cm² in size. It is therefore essential that pharmaceutical physicians understand and can apply these rules to avoid breaches of the Medicines Act or the Code of Practice. The PMCPA will readily provide training and guidance with respect to promotional material.

Many pharmaceutical companies also publish newsletters on the proceedings of conferences, congresses and their satellite symposia. These may provide information and commentary on clinical trials and other product data, using academic or clinical opinion, or interviews relevant to particular therapeutic areas. Such printed materials must also be reviewed for format, content and style according to SOPs governing the approval of ethical promotional material. Quotations from the literature or personal communication must be reproduced exactly, although modification is permitted to comply with the Code. Care is warranted that they represent the current views of the author or speaker and permissions must be gained.

Published data and company 'data on file' provide the main references for printed promotional material. Pharmaceutical physicians must be able to understand and interpret these data and then to advise on how those data may be incorporated into promotional copy without loss of context or being open to misunderstanding or misleading. A claim or highlighted item may be perfectly clear to the writer but may be interpreted quite differently by the reader. There are practising physicians and pharmacists who take a particular interest in the way that pharmaceutical companies promote their products and in ensuring that they obey the rules.[30] However, most physicians are fair-minded about promotion, and complaints are generally made by doctors who feel that companies are overstating their case or are taking unfair advantage. Pharmaceutical physicians must have an eye for these possibilities before distribution of the printed material.

Marketing and medical staff from competitor companies are also highly sensitive to promotional material from a competitor in an area where they may have a similar product. Complaints about printed promotional material and promotional behaviour are not infrequent between companies. Again, these are mainly with respect to 'breaking the rules' or taking unfair advantage. The Code of Practice rules that information, claims and comparisons are accurate, balanced, fair, objective and unambiguous, and reflect the current data clearly. Moreover, they must be capable of substantiation, and such evidence must be provided within 10 days of a request. The Code provides specific guidelines on the standards, presentation and wording of information, claims and comparisons, which may not be immediately realised by those producing the copy. In the event of materials found to be in breach of the Code, companies must ensure that they are quickly and entirely withdrawn from use.

Promotional material may only be distributed to health professionals and others with a need of or interest in such information. Additionally, there are restrictions on the volume of material distributed and the frequency with which it is sent. No more than eight mailings may be sent to a health professional in a year, although there is no limit to those reporting safety issues and price changes only.

12.3.1.3 Audio-visual promotion

Audio-cassette, video recording, film, DVD and CD-ROM, as well as electronic and web-based materials, all provide means of promotion. Clinicians, seeing it as a form of teaching, can be interviewed, and actors can be hired for the quality of their voices for introductions, link-pieces, voiceovers and even the actual promotion. Audio-visual items are treated similarly to more conventional forms of promotional material. Pharmaceutical physicians should review the complete script and then listen to the audio-tape or watch the film to ensure that products have been promoted in a balanced way, that rules have not been inadvertently breached and that the item has not been inappropriately edited or taken out of the context intended by the speaker. Invited clinical or scientific speakers should review and approve the use of their own text, and the finished item should then be certified according to company procedure.

Scientific congresses often attract television, radio or newspaper journalists interested in new medical discoveries or the financial performance of companies. Pharmaceutical physicians must be cautious when being interviewed because what they say may be construed as promotion by a third party. Those likely to find themselves in this position should be media-trained to minimise the risk inherent in on-the-spot interviews. Companies may find these materials useful from a promotional point of view but they should be assessed and formally approved before use.

Electronic data communications, including telephone, text messages, email, telemessages, facsimile and automated calling systems, must not be used for promotional purposes, except with the prior permission of the recipient.

12.3.1.4 The internet

The internet represents one of the best methods of disseminating information, providing opportunities for commerce, advertising and promotion. Unsurprisingly, the pharmaceutical industry has taken advantage of these opportunities for its medicinal products. Regulatory authorities have also adjusted to include promotional materials available transnationally on the internet. The situation is not simple due to differing legislation between countries. Direct-to-customer advertising is not permitted in the European Union and many other countries, whereas it is permitted in the USA. The US Food and Drug Administration is able to inspect and enforce for material that originates in the USA. Likewise, the UK authorities and codes of marketing practice have accommodated information on the internet by applying the same principles as with other materials.

The Medicines Act and Code of Practice prohibit the advertising of prescription medicines to the public (i.e. patients). To avoid public access to promotional materials about POMs, the ABPI and MHRA recommend a company-sponsored website be either access-limited or provide information for the public as well as promotion to health professionals, with the sections for each target audience clearly separated and the intended audience identified. Additionally, each page should include a statement identifying the intended audience. The majority of pharmaceutical company websites contain SPCs, patient information leaflets (PILs) and public assessment reports (UK and European) and as their sources of information for their POM products. All information must be presented in such a way as not to be promotional. It is hoped that adequate non-promotional information to the public discourages and dispels the need to access materials intended for health professionals. It is also intended that users avoid the need to access non-UK websites to obtain basic information. However, it should be clear to the user when they are leaving the company-sponsored site, as sites linked via company sites are not necessarily covered by the Code.

Reassuringly, while continuing to target their promotion to health professionals, company promotion to patients and/or their relatives appears to be responsible and informative. Companies appear to have understood that the provision of information about medical conditions, medicinal treatments, and the medicines themselves, to patients, relatives and carers, as well as health professionals, is necessary. It is also clear that the MHRA supports the supply of balanced informative material.

12.3.1.5 Meetings and conferences

Many scientific meetings and congresses are financed substantially by the pharmaceutical industry. The large international and national medical societies could not afford to hold their annual meetings without such company sponsorship. In return for this investment, promotional stands and exhibits are commonplace at conferences. Clinicians are expected and encouraged to visit a sponsor's stand or exhibit, and companies make use of the opportunities presented for promotion of their medicinal products. Companies also sponsor individual attendance at such meetings, which provide a level of medical education, debate and information that cannot readily occur elsewhere. Pharmaceutical physicians provide valuable support to marketing colleagues by being available to discuss product information and data. They can also bring clinicians to the stand to meet marketing people or to use the facilities and services provided by the company, including on-line literature search facilities, reprints and promotional material, and even hot beverages or soft drinks. These activities, which support product promotion, are legitimate and merely need care to adhere to the rules.

However, product licences may differ between countries and some products may not have marketing authorisation in all countries. Promotion of medicines that do not have a valid marketing authorisation, and indications not covered by the marketing authorisation, are prohibited. Materials relating to products that do not hold UK marketing authorisations are permitted provided that a significant number of attendees are from countries where the product is licensed. Accordingly, the regulatory status of a particular product should be made clear to clinicians at international congresses. To avoid being misleading, promotional materials for a medication or indication that does not have marketing authorisation in the host country must be clearly labelled to that effect.

12.3.1.6 Promotional gifts and prizes

Gifts to prescribers are not forbidden but must conform to certain sensible rules.[10] They should not cost the donor more than £6 excluding VAT and they must have some relevance to the practice of medicine. Marketing colleagues, whose job it is to create a rationale for a particular promotional gift and its relevance to medical practice, and the pharmaceutical physician, in approving such an item, must be aware as to what is reasonable. Items of general utility such as stationery (e.g. pens, pads) and clinical items (e.g. surgical gloves, tissues) are acceptable, whereas items of personal benefit or for use in the home or car are not. In deciding what is reasonable, it is prudent to consider whether the item would uphold a complaint made to the CPP or CPAB. Items provided on long-term or permanent loan to a prescriber or practice are also regarded as gifts and subject to the same Code requirements. Competitions and quizzes, and the giving of prizes, are unacceptable means of product promotion.

12.3.1.7 Promotional hospitality

Hospitality provided for the health professions is open to misinterpretation. Complaints arise when hospitality is clearly inappropriate. Companies may provide hospitality to health professionals only in association with meetings with an educational content. These range from small lunchtime presentations in a group practice through to large international conferences. The medical or scientific purpose of a meeting where hospitality is offered or arranged should always be more important than the hospitality itself, which should always be secondary to the purpose. For example, meetings should not be mainly social or sporting occasions. Moreover, there is no obligation to provide hospitality or a benefit in lieu of it. In determining whether hospitality is acceptable, it is useful to consider if you or the company would be willing to have the arrangements generally known. In particular, the value of the hospitality should not exceed the value of the purpose of meeting. Thus, inappropriate costs of refreshments, accommodation and travel, inappropriate venues, and the presence of spouses when the company is paying constitute breaches of the Code of Practice. However, guests are often key opinion leaders and inappropriate hospitality of poor quality would not be appreciated.

Meetings and their associated hospitality organised by pharmaceutical companies at venues outside the UK are allowed but there must be logistical sense for doing so. For example, a venue abroad would be appropriate if most of the invitees are from other countries or the resources/expertise that is the meeting focus are located outside the UK. Such meetings are bound by the rules governing those held within the UK.

12.3.1.8 Sponsorship

Companies, through the marketing department, medical grants committees or the medical department, are regularly approached for the provision of financial and non-financial support or sponsorship. Requests come from a range of sources, including charitable organisations, learned societies and individuals. They vary widely from financial support for schemes and activities, travel to meetings, or a salary or research post, to non-financial support such as supplies of drugs and other company products for personal research. Most companies have a budget for such sponsorship. Pharmaceutical industry managers, including the medical director, have to regard all sponsorship as a form of investment, which is therefore promotional whether it is of the company's name or products.

As with other forms of promotion, sponsorship is regulated. Pharmaceutical companies may accede to sponsorship but they must ensure that their involvement is made clear from the outset. This includes company-sponsored meetings, and materials relating to medicines and their uses. Interaction with patient or other user organisations requires a written agreement setting out what exactly has been agreed and all arrangements must comply with the Code of Practice. Clearly, companies should not influence text of an organisation's materials to its benefit or use their logo without permission. Schemes, charities or activities are acceptable as long as there is no associated element of promotion of an individual product.

12.3.1.9 Provision of medicines and samples

Companies frequently wish to assist prescribing health professionals in gaining familiarity with a medicinal product by making samples available. A sample must be marked 'free medical sample – not for resale', no larger than the smallest presentation on the UK market, and must not be a medicine that has been on the market for more than 10 years. Titration packs, free goods and bonus stock provided to pharmacists and to others are not samples. Neither are 'starter packs', which are small packs provided to allow a doctor to initiate treatment in an emergency situation. While providing an opportunity for promotion, samples must not be provided as an inducement to prescribe and supply. The Code of Practice lays down strict rules as to how and on what scale samples may be provided. In particular, samples may only be supplied in response to a written request from a health professional, who must sign and date any request card. No more than 10 samples of a particular product may be given to a particular recipient in the course of a year. Adequate company systems of control and accountability must be in place.

Like trials in phases I–III, phase IV (post-marketing) trials must be genuine investigations that are properly conducted and the data analysed. Guidelines for Company Sponsored Safety Assessment of Marketed Medicines (SAMM) state that SAMM studies should not be undertaken for the purposes of promotion.[31] Free drug must be made available for phase IV trials approved by the ethics committees. However, free drug may not be given to doctors solely to use as they think fit.

12.3.1.10 Services to doctors and patients

Provision of medical and educational goods and services to doctors that will enhance patient care or benefit the NHS is an accepted form of promotion if their provision is not connected with promotion. Many companies take advantage of this as such services create a favourable impression of a company and its products in the minds of health professionals and patients. For example, a DVD on the correct operating procedures for a nebuliser can be made available to patients through the doctor or asthma nurse by the manufacturers of a nebuliser solution. Similarly, funding practice nurses to be trained in the clinic management of hyperlipidaemia facilitates referral of the patient by the trained nurse to the doctor for treatment.

While such activities are provided by companies wishing to promote use of their products, provision of goods and services should neither be linked to the promotion of company products nor be dependent on their use. The General Medical Council[32] advises doctors to act in the interest of their patients and not to accept anything that may affect or be seen to affect patient management. There are specific rules regarding the role of company medical/generic representatives and the provision of goods and services.[10] Depending on the nature of the goods and services provided and method of provision, companies should consider using other staff or appropriately qualified persons such as a sponsored registered nurse. Importantly, confidential data must not be known to third parties. Thus, patient contact, either directly or by identification from patient records, is not permitted by representatives. Only an appropriately qualified person may undertake activities relating to patient contact or identification.

The Medicines Act and Code of Practice prohibit the advertising of prescription medicines to patients and their relatives or carers. Non-promotional information may be disseminated if it is factual, balanced and does not encourage patients to ask health providers to prescribe a specific medication. Information to the public falls into one of three categories depending on its purpose, how it is supplied, and how the public are made aware of the information. Thus, proactive information is supplied to the public with a direct request (e.g. booklets on diseases and/or medicines); reference information is intended to provide a current resource available on a website or by other means; and reactive information is supplied in response to and restricted to a specific request.

12.3.1.11 Market research

Market research is not exempt from following certain guidelines[33] and, like all promotional activities, may not be disguised promotion. However, unlike other materials, market research material need not reveal the name of the company but must state that it is sponsored by a pharmaceutical company.

12.4 Information

It is mandatory that pharmaceutical companies have a scientific service responsible for compiling and collating all information about the medicines and products that they market. The ABPI Code of Practice[10] states this clearly and, appreciating the need for high standards in the provision of information, the Pharmaceutical Information Pharmacovigilance Association (PIPA) has also published guidelines.[34] Prescribers and qualified suppliers of medicines must have access to neutral and objective information about the available products, and companies respect that an information service department (more usually termed medical information department) is a necessary and responsible facility. These are usually staffed and managed by qualified pharmacists, information scientists, others with a life sciences degree, and nurses. In general, they form part of the company's medical department so that impartial advice is provided. Such a service can only be maintained if its staff are trained in information database searching and other aspects of information provision, and have access to the company's product database and major external scientific literature databases.

The medical information department may also administer the company's product safety database, handling spontaneously reported adverse events, which may or may not be related to the company's product. It may also have access to the MHRA's anonymised database of reported adverse events and reactions. Usually, the medical information department receives adverse drug reaction reports as part of general enquiries from health professionals or the public, or from the company's medical representatives. These are generally then passed on to the company drug safety or pharmacovigilance department that more usually manages the company's product safety database and the entry of spontaneously reported adverse events on to the MHRAs database.

Information regarding medicinal products is available to health professionals from a variety of external and independent sources, including:

• *Drug and Therapeutics Bulletin (DTB)*;
• *British National Formulary (BNF)*;
• *Electronic Medicines Compendium (eMC)*;
• *Monthly Index of Medical Specialities (MIMS)*;
• *Medicines Resource Centre (MeReC)*;
• *Medicines Information Service (MIS)*;
• *Medicines and Healthcare products Regulatory Agency (MHRA)*;
• *European Medicines Evaluation Agency (EMEA)*;
• *European Public Assessment Report (EPAR)*;
• *Bandolier*.

The scale and scope of medicinal product information generated and provided either mandatorily or on demand by pharmaceutical companies is as follows.

12.4.1 Summary of product characteristics

The SPC is one of the key documents that must be submitted in draft by pharmaceutical companies to the competent authority(ies), such as the MHRA or the EMEA, upon application for a marketing authorisation. The regulatory authority, i.e. competent authority(ies) or the EMEA, to which the SPC is submitted, is dependent on the regulatory procedure being followed. Once approved, it is the definitive statement between the competent authority(ies)/EMEA and the company on the medicinal product and forms part of the marketing authorisation. The content can only be changed with the approval of the relevant competent authority(ies)/EMEA.

Additional to forming part of the marketing authorisation, the approved SPC is the basis of information for health professionals on how to use the medicinal product safely and effectively. It is not in the SPCs remit to give general advice on the treatment of particular medical conditions but it should mention specific aspects of the treatment related to use of the medicinal product or its effects.

The SPC also sets the boundaries for promotion of the product; forms the basis of the prescribing information/essential information that must appear on almost all promotional material; and is the source document for labelling, PILs and professional leaflets. It is often included in relevant published compendia (e.g. the eMC), or used as the source document for entries into other information sources (e.g. the BNF). Representatives must provide, or have available on request, a copy of the SPC for each medicine that they are to promote.

In October 2001, the European Commission published its proposals to amend the body of legislation covering the EU medicines regulatory regime, including the Council Directive 2001/83/EC[11] on the Community code relating to medicinal products for human use that details the required information for the SPC.[35] The agreed texts were adopted by the Council and the European Parliament in March 2004 as Council Directive 2004/27/EC (amending Directive 2001/83/EC on human medicines).[12]

The sequence of particulars on the SPC is listed in Box 12.1, and is detailed further in Article 11 of Council Directive 2001/83/EC as amended.[12] The European Commission's guideline on the SPC[36] provides advice on the presentation of information. Reference should also be made to Volume 3 of 'The rules governing medicinal products in the European Union'[37] where there are further SPC guidelines on specific therapeutic areas and pharmacological groups.

12.4.2 Patient information leaflets and labelling

While information on how a medicine should be used is provided to doctors and pharmacists in the SPC, information to patients or consumers is provided on the label and, unless all the necessary information can be included on the label, by PILs. Provision of good quality patient information is intended to supplement but not replace advice given to patients by health professionals. Every patient should receive a PIL with each medicine regardless of whether these are purchased OTC, supplied on prescription or administered by a health professional. The PIL must be non-promotional and consistent with the SPC.

Council Directive 92/27/EEC[38] concerning the labelling of medicinal products for human use and package leaflets came into force in March 1992. The Directive dealt first with the particulars required either on the outer packaging or, if none, on the immediate

---

BOX 12.1 The sequence of particulars on the summary of product characteristics (SPC)

1. NAME OF THE MEDICINAL PRODUCT
2. QUALITATIVE AND QUANTITATIVE COMPOSITION
3. PHARMACEUTICAL FORM
4. CLINICAL PARTICULARS
   4.1. Therapeutic indications
   4.2. Posology and method of administration
   4.3. Contraindications
   4.4. Special warnings and precautions for use
   4.5. Interaction with other medicinal products and other forms of interaction
   4.6. Pregnancy and lactation
   4.7. Effects on ability to drive and use machines
   4.8. Undesirable effects
   4.9. Overdose
5. PHARMACOLOGICAL PROPERTIES
   5.1. Pharmacodynamic properties
   5.2. Pharmacokinetic properties
   5.3. Preclinical safety data
6. PHARMACEUTICAL PARTICULARS
   6.1. List of excipients
   6.2. Incompatibilities
   6.3. Shelf life
   6.4. Special precautions for storage
   6.5. Nature and contents of container
   6.6. Special precautions for disposal
7. MARKETING AUTHORISATION HOLDER
8. MARKETING AUTHORISATION NUMBER(S)
9. DATE OF FIRST AUTHORISATION/RENEWAL OF THE AUTHORISATION
10. DATE OF REVISION OF THE TEXT
11. DOSIMETRY FOR RADIOPHARMACEUTICALS (if applicable)
12. INSTRUCTIONS FOR PREPARATION OF RADIOPHARMACEUTICALS (if applicable)

---

human use.[39] This conferred standards to the requirements of eligible, comprehensible and indelible information regarding content and format, and represents a determined effort to ensure that patients can understand the medical content of the information given.

The requirements for labelling and PILs are now are set out in Title V of Council Directive 2001/83/EC as amended by Council Directive 2004/27/EC.[11,12] Pharmaceutical companies are required to submit labels and PILs, along with mock-ups, for assessment and approval by the relevant competent authority when the marketing authorisation application is submitted. As for SPCs, changes to labels and PILs also require authority approval, although there are a few exemptions.[40] This Directive also specifies that 'The package leaflet shall reflect the results of consultations with target patient groups', often referred to as 'user testing'. Additionally, the European guideline concerned with excipients used in the medicinal product formulation should be consulted when preparing labels and leaflets.[41]

Further guidance on how to produce good quality information for provision with medicines to meet patients' needs has been produced by the MHRA.[42] The MHRA guidance and appendices are essential reading for those required to write PILs, who are generally members of the medical department. The guideline represents a determined effort to ensure that patients can understand the medical content of the information given. The sequence of particulars on the PIL is listed in Box 12.2.

In addition to providing good quality PILs, clear labelling is crucial for the safe use of all medicines. The primary purpose of labelling is for the clear and

packaging of the product and, secondly, with the contents of the package leaflet (PIL). Mock-ups of the packaging and the draft PIL had to be submitted by the pharmaceutical company for approval by the regulatory authority when the marketing authorisation application was submitted or, if the product was already authorised, when advised by the regulatory authority. Statutory Instrument 1994/3144[13] adopted the Council Directive 92/27/EEC[38] into UK legislation from January 1995, providing comprehensive regulations regarding medicines for human use.

From January 1999, labelling and package leaflet information was also assessed according to the European Commission guideline on the readability of the label and package leaflet of medicinal products for

---

BOX 12.2 The sequence of particulars on the patient information leaflet (PIL)

1. Identification of the medicinal product
2. Therapeutic indications
3. List of information that is necessary before taking the medicinal product
4. Necessary and usual instructions for proper use
5. Description of the adverse reactions
6. Reference to the expiry date indicated on the label, with storage conditions and further information on product composition, presentation, marketing authorisation holder, manufacturer
7. Where the medicinal product is authorised (if applicable)
8. Date of last revision of the PIL

---

unambiguous identification of the product and conditions for safe use. The MHRA has published guidance for those involved in the design and layout of labelling to help improve the way in which information is presented to health professionals and patients.[43] The guidance helps to ensure that the critical information necessary for the safe use of the medicine is legible, easily accessible and that users are assisted in assimilating the information so that confusion and error are minimised. Those involved in the design of labelling and packaging components should ensure adherence to the guidance before submission to the MHRA. The MHRA considers the guidance when assessing the labelling provided with mutual recognition and national licence applications; full justification for any deviation should be provided with the application. Once approved, amended components will be expected to be introduced ideally within 3 months but within 6 months at most. The guidance applies primarily to POMs but the principles also apply those available OTC.

The particulars listed in Box 12.3 should be on the outer packaging of medicinal products or, where there is no outer packaging, on the immediate packaging.

Homeopathic medicinal products are subject to the requirements of Council Directive 2001/83/EC as amended by 2004/27/EC.[11,12] Specific provisions for registration, authorisation and labelling are applicable to homeopathic medicinal products manufactured and placed on the market within the European Community. Specific guidance is given by the MHRA on labelling homeopathic medicines.[44] In particular, the clear mention of the words 'homeopathic medicinal product' is required, and both labelling and the PIL for the product are also required to state 'Homoeopathic medicinal product without approved therapeutic indications'. The supply of a PIL with a registered homeopathic product is optional although, if supplied, it must contain all of the specific particulars defined in the MHRA guidance and no other information.

While English is the only MHRA-approved language, other language versions may be used upon certification of identical content.

12.4.3 Medical information department

In general, the provision of product information is the responsibility of the medical information department in so far as the information sought and provided is non-promotional in nature. Companies vary in how this department is integrated within the medical division but the principles underlying the provision of the service are relatively consistent. The qualifications of those who provide medical product information are based on medicine, pharmacy, nursing, information science or a life science. The company physicians, pharmacists and information scientists are best placed to inform and discuss the company's medicinal products and will have the product development database readily available to them.

Information science is a specialist discipline. It arose with the increasing complexity of searching for specific information using specific command languages within rapidly expanding medical and scientific databases. Information scientists will either have a scientific qualification from a college or university and then learn information science as postgraduate training or, increasingly, will have taken a specific undergraduate course in information science at a recognised institution. With the advances in computers and reduced use of specific command languages, information searches have become easier for health professionals and the public to perform. However, the information scientist is still required to perform more specialised searches and, indeed, to interpret the findings. These professionals must receive training appropriate to their level of responsibilities. The Institute of Information Technology and PIPA

BOX 12.3 Particulars on the packaging

1. Name of the medicinal product[a,b]
2. Active substances
3. Pharmaceutical form and contents[b]
4. List of excipients known to have a recognized action or effect or all excipients (for injectable, topical or eye preparation)
5. Method and, if necessary, route of administration[b]
6. Special warning to store out of the reach and sight of children
7. Special warning (if applicable for the product)
8. Expiry date[a,b]
9. Storage precautions
10. Disposal precautions
11. Name and address of the holder of the authorisation[a]
12. Marketing authorization number
13. Manufacturer's batch number[a,b]
14. Instructions on product use (in the case of non-prescription products)

Particulars that should, at least, appear on: a, immediate packagings which take the form of blister packs and are placed in an outer packaging; b, small immediate packaging units on which other particulars cannot be displayed.

provide support to information scientists in the industry.

Medical information departments usually provide medical product information to external enquirers and scientific information within the company to those planning and designing clinical trials and developing product strategies and promotional material. The department must have a minimum set of up-to-date information resources to enable them to provide comprehensive information on all products for which they are responsible. Logically, the company library will be managed by the medical information department, as will the archives of published and unpublished reports relating to the company's medical products. However, with data and medical/scientific journals readily accessible through the internet as well as storage restrictions, increasingly, the trend is towards a 'virtual' library. The medical information department, in collaboration with a drug safety or pharmacovigilance department, may also manage spontaneous reports of adverse events or reactions associated with the use of the company's medicinal products.

Medical information together with 'medical affairs', usually two departments of the medical division, provide medical product information to those seeking information. All companies are familiar with day-to-day contact by telephone and letter directly from pharmacists and prescribing physicians, or through the company sales representatives. In the UK, the information department of a moderate-sized pharmaceutical company can expect to receive several thousand telephone calls per annum. Standard procedures should be in place for handling telephone calls, including speed of response, enquiry details and cover. Questions posed may relate to the chemistry or pharmaceutics of the product, or its use in conjunction with other medicines, in patients with severe organ dysfunction or in ways that are not covered by the SPC. A doctor or pharmacist using a medicine may want to know about the risk of side effects in particular circumstances. Conversely, upon encountering a particular side effect or adverse event, they may wish to know whether the event has been recorded previously. Product physicians, pharmacists and information scientists become adept at responding proficiently to such questions and acquire a substantial knowledge of their products as a result. As patients become increasingly aware and involved in their care, they may also contact companies and such enquiries from the public must be handled with care and judgement and according to the Code of Practice.

Finally, because some of the questions posed to medical information departments are of medicolegal importance (e.g. adverse event reporting and/or management and liability or high risk prescribing), information scientists will normally seek the support or advice of the company physician or pharmacist, or even the legal department, in providing a response. The company physician or pharmacist should be prepared to respond personally to the health professional who is making the enquiry, especially at the request of a non-medical colleague.

12.4.3.1 Information on the unlicensed use of medicines

Medicines licensed for one (or more) indication(s) are often used for indications for which they do not have a product licence. This may be either because data exist showing the medicine to be beneficial or because of ongoing clinical trials in new indications. The medicines legislation and the Code clearly state that no medicine may be promoted for an indication for which a product licence has not been obtained. However, the medicines legislation accepts that doctors may prescribe any agent that they believe may be of benefit to their patients while remaining professionally responsible.

The industry, while endeavouring to behave in an ethical fashion, has also made available unlicensed experimental drugs for patients whose condition is not responding to currently available medication. Experimental drugs may be supplied for compassionate use in, for example, cases of HIV or cancer, when a real need has been demonstrated. A product unlicensed in the UK but available in another country may be available through an international wholesaler, such as IDIS; this will then be available for 'named patients' and will involve import of the product under SI 2005/2789.[45]

Generally, doctors are not encouraged to prescribe medicines unlicensed in a particular indication. Management of prescribing has become more practical with the advent of evidence-based medicine and the concept of systematic review (e.g. the Cochrane Library). However, there is an obligation upon companies to provide published information regarding the investigation of their medicinal products in unlicensed or experimental indications and to be able to provide medical advice on how to use such agents and under what circumstances. Information pharmacists and product physicians can invariably provide such information as is at their disposal without being promotional.

12.4.3.2 Formulary packs and product monographs

Unfortunately, editors of peer-reviewed journals do not have the space to publish all pharmaceutical company data collected for obtaining product licences. Additionally, reviewers are becoming more stringent in their acceptance of manuscripts. Conversely, editors and others are demanding the publication of negative trials and refusing to publish trials unless they are managed independently of the sponsors by academic physicians and scientists. Equally, companies are criticised for subscribing to journal supplements or for paying to have clinical data reported in journals that operate for that purpose. Thus, when a new product is launched commercially much of the company's database is not published in medical journals that are read by the majority of prescribing physicians. However, the MHRA and the Committee on Safety of Medicines do review the entire company product database before reaching a decision as to whether a product should be licensed and made available for prescription.

Acknowledging problems of data publication, most companies are willing to make 'data on file' available to physicians or pharmacists on request, and may quote such data in their product information. Typically, medical staff write reviews, summaries and monographs about the company products. These documents form part of the impartial and unbiased database that companies are willing to make available on a non-promotional basis and are increasingly expected to provide.

However, the ultimate hurdle for pharmaceutical companies is not registration of a medicinal product but acceptance by formulary committees and inclusion in a hospital or general practice drug formulary. While not required for regulatory purposes, comparative efficacy and safety of medicines have become part of development programmes, and cost–benefit and cost-effectiveness data are increasingly expected and available. There is now need to provide clinical and cost-effectiveness data to NICE, SMC and AWMSG, which will then report independently. The views of such bodies are highly influential to the success of a product, particularly if it is one of a kind or expensive to prescribe. Indeed, it is prudent for companies to have a department of professional staff specifically trained in health economics and outcomes research. Company professional staff will write review articles that are factual but also aimed at persuading a formulary committee to agree to include that product or product range.

12.4.3.3 Meetings and conferences

Meetings and conferences at both national and international level perform a dual purpose, being both promotional in nature as well as permitting the interchange of unbiased scientific information. Such meetings would not occur if pharmaceutical companies did not provide substantial sponsorship, and learned societies cannot expect to have meetings funded without allowing companies to promote their products and provide non-promotional information. Additionally, it is recognised by the European Union Advertising Directives that without industry sponsorship of scientific meetings and attendance by doctors at such meetings, the medical community would be less well informed. The quality of data presented at such meetings is generally excellent as companies would not knowingly report poorly conducted studies so publicly at major international congresses.

Pharmaceutical physicians must be alert to the fact that information becomes promotional when published by virtue of industry sponsorship. Both written and verbal materials to be disseminated as information or 'a service to medicine' should therefore be reviewed and the relevant rules observed (see section 12.5). Companies have been found in breach of the Code of Practice when so-called 'independent' speakers of known opinion have been used too frequently in support of a product.

12.4.4 Promotional information

The term 'promotion' means any activity undertaken by a pharmaceutical company (or with its authority) that promotes the prescription, supply, sale or administration of its medicines. According to the ABPI Code of Practice, promotional information includes journal and direct mail advertising; detail aids and other printed materials used by representatives, participation at exhibitions, audio-visual media and data systems. Naturally, all information supplied through a pharmaceutical company's marketing department will be regarded as promotional in nature, even if not in a promotional format. Reasonably, the information would not be disseminated unless it was designed to increase use of the medicinal products. Depending on its nature and purpose, information supplied through the medical department is more likely to be accepted as unbiased by prescribers. It is therefore prudent to make known that all information is produced and used with the support of the medical department.

To clarify, information is regarded as non-promotional if it forms a reply made in response to individual unsolicited enquiries or communications from health professionals, including letters published in professional journals, but only if they relate solely to the subject matter. It also includes informative announcements and reference material concerning licensed medicines (e.g. pack changes, adverse event warnings and price changes). Information supplied to national public organisations (e.g. NICE, AWMSG and SMC, the SPC), public assessment reports, labelling on medicines and associated package inserts, and information relating to human health or diseases without reference to specific medicines are also considered non-promotional. Clearly, such information must be scientific, accurate and factual, and neither misleading nor promotional in nature.

12.5 Procedural aspects relating to information and promotion

To ensure conformity to the regulations relating to information and promotion, pharmaceutical companies act by SOPs for the preparation and approval of ethical promotional material. These written procedures cover the multiple steps in the preparation and approval of promotional copy and in so doing minimise the risk of mistakes and subsequent complaints.

There are two stages inherent in developing promotional material: generation and approval. Typically, the company brand team give a detailed brief to a specialist medical communications agency. The materials generated are then circulated as 'hard' copy or electronically, together with the references used to substantiate the data and claims. It is prudent to insist that evidence in the references is highlighted, as this saves the reviewers' time in finding the relevant text. Materials are first circulated to the product manager, product physician, scientific adviser and regulatory affairs professional, who collate their comments and request the agency to action any necessary changes. These individuals have key roles in material development: the product manager coordinates the exercise; the product physician reviews the relevant clinical data and ensures conformity with the ABPI Code of Practice; the scientific adviser focuses on the scientific content; and the regulatory affairs professional ensures the material conforms to the product licence.

All necessary prior discussion between product managers and their medical and scientific counterparts as to what the marketing department wishes to say is valuable in avoiding mistakes. A balance is usually found between that expected and that acceptable – the marketing department expects the medical department to interpret the data to permit the maximum exploitation permissible, while the medical department opposes claims or statements that the data do not support. It is essential that these individuals consider the material carefully, agree the contents and are in accord that it can be recommended to the official signatories for certification.

The product physician, medical adviser, scientific adviser and the regulatory affairs professional should treat the reading of promotional material and its references a priority. They should not be pressured into agreeing with material without due time for consideration. Up to 48 h each would seem a minimum to read and consider the promotional material and the accompanying reference documents. When the regulator is involved, the PMCPA allows 5 working days for comment. All of those involved in the creation of promotional material must be alert to possible misinterpretations or over-interpretations of claims and statements by the company, and that the material must not mislead. Protection is conferred by having several persons review and comment on what is being written, and this can be documented if the process of creating material follows a routine procedure.

Promotional material must not be issued unless the final form has been certified by two persons, one of whom must be a registered medical practitioner or, if the product or indications have been on the UK market for more than 1 year and are not part of a new promotional campaign, a registered pharmacist. The second person certifying on behalf of the company must be an appropriately qualified person (either of the company or whose services are retained for that purpose) or senior official of the company, such as the marketing director. These signatories examine the materials for accordance with the Code of Practice and relevant advertising regulations, for consistency with the marketing authorisation and SPC, and for fair presentation of the facts about the medicine.

An SOP or set of guidelines regarding the dissemination of promotional and non-promotional information is also likely to exist within companies. All information sent out by the company may be subject to the Code of Practice. Additionally, all information received from a pharmaceutical company may be considered to be promotional. Thus, if companies wish to have a trustworthy reputation they should ensure that any non-promotional information is truly non-promotional and factual. Promotional material should only be sent to people who are likely to have a need or interest in such information. Mailing lists must be current and exclude any persons who have requested not to receive such literature.

It is up to individual companies via their managing, marketing and medical directors, as to how formally they wish to proceed with respect to promotional material and the dissemination of information. The remit of all medical directors includes avoidance of complaints regarding the promotion of medicinal products. SOPs and appropriate guidelines in the management of promotion and information are not only very helpful to medical and marketing, but may be key elements in the successful sales of medicinal products.

References

1 House of Commons Health Committee. *The Influence of the Pharmaceutical Industry*. Fourth Report of Session 2004–5 H C 42–I (Incorporating HC 1030 i–iii). London: The Stationary Office, 2005.

2 Kesselheim AJ, Avorn J. Pharmaceutical promotion to physicians and first amendment rights. *N Engl J Med* 2008;**358**:1727–32.

3 *The Medicines Act*. London: HMSO, 1968.

4 Medicines (Advertising) Regulations 1994 (SI 1994 No. 1932). London: HMSO, 1994.

5 Medicines (Monitoring of Advertising) Regulations 1994 (SI 1994 No. 1933). London: HMSO, 1994.

6 Committee of Advertising Practice. *The British Code of Advertising, Sales Promotions and Direct Marketing*. London: Committee of Advertising Practice, 2003.

7 Proprietary Association of Great Britain (PAGB). *Code of Practice for Advertising Over-the-Counter Medicines, incorporating the PAGB Consumer Code and the PAGB Professional Code*. London: PAGB, 2004.

8 Independent Television Commission (ICT). *Code of Advertising Standards and Practice*. London: ICT, 1998.

9 Radio Authority. *Code of Advertising Standards and Practice and Programme Sponsorship*. London: Radio Advertising Clearance Centre and Commercial Radio Companies Association, 1991.

10 Association of the British Pharmaceutical Industry (ABPI). *Code of Practice for the Pharmaceutical Industry; together with the Prescriptions Medicines Code of Practice Authority Constitution and Procedure*. London: ABPI, 2008.

11 Council Directive 2001/83/EC of the European Parliament and of the Council of 6 November 2001. The Community Code relating to medicinal products for human use. *Official Journal* L 311, 28/11/2001 P.0067–0128.

12 Council Directive 2004/27/EC of the European Parliament and of the Council of 31 March 2004 amending Directive 2001/83/EC on the Community Code relating to medicinal products for human use. *Official Journal* L 136, 30/04/2004 P.0034–0057.

13 Medicines for Human Use (Marketing Authorisations) Regulations 1994 (SI 1994 No. 3144). London: HMSO, 1994.

14 Council Directive 2004/24/EC of the European Parliament and of the Council of 31 March 2004, amending as regards traditional herbal medicinal products for human use. *Official Journal* L 136, 30/04/2004 P.0085–0090.

15 Medicines (Advertising and Monitoring of Advertising) Amendment Regulations 2005 (SI No. 2787). London: HMSO, 2005.

16 *Trade Descriptions Act*. London: HMSO, 1968.

17 Control of Misleading Advertisements Regulations (SI No. 915). London: HMSO, 1988.

18 *The Broadcasting Acts*. London: HMSO, 1990, 1996.

19 *The Communications Act*. London: The Stationery Office, 2003.

20 Medicines Control Agency. *Advertising and Promotion of Medicines in the UK* (MHRA Guidance Note No. 23). London: The Stationery Office, 2005.

21 Association of the British Pharmaceutical Industry. *Code of Practice for the Pharmaceutical Industry*. London: ABPI, 2006.

22 European Federation of Pharmaceutical Industries' Associations. *European Code of Practice for the Promotion of Medicines*. Brussels: EFPIA, 2004.

23 European Federation of Pharmaceutical Industries' Associations. *European Code of Practice on Relationships between the Pharmaceutical Industry and Patient Organisations*. Brussels: EFPIA, 2008.

24 Health Food Manufacturers' Association (HFMA). *Guidelines for Good Manufacturing Practice*. Surrey, UK: HFMA, 1997.

25 British Dental Trade Association (BDTA). *Code of Practice*. 1998. Available at www.bdta.org.uk [Accessed 22 September 2008.]

26 National Office of Animal Health. *Code of Practice for the Promotion of Animal Medicines*. Enfield: NOAH, 1987.

27 International Federation of Pharmaceutical Manufacturers' Associations (IFPMA). *Code of Pharmaceutical Marketing Practice*. Geneva: IFPMA, 2007.

28 *World Health Organization Ethical Criteria for Medicinal Drug Promotion*. Geneva: World Health Organization, 1988.

29 *International Pharmaceutical Congress Advisory Association Code of Conduct*. Basel, Switzerland: International Pharmaceutical Congress Advisory Association, 2003.

30 Herxheimer A, Collier J. Promotion by the British Pharmaceutical Industry, 1983–8; a critical analysis of self regulation. *BMJ* 1990;**300**:307–11.

31 Guidelines for Company-Sponsored Safety Assessment of Marketed Medicines. Medicines and Healthcare products Regulatory Agency, Committee on Safety of Medicines, Royal College of General Practitioners, British Medical Association, and Association of British Pharmaceutical Industry (November 1993). *Br J Pharmacol* 1994;**2**:95–7, 22.

32 General Medical Council. *Good Medical Practice*. Available at: www.gmc-uk.org/guidance/good_medical_practice/index.asp [Accessed: 6 September 2008].

33 British Healthcare Business Intelligence Association and Association of British Pharmaceutical Industry. *The Legal and Ethical Framework for Healthcare Market Research*. 2008. Available at: www.bhbia.org.uk/library/EthicalandLegalFrameworkBHBIAGuidelines/tabid/143/Default.aspx [Accessed: 6 September 2008.]

34 Pharmaceutical Information and Pharmacovigilance Association (PIPA). *UK Guidelines on Standards for Medical Information Departments*. (Revised 2006). Available at: www.aiopi.org.uk/downloads/guidelines_revision2006.pdf [Accessed: 6 September 2008.]

35 Medicines and Healthcare products Regulatory Agency. *Review of EU medicines legislation ('2001 Review')*. Available at: http://www.mhra.gov.uk/Howweregulate/Medicines/ReviewofEUmedicineslegislation(2001Review)/index.htm [Accessed: 6 September 2008].

36 European Commission. *Notice to Applicants – A guideline on Summary of Product Characteristics*. October 2005. Brussels: European Commission. Available at: http://ec.europa.eu/enterprise/pharmaceuticals/eudralex/vol-2/c/spcguidrev1-oct2005.pdf [Accessed: 6 September 2008].

37 European Commission. *The rules governing medicinal products in the European Union*. Volume 3. Available at: http://ec.europa.eu/enterprise/pharmaceuticals/eudralex/vol3_en.htm [Accessed 22 September 2008.]

38 Council Directive 92/27/EEC of 31 March 1992. *Official Journal of the European Communities*. L1113/912.

39 European Commission. *A guideline on the readability of the label and package leaflet of medicinal products for human use*. Brussels European Commission 1999.

40 Medicines and Healthcare products Regulatory Agency. *Guidance on changes to labelling and patient information leaflets for self certification*. MHRA/selfcertification guidance/labelling/0108. MHRA, 2008.

41 European Commission. *Guidelines. Excipients in the label and package leaflet of medicinal products for human use*. Revision 1. Volume 3B. Brussels: European Commission, 2003.

42 Medicines and Healthcare products Regulatory Agency. Committee of Safety of Medicines. *Always read the leaflet – getting the best information with every medicine*. London: The Stationery Office, 2005.

43 Medicines and Healthcare products Regulatory Agency. *Best practice on labelling and packaging of medicines* (MHRA Guidance Note No. 25). London: The Stationery Office, 2003.

44 Medicines and Healthcare products Regulatory Agency. UK Homeopathic Registration Scheme Guidance Notes. *Note on labelling requirements for homeopathic products*. London: MHRA, 2004.

45 Medicines for Human Use (Manufacturing, Wholesale Dealing and Miscellaneous Amendments) Regulations 2005 (SI 2005 No. 2789). London: HMSO, 2005.

13 The supply of unlicensed medicines for individual patient use

Ian Dodds-Smith and Silvia Valverde

Arnold & Porter (UK) LLP, London, UK

13.1 Introduction

The general principle underlying the regulatory regime in the EU is that a product can only be placed on the market if its quality, safety and efficacy for its recommended use(s) have been subject to independent scrutiny. Such scrutiny will lead to national marketing authorisation being issued by the competent authorities [in the UK, by the Licensing Authority operating through the Medicines and Healthcare products Regulatory Agency (MHRA)] or by a centralised authorisation being issued by the European Commission (EC) on the advice of the European Medicines Agency (EMEA).

Nevertheless, the procurement by or supply to the medical profession of medicines with no current marketing authorisation is not forbidden in the UK, but it raises various regulatory and liability issues. Setting aside use in a clinical trial, such unlicensed products are frequently used to treat the particular clinical needs of individual patients. This is known variously as 'named patient', 'particular patient', 'individual patient' or 'compassionate use' supply. The first of these terms is misleading, because there has never been any requirement to identify a particular patient and for the purposes of this chapter the term 'individual patient' supply is used instead. Coordinated programmes for supply of unlicensed medicines to individual patients are sometimes called compassionate use programmes. In the UK these do not raise special considerations, except to the extent that they are affected by new EU rules now contained in Regulation 726/2004.

Supply on an individual patient basis encompasses various categories of use of medicinal products. A product may be unauthorised because it has been specially formulated for use; or it may be in the clinical trial stage of its development but is requested by doctors for use outside a trial; it may have been authorised previously and then withdrawn from the market for commercial reasons, or because of safety, efficacy or quality concerns. In addition, it may be authorised in no country or only authorised in a different country.

The British Pharmacopoeia (BP) has, in the past, been focused upon standards for authorised medicinal products. However, in 2007, for the first time and because of the significant usage of unlicensed medicines in the UK, the BP was asked to include a section on unlicensed medicines. It provides guidance to manufacturers and suppliers on the legal requirements for unlicensed medicines including the necessary standards for manufacture of unlicensed medicines. In addition, it provides some guidance to prescribers on ethical, as well as legal, considerations. The BP of 2008[1] explains that the use of unlicensed medicines is widespread in the UK, mainly in the hospital sector. It is said that the reasons for this include the requirements for liquid formulation for paediatric and geriatric populations, discontinued supply of licensed medicines, the need for specialist and novel products for use in hospital and the lack of authorised critical care products because of low demand.

Against that background, this chapter describes the regulatory framework in the UK covering the supply of medicinal products to meet the special needs of individual patients. In summary, there are provisions allowing manufacture in the UK of 'specials' to treat special clinical needs and a related import notification scheme where a finished, but unauthorised, product is available outside the UK and the product is imported to the order of a health professional. This framework is the outcome of the balancing by regulators of two

The Textbook of Pharmaceutical Medicine. Edited by John P. Griffin. © 2009, ISBN: 978-1-4051-8035-1.

important, but conflicting, principles. On the one hand, there is the need to ensure that patients are not exposed to any unnecessary risks, hence the extensive legal framework regulating the placing on the market of medicinal products. On the other hand, there is the desire to respect the clinical freedom of medical practitioners to determine the most appropriate treatment for their patients.

The regulatory framework in the UK does not control the use by doctors of authorised products for uses or in doses or patient populations that are not approved. Such 'off-label' prescribing is a matter purely for the doctor's clinical judgement. This issue is therefore not discussed in detail, although liability issues relating to use of unlicensed products or use of licensed products 'off label' are similar.

13.2 EC law

13.2.1 Directive 2001/83/EC – supply of unlicensed products to meet special needs
There is only limited EC legislation dealing with the supply of medicinal products for individual patient use and there were no relevant provisions prior to 1989. Article 6.1 of Directive 2001/83/EC (previously Article 3 of Directive 65/65/EEC) sets out the general rule that a medicinal product must have a marketing authorisation before being placed on the market. However, Article 5.1, which repeats wording introduced by Directive 89/341/EEC, provides an exception from this general rule:

A Member State may, in accordance with legislation in force and to fulfil special needs, exclude from the provisions of this Directive medicinal products supplied in response to a bona fide unsolicited order, formulated in accordance with the specifications of an authorised health-care professional and for use by an individual patient under his direct personal responsibility.

This provision allows Member States, if they wish (there is no obligation to do so), to make national arrangements for the supply of unlicensed medicines for individual use, but only in the narrow circumstances specified by the Directive. This provision is without prejudice to the right of Member States to authorise temporarily the distribution of unlicensed medicines to meet specific threats to public health e.g. the spread of pathogenic agents (Article 5.2) or the authorisation by a Member State on public health grounds of a product approved in another Member State but not in the UK (Article 126a).

13.2.2 Volume 9A of Notice to Applicants
The only other reference to such use at a European level appears in Volume 9A (March 2007) (Pharmacovigilance) of the Notice to Applicants issued by the European Commission. The Notice to Applicants does not have the force of law, but represents best practice and is frequently referenced by the European Court of Justice as a persuasive document when interpreting the scope of the EU regulatory framework. Section 5.7 states:

Compassionate or named-patient use of a medicine should be strictly controlled by the company responsible for providing the medicine and should ideally be the subject of a protocol.

Such a protocol should ensure that the Patient is registered and adequately informed about the nature of the medicine and that both the prescriber and the Patient are provided with the available information on the properties of the medicine with the aim of maximising the likelihood of safe use. The protocol should encourage the prescriber to report any adverse reactions to the company, and to the Competent Authority, where required nationally.

Companies should continuously monitor the risk–benefit balance of medicines used on compassionate or named-patient basis (subject to protocol or not) and follow the requirements for reporting to the appropriate Competent Authorities. As a minimum, the requirements laid down in Chapter I.4, Section 1 apply.

13.2.3 Directive 2001/83/EC – supply of products specially prepared by pharmacists
In contrast to the right of Member States to exclude from the provisions of the Directive products supplied at the request of a doctor to meet a special patient need, Article 3.1 of the Directive excludes *ab initio* from its requirements any medicinal product prepared in a pharmacy in accordance with a medical prescription for an individual patient. This is sometimes known as the magistral formula exception. Similarly, under Article 3.2, any medicinal product that is prepared in a pharmacy in accordance with the prescriptions of a pharmacopoeia and is intended to be supplied direct to the patients served by the pharmacy (commonly known as the officinal formula dispensing) is excluded from controls of the Directive. Member States control such supplies in different ways through a mixture of national law and professional guidelines and standards.

13.2.4 Regulation (EC) No 726/2004 – compassionate use schemes

In 2004, changes were made to the rules governing the centralised authorisation procedure. For the first time, specific provisions dealing with what the legislation calls 'compassionate use' were introduced. These are set out in Article 83 of Regulation (EC) No 726/2004 (these came into force on 20 November 2005). Article 83.9 states that the operation of this Article is without prejudice to the operation of the Clinical Trials Directive 2001/20/EC and the national provisions for individual patient supply/compassionate use in Article 5.1 of Directive 2001/83/EC.

Recital 33 of the Regulation states that a common approach should be followed, whenever possible, regarding the criteria and conditions for the compassionate use of new medicinal products under Member States' legislation.'

Article 83.1 confirms that Member States may make a medicinal product falling within the scope of the requirements for centralised assessment by the EMEA and grant of marketing authorisation by the Commission available for compassionate use.

Article 83.2 defines 'compassionate use' as meaning:

Making a medicinal product [falling within the scope of the Regulation] available for compassionate reasons to a group of patients with a chronically or seriously debilitating disease or whose disease is considered to be life-threatening, and who can not be treated satisfactorily by an authorised medicinal product. The medicinal product concerned must either be the subject of an application for a [centralised] marketing authorisation or must be undergoing clinical trials.

If a Member State 'makes use of the possibility provided for in paragraph 1', it is obliged to notify the EMEA under Article 83.3. Article 83.4 states that the Committee for Medicinal Products for Human Use (CHMP), acting on behalf of the EMEA, may, after consulting the manufacturer or the applicant, adopt opinions on various matters such as the conditions for use, the conditions for distribution and the patients targeted. The opinions must be updated on a regular basis. Under Article 83.6, the EMEA is required to keep an updated list of such opinions and publish that list on its website. Article 83.6 also states that Articles 24(1) and 25 (which set out adverse reaction reporting requirements for centrally authorised products) will apply to products supplied for compassionate use.

While it is mandatory for the competent national authorities to notify the EMEA of proposed supply,

the opinions of the CHMP are advisory only; Article 83.5 merely requires Member States to 'take account' of any available opinions. Article 83.7 makes it clear that the fact that an opinion has been obtained from the Committee will not affect the civil or criminal liability of a manufacturer or an applicant.

The legislation includes specific provisions concerning supply of unlicensed medicines for the period between authorisation and launch onto the market. In some Member States, where it is necessary to obtain approval for price or reimbursement arrangements, this may entail a delay of some months. During this time, where a compassionate use programme has previously been set up, Article 83.8 states that 'the applicant shall ensure that patients taking part also have access to the new medicinal product'. There is nothing in the final version of this article relating to costs. Early drafts of this article had proposed that supply should be free of charge, but this was removed and the position is therefore that companies may charge for such supplies.

Several points are worth noting. First, the Article seems to be broader in scope than Article 5.1 of Directive 2001/83/EC, because what is envisaged is a properly coordinated, pro-active approach to use the product (rather than a passive system relying on requests from individual doctors). Secondly, the provision only applies to a small category of products. For products not falling within the scope of the centralised procedure, the national rules will remain and there will be no harmonisation of the conditions of supply in individual Member States. Thirdly, the wording of Article 83 leaves open a number of questions on how Member States will operate this provision.

On 19 July 2007 the EMEA issued a guideline on such compassionate use and a questions and answers document clarifying the EMEA's role in relation to compassionate use. The guideline states that the objective of Article 83 is threefold:

1. Facilitating and improving the access of patients in the European Union to compassionate use programmes;
2. Favouring a common approach regarding the conditions of use, the conditions for distribution and the patients targeted for the compassionate use of unauthorised new medicinal products; and
3. Increasing transparency between Member States in terms of treatment availability.

The guideline also provides recommendations for use of a medicinal product in the period between adoption of a CHMP opinion relating to compassionate use and a CHMP opinion relating to grant of a marketing authorisation and in respect of the period between the latter and the Commission Decision granting an authorisation to the product and its subsequent placing on the market. The guideline also clarifies the meaning of the key terms used such as 'group of patients', 'chronically or seriously debilitating disease or whose disease is considered to be life-threatening', 'patients who cannot be treated satisfactorily', 'patients targeted' and 'conditions for use'.

The guideline also makes it clear that Article 83 is not applicable (even for medicinal products eligible for the centralised procedure) if: (a) the compassionate use envisaged is on an individual patient supply basis (as described in Article 5 of Directive 2001/83/EC) or; (b) if the compassionate used relates to a medicinal product which has already been authorised via the centralised procedure, even if the proposed conditions of use and target population are different from those approved in the marketing authorisation.

13.3 UK law

13.3.1 UK law prior to 1 January 1995

UK legislation has for many years permitted individual patient supply in specified circumstances. The original provisions date back to the early 1970s. Under section 7(2) of the Medicines Act 1968, it was necessary to hold a product licence in order to sell, supply, export or import a medicinal product, or to procure those activities, or the manufacture or assembly of the product. However, various exemptions from the licensing requirements, including those relating to individual patient supply, were provided for in the Act and in related statutory instruments. The most important exemptions were contained in sections 9 and 13 of the Act, the Medicines (Exemption from Licences) (Special and Transitional Cases) Order 1971,[2] the Medicines (Exemption from Licences) (Special Cases and Miscellaneous Provisions) Order 1972[3] and the Medicines (Exemptions from Licences) (Importation) Order 1984.[4]

The exemptions from the Directive's provisions concerning preparation of medicines by pharmacists, contained in Article 3, are reflected in the Medicines Act. In the UK, the preparation by pharmacists of unlicensed medicines in accordance with the prescription of an authorised health care professional, where there is no licensed product available or where the specific formulation of the authorised products is

not appropriate for the patient, it is usually referred to as 'extemporaneous preparation'. An exemption for such activities is contained in section 10 of the Medicines Act. The BP of 2008 suggests that batch manufacture should be undertaken only in licensed units holding a 'specials licence' and that manufacture under the section 10 exemption should only apply to the preparation of products for individual patients to fulfil specific prescriptions. However, it is recognised that batch preparation is technically possible under the section 10 exemption. The advice that batch manufacture should take place only in licensed units reflects the fact that these units are inspected by the MHRA for compliance with Good Manufacturing Practice (GMP). In contrast, the preparation activities of individual pharmacists are not inspected.

13.3.2 UK law from 1995 onwards

Significant changes to the legal basis for the exemptions, rather than to their scope, were introduced by the Medicines for Human Use (Marketing Authorisations Etc.) Regulations 1994,[5] which came into force on 1 January 1995. These Regulations sought to create a single instrument under which EU regulatory requirements could be implemented and updated. Prior to that time, rules derived from EU Directives were laboriously implemented through changes to the Medicines Act and statutory instruments made under it. The 1994 Regulations disapply much of the Medicines Act for 'relevant medicinal products', including the licensing provisions contained in section 7 (and consequently all exemptions relating to section 7).

Relevant medicinal products are defined in the 1994 Regulations as those medicinal products for human use to which the provisions of Directive 2001/83/EC apply. This broad definition includes most medicinal products, but excludes products prepared in a pharmacy for dispensing to an individual patient. Therefore, the pharmacy preparation exemption contained in section 10 of the Act remains in force. The other exceptions are medicinal products for clinical trial use, intermediate products, registered homeopathic products, non-industrially produced herbal remedies and some products that are not medicinal products within the meaning of the Directive, but which by Order have been made subject to control under the Medicines Act 1968. For products designated under such an Order, the old provisions on individual patient supply are still applicable. In practice, there are very few such products.

Regulation 3(1) of the 1994 Regulations states that no medicinal product may be placed on the market or distributed by way of wholesale dealing unless it has a marketing authorisation. This replaces the product licence requirement in section 7 of the Act. The exemptions to this requirement, and therefore the provisions relating to individual patient supply, are contained in Regulation 3(2) and Schedule 1 to the Regulations. They permit supply for individual patients and also enable practitioners to hold limited supplies of stocks of unauthorised medicines. The provisions apply equally to doctors, dentists and supplementary prescribers. The MHRA has issued a Guidance Note 14 that provides guidance on the scope and application of these rules.[6]

13.3.3 Scope of exemptions

The supply of unlicensed medicinal products for individual patients is governed by paragraph 1 of Schedule 1 to the Regulations. The text follows the wording of the Directive quite closely, although curiously it omitted any reference to the requirement 'to fulfil special needs' until 2005, when it was inserted by SI 2005/2759, Regulation 2(1), (13)(a). The current wording of this provision reads as follows:

Regulations 3(1) shall not apply to a relevant medicinal product supplied in response to a bona fide unsolicited order, formulated in accordance with the specification of a doctor, dentist or supplementary prescriber and for use by his individual patients on his direct personal responsibility, in order to fulfil the special needs of those patients, but such supply shall be subject to the conditions specified in paragraph 2.

The conditions specified in paragraph 2 are:
(a) The relevant medicinal product is supplied to a doctor, dentist or supplementary prescriber or for use in a registered pharmacy, a hospital or a health centre under the supervision of a pharmacist, in accordance with paragraph 1;
(b) No advertisement or representation relating to the relevant medicinal product is issued with a view to it being seen generally by the public in the UK, and that no advertisement relating to that product, by means of any catalogue, price list or circular letter, is issued by, at the request or with the consent of, the person selling that product by retail or by way of wholesale dealing or supplying it in circumstances corresponding to retail sale, or the person who manufactures it and that the sale or supply is in response to a bona fide unsolicited order;
(c) Manufacture or assembly of the relevant medicinal product is carried out under conditions which ensure that the product is of the character required by,

and meets the specifications of, the doctor, dentist or supplementary prescriber who requires it;
(d) Written records of manufacture and assembly are made, maintained and kept available for inspection by the licensing and enforcement authorities;
(e) The product is manufactured, assembled, or imported into the EU by the holder of the authorisation referred to in Article 40 of Directive 2001/83/EC (for products manufactured or assembled in the EU, a manufacturer's authorisation (often called a 'specials' licence in the UK); for products imported in finished form into the EU, a wholesale dealer's (importation) licence);
(f) The product is distributed by way of wholesale dealing by the holder of a wholesale dealer's licence.

Paragraph 3 extends the exemption to the supply of product for limited stocks, subject to a number of conditions:
1(a). The medicinal product is specially prepared by a doctor or dentist, or to his or her order, for administration to one or more patients. Where that doctor/dentist is a member of a practice group working together to provide general medical or dental services, the proposed recipients can be the patients of any other doctor or dentist in that group; or
(b) The manufacture/assembly of such stocks is procured by a registered pharmacy, a hospital or health centre, where this is done by or under the supervision of a pharmacist;
2. The product is manufactured and assembled by the holder of the appropriate licence (see above);
3. Only limited stocks of such products are held: no more than 5 L of fluid and 2.5 kg of solid of all such products per doctor or dentist.

Paragraph 4 sets out an exemption in certain circumstances for medicinal products not requiring a prescription for sale or supply, which are prepared by or under the supervision of a pharmacist and are sold or supplied to a person exclusively for use by him or her in the course of business for the purpose of administration to one or more persons. Paragraph 5 contains an exemption for radiopharmaceuticals prepared from an authorised kit, generator or precursor in respect of which there is a marketing authorisation in force, subject to certain conditions.[7] New Paragraph 5A covers by this exemption medicinal products authorised in accordance with Article 126a of the 2001 Directive (i.e. authorisations to place on the market for 'justified public health reasons').

Paragraph 6 requires any person selling or supplying a relevant medicinal product to maintain, for a period of at least 5 years, records showing:

(a) The source from which that person obtained the product;

(b) The person to whom, and the date on which, the sale or supply was made;

(c) The quantity of each sale or supply;

(d) The batch number of the product sold or supplied; and

(e) Details of any suspected adverse reaction to the product sold or supplied of which he or she is aware. However, this does not require a supplier to search the literature for reports concerning the substance.

Paragraph 7 requires that person to notify the licensing authority of any such suspected serious adverse reaction and to make available for inspection, at all reasonable times, the records required to be kept under the previous paragraph.

13.3.4 Products manufactured outside the UK

The Medicines (Exemption from Licences) (Importation) Order 1984 originally set out additional conditions to be complied with in the case of unauthorised medicinal products imported for individual patient supply, but that Order was disapplied by the 1994 Regulations. There were no provisions in the 1994 Regulations to parallel the 1984 Order and consequently the controls on imported unlicensed products were reduced to the level of those on products manufactured in the UK.

This was clearly the result of legislative oversight and additional controls were reinstated in February 1999 by the Medicines (Standard Provisions for Licences and Certificates) Amendment Regulations 1999.[8] These Regulations introduced a number of amendments to Schedule 3 (standard provisions for wholesale dealer's licences) of the Medicines (Standard Provisions for Licences and Certificates) Regulations 1971,[9] They were replaced, with respect to relevant medicinal products, by the Medicines for Human Use (Manufacturing, Wholesale Dealing and Miscellaneous Amendments) Regulations 2005.[10]

The 2005 Regulations reproduce the relevant wording from the Directive (including the reference to 'special needs'). Supply of an 'exempt imported product' falling within the scope of this wording is only permitted provided certain conditions are complied with:

(a) At least 28 days prior to each importation, the licence holder must give written notice to the licensing authority, together with certain specified details relating to the product, the quantity to be imported and the manufacturer/assembler/supplier;

(b) If, within 28 days of acknowledgement of receipt of the notice by the licensing authority, it notifies the licence holder that the product should not be imported, the licence holder must comply with this notification; if, within this period, he or she has received notification that the product may be imported, he or she may proceed with the importation;

(c) In addition to the usual record keeping requirements for wholesale dealers, the authorisation holder must keep records of the batch number of the product and of any adverse reaction of which he or she becomes aware;

(d) The licence holder may import on each occasion no more than is sufficient for 25 single administrations or for 25 courses of treatment not exceeding 3 months; he or she must not import more than the quantity referred to in the notice. However, there is no rule against multiple sequential notifications;

(e) The licence holder must inform the licensing authority forthwith of any matter coming to his or her attention which might reasonably cause the authority to believe that the product can no longer be regarded as safe for administration to humans or as of satisfactory quality for such administration; the licence holder must cease importation or supply if he or she receives a written notice from the licensing authority requiring cessation;

(f) The licence holder must not issue any advertisement, catalogue, price list or circular, or make any representations, relating to the exempt imported product.

It follows that the 'import scheme' involves greater regulatory oversight of proposed supply (including a right to refuse consent to import on grounds of safety) than is the case with unlicensed products manufactured in the UK. It is difficult to see the public health justification for this, particularly as the imported product may have a marketing authorisation in the source country (often the USA) and, therefore, may have undergone a rigorous regulatory review of a type entirely lacking in respect of 'specials' manufactured in the UK. Specification could be taken to ban sale of a product manufactured in the UK under Section 62 of the Medicines Act 1968; but that is a blunt instrument rarely used.

13.4 Particular issues relating to supply of unlicensed medicines

13.4.1 Advertising

Paragraph 2(b) of the Schedule to the 1994 Regulations makes it clear that no advertisement or representation may be issued to encourage the sale or supply of medicinal products for individual patient use. Sale or supply must be in response to a bona fide unsolicited order from the doctor. While the paragraph prohibits issuing catalogues, price lists and circulars referring to relevant medicinal products, it does not prohibit the advertising of a specials manufacturing facility, or a business of importing or wholesaling unlicensed medicines, provided no specific products are mentioned. A manufacturer may also respond to an enquiry as to whether or not a particular product could be supplied. The MHRA guidance note on the supply of unlicensed relevant medicinal products for individual patients, of January 2008, adds internet notices to the list of items that would be considered as advertisement.

This raises the question of whether the rules prevent the supplier giving the doctor, at the time of supply, purely factual, technical information on the use of that product. Because the rationale for individual patient supply is that the doctor has requested the product of his or her own accord and is acting on his or her direct personal responsibility, it would seem reasonable to assume that he or she is familiar with its use and should not need any further information. On the other hand, particularly where there are known to be significant risks associated with the use of the product, it may be prudent to issue safety information to minimise the product liability exposure of the supplier. As noted above, the provision of such information is also recommended by the European Commission in Volume 9A of its Notice to Applicants. It seems unlikely that the MHRA would consider this to be advertising, although no formal guidance has been issued on this point. If a company does decide to provide such information, it must ensure that the wording cannot be said to be an invitation to the doctor to order further supplies of the product, because that would arguably amount to illegal promotion through soliciting subsequent orders.

In addition to the specific prohibitions set out in the Regulations, companies must have in mind the more general provisions against the advertising of unauthorised medicinal products. It is a criminal offence under Regulation 3(1) of the Medicines (Advertising) Regulations 1994[11] to issue an advertisement for a relevant medicinal product in respect of which there is no marketing authorisation in force and, under Regulation 3A, to issue an advertisement which does not comply with the particulars listed in the summary of product characteristics. These Regulations implement Directive 92/28/EEC on the advertising of medicinal products for human use (now Title VIII of Directive 2001/83/EC). Corresponding restrictions

upon the use of promotional materials also appear in the Code of Practice of the Association of the British Pharmaceutical Industry.

The MHRA has, since December 2003, published on its website the results of its scrutiny of questionable advertising. It would appear that, up to September 2008, 11 cases (out of 224) concerned unlicensed medicines. The cases included website or journal advertising to the public of unlicensed medicines by pharmacies and others to the public such as for single component measles, mumps and rubella vaccine (see MHRA report of 3 September 2008). The reports also refer to companies trading in unlicensed medicines pro-actively notifying health professionals of the availability of particular unlicensed products (see MHRA reports of 3 September 2008). Usually, the MHRA warn the person concerned as to their obligations and require an immediate end to the promotion in question. Prosecution is possible, but rare. Where unlicensed medicines are promoted in meetings of health professionals, the MHRA is likely to require the issue of a corrective statement to all attendees and may require pre-vetting of all future communications concerning the product in question (see, for instance, MHRA report of 21 November 2007 on a complaint concerning promotion of an unauthorised presentation of botulinum toxin).

On several occasions the MHRA has investigated the circumstances in which articles in the national press have discussed the potential benefits of products as yet not authorised. The information given by a manufacturer to journalists writing such articles may be called for and scrutinised, to establish whether the material merely notifies progress in research and development or actually promotes the unauthorised product. Guidance on what is legitimate, and what is not, is contained in the supplementary information to clause 22 of the Association of the British Pharmaceutical Industry Code of Practice for the Pharmaceutical Industry (2008).

13.4.2 Quantity

The Regulations do not expressly impose any limit on the amount of medicinal product which the company may supply for use by the doctor's individual patients under paragraph 1 of the Schedule. In view of the specific provisions upon stock held by a doctor or dentist set out in paragraph 3 (a total of 5 L fluid and 2.5 kg of solid of all such products per doctor or dentist), it is likely that supply under paragraph 1 should be limited to a reasonable course of treatment for a specific patient for whom the doctor is prescribing the product. Companies should always be suspicious of large orders from doctors and should enquire why such large quantities are being sought.

13.4.3 Doctor's specification

Supply must be 'formulated in accordance with the specification' of a doctor, dentist or supplementary prescriber. Strictly, this means that the a product should be made up, or imported, in accordance with the doctor's specification and must not be manufactured in advance of any order being received, unless that product is already on the market in a country from which it is being sourced. As a matter of practice, it is rarely the case that a product is formulated in response to a detailed specification provided by a doctor.

13.4.4 Special needs and cost

Directive 2001/83/EC requires supply to be to 'fulfil special needs'. Curiously, this condition was omitted from paragraph 1 of Schedule 1 to the UK Regulations until 2005. This condition means that the exemption should only be available where there is no equivalent product containing the same active ingredient already authorised and on the market in the UK. This view has been endorsed in the Guidance Note issued by the MHRA.[6]

It is necessary to analyse the meaning of 'special needs'. It is difficult to see how such needs can exist where there is a licensed version of the product on the market for the physician to use. However tempting it may be for medical institutions to save costs by requesting an unlicensed version of a licensed product, economic needs should never be special needs in this context. This accords with the rationale underlying the Directive, which requires only authorised medicinal products to be place on the market, unless exceptional circumstances apply. The MHRA accepts that where a licensed medicine is likely to be unavailable for a significant period, such as because of a manufacturing interruption, a 'special need' may exist, as also will be the case where a licensed product is discontinued only for commercial reasons.

13.4.5 Special needs and differences between authorised products and available unauthorised products

A more difficult question arises where the product to be manufactured or imported differs in some way from the licensed version. Issues may arise, in particular, where a product has been available only in unlicensed presentations and then a different company obtains a marketing authorisation in respect of it.

Normally, it will be marketed at higher cost, because the authorisation holder will have had to make a substantial investment in tests and trials and bringing the product to market. Such cases are increasing because the Orphan Drug legislation within the EU offers rewards to manufacturers prepared to seek authorisations for products that would previously have been uneconomic to develop and market. Such rewards include market exclusivity for 10 years (or 12 years if paediatric research to an approved plan has been conducted) and during this period competing products cannot be approved, save in defined cases. In such circumstances, manufacturers will have a legitimate concern if equivalent, but unauthorised, medicines are allowed on the market under the 'special needs' or 'pharmacy preparation' exceptions.

The Guidance Note issued by the MHRA[6] states that unlicensed products that are the 'pharmaceutical equivalent' of available licensed medicinal products will not be permitted. A medicinal product will be regarded as a 'pharmaceutical equivalent' where it contains the same amount of the same active substance(s), or in the case of liquid dosage forms the same concentration; and it is in the same dosage form; and it 'meets the same or comparable standards considered in the light of the clinical needs of the patient at the time of use of the product'. In the light of this guidance, a different formulation of an authorised substance (e.g. one specifically formulated for children or the elderly, or those with an allergy to a particular excipient) might satisfy the principle of fulfilling special needs. Differences in strength are less likely to justify a special need and, in principle, the fact that a product equivalent to a product authorised in the UK, is approved outside the UK for a different indication is irrelevant. It should be noted that the ability of the MHRA to question whether a 'special need' exists is, in practice, much greater where the product is to be imported than where it is procured from a 'specials' manufacturer in the UK, when the MHRA will only investigate when a particular issue or complaint is raised.

The MHRA actively encourages doctors and pharmacists to prescribe and supply licensed products in preference to unlicensed products meeting the same clinical needs. For instance, in 2008 the research-based company, Lundbeck, made available in the UK a licensed product called Circadin which is a modified-release product containing melatonin which was previously only available as an unlicensed product. Melatonin products were reported by the MHRA to be the largest category of unlicensed products imported into the UK (the Agency apparently received 1053 notifications of imports of these products in the 6 months to June 2008). The MHRA issued a press release to notify the availability of a licensed product and asked doctors to prescribe and pharmacists to supply only licensed product. It also gave notice that approval to import unlicensed product would only be given where the prescriber gave written details of the special clinical need to the importer (such as where an alternative dosage form was required) which, in turn, would be submitted to the MHRA. The MHRA may recommend that manufacturers granted a marketing authorisation for a product previously widely supplied as an unlicensed medicine should give notice to those manufacturing or importing the unlicensed product of the change in the regulatory environment that would arise on launch of the authorised product.

13.4.6 Controlled drugs

Where the medicinal product in question is a controlled drug within the Misuse of Drugs legislation,[12] additional controls will apply. Drugs are classified in various Schedules according to their perceived risk of harm. In the case of most of the products covered by the legislation, it will be necessary to obtain a licence from the Home Office in order to import the product from another country.

13.4.7 Patients ordering products over the internet

Where a patient orders a product for his or her own use direct from a supplier in another country, that will not normally be caught by the rules on individual patient supply, because the product will not be 'placed on the market'. However, it is possible that the supplier of that product (which is likely to be a prescription-only medicine) will be committing an offence in the country in which it operates, particularly if it has advertised the product or supplied it otherwise than in response to a prescription.

13.4.8 Labelling

Confusion remains on the rules covering the labelling of unauthorised medicines. Special provisions were contained in Regulation 11 of the Medicines (Labelling) Regulations 1976.[13] The Medicines for Human Use (Marketing Authorisations Etc.) Regulations 1994 disapplied the 1976 provisions, but did not introduce replacement provisions for medicinal products without a marketing authorisation. In the absence of further legislation on this point, many companies are

continuing to label their products in compliance with regulation 11 of the 1976 Regulations on a voluntary basis.

The BP notes that the labelling of medicines is a critical contributor to patients' safety. It confirms that there are no specific legal requirements for labelling, but suggests that best practice is to ensure that critical items of information should appear on the pack in the same field of view. Such information is said to include, name, strength, route of administration, dosage and warnings.

13.4.9 Charging for supply

The Regulations do not deal with this point. Companies may charge doctors for products supplied to them on a individual patient basis. There are no general Department of Health restrictions on levels of price or price increase, as the Pharmaceutical Price Regulation Scheme agreed between the Department of Health and the Association of the British Pharmaceutical Industry only governs products with a marketing authorisation.

13.4.10 Manufacture of, and wholesale dealing in, unlicensed medicines

The rules described above provide exemptions from the requirement to hold a marketing authorisation, but other activities involved in the supply of medicines on a individual patient basis need to be carried out under the appropriate authorisations. Accordingly, in relation to manufacture section 8(2) of the Medicines Act 1968 requires those involved in the manufacture or assembly of a medicinal product to hold a manufacturer's licence. Section 23 of the Act prohibits the manufacture of a medicinal product unless that product has a marketing authorisation, or is exempt from the marketing authorisation requirement. Schedule 1 to 1994 Regulations requires the manufacturer/assembler in the UK of an unlicensed product for individual patient supply to hold a particular type of manufacturer's licence (a manufacturer's 'specials' licence). This requires compliance with GMP and facilities are subject to MHRA inspection.

Likewise, section 8(3) of the Act requires those involved in the wholesale dealing of a medicinal product to hold a wholesale dealer's licence. If the product is imported from another Member State, a wholesale dealer's licence will be required. If it is imported from a country outside the EU, a wholesale dealer's (importation) licence will be required. Schedule 1 to the 1994 Regulations confirms that these provisions apply equally to individual patient supply.

In relation to manufacture, the BP states[1] that because specials are manufactured in accordance with GMP, there is some assurance of the manufacturing quality, but the intrinsic safety and efficacy of specials are not assessed and are the responsibility of the prescriber and the supplier. It is noted that imported unlicensed medicines are outside the scope of the General Monograph on Unlicensed Medicines, but where an individual monograph exists for an imported unlicenced medicinal product, the product must comply with the monograph. In relation to the position of doctors and pharmacists, it is emphasised that the prescribing doctor and the pharmacist owe a duty of care to the patient receiving the medicine with the result that:

'An appropriate risk assessment should be undertaken, which includes consideration of the suitability and fitness for purpose of the drug product. The risk assessment should also consider the contribution of the excipients to the safety profile of the unlicensed medicine.'

The BP goes on to state that manufacture or preparation of unlicensed medicine:

Should only be undertaken by competent staff within suitable facilities and using equipment appropriate for the scale of manufacture and specific dosage form. Where such a monograph is available, the medicinal substance and any excipients must comply with the specific monograph requirements of the Pharmacopoeia. The medicinal substance and any excipients must also comply with the General Monograph for Substances for Pharmaceutical Use and, where appropriate, the provisions of Supplementary Chapter IVj on the Control of Impurities in Substances for Pharmaceutical Use and the General Monograph for Products with Risk of Transmitting Agents of Animal Spongiform Encephalopathies. Unlicensed medicines must comply with the requirements of the General Monograph for Unlicensed Medicines and with the requirements of the relevant General Monograph for the specific dosage form. Where a BP monograph for a formulated preparation is available, the product must comply.

13.4.11 Unlicensed medicines for children
The significant demand for unlicensed medicines to treat children is often the subject of comment. New EU legislation relating to paediatric research[14] seeks to obviate the need for use of unlicensed medicines longer term, but in the meantime the Joint Committee of the Royal College of Paediatrics and Child Health and the Neonatal and Paediatric Pharmacists Group has published a statement providing guidance

to health professionals and parents who prescribe, dispense or administer medicines for children.[15]

13.4.12 NHS health care standards
In relation to health care systems and medicines management in England, the Healthcare Commission's Standard 4d requires NHS organisations to have in place systems for handling medicines safely and securely, including unlicensed medicines. It is envisaged that Trusts will produce an annual report on medicines management. In addition the National Patient Safety Agency has responsibilities in relation to the use of medicines by patients and issues patient safety alerts to the NHS which may cover aspects of unlicensed medicines use.

13.4.13 Clinical trials
The widest use of unlicensed medicinal products is in the course of clinical trials. It is important to distinguish between clinical trial use and individual patient use, as very different rules govern these different types of use.

The rules governing clinical trials in the UK are set out in the Medicines for Human Use (Clinical Trials) Regulations 2004,[16] which implement Directive 2001/20/EC on Good Clinical Practice in the conduct of clinical trials. Clinical trials require advance approval from an ethics committee and from the MHRA. They also have different manufacturing and labelling requirements. European law forbids charging for clinical trial products, although the MHRA interprets this as allowing institutions to be charged (such as for doctor initiated studies) provided the patient is not charged.

Clinical trials are sometimes continued for an open extension period. This is permissible, provided there are genuine scientific reasons for continuing the study (rather than commercial reasons, such as attempting to create demand for the product) and that the appropriate regulatory clearance has been obtained. If the company does not wish to do this, it would be open to the doctor to request further supplies of the product, but the company must not invite him or her to do this. Any further supply to the doctor would then need to comply with the provisions regarding individual patient supply, unless the doctor decided to carry out his or her own clinical trial.

The distinction between supply for use by particular patients and supply for use in a clinical trial is therefore important, particularly because the rules in the latter case are stricter, and companies must be certain about the basis upon which supply of unlicensed products is made. Various factors are relevant in determining the basis of supply, such as the purpose of the administration (individual patient supply is concerned with treatment; clinical trials are primarily concerned with testing the effects of treatment), the number of patients being treated and the degree of organisation and coordination between physicians treating patients.

The EMEA guidelines on compassionate use under Article 83 of Regulation 726/2004 provide that compassionate use supply should not slow down the initiation or continuation of clinical trials intended to provide essential information relative to the benefit–risk balance of a medicinal product. It advises that patients should always be considered for inclusion in clinical trials before being offered compassionate use programmes.

13.5 Product liability issues

13.5.1 Doctors and pharmacists

Article 5.1 of the Directive refers to the personal responsibility of the doctor treating a patient with an unlicensed medicines. Consistent with this, paragraph 1 of the Schedule to the 1994 Regulations states that the supply of the unlicensed product must be for use by a doctor's or dentist's individual patients on his or her direct personal responsibility. Doctors should be aware of the product liability implications of using such products, even though both the health care institution and the MHRA (e.g. approving the import of a product) may, in certain circumstances, share responsibility with the clinician treating the patient.

The physician owes the patient a duty of care to act with appropriate skill and caution in advising upon and administering a treatment. Health authorities or, in the private sector, the corporation running the hospital will be vicariously liable for the negligence of those who they employ to provide care to patients. The liability of a physician will normally be based in negligence. The tort of negligence is based on the omission to do something that a reasonable man, guided by the considerations that ordinarily regulate appropriate conduct, would do, or doing something that a reasonable man would not do.

In the private sector it may be possible to frame a case in contract. As the courts will imply a contractual term that the physician will use reasonable skill and care in his or her treatment of a patient, the extent of the duty of care can in practice be treated as identical to that imposed by the tort of negligence. However, a claim in contract may be advantageous where a contract for private treatment also involves the supply of a particular drug. It may be easier to argue that an unlicensed product was not 'reasonably fit for its purpose' under legislation relating to the supply of goods and services. A claim against the authority or company controlling the institution where the treatment is provided might more readily be made on this basis than against the producer of the product on the grounds that it is defective for the purposes of the Consumer Protection Act 1987.

For the purposes of strict liability under the 1987 Act, a product is not defective if it offers the safety persons generally are entitled to expect having regard to matters such as presentation and the purposes for which it might reasonably be used. The concept of reasonable use can readily be related to the licensing status of the product. Unless the producer was wrongly promoting the unlicensed product, he or she would no doubt argue that the product is not defective because its unlicensed status necessarily qualifies the safety profile that can reasonably be expected. In contrast, the institution providing private care has a primary obligation in contract for injury flowing from the supply of a product in breach of the implied term of 'fitness for purpose'.

The same basic standard of care applies in respect of a physician's conduct regardless of whether the treatment is being made privately under contract or under the NHS (such that a claim does not arise out of a contract, but must be made in the tort of negligence). The legal standard is encapsulated in the so-called Bolam test:[17]

A doctor is not guilty of negligence if he has acted in accordance with the practice accepted as proper by a responsible body of medical men skilled in the particular art. . . . Putting it the other way round, a doctor is not negligent, if he is acting in accordance with such a practice, merely because there is a body of opinion which takes a contrary view.

Minor modifications of the test have been made in case law to reflect the fact that the Court defines the standard and therefore inappropriate conduct cannot be justified by the mere fact that a body of health professionals acts similarly. The practice must 'rightly' be supported by an appropriate body of medical opinion.[18] The standard of care to be achieved is affected by the apparent level of specialisation of the physician in question. A consultant is required to show the skill and care of persons operating in that specialist field and not that of a general practitioner.

The Bolam test governs all aspects of the doctor–patient relationship. Accordingly, in counselling a patient, the Bolam test will be applied in relation to the physician's recommendation to treat the patient with an unlicensed medicine (or indeed with a licensed medicine, but for an unauthorised use).

It follows that where use of an unauthorised medicine can be shown to be consistent with the conduct of a responsible body of relevant medical opinion, any claim by the patient may well fail. In contrast, if it can be shown that no relevant body of responsible physicians would, on the facts of the case, rightly advise treatment with an unauthorised product, the claim may succeed, unless it cannot be shown that the injury actually resulted from such use, for example, if the adverse event would have arisen even if an authorised product had been used.

There are few English cases directly concerned with the exposure of physicians in relation to unlicensed use. In one case[19] a Registrar was found to have failed in her duty to explain to the patient at the beginning of treatment with an unlicensed allergen that there were certain risks attaching to treatment. In this context it was noted that it was incumbent upon clinicians dispensing an unlicensed treatment to exercise caution and to be alert to any reports of possible adverse events surrounding such use, even more so than when using licensed products which have undergone extensive clinical trials for their indication. It was also said that it was the duty of the physician to provide the patient with information which enabled the patient to make a balanced judgement about treatment.

In contrast, and consistent with the Bolam test, in another case,[20] the High Court found a physician not to be negligent where a patient suffered injury after treatment with gentamicin despite the fact that the physician had used a dose in excess of that approved in the product information. The physician was able to produce evidence to indicate that the dose he used was consistent with a body of medical opinion which took the view that the approved data sheet erred on the side of caution.

Medicines Act Leaflet 30 (1985) is no longer in force, because of changes in the regulatory framework, but it is instructive that the original guidance of the Medicines Control Agency (now the MHRA) on the provisions of the legislation affecting doctors and dentists, stated that:

It should be remembered that a practitioner prescribing an unlicensed medicine does so entirely on his own responsibility, carrying the total burden for the patient's welfare and, in the event of an adverse reaction, may be called upon to justify his actions. Under these circumstances it may be advisable for the practitioner to check his position with his medical defence union before prescribing such unlicensed products.

This remains a relevant statement under the revised rules. The MHRA has suggested in its consultation paper on possible changes in the regime for unauthorised products discussed below, that the increased responsibility and potential implications for the doctor's professional indemnity arrangements might be unfair, if the NHS, for some reason, positively encourages clinicians to make use of an unlicensed product. Nevertheless, the increased exposure of doctors using unlicensed products is widely accepted.

A lead article in the *Drug and Therapeutics Bulletin*[21] (DTB) entitled 'Prescribing unlicensed drugs or using drugs for unlicensed indications' notes that the Medicines Act and European legislation preserves a doctor's clinical freedom to act as he or she sees to be in the best interests of the patient and that products prescribed by doctors outside the licence can be dispensed by pharmacists. However, the DTB goes on to emphasise the increased responsibility of the physician:

The responsibility for prescribing any medicine falls on the doctor, but if the prescription is for an unlicensed medicine, or for an unlicensed indication, the prescriber could be particularly vulnerable.

In relation to the practical implications the DTB makes the following statements which are consistent with the analysis of the law set out above:

In using an unlicensed drug, or a drug in a way incompatible with the data sheet, the doctor must act responsibility and with reasonable care and skill. When prescribing outside a licence it is important the doctor does so knowingly, recognises the responsibility that such prescribing entails and when obtaining consent to treatment should, where possible, tell the patient of the drug's licensed status, and for an unlicensed product that its effects will be less well understood than those of a licensed product.

The article concludes:

Doctors may prescribe unlicensed medicines or depart from the prescribing directions given in the data sheet of licensed medicines. Such prescribing should be done knowingly, and where possible the position explained to the patient in sufficient detail to allow them to give informed consent. Prescribing outside the licence alters, and probably increases, the doctor's professional responsibility.

13.5.2 Manufacturers and suppliers

In theory, therefore, the practitioner, as a professional person, is best able to assess the risks and potential benefits to his or her patient, and to decide that the balance of advantages and disadvantages lies in favour of the use of a particular unauthorised product. It follows that a company receiving a request from that practitioner is entitled to assume that the doctor understands the properties of the product and will exercise reasonable care and skill in using it so as to avoid causing injury to his or her patient. However, the principle that procurement is the doctor's sole responsibility does not provide companies with total protection against liability where a patient is injured. A manufacturing defect could give rise to a claim as could answering a request for product information in a way that is later found not to reflect accurately the state of scientific and technical knowledge. At the operational level, manufacturers must apply proper care and rigorous quality controls during production, to ensure that they supply unlicensed medicinal products of the highest quality.

More generally, companies should respond with great care to requests for unlicensed products from practitioners, bearing in mind that there is no legal obligation to comply with such requests. If they do not act with caution, companies risk becoming involved in a negligence claim, or in a product liability action under the Consumer Protection Act 1987 for supplying a defective product.

Where a company suspects that the product is to be used in a way that is not safe for patients, its duty to those patients may involve warning the doctor that it considers the proposed use to be hazardous and, if necessary, refusing or terminating supply. While there is no general obligation to provide product information with unlicensed medicines (and, as noted above, the use of promotional material is prohibited), from a product liability standpoint, the provision of basic safety information about the product is a sensible precaution. As noted earlier, such a practice is also effectively endorsed by the European Commission in Volume 9A of the Notice to Applicants.

Companies are advised to have in place a standard operating policy for dealing with and recording requests for individual patient supply, even though this can never act as a guarantee against a patient making a claim at a later stage. As part of this, it is useful to have a standard supply and consent form for

the physician to sign, which highlights the unlicensed status of the product and reminds the requesting physician that he or she has a personal responsibility for his or her use of the product. It can usefully require him or her to agree to counsel the patient on the regulatory status of the product, to keep records of such counselling and return any unused product and to report any adverse events occurring. It can also be useful to explain (if product is being supplied free) that there is no obligation to continue to supply product for the patient if and when marketing authorisation is granted.

A further possibility is for the company to provide a form for patients to sign, recording their consent to treatment with the unauthorised product. As a matter of English law, such a consent form could not exclude the manufacturer's liability for personal injury for negligence or under the Consumer Protection Act 1987.[22] Nevertheless, it might be helpful in qualifying the patient's expectations of safety from the product and reduce the risk of a claim being made.

13.5.3 Hospitals

In its Guidance Note,[6] the MHRA states that hospital trusts, and independent hospitals, should have clear policies on the use of unlicensed medicines, explaining liability considerations and requiring all those involved in the supply chain to ensure that the unlicensed status of a product is communicated to the patient and fully understood.

13.6 Professional guidance

13.6.1 Doctors

The practice of competent practitioners is influenced by the guidance that the profession provides to its members. It is, therefore, relevant to look at the guidance provided by the General Medical Council (GMC). Under Section 35 of the Medical Act 1983, the GMC has powers to provide advice for doctors on standards of professional conduct. The GMC provides quite detailed guidance to doctors in the form of booklets and on its website. It has issued guidance for doctors entitled *Good Practice in Prescribing Medicines* (2008). This includes, at paragraph 18, guidance on prescribing unlicensed medicines. It states that doctors can prescribe unlicensed medicines but that if they decide to do so they must meet the following requirements:

1. Be satisfied that an alternative, licensed medicines would not meet the patient's needs;

2. Be satisfied that there is a sufficient evidence base and/or experience of using the medicine to demonstrate its safety and efficacy;

3. Take responsibility for prescribing the unlicensed medicines and for overseeing the patient's care, including monitoring and any follow-up treatment (see also paragraphs 25–27 on prescribing for hospital outpatients);

4. Record the medicine prescribed and, where you are not following common practice, the reasons for choosing this medicine in the patient's notes.

The guidelines go on to state at paragraphs 21 and 22 that it is good practice to give as much information as patients require or which they may see as significant. At paragraph 23 it is said that the doctor should explain the reasons for prescribing a medicine that is unlicensed.

The theme of this advice is also reflected in the *British National Formulary* (BNF). It includes a reference to unlicensed medicines:

Where an unlicensed drug is included in the BNF, this is indicated in brackets after the entry. Where the BNF suggests a use (or route) that is outside the licensed indication of a product ('off-label' use) this too is indicated. Unlicensed use of medicines becomes necessary if the clinical need cannot be met by licensed medicines; such use should be supported by appropriate evidence and experience.

It follows from the above that, where there is an appropriately licensed alternative, the GMC does not deem it good practice to use an unlicensed product or use a product outside the terms of its authorisation, unless a cogent case can be put forward that it better serves the needs of the particular patient. Regardless of the evidence base, it can be argued that cost alone is not a justification for declining to use a licensed product that meets the same clinical need. However, the position is not clear-cut because of the vagueness of what is said about the relevance of cost in prescribing. The GMC states, in other general guidance, that physicians must have regard to costs in the sense that physicians should 'make efficient use of the resources available' to them. However, it seems unlikely that this can properly be viewed as requiring use of unlicensed products, where the needs of the patient can be met by use of a licensed product.

13.6.2 Pharmacists

The Royal Pharmaceutical Society of Great Britain has developed guidelines on the use of unlicensed medicines in pharmacies. The guidelines note that if a patient suffers injury following administration of an unlicensed medicine, the pharmacist may have some exposure to liability, along with the prescribing doctor and that the extent of this exposure will vary depending upon the facts of the case. It is said that the pharmacist should supply a product with a marketing authorisation where such a product is available in a suitable formulation, in preference to an unlicensed product or a food supplement. In addition, in relation to extemporaneous preparation, it is said that a product should be so prepared only where there is no product available with a marketing authorisation and where certain conditions are met including that the product is capable of preparation in compliance with accepted standards, the particular staff are competent to undertake this task, appropriate facilities and equipment exist, records are kept, the product is appropriately labelled, and the pharmacist is satisfied as to the safety and appropriateness of the formula of the product.

13.6.3 Attitude of the protection societies

The Medical Defence Union (MDU) and Medical Protection Society (MPS) indemnify doctor members in relation to claims of negligence brought against them. They do not act as insurance companies and, strictly speaking, the benefits provided are discretionary. The fact that they are discretionary gives the organisation some ability to forewarn doctors of cases where it is unlikely that the discretion will be exercised in their favour. Surprisingly, neither the MDU nor the MPS appears to have published specific material addressing prescription of unlicensed products or off-label prescription.

However, in the past in personal communications to the authors the MDU has advised that, in its view, the Bolam test applies with respect to the doctor's liability. The usage, therefore, has to conform with a responsible body of medical opinion. However, the MDU noted that the patient should be informed that the product or (as the case may be) the indication is not licensed. This is justified on the basis that, even if the product is not necessarily dangerous to use in the situation in question, the side effects would not be as well known as for a licensed product or indication. The MDU also noted that the doctor should record in the patient's records that the patient has been advised of the status of the product. The MDU observed that recent case law has tended to expand the requirements of counselling to obtain properly informed consent. Likewise the MPS has endorsed the Bolam test. Interestingly, the MPS stated that if the doctor is an employee of the institution he or she should obtain prior authorisation of his or her employers as there could be product liability issues in relation to the liability of the institution.

13.7 Review of the regulatory framework by the MHRA

In February 2008, the MHRA announced a review of the regulatory arrangements relating to supply of unlicensed medicines.[24] An informal consultation process began and responses were invited by end of June 2008 with the aim of developing specific proposals to amend the current regime. The MHRA suggests a need to determine the specific role and responsibilities of clinician, health care institution and the MHRA in relation to protecting the patient and notes the inconsistencies between the level of regulatory oversight in relation to unlicensed products manufactured in the UK and those imported. The MHRA explains the factors that can significantly affect the need for and use of unlicensed medicines. It states:

Changes in the overall regulatory burden of the medicines licensing system and trends in the rationalisation of companies in the pharmaceutical sector, are among factors that can have a strong effect at the margins as to whether it is considered commercially viable for a company to seek or maintain a marketing authorisation for products for which there is a lower demand. By the same token significant changes in the regulatory burden relating to unlicensed medicines may have the effect, intended or otherwise, at the margins of shifting the balance of demand between licensed and unlicensed medicines. It will be important to ensure that any proposed changes recommended by this review do not undermine the medicines licensing system and the safeguards if (sic) gives to patients on safety, quality and efficacy.

The MHRA notes that the use of unlicensed products appears to be increasing. Notifications for import were under 20,000 in 2000, but by 2006 had risen to approximately 180,000. Curiously, when fees for notifications were introduced in 2007, the figure for notifications fell to 60,000, although the 'special needs' of patients will surely not have evaporated. The MHRA notes that it has no accurate data on the size of the 'specials' market, but believes it to have increased.

These considerations and trends, together with the age and patchwork nature of the existing legislation, have encouraged the MHRA to review the rules and assess whether they meet the expectations of stakeholders, could provide clearer accountability and, in particular, could determine the extent to which the MHRA should be able to 'second guess' the judgement of the clinician on whether a patient genuinely has a 'special need' or whether, for instance, there is merely a desire to access less costly (but unauthorised) products. The review also will examine whether the current balance between regulatory intervention by the MHRA and professional guidance and governance arrangements in the NHS and private health care is appropriate.

In May 2009 the MHRA issued its Interim Report on the review. It identifies three main areas for possible amendment of regulatory requirements that it believes will enhance public health protection and upon which further consultation will now take place. These are quality standards, patient information and pharmacovigilance. An important proposal potentially relevant to liability issues is that all unlicensed medicines be supplied with a patient information leaflet and a technical information leaflet directed at the healthcare professional. The MHRA also propose that specific labelling requirements be introduced. In relation to pharmacovigilance it is proposed that all suspected adverse reactions be notified to the MHRA and not just serious reactions. More generally the MHRA propose a new regulatory fiamework based either on a revised notification system or a list system that would indicate products for which no notification is required. In either case, the system would apply to both UK manufactured and imported products.

13.8 Conclusions

There are compelling pragmatic reasons for allowing the supply of unauthorised medicines for individual patient use. Doctors are able to select the treatment that they consider most appropriate for each patient, even though that treatment may not have a marketing authorisation. Doctors increase their liability exposure using unlicensed products, but whether this is material depends upon the facts of each case. Companies are permitted to respond to requests for such products, provided that they, and the doctors, comply fully with the applicable regulatory requirements. Where the product in question has the potential to cause significant adverse reactions or requires very careful monitoring, the company must ensure that it takes particular care in order to avoid exposing itself to an increased risk of personal injury claims.

Any failure to comply with the 1994 Regulations could be prejudicial in any such litigation.

The regulatory framework in the UK is old and exhibits several inconsistencies between the treatment of unlicensed products manufactured as 'specials' in the UK and those imported from outside the UK. The MHRA is currently considering amending the regulatory requirements and therefore one must anticipate changes in the near future.

References

1 BP 2008: Supplementary Chapter V ('Unlicensed Medicines') at A 760.
2 Medicines (Exemption from Licences) (Special and Transitional Cases) Order 1971 (SI 1971/1450).
3 Medicines (Exemption from Licences) (Special Cases and Miscellaneous Provisions) Order 1972 (SI 1972/1200).
4 Medicines (Exemption from Licences) (Importation) Order 1984 (SI 1984/673).
5 Medicines for Human Use (Marketing Authorisations Etc.) Regulations 1994 (SI 1994/3144).
6 MHRA: The Supply of Unlicensed Relevant Medicinal Products for Individual Patients (Revised January 2008).
7 Medicines (Administration of Radioactive Substances) Regulations 1978 (SI 1978/1006).
8 Medicines (Standard Provisions for Licences and Certificates) Amendment Regulations 1999 (SI 1999/4).
9 Medicines (Standard Provisions for Licences and Certificates) Regulations 1971 (SI 1971/972).
10 Medicines for Human Use (Manufacturing, Wholesale Dealing and Miscellaneous Amendments) Regulations 2005 (SI 2005/2789).
11 Medicines (Advertising) Regulations 1994 (SI 1994/1932).
12 Misuse of Drugs Act 1971; the Misuse of Drugs Regulations 2001 (SI 2001/3998).
13 Medicines (Labelling) Regulations (SI 1976/1726).
14 Regulation (EC) No 1901/2006 of 12 December 2006 (as amended).
15 The use of unlicensed medicines or licensed medicines for unlicensed applications in paediatric practice, February 2000, Royal College of Paediatrics and Child Health.
16 Medicines for Human Use (Clinical Trials) Regulations 2004 (SI 2004/1031).
17 Bolam v Friern Hospital Management Committee 1957 2 All ER 118.
18 Bolitho v City and Hackney HA [1997] 3 WLR 1151.
19 Kennedy v Queen's Medical Centre, University Hospital NHS Trust (Unreported, but of 12 January 2001).
20 Vernon v Bloomsbury Health Authority [1995] 6 Med LR 297.
21 Volume 30, No 25 of December 1992.
22 Unfair Contract Terms Act 1977, section 2; Consumer Protection Act 1987, section 7.
23 Code of Ethics for Pharmacists and Pharmacy Technicians together with Professional Standards and guidance for the sale and supply of medicines. Royal Pharmaceutical Society of Great Britain (August 2007) and Legal and Ethical Advisory Service Fact Sheet: Five. *The Use of Unlicensed Medicines in Pharmacy* (September 2007).
24 MHRA. Informal consultation paper on the review of the regulation of unlicensed medicines. 28 February 2008.

14 Human experimentation – ethics of first human exposure

Duncan W. Vere

University of London, UK

14.1 Introduction

When faced with the mass of detailed and costly rules for ethics submission it might seem easy to think that they are what matter most. Not so, the most important duty is to imagine what the most likely risks may be to human volunteers and to plan how best to minimise these, even though they cannot be known at the planning stage.[1]

Situations that have been known to increase these risks are:

- Hurried initial tests, perhaps to reduce times or costs, following a routine protocol;
- When a novel group of compounds come to first testing;
- When the new drug is a biological derivative (e.g. a new antibody), whether in whole or in part, a vaccine, or bound to a peptide or protein;
- When volunteers fail to disclose, for whatever reason, some personal details about prior illness, medication or adverse reactions;
- If the environment of the studies is inadequate by reason of equipment, available staff or emergency facilities.[2]

14.2 Drug doses

A group of volunteers should not be dosed at the same time and at the same dose level, because when adverse events occur they should be dealt with singly; new symptoms can then be evaluated carefully in that individual and steps taken to minimise risk.[3]

The first dose should be very small compared to the expected effective dose range predicted from animal studies, and dose increments should be made on successive days for any one volunteer, rising in arithmetic (not logarithmic) steps.[2]

14.3 Symptoms and signs

The symptoms caused by novel drugs can be unusual and unexpected. This is true whether their significance is trivial or major. The only way to evaluate them is to elicit them, not to wait for volunteers to express them spontaneously. At times these symptoms have been unexpected or bizarre; it is important to avoid leading questions but to give the volunteer an opportunity to mention them, allowing time for delayed effects. The symptom inventory can be verbal or written, but must not suggest responses to the volunteer; it should use open-ended questions. It is important to measure vital functions whether these are expected to relate to the particular drug exposure under study or not. For example, some drug actions are silent (hypertension, prolongation of QTc interval).

The preclinical animal studies should be made available to the clinical investigators and should be read carefully by them, not just accepting the opinions of others about their interpretation. For example, cardiac arrhythmias which have been thought to be peculiar to the dog have been predictive of human arrhythmia on drug exposure. In general, animal toxicity is poorly predictive for humans, but there are exceptions. Unless one is prepared to take the unexpected seriously its predictive value for later hazard is lost.

Even so, the predictive value in general of phase I studies for adverse effects is small, and non-existant for idiosyncratic adverse effects, because the numbers

The Textbook of Pharmaceutical Medicine. Edited by John P. Griffin. © 2009, ISBN: 978-1-4051-8035-1.

of volunteers are so small. However, adverse effects have occurred to individuals and this is why particular care is appropriate.

14.4 Eliciting volunteers and informed consent

It is here that most ethical problems arise. A full description of the proposed tests must be given to possible volunteers with an opportunity for them to discuss the information. This must include some information about the nature of likely effects and purpose of the compound under test and its formulation. Its potential effects, possible interaction and incompatibility with other medication that they are taking or have taken until recently must be taken into account and mentioned to the volunteer.

The sites and times of tests must be disclosed and the safeguards present at these. The cost to volunteers must be fully disclosed, whether in terms of time lost, financial costs with likely risks, or costs of travel, meals or lost opportunity, and the amount and nature of reimbursement for these. They must be asked about previous drug reactions, idiosyncrasies and illnesses.

It is particularly important to avoid inducements to volunteering, such as offered presents or privileges; it must be remembered that there are vulnerable groups (e.g. students) who by reason of youth or poverty are eager to volunteer and may minimise risks so as to obtain money. They may volunteer for several drug studies synchronously, so it is wise to ask if they are involved with studies elsewhere.

Some areas of drug development require studies of a radically different kind (e.g. mitotoxic drugs, anti-cancer drugs, remedies for allergies) and this discussion does not apply to these; different trial conditions must be used. In general, in these cases drugs are not given to healthy volunteers but to volunteer patients with the illness they are aimed to benefit.

14.5 Environment of phase I studies

These should only be performed in a dedicated space within a fully equipped clinical environment. Safety, resuscitation and antidote drugs and equipment should be to hand immediately, with personnel who are skilled in their use present or within immediate on call for the site; they must be told where and when tests are to begin. This should be done in writing.

Thought must be given not only to early or immediate drug effects but also to possible late drug actions (e.g. sedation, disinhibition, postural hypotension, drug interaction). Volunteers should be given a telephone number for post-testing contact should they have queries or need further information.

Before tests begin volunteers' general practitioners should be contacted with details of the tests proposed and asked whether they can see any reasons in their patients' case why they should not volunteer.

All of the information just listed should form part of a written protocol, divided up into clearly headed sections; the local research ethics committee will certainly want to see this as part of the submission made by the investigators.

There should be a lead investigator who is the named individual responsible for the design and execution of the study, and also a nominated clinician caring for the trial volunteers, whether they are healthy (the usual case) or with a prescribed illness for which the drug under test is not a treatment although it may need to be given later to such patients for another reason.

Potential volunteers should be given a careful written account of the proposed study before they volunteer; it should include details of times of attendance, fasting or other dietary advice, tests they will be asked to undergo and drug safety in as far as it may already be known. The language used must be non-technical and such that the potential volunteers can understand. They must be given opportunity to ask questions, and for their understanding of it to be assessed.

Investigators' attitudes are very important. There were times when initial testing of new drugs was treated in a cavalier way by many; novel medicines should be regarded with similar respect to that needed in ordinary medical practice, but enhanced by the realisation that in ordinary practice much is known about the remedies used whereas here nothing can be known beforehand.[4] Good Clinical Practice (GCP) applies here as much as in ordinary medicine or in later stages of clinical drug testing.[5]

14.6 Tests of compliance, comprehension and conduct

In phase I studies, compliance tests are usually not needed because the researcher gives the doses to the volunteer singly. Even so, a drug given orally or by inhalation may not be taken adequately and a chewable formulation may be swallowed. Often, the only way to monitor absorption is by plasma or urine tests. This needs the development of methods of drug analysis in human plasma or urine before the human studies start. This raises the question of what, if any part of ADME (drug action, distribution, metabolism and excretion) studies should precede phase I tests, however simple and non-quantitative those tests might be. If carried out at all they would usually be tests of a simple kind for the presence of the drug.

14.7 General ethical problems

Because volunteers in phase I studies are healthy, two problems arise directly; the studies will be of no direct benefit to the volunteers, only risk is present for them. The potential risks, although seldom observed, are unknown. None of the knowledge gained will benefit them, at least at present. Also, volunteers may be driven to take part for unhappy reasons, be they impecunity, risk-taking or adventure or perhaps to experience new drug effects or to find out about them in curiosity. Tests in animals cannot predict some areas of human toxicity (e.g. reproductive or neuro-psychiatric toxicity, or effects on tissues which are not required to be examined by regulation), hence there are three areas of particular difficulty: tests in women, endocrine toxicity and interaction between a novel drug and others that volunteers have taken or be taking. It is right, therefore, to empanel women volunteers only after they have agreed to a pregnancy test and this has proven negative, unless they are menopausal. Urine tests for drugs of misuse should precede even phase I testing, and because minimal levels of intolerance are unpredictable a careful history of allergic reactions and especially anaphylaxis should be taken, whether to drug or other substances.

The care of volunteers during and after phase I trials is very important. Studies should be performed in the presence of staff trained and competent in resuscitation and the apparatus to hand should include resuscitation drugs and equipment. The instructions to volunteers should include details of when and how they should leave the test site and they should consent to these rules. Late effects which may cause problems include drowsiness (better to travel home by train or bus than drive a car or ride a bike) and postural hypotension, neither of which may trouble someone until they are well away from the site of testing. Volunteers may need to agree to stay for a while until it is safe for them to go home, and they may need food

before they go if the study has involved fasting before dosing. A difficult question is how much may payments to volunteers act as an inducement. Certainly, expenses should be paid, but inducement by offers of money or other gifts or privileges should be avoided as should payments for risks taken.

14.8 Regulations relating to ethical practice in phase I (healthy volunteer) studies of new drugs and treatments

14.8.1 Good Clinical Practice
Good Medical Practice (GMP) is published as guidance for doctors by the General Medical Council (GMC)[5] and contains specific information about research, financial and commercial dealings with patients and conflicts of interest. However, the GMP Guidelines do not refer to healthy volunteers but only to patients. The GMC is soon to issue similar advice relating to healthy volunteer tests. Good Clinical Practice (GCP) relates to this closely, but is more specifically concerned with clinical trials of remedies.[4]

14.8.2 UK Medicines for Human Use (Clinical Trials) Regulations 2004[6]
Volunteers can only be sought or recruited for any kind of trial when the proposed protocol has been approved by a recognised research ethics committee, which must have both lay and expert members. Failure to comply with this regulation is a statutory offence.[3]

14.8.3 Submissions to local research ethics committees
All proposed human experimentation must be submitted to a local research ethics committee (LREC). In academic institutions there is usually a local research committee to which submissions should go also, although this does not exempt the proposal from LREC submission.

Multicentre research in the UK must be submitted to the multicentre research ethics committee (MREC) and after their approval proposals must also go to the LREC, which will set about its assessment in ways set out by the Department of Health in 1998.

However, this whole process has been simplified greatly by a form for nationally standardised electronic submission online, published by the Central Office for Research Ethics Committees (COREC), version 5.3. This form makes submission to any ethics committee easier by setting out a series of questions.

Part A covers the scientific reasons for the study, the methods proposed, the funding, data monitoring and potential conflicts of interest. Part B requires details of medicinal products or devices to be used, human biological materials and radiation sources. It includes mandatory details of application to the Medicinal Healthcare products Regulatory Agency (MHRA). Part C has questions about the suitability, qualifications and research experience of the local investigator and details of the proposed site for the tests. When an investigation has to be extended to include more than one Health Service Trust then the online form must be extended to include a Site Specific Assessment (SSA) for each Health Trust which it is proposed to involve. Most Trusts will want a researcher to have at least an honorary contract with a Trust in order to conduct studies in its area, but other researchers who have a contract already in that Trust can join the team for a multicentre study. Where several Trusts are involved the various Part C forms (Site Specific Information forms) can be printed out separately and only the part relevant to each Trust sent to their LREC.[7,8]

Many forms for submission to ethics committees ask what is the hypothesis to be tested in the research. It is not the primary task of LRECs nor of the MREC to assess the scientific value or methodology of proposed research, although to be ethical an experiment must be capable of generating data that can answer a discernable set of questions. However, first human drug exposures are not experiments, nor do they test an hypothesis; they are solely carried out to assess a likely range of effective doses, tolerability at those doses and to detect surprising or even potentially hazardous effects from them. They also assess the tolerability and practical usage of the dose formulations of a novel medicine. Hence, the formulation of the test doses should in so far as is possible reproduce those that will be issued as the new remedy, and the apparatus and the environment used to assess the drug responses should mimic those in which the drug is likely to be used should it be marketed.

References

1 Bickerstaffe R, Brock P, Husson J-M, Rubin I et al. Guiding Principles for Pharmaceutical Physicians from the Ethical Issues Committees of the Faculty of Pharmaceutical Medicine of the Royal Colleges of Physicians of the UK. *Int J Clin Pract* 2006;**60**:238–41.

2 Mant TGK. Ethics and pharmaceutical research. *Faculty Pharm Med Newsl* 2006;**20**:5.

3 Carson AP, Davies JE. *Ethics in Pharmacology*. J.E. *pA2*, vol. 4(3), September 2006. Newsletter of the British Pharmacological Society. Ed. V. Raman http://bps.ac.uk

4 Hargreaves R. Understanding the requirements of the Clinical Pharmacology module of Pharmaceutical Medicine Specialty Training (PMST). *Faculty Pharm Med Newsl* 2007;**21**:6.

5 General Medical Council. Good Medical Practice. 13 November 2006. www.gmc-uk.org/guidance

6 Medicines for Human Use (Clinical Trials) Regulations. Geneva, Switzerland, 2004. http//www.opsi.gov.uk/si2004/20041031.htm

7 Abozguia K, Phan TT, Shivu GN et al. Insights into how to conduct a clinical trial in the UK. *J R Soc Med* 2007;**100**:469–72.

8 Central Office for Research Ethics Committees (COREC) version 5.3 of the NHS REC Application Form. January 2007. https://www.corecform.org.uk/AppForm/

15 Legal and ethical issues relating to medicinal products

Nick Beckett[1], Sarah Hanson[1], Christopher J.S. Hodges[2] and Shuna Mason[3]

[1] Partner CMS Cameron McKenna LLP, London, UK
[2] Head of the CMS Research Programme on Civil Justice Systems, Centre for Socio-Legal Studies, University of Oxford, Oxford, UK
[3] Head of Regulatory, CMS Cameron McKenna LLP, London, UK

15.1 Introduction

Other chapters in this book deal with the evolution of the legal and ethical controls over medicinal products and their development as well as the structure of the European Union regulatory systems set up to authorise business activities and dealings in these products, and to enforce the rules and restrictions the law places upon them. This chapter aims to select some specific legal and ethical issues that arise in relation to product development, authorisation and sale and supply both within the UK and within the context of the European systems.

15.2 Chronology of production, development and marketing

The laws and ethical codes that apply to the various stages of pharmaceutical product development are aimed at controlling and placing limits upon defined activities, thereby maximising the protection of the public. In practice, these objectives are supported not only by powers granted to competent regulatory authorities to enforce compliance with medicines laws through compulsory action, but also by the application of relevant principles of the general criminal and civil law.

15.2.1 Development

In the course of product development, testing in both animals and humans is subject to varying degrees of legal control, supplemented by a significant quantity of ethical or 'good practice' guidelines.

The Textbook of Pharmaceutical Medicine. Edited by John P. Griffin. © 2009, ISBN: 978-1-4051-8035-1.

15.2.1.1 Animal testing

The legal controls on animal testing were introduced at the European level by a Directive in 1986.[1] At the time of writing this is still undergoing a lengthy revision process which started in 2006. The central objectives cited in the formulation of the controls were: to avoid disparities in the controls applied across Member States that might affect the functioning of the common market, and also to limit to a minimum the number of animals used in product development whose use was necessary to meet testing requirements, and to ensure, as far as possible, the best care and treatment of the animals during the conduct of the research and in the method of their disposal: 'whereas such harmonisation should ensure that the number of animals used for experimental or other scientific purposes is reduced to a minimum, that such animals are adequately cared for, that no pain, suffering, distress or lasting harm are inflicted unnecessarily and to ensure that where unavoidable, they should be kept to a minimum. Whereas, in particular, unnecessary duplication of experiments should be avoided.'

In summary, Directive 86/609/EEC requires the premises in which animal research is undertaken and persons conducting such research to be subject to local registration and inspection and imposes limitations upon the breeding and supply of experimental animals. There are specific provisions regarding the care of experimental animals, including, for example, minimum caging and temperature requirements. As a Directive, 86/609/EEC required implementation in each Member State to take effect at national level (cf. Regulations which are immediately effective at national level without the need for national legislative or administrative action). Therefore, the systems for applying the requirements of the Directive vary from country to country; the function of the Directive being to achieve a harmonisation of the principles, aims and objectives to be achieved at local level. Accordingly, enforcement, monitoring and inspection are all matters of local control and design.

In the UK, by the time of the adoption of the Directive, the authorities had already introduced legislation for the control of animal experimentation in the form of the Animal and Scientific Procedures Act 1986. Its content and coverage was already relatively comprehensive so relatively little needed to be done to bring the UK law in line with the European provisions.

The conduct and control of animal experimentation are matters that give rise to strong public feeling. During 1996/1997, extensive UK media coverage of the conditions in testing facilities put the issue of experimentation and effective controls in the public eye, leading to increased animal rights activism and ultimately to the introduction of legislation to combat economic sabotage in the UK in 2005.[2] For the product developer using external facilities to generate the preclinical data necessary to make an application for a marketing authorisation (MA), the cost and time of the developmental process are too high for risks to be taken with the acceptability of data for regulatory purposes, whether generated in animal or human experiments. Delays are always costly. Under the European rules specifying the content of a MA application (Directive 2001/83/EC[3]), compliance with testing rules is essential because the preclinical data that are submitted must have been generated from studies complying with Directive 86/609/EEC and with Good Laboratory Practice.[4] Under these, compliance with the animal testing directive is mandatory. Any evidence to suggest that the data have not been properly generated will lead a competent regulatory authority to discount them in the evaluation of the MA application.

It is now a well-known theme in European pharmaceuticals legislation that the use of animals should be minimised as far as possible: 'The Commission and Member States should encourage research into the development and validation of alternative technologies which could provide the same level of information' (86/609/EEC Article 23).

Public opinion, including that of the European Parliament,[5] is strongly supportive and there are several initiatives looking at the potential for conducting tests *in vitro*, where an animal model may previously have been used, but may not be essential to generate useful data. Although the Commission has indicated in the context of the revision of Directive 86/609 that a

fixed timetable to phase out the use of all non-human primates in biomedical research is not feasible, in view of current scientific knowledge and the requirements of several vital disease research programmes, it is considering banning the use of great apes and possibly that of animals caught in the wild (subject to only limited exceptions). It is also considering introducing mandatory authorisation and ethical evaluation for all animal studies.[6]

The law tends to follow developments in public moral and ethical thinking and it is not surprising therefore that the same theme arises in different sectors of the European law. In the cosmetic sector, the use of animals for further substance testing is now prohibited. In the pharmaceutical sector, a complete ban – at least for the foreseeable future – remains highly unlikely where there is no other means of generating the required data. However, the inadequacy of most animal models for predicting human response is a recurrent issue and inescapable fact. Accordingly, many of the provisions concerning the generation of preclinical data, and particularly those set out in the amended Annex to Directive 2001/83/EC, leave considerable discretion to the developer to design and justify studies appropriate to the product concerned. In many cases, it is possible for the applicant to justify objectively the omission of certain studies, or the conduct of studies in only one, rather than two, species. The conduct of tests simply for the sake of following a 'traditional', or general, approach without evaluating what the product and the objective justify is wasteful and may not be either scientifically, morally or legally justified.

15.2.1.2 Testing in human beings

The conduct of clinical research in humans raises numerous legal and ethical issues of significant importance. A common legal framework for conducting clinical trials in Europe and providing a legal basis for compliance with Good Clinical Practice (GCP) has now been established. The Clinical Trials Directive[7] and the associated Commission Directives were required to be implemented in Member States' national laws over the period from May 2004 to January 2006. The latter Directives detail the principles and guidelines for GCP and the manufacture and importation of investigational medicinal products[8] and extend the principles and guidelines of Good Manufacturing Practice (GMP) to the use of these products in clinical trials.[9] Interpretation and enforcement remain a local matter. Although the legislation is fairly recent, its harmonising impact upon clinical trial regulation across the European Union has been hampered in consequence of different interpretations and implementations by the Member States, which has complicated the conduct of multicentre multinational research projects in particular, with consequent impact on costs and time. It has been suggested that some of the difficulties can be resolved by providing additional clarification and guidance although other changes would need to be addressed through changes to the legislation.[10]

The Clinical Trials Directive has introduced a legal requirement for clinical trials to be designed, conducted, recorded and reported in accordance with GCP, which the Clinical Trials Directive refers to as a 'set of internationally recognised ethical and scientific quality requirements'.[11] This dovetails with the pre-existing requirement upon applicants for MA to confirm that clinical trials performed outside the European Union meet the ethical requirements of the Clinical Trials Directive in order for that data to be taken into account.[12] Although it was not specifically adopted as the GCP standard by the Clinical Trials Directive – and there are several GCP standards around the world – the obvious GCP standard for European clinical trials is the international guideline (in use since 1997) developed within the International Conference of Harmonisation (ICH), to which European Union, US and Japanese regulators and industries subscribe.[13] Although the principles and guidelines of GCP are now enacted in the GCP Directive, the ICH standard should be taken into account. In addition, the introduction at the end of 2007 of specific legislation on advanced therapy medicinal products[14] has also led to the development of a detailed GCP standard specific to these products, which is the subject of a Commission consultation at the time of writing.

In addition, the GCP Directive specifies that all clinical trials must be conducted in accordance with the Declaration of Helsinki, 1996 version. That Declaration distinguishes between research that has the potential for therapeutic effect in the volunteers recruited and research conducted for the greater good (i.e. the expansion of knowledge without the expectation of direct benefit to the human volunteers), as well as the requirement for research projects to be subject to independent ethical review.[15]

Directive 2001/20/EC was designed to address the functioning, structure and funding of ethics committees across Europe. In the UK, prior to 1 May 2004, as a matter of law, it was not a universal requirement that all research (whether concluded for the purposes

of obtaining an MA by or on behalf of a pharmaceutical company, or by doctors or academics) should be subject to prior ethical review. This situation changed with the implementation of the Clinical Trials Directive and the associated GCP and GMP Directives by the Medicines for Human Use (Clinical Trial) Regulations 2004, as amended.[16] There are now extensive provisions relating to the requirement for and obtaining of an ethics committee opinion and regarding the establishment and registration of ethics committees.

Pharmaceutical company-sponsored research conducted in the UK (and other Member States) for purposes of regulatory submission has always been affected by the requirement that the data derived from studies in humans, which are submitted as part of an authorisation application, must have been generated in a study conducted according to standards of GCP. The UK implementing legislation also refers to the GCP provisions in the GCP Directive. Compliance with GCP is enforced by GCP inspections of trial and other related sites by competent authorities which are mandated by the Clinical Trials Directive. A further sanction provided by the law is that the competent authorities may discount any data not generated in accordance with good practice standards during their evaluation of a product. (This would clearly include studies that had not been ethically reviewed.) In the case of a pivotal study, this could be crucial to the success of the application, and therefore constitutes a strong incentive to comply with the practice standards set out in the guidelines.

GCP is also relevant in the context of any claims for personal injury. In the assessment of whether negligence has occurred, compliance with accepted practice guidelines is relevant to judging whether a sponsor (or investigator) has acted reasonably or in a manner that falls below accepted current standards of conduct, which, as stated, are likely to be the EU-adopted ICH guidelines for trials conducted in the European Union and the GCP Directive. As stated, law and ethics coincide in their aim to protect the interests of volunteers recruited for clinical research purposes. The issues of consent, confidentiality and access to compensation for personal injury tend to be uppermost in the minds of lawyers and ethicists, while the need to design and perform clinical trials with a view to generating cost-effectiveness data which can be submitted for purposes of health technology assessment (rather than just regulatory evaluation) is increasingly an important consideration for pharmaceutical companies.

15.2.1.3 Consent

In both legal and ethical terms, the consent of an individual to his or her participation in research is fundamental. There are few exceptions to this 'golden rule'. For research performed within the NHS the *Research Governance Framework for Health and Social Care*[17] reiterates this principle and requires prior consent to be obtained from participating patients in most cases. The Clinical Trials Directive (Articles 3–5) and the UK implementing legislation lay down a specific requirement for the consent of the trial subject or his or her 'legal representative' to participation in any 'clinical trial' (as defined widely by the legislation). In the UK, failure to adhere to the principles of GCP, which include the requirements for consent, is a criminal offence. Failure to obtain consent could also give rise to civil claims for damages, for example, on the basis of assault and battery, or trespass to the person. Failure adequately to inform a participant about a study may also undermine the consent given and constitute negligence, for which, again, a claim for damages in respect of any personal injury suffered as a consequence may lie. In these cases, the individual would have to show that the receipt of more complete information would have resulted in their withholding consent, thereby avoiding exposure to the risk of the hazard that in fact materialised.

For consent to be legally valid, a volunteer (or legal representative) must be competent to assess the proposed research and to make a considered decision. They must be properly informed (the term 'informed consent' is often used although, strictly speaking, it is tautologous, as it is not possible to have consent that is legally recognised, which is uninformed in the legal sense), that is, they must have been given 'sufficient' accurate information to appreciate the nature of the study: what would be involved in participation and what hazards and level of risk attach to the project in question. The decision must be made voluntarily without the exertion of any pressure, or influence from other persons. There must be no incentive offered that would encourage an individual to agree to what, in other circumstances, he or she would refuse. Reliable 'evidence' that a consent process has been properly followed and consent properly obtained is valuable for legal and ethical reasons. The Clinical Trials Directive defines informed consent as a 'decision which must be written' (Article 2(j)) and makes consent in writing the norm, except in 'exceptional cases as provided for in national legislation' (Article 3.2(d)).

There are, of course, some cases where the consent of the trial subject cannot be obtained. This may be because the individual is not competent to make a decision, either because of some mental illness or intellectual deficit, or because of injury resulting in unconsciousness. The legislation addresses the position of both incompetent minors (under-16s in the UK) and incompetent adults, setting specific conditions that must be met and the requirements for obtaining the consent of a legal representative. In the UK, the concept of a legal representative who may consent on behalf of an incompetent adult is a new one and applies only in the field of research and not, as yet, in relation to cases of treatment and therapy.

The rules in the UK for consent on behalf of minors to participation in research are now different from those that apply to consent to treatment. The law in relation to research classifies minors as under 16 years and requires the consent of a person with parental responsibility or other legal representative, although the 'explicit wish' of a minor should be considered by an investigator, there are no 'Gillick competent' minors capable of consenting in their own right in the legislation. In the Gillick case[18] (concerning the prescribing of contraceptives to teenage girls), the UK courts accepted that minors might be fully capable of consenting in their own right to treatment procedures, provided that, in the view of the doctor concerned, they had grasped the nature of the treatment and its potential benefits and risks and were sufficiently mature intellectually and emotionally to make a judgement.

15.2.1.4 Confidentiality

It is a clear ethical principle that the privacy of the individual should be respected and maintained. The law too, both in common law (i.e. judge-made law) and through certain statutory provisions (specifically Member States' implementation of the 1995 Directive on the protection of personal data 95/46/EEC), recognises a right to confidentiality in personal data. In the UK, there have been practice rules[19] within the NHS for several years and more recently, legislation has been enacted (to address issues concerning health data stored in special registries and databases) concerning the treatment and confidentiality of medical records. All electronically recorded data must be stored and handled by persons or institutions registered under the Data Protection Act of 1998. The 'processing' of such data (which is widely interpreted to include the act of anonymisation) must be performed in compliance with the principles of good practice that the Act lays down. The Clinical Trials

Directive also makes specific the need to adhere to the rules of personal data protection in the clinical trial context (Article 3.2(c)).

At common law, a right to confidentiality can arise either because of:

1. The nature of the information;
2. The circumstances in and conditions under which it is imparted; or
3. The status of the person to whom the information is given (e.g. a doctor).

The concern is with data that identify an individual, or from which an unnamed person could be identified. The common law upholds the right to confidentiality by providing that disclosure of confidential information, without the consent of the person concerned, is a breach of that right and may be subject to civil penalty (e.g. damages or even an injunction to prevent disclosure, i.e. breach). In cases where the maintenance of confidentiality in certain data is a contractual obligation, such as in employment contracts, a breach of confidence may lead to disciplinary action and/or loss of employment. Professional codes of conduct may also give rise to other sanctions (e.g. General Medical Council proceedings).

There are a few circumstances in which confidentiality will not be deemed to have been breached so as to give rise to legal sanctions. These include situations where disclosure is warranted as a matter of public interest (although this is interpreted restrictively) and also where disclosure is ordered within court proceedings.

In the context of research in individuals, all personal data should be safely and securely stored and handled. Confidentiality should also be assured by ensuring that no publication of study results includes any identifying personal information with regard to study subjects. Participants should be well aware, from the outset, of the extent of disclosure that will be necessary with regard to their 'sensitive' personal data, to whom it will be disclosed and for what purpose, and should agree to this when they sign a consent form after being given full information about the project. Where the subject agrees to disclosure to identified persons, disclosure will not constitute a breach of confidence. For this reason, specification of the scope of disclosure, the purpose and the types of people who may need to have sight of trial data, is extremely important. With express consent, there is no issue with regard to breach of an individual's confidence. However, in some cases data obtained may subsequently have value in the context of a different piece of secondary research. The issue then is whether the original consent obtained was sufficiently broad to cover use for the further purposes. This will be a matter of the wording used previously (and, possibly, what might be implied), but consent is referable only to the matters disclosed (whether specifically or generally) to the individual. In most research, where individuals are recruited to a study, issues of confidentiality should not create practical, ethical or legal problems. However, in pure records-based research, where gathering large numbers of individual consents is not practical and in the absence of specific enabling provisions in legislation, there remain issues surrounding the protection of confidentiality. Anonymisation of data is a possible solution or conduct of studies under the limited provisions of the National Health Act 2006 (applicable in England and Wales only) which permit patient confidentiality to be overridden in the context of records-based research that meets criteria laid out in the statute and that has been specifically authorised.

15.2.2 Conditional marketing authorisations

The requirement in the legislation for acceptable clinical data to support an MA application has certain limited flexibility. Since April 2006, Regulation 507/2006 has permitted conditional MAs of 1 year's validity (and for restricted categories of products) in cases where there are unmet medical needs and where the benefits of immediate availability outweigh the risks inherent in the absence of a full clinical data set. The legal basis for conditional MAs was already present in Regulation 726/2004.[20] Regulation 507/2006, however, fleshes out the provisions for granting and renewing such authorisations.

Although it remains possible to grant an MA subject to certain conditions, such as obligations to perform specified post-market clinical safety studies, the provisions for conditional MAs give some further degree of flexibility to authorise products at a Community level, where, despite a positive risk–benefit balance, complete data are not available at the date of the application for MA (i.e. in circumstances where the application would otherwise fail). Conditions include requirements that the conditional MA holder completes or initiates certain studies with a view to providing the outstanding data; enhanced pharmacovigilance and also risk management obligations. Conditional MAs are therefore not intended to remain conditional indefinitely, but rather to be replaced by a full MA once the missing data are provided and found acceptable.

15.2.3 Paediatric Use Regulation

The Paediatric Use Regulation 1901/2006 has imposed significant clinical testing and filing obligations for innovator companies. The Regulation came into force with direct effect in January 2007 with the aim of facilitating the development and accessibility of medicinal products for children. This followed a long debate concerning the relative ethics of testing drugs on children – who are not legally competent to give informed consent or possibly to realise the significance of risk–benefit – and the risk of prescribing drugs for children on a largely off-label basis, which in consequence may not be effective or may not be administered at an appropriate dose in view of the lack of clinical information concerning the use of those products in children.

Companies with new products not previously authorised in the Community must file paediatric study results in accordance with a Paediatric Investigation Plan, previously agreed with the Paediatric Committee (PDCO) at the European Medicines Agency (EMEA), or proof of a waiver or deferral for filing this data when they apply for an MA. Similarly, companies with authorised products which are covered by a supplementary protection certificate (SPC) or by a patent which is eligible for a SPC, must file comprehensive paediatric use data when applying for any variation or extension of an MA concerning a new indication, pharmaceutical form or route of administration.

The Paediatric Use Regulation is representative of the observable trend in EU products regulation towards increased transparency and disclosure obligation upon producers. As well as obligating innovator companies to disclose all paediatric studies related to products authorised in the Community by January 2008, there is also an obligation for details of paediatric studies which are conducted outside the European Economic Area in accordance with a Paediatric Investigation Plan, to be included on the EU's clinical trials data base, EudraCT. In addition, all results of clinical trials on the paediatric population are to be public.

As well as increased filing obligations upon companies and a new form of paediatric use MA (PUMA), the EC Regulation did introduce certain restricted rewards for performing relevant studies and filing the data. The potential rewards available to eligible innovator companies include extensions to the SPC for qualifying patents, data exclusivity and extensions to orphan drug market exclusivity (see also Chapter 19).

15.3 Contractual arrangements in clinical research

15.3.1 The legal background

The arrangements made for the conduct of clinical research will usually give rise to a number of legal contracts. For example, there will be a contract between a sponsor and any contract research organisation (CRO) as well as between the sponsor or CRO and the investigator and/or the institution in which the investigator works.

It would be unusual for there to be a contract between a patient participant and the sponsor or investigator, although this may arise where the participant is a private patient of the investigator. However, in the UK, in non-therapeutic research that is conducted in accordance with the Association for the British Pharmaceutical Industries (ABPI) guidelines (e.g. *Guidelines for Phase I Clinical Trials* and *Good Clinical Trial Practice*), there would normally be a written contract between the sponsor and the participant, in which the obligations on both sides are recorded, including the undertaking by the sponsor to provide compensation to a research subject in the event of trial-related injury, irrespective of fault.

15.3.2 General contractual principles

Under English law, it is not generally necessary that a contract should be in writing for it to be legally enforceable. Therefore, an oral agreement (e.g. by telephone) between a sponsor, CRO or investigator, may be valid and enforceable. However, it is always preferable to have a written agreement, as it may be very difficult to prove what the terms of an oral agreement were, and individual recollections may differ greatly.

Whether an agreement is written or oral, there are certain legal elements that must be satisfied before any agreement may be deemed to be legally enforceable. The following points form the basic requirements of a contract:

1. There must be an agreement. The normal approach to determining whether an agreement has been reached is to identify whether an 'offer' has been made by one party and accepted, on its terms, by another. The test is objective. Communications that are merely preliminary, such as requesting or giving information, or constituting merely an 'invitation to treat' (meaning encouragement given to another to make an offer), do not constitute an offer.[21] The acceptance must be a final and unqualified expression of agreement to the terms of the offer.[22] Acceptance may be

implied by conduct, but it must be communicated to the offerer.[23] A rejection terminates an offer, as does a counter-offer.

2. There must be certainty of terms. The terms of the agreement must be clear and enable the parties to ascertain their obligations.

3. There must be 'consideration'. As a rule, a promise is not binding in English law unless it is either made by deed or supported by some form of 'consideration'. Consideration can be shown if both parties are each bound to contribute 'something of value'. This is usually money, goods or services.[24] It is normally not difficult to identify the consideration flowing between the parties to commercial transactions. In the context of clinical research, a sponsor will, among other promises, provide information, pay fees and disbursements and provide products, while the investigator will give professional services.

4. There must be an intention to create legal relations. The parties must intend their agreement to be legally binding. This is not usually an issue in commercial transactions.

It is not essential that the legal contract is contained in a single document. Quite often, for example, a research agreement will cross-refer to a protocol and standard operating procedures (SOPs), which are to be treated as being incorporated into the terms of the agreement. However, it does simplify matters by having the terms in one document, particularly if a query or dispute arises.

In order to ensure minimum standards are adhered to, certain terms are implied by law into any contract for the supply of goods or services unless they are expressly excluded.[25] The actual terms of the agreement may 'exceed' the minimum standards implied. For example, it would be implied by statute that services supplied in the course of a business must be carried out with reasonable skill and care. These terms may be substituted by more specific terms agreed between the parties or by a course of dealing.

One further basic point, which is an important principle in contract terms, is that, in general, English law applies a doctrine of 'privity' to contracts. This means that a contract only binds the parties to it. Therefore, a contract between sponsor and CRO does not bind the investigator or any other person. Historically, only the parties (or their appointed representatives or legal substitutes) could enforce or sue upon an agreement. However, this has been changed by the Contracts (Rights of Third Parties) Act 1999, which enables an entity that is not a party to the agreement to enforce or sue upon the agreement in circumstances where either the contract expressly provides that they can do so or the terms of the agreement are intended to confer a benefit on them.[26]

15.3.3 Background to the standard clinical trial contract

Clinical trials supported by the pharmaceutical and biopharmaceutical industry are generally categorised in two ways:

1. *Contract Clinical Trials* are defined as commercial industry-sponsored trials of investigational medicinal products, involving NHS patients, undertaken in NHS hospitals, usually directed towards pharmaceutical product licensing;

2. *Collaborative Clinical Research*, on the other hand, is primarily carried out for academic rather than commercial reasons and is not usually directed towards product licensing.

Contracts dealing with collaborative clinical research are generally still individually negotiated between the company providing resources for the trial (which may, for example, include financial support or the provision of drug supplies) and the holder of the investigator's substantive employment contract. However, contracts for commercial clinical trials that involve current NHS patients and that are conducted in NHS hospitals, between the sponsor and the NHS site or 'trust', have in recent years been standardised.

The Department of Health and the ABPI, amongst others, drew up a model clinical trial agreement in 2003,[27] which was updated in 2006, for use in the UK (mCTA 2006).[28] This is a standard form of contract between the NHS trust and the pharmaceutical company, the 'sponsor', concerning commercial clinical trials, other than phase 1 trials involving healthy volunteers, taking place in NHS hospitals with NHS patients. In addition, a tripartite agreement between the NHS trust, sponsor and CRO as parties was released in 2007 (mCTA 2007).[29] The mCTA 2007 covers the same provisions as the mCTA 2006 except that these trials are managed by CROs.

The templates were created with the aim of decreasing the time to market for new medicinal products and to make the UK a more competitive location for clinical research. The assumption was that parties would not have to spend so much time and money in negotiating the clinical contract and so trials could be set up faster and more cheaply.

The balance between the NHS trust and the sponsor has been altered in the mCTA 2006 and mCTA 2007 from that set out in the 2003 template, especially with regards to intellectual property (IP) rights and risk allocation. This has made some sponsors wary of using unamended mCTAs. However, some NHS trusts will not accept modifications to the mCTA, so sponsors who are not willing to take on further risks have been forced to leave trial sites. There are not enough data yet to speculate with any certainty whether the use of the templates as unamended contracts will take hold across the industry.

Although the use of mCTA 2006 and mCTA 2007 is not mandatory, the Department of Health, the ABPI and the BioIndustry Association (BIA), amongst others, recommend that the templates are used without modification. However, the use of standard form contracts is not always appropriate. The relevant parties will need to consider whether it is sensible to use the mCTA 2006 or mCTA 2007 given the specific arrangement between the parties, and, if so, whether any amendments are required. In particular, parties should take care when choosing to use the tripartite mCTA 2007 over the bipartite mCTA 2006, as the sponsor might not want the CRO to have all the rights outlined for it in the mCTA 2007.

Whether the parties adopt one of the standard mCTA templates or not, the parties should consider the following non-exhaustive list of matters when drafting any clinical trail agreement.

15.3.4 Issues the parties should consider when negotiating a clinical trial agreement

15.3.4.1 Parties to the clinical trial agreement

Under the mCTA 2006, the parties are the sponsor and trust. While the sponsor will not enter into a contract with the investigator of the trial, the sponsor will want to make it clear what is to be expected of the investigator and so their duties will be stipulated in the CTA. Responsibility will generally devolve on the trust to ensure the investigator does what he or she is required to do under the CTA and the trust shall seek to carry out this duty by incorporating such responsibilities into the investigator's employment contract. Where the investigator is not the employee of the relevant NHS trust, the trust must inform his or her employer and get the employer's permission to participate in the conduct of the trial.

Under the mCTA 2007 the parties are the sponsor, the trust and the CRO. There are further provisions in the mCTA 2007 outlining how the duties are to be divided between the sponsor and the CRO and to which body the trust should refer certain matters. These duties tend to be tailored in each case.

15.3.4.2 Clinical trial governance

Clinical trials must be conducted in accordance with a number of laws and regulations, such as the Data Protection Act 1998, the Medicines Act 1968 and the Medicines for Human Use (Clinical Trial) Regulations 2004. In addition, the sponsor should comply with all ABPI guidelines, in particular those entitled Clinical Trial Compensation Guidelines (1991). Consequently, there must be a clause in the CTA that obliges the parties to follow these laws, regulations and guidelines and in particular to make clear whether adherence is confined to those laws that are domestic or extend to foreign laws as well; for example, when the trial is to be conducted as part of an investigational new drug (IND) (i.e. connected to an application for licensing by the US Food and Drug Administration).

There will be a clinical trial protocol, the Protocol, which provides very good guidance and structure as to how the trial should be conducted. In general, if there is any ambiguity in the CTA, the parties should be made to refer to the Protocol for guidance and the Protocol should prevail over the terms of the CTA in such scenarios. However, the mCTA 2006 gives precedence over the Protocol to its own provisions in respect of certain issues, such as liabilities/indemnities, confidentiality, data protection, freedom of information, publication and IP. It must be borne in mind, however, that any obligations the ethics committee places upon the conduct of the trial should take precedence over both the Protocol and the CTA.

15.3.4.3 Obligations of the parties

The sponsor and the trust want to get trials up and running as quickly as possible, but this has led to problems with trials being commenced before all the necessary authorisations have been secured. One of the aims with developing the mCTA 2006 was to resolve this issue. Consequently, the mCTA 2006 provides that sponsors cannot supply the investigational medical product (IMP) to the site until all the approvals are obtained and the ethics committee has sanctioned the trial. It also states which parties should be seeking what clearance and who should be monitoring the obtaining of necessary authorisations.

Generally, parties to a clinical trial will want some flexibility with regards to how they wish to conduct the trial. As the trial progresses, an issue may arise that means parts of the Protocol and CTA need to be amended. The danger of altering the trial structure is that the financial arrangements for the trial might not be simultaneously adjusted to meet the new outline.

Thus, in the mCTA 2006 there is a dual process whereby when the investigator initiates changes, the sponsor must restructure the finances at the same time.

Other general obligations of the parties throughout the trial should also be dealt with. For example, the mCTA 2006 states that the trust will probably be required to use its best endeavours to ensure that the investigator recruits a sufficient number of patients. It also states that the IMP can only be used for the conduct of the trial and any unused IMP must be disposed of as outlined in the contract. For all the obligations it is good to have a realistic timeline so the parties have some structure to work to. This could specify how the sponsor and trust are to divide responsibilities and what the parties are to do if timings are not met.

15.3.4.4 Provision of indemnity

The sponsor should consider indemnifying the trust in relation to a claim for compensation for personal injury that may be made against the trust by a research subject in the event of trial-related injury or death. Under the mCTA 2006, if a claim for personal injury is made, the sponsor shall indemnify and hold the trust and its employees and agents harmless against all such claims: (a) brought by, or on behalf of, research subjects taking part in a study; and (b) arising out of, or relating to, the administration of the product(s) under investigation, or any clinical intervention or procedure provided for or required by the Protocol, to which the subject would not have been exposed, but for his or her participation in the study. Among other things it is conditional upon compliance with the Protocol, there having been no negligence or other default on the part of the investigator, staff, institution, etc., and upon the sponsor being promptly informed of claims (actual and potential) and having the right to conduct the claims.

15.3.4.5 Limitations of liabilities

The issue of liability must be dealt with because of the likelihood of damage that could occur to the property and facilities of the parties during the trial. Trusts will be particularly wary of facing unlimited claims by the sponsor for breaches of issues such as IP rights so a solution has been attempted in the mCTA 2006 by introducing a two-tiered structure for any liability claims. First, for wilful or deliberate breaches of the CTA and any breach of clauses relating to confidentiality, publication and IP, the trust's liability to the sponsor will be limited to a maximum of twice the value of the contract. The value of the contract is the sum of total payments to be made by the sponsor to the NHS if all the target number of patients are recruited to trial. Secondly, for all other breaches, the trust's liability to the sponsor is capped to no more than the value of the agreement.

From the perspective of the sponsor, the mCTA 2006 liability structure is problematical. The sponsor could end up without adequate compensation cover if its IP rights are breached or if the trial is not conducted according to the necessary regulations, so the results cannot be used as extensively as the sponsor intended.

15.3.4.6 Confidentiality and freedom of information

The parties must work out how to look after and store confidential information and how the information will be used. Generally, the parties will agree to adhere to the principles of medical confidentiality in relation to the patients in the clinical trials. Personal data will not be disclosed to the sponsor by the trust unless this is required under the Protocol or in order to monitor adverse event reporting. In addition, the trust will be subject to the Freedom of Information Act 2000 (FOIA). Sponsors will not want to disclose sensitive information, so the trusts and hospitals must consult with them about any requests for information that they receive. Consequently, the parties should agree on a process with regards to giving the sponsor notice of a FOIA request and to what extent the sponsor can reasonably restrict information that is requested. The mCTA contains an outline about how to deal with such requests.

However, certain information will need to be disclosed. For example, the trust and investigator must publish results under the *Research Governance Framework for Health and Social Care*.[17] There should be a clause in the CTA that acknowledges that the parties must comply with these guidelines.

15.3.4.7 Intellectual property

The sponsor and the trust should consider carefully who will have what rights to any IP generated during the course of the trial. Under the mCTA 2006 there are a few basic principles that have been adopted. First, each party retains ownership of any pre-existing IP owned by it or licensed to it. Secondly, any IP generated at the trial site that relates to the clinical trial, IMP or the Protocol (but excluding any clinical procedure or related improvements) shall be owned by the sponsor. Thirdly, clinical procedures and related improvements are owned by the trust and depending on the inventor's employer, could be protected and exploited accordingly. Finally, the trust also has the right to use know how obtained during the trial in its normal clinical work, provided it does not result in disclosure of the sponsor's confidential information.

15.3.4.8 Term of the CTA and early termination

The CTA should make clear what the term of the agreement will be and specifically what will be the grounds for early termination. Typical grounds for termination under any contract would include failure by one party to carry out its obligations or insolvency. Additional scenarios in the context of a CTA would include that covered by the mCTA 2007, namely that both the CRO and the sponsor can terminate the contract if the clinical investigator leaves and no satisfactory replacement is found. The CRO should have a right to terminate the agreement, presumably acting upon the instructions of the sponsor. However, this right creates issues as the CRO also has the right under the mCTA 2007 to object to a replacement investigator. If the CRO can block the replacement of an investigator and then terminate the contract should no replacement be appointed, this means the CRO has a unilateral termination right when an investigator leaves.

15.4 Post-authorisation – controls and protection of investment

15.4.1 Regulatory controls

After a product has been authorised, the regulatory system operates to keep the quality, safety and efficacy of that product under review and to control the way in which it is manufactured, marketed and distributed. The pharmaceutical legislation in Europe was consolidated in 2004 and the majority of the amendments came into effect in October/November 2005. Since then the Advanced Therapy Medicinal Products Regulation (1394/2007), which will come into effect between the end of December 2008 and the end of December 2011, has introduced intensified post-authorisation controls for products within its scope, especially in the area of traceability, post-authorisation follow-up, pharmacovigilance and risk management.

Manufacturers of medicinal products (this includes those who undertake full or partial manufacture of the product, and those who package or 'assemble' the product) must have site-specific manufacturing authorisations and are subject to regular plant and system inspections where they are judged against appropriate standards, in particular GMP rules under Commission Directive 2003/94/EC and are subject to GMP inspections by competent authorities. Any subcontracting undertaken by a manufacturer of a manufacturing process (or any part of it) must be subject to a detailed technical agreement between the parties, setting out the specification for the work and the responsibilities, as they are divided between the parties, so as to ensure that all aspects of the process are properly conducted in compliance with the legal and regulatory requirements. Manufacturers of active pharmaceutical ingredients (APIs) do not generally require a manufacturing authorisation but MA holders are legally obliged to source APIs only from API manufacturers that operate in accordance with API GMP guidelines.

Those undertaking wholesale dealing activities must similarly hold an appropriate authorisation[30] and are also subject to site and system inspection to ensure that they are operating in accordance with legal requirements, including Good Distribution Practice (GDP) rules established under Directive 2001/83/EEC (Article 76–85). Specified paperwork and records must be kept (in particular to facilitate tracing of product and batch recall) and proper systems and operating procedures must be adhered to.

For the MA holder, there are numerous obligations and conditions attaching to the authorisation and, as with all authorisations held under pharmaceutical legislation, failure to comply will lead to regulatory enforcement action. Although this is still largely undertaken at Member State level, the introduction of the Financial Penalties Regulation (see section 15.4.1.8) for centrally authorised products means Community MA holders may additionally face regulatory enforcement action at an EU level for infringements of conditions attaching to a Community MA.

There is a tendency in European pharmaceutical legislation to assign compliance duties to an identified service or a particular individual operating on behalf of, or within the MA holder's organisation. For example, a manufacturer must have 'permanently and continuously at his disposal' a 'qualified person' whose personal responsibility it is to test product and certify it as conforming to the authorised specification before it is placed on the EU market. In some Member States, where breach of certain regulatory requirements is subject to criminal sanction, this approach has an obvious 'advantage' in terms of enforcement and in encouraging compliance. For example, MA holders must also have a person established within the Community who will take responsibility for the system for conducting pharmacovigilance and safety monitoring of the MA holder's products in the market. This involves collecting and reviewing data, making reports to the competent authorities and generating corporate decisions about how best to respond to signals arising as a result of safety monitoring (e.g. whether to make labelling changes to include new or stronger warnings, contraindications, precautions) or whether a problem warrants the restriction of the product in the marketplace (e.g. sales to hospitals and specialist clinics only) or the total or partial removal of the product from the distribution chain.[31]

MA holders must also establish 'within' their organisation an information and scientific service to serve the needs and requirements of the competent authorities and health care professionals using, prescribing and supplying product.[32] Although the legal text does not require the naming of a specific individual, nevertheless the identification of the service and its location and capabilities is becoming part of the information requirements of the competent authorities in considering the suitability of an application for an MA, and of the applicant as a potential MA holder (see Application Form Module in Notice to Applicants Part 2B, of the Rules Governing Medicinal Products in the European Union). The trend in pharmaceutical legislation (in part designed to try to achieve levels of harmonisation across Member States in the interests of promoting free movement of pharmaceutical goods) is to streamline the production and supply of product and to ensure public health protection by requiring the responsible party to be accessible to the authorities and readily identifiable within the Community.

15.4.1.1 Safety

The handling of product safety crises is generally handled at Community level. Serious concerns with regard to product safety – where the product is on the market of more than one Member State – will be considered at European level. Centralised product issues are automatically a matter for the EMEA and therefore the Committee for Medicinal Products for Human Use (CHMP), including its working parties. In respect of products that may have been authorised nationally (including through mutual recognition), the legislation (Regulation 726/2004 and Directive 2001/83/EC) mainly provides for references to the CHMP for the resolution of European concerns and the implementation of an EU-wide solution.

15.4.1.2 Relationship between local and European laws

All national legislation must be consistent and read in line with European legislation. National legislation that is at odds with European law cannot generally be relied upon locally. EC law now covers almost all aspects of pharmaceutical development, manufacture and supply. However, there is still variation in the approach of Member States to the determination of whether a product is a 'medicinal product' falling within the European pharmaceutical legislation, or whether it should be classified as some other product type (e.g. a food, medical device or cosmetic), despite the existence of the definition of 'medicinal product' in Article 1.2 of Directive 2001/83/EC. Within the Community, it still remains possible to see the same products accorded different classifications, and therefore supplied subject to the rules of different regulatory regimes, in different Member States.

15.4.1.3 Advertising, labelling and legal status

There are specific sets of European controls, implemented by national laws, concerning product advertising, labelling and leafleting, and their legal status for purposes of supply (see Directive 2001/83/EC Titles VIII, VIIIa, V and VI, respectively).

15.4.1.4 Advertising

There have been European controls on the advertising of medicinal products for human use since the early 1990s and these are currently contained in the amended Directive 2001/83/EC. In the light of disparities in practice concerning patient access to information about medicinal products, the Commission has consulted during 2007–2008 on this issue with a view to putting forward legislative proposals by the end of 2008. At the time of writing, these proposals appear likely to aim at harmonising practices across the Member States on the provision of information to patients (including via the internet) and creating a framework for companies to provide specified non-advertising information on medicines to the public, subject to specific quality criteria and to monitoring by national co-regulatory bodies overseen by national competent authorities and possibly also by an EU advisory committee to facilitate harmonised practice across Europe.[33]

Particular objectives in the current legislation involve the moderation of advertising directed at members of the public and the setting of high standards with regard to advertising and promotion directed at 'health care professionals' (a term that is broadly interpreted in the UK to include, for example, administrators with purchasing responsibility in hospitals and clinics). There are also limits upon the supply of free samples by companies, and requirements to ensure that companies have the resources to provide objective information to those health care professionals who require it. It also requires Member States to set up systems through which to monitor and enforce the advertising controls.

The important first principle with regard to advertising and promotion is that it cannot be undertaken in respect of any unauthorised product. Not only does this include products in respect of which there is no authorisation to market at all, but it also means that there can be no advertising of products for unauthorised indications; for those purposes, products are treated as being without a registration.

Further, the term 'advertising' is very broadly defined[34] and the intent behind an activity – that is, whether it is 'designed to promote the prescription, supply, sale or consumption of medicinal products' – is material in assessing an activity or printed material. Certain items are specifically excluded from the scope of the Directive: labelling and package leaflets; correspondence and material of a non-promotional nature needed to answer a specific question about a product; factual and informative announcements; reference material relating to pack changes; adverse reaction warnings, etc.; and statements concerning health and disease that are not referable (even indirectly) to individual medicinal products. The Commission proposals due in 2008 may further clarify the distinction to be drawn between advertising and information.

There can be no advertising to the public of products available on prescription only or that are intended and designed for use only with the intervention of a medical practitioner. There can also be no supply of samples to the public for promotional purposes. The Directive also produces a very significant list of 'don'ts' with regard to the content of advertising material.

Some of the more controversial provisions are contained in the sections of the Directive relating to advertising to health professionals, and in particular the extent to which pharmaceutical companies may support and sponsor pharmaceutical conferences and offer hospitality, gifts, etc. in the promotional context. The fundamental limitations that the EC legislation introduces include the following:

1. All advertising to health professionals must include certain 'essential information compatible with the summary of product characteristics or SPC'.

2. Medical sales representatives must be given adequate training and must have SPCs available for the products they promote at all visits to medical practitioners. They are also under an obligation to pass on information they receive with regard to the use of the product, and in particular suspected adverse reactions, to their employers.

3. No gifts, 'pecuniary advantages' or benefits in kind may be supplied, offered or promised to health care professionals 'unless they are inexpensive and relevant to the practice of medicine or pharmacy'.

4. Hospitality available at sales promotions must always be reasonable in level and secondary to the main purposes of the meeting. It may be offered only to health care professionals.

5. No health care professionals may solicit or accept inducements prohibited by the Directive.

6. Hospitality may be offered at events for professional and scientific purposes provided it is reasonable in level and subordinate to the scientific objective of the meeting. Again, it cannot be extended to persons other than health care professionals.

7. There are limits on the number of free samples for prescription-only products that may be left with practitioners each year and, in any event, these must be supplied in response to a written request from the recipient.

The current trend in the UK is for regulators to seek to take a restrictive line in the enforcement of advertising controls. In particular, since late 2005 and following a Parliamentary committee report, the UK competent authority (MHRA) has undertaken pre-vetting of advertising for all new active substances for 3–6 months following launch. In the UK, it has long been the case that the ABPI (for 'ethicals' manufacturers) and the Proprietary Association of Great Britain (PAGB) (for the over-the-counter (OTC) products manufacturers) have each participated in a voluntary 'system' of advertising review, monitoring and control. In the case of the ABPI, which has its own detailed Code of Advertising Practice, a quasi-judicial process for reviewing and dealing with complaints against member companies with regard to advertising practices is operated by the Prescription Medicines Code of Practice Authority (which is independent of the ABPI), to whom complaints are directed, whether from industry, practitioners or other individuals. The PAGB is organised to pre-vet advertising and promotional material with a view to averting breaches of advertising rules in the UK. Advertising regulations to implement EC law were introduced into the UK in 1994 (see also Chapter 12).[35]

15.4.1.5 Labelling

Leaflets and labelling requirements are part of Directive 2001/83/EC (with adapted requirements for advanced therapy medicinal products being set out in Regulation 1394/2007). These require patient information leaflets to be placed in all product packaging, and specify the content and the order of the content for such leaflets. They also require MA holders to consult with target patient groups when developing package leaflets in order to promote 'readability' by patients.[36]

The function of a leaflet is twofold: to help a patient to recognise the fact, and to cope with the consequences in the event, of side effects or problems arising; but also to allow them to decide whether to take or continue to take a product in the light of information provided. There are also specific requirements for the labelling of external, 'immediate' and container packaging for all pharmaceutical products (including Braille labelling), with the particular concern that the patient should be able to identify the product and the responsible source of the product within the European Community.

The provisions with regard to labelling do allow for differences between labels for products destined for different Member States. Such variations are intended to be located in one place on a product label, which has come to be known as the 'blue box'. Within the blue box, Member States are allowed to require information about the price of the product, reimbursement conditions, legal status and other information that goes to product 'identification and authenticity'. This permissive aspect of the Directive is notable, as it means that even in relation to products that have been authorised through the centralised procedure, where the authorisation is in all other respects identical, it is rarely possible to produce one label that (when translated) is acceptable and appropriate for every Member State in which the product will be marketed. It also tends to make less attractive the multilanguage label, where the combination of two or more languages and the different information required in the blue box, make design and printing overly complicated, expensive and/or impractical.

In the UK, the leaflet and labelling requirements are incorporated into UK law through the Medicines for Human Use (Marketing Authorisations Etc) Regulations 1994.[37] Under Regulation 4:

Every application for the grant renewal or variation of a [UK] marketing authorisation for a relevant medicinal product shall be made in accordance with the relevant Community provisions … and the applicant shall comply with so much of the relevant Community provisions as impose obligations on applicants as are applicable to the application or the consideration of it'. [Under Regulation 7] every holder of a [UK] marketing authorisation for a relevant medicinal product shall comply with all obligations which relate to him by virtue of the relevant Community provisions (apart from Regulation 726/2004) including in particular obligations relating to providing or updating information to making changes to applying to vary the authorisation to pharmacovigilance and to labels and package leaflets.

This represents a fairly common approach in the UK to the implementation of European legislation, which is either to cross-refer to the relevant European provisions, as here, or to 'import' the text of the European provisions directly and without alteration into the relevant implementing local statutory instrument. From a legal point of view, this approach can give rise to some difficulties in the event of complaints or disputes, as the drafting of European legislation is undertaken on a rather different basis from that in the UK, where a very literal approach is taken to the interpretation of precise wording. By contrast, European provisions are written more loosely and are intended to be read in line with the stated rationale of the legislation (i.e. the recitals in the Directive or Regulation), rather than by strict reference to the wording used. It is a fact of life that the implementation of European legislation can result in rather different provisions across Member States, each of which interprets the legislation according to its own understanding.

From a liability point of view, MA holders need to bear in mind that the way they present a product (not just its standard of manufacture or inherent design), both to the professionals and to patients, whether through direct advertising to patients of OTC products or through the label and patient information leaflet, is an area upon which focus will be placed in the event of a claim for personal injury that appears to have been caused or contributed to by shortcomings in product presentation or information. Such shortcomings can amount to a 'defect' in the product and/or to a manifestation of negligence, and could be sufficient to justify a claim for damages.

15.4.1.6 Status

The classification provisions at Title VI of the amended Directive 2001/83/EC lay down the criteria to be applied in determining whether a product should be available on prescription only (or subject to restricted limited supply) or available without prescription. These provisions continue to allow Member States to preserve multitier categorisation of product, such as applies in the UK, where a product may be prescription only, pharmacy only or on 'general sale'.

15.4.1.7 Civil litigation

The health care industries have historically seen a very high level (relatively speaking) of personal injury suits (often multiparty), with claims based both on negligence and under the Consumer Protection Act 1987 (which implemented the Product Liability Directive of 1985). The cases tend to be complex scientifically, with causation being a particular issue, both as to the general and to the specific arguments; that is, can the product in question cause the injuries alleged and, if so, did the product cause the injuries in the specific case? The changes made in the UK to the process of litigation pursuant to the Woolf Report; the increasingly controlled availability of legal aid and conditional fees will all have an impact upon the incidence of claims in years to come. However, in ensuring regulatory compliance, in determining corporate policy and practice, and in all aspects of manufacturing and sales, companies seek to limit the public's exposure and hence their own exposure to the risks of avoidable personal injury.

15.4.1.8 Financial penalties

Although most regulatory compliance enforcement still occurs at Member State level, the Commission has powers to impose fines upon Community MA holders, which resemble those granted to the EU competition authorities. In June 2007, the Commission adopted Regulation 658/2007 which details how the powers, already granted to it under Regulation 726/2004 to impose financial penalties for infringement of certain obligations in connection with Community MAs, may be exercised. These powers relate to infringements by the Community MA holder which are either intentional or derive from negligence and which belong to one of the following categories:

1. Inaccurate submissions to the EMEA;
2. Breach of the conditions and obligations contained in the MA;
3. Breach of post-marketing obligations; or
4. Breach of pharmacovigilance obligations.

The decision to initiate the required prior inquiry procedure lies with the EMEA, although this can be in response to requests received from Member States or the Commission as well as upon its own initiative.

Where the Commission finds that the Community MA holder has committed, intentionally or negligently, an infringement, it may adopt a decision imposing fines up to specified maximum percentages based upon average annual (or, in the case of continuing infringements or a failure to cooperate during the preceding inquiry procedure, average daily) Community-wide turnover during the preceding business year. A further concern to companies is the potential for 'double jeopardy', as in some cases the same infringement can be penalized at both EU level under this Regulation as well as under Member States' national laws.

15.4.2 Protecting investment

15.4.2.1 Intellectual property

There are other aspects to the maintenance of a product in the market. The ability to protect and recoup investment is vital if new products and the development of existing products are to be sustained. IP rights provide various methods of protecting products and can be an important and a valuable asset in providing legitimate barriers against domestic and foreign competition.

The principal method of protecting 'novel' products and processes is by patents. A patent confers an absolute monopoly on the holder in the territory for which it is granted, but in order for the patent to be valid, everything covered by the patent claim must be a new invention. Patents generally last for 20 years from the date of application.

The adoption and registration (where possible) of trade marks is another important commercial decision. Any words or symbols, and in some cases sounds, smells and colour codings (e.g. the colour of capsules), that identify the goods of one manufacturer or trader and that are distinctive of those goods may be protected. A trade mark may be registered in respect of goods or of services, but will generally be protectable only if it is used, or is to be used, in the course of trade by the owner. Even an unregistered trade mark can confer a level of protection upon its holder, who may be able to bring a 'passing-off' action against a competitor using the mark in order to benefit from the reputation built up by its owner.

Copyright applies automatically to literary and artistic works, including industrial designs, plans and drawings. In the pharmaceutical industry, copyright is likely to be of lesser importance than the levels of protection afforded by patents or registered trade marks. However, copyright may be relevant to the packaging used for pharmaceutical products, both as to the layout (artistic copyright) and to the text itself as well as patient information leaflets and related material. The right exists to prohibit the unauthorised copying of the whole or a substantial part of a protected copyright work.

Finally, registered and unregistered designs should be mentioned, although they again may be of less relevance to pharmaceutical products themselves. Nevertheless, it may be possible to obtain a degree of protection for some goods by registering the designs for the packaging in which they are sold, or the shapes of the products themselves in addition to logos, typefaces and 'brand features'. The cheapest and simplest method of obtaining European Community-wide protection for a design is by registering a Community design. Because the European Community is now a full member of the World Intellectual Property Organisation (WIPO) it is now relatively easy to extend design protection across most industrialised countries.

European law applies a doctrine of 'exhaustion of rights' in relation to the use of intellectual property rights. In effect, once the right has been used with respect to a particular product by its owner (e.g. to put a patented product on the market in a Member State), the owner may not assert that right to prevent the product moving round the community thereafter. This principle limits the circumstances in which these rights may be enforced in respect of onward trade in the EU (e.g. in relation to parallel imports).

Copycat or look-alike products are of particular concern to the pharmaceutical industry. Apart from the obvious impact on the brand holder, look-alike products can distort the market and lead to confusion for consumers. The law seeks to strike the right balance between allowing genuine competition and preventing misrepresentation, deception and the gaining of an unfair advantage. There are a range of potential legal causes of action that may be open to a brand holder, including for passing off, unfair competition and infringement of trade marks, designs and/or copyright.

15.4.2.2 Patents in the UK

In order to be patentable a product or process must:
- Be new;
- Involve an inventive step;
- Be capable of industrial application; and
- Not be otherwise excluded.

To be new, the invention must never have been disclosed publicly in any way, anywhere, before the date on which an application for a patent is filed.

To have an inventive step the invention must not be obvious when compared with what is already known,

to someone with good knowledge and experience of the subject – generally referred to in the trade as the person 'skilled in the art'. Further, it must be capable of being 'industrially applied'. Patents will thus often protect an apparatus or device, a product or substance, or an industrial process or method of operation.

Various things are excluded from patentability, for example, a mathematical method, a scientific theory or a mere discovery. Also excluded are methods of treatment of humans and animals (e.g. by surgery or therapy), these being deemed to be not 'capable of industrial application'. Nevertheless, a patent may be obtained for the use of a substance/composition in any such method, if this use is otherwise novel and inventive. There are issues surrounding the patentability of various types of biotech and chemical inventions, such as stem cells, diagnostic processes, bioinformatics, second medical uses, three-dimensional protein and crystalline structures, dosing regimes, classes of compound, DNA sequences and animals.

15.4.2.3 Application for a patent

Applications can either be made separately in every country where protection is sought or under one of the international conventions that exist. The one most relevant to applicants in Europe is the European Patent Convention (EPC). Under this, an application is made to the European Patent Office, designating the signatory states in which a patent is required. This replaces the procedures in the National Patent Offices and results, upon acceptance of the application, in separate national patents in each of the designated states. All European Community Member States, amongst others, are parties. It should be noted that there is no single unitary patent available for all the European Community countries: a so-called 'Community Patent' is envisaged for the future, but is still some way off. The London Agreement has lowered the costs associated with translation for the European patent system. This is because it is no longer necessary to translate the patent into the national languages of all countries where the patent is to come into force.

The European Patent Litigation Agreement (EPLA) is a voluntary agreement, yet to be ratified by the signatories to the EPC, which would create a central European Patent Court. This would harmonise patent litigation across Europe, preventing the current patchwork of protection whereby patents can be found valid or infringing in one member state and not another.

Another relevant convention is the Patent Cooperation Treaty, to which the UK is a party along with more than 80 other members in both North and South America, Africa, Asia and the Pacific, as well as most of the EPC countries and other European countries. This facilitates making many national applications by filing in a single Patent Office. Thereafter, the individual national procedures operate independently, leading again to separate national patents.

Generally speaking, every patent application must include sufficient disclosure of the invention for it to be capable of being put into practice by the person 'skilled in the art' after its expiry. The price of a temporary monopoly is the disclosure of the invention for later general use. There is invariably a considerable delay between the date of filing an application and the eventual patent grant, during which the relevant examining officers make searches and report any relevant prior documents they may find to the applicant. The applicant may then amend the specification to take these into account to avoid claiming what is known or obvious, which leads to a further examination of the specification as amended to ensure it meets the requirements of novelty and inventive step.

A patent gives the patentee a monopoly protection during its life, but it is up to the patentee to enforce his or her rights by detecting whether someone is infringing the patent, and then initiating legal action if the matter cannot be settled.

15.4.2.4 Trade marks in the UK

A trade mark is a means of identifying the origin of goods or services. It is a symbol, whether in words or a device, or a combination of the two, that a person uses in the course of trade so that his or her goods may be readily distinguished by the purchasing public from similar goods of other traders. To achieve this, the trade mark must be distinctive in itself. Broadly, the more descriptive a trade mark is in relation to the goods to which it is applied, the less distinctive it is likely to be. The more a mark is likely to fall into common use by persons trading in goods of a similar description, the less likely it is to be distinctive. Therefore, trade marks that are increasingly used as generic descriptions of classes of goods generally lose their special qualities and protection as trade marks.

Registration of a trade mark confers a statutory monopoly over the use of that trade mark in relation to the class of goods for which it is registered (e.g. pharmaceuticals), and the registered owner has the right to sue in the courts for infringement of that mark by a person seeking to apply it, or something confusingly similar to it, to his or her own goods or services. Because registration confers this statutory monopoly, it is clear that it would not be right to allow the registration of trade marks that are identical, or that can be confused with words or symbols, which other traders in the same class of goods should be free to use in the ordinary course of business.

Goods and services are divided for registration purposes into classes, in respect of which a mark may be registered. Pharmaceuticals fall within Class 5, but the scope of many of the classes (of which there are 45) is very wide. Class 5, in fact, covers pharmaceuticals, veterinary and sanitary substances, infant foods, plasters, material for bandaging, material for filling teeth and dental wax, disinfectants and preparations for killing weeds and destroying vermin.

The simplest and cheapest way to obtain trade mark protection across the European Union is to apply for a Community Trade Mark (or CTM). The CTM system is administered through the Office of Harmonisation for the Internal Market (OHIM), and a CTM application can be made directly to OHIM in Spain, or through a national trade mark office (e.g. the UK Trade Marks Registry). Once granted, the CTM is a unitary right that takes effect throughout the EU, and EU-wide relief can be obtained against infringement.

However, opposition to a CTM application is more likely than a national application, and if the mark is refused on the basis of an earlier right in one member state it will be refused for the whole EU. Individual national registrations give greater flexibility to the applicant, but are more complex.

In many cases it will not be possible to obtain a registration of the same trade mark in all countries, for various reasons, such as the existence of conflicting marks already held by others in those countries, or owing to unfortunate associations arising in particular languages. This variation in registration opportunities means that the same product may be marketed in different parts of the European Community under different trade marks (e.g. Septrin and Eusaprim). Regulatory authorities will also review and, if acceptable, approved proposed trade marks for use with pharmaceutical products.

A registered trade mark will not generally be infringed by its use in goods that have been put on the market in the European Economic Area under that trade mark, either by the proprietor or with its consent. This prevents the trade mark proprietor from stopping further circulation of goods bearing its trade mark, once it has allowed them to be placed on the market.

However, this will not apply where there are 'legitimate reasons' for the proprietor to oppose further dealing in the goods, such as where the goods have been altered. Repackaging gives rise to difficult issues. In the pharmaceutical industry it may be necessary to repackage or relabel goods to market them in other EU countries. The courts have sought to strike a balance between the interests of the trade mark proprietor in not allowing the reputation of its trade mark to be damaged, with the principle of free movement of goods within the EU.[38] The European Court of Justice (ECJ) has laid down a set of conditions that a parallel importer must follow in order to avoid infringing the trade mark when repackaging.[39] It must be necessary to repackage to market the product; there can be no effect on the original condition of the product or instructions; the repackaging must include clear identification of manufacturer and importer; the presentation must be non-damaging; and notice must have been given to the trade mark owner before importing the repackaged goods. These conditions have been the subject of much litigation before national courts and the ECJ over recent years.

15.4.2.5 Supplementary protection certificate

Patent protection usually lasts for a period of often more than half its term 20 years. This creates a difficulty in relation to medicinal products, as it can take many years for the products to undergo research, development, the extensive clinical trials that are required in order to obtain a marketing authorisation and the authorisation process itself. These steps are also extremely expensive. The amount of time that remains during which the patent holder can exploit his or her patent and recoup his or her massive investment can be severely curtailed in relation to medicinal products. For this reason, the European Community has provided a form of additional patent-related protection for medicinal products authorised within the European Community, by means of a Supplementary Protection Certificate (SPC). A patent holder may apply for a certificate that takes effect at the end of the term of the basic patent, for a period equal to the period that elapsed between the date on which the application for the basic patent was lodged and the date of the first authorisation to place a product derived from the patent on the market in the Community, reduced by a period of 5 years. The maximum duration of the certificate is 5 years. The certificate applies to all medicinal products derived from the basic patent, but the additional time that can be obtained under the SPC is calculated in relation to the first product derived from the patent, authorised in the EU.

Example	Product A	
Patent application	1990	
Patent granted	2000	
First MA in the EU	2004	
SPC: 2004–1990	14 years less 5 years. Leaves SPC of 9 years, rounded down to the maximum 5 years, to run from 2010.	

The ECJ has ruled that an SPC will not be granted for a product that has a combination of two substances in which only one of the substances has a therapeutic effect but is already known, while the other acts to increase this therapeutic effect.[40]

However, where a medicinal product is protected by a number of basic patents, the ECJ has stated that an SPC may be granted to each holder of a basic patent.[41] This is in contrast to the US system, which only allows one extension per product.

There is an additional possible 6-month extension to an SPC as a reward for compliance with the new Paediatric Regulation.[42] This includes a requirement for data on the use of the medicine in children to be submitted at the time of applying for MA, and subject to fulfilling the conditions, the extension will be granted whether or not the drug is actually shown to be efficacious in children.

15.4.2.6 Data and market exclusivity

Irrespective of patent law, the MA holder may be afforded a period of data and marketing exclusivity under the European regulatory provisions, that is, a period of freedom from competition and competitors, who do not themselves propose to generate and submit their own full data set in order to obtain an MA. A company that applies for an MA will normally be required to produce the results of pharmacological and toxicological tests and the results of clinical trials at the cost of considerable time and expense. Similarly, in order to benefit from the usual data and market exclusivity protection, companies applying for a PUMA, introduced under the Paediatric Use Regulation (1901/2006), must submit the results of paediatric studies supporting the paediatric indication which have been performed in relation to an off-patent product in accordance with an agreed Paediatric Investigation Plan.

Under the abridged application procedure for MA, a generic drug applicant can submit an application relying on preclinical and clinical data submitted by an innovative drug manufacturer once the data exclusivity period relating to a particular drug, which has been authorised in the EU (the European reference medicinal product), has expired. The amended Directive 2001/83 and Regulation 726/2004 standardise the data exclusivity period across the EU to 8 years from the date of initial authorisation in the Community for all innovative medicinal products where the authorisation application was submitted after 30 October 2005 and authorisation applications submitted after 20 November 2005 for centrally authorised products.[43] Previously, periods of either 6 or 10 years (and in some cases even 0 years beyond patent expiration) were in force across the various EU member states. These periods will continue to apply for reference products already authorised in October/November 2005.

Although data exclusivity expires after 8 years, there then follows an additional 2 years of market exclusivity, meaning an MA application may be submitted but a generic product cannot be placed on the market until 10 years after the initial authorisation of the reference medicinal product.

Where a medicinal product has been granted an initial MA, 'any additional strengths, pharmaceutical forms, administration routes, presentations as well as variations and extensions shall be granted an authorisation', but 'shall be considered as belonging to the same global MA'. Therefore, there is no separate data or market exclusivity periods for line extensions. However, the market exclusivity period for the reference medicinal product, including any line extensions, may be extended by a maximum of 1 year if during the data exclusivity period the MA holder obtains an authorisation for one or more new therapeutic indications that provide a significant clinical benefit. Companies considering applying for this extension which are also (or will be) eligible for a 6-month SPC extension under the Paediatric Use Regulation must choose between the potential benefits of these two rewards.

The new European system of market exclusivity is informally known as the '8 + 2 + 1' regime, with the initial 8-year period of data exclusivity followed by 2 years of marketing exclusivity, with a possible extra year if additional therapeutic indications can be found.

The EU finally launched an orphan drug policy in 2000 aimed at stimulating research and availability of drugs for diseases or conditions defined as low prevalence or as likely to result in low profitability for the products in question.[44] Such products became subject

to the normal MA centralised evaluation procedures under Regulation 726/2004 in November 2005. The main regulatory incentive to pharmaceutical companies to develop and market drugs for rare diseases and conditions in the EU is a 10-year market exclusivity period during which time applications for authorisation (or extension of authorisation) of other similar products for the same orphan indication can neither be accepted nor granted other than in very limited circumstances. Thanks in part to this 10-year market exclusivity period and to a reduction in fees payable to the EMEA and other available incentives, the 5-year report on the programme in June 2006 showed that 22 designated medicines had received MAs for the treatment of 20 life-threatening or chronically debilitating illnesses while a further 170 products with an orphan designation were still in clinical trials. Since then the Paediatric Use Regulation (1901/2006) has created the possibility of a further 2-year extension to this 10-year period for companies that perform the agreed paediatric studies in relation to an orphan product in accordance with an agreed Paediatric Investigation Plan.

15.5 Compensation liability

Various laws provide for compensation (damages) to be paid to a person who suffers injury or loss as a result of using a medicine or medical device. These laws are not specific to medical products, but apply generically to all conduct or products. Three broad legal theories are relevant: breach of contract, negligence and strict product liability. Liability under each of these theories is not automatic, but depends on the claimant proving a legal right (a legal duty owed to take reasonable care or a defect in the product), causation (that the act or product caused the specific damage) and the extent of damage claimed (quantum).

The following is a brief overview of the legal rules. The laws are similar in all European jurisdictions. The main structural difference is that laws on contract and negligence (fault) are contained in codes in continental 'civil law' states, and are a mixture of legislation and court-made law in the 'common law' states of the UK and Ireland. Strict liability law in each European state conforms to the European 'Product Liability Directive'.[45] Each state has different rules on litigation procedure, causation, quantum of claimable damage, amounts awarded and 'limitation periods' after which a claim may no longer be brought.

15.5.1 Breach of contract

A claim for breach of contract can only be brought where a contract exists, and where its terms have been breached. However, there is no contract between NHS patients in the UK and the providers of NHS care, and this inhibits legal claims to the more difficult basis of negligence. Private patients may, of course, bring breach of contract claims in respect of claimable injury that occurs. Such a claim must be brought against the health care professional or entity (e.g. hospital) with whom the patient has a contract. That defendant entity may, in turn, seek to claim against those with whom it has a contract in respect of breach of, for example, a contract to supply products of a specified quality. Standard NHS supply contracts, for example, provide terms that products supplied must be of satisfactory quality.

Hence, chains of contracts usually exist along the chains of supply of products and services, and the individual terms of each one must be examined separately to see if its terms have been broken, or if it includes any terms that exclude or limit liability. At the end of each contract chain, a supplier or manufacturer will usually hold a contract of insurance with an insurer, which will provide financial cover, again depending on its terms.

15.5.1.1 Clinical research injuries

Ethical evaluation of a study automatically involves consideration being given to the provision made for the payment of compensation (if any), and the basis upon which it may be payable to a subject injured by participation in proposed research. The Clinical Trials Directive makes it a prerequisite for conducting a trial that 'provision' for insurance or indemnity has been made (Article 3.2(f)). Unlike the above position in relation to normal NHS care with licensed medicines, particular 'no fault' arrangements apply in the UK to compensation of research subjects who are injured as a result of taking part in research. Most UK ethics committees will look for confirmation of the intention to apply the ABPI Guidelines[46] in the case of company-sponsored studies, even from non-member companies and this common practice is reflected by the inclusion of the 1991 ABPI Guidelines in the model clinical trial agreement templates, which have been developed jointly by the ABPI and the Department of Health, and which are commonly employed for phase II and III clinical trials involving NHS patients in the UK.

Companies that sponsor research in phase I are required as a matter of ethical practice to enter into a written contract with each healthy volunteer research subject, including terms that the company will compensate the research subject if he or she suffers injury as a result of taking part in the trial. Where products are being investigated for unlicensed indications in phases II or III, the sponsoring company is ethically required to provide an undertaking, verified as part of the ethical review process, to provide compensation. In all phases, the amounts of compensation are to be the same as would be awarded by a court. The sponsor will also be required to enter into a standard form indemnity with the NHS entity that controls the research.[47]

Where potential claims arise in industry-sponsored research (which is relatively uncommon), experience indicates that they tend to be dealt with under the applicable ABPI Guidelines. However, gaps can occur, as demonstrated by the lack of adequate compensation available for the six injured healthy volunteers in the 2006 Northwick Park 'first time in humans' clinical trial, where the early termination of the trial was quickly followed by the insolvency of the sponsor and where the clinical trial insurance (£2 million) was inadequate.

In the absence of any 'no fault' scheme, the participant who suffers injury and believes it to be trial-related must rely only on his or her ability to claim compensation through the courts – often a difficult and lengthy process. Most ethical guidelines require a study participant to be told in advance what provision has been or will be made – if any. However, in practice some ethics committees are unhappy that there are different approaches applicable to compensation in research, depending upon the identity of the sponsor/initiator.

15.5.2 Negligence

Any person in a chain of supply of medicinal products or medical services might act, or fail to act, in such a way that he or she breaches a duty of care towards a patient, and this causes damage. This is negligence liability. The law requires the existence of a legal duty of care (which usually exists between product manufacturers and patients), breach of the duty (conduct falling below the reasonable standard of care that the law requires), recoverable damage and causation (the breach caused the foreseeable damage).

Negligence can be difficult and costly for claimants to prove, especially in medical situations. Standards of testing, manufacture, labelling, supply and safety are generally high in the pharmaceutical sector, and extensively controlled and documented, so it should be rare that the conduct of manufacturers or suppliers falls below the required level of reasonableness. Liability will be clearer if a product contains a contaminant as a result of a substandard manufacturing process. The area that causes most problems is where an adverse drug reaction occurs that was not listed in the safety labelling: the argument will be whether the risk should have been identified earlier or more clearly, whether the doctor knew but did not pass the information on (the 'learned intermediary defence') or whether the patient knew and accepted the risk.

15.5.3 Strict liability

The producer of a defective product will be liable for damage that it causes. There may be more than one 'producer' of a product, encompassing the product's manufacturer, the owner of a name or trade mark that appears on it and appears to be the producer, or the entity that undertakes the first import of a product from outside the EU. Where there is no identifiable producer, a person in the chain of supply may be liable unless he or she identifies a producer or the person who supplied him or her. A product is 'defective' if it does not provide the safety that a person is entitled to expect, taking all the circumstances into account, including the product's presentation, the use to which it could reasonably be expected that it would be put, and the time when it was put into circulation.[48]

There are certain specified defences, the most well known of which is where the state of scientific and technical knowledge at the time that the producer put the product into circulation was not such as to enable the existence of the defect to be discovered (the 'development risks' defence).[49] In Germany, product liability compensation for death or injury resulting from the administration of a medicinal product is dealt with under a specific strict liability regime established under the Pharmaceutical Products Act (Arzneimittelgesetz), which predated and has remained untouched by the Product Liability Directive. The German Pharmaceutical Products Act caps the amount of damages that can be recovered by an injured person and cuts off all claims under the Product Liability Directive. It does not, however, include an equivalent 'development risks' defence.

15.5.4 Alternative schemes

In order to avoid the cost, delay and publicity of court procedures, some alternative approaches can exist. Product liability claims in Sweden, Finland, Norway and Denmark are dealt with under the admirable national 'no fault' pharmaceutical injury insurance schemes.[50] It has so far appeared to be too expensive to introduce similar schemes elsewhere. In Germany, a mutual top-up insurance scheme (Pharmapool) exists to cover very expensive claims. Certain countries are introducing national schemes to cover medical accidents, which may (the French Office National d'Indemnisation des Accidents (ONIAM) scheme)[51] or may not (the English NHS Redress scheme)[52] also include product manufacturers. In other Member States there have been specific legal provisions in place with regard to the compensation of research subjects (e.g. in Ireland under the Controls of Clinical Trials and Drugs Act 1990) for some time and also with regard to the means of ensuring that adequate funds are available to meet such claims, such as by insurance.[53]

References

1 Animal Testing Directive 86/609/EEC.
2 Serious Organised Crime and Police Act 2005.
3 Directive 2001/83/EC Annex (as amended).
4 'GLP': Directives 2004/10/EC and 2004/9/EC.
5 European Parliament's Written Declaration 0040/2007 on primates in scientific experiments adopted on 25 September 2007.
6 Response by the European Commission to the European Parliament's Written Declaration 0040/2007 adopted on 25 September 2007.
7 Directive 2001/20/EC.
8 'GCP' Directive 2005/28/EC.
9 'GMP' Directive 2003/94/EC.
10 Report on the October 2007 European Commission–European Medicines Agency Conference on the Operation of the Clinical Trials Directive (Directive 2001/20/EC) and Perspectives for the Future.
11 Directive 2001/20/EC, Article 1(2).
12 Directive 2001/83/EC, Article 8(3)(ib) and the Annex to Directive 2001/83/EC, as amended.
13 ICH guideline: adopted in the EU by the CPMP (now CHMP) 135/95/EEC.
14 EC Regulation 1394/2007.
15 Declaration of Helsinki (amended 1975,1983,1989, 1996, 2000, 2002 and 2004). Ferney-Voltaire, France: World Medicinal Association.
16 SI 2004/1031 as amended.
17 Research Governance Framework for Health and Social Care, 2nd edn. Department of Health, April 2005.
18 Gillick v West Norfolk and Wisbech AHA (HL) [1986] AC 112.
19 Confidentiality: NHS Code of Practice (November 2003); see also The Caldicott Guardian Manual 2006.
20 Article 14.7 of Regulation 726/2004.
21 Harvey v Facey [1893] A.C. 552.

22 Peter Lind & Co Ltd v Mersey Docks and Harbour Board [1972] 2 Lloyd's Rep. 234.

23 Harvey v Johnston (1848) 6 CB 295.

24 Currie and Others v Misa (1874–75) L. R. 10 Ex.153.

25 Supply of Goods and Services Act 1982: section 11(1).

26 Contracts (Rights of Third Parties) Act 1999: section 1(1).

27 Model Clinical Trial Agreement 2003. Department of Health and ABPI, February 2003.

28 NHS/ABPI/BIA Model Clinical Trial Agreement 2006: Clinical Trial Agreement for Pharmaceutical and Biopharmaceutical Industry Sponsored Research in NHS Hospitals.

29 NHS/ABPI/BIA CRO Model Clinical Trial Agreement 2007: Tripartite Clinical Trial Agreement for Pharmaceutical and Biopharmaceutical Industry Sponsored Research in NHS Hospitals, Managed by Contract Research Organisations.

30 Directive 2001/83/EC Title VII.

31 Regulation 726/2004 Articles 21 *et seq* and Directive 2001/83/EC Articles 101 *et seq*.

32 Directive 2001/83/EC Article 98.

33 Commission Public Consultation: Legal Proposal on Information to Patients. February 2008.

34 Article 86.1 2001/83/EC.

35 Medicines (Advertising) Regulations 1994 and Medicines (Monitoring of Advertising) Regulations 1994, both as amended.

36 Directive 2001/83/EC, as amended, Articles 59 and 61.

37 SI 1994/ 3144 as amended.

38 Article 28 of the EC Treaty.

39 Bristol-Myers Squibb v Paranova [1996] ECR I-3457.

40 Massachusetts Institute of Technology (C-431/04).

41 Biogen v SmithKline Beecham (C-181/95).

42 Regulation (EC) No 1901/2006.

43 Directive 2001/83/EC, as amended by Directive 2004/27/EC, Regulation 726/2004 and Volume 2A of the Rules Governing Medicinal Products in the European Union.

44 EC Reg. 141/2000 and Commission Reg. 847/2000.

45 Directive 85/374/EEC. The UK implementing legislation is the Consumer Protection Act 1987, Part I.

46 Guidelines for Compensation in Clinical Trials (ABPI 1991). *The Use of Healthy Volunteers in Research* (ABPI 1988) as amended.

47 Appendix 4 of mCTA 2006; Form of Indemnity for Clinical Studies at http://www.abpi.org.uk/publications/word_documents/indemnityf%20england%20&%20wales.doc

48 Directive 85/374/EEC, article 6.

49 Directive 85/374/EEC, article 7 (e).

50 Hodges C. Nordic compensation schemes for drug injuries. *J Consum Policy* 2006;29:143–75.

51 Office National d'Indemnisation des Accidents Médicaux.

52 NHS Redress Act 2006. For the previous history see *The NHS Plan, A plan for investment, a plan for reform* (2000) Cm 4818, at http://www.dh.gov.uk/assetRoot/04/05/57/83/04055783.pdf; *Making Amends. A consultation paper setting out proposals for reforming the approach to clinical negligence in the NHS: A report by the Chief Medical Officer* (2003) at http://www.dh.gov.uk/assetRoot/04/06/09/45/04060945.pdf

53 Spanish Law No. 29 of 2006 and subordinate Decrees.

16 The safety of medical products

A. Peter Fletcher[1] and Susan Shaw[2]

[1] Independent Consultant Little Maplestead, Essex, UK
[2] Chelsea and Westminster Hospital, London, UK

16.1 Introduction

The pharmaceutical industry presents many new challenges to the pharmaceutical physician which include the interface with pharmacy and pharmacology, toxicological research, human volunteer studies, clinical trials and post-marketing surveillance to name just a few. Product safety is a factor that impacts on all of those endeavours and the pharmaceutical physician will be expected to work and provide advice within that framework. It will be clear to anyone that evidence of lack of safety in a medical product is not good news for the company concerned and that some level of protective action will often be required which in extreme circumstances may involve product withdrawal. It is, therefore, essential that the pharmaceutical physician should be absolutely clear what constitutes lack of safety in relation to the intended use of the product.

Unfortunately, the public perception of such concepts as safety, risk, hazard, tolerance, toxicity are notoriously inconsistent in that the same person may consider a drug unacceptably hazardous if it is associated with serious adverse reactions that are slightly more frequent than 1 in 10,000 exposures and yet they will go hang-gliding at weekends without a qualm. On the other hand, patients with troublesome joint pain may be willing to take high doses of non-steroidal anti-inflammatory drugs (NSAIDs) even though their pain poses minimal risk to life whereas the drug may rarely cause a fatal outcome from gastrointestinal haemorrhage.

Nevertheless, pharmaceutical physicians will have to take in their stride these irritating whims when they are faced with a new publication describing 20 cases of cardiac dysrrhythmia apparently triggered by their drug. Dealing with such a problem will require careful judgement based upon a comprehensive review of all the available evidence. Experience tells us that almost always jumping to conclusions is unwise, whether that is a declaration of the product's 'complete' safety or instant withdrawal from the market.

What is 'safe' may be quite different from the points of view of the patient, the doctor in charge of the case, the regulatory authority or the pharmaceutical company. Responsibility for ensuring acceptable safety lies mainly with the pharmaceutical company and/or the licence holder who may or may not be the same. However, to a not inconsiderable extent, that burden is shared by the regulatory authority which determines the granting of marketing authorisation and the terms under which the product may be used. The doctor trusts the drug development capabilities of the company and the judgement of the licensing authority when he prescribes the product within the terms of the licence. The patient trusts the doctor to prescribe the product appropriately. Sometimes the effect on the patient is an adverse reaction which is out of proportion to any amelioration or cure of the condition being treated. The cause and consequences of such an event may lead to much arduous work for the pharmaceutical physician.

At one end of the spectrum, the event may be a simple dosage problem which could be an error on the part of the prescriber or an unanticipated hypersensitivity for that particular patient. At the other end of the spectrum is an uncommon, serious adverse reaction not revealed in premarketing clinical trials. Somewhere between those two extremes are more or less serious adverse events which are not entirely unexpected but appear to be more common than is accepted for comparable products in the same

The Textbook of Pharmaceutical Medicine. Edited by John P. Griffin. © 2009, ISBN: 978-1-4051-8035-1.

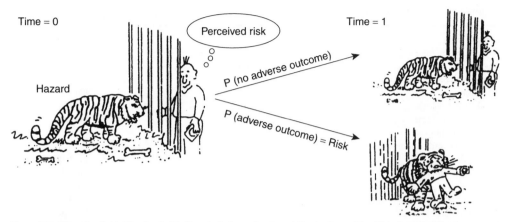

Figure 16.1 Hazard and risk. The tiger behind bars is the hazard, as it could lead to harm. The risk is the probability that an adverse outcome will occur in unit time, or for some other specified denominator, such as 'per caged tiger'. The perceived risk is the man's intuitive estimate of the risk. He may express it ('more dangerous than crossing the road') or reveal it, by avoiding the tiger's cage, even if he risks falling into the penguins' pool.

therapeutic category. This may be a real increase in frequency or may be due to patient selection bias. The latter has arisen with new products that claim a lower incidence of certain adverse reactions, which encourages doctors to prescribe them preferentially for patients who have had such reactions with older products.

16.2 The concept of safety

All activities in life are associated with some level of risk, although in most circumstances the potential dangers are so small that we are unaware of their existence.[1] For example, when, on a sunny day, we take a stroll along a sandy beach listening to the distant cries of seagulls and the gentle sound of waves lapping on the shore the awareness of danger (risk) is far from our minds, and yet a boulder may fall from the cliff above us and have serious consequences. There is no such thing as absolute safety, and we live in a world where we continually make judgements on the level of risk we are willing to accept.

This inconsistency also applies to our perception of risk associated with medicinal products, even though most are remarkably safe. This is not the impression given by reports in the popular press and in television programmes which purport to provide the public with a factual view of medicine but which in fact emphasise the most sensational aspects and spread alarm. A useful review of safety and risk may be found in *The BMA Guide to Living with Risk*,[2] which brings

into perspective the dangers encountered in everyday life.

The Office of Health Economics has also published a review entitled *What are My Chances Doctor?*[3] which takes into account not only treatment by drugs but also the hazards of surgery. People perceive risk in many different ways that would seem to the objective scientist alarmingly irrational. The distinction between risk and hazard has been nicely illustrated by Ferner[4] (Figure 16.1), who has defined risk as 'the probability that a particular adverse outcome occurs during a given quantum of exposure to a hazard'.

The risks of dying in any particular year (Table 16.1) from a variety of causes gives some idea of the relative risks of a variety of life events, but in the case of drugs it is not only death that is a concern, it is the possibility of survival with long-term or permanent disability. The mortality risks from a number of diseases (Table 16.2) make useful comparisons when considering the relative risks of taking medication. Similar tabulations of the risks associated with life events (Table 16.3) in the USA shows the estimated effects of certain common activities when continued for defined periods of time.

In a somewhat arcane context, Chapman and Morrison,[5] in the scientific journal *Nature*, have provided a list of comparative risks of death in the USA (Table 16.4) from a number of causes. The purpose of their paper was to assess the hazard of an asteroid or comet impact on the Earth. Such an event does not immediately come to mind when considering the safety of medicines, but according to their estimates

Table 16.1 Risk of dying in 1989 in England and Wales by cause

Cause	In 1989	Due to a given cause
Any cause	1 in 88	1 in 1
Disease of the circulatory system	1 in 190	1 in 2.2
Neoplasm	1 in 350	1 in 4
Accident and violence	1 in 3000	1 in 33
Motor traffic accidents	1 in 10,000	1 in 130
Poisoning by drugs	1 in 30,000	1 in 330
Toxic effect of carbonmonoxide	1 in 40,000	1 in 450
Fire and flames	1 in 90,000	1 in 1000
Poisoning by antidepressants	1 in 160,000	1 in 1899
Homicide	1 in 180,000	1 in 2000
Toxic effect of ethanol	1 in 420,000	1 in 4800
Railway accidents	1 in 700,000	1 in 8000
Poisoning by salicylates	1 in 800,000	1 in 9500
Assault by poison	1 in 4,200,000	1 in 48,000
Any cause	2 in 88	2 in 1

Source: Based on 1989 Mortality Statistics for England and Wales. DH2 No 16, Office of Population Censuses and Surveys.

Table 16.2 Selected mortality risk levels, England and Wales 1984

Cause	Number of deaths in 1984	Probability of mortality
All causes	566,881	1.0×10^{-2}
Cancers	140,101	2.8×10^{-3}
Coronary heart disease	157,506	3.2×10^{-3}
Strokes	14,211	2.9×10^{-4}
Diabetes	6369	1.3×10^{-4}
Asthma	1764	3.5×10^{-5}
Cirrhosis	2280	4.5×10^{-5}
Ulcers (stomach and duodenum)	4483	9.0×10^{-5}
Pregnancy	52	1.4×10^{-6}
Measles	10	2.0×10^{-8}
Whooping cough	1	4.0×10^{-8}

the chances of being killed by an asteroid or comet impact are about the same as dying in an air accident, which is about 1 in 20,000. This is, of course, a somewhat misleading figure because it refers to an extremely rare event that carries the probability of killing many thousands of people at one time; however, it is interesting that the risk of death from chloramphenicol is about the same.

16.2.1 The quantification of risk

A previous Chief Medical Officer in the UK has expressed concern that the public's perception of risk with respect to adverse drug reactions (ADRs) is not consistent with other kinds of risk to which people are exposed on a day-to-day basis. In a paper entitled 'Risk language and dialects', published in the *British Medical Journal*, Calman and Royston[6] proposed a logarithmic scale for risk probabilities that may be relevant in the UK. This is probably a good way of presenting numerical information that covers a very wide range of values, even though the concept may be rather too mathematical for the general public. We live in an age in which people are constantly reminded of the many hazards they may encounter, and the media waste no time in sensationalising all manner of disasters. The fact that there is no such thing as zero risk is curiously difficult to transmit, in spite of the fact that virtually every action we take involves some kind of hazard. Calman and Royston[6] advocate the idea of 'negligible risk' even though it begs the question

Table 16.3 Risks estimated to increase chance of death in any year by one part in a million (USA)

Activity	Cause of death
Smoking 1.4 cigarettes	Cancer, heart disease
Drinking 0.5 L wine	Cirrhosis of liver
Spending 1 hour in a coal mine	Black lung disease
Spending 3 hours in a coal mine	Accident
Living 2 days in Boston or New York	Air pollution
Travelling 6 min by canoe	Accident
Travelling 10 miles by bicycle	Accident
Travelling 150 miles by car	Accident
Flying 1000 miles by jet	Accident
Flying 6000 miles by jet	Cancer caused by cosmic radiation
Living 2 months in average stone or brick building	Cancer caused by natural radioactivity
One chest X-ray in a good hospital	Cancer caused by radiation
Living 2 months with a cigarette smoker	Cancer, heart disease
Eating 40 tablespoons of peanut butter	Cancer caused by aflatoxin B
Drinking 30 cans of diet soda	Cancer caused by saccharin
Living 150 years within 20 miles of a nuclear plant	Cancer caused by radiation

Table 16.4 Chances of dying from selected cause as lifetime risk (USA)

Causes of death	Chances
Motor vehicle accident	1 in 100
Murder	1 in 300
Fire	1 in 800
Firearms accident	1 in 2500
Asteroid/comet impact (lower limit)	*1 in 3000*
Electrocution	1 in 5000
Asteroid/comet impact	*1 in 20,000*
Passenger aircraft crash	1 in 20,000
Flood	1 in 30,000
Tornado	1 in 60,000
Venomous bite or sting	1 in 100,000
Asteroid/comet impact (upper limit)	*1 in 250,000*
Fireworks accident	1 in 1 million
Food poisoning by botulism	1 in 3 million
Drinking water with EPA limit of TCE	1 in 10 million

EPA, Environmental Protection Agency; TCE, trichloroethylene.

of what is negligible in any particular situation. Griffin[7] has commented on the Calman paper and questioned whether or not risk assessment is an achievable goal. If serious concern exists with respect to fatal or life-threatening adverse reactions occurring at a rate of 1 in 50,000 to 1 in 100,000, then there are very few drugs with prescription volumes sufficiently large for such reactions to be detected even under the most favourable circumstances. Moreover, it is not simply the perception of level of risk that is difficult to convey realistically to patients, but also the severity of an adverse reaction. These problems are compounded by the fact that everyday life frequently involves appreciably greater risks than those posed by treatment with drugs. People do not stop driving cars, riding motorcycles, taking skiing holidays or smoking even when they know the risks they are taking.

If the risk of death from a road traffic accident is taken as some sort of 'gold standard' then we have to assume that most people are willing to accept a 1 in 10,000 chance of death in a single year, or 1 in 300 over a lifetime without great concern. So how does this picture match up with people's view of medicines?

If products intended for use in clinical conditions that are not life-threatening in the relatively short term, then experience suggests that regulatory authorities start to be concerned at a potentially drug-related death rate of about 1 in 10,000 exposures. NSAIDs, minor tranquillisers or products for the relief of common acute gastrointestinal disorders would come into this category; so, in such cases, patients' expectations of safety are approximately the same as in circumstances that are acceptable in everyday life. It has to be questioned whether or not this is a realistic expectation and, in particular, whether methods are available for detecting, measuring and assessing risks at that level.

16.2.2 Balance of benefit and risk in modern society

The fact that the public, the media, patients and probably the medical profession itself, have a distorted view of the risks involved in taking medicines does not in any way diminish the need for continuing research into the safety of drugs. The fact that the major drugs advisory body in the UK is called the Committee on Safety of Medicines is not without significance. The Medicines Act (1968) charges the committee with the assessment of the quality, safety and efficacy of drugs before they are granted a product licence.

It is clear that continuing awareness of ADRs, as a major problem in the treatment of most diseases, by doctors, patients, pharmaceutical companies and national regulatory authorities has had little effect in improving safety evaluation over the past 20–30 years. During the period covered by the last two editions of this chapter, drug withdrawals, exemplified by the hypo-glycaemic agent, troglitazone, and the cholesterol-lowering agent, cerivastatin, have continued to the dismay of patients, doctors and the pharmaceutical industry. At the time of the present edition, the COX-2 inhibitor rofecoxib (Vioxx) has been withdrawn as a consequence of cardiovascular adverse reactions. It is disheartening that all the efforts made to develop new methods of safety evaluation should have failed yet again. It has to be questioned whether this failure is a consequence of not using the most appropriate methods available, or whether the detection of such adverse reactions is inherently unattainable. It seems obvious that premarketing clinical trials, which seldom study more than a few thousand patients, are incapable of evaluating safety for any but the most common adverse reactions of short latency, and that spontaneous reporting, which is so inefficient that a 10–15% reporting rate would be considered quite exceptional, is not an appropriate method for new drugs.

From the pharmaceutical industry's point of view, the evaluation of safety for a new product begins from the time that it is first tested in living material. It is for this reason that the great majority of potential new drugs are abandoned before they go beyond animal toxicology. At the first sign of unacceptable toxicity it is highly likely that all research will be stopped, and other related compounds investigated in the hope that they will be less toxic. This is undoubtedly a wasteful process, and it is certain that drugs that would ultimately prove to be safe and effective are abandoned unnecessarily. An excessive concern with safety is certainly part of the problem, but the lack of predictive precision of animal tests[8] and the inability to identify groups of patients that may be at high risk ensure that a very cautious attitude prevails.

The great majority of ADRs are dose related and may be readily understood as excessive responses to the expected pharmacological and physiological effects of the substance. A very small number of reactions do not fall into this category and, although they are rare, create considerable alarm because they are sometimes serious and always unexpected.

Potential new drugs that show acceptable toxicity in animals are usually first tested in healthy human volunteers before being investigated in patients. Chapters 3–6 deal with these aspects of new drug development, and it is the purpose of this chapter to consider how safety should be evaluated at the time of the product licence application and in the post-marketing phase.

16.3 General considerations

By the time that an application for a product licence is ready, a certain amount of evidence on the safety of the drug will be available. In a review of product licence applications to the Committee on Safety of Medicines (CSM), Rawlins and Jefferys[9] presented data on the number of patients who were available for the assessment of safety and efficacy (Table 16.5). When

Table 16.5 Median numbers (range) of volunteers and patients exposed to new active substances during premarketing studies[9]

	Healthy volunteers	Efficacy studies	Safety database
All applications	60 (0–819)	861 (41–4906)	1171 (43–15,962)
Successful applications	92 (0–819)	1126 (122–4906)	1480 (129–9400)
Unsuccessful applications	64 (0–431)	785 (41–4786)	1052 (43–15,962)

it is considered that many of the patients included would have been in short-term clinical trials (up to 28 days), and that other trials would have been conducted on formulations and doses that were different from those recommended in the product licence application, then the relevant numbers are substantially reduced.

In addition, some patients could well have been studied for conditions other than those finally selected, thereby reducing the numbers still further.

If data are available on 1000 patients, then on the assumption that there were no confounding factors, an adverse effect with an incidence of about 1 in 300 might be detected. If there were confounding factors, such as a significant background level of the adverse drug event (ADE), not associated with the drug, then the level of detection could fall to 1 in 100 or even less. Most ADEs that have caused problems occur less frequently than 1 in 1000 patients, and may be as rare as 1 in 10,000 or 50,000, so the evidence available in the product licence application is wholly inadequate for such an assessment. The need for the continuing evaluation of safety is, therefore, a matter of considerable importance, and has been the subject of numerous publications.[10–24]

Many of the major new products reaching the market in the last few years will have had total databases of 5000 or more patients, but when the subtractions are made for formulation, dose and indications that are no longer relevant, then, perhaps, no more than 2500–3500 remain. This is still far short of the number required to make an assessment of safety that would be appropriate for its expected performance when it reaches the market.

There are many uncertainties in the information available on ADEs, as estimated from premarketing clinical trials, and even the 'incidence' figures quoted are frequently guesses rather than precise quantitative estimates. Indeed, many words – 'incidence', 'prevalence', 'frequency' and so on – that have specific definitions are used indiscriminately without considering their precise meaning. They are used to suggest some sort of magnitude of risk by which the acceptability of the drug may be judged. There is no harm in this so long as the lack of precision is understood. A major problem is that the chances of experiencing an ADE from a particular drug depend on a number of factors that may be specific to that drug or that class of drug, and not to others. Such factors might be duration of administration, route of administration, need for dose titration, and a whole range of precautions in special groups of patients.

16.4 Methods of post-marketing safety evaluation

Many methods have been used for the evaluation of safety in the post-marketing period, but these can be reduced to five basically different approaches to the problem:

- Clinical trials;
- Spontaneous reporting;
- Computerised databases;
- Prescription event monitoring (PEM);
- Ad hoc methods.

Each group of methods will be considered in some detail in order to identify their strengths and weaknesses, and to determine those circumstances in which their use is most appropriate. There has in the past been a hope that some new method – a 'holy grail' – might be discovered that would fulfil all the requirements for post-marketing safety evaluation but, not surprisingly, this has not been realised, and it is now accepted that each situation has different needs and the most appropriate method or methods have to be determined according to the circumstances.

A continuing problem is the lack of attention that has been paid to the capabilities of each method. Too often the temptation to accept the currently fashionable method has taken precedence over a well-considered appraisal of what is available, resulting in a study that fails to measure up to the requirements. Each of the methods has serious defects; numbers of patients and costs are negative factors for cohort studies; completeness of data and validation are problems for computerised systems; and lack of a clear hypothesis or poorly defined diagnostic criteria are incompatible with high-quality case–control studies. Clinical trials pose even greater problems with respect to patient numbers, cost and the logistics of conducting large-scale controlled studies on a multicentre basis. To a great extent this lack of discrimination is a consequence of the predominant influence of clinical trial methodology on clinical research. For example, it has proved difficult to persuade clinical trialists that purely observational studies do not have 'dropouts': they merely have patients who discontinue or change their medication. The patients are still being observed and are therefore still in the study. There are no 'protocol violations' in observational studies because there are no exclusive or inclusive criteria, and it is just medical practice in the real world that is being recorded. Another factor that is often overlooked is time. This is a vital matter in the premarketing phases of new drug development, when the time taken to achieve marketing authorisation is par-amount. However, it is also frequently forgotten that the safety of a new product and supporting its position on the market should not be the subject of undue delay.

A recent editorial in the *BMJ* by Ioannidis et al.[25] has questioned the widely held view that the only scientifically acceptable studies are randomised con-trolled clinical trials, and that observational studies are unreliable and unreproducible. They cite two papers[26,27] reviewing more than 20 studies which show that the correlation between observational and randomised controlled studies was remarkably close, and that the reproducibility of observational studies was good.

In the following sections the case of an orally administered drug intended for long-term use in a commonly occurring condition will be taken as the classic example. Drugs administered by different routes, for acute conditions, for life-threatening diseases or in other special circumstances will require modifications not only in study design but also in analysis and inter-pretation. The way in which post-marketing safety will be monitored in the new 'biotech' products and gene therapy has yet to be determined, but will cer-tainly involve the development of new methods. It has already been suggested (MD Rawlins, personal communication, 1993) that patients receiving gene therapy will have to be monitored for the rest of their lives. It might also be thought necessary to monitor any children they may have in the same way.

16.5 Clinical trials

The vast subject of clinical trials in new drug develop-ment is the subject of Chapter 6 and will be dealt with here only with respect to their use after marketing for the further evaluation of safety.

Clinical trials are specifically designed as experi-ments to test the many and various aspects of a new drug's characteristics, in particular the determination of appropriate diagnostic indications and the correct dose and dosage regimen. There are clear-cut patient inclusion and exclusion criteria, there may be strin-gent requirements to confirm the diagnosis, and there will be specific limitations on dosage and duration of treatment. In most clinical trials, a control or com-parator group will be included, and patients will be randomly allocated to either the treatment or the control group. These requirements, therefore, create an entirely artificial set of circumstances which are quite unlike the situation that exists in the real world

of clinical practice. Such trials are essential in drug development, when efficacy and dosage determina-tion are dominant factors. They are of much less value in the evaluation of safety.

As has already been stated, major new drugs intended for long-term use in common conditions may have been tested in several thousand patients by the time marketing permission is granted. This may seem to be a substantial number but, as has already been pointed out, many of the patients will have been in relatively short-term trials and many will have been in studies conducted on different doses, different dosage regi-mens and for different indications from those finally agreed upon for marketing. Many other patients may also have been studied in countries in which the standards of clinical research are below an acceptable level. A survey of 118 product licence applications considered by the CSM[9] found that the median number of patients included in the safety database was 1480 (range 129–9400) which, when corrected for studies involving inappropriate formulations, doses and indications and short durations of treatment, would only be able to detect adverse reactions occur-ring more frequently than 1 in 1000 at the very best. In the great majority of cases the detection capability would be as low as 1 in 2–300, which by any standards is totally inadequate. The reader is referred to some examples of large-scale clinical trials used mainly for the evaluation of safety, but also for better defining drug use.[28–32]

It will be seen that the use of controlled clinical trials to evaluate safety in new drugs is very limited, both from the point of view of the relatively small number of patients that can be studied and because they are, of necessity, conducted in an artificial, experi-mental setting. The more common conditions may be detected in this way, but ill-defined and less com-mon adverse events will usually be missed, and will not be discovered until the drug has been used by large numbers of patients in the real world of everyday clinical practice. It is not just that increasing the size and range of controlled clinical trials is impractical for reasons of cost and the time involved in their comple-tion, but because they are essentially experimental in nature they can never provide information on the way in which a drug will be used in the real world. It is well known that even in the best of circumstances drugs are used in ways that are not recommended in the official literature. Dosage levels and dosage regi-mens, diagnostic indications and durations of treat-ment, to mention just a few examples, are frequently extended beyond what is permitted in the licence. It is in just these, unapproved, circumstances, which are excluded from clinical trials, that adverse drug-related events are most likely to occur.

The great majority of new drugs will therefore come to the market with only a superficial evaluation of safety. As a consequence, it is now universally agreed that the assessment of safety must be continued into the post-marketing phase, and probably for the entire life of the drug. This is a major challenge for the pharmaceutical industry, all those involved in clinical research and the regulatory authorities. A serious legal problem arises from the fact that drug law in most countries, and in particular the Medicines Act (1968) in the UK, has little power after a product licence has been granted. It is true that there are requirements for companies to submit any new information that may become available in the post-marketing period if it has relevance to the quality, safety or efficacy of the product, but there are no formal powers to demand specific studies for the evaluation of safety. If a product should become the subject of serious adverse event reports or other evidence that its safety is in doubt, then the licensing authority may request further information on which to base regulatory action if it should be appropriate. It has long been hoped that formal studies continued into the post-marketing period might counteract the ever-present demand for bigger and longer clinical trials, but unfortunately this has never been put into effect. A combination of the legal limitations of the regulatory authorities and a lack of will on the part of the pharmaceutical industry has effectively blocked any progress in this direction.

The granting of a product licence in the UK, or its equivalent in other countries, is a dividing line that places firm constraints on what studies can and cannot be done in the pre- and post-marketing periods. Because it would be medically and ethically unacceptable to permit doctors (investigators) to use an unapproved drug in unrestricted circumstances, it is essentially impossible to conduct clinical trials that would mimic real-world use rather than a controlled experimental situation. The result is obvious. The real world is inaccessible in the premarketing period. Conversely, once in the post-marketing phase, it is difficult or impossible to constrain drug use to the situations that were defined in clinical trials.

It is no exaggeration to say that nearly 30 years have passed since the Medicines Division, as it was then called, began a campaign to encourage the pharmaceutical industry to continue premarketing safety evaluation into the post-marketing phase, which, on

the one hand, would provide the licensing authority with greater assurance of safety and on the other would safeguard the licence holder from the possible disaster of unexpected adverse reactions. This incentive to self-regulation has never been more than moderately successful and it may well be that this will not be achieved until the post-marketing period is included in the legally recognised period of new drug development. When post-marketing safety evaluation becomes an integral part of the research and development process, a more uniform approach may be achieved.

It is now necessary to consider the various methods that are available for studying drugs in the context of actual clinical practice with the assessment of safety as a primary objective.

16.6 Spontaneous event reporting

Spontaneous adverse event reporting may be defined as any system of safety data collection which, in the UK, relies upon certain health care professionals, physicians, dentists, other health care workers and sometimes patients[33] to report adverse clinical events which, they suspect, may be causally related to the administration of a drug or drugs. The present Yellow Card scheme invites such reports from doctors, dentists, pharmacists, coroners, radiographers, optometrists and nurses. Discussions are in progress to include patient reporting, and pilot studies will be evaluated to determine their effectiveness. It is these systems that are sponsored by the governments of virtually all developed countries and, increasingly, by developing countries as well. For the physician in the pharmaceutical industry it is this method of safety evaluation that will most frequently be encountered and, in spite of its numerous defects and limitations, will take up much working time.

It is one of those illogical quirks of new drug development that a method which is almost universally agreed to be seriously inadequate is, nevertheless, a major consideration in the organisation and running of the pharmaceutical company medical department. For this reason alone it is necessary to look into spontaneous reporting systems in some detail. Misunderstanding and confusion start at the very beginning. Is the clinical condition that is the subject of a report an event or a reaction? At the very least, in the eyes of the reporter it is potentially an adverse reaction, as there was the suspicion of a causal relationship with a drug or drugs. For the personnel of a regulatory agency, who receive thousands of such reports each year, the perception may be totally different, knowing that the reporting doctor usually has little evidence to support an attribution of causality. This is no fault of the doctor, as the well-known common ADRs are of little interest and the uncommon ones are so infrequent that any individual doctor may only observe a handful in his or her entire career. The reporting doctor thus has no frame of reference by which to assess possible causality and has to fall back on clinical judgement, which is largely subjective.

The entire basis of medicine is, quite properly, moving from the 'art of medicine' to the 'science of medicine', and the reporting of clinical events observed while a patient is receiving a drug should reflect this change of attitude. At the time of observation, apart possibly from a temporal relationship between the administration of a drug and the event, there may be no other evidence on which to base an attribution of causality. In these circumstances, it would be correct to term the observation an 'event' and not a 'reaction', the latter term being strictly reserved for the situation in which a causal relationship has been reasonably established. The vast majority of spontaneous reports, apart from those recording well-established ADRs, are therefore, with respect to clinical events, not reactions. The next stage of the process may be aimed at collecting further data which could provide evidence of causality, particularly when the event is either serious or unexpected or both.

At the present time, several countries have well-organised and experienced spontaneous reporting systems which contribute the bulk of ADE reports. In particular, the USA, the UK, France and the Scandinavian countries have records going back several decades, and can claim to have in their possession data of reasonable quality. The section on p. 400 considers the various methods of causality assessment that are available and the data that are required for their application.

In Europe, the term 'pharmacovigilance' is now used to cover the continuing evaluation of safety into the post-marketing period, and is intended to include all methods of data collection. In practice this has not happened, and 'pharmacovigilance' is almost always used synonymously with spontaneous reporting, which further adds to the existing confusion over definitions and terminology. A mythology now surrounds spontaneous reporting that is disproportionate to its true value and which allows conclusions to be drawn and decisions to be made which, in any other science,

would be rejected as unjustifiable speculation. This is not to say that spontaneous reporting is valueless: it has its proper place in safety evaluation but must be used appropriately and its capabilities and limitations recognised. The recently published EU document 'Notice to Marketing Authorisation Holders – Pharmacovigilance Guidelines No PhVWP/108/99' is now the principal source of information and instruction on the reporting of suspected ADRs in the European Union (EU).

In the UK, the present Yellow Card system had its origins in 1965, when Witts,[23] who was then a member of the Committee on Safety of Drugs (the precursor to the CSM), published a method for the collection of suspected adverse reactions to drugs.

The thalidomide tragedy[34-38] was a powerful stimulus for the setting up of an effective system of adverse event monitoring. An excellent early publication which set out many of the basic principles and definitions of terms and procedures is that of Finney.[39]

Since then there have been many publications and reviews of the UK Yellow Card system and spontaneous reporting systems internationally.[40-49] A summary of the capabilities and limitations of the method is given in Table 16.6. Although these have been discussed in the greatest detail over the past three decades, the obligations that exist for pharmaceutical companies in the reporting of adverse events to the regulatory authorities at both national and international levels make it essential to review them in this chapter.

The European Pharmacovigilance Research Group (EPRG) sponsored by the EU Biomed Programme, which has now been discontinued, examined methods of ADE reporting that would be appropriate for multinational studies within the EU. As part of the programme an attitudinal survey was carried out in Denmark, France, Ireland, Italy, the Netherlands, Portugal, Spain, Sweden and the UK to investigate the reporting characteristics of health care professionals in those countries. EPRG recognised that underreporting is a universal problem for spontaneous reporting systems, and sought to identify the factors that discouraged reporting. The survey was conducted by sending self-administered questionnaires to approximately 1% of medical practitioners in each country. There was a large variation in response from country to country, as might have been expected, although inhibitory factors seemed to be more similar. Lack of availability of report forms was a common problem, as was the lack of address and telephone number of the reporting agency. Inadequate information on

Table 16.6 Spontaneously reported adverse reactions in WHO database from EU countries

Country	1985	1986	1987	1988	1989	Mean
Belgium	54	52	53	47	36	48
Denmark	213	379	372	346	160	294
France	5	44	95	108	53	61
German Fed. Rep.	38	41	48	23	1	30
Ireland	293	336	227	147	74	215
Italy	17	21	21	17	3	16
The Netherlands	69	68	65	24	6	46
Spain	30	42	58	57	28	43
UK	217	273	301	314	254	272

how to report and shortage of time in which to report were also general complaints. Issues that did not discourage reporting included concern about patient confidentiality, fear of legal liability or appearing foolish, reluctance to admit that harm had been caused to a patient, or ambition to collect and publish a personal series of cases.

Another disincentive to reporting is uncertainty in the mind of the doctor or other health professional in judging the seriousness or severity of a suspected adverse reaction. Serious reactions are those that are fatal, life-threatening, disabling, incapacitating or which result in prolonged hospitalisation and/or are medically significant. On the other hand, severe reactions may be those that are not life-threatening or disabling but in individual patients are extreme.

16.6.1 Underreporting

It has always been known that only a very small proportion of adverse events were ever the subject of spontaneous reports. There are various reasons for this, the most common probably being a lack of enthusiasm on the part of the doctor, although more serious disincentives may be a fear of criticism, a fear of displaying ignorance or a genuine and entirely understandable failure to recognise a potential ADR when it occurs. Various estimates, usually based on the known number of reporting doctors taken as a proportion of the total, suggest that reporting levels are seldom, if ever, higher than 10% and are almost always much lower.[50] The Nordic countries have claimed levels of 15%, which may be possible in countries with small populations, socialised medicine, legally enforceable requirements and constant motivation by the authorities.

Estimates based upon data from large-scale observational cohort studies[51,52] which involved data collection by event monitoring and spontaneous reporting suggest that the level is more often in the region of 5%, and is frequently below 2%. These are estimates taken across the full range of ADE reports, which include a high proportion of irrelevant observations relating to trivial, symptomatic conditions that are dubiously related to the administration of drugs. There has always been an optimistic hope that the more serious, pathologically distinct conditions may be more frequently recorded and reported as potential ADRs. The papers referred to above do not support that view, but seem to show that many relatively serious conditions, such as photodermatitis, hyperthyroidism and hypothyroidism, Cushing's syndrome and extrapyramidal symptoms are only rarely reported, even though they have all been identified as occasionally being causally related to particular drugs. It seems possible that high-profile, well-publicised serious ADRs, such as aplastic anaemia or acute hepatic failure, which have come to be regarded as drug-associated conditions, may be much less affected by underreporting.

Another contributory factor in underreporting is the background incidence of the condition in the overall patient population. The chances of identifying a clinical condition that occurs in the population only extremely rarely as a drug-related event is clearly much greater than if it occurred commonly. The case of thalidomide is the classic example, phocomelia being exceptionally rare as a background condition, which permitted the detection of an increased incidence at an early stage. Had the defect been one of a variety of minor abnormalities that are relatively common, then the detection of the thalidomide problem might have taken much longer. In order to detect ADRs that may be confused with commonly occurring conditions it is essential to use a monitoring method that can provide data containing precise denominator values, so that incidence may be calculated. It is also necessary to know the background incidence with which to compare the ADR data. These requirements are seldom met, and usually the situation remains inconclusive.

An example of this involved the combination product Debendox (Bendectin in the USA), which was indicated for the relief of vomiting in pregnancy. In the formulation that was marketed in the UK, Debendox contained dicyclomine hydrochloride, doxylamine sulphate and pyridoxine, but in formulations used in some other countries the dicyclomine hydrochloride was left out. In 1983, the company withdrew the product from the market because of increasing media pressure and the risks of litigation arising from unfounded suspicions that it was associated with birth defects. No specific defect was referred to, although it was implied that there was a general increase in minor midline and skeletal abnormalities. These occur sporadically, with a total incidence that is estimated to be about 1% of live births. Numerous large-scale studies were conducted,[53-59] which failed to demonstrate any association with Debendox. From the regulatory point of view, the drug was no longer under suspicion, but for the company it was off the market. In the period leading up to its withdrawal from the market, regulatory action had reduced the pregnancy indications to severe hyperemesis gravidarum, which is a relatively uncommon condition and is itself associated with an increase in birth defects. In this situation there was, quite literally, no way in which a possible association between Debendox and birth defects could ever be proved. Even if every use of the product were to be monitored the numbers would have been insufficient to reach a statistically significant conclusion. It cannot be stressed too strongly that there are occasions when the size of the total patient population relevant to the problem is too small to provide any answers.

Another serious deficiency with spontaneous reporting is the possibility of bias in the data. The problem is particularly difficult because, often, it is not possible to detect the existence of bias until the lengthy process of collecting additional data has been completed. Increases or decreases in reporting levels may result from numerous external and largely uncontrollable factors. At the 'macro' level it is known that reporting levels differ greatly from country to country as a consequence of social, medical, religious and other national influences.[43] At the 'micro' level, publications in the medical literature, media pressure, regulatory

agency activities and a host of other ill-defined factors may enhance or inhibit reporting. To add to the difficulties, these biases are capricious in their effects, sometimes causing a flood of reports relating to a particular drug or clinical condition and on other occasions apparently demotivating doctors in reporting.

Other factors causing bias are related to the particular drug or class of drugs, and to the particular clinical condition or organ system involved. As an example, in the UK the class of NSAIDs has always been heavily overrepresented in the Yellow Card figures, possibly as a consequence of a high level of regulatory activity and media pressure. Many of these biases are shown in the spontaneous reports held on the World Health Organization (WHO) Collaborative Centre database in Uppsala, Sweden, particularly when comparisons are made between country, drug and clinical condition[24,60] (IR Edwards, personal communication) (Tables 16.6–16.9). Potential dangers are involved in combining spontaneous reporting data when it derives from different sources, at different times, for different drugs and relating to different clinical conditions. The current developments in the EU, with the establishment of a central agency and an increasingly integrated approach to drug registration and post-marketing safety evaluation, will have to proceed with caution if erroneous decisions are to be avoided. A similar trend towards the extrapolation of data derived from one source to problems occurring in another area is happening in the USA and Canada, where the large multipurpose databases are being used in this way.

16.6.2 The need for denominators

Underreporting and bias are both serious problems, but the greatest deficiency of spontaneous reporting is its lack of denominator values. This means that, without recourse to information derived from other sources, spontaneous reporting can only provide absolute numbers. It may be true that there are rare circumstances when absolute numbers are all that is required to make a regulatory decision. This might happen when a drug with no exceptional benefits in a non-life-threatening condition is shown to have a causal relationship to a serious and potentially fatal condition. In such circumstances, three or four well-documented reports may be sufficient to withdraw the product from the market. In all other circumstances, it is necessary to use one or more denominator values in order to calculate an incidence for the suspected ADR.

Table 16.7 Adverse reaction reports in WHO database from EU countries. Distribution of reports per therapeutic drug group as percentage of total number of reports

Country	ATC groups			
	Cardiovascular	Anti-infective	Musculoskeletal	CNS
Belgium	22.2	13.9	11.8	17.8
Denmark	17.4	17.1	10.1	13.7
France	18.2	4.2	9.5	19.2
German Fed. Rep.	9.6	22.5	11.1	10.8
Ireland	17.7	15.7	10.1	15.1
Italy	9.5	16.6	14.4	15.3
The Netherlands	20.7	12.6	8.8	14.1
Spain	16	20.8	9	15.2
UK	19.9	15	17.5	13

Table 16.8 Adverse reaction reports in WHO database from EU countries. Distribution of reports per body system organ class as percentage of total number of reports

Country	Body system organ class			
	Skin	CNS	Gastrointestine	Liver
Belgium	19.2	11	10.8	4.5
Denmark	30.3	7.7	8.9	4.3
France	17.6	9.1	8	8.4
German Fed. Rep.	12.4	10.1	15	2.5
Ireland	13.9	13.1	15.4	1.6
Italy	17.7	8	18.2	1.9
The Netherlands	17.5	10.6	9.3	5.4
Spain	18.6	11.9	17.2	1.7
UK	20.7	11.1	12.9	2.4

Table 16.9 Adverse reactions in WHO database from EU countries

Country	Skin reactions				
	Rash	SJS	Total	R/T (%)	S/T (%)
Belgium	257	4	642	40	0.6
Denmark	2086	0	3241	64.4	0
France	2290	69	4778	47.9	1.4
German Fed. Rep.	1872	22	4348	43.1	0.5
Ireland	549	9	956	57.4	0.9
Italy	578	8	1207	47.9	0.7
The Netherlands	468	4	969	48.3	0.4
Spain	1445	20	2757	52.4	0.7
UK	12,645	203	24,382	51.9	0.8

Rash/total (R/T), Stevens Johnson Syndrome (SJS), SJS/total (S/T).

The choice of a suitable denominator may not be simple, as the aetiology and pathology of the adverse effect have to be taken into account and these may not be known with any certainty. For example, a particular adverse event may only occur after the drug has been taken for an extended period, and is related to the total amount of drug administered. It could be that only a small minority of patients are in that category, and for whom the risk is high. For the great majority, who only take the drug short term, the risk may be negligible. Similarly, the adverse effect may only occur in a subgroup of patients who, coincidentally, have another pathological condition which predisposes to the ADE. In this case, the incidence in those at risk depends on the selection of an appropriate denominator.

The absolute numbers of spontaneous reports relating to any particular clinical event are dependent on a number of fairly obvious factors. The extent to which a drug is used is clearly important, but may be complicated by the pathological mechanism of the adverse reaction. The significance of prescription volume is different for reactions associated with the initiation of treatment from reactions that do not become apparent until the drug has been taken for an extended period.

The extent to which a drug is used is at least partly dependent on the success of the pharmaceutical company's promotional programme, but also on the total number of patients with the relevant clinical indications, which in turn is dependent on the population of the country concerned. For some rare ADEs, small countries such as Belgium or Denmark, which have fewer than 15 million inhabitants, may never have enough patients to make detection possible. In these cases the serious problems involved in using data from other countries arise, and great care must be exercised before conclusions are drawn.

The problem is further complicated by the fact that drug use is spread unevenly over the patient population, with age and sex having a strong influence on prescribing patterns.[61] For example, if age is split into decades, then in general there is a predominance of first prescriptions in the first three decades and a predominance of repeat prescriptions in the sixth, seventh and eighth decades. The proportion of people who are patients also differs from decade to decade, and this may be an important factor to take into account. On the day of our birth virtually 100% of us are patients, and the same is true on the day of our death, but between these two extremes there is a varying proportion of people

who are patients to people who are not patients. It is possible to imagine a number of scenarios in which this might be of decisive importance in assessing the importance of an adverse reaction. For example, over the total patient population, and taking into account total drug use, a serious ADR may appear to be at an acceptable level. However, further investigation might show that 90% of drug use was in patients in the first five decades of life, whereas 90% of the ADRs were in patients in the seventh, eighth and ninth decades. This would almost certainly arouse great concern and require major changes in the package insert or data sheet.

These denominators may be regarded as scaling factors by which the clinical, regulatory, ethical or social importance of an ADR may be measured, but they are still inadequate if truly balanced decisions are to be taken. Within these constraints there are the ever-present problems of underreporting and bias that have already been discussed. Unfortunately, these two defects of the system are not evenly spread across disease, drugs or patients, making it impossible to apply any simple, generally applicable correction factor. In recently published appraisals of spontaneous reporting,[51,52] it was shown that, within the limitations of the studies reviewed, there were wide variations in underreporting, depending on the clinical event reported. The range probably extends from about 15% at best (85% underreporting) to less than 1% (99% underreporting) at worst. The problem of bias is even more difficult to quantify, and apart from the certain knowledge that it exists there is little objective evidence on its extent.

Overall reporting levels in differing circumstances are an essential requirement if comparisons are to be made between countries, or even comparisons between drugs in a particular class. In the first case it is clear that different correction factors would have to be applied if data from a country with an overall reporting rate of 10% were to be compared with those from a country with a rate of only 5%. The second case would be exemplified by a drug such as triazolam, which has been the subject of high-profile media and regulatory attention, compared with a similar drug such as temazepam, which has not been so closely scrutinised.

The selection of a relevant denominator or denominators is thus a matter for careful consideration. The following factors should be taken into account and, wherever possible, quantified so that appropriate corrections may be made:

• Total population of country;

- Total patient population for the indicated clinical condition(s);
- Total prescriptions over a defined period of time;
- Number of first prescriptions over a defined period of time;
- Overall reporting rates for country, clinical condition, drug, etc.

The above factors should be subdivided by sex and age (in decades or other appropriate bands).

16.6.3 Special circumstances

There are a number of situations in which spontaneous reporting is essentially inappropriate for the detection of ADEs. Occasionally, the appearance of an ADE is delayed for an extended period after the initiation of treatment with the drug in question. These ADEs of long latency have been reviewed by Fletcher and Griffin,[62] and in none of the examples cited had they been detected by spontaneous reports. Attention was most often first drawn to the possible drug association by individual case reports in the medical literature. Indeed, it may be that this is the route by which knowledge of potential new ADRs is most commonly gained, whether they are of long latency or immediate. Up to a few years ago no other method had been available for the detection of delayed ADEs, but now, with the development of computerised systems for recording patient information in the doctor's surgery, it is possible to conduct retrospective surveys of drug use over relatively long periods. Many of the important drug disasters of the past three decades, such as thalidomide (drug taken during pregnancy causing phocomelia in the newborn), stilboestrol (drug taken during pregnancy causing carcinoma of the vagina in daughters)[63] and practolol (causing the oculomucocutaneous syndrome many months after administration)[64–66] have been of this type of ADR.

Carcinogenicity is always a concern with drugs that are administered chronically, and as the lag period before the development of a detectable tumour and first administration may be as long as 20 years this is a particularly severe problem. It seems unlikely that conventional prospective drug monitoring could ever be a practical method in these circumstances. The problem would more likely be seen as an unexplained rise in the incidence of a particular neoplasm. Surveys conducted by the National Cancer Institute[67,68] in the USA and by others[69] have investigated the possible carcinogenicity of an extensive list of drugs. The effective use of aggressive chemotherapy in conditions such as Hodgkin's disease is now known to be associated with an increase in second primary malignancies.[69]

Another situation in which spontaneous reporting is unlikely to be of help is when the ADE closely resembles another common disease and the prescribing doctor is unable to distinguish between them. In order to recognise such an ADE it is necessary to know the background incidence of the condition, and also to be in a position to see an otherwise unexplained increase in its incidence. Needless to say, these conditions are seldom met, and it is only after long experience with the drug that an increase in ADEs may be detected. Large-scale cohort studies involving 10,000 or more patients are probably the most powerful way of discovering and quantifying such ADEs, provided they occur more frequently than about 1 in 1000 patients taking the drug. This is the situation for many of the better-known examples, such as cough with angiotensin-converting enzyme (ACE) inhibitors, tremor with beta-agonists and debility with beta-blockers, so there is a real place for the cohort study in post-marketing safety evaluation. The wealth of other clinical data provided by cohort studies is an additional benefit in the continuing evaluation of the drug.

The advent of computerised databases that link the prescribed drug to diagnosis and record patient histories over extended periods provides another method by which the incidence of the more common ADEs may be estimated.

Related to the ADE that mimics another condition is the ADE that is a deterioration or alteration of the disease being treated. In this case, it is necessary to know the natural history of the disease when treated by established therapies, and to be in a position to observe an alteration in that process. Once again, these conditions are not often met and so detection may be long delayed.

A failure to detect these classes of ADE may have serious consequences, as the ADE itself may be disabling or even life-threatening, but even when it is relatively trivial it may be a reason for the patient's discontinuing effective treatment, which in turn may cause a deterioration in their condition. An example would be the patient who discontinues the treatment of his or her asthma with a beta-agonist because of tremor and then goes into status asthmaticus, with fatal consequences.

The UK Medicines and Healthcare products Regulatory Agency (MHRA) has recently drawn special attention to several areas of interest and have highlighted adverse reactions in children and the elderly. Children pose a particular problem because they are seldom studied in clinical trials that form the basis of marketing authorisation submissions. The consequence of this is that children are prescribed medicines that are not licensed for their age group and little experience of possible adverse effects is available. The elderly are also underrepresented in premarketing clinical trials and are also subject to diminished metabolic activity in respect of numerous commonly used drugs.

The preoccupation of many regulatory agencies with rare and serious ADRs as detected by spontaneous reporting systems may provide partial protection against the political and media excesses of the classic drug disaster, but are of little help in detecting the kind of drug-related conditions that endanger patients by limiting effective therapy and preventing optimal drug treatment. It should be remembered that the health of nations is unaffected by rare and exotic ADRs, which may be fascinating for the collector but are of little value in the better treatment of patients. On the other hand, the health of nations is affected by the common, but sometimes less serious, drug-related clinical conditions that place constraints on the most effective treatment.

16.6.4 Can spontaneous reporting be improved?

Much time and discussion has gone into this question over the past several years.[70–74] The cynics would say that more is already being expected of spontaneous reporting than it can ever deliver, and that it has probably reached its limits. The more optimistic – or possibly the more naive – would say that improvements are possible and that we should set about achieving them.

Broadly speaking, there are two areas where improvement might be possible. First, there is the input side[75] of the ADE report that is provided by the prescribing physician, and secondly, there is the output – the analysis and evaluation of the report.

Anyone who has examined a few hundred spontaneous reports will know that there is great variability in both the quantity and the quality of their content. The reports range from the totally useless to excellent records of important clinical observations. In between, the great majority reflect the real dilemma faced by the reporting physician. Is the observation worth reporting or is it just an irrelevance? Is this going to cause trouble for me, for the company, for the authorities, for the patient? How is it possible to judge potential causality?

The answers are elusive, and although virtually all regulatory agencies limit their requirements to events that meet the accepted definition of 'serious',

in the real world this definition is inadequate. For example, is abdominal pain serious? According to the definitions, if it is disabling, life-threatening, causing hospitalisation, etc. it is, but not otherwise. If it did not come into any of the defined categories the doctor would not be required or expected to report the event even though it might herald the perforation of a peptic ulcer. There are, similarly, many other symptomatic drug-related events that, although not serious by definition, are nevertheless important indicators of potentially serious conditions. Improving the quality of the input, however desirable, is not a simple matter, as it inevitably relies to a considerable extent on the clinical judgement of the reporting doctor. Improving the education of physicians may help, but there would seem to be a limit to what is possible.

Assuming that the quality of the input is maximal then improving the output will be dependent upon the analysis and evaluation of the data. Because the spontaneous report alone will seldom, if ever, contain sufficient information to determine causality satisfactorily, it is usually necessary to seek additional data which may be available from hospital records, laboratory investigations or post-mortem reports. It is highly desirable that comparable methods and formats of reporting should be used as widely as possible, particularly if international comparisons are to be made. A major benefit of formalised systems of causality assessment, which will be considered in greater detail later in this chapter, is the element of standardisation that is brought to the process of interpretation.

16.6.5 Cohort studies

The basic essentials of a cohort study are a group of patients of defined size, a system of data collection over a defined period, and a system for handling, analysing and presenting the findings. The methods available range from paper-based manual systems to fully computerised technology for all stages of the process. Phase IV clinical trials are a special kind of cohort study which have been dealt with separately, leaving this section to cover purely observational, non-interventional studies. The main objective of observational studies is to monitor drug use in the actual circumstances of everyday clinical practice. Study design should make all possible provision for data collection to proceed without influencing the normal course of treatment. Observational methods will, of course, record inappropriate as well as appropriate drug use, in contrast to clinical trials which involve patient selection and defined dosages and durations of treatment. Observational cohort studies are therefore also capable of monitoring for those ADEs that are predominantly associated with misuse of the product. By definition, such ADEs are inaccessible to clinical trials. It is for this reason that, in the case of a potential drug disaster, there is little to be gained by simply conducting more, longer and larger clinical trials, which can only measure the effects in an artificial, experimental situation. In fact, it should be emphasised that patient exclusions or drug use limitations should never be included in observational study plans unless there are exceptional circumstances. Provision of the package insert or summary of product characteristics (SPC) is an adequate way of bringing the attention of the doctor to the correct use of the product. In principle, limitations beyond those in the manufacturer's approved literature should always be excluded unless there are compelling safety requirements to be observed. If such compelling requirements do exist then their inclusion in the data sheet should be considered.

A critical review[76] of observational cohort studies conducted by, or on behalf of, pharmaceutical companies in the UK drew attention to a number of deficiencies in study design which, in certain cases, limited the value of the study. The authors, from the Medicines Control Agency (MCA) and the CSM, were motivated by the wish to improve the standard of post-marketing cohort studies, but they failed to distinguish between the good and the bad studies that were included in their review, and in doing so created the impression that the observational cohort study as a method was of little value in the assessment of safety. It is unfortunate that none of the good studies (there were at least three that met the highest standards) was cited in greater detail to emphasise that it is not the method which is at fault but the adequacy of the performance. As a consequence of these failings the paper has had a powerful inhibiting effect on companies' enthusiasm for all kinds of post-marketing safety studies. There is little doubt that, quite unintentionally, a great deal of damage has been done, and that some long time may elapse before a more balanced view is regained.

One aim of this paper, which has been achieved, was to stimulate the revision of the existing post-marketing surveillance guidelines which, it was hoped, would improve the overall standard of cohort studies. The new guidelines, which are entitled 'Guidelines for Company Sponsored Safety Assessment of Marketed Medicines (SAMM)', have had a mixed reception from the industry and their effect on the conduct of relevant studies has yet to be assessed. Ten years on from the MCA/CSM paper[76] there is little interest in observational cohort studies. Whether this has been because of an inhibitory effect of the paper or to a real disenchantment with the method is difficult to assess, but the result has been the virtual loss of a valuable way of assessing post-marketing safety. A recent overview by Linden[77] has drawn attention to the importance of observational studies for research into the actual treatment of patients in everyday clinical practice, in contrast to the highly restricted circumstances of randomised controlled clinical trials. In the same journal, Schafer[78] also points out the shortcomings of premarketing clinical trials and advocated the use of large-scale observational studies conducted in routine medical practice.

The strengths of observational cohort studies are the depth and quality of data that may be collected. Even though these studies are unstructured in the sense that there are no limiting criteria in respect of patient, drug or dosage, they are defined in size and duration and data collection methods, whether on paper forms or on computer screens, and they can draw the attention of the participating doctor to particular pieces of information that are highly desirable. Should data be deficient or inconsistent then it is a relatively simple matter to go back to the doctor for clarification.

Of considerable importance is the possibility of collecting data on other clinical conditions the patient may have and other drugs that may also be prescribed. It must be emphasised that the elderly are the largest users of drug therapy, they frequently have more than one pathology and they are consequently often being treated with a multiplicity of drugs. It is in these circumstances that ADEs are most likely to occur, and so data covering concomitant disease and medication are an essential part of safety evaluation.

The weaknesses of cohort studies are limits on the numbers of patients that may be included, organisational difficulties, the handling of vast quantities of complex data, and the often quoted but less well-quantified high costs. It is a strange thing that although when companies are faced with the need to conduct a large post-marketing study the first question often concerns cost, remarkably little information is available for each of the different methods.

There are undoubtedly fairly severe problems of a practical nature in conducting cohort studies on numbers of patients in excess of 10–15,000. It is certainly true that larger studies have been carried out, but usually on drug classes or disease areas where adequate numbers of patients are more readily available. In the case of a drug newly introduced to the market, it is a major challenge to enlist a cohort of 10,000 patients within 2 years of launch unless it is one of the few 'blockbuster' products that will be used in hundreds of thousands of patients. These, and the problems of organisation and data handling, are practical matters rather than scientific ones, and the benefits of plentiful high-quality data have to be balanced against the methodological limits that exist. For the identification and quantification of both expected and unexpected ADEs that occur at a frequency of more than 1 in 3000 patients, and to have the capability of assessing the possible influences of concomitant disease and concomitant medication, the prospective observational cohort study is the best method available.[79,80]

The SAMM guidelines have been supplemented by a useful review entitled 'International guidelines on postauthorisation research and surveillance' by Herbold.[81]

16.7 Computerised databases

In the UK, approximately 80% of general practices are computerised, about half of which use their computers for maintaining patient records as well as for practice management, and there is little doubt that these numbers will continue to increase in the years ahead. The existence of detailed patient records extending over prolonged periods is a new resource for a broad range of clinical and related health care research. Perhaps their greatest value lies in the area of retrospective observational studies, where information on actual clinical practice is required. As these databases are the records of patient health care at the time of general practitioner (GP)–patient contact, the normal course of treatment is uninfluenced by the conduct of the study itself. Indeed, it is probably true to say that for the long-term evaluation of drug safety, which is one of the more important research applications of these new systems, there is no other method that could provide years of continuous data together with a wealth of information on morbidity and comedication. The databases may also be used for prospective studies by identifying patients currently receiving health care and following their clinical courses at defined future time points.

Because of their recent development, the full range of their research potential has not, as yet, been exploited or even explored. The evaluation of drug safety has already been mentioned, and it is a small step for studies that investigate the consequences of non-serious but troublesome side effects on the continuity of drug treatment and drug switching.[82,83] The importance of factors that adversely affect drug compliance and which therefore have both therapeutic and economic consequences has been sadly neglected, to the detriment of both patients and health care providers. Applications to research in the fields of epidemiology, the natural history of disease, case–control studies and pharmaco-economics, to mention just a few, have yet to be developed.

The fact that the great majority of the data needed for a retrospective study are already present in the database demands an entirely new conceptual approach. The situation can be compared to that of a sculptor faced by a massive block of stone from which he plans to carve a much smaller but absolutely precise statue. The sculptor has to cut away all the unwanted stone so as to leave just those parts that are required for the statue. A large computerised database contains the elements of the study, and all that has to be done is to strip away the unnecessary data. To do this, the required data must be selected by carefully defining those elements as accurately as possible. This may sound simple, but in practice it is frequently extremely difficult to achieve. A single data element, such as an age in years, a diagnosis or a particular drug, presents no problem, but millions of data elements related in extremely complex chronological ways are a completely different matter. To obtain the maximum value from these new systems, it is desirable to utilise their full potential. This means drawing upon the complete range of demographic, diagnostic and therapeutic data, and their chronological relationships. Any study that fails to incorporate all the data elements in the database that are relevant to the investigation runs the risk of reaching incomplete or erroneous conclusions.

In the randomised controlled clinical trial the structure of the study is determined by the preparation of a detailed protocol, which is designed to ensure that all essential data elements will be provided. In the case of studies conducted with computerised patient databases, the study has to be designed within the limitations of the data already in the database. These existing data may be supplemented by seeking extra information from the doctor, as has been done in several studies conducted by Jick and co-workers,[84–87] but this adds to the cost and the time taken to complete the study. The fact that patient demographics, diagnosis, drug(s) prescribed, dosage, duration of treatment, laboratory investigations and many other factors have already been determined and are in the past, which demands a major new conceptual approach.

In the USA, there are several computerised health care systems, sometimes referred to as multipurpose databases, which have been used for post-marketing surveillance purposes. The best-known include Group Health Cooperative of Puget Sound, Kaiser-Permanente, Medicaid, Rhode Island and the Saskatchewan database in Canada.[88–103]

Some confusion exists because these databases may be used in two essentially different ways. Most commonly, they have been used to investigate in greater detail previously identified clinical conditions that are suspected of being drug related. A recent example would be the suspicions raised by several reports in the medical literature that the use of human insulin was associated with an excess of hypoglycaemic episodes in the absence of prodromal signs or symptoms, compared with the use of animal insulins. In this case, databases could be searched retrospectively to find all insulin-dependent diabetics being treated in a defined period, and then to determine how many were on each of the two kinds of insulin and the number of hypoglycaemic episodes experienced by each group. Similar database searches could be made starting, for example, from the identification of all patients being prescribed short-acting benzodiazepines and then determining all adverse clinical events associated with their administration. The identification of patients with particular characteristics for cost–control studies, which are considered in the next section, may be facilitated by computerised database searching.

The second way in which the databases may be used is to identify all patients on a particular drug or with a particular clinical condition and then to follow them up over a defined period to determine what clinical events subsequently occur. For all practical purposes this method is a cohort study conducted through a computerised database, using screens and electronic data transmission rather than paper.

The advantages and disadvantages of computerised systems may be summarised as follows.

16.7.1 Advantages

1. In the right circumstances, very large patient groups may be identified and studied, retrospectively, over extended periods.
2. Retrospective database searching has no influence on the treatment of the patient and is thus free from any inducements to change treatment for the purposes of the study.
3. Data collection and management may be quicker, more efficient and more sophisticated than by other methods.

4. The database is continually being added to and is thus an increasing resource for research.
5. Comparator data may be readily available.
6. It is possible to conduct case–control studies by identifying the relevant groups of patients from the database.

16.7.2 Disadvantages

In the case of retrospective studies, the data items that have been entered into the database are, essentially, the data that are available. If data items are missing, then for all practical purposes they are not available for the study. It is possible to go back to the physician in the hope that other records or memory may be of help, but after months or years this could be a costly and unprofitable procedure.

1. In the absence of intensive training programmes, with their considerable cost implications, the quality of data is highly variable from doctor to doctor.
2. Within any computerised system the physicians involved are a fixed group with its own idiosyncrasies and limitations in number.
3. Any particular system may contain certain fixed biases. In some of the US systems, patients may be predominantly of particular age groups, of particular social classes or in other ways atypical of the total population.
4. The multiplicity of hardware and software that is available creates incompatibilities between systems, which in turn makes the combination or comparison of data difficult or impossible.

Since the first edition of this book, developments have continued in this area, particularly with respect to computerised databases as a source of detailed and reliable data for use in the pharmaco-economic assessment of new drugs. The creation of specialised databases, such as HIV Insight, which contains the detailed clinical records of about 2500 patients who are either HIV seropositive or have the disease AIDS, has been very successful and plans are being made to develop other specialised databases in diabetes, oncology, Alzheimer's, osteoporosis and other similar chronic diseases.

16.8 Case–control studies

These studies are of greatest value when a potential ADR has already been identified (i.e. they are hypothesis testing rather than hypothesis generating). The case–control method has been used in a wide range of circumstances where risks to health have been identified. The classic examples are the relationship between smoking and bronchial carcinoma, and the association of the oral contraceptive with thromboembolic disorders. Case–control studies have also been used when no potential ADE has been identified, but these can be little more than 'fishing trips' conducted in the hope that something of interest may be caught.

The foundations of the method were laid by Cornfield, Dorn, Mantel and Haenszel[104–108] in the 1950s, and it was rapidly adopted by epidemiologists as a major new technique. An interesting historical account of case–control studies has been given by Lilienfeld and Lilienfeld,[109] who trace the method back to Louis and his study of tuberculosis in 1844.[110] Later developments have been reviewed by Cole,[111] who provides a useful assessment of the strengths and weaknesses of such studies. Emphasis is placed upon the need for precise case definition and the futility of attempting to get meaningful results in studies on broad diagnostic descriptions, such as depression or bone cancer. Further methodological problems have been addressed by Feinstein,[112] and the particularly serious problem of bias was reviewed by Sackett.[113]

There is little doubt, on the one hand, that case–control studies have a valuable place in pharmaco-epidemiology, and therefore in the evaluation of drug safety. There is also little doubt that without minute attention to detail and, possibly, a little luck, the method may be unreliable or even completely misleading. A list of 56 topics was reviewed by Mayes et al.[114] because the case–control studies on them had provided conflicting results. A total of 265 studies were considered, of which 137 were supportive of the hypothesis and 128 were not. On this basis it would be unwise to draw conclusions from a single case–control study, it being prudent to wait until further studies confirm or refute the original findings.

The basic principle of the method is simple. A cohort of patients with the disease in question is identified, and then a cohort of patients without the disease (usually two to three times as many) is matched with respect to a number of critical characteristics and used as the control group. Differences between the two groups with respect to exposure to the suspected causative agent are then measured. A major advantage is that uncommon or rare conditions are accessible to study, which is not the case for cohort studies or for computerised systems, where the total number of patients available is less than the several millions that might be needed.

In practice, the method is considerably more difficult than the simplicity of the design suggests. The series of studies conducted on the possible relationship of the Rauwolfia derivatives to various cancers is testimony to the conflicting findings that may result. Indeed, the 11 case–control studies[115–126] on reserpine and other Rauwolfia alkaloids reviewed by Labarthe,[127] and the additional study by Friedman,[128] could well be regarded as the classic example of the uncertainties inherent in this method of safety evaluation. The first three studies to be published strongly suggested a causal association between reserpine and breast cancer, although each of them urged caution in their interpretation. In spite of this plea for a carefully considered approach there was a flurry of regulatory activity by both the Food and Drug Administration (FDA) in the USA and the CSM in the UK. Both agencies considered the possibility of removing the products from the market, but decided to await further studies before coming to a final conclusion. Later studies did not confirm the original findings, no regulatory action was taken, and it was concluded that a causal relationship between reserpine and breast cancer was unlikely.

It is not the purpose of this chapter to analyse in detail the shortcomings of the original studies which resulted in weeks of work for the FDA and CSM, but there are one or two important lessons to be learnt. The importance of case definition referred to earlier was clearly not heeded in these studies. The condition studied was 'breast cancer', which is almost certainly too broad as a diagnostic classification.

Depending upon the pathology textbook of your choice, somewhere between 15 and 20 different kinds of malignant tumours of the breast are recognised, all of which would fall within the description 'breast cancer'. There is an enormous variation in the characteristics of these tumours with respect to originating tissue, histological type, malignancy, hormone dependence and tendency to metastasise. It is highly unlikely that any single agent could be the cause of such a wide variety of neoplasms. The most common malignant breast tumour is the scirrhous adenocarcinoma, which is usually very slow growing. It is known to have low growth fractions, with cell production exceeding cell loss by only about 10%, with the consequence that many years may pass from the time of tumorigenesis to the point at which the tumour becomes detectable. In the Boston Collaborative study six out of the 11 cancer cases had first been exposed to reserpine 5 years or less before the diagnosis. From these facts alone the role of reserpine as a carcinogen would seem to be very unlikely, and fully justified the cautious approach taken by the FDA and CSM.

In the assessment of causality, Bradford Hill[129] cited biological plausibility as a major factor to take into consideration. If existing knowledge of physiological or pathological mechanisms is difficult to reconcile with the findings of a study, then much thought should be given to any attribution of causality.

Even in situations in which the diagnosis is straightforward, difficulties may arise if an assessment of severity or the presence of associated disease is required. However, it is in the selection of control cases that major difficulties occur. There is the assumption, in the methodology, that all the relevant criteria for matching cases to controls are known, which in some cases is certainly not true. The hope is that cases and controls will be the same for all essential characteristics except the presence or absence of the disease. The finding that the test group exhibited excess exposure to the suspected toxin would then be interpreted as a positive result and the existence of a causal relationship inferred.

Case–control studies are powerful tools for the further investigation of suspected rare and uncommon ADEs, provided the factors discussed above are carefully controlled. The literature contains numerous examples of the method which should be evaluated critically.[130,131]

16.9 Prescription event monitoring

This form of adverse event monitoring was pioneered and developed by the Drug Safety Research Unit (DSRU) in Southampton. The aim is to monitor all new products that are expected to be widely used in general practice, with studies starting as soon as possible after the drug is first launched in the UK. Prescription event monitoring (PEM) can be used to generate safety signals about new medicines that participating doctors may not have suspected to have been caused by the drug.

All patients who are prescribed the drug are identified from prescriptions submitted to the Prescription Pricing Authority (PPA). Copies of the prescriptions are sent to the DSRU to provide exposure data on patient and prescribing doctor. After a certain interval, typically 12 months, each GP is contacted and asked to complete a simple questionnaire (the 'green form') describing any 'event' that might have been recorded since the first prescription to the individual patient.

An 'event' is defined as a diagnosis, sign or symptom, accident, operation, change of treatment or any other incident that the doctor had considered important enough to enter into the patient's notes. For example, a fall would be considered an event, but not necessarily an ADR. The GP is not required to decide whether events are drug related or not.

The green forms are returned, scanned and the data entered on to computer. Important medical events, serious possible ADRs, all deaths from uncertain causes, pregnancies and events of interest are followed up. The response rate from green forms is very high (55.75%) compared with spontaneous reporting (Yellow Cards). The incidence densities (IDs) are then calculated for all the events occurring during treatment with the drug during a specified time period (t). The figures are expressed as ID per 1000 patient-months of treatment:

$$\mathrm{ID}_t = \frac{\begin{array}{c}\text{Number of reports of an event}\\ \text{during treatment for period } t\end{array}}{\begin{array}{c}\text{Number of patient-months of}\\ \text{treatment for period } t\end{array}} \times 1000$$

Event rates are compared between the first month of treatment and the second to sixth months, and also during and after drug exposure. 'Reasons for stopping' are identified and medically qualified staff assess the causal relationship between the drug in question and selected events, using the following categories: probable, possible, unlikely or not assessable. The incidence of a particular event in patients who have not been exposed to the drug is examined (easier in those illnesses that are rarer), and event rates are compared between drugs of the same class and with similar indications. Safety signals, if present, can then be generated.

The system has several qualities that are very desirable in observational studies which include access to a large and widely distributed patient population and applicability to most new and generally used medicines. Reporting can be commenced as soon as the product reaches the market and observation may be extended over relatively long time periods. Disadvantages are the probability that there is considerable bias resulting from self-selection or exclusion by the doctor, impracticality of providing comprehensive clinical information on many chronically ill patients, recent low response rates, concerns in respect of confidentiality and increasing time constraints on GPs. Two recent studies[132,133] have also suggested that response rates may be affected by the extent of prescribing for non-approved indications which would be perceived as increasing liability for the prescriber. An example of this is the widespread use of NSAIDs as general analgesics even when particular products are not licensed for those indications.

Examples of recent work carried out by the DSRU includes the examination of mortality rates and cardiac arrhythmias between sertindole and two other atypical antipsychotics, olanzapine and risperidone.[134] Tolterodine, an agent often used for urinary frequency and bladder instability, is the latest drug to be examined by the DSRU.[135]

16.10 Some examples

It would be useful for pharmaceutical physicians to have some examples of medical products that have been the subject of serious adverse reactions requiring regulatory action. In the following subsections a number of products have been selected that illustrate different drug safety problems. Major attention has been paid to psychotropic agents because they are widely used and have been the subject of regulatory evaluation and action over the past several years which has resulted in restrictions to use and in some cases withdrawal from the market.

16.10.1 Psychotropic agents

Before the late 1980s there were very limited options in terms of pharmaceuticals for the psychiatric patient. With the advent of fluoxetine (Prozac), which was first launched in Belgium in 1986, the whole area of neuroscience became of much greater interest, especially given the fact that it was an area that had been relatively neglected up until that point. Options for treatment are now much more varied and offer the psychiatrist and patient far more choice. However, this has come at a price; several drugs have had to be taken off the market while some remain available but with restricted use. In this section, antidepressants and antipsychotics are examined.

16.10.1.1 Clozapine

Clozapine is considered to be the gold standard of treatment of schizophrenia with patients usually moving onto it after treatment failure with two other antipsychotics. Yet its history is quite chequered. When it was first introduced onto the European market in 1975 it was used freely with no restrictions on use. Following the death of eight patients in Finland from agranulocytosis, a very rare (<1%) but often fatal condition occurring normally within the first few months of use, it was voluntarily taken off the market.

Thirty years later it is widely used throughout the UK and is growing in popularity. Further trials were carried out showing that up to 60% of patients who had been unresponsive to other antipsychotic treatment, did respond to long-term clozapine therapy. In 1990, clozapine gained a product licence and was relaunched with concurrent weekly monitoring of the white cell count for the first 16 weeks followed by fortnightly monitoring for the first year. Stringent measures were introduced such that hospital pharmacies were not permitted to dispense the drug until they had received notification of a 'green' result from the clozapine patient monitoring service (CPMS). An amber result (white count lowered) requires a repeat result which must be green before dispensing can take place, and a red result means that the patient has to stop the drug immediately. With such monitoring the incidence of agranulocytosis is 0.38%.

The successful relaunch of clozapine illustrates how life-threatening side effects can be managed as long as:
1. They are detected quickly enough both in clinical practice and in pre-registration clinical trials; and
2. Stringent enough measures are put in place to prevent dispensing of drugs if necessary.
It is interesting to note that clozapine now prevents more deaths from suicide in patients with schizophrenia than it does in causing death from agranulocytosis.

16.10.1.2 Cardiac dysrhythmias associated with antipsychotics

Sertindole, an atypical antipsychotic, was introduced into the UK market in 1996 and initially it appeared that the drug would be useful, despite recommendations for ECG monitoring before and during sertindole therapy. QTc prolongation (rate corrected QT interval) was known to effect approximately 2% of patients in clinical trials. The drug was voluntarily suspended in 1998[134] following reports of sudden unexpected deaths and is now only available on a named-patient basis for those patients already stabilised on it, for whom other antipsychotics are inappropriate. Although 2% might seem a relatively insignificant figure for a side effect, given the fact that the consequences of a prolongation of the QT interval can be fatal, the pharmaceutical physician needs to be mindful of the type of side effect and potential seriousness of it. A side effect of perhaps 10% of patients experiencing headache would not potentially lead to the withdrawal of a drug, unlike a 2% risk of QTc prolongation or a 1% risk of agranulocytosis.

Reilly et al.,[136] in their seminal review of antipsychotics and QTc-interval prolongation, further highlighted the potential risks of such drugs. They noted that thioridazine and droperidol were at higher risk of causing such abnormalities. Thioridazine had been used for many years both with psychiatric patients and the elderly as a means of sedation. It is likely that many elderly patients may have died as a result of the drug because 'old age' was thought to be the cause. It is now available as a second-line treatment, under specialist supervision only. Droperidol is a long-established antipsychotic of high potency which was used in the control of schizophrenia and for acutely agitated patients. Droperidol was withdrawn for use in the UK in 2002. Ziprasidone,[137] another atypical antipsychotic which can cause QT interval prolongation, although available in the USA, has never received approval in the EU.

16.10.1.3 Antipsychotics and stroke

Risperidone and olanzapine have been widely used in patients with dementia exhibiting behavioural problems. Following the withdrawal of thioridazine from the market, psychiatrists and GPs working with the elderly were increasingly prescribing atypical antipsychotics, in particular risperidone as it was the only atypical that had been examined in randomised clinical trials with the elderly. In 2004, the CSM[138] advised that both risperidone and olanzapine caused a three-fold increased risk of cerebrovascular events in elderly patients with dementia compared with placebo. Consequently, the CSM advised that these drugs should be used with caution in patients with risk factors for cerebrovascular disease and many thousands of patients have now been taken off the atypical antipsychotics.

16.10.1.4 Antipsychotics and diabetes/hyperlipidaemia

Atypical antipsychotics[139,140] have also been linked with the development of type II diabetes and hyperlipidaemia in patients with schizophrenia. In several studies, olanzapine[141–143] has been more strongly linked than risperidone and there is a caution for use in patients with diabetes. Many psychiatrists now carry out a baseline glucose before initiating patients on it. The development of diabetes and hyperlipidaemia is of great concern, as patients with schizophrenia often neglect their physical health, smoke heavily and are at greater risk of developing diabetes than the normal population, even before they start to take antipsychotics. It is a problem that has emerged over several years and thus illustrates the importance of Yellow Card reporting and the pharmaceutical physician paying close attention to case reports and the company database. Side effects that can seem relatively minor in clinical trials can take on a much greater significance once a drug has been on the market for several years and had huge patient exposure, and thus increasing numbers of cases.

16.10.1.5 Selective serotonin reuptake inhibitors and major depressive disorder in children and adolescents

In 2003, the CSM[138] advised that paroxetine and venlafaxine should not be used in children under the age of 18 to treat depression, following advice that the risks of self-harming behaviours outweighed the benefits of treatment. An expert working party was then set up to examine the safety and efficacy of the other selective serotonin reuptake inhibitors (SSRIs). All the clinical trial data available for citalopram, escitalopram, sertraline, fluvoxamine and fluoxetine were examined. Only fluoxetine was shown to have a favourable risk–benefit ratio in children and adolescents and is now the only SSRI recommended for use in this age group. In the other SSRIs, clinical trial data did not demonstrate efficacy in this age group and were associated with serious side effects such as suicidal thoughts and an increased rate of self-harm. Given that approximately 20,000 children under the age of 18 were estimated to be taking SSRIs other than fluoxetine at the time of this advice, clearly this had huge implications for treatment and confidence in the use of these drugs.

Thus, the psychiatric drugs which showed so much hope when they were initially launched, and indeed for some years afterwards, are now increasingly being linked with serious and potentially fatal side effects. Clinical trials either do not detect these problems or detect it in such small figures that problems do not emerge until widespread use. This is the reason that extremely large phase IV trials which are naturalistic are so vital in order to be able to detect these types of side effects. Phase IV trials are, of course, costly but necessary, if useful drugs can be made available to patients in a safe manner. Clozapine is one such drug that illustrates well how a potentially lethal drug can still be prescribed with confidence by the clinician. The pharmaceutical physician must be alert to these potential problems and be creative in advising how they can be managed.

For instance, if patients taking olanzapine are obliged to be warned of these serious side effects before taking the drug and health advice is given initially, the weight gain usually seen in the first few months may be prevented and hence the onset of type II diabetes, which is associated with obesity. As ever, the risks and benefits of drugs must be weighed up and not ignored, even if it leaves the treating clinician with few options.

16.10.2 Safety of medicinal products intended for use by healthy patients

16.10.2.1 Hormonal contraceptives

The foremost medicinal products in this unusual class are the hormonal contraceptives followed by vaccines and a number of products, such as antimalarials, which have a clear preventative clinical function. Then there are other drugs, such as hypnotics, which are predominantly used for the treatment of disorders that are troublesome but are not associated with serious morbidity or mortality.

The benefit : risk assessment of these medicines demands that product safety very firmly holds the balance. Even extremely low incidence of serious adverse reactions might outweigh the benefits in all but exceptional circumstances.

The hormonal contraceptives first became available as prescription products in 1960 with the combined oestrogen–progestogen product, trade name Enovid, in the USA. A year later a similar oestrogen–progestogen product, trade name Anovlar, with lower hormonal dosage was introduced in Europe. The efficacy of these new oral contraceptives was unrivalled although it soon became apparent that activation of the renin–angiotensin system caused serious hypertension in a subset of women. Further lowering of both hormonal components and the development of different oestrogens and progestogens were successful in lowering the incidence of adverse effects.

Nearly 50 years after the first hormonal contraceptives were introduced we have reached a new era of 'third generation oral contraceptives' which have been the subject of litigation in respect of possible increased risk of venous thromboembolism in comparison with previous products. This case was heard in the High Court and the judge concluded that there was no significant excess risk associated with the third generation products in comparison with second generation.

This concern with safety has demanded intensive research in both animal and human studies. During the years since 1960 several 10-year carcinogenicity studies in primates have been conducted in addition to numerous similar long-term studies in dogs and

tens of thousands of patients in clinical trials making the oral contraceptives (OCs) by far the most intensively investigated medicinal products. Needless to say, even though safety evaluation began long ago, our concerns in respect of administering powerful hormonal materials to healthy women has continued to be an important issue.

In 1987 the Special Program of Research Training in Human Reproduction run by the WHO reviewed the results of animal and human studies analysing contraceptive steroids.[144] These studies covered a broad range of safety matters including breast disease, gallbladder disease, congenital malformations and several other topics. It was concluded that the investigation of safety involved the joint responsibility of experimental toxicology and clinical pharmacology and that extensive studies should be conducted in several animal species. It was also recommended that both *in vivo* and *in vitro* tests should be included to investigate mutagenic potential. The report finally stated that post-registration surveillance was an integral part of the risk assessment process.

McKenzie[145] has stated that the OC steroids have been subjected to preclinical and clinical investigations unprecedented in medical history. The need for extra vigilance in respect of pharmaceutical products intended for healthy individuals were emphasised by McKenzie – 'The initial requirements for the safety evaluation of OCs were identical to those of other drugs. There were no explicit requirements for OCs although it was generally felt that the requirements should be more stringent because OCs were being used in otherwise healthy women for long periods of time and with minimal medical supervision.'

Clinical investigations on the steroid contraceptives have mostly been limited to epidemiological design studies because randomised controlled trials are essentially unable to be used because the incidence of cardiovascular and thromboembolic diseases in women of reproductive age is generally very low. Hannaford[146] has emphasised the importance of interpreting data from epidemiological studies very carefully, particularly in respect of potential biases or sources of confounding. Furthermore, findings from these sources should always be evaluated in comparison with other non-epidemiological methods of clinical investigation and with animal studies.

More recently, the possible interaction of hormonal contraceptives with new medicinal products has become a matter of concern such as antiretroviral treatment of HIV-infected women.[147,148] It is thus clear that the hormonal contraceptives have been the subject of intensive clinical and animal safety studies since the time of their introduction in 1960.

16.10.2.2 Vaccines

A contrasting class of medicinal products administered almost entirely to healthy individuals are the vaccines. These are characteristically administered as a single initiating dose with varying programmes of follow-up booster doses. Although this is clearly different from chronically administered daily doses as is the case for the OCs the clinical effect of vaccines is commonly lifelong, meaning that physiological changes brought about by a few administrations may be the cause of adverse effects later in life.

The history of vaccination is beyond the scope of this chapter but it is an aspect of preventative medicine which is commonly claimed to have originated with Edward Jenner's use of cowpox-infected material to prevent smallpox at the end of the eighteenth century. It became immediately clear that this was effective in the prevention of the disease but it was equally clear that serious adverse effects, including death, were not uncommon. Over the past 200 years many infectious diseases have been satisfactorily controlled by the development of specific vaccines. There is little doubt that the safety testing of these vaccines has fallen short of the intensive investigations conducted on the hormonal contraceptives. This is certainly in part because preclinical testing in animals is severely limited by major differences in their immune systems when compared with humans but also because clinical trials of appropriate size have been difficult to conduct.

During the past decade, the safety aspects of several vaccines, those intended for administration to children in particular, have been questioned and, in some cases, become the subject of litigation. This chapter is not the appropriate place to analyse the details of these cases but should address some general aspects of vaccine safety. As with all medicinal products the balance between benefits and risks is of paramount importance. Even the briefest literature search reveals that there are many thousands of publications concerning the efficacy and safety of vaccines but closer examination indicates a vanishingly low number or even absence of research papers that are both authoritative and substantial. A mistaken belief is that adverse reactions to vaccine administration all occur within a week or so of the injection which has led to studies limited to very short surveillance periods. That this is wrong is evidenced by recent reports strongly supporting an increase in later life of herpes zoster after prior vaccination against varicella. It is clear that this adverse effect could be delayed by many months or even years after the administration.[149–151]

The benefit–risk balance is also profoundly influenced by the dramatic improvements in social conditions and health care in affluent developed countries. For example, in the first decade of the twentieth century in the UK annual mortality from measles was approaching 10,000; in the decade prior to the introduction of measles vaccine this had fallen to less than 100 (99% reduction). From these figures there is no doubt that social conditions and the standards of health care are predominant factors in mortality rates due to infectious diseases. This is of particular importance for developing countries where those conditions are incomparably lower. In circumstances in which high mortality rates prevail even serious adverse reactions to vaccines may be acceptable if there are overwhelming benefits. The converse is the case in countries such as the UK where background mortality rates are very low which require minimal serious adverse reactions attributable to vaccines if benefits are to exceed risks.

Recent years have seen a substantial increase in the administration of multicomponent vaccines each containing five or more immunogens. At the present time no convincing safety research has been conducted to compare single-component vaccines with multicomponent products. It has been assumed that the simultaneous administration of several immunogens carries no excess risk while providing the benefits of fewer injections. Because this assumption has no acceptable supporting evidence it has to be regarded as unjustified.

16.10.3 Biological and biotech products

The safety evaluation of these products presents many difficult problems which are still poorly defined and shrouded in uncertainty at the present time in spite of numerous conferences, working parties and other guideline groups in the UK, EU and USA. It has to be said that most safety programs for biological and biotech substances have to be regarded with caution.

A healthy volunteer study on TGN 1412 conducted in March 2006 had catastrophic consequences for the six volunteers who were administered the material. Even though the dosage administered was 500 times lower than that found safe in animals, four of the subjects suffered multiple organ dysfunction. It was fairly clear that the findings in animals were not relevant to toxicity in humans which has been tentatively diagnosed as a cytokine release syndrome.[152]

This exceptional and unexpected adverse reaction stands as a most serious warning of possible fundamental differences between immunological effects in animal models and effects in healthy human subjects. It has demonstrated most forcefully that even extremely low multiples (i.e. less than 500 times lower) may still be of near lethality to human subjects.

16.10.4 Rofecoxib (Vioxx)

The cyclo-oxygenase 2 (COX-2) inhibitors were first licensed for sale at the end of the 1990s as more effective and better tolerated NSAIDs which, it was hoped, would provide improved therapy for patients with rheumatoid and osteoarthritis. One of the first of those was rofecoxib which quickly achieved dominance in the market and seemed to have lived up to its expectations over its first 2 years. Other similar agents, valdecoxib, celecoxib and meloxicam, were granted product licences and became competitor products. As might be expected, the major comparative clinical trials which were conducted in support of the products concentrated almost exclusively on gastrointestinal adverse effects which are generally accepted as being limiting factors in the use of earlier NSAIDs. Two of the studies concerned (CLASS and VIGOR[153,154]) demonstrated clear gastrointestinal advantages but only VIGOR noted a lower incidence of myocardial infarction in the comparator group although the authors stated that the overall mortality from cardiovascular causes was not increased.

In September 2001, however, a news item in the *British Medical Journal*[155] reported that further analyses confirmed the increase in rates of myocardial infarction and questioned whether this was an adverse reaction affecting the whole class of COX-2 drugs. The debate continued for the next 3 years with the main emphasis remaining on gastrointestinal toxicity. A PEM study[156] that included more than 15,000 patients made no mention of cardiovascular adverse events. However, a second paper[157] compared rofecoxib and meloxicam with respect to thromboembolic events which showed that both, to a variable extent, were associated with cardiovascular, cerebrovascular and peripheral venous pathology. A meta-analysis published recently in *The Lancet*[158] suggests that Merck,

the licence holder for Vioxx, was aware of cardiovascular problems as early as 2000 and there is the implication that the US FDA failed to act on the basis of this information. Indeed, there are growing doubts concerning the independence and impartiality of drug regulatory authorities in general. The Vioxx saga culminated in the withdrawal of the product from the market by Merck in September 2004 with disastrous results for the company.

16.10.4.1 Overall conclusions

The above examples have been selected to illustrate the complexity of managing suspected and actual adverse reactions to medical products. The pharmaceutical physician should take careful note of two vital factors. First, the initial recognition that a product may be related to a series of adverse event reports could be a slow process extending over months or even years and, secondly, that proof of causality is usually difficult and frequently impossible. This does not mean that regulatory action is not required or that a legal case may not follow. However, what is certain is that a potentially developing situation must not be neglected and every effort should be made to investigate the problem as scientifically as possible. The case of the measles–mumps–rubella (MMR) vaccine illustrates very well the regrettable fact that epidemiologically based studies may not be capable of recruiting a sufficient number of patients to provide statistically significant conclusions. This is a particularly serious problem for vaccines that are commonly administered to a major proportion of the relevant population which results in comparator groups that are too small to permit meaningful results.

It has long been recognised that individual patient susceptibility may be a major factor in the causality of adverse reactions. Recent advances in human genetics hold out the promise of identifying individuals or families that may be at greater risk but the application of these opportunities to improved prescribing has been extremely disappointing. It is clear from simple observational studies that ADRs occur in only relatively small subsets of the patient population leaving the majority unaffected. The unfortunate subset remains undetected until after the event.

There has never been any incentive for the pharmaceutical industry to pursue research along these lines even though, as in the case of Vioxx, the end results of neglecting adverse effects may be very costly. The aim of the industry has usually been to extend the market size irrespective of potential risk and attempts to implement effective post-marketing surveillance has received little enthusiasm. It is to be hoped that company medical departments and pharmaceutical physicians will continue to support the need for a broad range of safety evaluation studies to be conducted on new medicinal products.

16.11 Causality assessment

Lack of safety in medicinal products arises from the recurrence of undesired adverse effects associated with their use. The first requirement for the assurance of safety is the ability to detect such adverse effects. This has been dealt with in an earlier section of this chapter. Once detected, it is highly desirable that a significantly convincing causal relationship between the use of the product and the adverse effect should be established.

In previous editions of this textbook a number of methods of determining causality have been described and an attempt made to evaluate their relative reliability and validity. It has to be understood that such statistically based methods have, over several decades, been in competition with common observation and 'inspired guesswork' for the assessment of adverse effects in respect of the need for regulatory action. This is not just a matter of idiosyncratic personal preference but is frequently imposed by the clinical and numerical evidence available.

The most familiar story of a new and unexpected adverse effect starts in a dense fog of uncertainty. The pharmaceutical company may have received a few reports from doctors or other health care workers, there may be a letter in the medical press describing six or so cases of a suspected adverse effect or the regulatory authority may tentatively draw attention to a possible problem. The pharmaceutical physician may, quite reasonably, assess the small number of reports and conclude that they are slightly worrying but probably chance associations. Time passes and similar reports accumulate and the level of concern rises. This increasing concern may well be more apparent in the medical departments than those responsible for sales, and the pharmaceutical physician should not be inhibited from further investigations. A point is reached as the numbers increase, $20, \ldots, 30, \ldots, 40, \ldots, 50$ at which chance becomes a receding explanation. The physician may question him or herself, 'Can I realistically believe that all these reports are spurious, that not a single one is a true bill?' This has little to do with objective clinical science but it has

a real impact on further action. If the answer is 'no' then numbers, in themselves, have assumed the status of evidence.

This turning point in the decision process anticipates the continuing accumulation of case reports which may provide the quantity of data required by objective statistical methods. In the case of medical products that are in widespread use for common, well-understood clinical conditions this may be readily available but for products not having these attributes the data demanded for scientifically supported causality may be unobtainable.

The aims of causality assessment are manifold. Adverse events need to be classified, a decision needs to be made whether a drug has caused this event, regulatory requirements need to be satisfied, signal recognition can be aided, and finally, at the end of this process, a label change may be necessary.

Attributing causality is a major problem with spontaneous reports of suspected drug-related events. Clinical event reports arising from cohort studies or from computerised databases may also raise similar problems, particularly when they are in isolation or in such small numbers that a conventional statistical approach is not appropriate. If ADRs occur a long time after the original use of the drug, or there are delayed consequences of long-term use (e.g. tardive dyskinesia with the use of typical antipsychotics), then detection becomes difficult. In addition, clinical trials often do not include special populations, such as pregnant women, the elderly, children or patients with severe hepatic or renal disease, who may be at special risk of an ADR.

In the time that has elapsed since the previous edition of this book, it has been the authors' impression that enthusiasm for formal methods of causality assessment has decreased to the extent that few, if any, pharmaceutical companies still use them. Nevertheless, brief comments on methods that have been developed over the years are needed to complete the picture.

In a typical situation, two or three individual case reports may be published in the medical literature, to be followed by another half dozen spontaneous reports (Yellow Cards) to the regulatory agency that draw attention to a possible ADR to a particular product. The scientific value of such reports ranges from situations in which a causal relationship is a near-certainty, to those in which any attribution of causality would seem to be a forlorn hope. The former would include reports on patients with a single disease, who are administered a single drug for the first time, with a clearly described adverse clinical event occurring within hours of administration and resolving on withdrawal of the drug. Even if the event occurs many years later, as in the cases of clear cell adenocarcinoma in young women exposed to stilboestrol, it can be detected if the rate of this illness in this population would otherwise be negligible. Needless to say, this is seldom the case. At the other end of the scale is the patient with multiple pathologies, on 10 or more drugs, who develops a vague symptomatic adverse event 10 days after the introduction of a new medication, with partial resolution after its withdrawal. Often, the reporting physician has no idea whether the drug in question has caused the effect or not. Even beyond such confused and nebulous accounts are reports of so little clinical or scientific value that they can only be described as frivolous and have to be disregarded as useless.

In between these two extremes lie the great majority of spontaneous reports for which the attribution of causality is at best doubtful, and always difficult. It is not surprising, therefore, that considerable work has been done to devise mathematical methods to give numerical values to the varying degrees of certainty or uncertainty. These methods are applicable to individual cases either singly or for relatively small groups of selected cases where there are high-quality data and few confounding factors. It may be questioned whether assigning numerical values, in which a degree of precision is implicit, to data which are, to a substantial extent, subjective in nature can produce better results than the clinical judgement of experts. Whatever the answer to this question may be, there is no doubt that the application of a formalised system of assessment to ADE evaluation may produce a level of consistency that would not be possible by clinical judgement alone.

Meta-analysis is a method often used to determine the effectiveness of a drug but to date it has rarely been used to assess safety. One case illustrates how this technique can help. Six studies examining the use of intravenous lidocaine for acute myocardial infarction did not, on an individual basis, give strong enough evidence to support the hypothesis that this technique could cause excess mortality. The meta-analysis, however, was able to demonstrate this.[159]

A useful review of causality assessment methods has been produced by Stephens,[160] one of which he has developed for use by Glaxo Group Research. Because most of the methods are relatively time-consuming and rely on high-quality clean data, they are not readily applicable to situations in which hundreds or even thousands of reports have to be assessed. It is possibly true to say that most pharmaceutical companies still rely heavily upon clinical judgement, with occasional use of one or other of the described methods of causality assessment. In many cases, the continuing accumulation of similar ADE reports becomes the most convincing evidence that some unexpected reaction is occurring. This may be scientifically unsatisfactory, but is a reminder of the uncertainties that are an inseparable part of clinical medicine.

Edwards and Aronson[161] have suggested a way of coding whether an adverse event is an ADR. This depends on factors such as the time relation between the use of the drug and the occurrence of the reaction being assessed; pattern recognition; dechallenge and rechallenge of the drug in question; and laboratory investigations.

Another system has been devised by Benichou and Danan[162] which assigns numerical values to factors of importance in the assessment of causality (Table 16.10).

In recent years, a method of causality assessment based on Bayes' theorem has been developed by a number of workers in the USA.[163–167] Its application to the evaluation of ADEs is shown in Box 16.1 and a practical method (from Hutchinson) is shown in Table 16.11 and Figure 16.2. This is probably the most sophisticated system developed so far, and it has been applied to a number of actual drug problems. An integrated approach to ADE assessment which permits the prediction of incidence extends the method beyond individual case evaluation.

In 1968, an international collaboration to identify rare adverse events not detected in clinical trials was set up under the auspices of WHO in Uppsala, Sweden. The Uppsala Monitoring Centre maintains an international database with data collected from 58 official member countries (those with a formally recognised national ADR monitoring centre) and six associate member countries (those with strong pharmacovigilance capacity but no formally recognised ADR monitoring centre).[168] Reports are published two or three times a year giving updated information on ADRs and the work of the centre (available online at http://www.who-umc.org). A new signalling process using Bayesian logic applied to data-mining, within a confidence propagation neural network, has been developed, with initial work suggesting that this approach has a high predictive value that can identify early signals of ADRs.[169]

Table 16.10 Method for causality assessment of adverse drug reactions

Criteria	Score
1. Time to onset of the reaction	
Highly suggestive	+3[a]
Suggestive	+2
Compatible	+1
Inconclusive	0[a]
If incompatible, then case 'unrelated'	
If information not available, then case 'insufficiently documented'	
2. Course of the reaction	
Highly suggestive	+3
Suggestive	+2
Compatible	+1
Against the role of the drug	−2
Inconclusive or not available	0
3. Risk factor(s) for drug reaction	
Yes	+1[b]
No	0
4. Concomitant drug(s)	
Time to onset incompatible	0
Time to onset compatible but unknown reaction	−1
Time to onset compatible and known reaction	−2
Role proved in this case	−3
None or information not available	0
5. Non-drug-related causes	
Ruled out	−2
Possible or not investigated	−1
Probable	−3
6. Previous information on the drug	
Reaction unknown	0
Reaction published but unlabelled	+1
Reaction labelled in the product's characteristics	+2
7. Response to re-administration	
Positive	+3
Compatible	+1
Negative	−2
Not available or not interpretable	0
Plasma concentration of the drug known as toxic	+3
Validated laboratory test with high specificity, sensitivity and predictive values	
Positive	−3
Negative	+3
Not interpretable or not available	0

[a] Qualifying terms in italics are not to be used for assessing acute drug-induced liver injuries.

[b] One additional point for each validated risk factor.

BOX 16.1 Hand-held Bayesian adverse drug reaction (ADR) assessment

Instructions

Case parameters

Read the case and write down those elements in the following categories that best describe the generic type of case and which most facilitate assessment of the prior. This may mean picking descriptions that fit with other cases reported in the literature or on which you have other sources of information

Clinical background – Usually includes patient's age, sex, underlying illness. It should include anything else that changes the likelihood for different causes of the event, but which will not be used later in the case findings

Adverse event type – Usually a general description of the event that would allow you to look it up in a reference source (e.g. acute renal failure, diarrhoea). Does not usually include all details of the event

Time to onset – The interval between starting the suspected drug and the occurrence or detection of the adverse event

Evolution of the event and drug withdrawal – What was there about the course of the event and its response (or non-response) to drug withdrawal that helped differentiate between the causes?

Rechallenge – As for behaviour of the event on restarting the suspected drug

Other – List other items that you feel have diagnostic value

Scoring

For each category of assessment consider the list of possible causes. Identify the one least likely to lead to the particular finding being considered (in the case of the prior, the finding is the adverse event type). Give this cause a score of 1 in that category. Identify the next lowest cause likely to lead to the findings and assign it a number between 1 and infinity that represents by how many times more likely it is to lead to the finding that the least likely cause. Proceed in this way for each cause using the cause that received a score of 1 in that category as the comparator in each case

Time horizon – An arbitrary time chosen to be longer than the actual time of occurrence and longer than expected timings for the drug cause being considered. Using these guidelines, choose the time that most facilitates the assessment

Possible causes – List the suspected drug, other drugs that you consider potential causes, and other possible causes (such as the patient's underlying disease). The list should include all the causes you consider possible. Note that if you consider a drug interaction a possible cause, this should appear as a separate item on the cause list

16.12 The legal framework and its implications for future international developments

In the premarketing phase of new drug development national regulatory authorities encourage and evaluate a broad range of experimental methods that come within the definition of clinical trials.

In the evaluation of safety in the post-marketing phase, regulatory agencies are greatly more restricted in their enthusiasm for data derived from some of the methods available than from others. Indeed, the EC national agencies separately and the Committee for Medicinal Products for Human Use (CPMP) collectively have developed a legislative framework that is predominantly concerned with spontaneous adverse event monitoring and which is, for all practical purposes, silent on the matter of safety data collected by other methods.

The starting point was set out in Directive 65/65/EEC which states:

The competent authorities of the Member States shall suspend or revoke an authorisation to place a proprietary medicinal product on the market where that product proves to be harmful in the normal conditions of use, or where its therapeutic efficacy is lacking when it is established that therapeutic results cannot be obtained with the proprietary product.

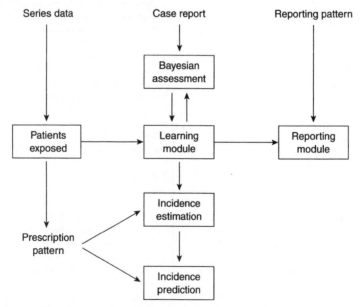

Figure 16.2 An integrated Bayesian system for predicting adverse drug reaction incidence.

Table 16.11 Hand-held Bayesian adverse drug reaction (ADR) assessment: data and scoring sheet

Case (DSD) number

Case parameters (used for assessing prior)	Case findings (for other assessment categories)
General background	Time to onset
Adverse event type	Specific background
Time horizon	Evolution of event
Possible causes	Rechallenge
Drug withdrawal	Other
	1.
	2.
	3.
	Possible causes

Assessment category	Drug	Other (1)	Other (2)	Other (3)
Prior				
Time to onset				
Specific background				
Evolution of event				
Drug withdrawal				
Rechallenge				
Other				
1.				
2.				
3.				
				Total
	+	+	+	=
Products				
Products ÷ total				

This is a very general statement, giving no guidance on what might be seen as harmful or what would constitute lack of efficacy.

In 1989, in Article 33 of Directive 89/341/EEC, the situation was dealt with in more detail.

1. Each Member State shall take all the appropriate measures to ensure that decisions authorizing marketing, refusing or revoking a marketing authorization, prohibit supply, or withdrawing a product from the market together with the reason on which such decisions are based, are brought to the attention of the Committee forthwith.

2. The person responsible for the marketing of a medicinal product shall be obliged to notify the Member States concerned forthwith of any action taken by him to suspend the marketing of a product or to withdraw a product from the market, together with the reason for such action if the latter concerns the efficacy of the medicinal product or the protection of the public health.

Member States shall ensure that this information is brought to the attention of the Committee.

3. Member States shall ensure that appropriate information about action taken pursuant to paragraphs 1 and 2 which may affect the protection of public health in third countries is forthwith brought to the attention of the World Health Organization, with a copy to the Committee.

4. The Commission shall publish annually a list of the medicinal products which are prohibited in the Community.

The term 'pharmacovigilance' has now been adopted by all Member States for the activities involved in the study and evaluation of drug safety. Although pharmacovigilance covers a broad range of data collection methods, it is the spontaneous reporting systems sponsored by all European governments to which the term usually refers.

Since the fourth edition, numerous lengthy documents have become available which address the ADR reporting requirements in greater detail and in a more comprehensible way. It is not the purpose of this chapter to review each of these individually, but the reader is recommended to become familiar with those listed below.

1. Directive 75/319/EEC (Amended) on the approximation of provisions laid down by law, regulation or administrative action relating to medicinal products.

2. Regulation (EEC) No 2309/93. Council Regulation (EEC) No 2309/9 of 22 July 1993 laying down Community procedures for the authorisation and supervision of medicinal products for human and veterinary use and establishing a European Agency for the Evaluation of Medicinal Products.

3. Regulation (EC) No 540/95. Commission Regulation (EC) No 540/95 of 10 March 1995 laying down the arrangements for reporting suspected unexpected adverse reactions which are not serious, whether arising in the Community or in a third country, to medicinal products for human or veterinary use authorised in accordance with the provisions of Council Regulation (EEC) No 2309/93.

4. Conduct of Pharmacovigilance for Centrally Authorised Products: European Medicines Agency (EMEA), April 1997.

5. Conduct of Pharmacovigilance for Medicinal Products: authorised through the mutual recognition procedure EMEA, June 1997.

6. ICH Topic E1A Population Exposure: the extent of population exposure to assess clinical safety.

7. ICH Topic E2A Clinical Safety Data Management: definitions and standards for expedited reporting.

8. ICH E2B(M) Clinical Safety Data Management: data elements for transmission of individual case safety reports.

9. ICH Topic E2C Clinical Safety Data Management: periodic safety update reports for marketed drugs.

10. CPMP Note for Guidance on Electronic Exchange of Pharmacovigilance Information for Human and Veterinary Medicinal Products in the European Union, August 1999.

11. CPMP Joint Pharmacovigilance Plan for the Implementation of the ICH E213 M1 and M2 Requirements Related to the Electronic Transmission of Individual Case Safety Reports in the Community.

Since the fourth edition of this book was published, a plethora of new updating information has become available on the internet. The sheer volume of this is such that it is beyond the reach of this chapter. Attempts to create a standard set of procedures and requirements in the new and enlarged EU have certainly made progress although the pharmaceutical physician will have to consult the most recent regulations and guidelines if errors are to be avoided. Even such basic concepts as a suspected 'serious' adverse reaction may vary between countries.

The following is a generally accepted listing of serious events:
• Fatal;
• Life-threatening;
• Results in persistent or significant disability and/or incapacity;
• Results in or prolongs hospitalisation.
This also includes congenital abnormalities and/or birth defects and serious adverse clinical consequences with use outside the terms of the SPC including overdoses or abuse.

The generally expected reporting requirements for serious adverse reactions (expedited reporting) are as follows. All such reports should be reported immediately and in no case later than 15 calendar days from receipt. The clock for expedited reporting starts as soon as one or more of the following has received the minimum information required for the submission of an adverse reaction report:

1. Any personnel of the marketing authorisation holder – including sales representatives.

2. The qualified person responsible for pharmacovigilance or persons working for or with this person.

3. Where the marketing authorisation holder has entered into relationships with a second company for the marketing of, or research on, the suspected product, the clock starts as soon as any personnel of the marketing authorisation holder receives the minimum information; however, wherever possible, the time-frame for regulatory submission should be no longer than 15 days from the receipt by the second company. Explicit procedures and detailed agreements should exist between the marketing authorisation holder and the second company to facilitate the achievement of this objective.

4. In the case of relevant worldwide scientific literature, the clock starts with awareness of the publication by any personnel of the marketing authorisation holder; the marketing authorisation holder is expected to maintain awareness of possible publications by accessing a widely used systematic literature review and reference database, such as Medline, Excerpta Medica or Embase, no less frequently than once a week, or by making formal contractual arrangements with a second party to perform this task; marketing authorisation holders are also expected to ensure that

relevant publications in each Member State are appropriately reviewed.

Some comments are required in respect of the document entitled 'Notice to Marketing Authorisation Holders – Pharmacovigilance Guidelines' and identified as MCA EuroDirect Publication No PhVWP/108/99. This guideline was issued from the European Medicines Evaluation Agency (EMEA) in January 1999 and probably has more practical importance for the reader of this book. It has to be said that it is not without a number of shortcomings that make it less clear than it should be. Nevertheless, it does outline the actual procedures involved in ADR reporting and the responsibilities of all those concerned. Like many other publications from the various European authorities it is likely to be the subject of revisions and amendments as time goes by, so vigilance is advised.

As in other areas in which self-regulation has been relied upon, the response has been disappointing. Even though all major companies would agree that the safety evaluation of new drugs should be continued into the post-marketing phase, remarkably little enthusiasm has been apparent when the time actually comes. The solution to the problem probably lies in the integration of post-marketing studies into the overall drug development procedure in such a way that new drug applications would only be considered if a detailed and realistic post-marketing plan were to be included.

Back in the mid-1970s the Association of the British Pharmaceutical Industry (ABPI) was very concerned by the increasing demands being made with respect to the numbers of patients in clinical trials and the duration of treatment. They entered into discussion with the CSM to see if there were ways in which the demands for the better assessment of safety could be met without enlarging clinical trials to the point where new drug development would be stifled. It was recognised nearly 20 years ago that there were limitations on what clinical trials could achieve, and that at the time of marketing the new product emerged from a very carefully controlled environment to the largely uncontrolled world of everyday clinical practice. It was at this time that the Medicines Division in the UK was becoming very active in creating the Yellow Card system, experimenting with monitored release, post-marketing surveillance and prescription event monitoring, and there were hopes that one or more of these systems would provide a solution to the problem.[160] It has to be said that those hopes have never been realised, and we are no further ahead than

we were then except that clinical trial demands have continued to increase, albeit probably more slowly than had been feared.

The hope had been that stopping escalating demands for bigger clinical trials could be offset by continuing large-scale studies into the post-marketing period. This could not be done, because the CSM had only limited powers after the granting of a product licence and so could not require post-marketing studies.

A similar pattern seems to have occurred in other countries of the EU, and it is now difficult to believe that progress could be made in this direction without fairly substantial changes in existing legislation. The insubstantial legal framework provides no incentives for companies to set up realistic post-marketing programmes. They will therefore continue to put their faith in spontaneous reporting systems and to receive unpleasant surprises when unexpected adverse events arise. The concentration of regulatory authority efforts on spontaneous reporting, which is essentially the only method envisaged in the present legal structure, focuses attention upon uncommon, bizarre and usually serious conditions and neglects more common problems which, although they may be less serious, are nevertheless limiting factors in drug treatment.

This policy may well be shortsighted, but competition is such that pharmaceutical companies would prefer to accept the risk and save the money. It is this attitude that is a major contributor to the poor image of the industry in the eyes of the public and the media. Unfortunately, in this and many other fields, self-regulation has not worked, so we probably have to look to strengthening legal framework and setting down requirements if improvements are to be made.

16.13 Other considerations and conclusions

There is no doubt that the continuing evaluation of the safety of medicines into the post-marketing period is an expanding and still developing area of research. Matters relating to safety spread over into efficacy, which together imply risks and benefits which, in the present international climate of health care provision, have consequences for outcomes and costs. A whole new field of research – pharmaco-economics – is in the process of development and it is to be anticipated that many of the methods used for safety evaluation will be modified and applied in this area.

Then there are questions of ethics, patient confidentiality, informed consent and ethics committee approval to be addressed, as well as the whole new range of legislation already referred to. At present, purely observational studies, which have no influence on the normal course of the patient's treatment, require neither informed consent nor ethics committee approval. Whether this will continue to be the case in the new Europe and internationally remains to be seen. There are certainly concerns for the privacy and protection of the patient as an individual, but there are also the broader questions of the delivery of efficient and effective health care to large populations, which depends on the continuation of high-quality clinical research.

Phase IV clinical trials and prospective observational cohort studies have been criticised as no more than promotional devices used by aggressive pharmaceutical companies. The fact that misuse has sometimes happened should not be allowed to obscure the greatly more important needs of safety evaluation and the further development of new and improved therapies. A set of guidelines[170,171] has been published in the UK which are specifically intended to provide the high standards of study design and methodology necessary for observational cohort studies. It is to be hoped that similar procedures will be adopted internationally.

In addition to the methods reviewed in this chapter there has been the development of a procedure known as 'meta-analysis',[172–174] which seeks to combine as many clinical studies as possible in a formal and structured way, so that patient numbers may be increased to a level at which conclusions may be drawn that would not be possible from single studies. Needless to say, there are strongly held views both for and against meta-analysis, but at present it would probably be true to say that the jury is still out.

Another area of research is growing within the established fields of biochemistry, metabolism, immunology and genetics which is aimed at the elucidation of mechanisms[175] involved in ADRs. The importance of this development is hard to over-emphasise when it is considered that the risk for patients not susceptible to a particular ADR is probably zero, whereas for the susceptible patient it approaches certainty. The detection of susceptible patients through knowledge of genetic or metabolic characteristics would be a major advance in knowledge.

Since the fourth edition of this book, the internet has become a valuable source of information on ADRs and pharmacovigilance. The various directives, regulations and guidelines referred to in this chapter are now readily available from this source, and the reader will be able to obtain the full versions of all such documents. A paper by Cobert and Silvey[176] contains much useful information and many internet addresses.

A hope for the future would be to limit the massive burden of premarketing testing of new drugs, which threatens the continuation of research in the pharmaceutical industry, and to establish methods of investigation in the post-marketing phase that would provide the necessary safeguards. It should be remembered that the cost of a patient in a controlled clinical trial may be 10–20 times greater than that of the same patient in an observational study. There is certainly a difference in the type and quantity of data available, but as a means of evaluating safety in the real-life situation the observational cohort study is the method of choice.

A recent editorial in the *BMJ* entitled 'Using drugs safely'[177] has reported that the Audit Commission found that nearly 1100 people had died in England and Wales in the previous 12 months as a result of medication errors or adverse reactions and that this was a fivefold increase in just 10 years. The editorial emphasises the need for improvements in medical education in order to foster good prescribing and an awareness of ADRs. It is a sobering observation in the revision of this chapter that so little progress has been made since the first edition.

References

1 Royal Society Study Group. *Risk Assessment.* London: Royal Society, 1983.
2 British Medical Association. *The BMA Guide to Living with Risk.* London: Penguin Books, 1987.
3 O'Brien B. *'What are My Chances Doctor?' A Review of Clinical Risks.* London: Office of Health Economics, 1986.
4 Ferner RE. Hazards, risks and reality. *Br J Clin Pharmacol* 1992;**33**:125–8.
5 Chapman CR, Morrison D. Impacts on the Earth by asteroids and comets: assessing the hazard. *Nature* 1994;**367**:33–40.
6 Calman KC, Royston HD. Risk language and dialects. *BMJ* 1997;**315**:939–42.
7 Griffin JP. Realistic risk assessment: an unachievable goal. *Scrip* 1997;March:22–4.
8 Fletcher AP. Drug safety tests and subsequent clinical experience. *J R Soc Med* 1978;**71**:693–6.
9 Rawlins MD, Jefferys DB. Study of United Kingdom product licence applications containing new active substances. *BMJ* 1991;**302**:223–5.

10 Inman WHW. Let's get our act together. In: Dukes MNG, ed. *Side Effects of Drugs Essay.* Amsterdam: Elsevier, 1990;115–35.

11 Lawson DH. Postmarketing surveillance of drugs. *Proc R Coll Physicians Edinb* 1990;**20**:129–42.

12 Mann RD. CSM monitoring today. *Pharm Med* 1988;**3**:275–89.

13 Rawlins MD. Spontaneous reporting of adverse drug reactions I: the data. *Br J Clin Pharmacol* 1988;**26**:1–5.

14 Rawlins MD. Spontaneous reporting of adverse drug reactions II: uses. *Br J Clin Pharmacol* 1988;**26**:7–11.

15 Rawson NSB, Pearce GL, Inman WHW. Prescription event monitoring: methodology and recent progress. *J Clin Epidemiol* 1990;**43**:509–22.

16 Tilson HH. *Postmarketing Surveillance: the Way Forward.* Centre for Medicines Research, MTP Press.

17 Venning GR. Identification of adverse reactions to new drugs. I: what have been the important adverse reactions since thalidomide? *BMJ* 1983;**286**:199–202.

18 Venning GR. Identification of adverse reactions to new drugs. II: how were 18 important adverse reactions discovered and with what delay? *BMJ* 1983;**286**:365–8.

19 Venning GR. Identification of adverse reactions to new drugs. III: alerting processes and early warning systems. *BMJ* 1983;**286**:458–60.

20 Venning GR. Identification of adverse reactions to new drugs. IV: verification of suspected adverse reactions. *BMJ* 1983;**286**:544–7.

21 Venulet J. Possible strategies for early recognition of potential drug safety problems. *Adverse Drug React Acute Poisoning Rev* 1988;**1**:39–47.

22 Winstanley PA, Irvin LE, Smith JC, et al. Adverse drug reactions: a hospital pharmacy-based reporting scheme. *Br J Clin Pharmacol* 1989;**28**:113–16.

23 Witts LJ. Adverse reactions to drugs. *BMJ* 1965;**2**:1081.

24 WHO Anniversary Symposium Proceedings. *Adverse Drug Reactions: A Global Perspective on Signal Generation and Analysis.* Uppsala, 1988.

25 Ionnidis JPA, Haidich A-B, Lau J. Any casualties in the clash of randomised and observational evidence? *BMJ* 2001;**322**:879–80.

26 Benson K, Hartz AJ. A comparison of observational studies and randomized, controlled trials. *N Engl J Med* 2000;**342**:1878–86.

27 Concato J, Shah N, Horwitz RI. Randomized, controlled trials, observational studies and the hierarchy of research designs. *N Engl J Med* 2000;**342**:1887–92.

28 Daneshmend TK, Hawkey CJ, Langman MJS, et al. Omeprazole versus placebo for acute upper gastrointestinal bleeding: randomised double blind controlled trial. *BMJ* 1992;**304**:143–7.

29 Ferguson J, Addo HA, McGill PE, et al. A study of benoxaprofen induced photosensitivity. *Br J Dermatol* 1982;**107**:429.

30 GREAT Group. Feasibility, safety, and efficacy of domiciliary thrombolysis by general practitioners: Grampian region early anistreplase trial. *BMJ* 1992;**305**:548–53.

31 ISIS–3. ISIS–3: a randomised comparison of streptokinase vs tissue plasminogen activator vs anistreplase and of aspirin plus heparin vs aspirin alone among 41299 cases of suspected acute myocardial infarction. *Lancet* 1992;**339**:753–70.

32 Jacobson SJ, Jones K, Johnson K, et al. Prospective multicentre study of pregnancy outcome after lithium exposure during the first trimester. *Lancet* 1992;**339**:530–3.

33 Campbell JPM, Howie JGR. Involving the patient in reporting adverse drug reactions. *J R Coll Gen Pract* 1988;**38**:370–1.

34 McBride WG. Thalidomide and congenital abnormalities. *BMJ* 1962;**5320**:1681.

35 Lenz W. Thalidomide and congenital abnormalities. *Lancet* 1962;**1**:45.

36 Lenz W. Malformations caused by drugs in pregnancy. *Am J Dis Child* 1966;**112**:99–106.

37 Lenz W, Knapp K. Die thalidomidembryopathie. *Dtsch Med Wochenschr* 1962;**87**:1232.

38 Burley DM. Thalidomide and congenital abnormalities. *Lancet* 1962;**1**:271.

39 Finney DJ. The design and logic of a monitor of drug use. *J Chronic Dis* 1965;**18**:77–98.

40 Edlavitch SA. Adverse drug event reporting. *Arch Intern Med* 1988;**148**:1499–503.

41 Faich GA. National adverse drug reaction reporting. *Arch Intern Med* 1991;**151**:1645–7.

42 Faich GA. Special report: adverse drug reaction monitoring. *N Engl J Med* 1986;**314**:1589–92.

43 Griffin JP. Survey of adverse drug reaction reporting schemes in fifteen countries. *Br J Clin Pharmacol* 1985;**22**:838–100S.

44 Griffin JP, Weber JCP. Voluntary systems of adverse reaction reporting. Part I. *Adverse Drug React Acute Poisoning Rev* 1985;**4**:213–30.

45 Griffin JP, Weber JCP. Voluntary systems of adverse reaction reporting. Part II. *Adverse Drug React Acute Poisoning Rev* 1986;**5**:23–55.

46 Griffin JP, Weber JCP. Voluntary systems of adverse reaction reporting. Part III. *Adverse Drug React Acute Poisoning Rev* 1989;**8**:203–15.

47 Lawson DH. The yellow card: mark II. *BMJ* 1990;**301**:1234.

48 Sachs RM, Bortnichak EA. An evaluation of spontaneous adverse drug reactions monitoring systems. *Am J Med* 1986;**81**:49–55.

49 Walker SR, Lumley CE. The attitudes of general practitioners to monitoring and reporting adverse drug reactions. *Pharm Med* 1986;**1**:195–203.

50 Lumley CE, Walker SR, Hall GC, et al. The underreporting of adverse drug reactions seen in general practice. *Pharm Med* 1986;**1**:205–12.

51 Fletcher AP. Spontaneous adverse drug reaction reporting vs event monitoring: a comparison. *J R Soc Med* 1991;**84**:341–4.

52 Fletcher AP. An appraisal of spontaneous adverse event monitoring. *Adverse Drug React Toxicol Rev* 1992;**11**:213–27.

53 Smithells RW, Sheppard S. Teratogenicity testing in humans: a method demonstrating safety of Bendectin. *Teratology* 1978;17:31–6.

54 Harron DWG, Griffiths K, Shanks RC. Debendox and congenital malformations in Northern Ireland. *BMJ* 1980;281:1379–80.

55 Jick H, Holmes LB, Hunter JR, et al. First trimester drug use and congenital disorders. *JAMA* 1981;246:343–6.

56 Mitchell AA, Rosenberg L, Shapiro S, et al. Birth defects related to Bendectin use in pregnancy. *JAMA* 1981;245:2311–14.

57 Cordero JF, Oakley GP, Greenberg F, et al. Is Bendectin a teratogen? *JAMA* 1981;245:2307–10.

58 Correy JF, Newman NM. Debendox and limb reduction deformities. *Med J Aust* 1981;1:417–18.

59 Clarke M, Clayton DG. Safety of Debendox. *Lancet* 1981;1:659–60.

60 Edwards IR, Lindquist M. The WHO database II. *Drug Inf J* 1992;26:481–6.

61 Mann RD, Rawlins MD, Fletcher P, et al. Age and the spontaneous reporting of adverse reactions in the UK. *Pharmacoepidemiol Drug Saf* 1992;1:19–23.

62 Fletcher AP, Griffin JP. International monitoring for adverse reactions of long latency. *Adverse Drug React Acute Poisoning Rev* 1991;10:189–210.

63 Herbst AL, Ulfelder H, Poskanzer DC. Adenocarcinoma of vagina: association of maternal stilboestrol therapy with tumour appearance in young women. *N Engl J Med* 1971;284:878–81.

64 Wright P. Skin reactions to practolol. *BMJ* 1974;2:560.

65 Wright P. Untoward effects associated with practolol administration: oculomucocutaneous syndrome. *BMJ* 1975;1:595–8.

66 Wright P. Ocular reactions to beta-blocking drugs. *BMJ* 1975;4:577.

67 Friedman GD, Ury HK. Screening for possible drug carcinogenicity: second report of findings. *J Natl Cancer Inst* 1983;71:1165.

68 Williams RR, Feinleit M, Connor RJ, et al. Case–control study of anti-hypertensive and diuretic use by women with malignant and benign breast lesions detected in a mammography screening program. *J Natl Cancer Inst* 1978;61:325–7.

69 Swerdlow AJ, Douglas AJ, Vaughan Hudson G, et al. Risk of second primary cancers after Hodgkin's disease by type of treatment: analysis of 2846 patients in the British National Lymphoma Investigation. *BMJ* 1992;304:1137–43.

70 McEwen J. Improving adverse drug reaction reporting. *Med Toxicol* 1987;2:398–404.

71 Council for International Organisations of Medical Sciences (CIOMS) Working Group. *International Reporting of Adverse Drug Reactions.* Geneva: CIOMS, 1990:45–7.

72 CIOMS. Standardisation of definitions and criteria of causality assessment of adverse drug reactions: drug-induced cytopenia. *Int J Clin Pharmacol Ther Toxicol* 1991;29:75–81.

73 CIOMS. Basic requirements for the use of terms for reporting adverse drug reactions. *Pharmacoepidemiol Drug Saf* 1992;1:39–45.

74 CIOMS. *Working Group II Final Report.* Geneva: CIOMS, 1992.

75 Edwards IR, Lindquist M, Wiholm B-E, et al. Quality criteria for early signals of possible adverse drug reactions. *Lancet* 1990;336:156–8.

76 Waller PC, Wood SM, Langman MJS, et al. Review of company postmarketing surveillance studies. *BMJ* 1992;304:1470–2.

77 Linden M. Phase IV research and drug utilisation observation studies. *Pharmacopsychiatry* 1997;30(Suppl):1–3.

78 Schafer H. Post-approval drug research: objectives and methods. *Pharmacopsychiatry* 1997;30(Suppl):4–8.

79 Fletcher AP. Profile of a large scale cohort study. *Drugs* 1990;40(Suppl 5):43–7.

80 Hill PL, Bridgman KM. A multicentre postmarketing surveillance study to evaluate the safety of bisoprolol in the treatment of hypertension and ischaemic heart disease. *Br J Clin Res* 1992;3:85–98.

81 Herbold M. International guidelines on post-authorisation research and surveillance. *Pharmacopsychiatry* 1997;30(Suppl):62–4.

82 Hall GC, Luscombe DK, Walker SR. Postmarketing surveillance using a computerised general practice database. *Pharm Med* 1988;2:345–51.

83 Johnson N, Mant D, Jones L, et al. Use of computerised general practice data for population surveillance: comparative study of influenza data. *BMJ* 1991;302:763–5.

84 Jick H. Use of automated databases to study drug effects after marketing. *Pharmacotherapy* 1985;5:278–9.

85 Jick H, Madsen S, Nudelman PM, et al. Postmarketing follow-up at Group Health Cooperative of Puget Sound. *Pharmacotherapy* 1984;4:99.

86 Jick H, Walker AM, Watkins RN, et al. Oral contraceptives and breast cancer. *Am J Epidemiol* 1980;112:577.

87 Jick H, Dinan BJ, Hunter JR, et al. Tricyclic antidepressants and convulsions. *J Clin Psychopharmacol* 1983;3:182.

88 Faich GA, Fishbein HA, Ellis SE. The epidemiology of diabetic acidosis: a population based study. *Am J Epidemiol* 1983;117:551.

89 Friedman GD, Collen MF, Harris LE, et al. Experience in monitoring drug reactions in outpatients: the Kaiser-Permanente Drug Monitoring System. *JAMA* 1971;217:2498.

90 Guess HA, West R, Strand LM, et al. Fatal upper gastrointestinal hemorrhage or perforation among users and nonusers of nonsteroidal anti-inflammatory drugs in Saskatchewan, Canada 1983. *J Clin Epidemiol* 1988;41:35.

91 Morse ML, LeRoy AA, Strom BL. COMPASS: a population-based post-marketing drug surveillance system. In: Inman WHW, ed. *Monitoring for Drug Safety*. Philadelphia: JB Lippincott, 1986.

92 Ray WA, Griffin MR. The use of Medicaid data for pharmacoepidemiology. *Am J Epidemiol* 1989;**129**:837.

93 Saskatchewan Health: International symposium on drug database uses, Regina, Canada, 7–8 November 1984. Proceedings. Regina: Saskatchewan Health, 1985.

94 Schnell BR. A review of the use of prescription drugs in Saskatchewan. *Can Pharm J* 1981;**7**:267.

95 Shapiro S. The role of automated record linkage in the post-marketing surveillance of drug safety: a critique. *Clin Pharmacol Ther* 1989;**46**:371–86.

96 Skoll SL, August RJ, Johnson GE. Drug prescribing for the elderly in Saskatchewan during 1976. *CMAJ* 1979;**121**:1974.

97 Stergachis A. Record linkage studies for postmarketing surveillance: data quality and validity considerations. *Drug Intell Clin Pharm* 1988;**22**:157.

98 Strand LM. Drug epidemiology resources and studies: the Saskatchewan database. *Drug Info J* 1985;**19**:253.

99 Strom BL, Carson JL, Halpern AC, et al. Using a claims database to investigate drug-induced Stevens–Johnson syndrome. *Stat Med* 1991;**10**:565–76.

100 Strom BL, Carson JL, Morse ML, et al. The computerised on-line Medicaid pharmaceutical analysis and surveillance system: a new resource for post marketing drug surveillance. *Clin Pharmacol Ther* 1985;**38**:359.

101 Strom BL, Carson JL, Morse ML, et al. Hypersensitivity reactions associated with zompirac sodium and other nonsteroidal anti-inflammatory drugs. *Arthritis Rheum* 1987;**30**:1142.

102 Carson JL, Strom BL, Morse ML, et al. The relative gastrointestinal toxicity of the nonsteroidal anti-inflammatory drugs. *Arch Intern Med* 1987;**147**:1054.

103 Tilson H. Getting down to bases: record linkage in Saskatchewan. *Can J Public Health* 1985;**76**:222.

104 Cornfield J. A method of estimating comparative rates from clinical data: application to cancer of the lung, breast and cervix. *J Natl Cancer Inst* 1951;**11**:1269–75.

105 Dorn HE. Some applications of biometry in the collection and evaluation of medical data. *J Chronic Dis* 1955;**1**:638–69.

106 Dorn HE. Some problems arising in prospective and retrospective studies of the etiology of disease. *N Engl J Med* 1959;**261**:571–9.

107 Mantel N, Haenszel W. Statistical aspects of data from retrospective studies of disease. *J Natl Cancer Inst* 1959;**22**:719–48.

108 Cornfield J, Haenszel W. Some aspects of retrospective studies. *J Chronic Dis* 1960;**11**:523–34.

109 Lilienfeld AM, Lilienfeld DE. A century of case–control studies: progress? *J Chronic Dis* 1979;**32**:5–13.

110 Louis PCA. *Researches on Phthisis: Anatomical, Pathological and Therapeutical* (Trans. by WH Wolshe). London: Sydenham Society, 1844.

111 Cole P. The evolving case–control study. *J Chronic Dis* 1979;**32**:15–27.

112 Feinstein AR. Methodologic problems and standards in case–control research. *J Chronic Dis* 1979;**32**:35–41.

113 Sackett DL. Bias in analytic research. *J Chronic Dis* 1979;**32**:51–63.

114 Mayes LC, Horwitz RI, Feinstein AR. A collection of 56 topics with contradictory results in case–control research. *Inf J Epidemiol* 1988;**17**:680–5.

115 Armstrong B, Stevens N, Doll R. Retrospective study of the association between use of Rauwolfia derivatives and breast cancer in English women. *Lancet* 1974;**2**:672–5.

116 Boston Collaborative Drug Surveillance Program. Reserpine and breast cancer. *Lancet* 1974;**2**:669–71.

117 Friedman GD. Rauwolfia and breast cancer: no relation found in long-term users aged fifty and over. *J Chronic Dis* 1983;**36**:367.

118 Heinonen OP, Shapiro S, Tuominen L, et al. Reserpine use in relation to breast cancer. *Lancet* 1974;**2**:675–7.

119 Laska EM, Siegl C, Meisner M, et al. Matched pairs study of reserpine use and breast cancer. *Lancet* 1975;**2**:296–300.

120 Lilienfeld AM, Chang L, Thomas DB, et al. Rauwolfia derivatives and breast cancer. *Johns Hopkins Med Bull* 1975;**139**:41–50.

121 Armstrong B, Skegg D, White G, et al. Rauwolfia derivatives and breast cancer in hypertensive women. *Lancet* 1976;**2**:8–12.

122 Aromaa A, Hakama M, Hakulinen T, et al. Breast cancer and use of Rauwolfia and other antihypertensive agents in hypertensive patients: a nation wide case–control study in Finland. *Int J Cancer* 1976;**18**:727–38.

123 Kewitz H, Jesdinsky HJ, Shroter PM, et al. Reserpine and breast cancer in West Germany. *Eur J Clin Pharmacol* 1977;**11**:79–83.

124 Mack IM, Henderson BE, Gerkins VR, et al. Reserpine and breast cancer in a retirement community. *N Engl J Med* 1975;**292**:1360–71.

125 Christopher LJ, Crooks J, Davidson JF, et al. A multicentre study of Rauwolfia derivatives and breast cancer. *Eur J Clin Pharmacol* 1977;**11**:409–17.

126 O'Fallon WM, Labarthe DR, Kinland LT. Rauwolfia derivatives and breast cancer. *Lancet* 1975;**2**:292–6.

127 Labarthe DR. Methodologic variation in case–control studies of reserpine and breast cancer. *J Chronic Dis* 1979;**32**:95–104.

128 Friedman GD. Rauwolfia and breast cancer: no relation found in long-term users aged fifty and over. *J Chronic Dis* 1983;**36**:367.

129 Hill AB. The environment and disease: association or causation. *Proc R Soc Med* 1965;**58**:295–300.

130 Jick H, Vessey MP. Case–control studies in the evaluation of drug-induced illness. *Am J Epidemiol* 1978;**107**:1–7.

131 Hine IK, Laird K, Hewitt P et al. Meta-analytic evidence against prophylactic use of lidocaine in acute myocardial infarction. *Arch Intern Med* 1980;**149**:2694–8.

132 Layton D, Heely E, Hughes K, et al. Comparison of the incidence rates of selected gastrointestinal events reported for patients prescribed rofecoxib and meloxicam in general practice in England using prescription-event monitoring data. *Rheumatology* 2003;**42**:622–31.

133 Layton D, Riley J, Wilton LV, et al. Safety profile of rofecoxib as used in general practice in England: results of a prescription-event monitoring study. *Br J Clin Pharmacol* 2003;**55**:166–74.

134 Wilton LV, Heeley El, Pickering RM, et al. Comparative study of mortality rates and cardiac dysrhythmias in post-marketing surveillance studies of sertindole and two other atypical antipsychotic drugs, risperidone and olanzapine. *J Psychopharmacol* 2001;**15**:120–6.

135 Layton D, Pearce G, Shakir S. Safety profile of tolterodine as used in general practice in England: results of prescription event monitoring 2001. *Drug Saf* 2001;**24**:703–13.

136 Reilly JG, Ayis SA, Ferrier IN, et al. QTc-interval abnormalities and psychotropic drug therapy in psychiatric patirents. *Lancet* 2000;**355**:1048–52.

137 Taylor D. Ziprasidone in the management of schizophrenia: the QT interval issue in context. *CNS Drugs* 2003;**17**:423–30.

138 Committee on Safety of Medicines: www.mca.gov.uk/aboutagency/regframework/csm/csmframe. htm

139 Gianfresco FD, Grogg AL, Mahmoud RA, et al. Differential effects of risperidone, olanzapine, clozapine, and conventional antipsychotics on type 2 diabetes: findings from a large health plan database. *J Clin Psychiatry* 2002;**63**:920–30.

140 Sernyak MJ, Leslie DL, Alarcon RD, et al. Association of diabetes mellitus with atypical neuroleptics in the treatment of schizophrenia. *Am J Psychiatry* 2002;**159**: 561–6.

141 Koro CE, Fedder DO, L'Italien GJ, et al. Assessment of independent effect olanzapine and risperidone on risk of diabetes among patients with schizophrenia: population based nested case–control study. *BMJ* 2003;**326**:283.

142 Meyer JM. A retrospective comparison of weight, lipid and glucose changes between risperidone and olanzapine-treated inpatients: metabolic out comes after 1 year. *J Clin Psychiatry* 2002;**63**:425–33.

143 Koro CE, Fedder DO, Ultalien GJ, et al. An assessment of the independent effects of olanzapine and risperidone exposure on the risk of hyperlipidemia in schizophrenic patients. *Arch Gen Psychiatry* 2002;**59**:1021–6.

144 Berry CL. Evaluation steroidal contraceptives: preclinical and clinical approaches. *Hum Toxicol* 1988;**7**:235.

145 McKenzie BE. Guidelines and requirements for the evaluation of contraceptive steroids. *Toxicol Pathol* 1989;**17**:377.

146 Hannaford P. The collection and interpretation of epidemiological data about the cardiovascular risks associated with the use of steroid contraceptives. *Contraception* 1998;**57**:137.

147 Watts DH, Parks JG, Cohn SE, et al. Safety and tolerability of depot medroxyprogesterone acetate among HIV-infected women on antiretroviral therapy. *Contraception* 2008;**77**:84.

148 Schwartz JI, Wong PH, Porras AG, et al. Effect of rofecoxib on the pharmacokinetics of chronically administered oral contraceptives in healthy female volunteers. *J Clin Pharmacol* 2002;**42**:215.

149 Hambleton S, Steinberg SP, Larussa PS, Shapiro ED, Gershon AA. Risk of herpes zoster in adults immunised with varicella vaccine. *J Infect Dis* 2008;**197**:S196.

150 Goldman GS. Universal varicella vaccination: trends and effects on herpes zoster. *Int J Toxicol* 2005;**24**:205.

151 Reynolds MA, Chaves SS, Harpaz R, Lopez AS, Seward JF. The impact of the varicella program on herpes zoster epidemiology in the United States: a review. *J Infect Dis* 2008;**197**:S224.

152 Investigations into adverse incidents during clinifcal trials of TGN 1412. (http://www.mhra.gov.uk/home/idcplg) MHRA Interim Report.

153 Silverstein FE, Faich G, Goldstein, et al. Gastrointestinal toxicity with celecoxib vs nonsteroidal anti-inflammatory drugs for osteoarthritis and rheumatoid arthritis: the CLASS study: a randomised controlled trial. *JAMA* 2000;**284**:1247–55.

154 Bombardier C, Laine L, Reicin A, et al. Comparison of upper gastrointestinal toxicity of rofecoxib and naproxen in patients with rheumatoid arthritis. VIGOR study group. *N Engl J Med* 2000;**343**:1520–8.

155 Gottlieb S. COX2 inhibitors may increase risk of heart attack. *BMJ* 2001;**323**:471.

156 Layton D, Riley J, Wilton LV, et al. Safety profile of rofecoxib as used in general practice in England: results of a prescription event monitoring study. *Br J Clin Pharmacol* 2003;**55**:166–74.

157 Layton D, Heeley E, Hughes K, et al. Comparison of the incidence rates of thromboembolic events reported for patients prescribed rofecoxib and meloxicam in practice in England using prescription event monitoring. *Rheumatology* 2003;**42**:1342–53.

158 Juni P, Nartey L, Reichenbach S, et al. Risk of cardiovascular events and rofecoxib: cumulative meta-analysis. *Lancet* 2004;**364**:2021.

159 Hine IK, Laird K, Hewitt P et al. Meta-analytic evidence against prophylactic use of lidocaine in acute myocardial infarction. Arch Intern Med 1980;**149**:2694–8.

160 Stephens MDB, Talbot JCC, Routledge PA. Detection of New Adverse Drug Reactions. 4th edn London: Macmillan Reference Ltd. 1998.

161 Edwards RI, Aronson JK. Adverse drug reactions: definitions, diagnosis and management. *Lancet* 2000; **356**:1255–9.

162 Benichou C, Danan G. Causality assessment in the European pharmaceutical industry: presentation of preliminary results of a new method. *Drug Inf J* 1992; **26**:589–92.

163 Hutchinson TA. Computerised Bayesian ADR assessment. *Drug Inf J* 1991;**25**:235–41.

164 Lane DA, Hutchinson TA, Jones JK, et al. *A Bayesian Approach to Causality Assessment.* University of Minnesota School of Statistics Technical Report No 472.

165 Lane DA, Kramer MS, Hutchinson TA, et al. The causality assessment of adverse drug reactions using a Bayesian approach. *Pharm Med* 1987;**2**:265–83.

166 Naranjo CA, Busto U, Sellers EM, et al. A method for estimating the probability of adverse drug reactions. *Clin Pharmacol Ther* 1981;**30**:239–45.

167 Naranjo CA, Lanctot KL. Microcomputer-assisted Bayesian differential diagnosis of severe adverse reactions to new drugs: a 4-year experience. *Drug Inf J* 1991;**25**:243–50.

168 Olsson S. The role of the WHO programme on international drug monitoring in coordinating worldwide drug safety efforts. *Drug Saf* 1998;**19**:1–10.

169 Lindquist M, Stahl M, Bate A, et al. A retrospective evaluation of data mining approach to aid finding new adverse drug reaction signals in the WHO international database. Drug Safety 2000;23:533–32.

170 Grahame-Smith DG. *Report of the adverse reactions working party to the Committee on Safety of Medicines.* London: Department of Health and Social Security, 1983.

171 Joint Committee of ABPI, BMA, CSM, and RCGP. Guidelines on postmarketing surveillance. *BMJ* 1988;**296**:399–400.

172 Eysenck HJ. Meta-analysis, sense or non-sense? *Pharm Med* 1992;**6**:113–19.

173 Huque MF. Experience with meta-analysis in NDA submissions. *Proc Biopharm Sect Am Stat Ass* 1988;2:28–33.

174 Spitzer WO. Meta-analysis: unanswered questions about aggregating data. *J Clin Epidemiol* 1991;44:103–7.

175 Rawlins MD, Thompson JW. Mechanisms of adveres drug reactions. Oxford: Oxford University Press, 1988; 18–38.

176 Cobert B, Silvey J. The Internet and drug safety: what are the implications for pharmacovigilence? *Drug Saf* 1999;20:95–107.

177 Maxwell S, Walley T, Ferner RE. Using drugs safely. *BMJ*;324:930–1.

Part III Regulatory aspects

17 History of drug regulation in the UK

John P. Griffin

Asklepieion Consulting Ltd, Herts, UK

17.1 Introduction

Our concepts on how medicines should be tested and regulated have evolved very gradually over time, perhaps dating back to 120 BC. This chapter is a brief account of some of the major events that have guided drug regulation to what it is today in the UK.[1]

Mithridates VI, 120 BC, King of Pontus, concocted a compound preparation called Mithridatium which was held as a panacea for almost every illness until the 1780s. Having investigated the powers of a number of single ingredients, which he found to be antidotes to various venoms and poisons individually, he evaluated them experimentally. The required 'clinical trials' were conducted on condemned criminals. Once an ingredient was found to be effective, Mithridates proceeded to incorporate it into his compound preparation, which included 41 individual components when fully formulated. Another formulation of Mithridatium, known as Galene, which included 55 components, was also available from the days of Andromachus (c. AD 50). 'Galene' means 'tranquility' and also became known as a theriac. The concoction took some 40 days to prepare, after which the process of maturation began. Galen considered 12 years as the proper period to keep it before use. The quality of Mithridatium and Galene was important because, as late as 1540, failure of their efficacy was attributed to the use of poor quality ingredients.

Mithridatium and Galene found their way into England, where, after the founding of the Royal College of Physicians in 1518, their manufacture was made subject to supervision under the Apothecary Wares,

Drugs and Stuffs Act of 1540. This Act was one of the earliest British statutes on the control of drugs. It empowered the physicians to appoint four inspectors of 'Apothecary Wares, Drugs and Stuffs'. (Stuffs included such items as wooden legs – which were to be 'of Oake and free of the worme'.) Section 2 of the Act gave the physicians the right to search apothecaries' shops for faulty wares with the assistance of the 'Wardens of the said mysterie of Apothecaries within the said City'. Defective wares were to be burnt or otherwise destroyed. The right of the Royal College of Physicians to conduct visitations of apothecaries' premises was withdrawn at the time of the implementation of the Food and Drugs Act 1875.[2] Details of the conduct of such inspections can be found in the *Royal College of Physicians: Visitation of Apothecary and Druggist Shoppes* in three volumes: I 1724–1731; II 1732–1747; III 1748–1754. The final volume also contains the records of four visitations made on 14 April, 21 June and 10 August 1756 at which William Heberden was one of the censors. The last recorded visitation was on 9 June 1757.[1]

Standards for the manufacture of Mithridatium and Galene were laid down in *The London Pharmacopoeia* in 1618 (Figure 17.1). The manufacture of these theriacs took place in public with much pomp and ceremony (Figure 17.2). It was commonly thought by those in authority that if Mithridatium did not produce the desired cure, this was a result of incorrect preparation (perhaps with adulterated or poor quality materials) or incorrect storage after use. However, Galen records that Marcus Aurelius consumed the preparation within 2 months of its being compounded without ill effect.

In 1665, during the Great Plague of London, Charles II turned to the Royal College of Physicians for advice. This advice recommended, among other measures, that the victims of the plague who developed buboes

The Textbook of Pharmaceutical Medicine. Edited by John P. Griffin. © 2009, ISBN: 978-1-4051-8035-1.

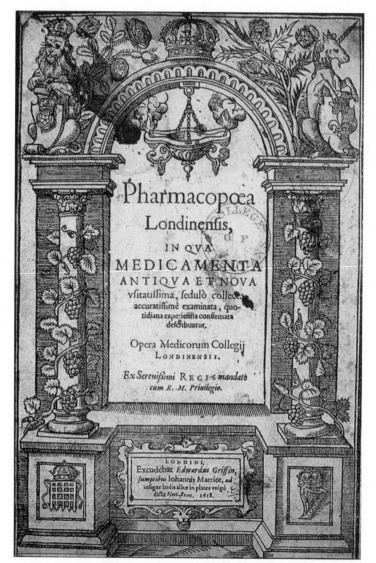

Figure 17.1 Frontpiece from *The London Pharmacopoeia*, 1618. (Reproduced with kind permission from the Hunterian Libraries, Royal College of Physicians, London.)

were to be treated with a plaster of either Mithridatium or Galene applied hot, thrice daily.

Many physicians in the early eighteenth century had doubts as to whether Mithridatium was the universal panacea of all illness as claimed. The ultimate mortal attack on the remedy came from Dr William Heberden (1710–1801) (Figure 17.3), best known for his description of the 'Heberden's nodes' in osteoarthritis. Consequently, the 1746 edition of *The London Pharmacopoeia* was the last in which references to

Mithridatium appear. With its disappearance, the long-used complex remedy attributable to an experimental toxicologist from the second century BC came to an end. Perhaps in the final analysis, the contribution of Mithridatium to modern medicine was that concerns about quality stimulated the earliest concepts of medicines regulation.

Concerns on the safety of medicines began to emerge when the laws on vaccination against smallpox were tightened in 1853 and later in 1871[2] when a House of

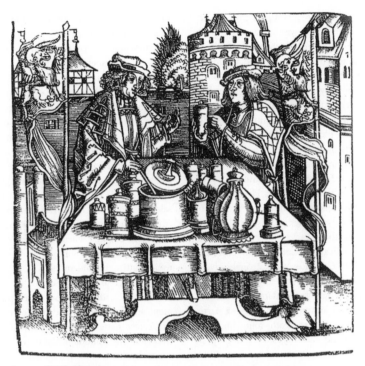

Figure 17.2 Manufacture of Mithridatium.

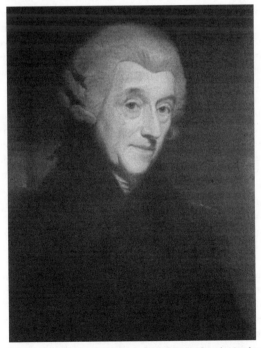

Figure 17.3 Dr William Heberden (1710–1801). To produce it each batch had to be submitted to the Medical Research Council (MRC) for approval before marketing. (Reproduced with kind permission from the Hunterian Libraries, Royal College of Physicians, London.)

Commons Select Committee investigating the efficacy of the compulsory system was concerned by Dr Jonathan Hutchinson's report of the transmission of syphilis in two patients by arm-to-arm inoculation.

Following the discovery and clinical use of chloroform in 1847, the Royal Medical and Chirurgical Society (later to become the Royal Society of Medicine) had already set up in 1864 a committee to inquire 'into the uses and the physiological, therapeutical and toxicological effects of chloroform'. There had been 109 fatalities following administration of chloroform. A critical relationship had been demonstrated between the dose and effect of this anaesthetic. The committee commented on the need for animal experiments to compare chloroform with ether and also on the relative cardiac safety of ether.

At the British Medical Association (BMA) meeting in Manchester in 1877, Spencer Wells strongly advocated urgent investigations into how anaesthesia, effective as it was, might be rendered safe for the future. The BMA too set up its own working party, in 1877, to investigate sudden deaths following chloroform anaesthesia and had suggested setting up an independent body to assess its safety. This BMA working party published its report in 1880 but this had little impact on generating public or political concern to set up a regulatory authority. The safety of chloroform was to resurface as late as 1978 (see below).

The stimulus to drug regulation ultimately came following the publications of two BMA papers entitled 'Secret Remedies' in 1909 and 'More Secret Remedies' in 1912. These prompted a Parliamentary Select Committee on Patent Medicines to be set up. This Select Committee reported in 1914, but the outbreak of war resulted in the shelving of all proposed legislation.[2] There was no further investigation into the pharmaceutical industry's activities until the report of the House of Commons Health Select Committee in March 2005.[3]

Following the discovery of arsphenamine (Salvarsan) in Germany in 1907, it was imported into the UK until the beginning of the First World War, when the Board of Trade issued licences to certain British manufacturers.

The forerunner to monitoring of adverse reactions can be traced to a recommendation in 1922 by the Medical Research Council (MRC) Salvarsan Committee. This Committee, set up to investigate epidemics of jaundice and hepatic necrosis following the use of Salvarsan, encouraged reporting 'to the Ministry of Health of details concerning such accidents, for it is only in the light of such information that investiga-tion and measures with regard to their prevention can be successfully undertaken'.

Following concerns on impurities and standardisation, the Therapeutic Substances Act was passed in 1925 with the aim of regulating the manufacture of biological substances, providing the standards to which they must conform and regulating their labelling. This Act recognised the significance of the manufacturing process and factory inspection and in-process controls played a large part in supervision by the Ministry of Health. This Therapeutic Substances Act was later consolidated and strengthened in 1956 when Part II was added, which dealt with control of sale and supply. Records of sale had to be kept and the container had to identify both the manufacturer and the batch. The first schedule to the 1956 Act included the substances commonly known as vaccines, sera, toxins, antitoxins and antigens.

The Venereal Disease Act of 1917 and the Cancer Act of 1939 had already prevented public advertisement and promotion of drugs for these conditions to protect patients from inadequate or unsuitable treatment and fraudulent claims (of efficacy).

Clearly, by the 1950s, fragments of legislation controlling the quality, sale and promotion of drugs had existed in the UK for many years but these had in general been disease-orientated and had little relevance to the therapeutic revolution that was taking place at the time. There seemed to be no major concerns in Europe with the way the drugs were manufactured, placed on the market and, in a broad sense, controlled.

In France, 102 people had died and 100 more were affected by paraplegia in 1957 as a result of the administration of Stalinon capsules for the treatment of boils. The Stalinon episode had resulted from a formulation error – Stalinon capsules for marketing contained 15 mg diiodoethyltin and 100 mg isolinoleic acid esters. Clinical trials were carried out with capsules containing only 3 mg diiodoethyltin (one-fifth of the marketed dose). Subsequent studies in animals and in humans confirmed the neurotoxicity of diiodoethyltin, which was characterised by intramyelinic vacuolation and astrocyte swelling with no evidence of neuronal degeneration. This tragedy, however, was a foretaste of an even greater disaster – that of thalidomide.

The thalidomide disaster in 1961 was to blow apart the complacency on regulation of drugs. The confidence in the therapeutic revolution promised by the pharmaceutical industry was shattered and there followed considerable public outcry.

17.2 The thalidomide disaster and its immediate aftermath

Thalidomide[4] was a sedative and a hypnotic that first went on sale in 1956 in West Germany. Between 1958 and 1960, it was introduced in 46 countries under 51 different trade names. It was first introduced in the UK market in April 1958 under the name Distaval. It enjoyed good sales because of its prompt action, lack of hangover and addiction observed with barbiturates, and apparent safety.

Following anecdotal reports of benefit in the treatment of vomiting in early pregnancy, it was heavily promoted for this purpose. This use in early pregnancy was soon followed by an epidemic of a previously unknown congenital malformation of the limbs, termed 'phocomelia' because of its resemblance to the flippers of a seal, and other associated internal malformations. The first cases were reported from Germany beginning in 1959 but the malformation also began to make an appearance in other countries where the drug was on sale. Curiously, among the West European countries the drug was not marketed in France, which was spared the tragedy. The Stalinon disaster had resulted in new regulatory requirements being published in February 1959 by the French Health Authority. The manufacturers had to have recourse to an officially appointed expert committee for the preparation of registration file. This registration file had to provide evidence of the therapeutic interest of the product and of its safety under normal conditions of use as well as of the manufacturing process associated with adequate testing to guarantee the quality of the product on an industrial scale.

Of considerable concern was the scale of the disaster resulting from its protracted marketing, the manufacturer continuing to deny all evidence of a causal relationship between these congenital abnormalities and the drug. Worldwide, there were an estimated 10,000 babies with phocomelia and other allied deformities, including more than 500 in England. The frequency of the malformations in Germany followed the absolute sales of the drug with a time lag of a little less than 1 year. The drug was withdrawn from the market in Germany in November 1961, in the UK in December 1961 and, over the next 10 months thereafter, from most countries of the world. After the withdrawal of the drug from the market, 8–9 months later the wave of the unique malformations disappeared as suddenly as it had appeared and with the same time lag that had followed the introduction of the drug. The drug was soon confirmed as a potent teratogen in a number of animal studies.

Governments throughout the Western world were now galvanised into introducing effective drug regulation. Even in the USA, despite the strength of the prevailing legislation on safety, news reports on the role of Dr Frances Kelsey, a medical officer at the Food and Drug Administration (FDA), in keeping the drug off the US market, aroused much public support for even strong drug regulation.

The UK government set up in August 1962 the Joint Subcommittee of the English and Scottish Standing Medical Advisory Committees, under the chairmanship of Lord Cohen of Birkenhead, with the following terms of reference to advise the Minister of Health and the Secretary of State for Scotland on what measures are needed:

1. To secure adequate pharmacological and safety testing and clinical trials of new drugs before their release for general use;
2. To secure early detection of adverse effects arising after their release for general use; and
3. To keep doctors informed of the experiences of such drugs in clinical practice.

17.3 Voluntary controls in the UK (1963–1971)

In its interim advice delivered on 2 November 1962, the Joint Subcommittee of the English and Scottish Standing Medical Advisory Committees, set up in the aftermath of the thalidomide disaster, made three main recommendations:

1. The responsibility for the experimental laboratory testing of new drugs before they are used in clinical trials should remain with the individual pharmaceutical manufacturer.
2. It was neither desirable nor practical that at this stage of their evaluation the responsibility for testing drugs should be transferred to a central authority.
3. There should be an expert body to review the evidence and offer advice on the toxicity of new drugs, whether manufactured in Great Britain or abroad, before they were used in clinical trials.

Following further consideration and consultations, the Joint Subcommittee proposed to formulate detailed advice on the composition and terms of this expert advisory body. On 6 November 1962, the Minister of Health announced that the government had accepted the first two recommendations and would await the advice on the third.

In the period intervening between its interim advice and its final report, the Joint Subcommittee received memoranda from and met representatives of the Association of the British Pharmaceutical Industry (ABPI), the British Medical Association (BMA), the Pharmaceutical Society of Great Britain and the College of General Practitioners.

Despite reservations expressed by a number of these bodies, the Joint Subcommittee took the view that public opinion was unlikely to be content with anything short of ministerial responsibility for verifying that adequate precautions had been taken to secure the safety of drugs, the more so because of the number and nature of new drugs.

The Joint Subcommittee issued its Final Report on 'Safety of Drugs'[5] in March 1963, which states in paragraph 10:

We think that a Committee on Safety of Drugs should be established with subcommittees to advise it on each of the three aspects, namely:
(i) toxicity
(ii) clinical trials and therapeutic efficacy and
(iii) adverse reactions.

17.3.1 Committee on Safety of Drugs

The three health ministers of the UK, in consultation with the medical and pharmaceutical professions and the ABPI, set up the Committee on Safety of Drugs (CSD) in June 1963. The three health ministers were the Secretary of State for Scotland, the Minister of Health and the Minister of Health and Social Services, Northern Ireland.

The Committee had the following terms of reference:
1. To invite from the manufacturer or other person developing or proposing to market a drug in the UK, any reports they may think fit on the toxicity tests carried out on it; to consider whether any further tests should be made and whether the drug should be submitted to clinical trials; and to convey their advice to those who submitted reports.
2. To obtain reports of clinical trials of drugs submitted thereto.
3. Taking into account the safety and efficacy of each drug, and the purposes for which it is to be used, to consider whether it may be released for marketing, with or without precautions or restrictions on its use; and to convey their advice to those who submitted reports.
4. To give to manufacturers and others concerned any general advice they may think fit.
5. To assemble and assess reports about adverse effects of drugs in use and prepare information thereon that may be brought to the notice of doctors and other concerned.
6. To advise the appointing ministers on any of the above matters.

The Committee consisted of a panel of independent experts from various fields of pharmacy, medicine and pathology, among others, with Sir Derrick Dunlop as its first chairman. In tribute to his personal charm, considerable skills and foresight, it soon became popularly known as the Dunlop Committee.

The Committee had no legal powers but worked with the voluntary agreement of the ABPI and the Proprietary Association of Great Britain (PAGB). These associations promised that none of their members would put on clinical trial or release for marketing a new drug against the advice of the Committee and whose advice they would always seek. In an attempt to make sure that the manufacturers adhered to this, the health ministers undertook, in a circular sent to all dentists and doctors in the UK, to inform the prescribers of any cases of drugs being marketed or put to clinical trials without the Committee's approval.

A number of subcommittees were also established to assist the main Committee. These were the Subcommittee on Toxicity and the Subcommittee on Clinical Trials and Therapeutic Efficacy. Against the background of the thalidomide tragedy, an important subcommittee established was the Subcommittee on Adverse Reactions. The memberships of the main Committee and its three Subcommittees when first established in 1963 are shown in Table 17.1. The Committee spent the first 6 months of its existence (the latter half of 1963) in completing its preparatory work. By 1 January 1964, the Committee was in a position to invite submissions (this is what they were called, and not 'applications') on drugs intended for clinical trials or about to be released for the market.

In 1967, the Subcommittee on Toxicity and the Subcommittee on Clinical Trials and Therapeutic Efficacy were merged because the interests of the two were shown by experience to overlap considerably. The new subcommittee, the Subcommittee on Toxicity, Clinical Trials and Therapeutic Efficacy, was chaired by Professor A.C. Frazer with Professor E.F. Scowen (later Sir Eric Scowen) as the deputy chairman.

17.3.2 Medicines Division of DHSS

The CSD was serviced by a professional secretariat of pharmacists and medical officers who undertook the assessment of the submissions and presented these to the Committee and its various subcommittees. The secretariat initially included three doctors and two

Table 17.1 Submissions to the Committee on Safety of Drugs (1964–1971)

	1964	1965	1966	1967	1968	1969	1970	1971
Clinical trial submissions	66	168	203	202	239	218	178	122
	(11.0%)	(19.2%)	(22.4%)	(26.4%)	(30.2%)	(25.7%)	(24.9%)	(22.0%)
Marketing submissions	534	706	705	563	552	630	536	432
Total (inc. NCEs)	600	874	908	765	791	848	714	554
	(55)	(69)	(66)	(56)	(56)	(66)	(69)	(??)
Approved	386	807	771	698	669	694	499	411
Rejected	15	19	24	36	36	33	53	38
	(2.5%)	(1.8%)	(2.4%)	(4.1%)	(4.1%)	(3.5%)	(6.3%)	(5.0%)
Withdrawn by applicant	32	119	86	70	83	86	79	66
	(5.3%)	(11.4%)	(8.6%)	(7.9%)	(9.5%)	(9.2%)	(9.4%)	(8.7%)
Further information	99	49	39	43	34	47	68	74
requested	(16.5%)	(4.7%)	(3.9%)	(4.8%)	(3.9%)	(5.0%)	(8.1%)	(9.7%)
Pending further consideration	68	47	84	41	53	75	137	170
Total	600	1041	1004	888	875	935	836	759

NCE, new chemical entity.

pharmacists. In 1965, the number of professional staff had been increased to six doctors and three pharmacists. The six doctors were Dr Denis Cahal, who headed the secretariat, and Drs J. Broadbent, M. Hollyhock, W.H. Inman, D. Mansel-Jones and C. Ruttle. The secretariat, known as the Medicines Division, was created as a branch of the Department of Health. The close collaboration between Dr Cahal and Sir Derrick Dunlop was pivotal in guiding the Medicines Act through Parliament in 1968 and setting the foundation of a system that became a model to the rest of the world for fairness and efficiency.

The Medicines Division was originally based at Queen Anne's Mansions, Queen Anne's Gate, London SW1, where the Committee and the Subcommittees also held their meetings. The secretariat was moved on 1 April 1971 to a new accommodation at Finsbury Square House, 33/37a Finsbury Square, London EC2A 1PP. In March 1980, it moved to its current imposing location, overlooking the River Thames, at Market Towers, 1 Nine Elms Lane, Vauxhall, London SW8 5NQ.

Each manufacturer was given a four-digit company number for identification and this number was to be used for all their product-related documents – a system that prevails even today. For example, Geigy (UK) Ltd was 0001, Glaxo Group Ltd was 0004, John Wyeth & Brother Ltd was 0011, Astra-Hewlett Ltd was 0017, Parke Davis & Co. was 0018, AB Kabi was 0022, ER Squibb & Sons Ltd was 0034, Abbott Laboratories Ltd was 0037 and, for those who are given to reminisce and remember it, Beecham Research

Laboratories was 0038. The order of the allocation of these numbers was determined by the order in which the submissions were received by the new regulatory body from the companies. Thus, Geigy (UK) Ltd was the first company ever to make a submission to the CSD. A second set of four-digit numbers followed the company number (i.e. 0000/0000) and related to the individual products licensed for sale to that company, again in a numerical order in which the submissions for marketing authorisations were received.

17.3.3 Legacy of the Committee on Safety of Drugs

Even in these embryonic days, the Committee was to establish many important principles that still dominate drug regulation today. The Committee had required, as a minimum, teratogenicity testing in two species, one of which should preferably be a non-rodent, for one generation only. They also recognised the limitations of teratogenicity tests in animals but emphasised that only in the most exceptional circumstances would they release any drug for clinical trial in women of child-bearing age until the appropriate tests on animals had been carried out satisfactorily.

The Committee also required a wider interpretation of the term 'new drugs' to include 'new formulations of existing drugs, drugs to be presented for a new purpose, and existing substances not previously used as drugs, covering virtually all new products introduced'. The Committee had clearly appreciated that new formulations ought to be subject to scrutiny because reformulation did occasionally introduce additional hazards.

Perhaps one of the most important years in drug regulation in the UK was 1965. That year, the manufacturers began to challenge the right of the Committee to require under its terms of reference evidence of efficacy of a drug. The Committee took the view that for serious diseases failure of efficacy constituted an unacceptable risk, while for trivial diseases where efficacy may be irrelevant, even a trivial safety hazard is not acceptable – the concept of modern day 'risk–benefit'. The Committee also emphasised that it was not concerned with efficacy and its clearance of a drug for the market did not necessarily imply its approval of the drug as a valuable remedy. The Committee also noted: 'Medicines are not sacrosanct however, simply because they have been in use for a long time.'

During the year there were a number of reports in the press of deaths associated with phenacetin. The Committee emphasised that the hazard was associated with the abuse of the drug (excessive doses taken over a long term) and reiterated that, consequently, no special action was necessary. Furthermore, because a drug (including phenacetin) could be marketed under different proprietary names, it could confuse a doctor. Therefore, the Committee decided that they would not consider an application by a manufacturer to market a new substance unless the applicant gave an assurance that an approved name had been obtained or applied for.

When considering new drug submissions, the Committee also paid attention to the claims and indications that the promoter intended to include on the label of a drug or in its promotional literature. Another significant step taken by the Committee related to labelling of the prescribed medicines by pharmacists. The practice of labelling the container as 'The Tablets' was no longer considered acceptable (unless the prescribing doctor specified otherwise). After canvassing the opinions of many professional bodies, including all Royal Colleges, the BMA and the Pharmaceutical Society of Great Britain had agreed by 1971 to the proposal of marking of prescriptions *nomen proprium*.

The period 1966–1967 was one of consolidation. The Committee had received considerable support for and re-emphasised all their previous recommendations. Between 1964 and 1967 the Committee received representatives from the World Health Organization (WHO) and many European and Far and Middle Eastern countries, as well as from Canada and the USA, to study its methods.

In 1966, the Committee made observations on a hazard that increasingly plagues many drugs even today – the problems of drug–drug interactions. The Committee noted:

It is now well known that the administration of one drug may considerably modify the actions of another being given at the same time. Both the toxicity and the metabolism of each drug may be affected by the other. This applies to combinations of drugs in one preparation as well as to those separately administered. However, it is still too readily assumed by some manufacturers that no additional hazard is incurred by combining two or more drugs in one preparation.

The first drug–drug interaction alert issued by the Committee in 1966 concerned the risks from interactions between preparations containing adrenaline or noradrenaline and monoamine oxidase (MAO) inhibitors used for the treatment of depression.

In its final report, in 1969–1970, the Committee expressed safety concerns arising from the names of products that differ, for example, only by a suffixed letter, and expressed a desire to see the naming of products put on a more rational basis.

It is interesting that for entirely new chemical entities, submissions in those early days of drug regulation were 'often voluminous: a submission containing over 1000 pages of reports, drafts and tables was not unusual'. Rejection of drugs outright was a comparatively minor part of the Committee's operations; by far the more important actions involved persuading manufacturers to make changes in their intentions (e.g. formulation, indication).

In 1965, the great majority of submissions had concerned reformulation of established drugs. The number of submissions for reformulated preparations of established drugs was even higher in 1966, a matter that concerned the Committee in respect of 'the extent to which the drug houses have tended to flood the market with so many similar preparations'. As a result, Mr C.A. Johnson (a pharmacist) and Dr D.F.J. Mason (a toxicologist) were then appointed to the Subcommittee on Toxicity. The work of the Committee during their tenure from January 1964 to 31 August 1971 in terms of submissions received and determined is shown in Table 17.1.

From time to time, the Committee received submissions related to vaccines or immunological products. When considering these, the Committee felt the need to seek advice of experts in that special field. Therefore, in November 1969 it was decided to set up a Vaccine Advisory Group. This initiative ultimately culminated in the establishment of the Subcommittee on Biological Substances, and the Biological Standards Act received the Royal Assent in February 1975. This Act provided for the establishment of a National Biological Standards Board to manage the activities carried out at the National Institute for Biological Standards and Control. The Institute undertook the control of testing of biological substances used for therapeutic, prophylactic and diagnostic purposes (e.g. vaccines, sera, antibiotics) to discharge their obligations under the Therapeutic Substances Act 1956 and the Medicines Act 1968.

In 1969, it came to the attention of the Committee that unidentified tablets of a drug purporting to be nitrazepam were being distributed in the UK. The Ministers issued a press statement warning those concerned not to use any other but the branded product that the Committee had cleared. Likewise, in early 1970 it came to public notice that one manufacturer was proposing to market *L*-dopa, a drug that at the time was still under clinical trial for the treatment of parkinsonism, without first making a submission to the Committee. The Department of Health responded by issuing a statement advising strongly against the use of this drug from any source that had not been approved by the Committee. By the end of 1969, the Committee was able to 'fast track' the only two submissions for approval of clinical trials with *L*-dopa for its use in parkinsonism. These manufacturers were encouraged by the Committee to submit the data early and it was possible to release some *L*-dopa preparations for marketing during the earlier part of 1970.

The membership of the CSD and its subcommittees changed further following the resignation of Sir Derrick Dunlop in May 1969, as a result of his appointment as the first chairman of the Medicines Commission (MC), established under the Medicines Act 1968.

Professor A.C. Frazer was appointed to succeed Sir Derrick but unfortunately he died shortly thereafter. During 1969, therefore, Professor E.F. Scowen succeeded Professor Frazer as the chairman of the Committee. In June 1970, the membership of the Committee was revised to correspond with that of the then newly established (under section 4 of the Medicines Act 1968) Committee on Safety of Medicines (CSM).

17.3.4 Voluntary adverse reactions reporting system: the Yellow Card scheme

The CSD had also started studies of adverse reactions to drugs (ADRs) by the beginning of 1964. Sir Derrick Dunlop wrote to all doctors (4 May 1964) and dentists

(15 June 1964), inviting them: 'to report to us promptly details of any untoward condition in a patient which might be the result of drug treatment'. They were assured that 'all the reports or replies that the Committee receive from them will be treated with complete professional confidence by the Committee and their staff. The Health Ministers have given an undertaking that the information supplied will never be used for disciplinary purposes or for enquiries about prescribing costs.'

This spontaneous adverse reaction reporting system was the brainchild of Professor Leslie Witts and was, and still is, based upon the submission of ADR reports by doctors and dentists by means of reply-paid yellow cards, and hence it is popularly known as the Yellow Card scheme.

In the first year, up to 100 Yellow Card reports were received each week. In the case of 'serious suspected adverse reactions that might call for action it is necessary, therefore, to have more information about the reported incident and a number of doctors have been appointed throughout the country who will help the Committee on a part-time basis by following up reports'. At the end of 1965, there were 35 such part-time doctors helping with the follow-up of serious reports. During the first 5 years, the number of reports received averaged about 60 per week, but the problem of determining number of prescriptions was soon recognised. The Committee needed to relate the number of reports with exposure. It concluded, 'it is possible to determine the ratio of adverse reactions only by asking a number of doctors who have prescribed a drug about their experience of it with special reference to the adverse reactions which, from reports, appear to be associated with its use'.

The Committee, as early as 1964, seemed to have anticipated prescription event monitoring as well as the need for compiling large databases. It thought of a scheme that 'involves taking a sample of prescriptions written by doctors for the drugs being investigated. In the United Kingdom the assembly of National Health Service prescriptions for pricing purposes offers a unique opportunity for this sort of analysis that is not available anywhere else in the world and the pricing bureaux have kindly offered their help.' Regarding large databases, it went on 'prescription scripts are not at present filed in a way which allows easy identification of particular drugs but with the cooperation of the pricing bureaux, the Committee are developing a satisfactory procedure'.

Because new drugs are often at first used in hospitals and 'it is at this stage that serious adverse reactions are likely to be noticed', a pilot scheme was set up with a number of hospitals for recording prescriptions and the Committee devised a 'list of specially monitored drugs' which at 'any time will contain all the new substances introduced during the previous 2 years and a number of older drugs that still need special observation'. This clearly was the forerunner to the present Black Triangle scheme that operates to identify drugs requiring intensive monitoring for at least 2 years.

When a safety problem was suspected, the promotion of information on safety of drugs was an important remit of the Committee and this they discharged by issuing a series of leaflets to all doctors and dentists in the UK. The first alert leaflet in this *Adverse Reactions Series* was issued by the CSD in February 1964. It dealt with reports of liver damage and blood pressure changes following the use of MAO inhibitor drugs. Nine such alert leaflets were issued over the next 5 years to December 1969. The contents of these alerts are summarised in an earlier account.[4]

In 1967, computer facilities were installed for handling the Yellow Card reports and, after consultation, a method of confidential feedback to the profession was designed. A doctor reporting an ADR was automatically sent a summary of all the reports received by the Committee on the drug and on similar drugs. Where possible, an estimate of the extent to which the drug was prescribed was also given.

By 1965, the value of the Yellow Card scheme was clearly established and two other countries had introduced a similar scheme. By the beginning of 1967, the Committee was also cooperating in the WHO's pilot study on the monitoring of ADRs at an international level. By the end of 1968, a total of 10 countries were participating in this pilot study. This study matured into the international WHO ADR Monitoring Centre based in Uppsala (Sweden), with a membership that now stands at 67 countries with six others enjoying associate status.

The Yellow Card scheme was soon beginning to pay dividends. In early 1966, the Yellow Card scheme had identified Methyl Dopa as a cause of haemolytic anaemia and appropriate advice was issued. Another success was the detection of a faulty batch of a particular product, which the manufacturer immediately withdrew, underlining the value of an efficient procedure for tracing a batch. During June 1967, the Committee distributed a leaflet on the use of aerosols in asthma. This was prompted by the death rate amongst asthmatic patients aged 5–34 years that had risen some 300% above the level in 1959–1960 when such preparations were introduced. By September

1968, the rate had dropped to only 50% above that seen in 1959–1960 despite sales having dropped only 20%.

Among the first three 'old' drugs to be withdrawn from the market during the tenure of the CSD were benziodarone, a vasodilatator launched in 1962 and withdrawn in 1964 because of reports of jaundice; pronethalol, a beta-blocker introduced in 1963 and withdrawn in 1965 because of animal carcinogenicity; and phenoxypropazine, an antidepressant introduced in 1961 and withdrawn in 1966 because of its hepatotoxicity.

The first major new drug to be approved and withdrawn from the market by the CSD was ibufenac, the first of the non-steroidal anti-inflammatory drugs (NSAIDs) to be marketed. Ibufenac was a precursor of ibuprofen and its use in the UK was associated with serious and frequent hepatotoxicity. Two other drug withdrawals (also approved during their tenure by CSD) were chlormadinone and fenclozic acid.

During 1969–1970, the nephropathic hazards of phenacetin again attracted much attention and the Committee made a seminal observation that has profoundly influenced our regulatory philosophy even today: 'It is the safety of drugs in normal usage that is the Committee's concern, and because all drugs have their hazards when abused, particularly by over-dosage, the Committee has not considered that it should take special action in connection with phenacetin.'

The 'demise' of the CSD was marked by a reception at Lancaster House in December 1971. It was attended by the Secretary of State together with the Health Ministers of Scotland, Wales and Northern Ireland as well as by the current and previous members of CSD, its first chairman, Sir Derrick Dunlop, the Presidents of the Royal Colleges and representatives of the medical and pharmaceutical professions and pharmaceutical industry. The CSD had already set the pattern for effective drug controls in the future.

17.4 Medicines Act 1968

The Joint Subcommittee of the English and Scottish Standing Medical Advisory Committee, chaired by Lord Cohen of Birkenhead, had included as its members seven distinguished clinicians and pharmacists of the day:[5]

• Professor S. Alstead, CBE, MD, FRCP, FRFPS;
• A.B. Davies, BSc, MD, ChB, MRCS, LRCP;
• Professor Sir Charles Dodds, MVO, MD, DSc, FRCP, FRS;

- J.B. Grosset, MPS, DBA;
- Sir Hugh Linstead, OBE, LLD, FPS, MP;
- Professor E.J. Wayne, MD, FRCP, FRFPS; and
- Professor G.M. Wilson, MD, FRCP.

The Joint Subcommittee had concluded that testing was the responsibility of the manufacturers and they appeared to favour a voluntary scheme of control.

Para 25: Sanctions under a Voluntary Scheme *While a voluntary scheme could have no formal legal sanctions, we think that the following measures might help, nevertheless, to ensure that new drugs were subject to adequate toxicity testing and clinical trials.*

However, the two eminent pharmacists, John Grosset and Hugh Linstead, appended to the report a lengthy note of dissent that was forceful and stated with uncompromising clarity:

Voluntary or Statutory Control of Toxicity Testing and Clinical Trials? *Our main disagreement with our colleagues lies in the answer to this question. They favour a voluntary system until time can be found for legislation. We believe that any voluntary system must have so many loopholes that it can offer no real additional safeguards to the public. In consequence, we consider that there is no satisfactory alternative to early legislation.*[5]

In their note, they also commented extensively on the deficiencies of a voluntary system. Grosset and Linstead concluded their note with a plea 'to set on foot, with or without further enquiry, the preparation of a comprehensive statute dealing with drugs and medicines that will bring the whole field, including the supervision of toxicity testing and clinical trials, under the responsibility of the Health Ministers advised by a central body of experts'.

Full voluntary cooperation was clearly not as assured as might have been anticipated. During 1965, the CSD itself seemed to articulate in its Annual Report a carefully concealed aspiration for the introduction of statutory controls on drug regulation. After a period of review and consultation, a White Paper 'Forthcoming Legislation on the Safety, Quality and Description of Drugs and Medicines' was published in September 1967 and the Medicines Act based on these proposals received the Royal Assent on 25 October 1968. The CSD 'welcomes the statutory provisions that provide a firm basis for the continued evaluation of drug safety in the future'.

The Medicines Act 1968 is a comprehensive set of measures replacing most of the previous legislation on the control of medicines for human use and for veterinary use in the UK. It is a consolidation into a single Act of the most desirable features of all previous rules, regulations and Acts in the UK and also includes controls on promotion and sale of drugs. The Act has 136 sections divided into Parts I–VIII and has a further eight schedules appended to it. Among the important sections for licensing and monitoring purposes are:

- Sections 18–24 regarding applications for, and grant and renewal of, licences with section 19 requiring evidence for safety, efficacy and quality when determining an application;
- Sections 28–30 in respect of suspension, revocation and variation of licences;
- Sections 31–39 on clinical trials;
- Sections 51–59 on sale and supply;
- Sections 85–88 on labelling and leaflets;
- Sections 92–97 on promotion and advertising;
- Sections 104–128 on enforcement.

Under section 118 of the Act, all data submitted by a company in support of an application to conduct clinical trials or market a medicinal product are confidential; indeed, even the existence of such an application is confidential. Breach of confidentiality attracts penalties and 'any person guilty of an offence under this section shall be liable (1) on summary conviction, to a fine not exceeding £400; (2) on conviction on indictment, to a fine or to imprisonment for a term not exceeding 2 years or to both'.

The Act has been frequently amended as appropriate to ensure that it is in line with the European Community legislation. Given the remarkable degree of similarity between the requirements under the Medicines Act 1968 and the legislations prevailing at the time in the USA and the European Economic Community (EEC), the existence of four major legislations, together with their amendments and consequential secondary legislations, is worth bearing in mind.

One was the Federal Pure Food and Drugs Act (also known as the Wiley Act) which was introduced in the USA in 1906. This law was enacted in response to revelations of worthless, impure and dangerous patent medicines that were claimed to cure almost anything. Another was the Federal Food, Drug and Cosmetic Act 1938 that had been passed following the Elixir Sulfanilamide disaster in the USA during 1937 in which 107 people (mostly children) had died from renal failure associated with its therapeutic use. As the drug was called 'elixir', implying that the preparation contained alcohol, the FDA could only make seizure of the product for misbranding. In reaction to this calamity, the US Congress passed the 1938 Act, which, for the first time, required proof of safety before release of a new drug. However, no proof of efficacy was required. Following the thalidomide tragedy in western Europe, a subsequent New Drug Amendment (the Kefauver–Harris Amendment) was introduced in 1962 that required the FDA to monitor all stages of drug development. As a result of the Kefauver–Harris Amendment, even investigational drugs then required comprehensive animal testing before extensive human trials could be started. Proof of efficacy and safety was mandatory and the time constraints for disposition of new drugs, previously deemed approved by default if the FDA had failed to consider the new drug application by 60 days, were removed.

The EEC had already in place the Council Directive 65/65/EEC on the approximation of provisions laid down by law, regulation or administrative action relating to medicinal products. Many of the requirements under Council Directive 65/65/EEC had already formed part of the Medicines Act. When Directives 75/318/EEC and 75/319/EEC were adopted by the Council of Ministers on 20 May 1975, they only supplemented and amended the original Directive 65/65/EEC. Therefore, when the UK joined the EEC in 1973, the provisions of these two new Directives did not substantially affect the licensing system that operated in the UK under the Medicines Act, although certain relatively minor amendments were necessary.

The first provisions laid down in the Medicines Act regarding licensing of medicinal products and other aspects of control came into effect on 1 September 1971 – the 'duly appointed day'. The Act was administered by the Health and Agriculture Ministers of the UK acting together as the Licensing Authority or in some cases acting separately as the health ministers or the agriculture ministers in respect of human and veterinary medicines, respectively. The Act allows for Orders and Regulations to be made implementing its provisions and 98 Statutory Instruments had been made by the end of 1977. The first four were made in 1970 (SI 1970/746, 1257, 1304 and 1256), establishing the Medicines Commission, Committee on Safety of Medicines, Veterinary Products Committee and the British Pharmacopoeia Commission, respectively. A full list of these is contained in the Annual Reports for 1976 and 1977 of the Medicines Commission and the section 4 Committees.

17.4.1 Licensing Authority

Under section 6 of the Medicines Act 1968, the Licensing Authority (LA) is the authority responsible for the grant, renewal, variation, suspension and revocation of licences and certificates. In 1971, the LA was constituted of a body of Ministers consisting of the Secretary of State for Social Services, the Secretary of State for Scotland, the Secretary of State for Wales, the Minister of Health and Social Services for Northern Ireland, the Minister of Agriculture, Fisheries and Food and the Minister of Agriculture in Northern Ireland.

17.4.2 Medicines Division (DHSS)

The day-to-day administration of the Act for human medicines was delegated to the Medicines Division of the Department of Health and Social Security (DHSS) and was managed jointly by an Under Secretary and the professional head of the division. The professional head of the Medicines Division held the rank of senior principal medical officer. The staff levels in the period 1976–1987 was a nominal 330 but the complement was seldom full.

Over the period, the successive professional heads of the Medicines Division have been Drs D.A. Cahal (1964–1970), D. Mansel-Jones (1970–1974), E.L. Harris (1974–1977), J.P. Griffin (1977–1984) and G. Jones (1984–1989). In 1989, when the Medicines Division was reorganised into the Medicines Control Agency (MCA; see section 16.7), Dr K.H. Jones was appointed the first director of the new agency.

Before the UK joined the European Union, the Medicines Division had developed close links with other authorities both within and outside the European Union. Notable among these were the Tripartite Meetings held biannually with the US FDA and the Canadian Health Protection Branch. These meetings, lasting a few days, discussed all areas of drug regulation generally and problems with specific drugs. Having first started in 1971, these meetings continued, while the EU system was evolving during the UK membership, until 1991 (apart from a very brief lull during the mid-1980s). By 1991, the International Conference on Harmonisation (ICH) initiative (see below) had fully matured into the first ICH meeting, to be held in Brussels in November 1991.

17.5 Statutory controls in the UK (1971 and thereafter)

17.5.1 Medicines Commission

The Medicines Commission, provided for in section 2 of the Act, was established by the Ministers to give them advice generally relating to the execution of the Act (SI 1970/746), with Sir Derrick Dunlop as its first chairman.

The scope of the functions of the Commission is very wide, but as defined in 1975 may be summarised as follows:

1. To advise the LA on matters relating to the execution of the Medicines Act;
2. To recommend to the Ministers, the number and functions of committees to be established under section 4 of the Act and to recommend such persons as they consider well qualified to serve as members of such committees; and
3. To advise the LA in cases where it consults the Commission, including cases where the LA arranges for the applicant for the grant of a licence to have an opportunity of appearing before, and being heard by, the Commission.

Sir Derrick Dunlop's tenure of office ended on 31 December 1971. The Medicines Commission has since been successively chaired by Lord Rosenheim (from January 1972 to 2 December 1972, when he died suddenly), Professor A. Wilson (acting chairman, December 1972 to the middle of 1973), Sir Ronald Bodley Scott (middle of 1973 to December 1975), Professor W.J.H. Butterfield (later Sir John Butterfield and later still Lord Butterfield, January 1976 to December 1981), Professor Rosalinde Hurley (later Dame Rosalinde Hurley, January 1982 to December 1993), Professor D.H. Lawson (January 1994 to December 2001) and Professor Parveen Kumar (January 2002 to October 2005).

The establishment of the Medicines Commission in May 1969 was followed by the establishment of a number of expert committees with specific advisory functions, appointed by Ministers after considering the recommendations of the Commission as proposed in section 4 of the Medicines Act. These expert committees, whose members are appointed by Ministers on the advice of the Medicines Commission, advise the LA and consist of independent experts such as hospital clinicians, general practitioners, pharmacists and clinical pharmacologists, and not the staff of the DHSS.

The relevant advisory committees with a remit for medicines for human use established under the Medicines Act 1968 were the Committee on Safety of Medicines (CSM), set up in June 1970 (SI 1970/1257) under the chairmanship of Professor E.F. Scowen and the British Pharmacopoeia Commission (BPC), also set up in June 1970 (SI 1970/1256) under the chairmanship of Dr F. Hartley (later Sir Frank Hartley). The Veterinary Products Committee (VPC), chaired by Professor C.S.G. Grunsell (with a remit for medicines for veterinary use and administered through the Ministry of Agriculture Food and Fisheries), was also established in June 1970 (SI 1970/1304). Other important bodies set up were the Joint Subcommittee on the Use of Antibiotics and Related Substances and Standing Joint Subcommittee on the Classification of Proprietary Preparations, both of which reported directly to the Medicines Commission.

The products already on the market on 1 September 1971, the date for implementation of the Medicines Act, were given the Product Licences of Right (PLR) which were subject to a review process at a later date. This proposal for review of PLRs is reminiscent of the FDA contract with the National Academy of Sciences/National Research Council (NAS/NRC) in 1966, to evaluate the effectiveness of some 4000 different drug formulations approved on the basis of safety alone between 1938 and 1962 – the year of the Kefauver–Harris Amendment.

In 1977, the Medicines Commission reached a significant milestone when the work on classification of medicines was completed. New arrangements provided for three categories of medicines according to their safety factor: those available on prescription only (POM); those sufficiently safe to be on general sale to the public through any retail outlet (GSL); and an intermediate category of those that should only be sold at pharmacies (P). Under section 59 of the Medicines Act, all new medicinal products, not previously on the market, are prescription only for the first 5 years. A conscious decision is made for reclassification of each before the 5-year period expires. This requires updating the Prescription Only Medicines (POM) Order or the General Sales List (GSL) Order.

Rule 13(1) of the Poisons Rules (1972) allowed a pharmacist to supply a POM without a prescription when, by reason of some emergency, a doctor was unable to furnish a prescription immediately.

Section 96 of the Medicines Act provided that after the duly appointed day (1 September 1971), no advertisement relating to medicinal products may be sent to a practitioner unless a data sheet had been sent some time in the previous 15 months. Final regulations on long-term arrangements for data sheets appeared in 1972. The issue of chloroform had surfaced again in 1978. In June 1977, a consultation letter was issued by the LA (MLX 90) introducing a proposal to make an Order under section 62 of the Act prohibiting the sale, supply and importation of any medicinal products containing chloroform (with certain exceptions such as its use as a preservative in pharmaceuticals). Many organisations, including the Joint UK Working Party on Chloroform, made representations and the Commission considered the safety of chloroform in the context of its alleged carcinogenicity in animals and safety in humans. It was concluded that chloroform was not mutagenic and hence did not present a carcinogenic risk to humans. It was also concluded that the upper permitted level of chloroform in medicinal products should be that of the saturated aqueous solution, which is 0.5% volume in volume. The exceptions to the prohibition included the use of chloroform as an anaesthetic agent, its use in dental surgery and the right of doctors and dentists to exercise clinical judgement to have prepared for their patients products containing a higher concentration.

Over the period, the Commission continued to discharge its functions and was pivotal not only in implementing the provisions of Medicines Act 1968, but also advising the Ministers on broader policies relating to public health and drug regulation in the UK. For example, apart from deregulating medicines from prescription control and to GSL, the Commission has deliberated and advised on sale, supply and administration of medicines by health professionals under patient group directions, administration of POMs by ambulance paramedics, review of the process for reclassification (change of legal status) of medicines in the UK, proposals for supplementary prescribing by chiropodists, physiotherapists, radiographers and optometrists and proposed amendments to the POM (Human Use) Order 1997 and access to the Yellow Card scheme.

The Commission had some 24 members (the Act required it to have a minimum of eight) and met five to six times per year. Members were appointed for 4-year terms. However, the work of the Commission has steadily diminished over recent years because of changes in licensing arrangements (e.g. the growth of EU licensing under the centralised and mutual recognition procedures) and other procedural changes within the Medicines and Healthcare products Regulatory Agency (MHRA) (e.g. reclassification procedures). For example, the Commission heard a total of three appeals in 2002 and none in 2003, compared with an average of four or five per year for the previous 10 years. Given also that there are profound changes in the European regulatory structure, environment and legislation (see section 17.9 and Chapter 18), Ministers therefore decided to implement the amalgamation of the functions of MC and CSM (see section 17.8.)

17.5.2 Committee on Safety of Medicines

The CSM, first chaired by Professor E.F. Scowen, replaced the previous CSD and first met on 25 June 1970. Its functions may be summarised as follows:

1. Giving advice with respect to safety, quality and efficacy, in relation to human use, of any substance or article (not being an instrument, apparatus or 'appliance') to which any provision of the Act is applicable.

2. Promoting the collection and investigation of information relating to adverse reactions, for the purpose of enabling such advice to be given.

A number of subcommittees assisted the main Committee. Originally, these were the Subcommittee on Toxicity, Clinical Trials and Therapeutic Efficacy; the Subcommittee on Chemistry, Pharmacy and Standards; the Subcommittee on Adverse Reactions; and the Subcommittee on Biologicals.

In order to permit a smooth transition, the two committees (that on Safety of Drugs and that on Safety of Medicines) met simultaneously from June 1970 onwards, the CSD continuing to appraise products for clinical trials and marketing while the CSM had been concerned with preparation for the implementation of the Medicines Act. On 1 September 1971, the 'duly appointed day', the CSM took over the work formerly carried out by the CSD and the applicants, responsible for submissions still awaiting consideration by the CSD on 1 September 1971, were invited to convert those submissions into applications for Clinical Trial Certificates or for Product Licences. The CSD, however, continued to meet several times after 1 September 1971 to deal with some residual matters arising directly from its own decisions.

Commensurate with the emphasis on drug safety, the terms of reference of the Subcommittee on Adverse Reactions were reviewed in 1971 and revised as follows:

1. To promote and assemble reports about possible adverse effects of medicinal products administered to humans;

2. To assess the meaning of such reports;

3. To recommend to the Committee any special or extended investigations that it considered desirable;

4. To keep under review the methods by which adverse reactions are monitored;

5. To make recommendations to the Committee based on its assessment of any action that it considers should be taken; and

6. To advise the Committee on communications with the professions relating to the work of the Subcommittee.

The LA was already empowered by the Medicines Act to suspend, revoke or vary licences under section 28 and to control clinical trials in patients under section 36. At the outset in 1971, the Committee recognised the need to adhere to the policy stated by the CSD in respect of considering efficacy but took a much firmer line in 1972, bearing in mind section 19 of the Act. The Committee stated explicitly that, in future, it would require applications to be supported by some evidence of efficacy before advising that a product licence should be granted.

Since its establishment, the CSM has been chaired successively by Professors E.F. Scowen (June 1970 to March 1976), G.M. Wilson (April 1976 to December 1976), E.F. Scowen (January 1977 to June 1980), A. Goldberg (later Sir Abraham Goldberg, July 1980 to December 1986), A.W. Asscher (later Sir William Asscher, January 1987 to December 1992), M.D. Rawlins (later Sir Michael Rawlins, January 1993 to December 1998), A.M. Breckenridge (later Sir Alasdair Breckenridge, January 1999 to March 2003) and G. Duff (April 2003 to the amalgamation of the Medicines Commission with the CSM and has chaired the amalgamated body to date).

17.5.3 Committee on the Review of Medicines and Committee on Dental and Surgical Materials

The proposed review of PLRs was already considered necessary by the UK but became a requirement when it joined the European Union. It was to correspond to the requirements under Directives 65/65/EEC and 75/318/EEC of the European Community that required that, throughout the Community, proprietary medicinal products granted licences before 22 November 1976 should be reviewed by 20 May 1990. All Member States of the European Community were similarly required to review the quality, safety and efficacy of products on their market.

Therefore, under the Act, the CRM was established in 1975 (SI 1975/1006), under the chairmanship of Professor E.F. Scowen with Professor O.L. Wade as the deputy chairman, to review all PLRs.

This Committee first met in October 1975. Initially, the review was organised in approximately 30 therapeutic categories such as analgesics, NSAIDs, psychotropics. The priority was antirheumatics first, followed by analgesics and psychotropics, the priority being determined by the fact that adverse reactions related to these drugs were reported frequently. Therefore, a number of subcommittees were established, such

as the Subcommittee on Anti-Rheumatic Agents, Subcommittee on Analgesics and Subcommittee on Psychotropic Agents. This approach proved slow and it was modified to a review of products of all companies, each company in two 5-yearly cycles. The Herbal Standards Subcommittee of the CSM also contributed to the review of PLRs.

In 1974, the Health Ministers consulted the UK Medicines Commission on a proposal to set up a committee under section 4 to advise the LA on applications for product licences for dental and other surgical materials.

The Committee on Dental and Surgical Materials (CDSM) was also established (SI 1975/1473) in 1975 under the chairmanship of Professor R.A. Cawson to advise on dental and ophthalmic products and surgical materials. It dealt with PLRs within its area of expertise and held its first meeting in October 1976.

These two main review Committees had their own dedicated professional secretariat with a remit to review the evidence of safety, quality and efficacy of all 39,035 PLRs. Of these, some 6000 PLRs related to homeopathic or blood products, vaccines, toxins, sera and radiopharmaceuticals that were excluded from review requirements because these were excluded from Directives EEC/65/65, 75/318 and 75/319 as they stood in 1976. Subsequently, however, the Extension Directive brought even these products within the scope of review.

The number of PLRs that were allowed to lapse by the manufacturers or were revoked or suspended in the UK in 1971–1982 was 22,376, and by 1988 this number had increased to 27,938. By 1982, the number of PLRs that were converted into full product licences was only 598. At the completion of the review in 1990, the number of applications received for full product licences was 6272 and of these just under 5300 were converted into full licences, most after changes had been agreed to the terms of the licences.[6] Of the 6272 applications, only 706 required referral to the CRM or CDSM for advice. The CRM was deemed to have completed its work in 1991 and was disestablished on 31 March 1992 (SI 1992/606) while similarly, the CDSM was disestablished on 31 December 1994 (SI 1994/15).

During their existence, the CRM and the CDSM had four chairmen each – Professors E.F. Scowen (October 1975 to December 1978), O.L. Wade (January 1979 to December 1984), W. Asscher (January 1985 to December 1986) and D.H. Lawson (January 1987 to March 1992) chairing the CRM, while Professors R.A.

Cawson (October 1976 to December 1979), R. Hurley (January 1980 to December 1981), C.L. Berry (later Sir Colin Berry, January 1982 to December 1992) and D. Poswillo (January 1993 to December 1994) chaired the CDSM.

17.5.4 Earlier controls on conduct of clinical trials in the UK

The Medicines Act 1968 included the definitions of a clinical trial and of a medicinal product. Clinical studies involving healthy volunteers did not meet this definition of a clinical trial and, as a result, did not come under the remit of regulatory controls. Such studies were subject to self-regulation by the pharmaceutical industry. Consequently, only the clinical trials in patients had to be covered by a clinical trial certificate (CTC). The LA did not lay down rigid requirements concerning the data that must be provided before authorisation could be given for a certificate for the clinical trial of a new drug. It did, however, issue guidelines for applicants.

In view of the regulatory delay that was caused by the need to apply for a CTC, a Statutory Order (SI 1974/498) was made during 1974, to provide an exemption from the need to hold a CTC in such cases, subject to certain conditions. This order applied to trials conducted by doctors and dentists on their own responsibility (DDX). The basis of the clinical trial exemption (CTX) scheme, introduced in 1981, to include studies initiated by the pharmaceutical industry, was that together with a detailed clinical trial protocol and summaries of chemical, pharmaceutical, pharmacological, pharmacokinetic, toxicological and human volunteer studies, a clinical trial in patients may proceed without the need for the additional details normally required for a CTC or product licence application. This exemption scheme was based on the requirements that:

• A doctor must certify the accuracy of the data;
• The applicant undertook to inform the LA of any refusal to permit the trial by an ethical committee; and
• The applicant also undertook to inform the LA of any data or reports concerning the safety of the product.

The LA had 35 days to respond to the notification to proceed with a clinical trial but could in exceptional circumstances require a further 28 days to consider the notification. If the CTX was refused, the applicant could apply for a CTC, in which case complete data had to be filed. If the CTC application was refused, the statutory appeal procedures came into play if the applicant company wished to avail itself of this provision.[7] These appeal procedures were identical with those applying to marketing applications. The CTX scheme proved highly successful in encouraging inward investment into research in the UK. In a sample of 42 companies, an increase in research investment of 10% or more was attributed to the scheme by 23 of them.[8,9] Its implementation was criticised by consumer groups and its effect was carefully monitored every 6 months to ensure that no added risk to patients had been introduced. This introduction of the CTX scheme is widely cited as an example of the benefits of deregulation. Australian drug regulatory authorities subsequently also introduced a similar scheme.

With a view to harmonising the conduct of clinical trials across the European Union, Directive 2001/20/EEC was finally agreed on 14 December 2000 and was formally adopted in May 2001 with a 3-year transition period for its implementation. The Directive is now fully implemented in the UK and further information on clinical trials there can be accessed at the MHRA website. Under the provisions of the Directive, all clinical trials now require a clinical trial authorisation (CTA). This is discussed in detail in Chapter 18.

17.5.5 CSM and monitoring adverse reactions

One of the most important aspects of the UK regulatory system is the scheme that provides for the voluntary reporting of adverse reactions to a marketed drug. Because most serious ADRs are rare events, they are unlikely to be detected in early clinical trials.

In order to stimulate a decreasing rate of reporting, the CSM in 1971 adopted a new version of the Yellow Card that was simple to complete but provided for more information to be included. The trial proved successful. In addition, to promote reporting of ADRs from general practitioners, the Subcommittee on Adverse Reactions convened a conference at the Royal College of General Practitioners in September 1973. In order to explore the ways of improving the dissemination of information about ADRs, a conference was also organised at the Royal College of Physicians in October 1975. Sustaining the efforts of the CSD, the CSM continued close cooperation with the WHO and with other regulatory authorities, in particular on matters relating to adverse reactions to medicinal products.

The first two safety letters from the CSM to the doctors were sent out in 1973. One in May dealt with a range of issues, including the reports of subacute myelo-optic neuropathy (SMON) in association with clioquinol (some 10,000 cases in Japan but in the UK none of SMON and only a few cases of reversible neurotoxicity following prolonged exposure) and vaginal adenocarcinoma in daughters of mothers who had taken stilboesterol during pregnancy (80 cases in the USA but none in the UK). The other dated 3 January 1974 reported on 130 cases (66 fatal) of halothane-induced jaundice, 94 of which were associated with repeated exposures to this anaesthetic.

Following reports of permanent brain damage in children who had received diptheria–pertussis–tetanus vaccine, these reports were collected by the Association of Parents of Vaccine Damaged Children (APVDC). These reports were examined by two committees set up by the Secretary of State for the purpose: the Advisory Panel on Serious Reactions to Vaccines and the Advisory Panel on the Collection of Data Relating to Adverse Reactions to Pertussis Vaccine.

The APVDC data consisted of information in documents of 555 children born between 1940 and 1975 who were thought to have sustained damage after receiving pertussis vaccine. These data were somewhat variable in scientific quality and ranged from accounts of incidents by parents, nurses or doctors which occurred soon after to a long time after the specific event. Further information was provided by Professor Gordon Stewart of Glasgow University.

The Advisory Panel on Serious Reactions to Vaccines examined only 50 case summaries selected on the basis that their documentation was reasonably good. The Advisory Panel on the Collection of Data Relating to Adverse reactions to Pertussis Vaccine examined the 50 cases above plus a total of 229 reports from the UK for the period 1970–1974. The most common neurological events from the 305 events reported for these 229 children were 115 cases of grand mal convulsion (38%), 47 infantile spasms (15%) and 25 cases of screaming (8%). This Panel eventually reported in 1981.

The need for two panels basically stemmed from the position taken by Sir Alistair Dudgeon, chairman of the Joint Committee on Vaccination and Immunisation (JCVI), who refused to believe in the ADR reports to Diptheria Tetanus Pertussis Vaccine (DTP) and had been appointed to chair the Advisory Panel on Serious Reactions to Vaccines.[10] The Secretary of State, David Ennals, later Lord Ennals, set up a vaccine damage compensation scheme.

During 1974, the Committee discussed the introduction of a special mark to identify recently introduced products. This resulted in the introduction in January 1976 of the Black Triangle scheme to identify drugs requiring intensive monitoring. This involves the product name to be followed immediately by an inverted black triangle (▼) as a superscript next to it in all product literature. Products requiring this symbol would include new drugs, established products having significantly new indications or new routes of administration and entirely novel combinations of potent medicinal substances. In 1977, the Committee also produced detailed guidelines for the improved post-marketing surveillance of drugs. Following consultations in 1978, final guidelines were agreed with the ABPI and BMA.

The controversy and disquiet following the suspension of the product licences for benoxaprofen in August 1982 (see below) led to a review of the efficiency of the Yellow Card scheme and to the establishment of a Working Party under the chairmanship of Professor David Grahame-Smith. The terms of reference of this Working Party were 'to consider how best the Committee on Safety of Medicines should fulfil its statutory functions of promoting the collection and investigation of information relating to adverse reactions, for the purpose of enabling it to give advice on safety, quality or efficacy of medicinal products; and to make recommendations'. The Working Party produced its first report in June 1983 and made 29 recommendations. The Grahame-Smith Working Party reconvened and its second report was published in January 1986 and made 13 recommendations. In general, these recommendations were only partially implemented.[11] One of the major points in the Grahame-Smith report was its emphasis on the large numbers of patients who need to be monitored to detect an ADR and the importance of an appreciation of the background incidence of that event in the population (Table 17.2). Proper monitoring could only be achieved with computerised record linkage schemes.

The Yellow Card scheme, at first restricted to receive reports from doctors, dentists and coroners, has been gradually expanded to receive reports from other sources. From October 1996, the scheme was extended to include reporting of suspected adverse reactions to unlicensed herbal remedies. In April 1997, the Yellow Card scheme was further extended to include hospital pharmacists as recognised reporters of suspected ADRs. In addition, there are specially targeted extensions of the scheme such as adverse reactions to HIV medicines and adverse reactions in children. The scheme has been gradually extended further to receive reports from community pharmacists

Table 17.2 Number of patients required to be monitored to show a given increase in incidence of an adverse event

Incidence (risk) of ADR	Spontaneous background incidence of adverse event	Minimum number of patients
1 in 100	0	360
	1 in 1000	730
	1 in 100	2000
1 in 500	0	1800
	1 in 1000	6700
	1 in 100	35,900
1 in 1000	0	3600
	1 in 1000	20,300
	1 in 100	136,400

ADR, adverse drug reaction.

and, in October 2002, from nurses, midwives and health visitors.

On 21 July 2003, the Parliamentary Under Secretary of State for Health (Lords), Lord Warner, announced an Independent Review of the Yellow Card scheme, under the chairmanship of Dr Jeremy Metters. Dr Metters convened a multidisciplinary Steering Committee and on 6 October 2003, undertook a 3-month public consultation on the potential implications of increasing access to Yellow Card data. The full report of the Independent Review is available at the MHRA website (http://medicines.mhra.gov.uk/ourwork/monitorsafequalmed/yellowcard/yellowcardreport.pdf). Among the 24 main recommendations contained in the report of the Steering Committee on access to the Yellow Card scheme was one to enable and encourage patients to directly report suspected ADRs to the MHRA. As a result, on 17 January 2005, a pilot scheme was initiated whereby patients too could report suspected ADRs. Thus, for the first time in the UK, the scheme was being opened to patients, parents and carers. The CSM/MHRA have set up a special Patient Reporting Working Group. Direct reporting of adverse drug reactions to national regulatory authorities has been possible in the USA and Germany since the mid-1980s.[12]

In compliance with data protection legislation and the General Medical Council (GMC) guidelines on confidentiality, the Yellow Card was updated in September 2000 to ask for an identification number for the patient (e.g. a practice or hospital number). The CSM no longer asked for personal patient identifiers on Yellow Cards; all that is now required is the patient's initials and age instead of their name and date of birth. The inclusion of the identification number enables the patient to be identifiable to the reporter but not to the CSM, thus allowing the reporter to know to whom the report refers for any potential future correspondence.

Apart from these changes necessary to keep pace with the changing times, the system has continued unchanged from when it was first set up, and the number of reports and fatal reactions each year of the scheme's operation to 2004 is shown in Table 17.3. By then, the CSM had received well over 450,000 reports since 1964. Despite relatively low reporting rates (a common feature of all spontaneous reporting systems worldwide), the UK Yellow Card scheme has enjoyed a remarkable success and international recognition and has been responsible for uncovering many important drug safety hazards.

Communication with the profession was at first maintained by continuing (until January 1985) the Adverse Reaction Series of leaflets started by CSD, and later by a regularly published bulletin on *Current Problems*. The first issue of *Current Problems* in September 1975 led with the adverse oculocutaneous effects and sclerosing peritonitis associated with β-adrenergic receptor blocking agents and also included items on loss of consciousness associated with prazosin and on the risks of anti-inflammatory agents and asthma.

Major drugs withdrawn between 1971 and 1982 for safety reasons included polidexide (introduced 1974, withdrawn 1975), oral formulation of practolol (introduced 1970, withdrawn 1976), alclofenac (introduced 1972, withdrawn 1979), tienilic acid (introduced 1979, withdrawn 1980), clomacron (introduced 1977, withdrawn 1982) and indoprofen (introduced 1982, withdrawn 1982).

Practolol illustrated not only the value of a spontaneous reporting system, but also the depth to which

Table 17.3 Annual number of total and fatal adverse drug reaction (ADR) reports to the Committee on Safety of Drugs (CSD) and Committee on Safety of Medicines (CSM)

Year	Total ADR reports	Total fatal reports	Fatal reports (% of total)
1964	1415	86	6.1
1965	3987	169	4.2
1966	2386	152	6.4
1967	3503	198	5.7
1968	3486	213	6.1
1969	4306	271	6.3
1970	3563	196	5.5
1971	2851	203	7.1
1972	3638	211	5.8
1973	3619	224	6.2
1974	4815	275	5.7
1975	5052	250	4.9
1976	6490	236	2.6
1977	11,255	352	3.1
1978	11,873	396	3.3
1979	10,881	286	2.6
1980	10,179	287	2.9
1981	13,032	303	2.3
1982	10,922	340	3.1
1983	12,689	409	3.2
1984	12,163	340	2.8
1985	12,652	348	2.8
1986	15,527	403	2.6
1987	16,431	390	2.4
1988	19,022	410	2.2
1989	19,246	475	2.5
1990	18,084	377	2.1
1991	20,272	541	2.7
1992	20,161	478	2.4
1993	18,078	480	2.7
1994	17,556	412	2.3
1995	17,748	467	2.6
1996	17,109	393	2.3
1997	16,637	455	2.7
1998	18,062	529	2.9
1999	18,505	560	3.0
2000	33,147	610	1.8
2001	21,467	650	3.0
2002	17,622	666	3.8
2003	19,257	737	3.8
2004	20,206	861	4.3
2005	21,831	NA	NA
2006	21,426	NA	NA
2007	21,464	NA	NA

the Committee would investigate a signal of a serious ADR. Practolol-induced eye damage first came to light as a result of a publication by an ophthalmologist. Prior to this, the Committee had received only one report over a period of nearly 3 years. Subsequent to the publication, more than 200 cases of eye damage were reported retrospectively. In January 1975, a warning leaflet in the Adverse Reaction Series was issued and the Committee continued to receive additional reports. Later that year, the manufacturer proposed restrictions in the use of practolol. Ultimately, the oral formulation was withdrawn from the market.

Benoxaprofen was launched in October 1980 in the UK for use as a NSAID, and was removed from the market in August 1982. It was known that the product was associated with photosensitivity reactions at the time the CSM considered the application for marketing approval. It was marketed by Eli Lilly under the name Opren. It was launched amidst massive publicity and its marketing was 'explosive'. However, reports of serious ADRs and associated fatalities began to appear in April and May 1982. Deaths were associated with hepatorenal failure (29 cases), liver damage alone (13 cases) or renal failure alone (11 cases). Liver biopsies showed intrahepatic cholestasis. It was noted that the fatal cases had received benoxaprofen for an average of 8.5 months and the non-fatal cases for an average of 6.9 months. The cases of hepatorenal syndrome were mostly in patients in their seventies and eighties.[13]

Experience with benoxaprofen and later with other drugs given to elderly patients was ultimately to result in a clinical guideline, adopted by the European Community's Committee for Proprietary Medicinal Products (CPMP) in September 1993, requiring the Investigation of Medicinal Products in Geriatrics, focusing on pharmacokinetics, pharmacodynamics and drug interactions as well as on the influence of renal or hepatic diseases on drug disposition. This also illustrates how guidelines frequently evolve with experience.

At the time the Yellow Card system celebrated its Silver Jubilee in 1989 at the Royal College of Physicians in London, the number of ADR reports in the CSM register was well in excess of 210,000. In relation to the size of the population, this represented a reporting rate in the UK that was among the highest in the world. The UK is a major contributor to the reports held by the WHO ADR Monitoring Centre in Uppsala, who have over three million reports in their database.[14] In 1991, the existing computer system was completely replaced by inauguration and introduction of ADROIT (Adverse Drug Reactions On-line Information Tracking), which was developed by the Medicines Control Agency (MCA). This system makes use of state-of-the-art information technology and highly interrelational databases including a medical dictionary designed by the agency staff. All major regulatory authorities now use this dictionary, MedDRA, for the purposes of monitoring and communicating information on ADRs. Data held on the previous system were transferred to ADROIT, which

allowed assessors to set up complex enquiries of the database and respond rapidly to emerging safety issues.

On 4 May 2004, the CSM/MHRA celebrated fortieth anniversary of the Yellow Card scheme.

However, the post-marketing surveillance systems in the UK failed to impress the House of Commons Health Select Committee who recorded in their Report published in March 2005 'PMS in the UK is inadequate' (see para 312 and the criticisms in paras 296–305 and the Summary) (see below).

17.6 Manufacturers' licences and Good Manufacturing Practice

Manufacturers' licences were issued by the UK Licensing Authority from the inception of the Medicines Act to cover all manufacturing operations, including those previously covered by the Therapeutic Substances Act. The Medicines Inspectorate laid down standards in its *Guide to Good Manufacturing Practice*, popularly known as the Orange Guide. The Orange Guide has been published in several editions since it was first published in the 1970s, the most recent edition appeared in 2008. Although the issue of manufactures' licences remains a national regulatory function, it is governed by the standards set in EC Commission Directive 91/356EEC which can be summarised as follows.

The Directive lays down the principles and guidelines of Good Manufacturing Practice (GMP) to be followed in the production of medicines, and requirements to ensure that manufacturers and member states adhere to it provisions. Manufacturers must ensure that production occurs in accordance with GMP and the manufacturing authorization. Imports from non-EU countries must have been produced to standards at least equivalent to those in the EU, and the importer must ensure this. All manufacturing processes should be consistent with information provided in the MA application, as approved by the regulatory authorities. Methods shall be updated in the light of scientific advances, and modifications must be submitted for approval.

17.6.1 Principles and practice of GMP

• *Quality management* – implementation of quality insurance systems.

• *Personnel* – appropriately qualified, with specified duties, responsibilities and management structures.

• *Premises and equipment* – appropriate to intended operations.

- *Documentation.*
- *Production* – according to pre-established operating procedures with appropriate in-process controls, regularly validated.
- *Quality control* – independent department or external laboratory responsible for all aspects of quality control. Samples of each batch must be retained for 1 year, unless not practicable.
- *Work contracted out* – subject to contract, and under the same conditions, without subcontracting.
- *Complaints and product recall* – record keeping and arrangements for notification of the competent authority.
- *Self-inspection* – by manufacturer of their own processes with appropriate record keeping.
- Good manufacturing standards are enforced by the Medicines Inspectorate of the MHRA. The UK has been involved in the Pharmaceutical Inspection Convention since its inception and, through the Orange Guide, set standards which are now reflected in the EU Directives.

17.7 Wholesale dealers' licences

This activity, established in the UK under the Medicines Act 1968, still remains wholly within the remit of the individual national EU regulatory authorities but in accordance with Directive 92/25EEC on the wholesale distribution of medicinal products for human use (Official Journal L113/1-4 30 April 1992).

17.8 General safety measures

The Commission and the CSM also made recommendations on the introduction of many other broad safety measures. These included the phenacetin prohibition order (SI 1974/1082), presentation of medicines in relation to child safety (SI 1975/2000) and declaration of alcohol in medicinal products on their package as active ingredient where this is likely to be pharmacologically active. Other labelling issues culminated in an order (SI 1976/1726) that set out the standard particulars that must be shown on the containers and packaging of medicinal products. Consultations on other generally applicable warnings on the labels of certain medicines to protect children and to ensure that more general advice and information is provided resulted in SI 1977/996.

In the USA, the FDA had first required patient information leaflets in 1970. Following consultations

with the Pharmaceutical Society, the ABPI, BMA, Health Council and other bodies, regulations on leaflets (SI 1977/1055) were introduced to make sure that the public had greater information on the medicines they were prescribed.

Concerns on promotion of drugs were beginning to emerge and regulations were introduced under section 95 of the Act to control advertising to practitioners (SI 1975/298 and 1326). The former dealt with the advertising of products covered by PLRs while the latter dealt with specifying the information that must appear in all advertisement, including succinct statements on contraindications, warnings and adverse effects relevant to the indications. In addition, the generic name and the NHS cost were also required to appear. Further regulations (SI 1978/41) were also introduced on 1 February 1978 in respect of advertising direct to the public. Part of this made it an offence to advertise any product for certain serious diseases.

In 1975, the Medicines Division set up the Advertising Action Group to monitor advertising. The group included doctors, pharmacists, lawyers and administrators. In 1977, agreement was also reached with the ABPI for voluntary control and monitoring of advertisements by the industry and the ABPI instituted a Code of Practice and a Committee to supervise its implementation. Although a number of small companies had been prosecuted by the LA for breaching the regulations on advertising, these cases attracted little attention or interest within the industry at large. However, in 1984, monitoring of advertisements reached its climax with the successful prosecution of a major pharmaceutical company in respect of its advertisement for its drug Surgam (tiaprofenic acid).[15] The outcome of this prosecution has greatly influenced the behaviour of the industry and strengthened the case for the professional independence and responsibilities of physicians working in the industry.

17.9 Scrutiny of functioning of the Medicines Division and the establishment of the Medicines Control Agency

The Review of Medicines produced an increasing workload on the Medicines Division, and the increase in resources were minimal and not commensurate with the increased demands. Resources were diverted from licensing of new drugs towards the review driven with EU time limits. This can be illustrated by the time taken to process a product licence for a new chemical entity (NCE). In 1971 the mean time was 8.4 months, by 1977 this had risen to 12.1 months, by 1979 to 16.8 months, by 1981 it was 15 months and in 1984 it was 23.0 months.

A similar situation affected the processing times for abridged applications. In 1982 an investigation by Sir Derek Rayner (later Lord Rayner) suggested that abridged applications should be dealt with within 2 months. At this time the Medicines Division received some 6000 applications for NCEs, abridged applications, variations to existing licences and included 2500 product licence applications for parallel importations (PLPI). This meant that if all the professional staff were directed to this they would have to process two applications per head per day in addition to dealing with CTCs and CTXs, adverse reaction reports and the review,[11] an impossible recommendation and clearly indicated the extent to which Medicines Division was under-resourced.

In the period 1985–1987, the pharmaceutical industry expressed concerns about the manner in which the UK Regulatory Authority conducted it business. The Secretary of State for Social Services set up an inquiry to be conducted by Dr J.B. Evans, a previous Deputy Chief Medical Officer in the DHSS, and Mr P.W. Cunliffe, chairman of the Pharmaceutical Division of ICI. In its evidence to the inquiry the ABPI wrote as follows:

The pharmaceutical industry would not dispute the need for, or the value of an effective national medicines regulatory authority. The interests of the medicines-consuming public and the innovative pharmaceutical industry are best safeguarded by the presence of an independent, professionally administered control over the process by which new medicines enter or are withdrawn from the therapeutic armamentarium.

However, the manner in which regulatory bodies conduct their business and the way in which their internal resources are allocated between the various activities they are required to perform, is seriously in question. Industry is not satisfied with delays inherent in present licensing procedures, whereby new products enter the market place and the licences of existing products are maintained.

The number of applications for product licences from 1981–1985 inclusive were 1043, 1282, 1158, 922, and 1365 respectively, of which the over-whelming majority, about 98%, were for abridged applications. The diversion of resources to the Review Process and parallel importing problem has increased the time taken to grant

a product licence for a major application for an NCE to some 2 years. This represents a marked increase over the years prior to 1984. The situation is worse for abridged applications.

The UK Licensing Authority were in Breach of Directives 65/65EEC and 75/319EEC regarding the time limits laid down for processing product licence applications. These EC Directives specify a period of 120 days to process an application, unless it is referred to an advisory committee by the licensing authority when a further 90 days is permitted; that is a total of 210 days. In a reply in the House of Lords (Hansard 20 May 1986) the DHSS admitted that of 565 applications issued with a product licence in 1985, 46% had taken longer than these stipulated time limits to process.

The ABPI also noted: 'Over the past 2 years the Licensing Authority has received well over 2500 applications for pharmaceutical product licences (parallel importing (PL/PI)). This considerably increased workload has been met without additional resources and has resulted in a diversion of Licensing Authority Resources.'

The ABPI submission was accompanied by 29 recommendations for management reform of the Medicines Division. In December 1987, the Evans–Cunliffe report made a total of 54 recommendations for improvement of the management and efficiency of the Medicines Division. In 1988, the DHSS was split into two departments: the Department of Health (DoH) and the Department of Social Security (DSS). Following the Evans–Cunliffe report, the Medicines Division of the DoH was reorganised in April 1989 to become the Medicines Control Agency (MCA) with Dr Keith Jones appointed as the first Director. A Joint Consultative Group to review management processes of handling of the applications (but no decisions relative to quality, safety and efficacy) was set up between the DoH and the pharmaceutical industry. The MCA was expected to be self-funding from fees commensurate with the services provided. In July 1991, the MCA became an Executive Agency of the DoH under the government's 'Next Steps' initiative. Dr Jones therefore became the Chief Executive and was thereafter accountable directly to the Secretary of State for Health.

In general, the servicing of industry needs had undoubtedly improved but at a significantly increased cost to the industry in terms of fees. The requirement for the MCA (and later the MHRA) to be self-funding and compete for fee income would become a matter of concern for the House of Commons Health Select Committee (see below).

The MCA was the competent national authority responsible for human medicinal products in the UK and continued to discharge the functions of its predecessor, the Medicines Division, in implementing the Medicines Act and all European legislation. As at January 2001, the total staff had increased to 530 of whom 153 were working in the licensing division and 152 in the post-licensing division. These 530 included 49 medical, 53 pharmaceutical and 85 preclinical or scientific staff.

The MCA continued to thrive and have a key role in Europe and also in all the regulatory and scientific activities of the European Committee for Proprietary Medicinal Products (see section 17.9) and all its Working Parties. Dr Susan Wood represented the UK at CPMP and until her death in 1998 was the first chairperson of its Pharmacovigilance Working Party. Dr P.C. Waller succeeded her as the UK representative at CPMP and also chaired this important working party. Mr A.C. Cartwright, from the UK, chaired the Quality Working Party. Over the period, the UK has remained among the leading regulatory authorities in the European Union in terms of rapporteurship for the applications going through the Centralised Procedure, acting as a Reference Member State for the applications intended to go through the Mutual Recognition Procedure and as a coordinator of scientific advice from the CPMP.

At a European level, the UK has continued to contribute extensively to the many subsequent EU Directives and Regulations that control drugs in the European Union. All these, once adopted, have been incorporated into UK national legislation. In the UK, for example, Council Directive 92/27/EEC of 31 March 1992 regulated labelling and leaflets while Council Directive 92/28/EEC of 31 March 1992 regulated advertising of medicinal products for human use.

17.10 Medicines and Healthcare products Regulatory Agency

The formal regulation of medical devices in the European Union began in the mid-1990s. Prior to that, the Scientific and Technical Branch (STB; established in the late 1960s) of the DHSS had been set up to improve the quality and safety of medical equipment. During the the 1980s the STB became part of the NHS Procurement Directorate, which was later split into the NHS Supplies Authority and the Medical Devices Directorate (MDD). The MDD in effect became the Medical Devices Agency (MDA) in 1994.

On the 12 September 2002, the Health Minister, Lord Philip Hunt, announced that the MCA and the MDA would merge with effect from 1 April 2003. The merged agency was to be known as the Medicines and Healthcare products Regulatory Agency (MHRA).

Effective from 1 January 2004, Professor Kent Woods, Professor of Therapeutics at the University of Leicester, was appointed Chief Executive of the MHRA.

Having been established under section 4 of the Medicines Act, 1968, the CSM advises on the safety, efficacy and quality of medicines for human use and to promote the collection and investigation of information relating to ADRs. Applications for national marketing authorisations cannot be refused by the LA on grounds of safety, efficacy or quality unless first referred to the CSM. Similarly, proposals to revoke or suspend a national authorisation on those grounds, or to refuse certain applications to vary a marketing authorisation, must be referred to the CSM. As a matter of practice, all applications for national authorisations for medicines containing new chemical entities are also referred to CSM. It is also the 'appropriate committee' that must be consulted on proposals to make regulations and orders under Part III of the Medicines Act 1968, which relates to the sale and supply of medicines. For example, the CSM is consulted on amendments to the POM (Human Use) Order 1997 when changes are required in relation to matters such as nurse prescribing, and on prohibition orders under section 62 of the Act. In addition, the views of the CSM are sought by the MHRA on those centralised applications to the European Medicines Agency (EMEA) where the UK is rapporteur or co-rapporteur, and also on applications received under the mutual recognition procedure where a marketing authorisation is sought in the UK. The CSM's views are also sought on matters relating to the safety of marketed medicines. To fulfil these roles, the CSM has created three subcommittees: the Chemistry, Pharmacy and Standards Subcommittee (CPS); the Biologicals Subcommittee; and the Subcommittee on Pharmacovigilance (SCOP), all of which report to the main Committee. In addition, the CSM creates working parties to deal with specific regulatory issues, usually relating to safety, and where it considers that it requires advice that is not available from within its membership. The CSM currently has 34 members and meets twice monthly, most members attending one meeting per month. Members are appointed for 3-year terms. The MHRA is planning amalgamation of the functions of the MC and CSM. The MHRA issued a Consultation Letter (MLX No 300) in February 2004 seeking wider views on the proposed amalgamation of CSM and MC.

In summary, from autumn 2005, the new advisory structure comprised:

1. A new Commission on Human Medicines (CHM) that amalgamates the responsibilities of the present MC and the CSM, which will advise Ministers directly on matters relating to medicines for human use.

2. A number of other committees established by Ministers, which will be able to advise Ministers directly on issues for which they are responsible. These are:

• The Advisory Board on the Registration of Homeopathic Products (ABRH);

• A new Herbal Medicines Advisory Committee (HMAC); and

• The British Pharmacopoeia Commission (BPC).

3. A number of Expert Advisory Groups (EAGs) that will advise the Commission, ABRH, HMAC and BPC on certain specific and technical matters.

4. A panel of experts (including toxicology and statistics) to provide specialist advice to the above bodies and EAGs if required.

5. A panel that brings together the lay (patient and consumer) representatives on the various bodies and EAGs.

17.10.1 House of Commons Health Select Committee Report March 2005

This very detailed report should be compulsory reading for all pharmaceutical physicians. The Select Committee was chaired by Mr David Hinchcliffe (MP for Wakefield) and had a total of 10 other MPs serving on the Committee.

The MHRA was the subject of serious criticism in this Select Committee Report entitled 'The Influence of the Pharmaceutical Industry'. In its 4-page summary the Select Committee state: 'this is the first major select Committee Inquiry into the pharmaceutical industry for almost one hundred years – the last was undertaken by the Select Committee on Patent Medicine which reported in August 1914'.

In this general summary the following criticisms were levelled at the MHRA:

The regulator, the Medicines and Health Care Products Agency (MHRA), has failed to adequately scrutinise licensing data and its post-marketing surveillance is inadequate.

The consequence of lax oversight is that the industry's influence has expanded and a number of practices have developed which act against the public interest.

We are concerned that a rather lax regime is exacerbated by the MHRA's need to compete with other European regulators for licence application business.

In Para 280 the report states: 'In its own interests the Agency (MHRA) need to keep a close eye on its market share of regulatory business, increasingly it competes with other European drug regulatory agencies to scrutinise drug licence applications.' More detailed criticism of the MHRA appears in the main body of this 126-page report.

17.10.1.1 Staff levels

The MHRA was stated to employ about 750 staff.

17.10.1.2 Fees

The annual income of the MHRA is stated in paragraph 98 to be £65 million. 'The MHRA's activities are 60% funded through licensing fees paid by those seeking marketing approvals and 40% through an annual service fee, also paid by the industry most of the income generated from the service fee is allocated to post-marketing surveillance and inspection as opposed to premarketing scrutiny of drug licence applications.' Paragraph 375 states: 'The MHRA, like many regulatory organisations, is entirely funded by fees from those it regulates . . . This situation has led to concerns that it might loose sight of the need to protect and promote public health above all else as it seeks to win fee income from companies.'

17.10.1.3 Scrutiny of data

Failure to scrutinise raw data in applications and undue reliance on expert summaries provided by the companies making the applications was a major source of criticism and is referred to in paragraphs 101, 283, 284, 342, 345, 346 and boxed tables 5 (page 87) and 7 (page 96). In paragraph 284 the Committee report, 'The evidence is that the MHRA examined (raw) primary data on drug effects only if it suspected some misrepresentation in the summary data supplied. It was argued that such trust in regulated companies goes too far: reliance on company summaries is neither sufficient nor appropriate.'

Griffin[16] goes further when he states, 'Regulatory approval of an application for marketing approval of a new medicine is a paper exercise based on the acceptance of the integrity of the data submitted and trust in the peer review system and those who operate it.' If the peer review does not involve the examination of raw data the system is merely an act of faith.

17.10.1.4 Post-marketing surveillance

Post-marketing surveillance was singled out for particularly harsh criticism in paragraphs 296–305. In paragraph 312 and paragraph 13 of the Summary it is stated: 'PMS in the UK is inadequate', giving as examples the drug-related adverse events related to the selective serotonin reuptake inhibitors and COX-2 inhibitors. The Select Committee is damning in its reference to 'regulatory inertia' in this context.

17.10.1.5 Good Clinical Practice inspection records

The Parliamentary Health Select Committee also referred to the ICH recommendations preventing the MHRA having routine access to Good Clinical Practice (GCP) reports in paragraphs 279 and 364. The Select Committee noted: 'surprisingly, the MHRA expressed no concerns about this issue'. In paragraph 364 the Committee stated: 'We are concerned that the MHRA is not permitted to routinely inspect audit reports for compliance with standards of Good Clinical Practice (GCP).'

17.10.1.6 General criticism

The Select Committee in paragraph 376 states: 'During this long enquiry we became aware of serious weaknesses in the MHRA. Worryingly in both its written and oral evidence the Agency seemed oblivious to the critical views of outsiders and unable to accept that it had any obvious shortcomings.'

While the Rayner Inquiry and the Evans–Cunliffe report raised issues of both level and allocation of resources by management to various tasks as well as funding issues, the Health Select Committee raised more fundamental issues of competence and diligence, with which the MHRA applied itself to its roles.

17.10.2 Commission on Human Medicines

The Commission on Human Medicines (CHM) was to be a newly appointed body rather than an amalgamation of the current bodies. Its membership would be subject to a full appointments exercise, with a view to appointing the chairman and members. On 27 July 2005, Professor Gordon Duff, previously the chairman of the last CSM, was appointed the first chairman of CHM, for a term of 4 years effective from 30 October 2005.

17.10.2.1 Functions of the new commission

The new commission took on the functions currently performed by the MC and the CSM in relation to medicines for human use. In particular the responsiblity for:

1. Advising Ministers and the Agency on policy matters relating to the regulation of medicinal products;
2. Advising on the safety, quality or efficacy of medicinal products (e.g. advising the Agency on those licensing applications that are currently considered by the CSM);
3. Promoting the collection and investigation of information relating to adverse reactions;
4. Advising on the establishment and membership of committees established under section 4 of the Medicines Act 1968. For example, the BPC and VPC would be retained.

17.10.2.2 Subcommittees and expert advisory groups

To facilitate the fullest participation in the new EU regulatory environment it is proposed that, in addition to the new commission, provision would be made for the establishment of EAGs in defined therapeutic areas. CHM or relevant section 4 Committee will make the appointments to the EAGs, expert panels and list of experts. These EAGs advise them on scientific issues which apply across therapeutic areas, or which relate to relatively self-contained substance types. The EAGs are expert groups set up to advise and make recommendations to the new CHM on specific issues, and they would not themselves have decision-making powers.

There is likely to be a continuing need for some subcommittees of the new commission, such as those which had previously served the CSM. Although their remit would not change under the new arrangements, it is proposed that these too should become known in the future as EAGs.

17.10.3 How the Commission and EAGs operate

The CHM and the EAGs operate under the following arrangements:

1. The CHM would comprises approximately 10–12 core members, appointed by Ministers. Rather than restricting membership within the areas currently specified in the Medicines Act for the MC, the CHM would need members with high level scientific expertise and an ability in critical appraisal, a capacity to contribute beyond individual speciality and, where possible, experience in the NHS clinical practice and the regulatory field.
2. A number of EAGs have been created by the new Commission, with members selected and appointed by them and comprising national experts.
3. Recommendations from EAGs to the new Commission would be in the form of either a paper or a

personal presentation by the EAG chairman who would attend as an invited member.

4. The majority of EAGs will exist as standing committees, each with certain members 'on retention'. Permanent members would include the chairman, and one or two permanent experts. MHRA would supply the secretariat and MHRA designated assessors may need to attend. Other experts would be invited for specific topics. Referrals from and between the various committees and groups are arranged as necessary.

5. It will be an important task of the secretariat both to manage the logistics of EAG membership and to ensure that appropriate issues are referred to EAGs for their timely consideration.

6. The Commission meets once monthly.

7. EAGs meet as required depending on the nature of the advice required by the Commission.

Initially, there will be EAGs in the following therapeutic areas and disciplines:

- Pharmacovigilance;
- Biologicals and vaccines (including clinical issues for vaccines);
- Pharmacy and Standards (including pharmacokinetics).

The chairs of the above three EAGs will also be full members of the CHM. In addition, there are likely to be EAGs for:

- Paediatrics;
- Cardiology, diabetes, renal;
- Respiratory and allergy;
- Oncology and haematology;
- Endocrine, obstetrics and gynaecology and bone metabolism;
- Gastrointestinal and hepatology;
- Anti-infectives and HIV/AIDS;
- Neurology and pain management;
- Psychiatry and psychiatry in the elderly;
- Rheumatology, immunology;
- Patient information; and
- Dermatology.

17.10.4 Other expert advice

For other areas where advice is less frequently required there will be panels of experts who may supplement the EAGs or be called upon by the CHM as experts for the day.

Under the proposed new arrangements, if a marketing authorisation for a product (or a certificate of registration) was refused by the licensing authority, after a hearing before the CHM, the applicant would still be able to appeal to a 'person appointed' as provided for in the legislation. In particular, there would

be scope for involving EAGs in clarification meetings to maximise predictability of outcome for companies and to resolve issues without the necessity of involving formal statutory appeals procedures.

In view of the increasing profile and use of herbal medicines, the European Union has established a Committee for Herbal Medicinal Products (see Chapter 18). The MHRA consulted and has also established a Herbal Medicines Advisory Committee (HMAC). This Committee would advise Ministers directly on areas for which the Committee is responsible. The remit of HMAC would be the registration scheme to be introduced under the Directive 2004/24/EC on Traditional Herbal Medicinal Products and unlicensed herbal medicines. However, CHM will be responsible for advice in relation to marketing authorisations for herbal medicines. Professor Philip Routledge was appointed the first chairman of HMAC, for a term of 4 years effective from 30 October 2005.

17.11 European dimensions

The UK joined the European Community in January 1973 but the data requirements for granting marketing authorisations have, since the implementation of the Medicines Act 1968, been in accordance with European Community Directive 65/65/EEC and the subsequent Directive 75/318 as amended, which elaborated on the requirements for preclinical testing, pharmaceutical quality and manufacture. It was vital that during 1973, following the entry of UK into the Community, the CSM also had the opportunity to consider and comment extensively on the two draft Directives (later to become 75/318/EEC and 75/319/EEC). Directive 75/318/EEC introduced the common dossier that harmonised the standards and requirements across the European Union while Directive 75/319/EEC established the CPMP, introduced the Mutual Recognition Procedure and brought in the requirements for expert reports.

The European Union's advisory committee, the CPMP, was set up in 1975 under Directive 75/319. The first meeting was held on 26 November 1976 and Mr Leon Robert from Luxembourg was appointed its first chairman. The Professional Head of the then UK Medicines Division, Dr E.L. Harris, who was also the UK Representative to CPMP, was elected a deputy chairman. Dr J.P. Griffin, initially his alternate but later the UK representative during 1977–1984, was appointed chairman of the CPMP Working Party on Safety. Dr N.M.G. Dukes from the Dutch regulatory authority was appointed chairman of the Efficacy Working Party at the same time. Dr Dukes was later succeeded by Professor J.M. Alexandre (from the French regulatory authority) who then proceeded to become the chairman of the CPMP (1995–2000).

The proposed review of PLR in the UK, already considered necessary, was to correspond to the requirements under European Directives. These Directives required that throughout the Community proprietary medicinal products granted licences before 22 November 1976 should be reviewed by 20 May 1990. Indeed, the UK was among the first to complete this review on time. This review eliminated from the market all medicinal products that were released for clinical use previously without scrutiny and that were ineffective, unsafe or that had an unacceptable risk–benefit ratio.

Much later, Directive 83/570 required the applicants to produce a draft Summary of Product Characteristics (SPC) as an integral part of the documentation. In September 1995, an order was made (SI 1995/2321) to the effect that, in the UK, data sheets were no longer required where a product had an approved SPC and also that data sheets no longer had to be sent to all doctors and dentists prior to advertising.

In the UK, healthy volunteer studies were subject to self-regulation by the pharmaceutical industry and consequently only the clinical trials in patients had to be covered by a CTC. However, clinical trials in the UK are now regulated under EU Clinical Trials Directive (2001/20/EEC) fully implemented in the UK.

The EU Clinical Trials Directive contains specific provisions regarding the conduct of clinical trials, including multicentre trials, on human subjects. It defines 'clinical trial' as any investigation in human subjects intended to discover or verify the clinical, pharmacological and/or other pharmacodynamic effects of one or more investigational medicinal product(s), and/or to identify any adverse reactions to one or more investigational medicinal product(s) and/or to study absorption, distribution, metabolism and excretion of one or more investigational medicinal product(s) with the object of ascertaining its (their) safety and/or efficacy and defines 'subject' as an individual who participates in a clinical trial as either a recipient of the investigational medicinal product or a control. Thus, healthy volunteer studies are included.

Further stringent requirements have evolved over time in respect of investigations to be carried out during the clinical development of drugs, the data required before they are approved for marketing, and subsequently the requirements for safety monitoring during the post-marketing period (pharmacovigilance).

The raft of rules, regulations, guidelines and procedures (both the European Union and ICH) governing the human medicinal products in the European Union can be found in the following five volumes published by the European Commission:
- Volume 1 – Pharmaceutical Legislation.
- Volume 2 – Notice to Applicants:
2A: Procedures for Marketing Authorisation;
2B: Presentation and Content of the Dossier;
2C: Regulatory Guidelines.
- Volume 3 – Guidelines:
3A: Quality and Biotechnology;
3B: Safety, Environment, and Information;
3C: Efficacy.
- Volume 4 – Good Manufacturing Practice.
- Volume 9 – Pharmacovigilance.
(Volumes 5–8 relate to veterinary medicinal products.)

Many of the Directives originally adopted have been frequently amended over the period. In the interests of clarity and rationality, a whole range of the latest versions of these Directives was codified by assembling them in a single text, Directive 2001/83/EC of 6 November 2001. Therefore, the reader should also cross-refer to this Directive, which codifies the following:

1. Council Directive 65/65/EEC of 26 January 1965, on the approximation of provisions laid down by law, regulation or administrative action relating to medicinal products.
2. Council Directive 75/318/EEC of 20 May 1975, on the approximation of the laws of Member States relating to analytical, pharmacotoxicological and clinical standards and protocols in respect of the testing of proprietary medicinal products.
3. Council Directive 75/319/EEC of 20 May 1975 on the approximation of provisions laid down by law, regulation or administrative action relating to proprietary medicinal products.
4. Council Directive 89/342/EEC of 3 May 1989 on immunologicals (vaccines, toxins or serums and allergens).
5. Council Directive 89/343/EEC of 3 May 1989 on radiopharmaceuticals.
6. Council Directive 89/381/EEC of 14 June 1989 on products derived from human blood or human plasma.
7. Council Directive 92/25/EEC of 31 March 1992 on wholesale distribution.
8. Council Directive 92/26/EEC of 31 March 1992 on classification for supply.
9. Council Directive 92/27/EEC of 31 March 1992 on labelling and package leaflets.

10. Council Directive 92/28/EEC of 31 March 1992 on advertising.

11. Council Directive 92/73/EEC of 22 September 1992 on homeopathic medicinal products.

Directive 2001/83/EC was subsequently amended by:

1. Directive 2002/98/EC of 27 January 2003, setting standards of quality and safety for the collection, testing, processing, storage and distribution of human blood and blood components;

2. Commission Directive 2003/63/EC of 25 June 2003, replacing Annex 1 of Directive 2001/83/EC (detailing scientific and technical requirements) with a new Annex (detailing scientific and technical requirements in CTD terms); and

3. Directive 2004/24/EC of 31 March 2004 as regards traditional herbal medicinal products.

Regarding all activities for the regulation of pharmaceuticals at the European Union level, Article 71 of Regulation EEC/2309/93 required that, 'Within 6 years of the entry into force of this Regulation, the Commission shall publish a general report on the experience of the procedures laid down in this Regulation, in Chapter III of Directive 75/319/EEC and in Chapter IV of Directive 81/851/EEC.' The tender for review was awarded to a consortium of Cameron McKenna and Arthur Anderson. The full report from Cameron McKenna, entitled 'Evaluation of the Operation of Community Procedures for the Authorisation of Medicinal Products', is a comprehensive and highly constructive document.

Following extensive discussions among all interested parties, such as the national authorities, the EC and the European Federation of Pharmaceutical Industries and Associations (EFPIA), the EC proposed comprehensive reform of the EU pharmaceutical legislation. The amending legislations are:

1. Directive 2004/27/EC of the European Parliament and of the Council of 31 March 2004, amending Directive 2001/83/EC, on the Community code relating to medicinal products for human use; and

2. Regulation (EC) No 726/2004 of the European Parliament and of the Council of 31 March 2004, laying down Community procedures for the authorisation and supervision of medicinal products for human and veterinary use and establishing a European Medicines Agency – thus replacing Regulation EEC/2309/93.

The adoption this reformed legislation just preceded the enlargement of the European Union on 1 May 2004 when the EU membership was increased from 15 to 25 Member States by the accession of 10 new Member States: Cyprus, Czech Republic, Estonia, Hungary, Latvia, Lithuania, Malta, Poland, Slovak Republic and Slovenia. Directive 2004/27/EC must come into force in all Member States by 30 October 2005, although Member States are able to implement early any of the provisions should they wish. Regulation 726/2004 has a transposition date of 20 November 2005, from which date its provisions will apply in all Member States.

Article 5 of Regulation (EC) No 726/2004 created a Committee for Medicinal Products for Human Use (CHMP) which shall be responsible for drawing up the opinion of the Agency on any matter concerning the admissibility of the files submitted in accordance with the centralised procedure, the granting, variation, suspension or revocation of an authorisation to place a medicinal product for human use on the market and pharmacovigilance. The CPMP therefore became the CHMP and consists of one member (with an alternate) appointed by each of the EU Member States, after consultation with the management board, for a term of 3 years, which may be renewed, and a chairperson. The Committee also includes one member appointed by each of the European Economic Area–European Free Trade Area (EEA-EFTA) States, for a term of 3 years, which may be renewed.

The Committee, in order to complement its expertise, has appointed five co-opted members chosen on the basis of their specific scientific competence, from among the experts nominated by Members States or the Agency. Co-opted members are appointed for the term of the committee, which may be renewed, and do not have alternates. The chairman of CPMP, Dr Daniel Brasseur was elected chairman of the CHMP during its inaugural meeting on 1–3 June 2004.

Article 55 of Regulation (EC) No 726/2004 created the European Medicines Agency, comprising of a Management Board, an Executive Director, a Secretariat, the CHMP, the Committee for Medicinal Products for Veterinary Use (CVMP), the Committee on Orphan Medicinal Products (COMP) and the Committee on Herbal Medicinal Products (CHMP). Thus, the former European Medicines Evaluation Agency (EMEA) became the European Medicines Agency. However, for technical reasons, it had to retain the acronym EMEA (the acronym EMA belongs to European Medical Association).

17.12 International dimensions

In June 1984, the Commission decided that a meeting with the Japanese authorities, attended by Mr

F. Sauer and the chairman and vice-chairman of the Safety Working Party, Dr J.P. Griffin and Professor R. Bass, respectively, and the chairman of the Efficacy Working Party, Professor J.M. Alexandre, should take place in Tokyo. The efforts following this initial meeting were ultimately to culminate in the ICH.

The main players at ICH are now the European Commission/EMEA, EFPIA, Japanese Ministry of Health Labour and Welfare (MHLW), Japanese Pharmaceutical Manufacturers Association (JPMA), US FDA and Pharmaceutical Research and Manufacturers of America (PhRMA). The WHO, Canadian Health Protection Branch and the EFTA countries enjoy an observer status at ICH meetings.

The ICH Steering Committee establishes expert working groups to discuss areas where harmonisation is possible and to produce universally acceptable guidelines. Thus, under the auspices of the ICH, a large number of guidelines have been issued in the areas of quality, safety and efficacy, with the objective of achieving harmonisation of requirements for registration between regulatory authorities and thereby reducing the need to duplicate studies. It must be made clear that these documents are guidelines and not requirements.

These guidelines may not be at the cutting edge of science but they represent acceptable compromises based on sound science. As of January 2004, there were at least 13 safety, 17 efficacy (clinical safety is included in these), 19 quality and 8 multidisciplinary guidelines accepted since the first meeting of ICH in Brussels in November 1991. Once adopted by the CPMP and published, the guidelines resulting from the ICH process are locally implemented and applied as EU Community guidelines.

Regarding pharmacovigilance, the cornerstone of post-marketing safety of drugs, there are a number of ICH/CPMP guidelines and a joint Pharmacovigilance Plan (CPMP/PhVWP/2058/99 Revision 1) for the implementation of the ICH guidelines E2B, M1 and M2. Two major advances were the acceptance of MedDRA (ICH topic M1) as a common medical dictionary for regulatory work and the acceptance of Periodic Safety Update Reports for marketed drugs (PSUR) (ICH topic E2C). The ICH pharmacovigilance guidelines adopted by the CPMP include ICH/135/95 [Good Clinical Practice, (E6)], ICH/285/95 [Guidance on Recommendations on Electronic Transmission of Individual Case Safety Reports Message Specification (M2)], ICH/287/95 [Guidance on Clinical Safety Data Management: Data Elements for Transmission of Individual Case Safety Reports (E2B)], ICH/288/95 [Guidance on Clinical Safety Data Management: Periodic Safety Update Reports for Marketed Drugs (E2C)], and ICH/377/95 [Clinical Safety Data Management: Definitions and Standards for Expedited Reporting (E2A)].

If harmonisation can be achieved across a broad range of areas in quality, safety and efficacy, there seems no logical reason why a Common Technical Document (CTD) or dossier could not be prepared that would be acceptable to all drug regulatory authorities. At the ICH meeting in November 2000 in San Diego (USA), an agreement was reached on a CTD that represented a common format for the submission of dossiers to the USA, the European Union and Japan. Effective from July 2003, the format of the EU dossier must conform to the CTD format. CTD is common to all the three major regions of drug regulation (European Union, USA and Japan) and most of the other major non-ICH authorities have also agreed to accept the dossier in this format. Information on the CTD 'Presentation and format of the dossier CTD' can be accessed from the EC website. This document also shows the correspondence of the previous format with the CTD format. It is important to appreciate that the introduction of CTD has not resulted in a change in the qualitative or quantitative nature of data required – only the format in which these data are presented has changed. Even applications for line extensions must be submitted using the new EU CTD format. However, references can be made to already assessed and authorised 'old' parts of the dossier, but only if no new additional data are submitted in these parts. In such cases, it is not necessary to reformat already assessed and authorised 'old' documentation.

In order to expedite and optimise drug development, clinical trials are now conducted in different parts of the world. Recognising that drug development is a global process and in order that the data from one ethnic group can be confidently extrapolated to another, an ICH guideline (CPMP/ICH/289/95) has been agreed taking into account the genetic and non-genetic influences on drug responses. Application of this and all other regional, national and international guidelines relevant to quality, toxicity testing and demonstrating efficacy in clinical trials has ensured that public safety is not compromised while still ensuring that safe and effective medicines are made available to the UK public without the need for repeating lengthy clinical trials.

17.13 Conclusions

This chapter has provided a brief but, it is to be hoped, interesting account of the events that have been responsible for the evolution of the present drug controls in the UK. Importantly, it highlights how the broad pattern of drug regulation was already set during the early period which led to the implementation of the Medicines Act in 1971 and how this pattern was consolidated during the three decades thereafter.

Contrary to what is generally believed, the need for an effective control was always recognised, and indeed demanded, and there was a sort of control. However, it was patchy, very limited in its scope, erratic in its implementation and of little relevance to the drugs that were beginning, and were likely in the future, to appear in the market as a result of progress in pharmacology and medicinal chemistry.

Thalidomide generated an outcry and a demand that could no longer be ignored, and spurred the government into not only consolidating all previous legislation and extending its scope, but also creating a formal regulatory structure by which to ensure that the legislation was adequately and fully implemented.

The Medicines Act, together with the associated EU legislation and EU and ICH guidelines, should ensure that the safety of drugs made to the highest quality, the acceptability of their risk–benefit ratio and the promotion of correct information to the prescribers and consumers are the dominant features of the controls that operate today. In the *Daily Telegraph Magazine* in April 2008 in an article entitled 'The pills that kill' in an interview with Mick Deats of the MHRA intelligence and enforcement unit, a former police Detective Chief Superintendent, counterfeit medicines reaching the patient was identified as a major issue facing the MHRA. It was stated that in 'Britain between August 2004 and the end of last year (2007) there were nine recalls of counterfeit medicines where there was clear evidence that fakes reached pharmacies and patients'. The problem of counterfeit medicines is an international issue and a growing one for regulatory authorities, legitimate manufacturers and patients. The WHO began collecting data on counterfeit drugs in the early 1980s; until 10 years ago they regarded this as a problem in developing countries. The situation has changed: 'by 2001 counterfeit versions of major prescription medicines have appeared all over Europe'.

References

1 Griffin JP. Venetian treacle and the foundation of medicines regulation. *Br J Clin Pharmacol* 2004;**58**: 317–25.

2 Penn RG. The state control of medicines: the first 3000 years. *Br J Clin Pharmacol* 1979;8:293–305.

3 House of Commons Health Select Committee. *The Influence of the Pharmaceutical Industry*. London: HMSO, 2005.

4 D'Arcy PF, Griffin JP. Thalidomide revisited. *Adverse Drug React Toxicol Rev* 1994;13:65–76.

5 Ministry of Health, Scottish Home and Health Departments. *Safety of Drugs*. Final Report of the Joint Sub-Committee of the Standing Medical Advisory Committees. London: Her Majesty's Stationery Office, 1963.

6 Winship K, Hepburn D, Lawson DH. The review of medicines in the United Kingdom. *Br J Clin Pharmacol* 1992;33:583–7.

7 Griffin JP, Long JR. New procedures affecting the conduct of clinical trials in the United Kingdom. *BMJ* 1981;2:477–9.

8 Speirs CJ, Griffin JP. A survey of the first year of operation of the new procedure affecting the conduct of clinical trials in the United Kingdom. *Br J Clin Pharmacol* 1983;15:649–55.

9 Speirs CJ, Saunders RM, Griffin JP. The United Kingdom Clinical Trial Exemption Scheme: its effects on investment in research. *Pharm Int* 1984;5:254–6.

10 Holgate JA. Adverse effects associated with vaccines. In: D'Arcy FF, Griffin JP, eds. *Iatrogenic Diseases*. Oxford: Oxford University Press, 1986;882–97.

11 Griffin JP. Clinical pharmacology in the UK, c1950–2000: industrial and regulatory aspects. In Reynolds LA, Tansey EM, eds. *Welcome Witnesses to Twentieth Century Medicine, Vol. 34*. London: Welcome Trust Centre for the History of Medicine at UCL, 2008.

12 Griffin JP. Survey of the spontaneous adverse drug reactions reporting schemes in 15 countries. *Br J Clin Pharmacol* 1986;22(Suppl 1):83S–100S.

13 Griffin JP, Walker SR, Goldberg A, eds. *Voluntary Reporting in Monitoring for Adverse Reactions*. Lancaster: MTP Press, 1984;21–30.

14 World Health Organization (WHO). *Pharmacovigilance: Ensuring the Safe Use of Medicines*. WHO Policy Perspectives on Medicines No 9. Geneva, October 2004.

15 Collier J, Herxheimer A. Roussel convicted of misleading promotion. *Lancet* 1987;i:113–4.

16 Griffin JP. Clinical studies in medical journals. *J R Soc Med* 2007;100:64.

Other sources of information

Committee on Safety of Drugs. Report of the Committee on Safety of Drugs for the year ended December 31, 1964. London: Her Majesty's Stationery Office, 1965.

Committee on Safety of Drugs. Report for the year ended 31 December 1965. London: Her Majesty's Stationery Office, 1966.

Committee on Safety of Drugs. Report for the year ended 31 December 1966. London: Her Majesty's Stationery Office, 1967.

Committee on Safety of Drugs. Report for the year ended 31 December 1967. London: Her Majesty's Stationery Office, 1968.

Committee on Safety of Drugs. Report for the year ended 31 December 1968. London: Her Majesty's Stationery Office, 1969.

Committee on Safety of Drugs. Report for 1969 and 1970. London: Her Majesty's Stationery Office, 1971.

Medicines Commission. First Annual Report to end of 1970. London: Her Majesty's Stationery Office, 1971.

Medicines Commission. Annual Report for 1971. London: Her Majesty's Stationery Office, 1972.

Committee on Safety of Medicines. Report for the year ended 31 December 1971. London: Her Majesty's Stationery Office, 1972.

Committee on Safety of Medicines. Report for the year ended 31 December 1972. London: Her Majesty's Stationery Office, 1973.

The Medicines Commission. Annual Report for 1973 (together with annual reports of standing committees appointed under section 4 of the Medicines Act 1968). London: Her Majesty's Stationery Office, 1974.

The Medicines Commission. Annual Report for 1974 (together with annual reports of standing committees appointed under section 4 of the Medicines Act 1968). London: Her Majesty's Stationery Office, 1975.

The Medicines Commission. Annual Report for 1975 (together with annual reports of standing committees appointed under section 4 of the Medicines Act 1968). London: Her Majesty's Stationery Office, 1976.

The Medicines Commission. Annual Report for 1976 (together with annual reports of standing committees appointed under section 4 of the Medicines Act 1968). London: Her Majesty's Stationery Office, 1977.

The Medicines Commission. Annual Report for 1977 (together with annual reports of standing committees appointed under section 4 of the Medicines Act 1968). London: Her Majesty's Stationery Office, 1978.

The Medicines Commission. Annual Report for 1978 (together with annual reports of standing committees appointed under section 4 of the Medicines Act 1968). London: Her Majesty's Stationery Office, 1979.

18 Regulation of human medicinal products in the European Union

Rashmi R. Shah[1] and Agnès Saint Raymond[2]

[1] Medicines and Healthcare products Regulatory Agency (MHRA), London, UK
[2] European Medicines Agency (EMEA), London, UK

18.1 Introduction

The history of pharmaceutical legislation in the European Union (EU) is intricately linked with legislation and harmonisation across other socioeconomic sectors as well as ever-increasing membership of the EU. The unique strength of the European system of licensing and monitoring medicinal products lies in the scrutiny a new drug, or the safety of an approved drug, receives from the national authorities of all its Member States. A major advantage of this pan-European system is that it can draw on the expertise of all its Member States and, invariably, each application is closely scrutinised by all the experts and advisory committees of each of its Member States. The EU system, through initiatives of its Member States, has provided important leads to other regulatory authorities of the world, either indirectly or formally through the International Conference on Harmonisation of Technical Requirements for Registration of Pharmaceuticals for Human Use (ICH).

Although at first it did not attract as much attention as do regulatory bodies in other parts of the world, the EU system of pharmaceutical regulation is probably among the best in the world in terms of transparency and consumer interests without being unfair to the sponsors. In matters of doubt, consumer interests take precedence. Naturally, the need to seek consensus among the Member States and reach a harmonised pan-European view necessarily takes time and this could be seen as a potential drawback of the EU system.

The websites of the EU and the European Medicines Agency (EMEA) include all legislation and guidelines as well as a vast amount of information related to pharmaceutical procedures and medicinal products.

In order not to distort the contents or the message, this chapter brings together the relevant legislation, guidelines and information, almost verbatim in many instances, from these websites. We gratefully acknowledge these sources at the outset and provide links to the appropriate locations of various documents on these websites when considered helpful to the reader. Because the legislation, the requirements and the procedures continue to evolve, the applicant should verify the latest position before making important decisions.

This chapter first sets out in brief the historical developments that underpin the EU followed by a review of the evolution of the prevailing pharmaceutical legislation and current regulatory procedures, requirements and expectations.

18.2 History of the European Union

The historical roots of the EU, today one of the three largest economic blocks in the world by population, surface area or wealth, lie in the Second World War. In 1949, Western Europe created the Council of Europe as a first step towards preventing further wars by setting up economic cooperation. However, six countries (Belgium, France, Luxembourg, Italy, the Netherlands and Germany – 'the Six') wanted to go further. In 1950, the French Foreign Minister, Robert Schuman, proposed integrating the coal and steel industries of Western Europe. In 1951, the Six countries signed the Treaty of Paris establishing the European Coal and Steel Community (ECSC or the 'High Authority') and, by February 1953, the Common Market for coal and iron ore was set in place. The Six removed custom duties and quantitative restrictions on these raw materials and, on 8 December 1955, the Council of Ministers of the Council of Europe adopted as its emblem the blue flag hosting 12 golden stars.

The Textbook of Pharmaceutical Medicine. Edited by John P. Griffin. © 2009, ISBN: 978-1-4051-8035-1.

On 25 March 1957, the Treaties establishing the European Economic Community (EEC) and the European Atomic Energy Community (EURATOM) were signed by the Six in Rome and are referred to as the 'Treaties of Rome', which came into force on 1 January 1958. The ECSC, EEC and EURATOM were set up in Brussels. The Parliamentary Assembly, and the Court of Justice both already set up in Luxembourg in 1952 were common to the three Communities (ECSC, EEC and EURATOM).

20 April 1958 saw the publication of the first *Official Journal of the European Communities*. Customs duties between the Six countries were completely removed on 1 July 1968.

From these beginnings the EEC established by the Six has gradually enlarged and the scope of areas of harmonisation widened. The Six were joined by Denmark, Ireland and the UK in 1973, Greece in 1981, Spain and Portugal in 1986 and Austria, Finland and Sweden in 1995. In October 1990, Germany was unified and former East Germany became part of the EU. This comprised the EU15. Later, in 2004, Cyprus, Czech Republic, Estonia, Hungary, Latvia, Lithuania, Malta, Poland, Slovakia and Slovenia joined the EU followed by Bulgaria and Romania in 2007, making the current membership of 27 sovereign states (and referred to as EU27). Croatia, the Former Yugoslav Republic of Macedonia and Turkey are also candidates for future membership.

In 1984, the Single European Act enshrined a single European market and, in 1993, the Treaty of the European Union (Maastricht) created the European Community. Areas of cooperation identified were defence, justice and home affairs. Later, in 1997, the Treaty of Amsterdam extended the harmonisation process into areas of employment and citizens' rights, improvement of employee and consumer protection, non-discrimination, removal of any remaining obstacles to free movement, cooperation between police forces and customs authorities, easier extradition of criminals between Member States and common minimum standard for rules and penalties for certain offences. The year 2002 saw the introduction of the 'Euro' coins and notes into circulation in the 12 Member States participating in the 'Euro Zone' (Austria, Belgium, Finland, France, Germany, Greece, Ireland, Italy, Luxembourg, the Netherlands, Portugal and Spain).

A small village in Luxembourg gave its name to the Schengen Agreement, which first came into force in March 1995 and is part of EU law, allowing people to travel across the frontiers of the participating Member States without having their passports checked at the borders. The membership of the 'Schengen countries' has grown from the original 7 to 22 Member States (the exceptions by derogation being Bulgaria, Cyprus, Ireland, Romania and the UK).

The above brief account provides only a flavour of the depth and breadth of harmonisation and cooperation across the EU but, against this background, it should come as no surprise that there has evolved Community-wide legislation that aims to harmonise regulation of pharmaceutical or medicinal products – both human and veterinary.

Through the European Economic Area (EEA) agreement of 28 May 1999, two European Free Trade Area (EFTA) states – Iceland and Norway – have adopted a complete Community *acquis* on medicinal products with effect from 1 January 2000. Where in this chapter a reference is made to Member States, this should therefore be read to include these EFTA states. The only exemption from this is that legally binding acts from the Community (e.g. the European Commission (EC) Decisions) do not directly confer rights and obligations in these countries but first have to be transposed into legally binding Acts in these states. Although Liechtenstein is also entitled to participate, it more frequently than not adopts the decisions made by SwissMedic – the Swiss agency responsible for regulation of therapeutic products. However, authorisations granted by SwissMedic are not viewed as Community authorisations because Switzerland is not a participating Member of the EU.

18.3 European pharmaceutical legislation

The EU has a set of legal instruments known as either the Regulations or the Directives. In addition, the European Commission (EC) issues communications to clarify its legal understanding of the legislation or requirements. There are also guidelines issued by various EU regulatory bodies.

A Regulation is a legal instrument which has a general application; it is binding in its entirety and is directly applicable in all Member States. As 'Community laws', Regulations must be complied with fully by those to whom they are addressed (individuals, Member States, Community institutions). Regulations apply directly in all Member States, without requiring a national act to transpose them into the national legislation, on the basis of their publication in the *Official Journal of the European Communities*. Regulations serve to ensure the uniform application of Community law in all Member States. At the same time, they prevent the application of national rules the substance of which is incompatible with their own regulatory purpose. National laws, Regulations and administrative provisions are permissible only in so far as they are provided for in Regulations or are otherwise necessary for the effective implementation of the Community Regulations. National implementing provisions may not amend or amplify the scope and effectiveness of Regulations.

A Directive is a legal instrument that is binding, as to the result to be achieved, upon each Member State to whom it is addressed. However, the national authorities are left the choice of form and methods to achieve their objectives. Directives may be addressed to individual, several or all Member States. In order to ensure that the objectives laid down in Directives become applicable to individual citizens, an act of transposition by national legislators is required, whereby national law is adapted to the objectives laid down in Directives. Individual citizens are given rights and bound by the legal act when the Directive is incorporated into national law.

Because Member States are only bound by the objectives laid down in Directives, they have some discretion in transposing them into national law, taking into account specific national circumstances. Transposition must be effected within the period laid down in a Directive. In transposing Directives, the Member States must select the national forms that are best suited to ensure the effectiveness of Community law.

Directives must be transposed in the form of binding national legislation that fulfils the requirements of legal security and clarity and establishes an actionable legal position for individuals. National legislation that has been adapted to EC Directives may not subsequently be amended contrary to the objectives of those Directives (blocking effect of Directives).

A guideline is a Community document that is either referred to in the legislative framework as intended to fulfil a legal obligation laid down in the Community pharmaceutical legislation or considered to provide advice to applicants or marketing authorisation holders, competent authorities and/or other interested parties on the best or most appropriate way to fulfil an obligation laid down in the Community pharmaceutical legislation. In the case of scientific guidelines, these are adopted after consultation with interested organisations and may relate to specific scientific issues reflecting a harmonised EU approach and based on the most up-to-date scientific knowledge. Although Commission guidelines do have a legal force, most scientific guidelines drafted within the framework of the pharmaceutical legislation to assist the applicants do not have legal force and the definitive legal requirements are those outlined in the relevant Community legislative framework (e.g. Directives, Regulations, Decisions) as well as appropriate national rules. However, scientific guidelines are to be considered as a harmonised Community position, which, if followed by relevant parties such as the applicants, marketing authorisation holders, sponsors, manufacturers and regulators, will facilitate the assessment, approval and control of medicinal products in the EU. Nevertheless, alternative approaches may be taken, provided that these are appropriately justified.

There are other documents referred to as 'concept papers' and 'points to consider' documents. Of late, the documents are no longer classified as 'points to consider' but as 'guidelines' or 'reflection papers'.

18.3.1 Early legislation and initiatives before January 1995

The scale of the thalidomide disaster during 1959–1961, described in Chapter 17, reached such proportions that not only was the drug withdrawn from the market worldwide but there was also a public outcry on the lack of controls on human medicinal products in Europe.

In France, 4 million capsules containing diethyltin diiodide were distributed during 1954 under the name of Stalinon for the treatment of staphylococcal infections. The disaster that followed during 1954–1957 (resulting in 102 deaths from neurotoxicity and 100 more affected by paraplegia from a formulation error) had already resulted in new regulatory requirements being published in February 1959 by the French Health Authority. The manufacturers had to have recourse to an officially appointed expert committee for the preparation of registration file. This registration file had to provide evidence of the therapeutic interest of the product and of its safety under normal conditions of use as well as of the manufacturing process associated with adequate testing to guarantee the quality of the product on an industrial scale. Not surprisingly, thalidomide was not marketed in France which was spared the tragedy.

The evaluation of marketed medicines in Germany from 1911 was the responsibility of the Congress of Internal Medicine, later known as Medicines Commission of the German Medical Profession (Arzneimittelkommission der deutschen Ärzteschaft). During 1958–1961, the Commission, which had then become the Scientific Expert Committee of the German Medical Association, reinforced the request for the submission of adverse drug reactions following the thalidomide birth defect tragedy. In 1961, the First German Medicines Act was passed and, in 1963, an adverse drug reaction form was introduced, to be forwarded to the Federal Board of Health.

The USA was essentially spared the thalidomide tragedy because of the concerns the Food and Drug Administration (FDA) had regarding the neurotoxicity of thalidomide. This had resulted in the application being stalled in the USA. The US Federal Pure Food and Drugs Act (1906) and the Federal Food, Drug and Cosmetic Act (1938) were already in place but following the thalidomide tragedy in Western Europe, a subsequent New Drug Amendment (the Kefauver–Harris Amendment), in 1962, called for the FDA to monitor all stages of drug development.

As a result, even investigational drugs then required comprehensive animal testing before extensive human clinical trials could be started. Under the Kefauver–Harris Amendment, proof of efficacy and safety was mandatory and the time constraints on the FDA for disposition of new drug applications were removed.

The thalidomide disaster was to provide the stimulus to the introduction, for the first time in most of Western Europe and elsewhere in the world, of regulatory control of drugs to be marketed for clinical use. In the UK, a voluntary system of control that was introduced immediately in 1963 gave way to a system of statutory controls effective from September 1971 when the Medicines Act of 1968 received the Royal Assent on 25 October 1968 and establishment of the Licensing Authority.

At the European level, the thalidomide tragedy resulted in the adoption of Council Directive 65/65/EEC of 26 January 1965 and its primary aim was set out in its preamble, which stated that:

The Council of the European Economic Community, having regard to the Treaty establishing the European Economic Community and in particular Article 100 thereof:
• Whereas the primary purpose of any rules concerning the production and distribution of medicinal products must be to safeguard public health;
• Whereas, however, this objective must be attained by means which will not hinder the development of the pharmaceutical industry or trade in medicinal products within the Community;
• Whereas trade in medicinal products within the Community is hindered by disparities between certain

national provisions, in particular between provisions relating to medicinal products (excluding substances or combinations of substances which are foods, animal feeding stuffs or toilet preparations); and whereas such disparities, directly affect the establishment and functioning of the common market;
• Whereas such hindrances must accordingly be removed; and whereas this entails approximation of the relevant provisions;
• Whereas, however, such approximation can only be achieved progressively; and whereas priority must be given to eliminating the disparities liable to have the greatest effect on the functioning of the common market; has adopted this Directive.

The breadth of the regulatory definition of a medicinal product defined the scope of this Community-wide legislation. The legislation defined a medicinal product as any substance or combination of substances presented for treating or preventing disease in human beings or animals or that may be administered to human beings or animals with a view to making a medical diagnosis or to restoring, correcting or modifying physiological functions in human beings or animals. Substance was further defined as any matter that may be of human, animal, vegetable or chemical origin.

In the EU, a medicinal product may only be placed on the market when the competent authority of a Member State has issued a marketing authorisation for its own territory (national authorisation) or when the EC has granted an authorisation for the entire Community (Community authorisation).

Subsequent to Directive 65/65/EEC, four other key legislations were adopted:
1. Directive 75/318/EEC of 20 May 1975 introduced the requirements relating to analytical, pharmacotoxicological and clinical standards and protocols in respect of the testing of proprietary medicinal products in order to establish their quality, safety and efficacy.
2. Directive 75/319/EEC of 20 May 1975 established the Committee for Proprietary Medicinal Products (now referred to as 'old' CPMP) and introduced the multistate procedure (known now as the mutual recognition procedure).
3. Decision 75/320/EEC of 20 May 1975 set up a Pharmaceutical Committee.
4. Directive 87/22/EEC of 22 December 1986 introduced the concertation procedure (known now as the centralised procedure) relating to the placing on the market of high technology medicinal products, particularly those derived from biotechnology.

This 'old' CPMP met on 26 November 1976 for the first time and on 13–14 December 1994 for the last time. Its Opinions were not binding on the Member States. It was chaired first by M. Leon Robert (Luxembourg) later followed by Professor Duilio Poggiolini (Italy) and later still by Professor Jean-Michel Alexandre (France). The CPMP had also established a Safety Working Party, Efficacy Working Party and Herbal Working Party. Whereas the former two have evolved into their present form, the last one was abandoned for a number of years and only re-established much later.

Since the above legislative requirements in the EU, further stringent legislation and requirements have evolved in respect of investigations during the development of a drug, data necessary for its approval, its promotion, and monitoring the safety of medicines during the post-marketing period (pharmacovigilance). Some of the key legislation and EC communications are listed below:

1. Council Directive 78/25/EEC of 12 December 1977 on colouring matters that may be added to medicinal products;
2. Commission Communication on parallel imports of proprietary medicinal products for which marketing authorisations have already been granted;
3. Council Directives 83/570/EEC of 26 October 1983 introduced the purpose and scope of Summary of Product Characteristics (SPC or SmPC);
4. Council Directive 86/609/EEC of 24 November 1986 on the protection of animals used for experimental and other scientific purposes;
5. Council Directives 87/18/EEC of 18 December 1986 and 88/320/EEC of 9 June 1988 on Good Laboratory Practice (GLP);
6. Council Directive 87/19/EEC of 22 December 1986 amending Directive 75/318/EEC relating to analytical, toxico-pharmacological and clinical standards and protocols in respect of the testing of proprietary medicinal products;
7. Council Directive 87/21/EEC of 22 December 1986 amended Directive 65/65/EEC on the approximation of provisions laying down by law, Regulation or administrative action relating to proprietary medicinal products;
8. Council Directive 89/105/EEC of 21 December 1988 relating to the transparency of measures regulating the pricing of medicinal products for human use and their inclusion within the scope of national health insurance systems and Commission Communication on the compatibility with Article 30 of the EEC Treaty of measures taken by Member States relating to price controls and reimbursement of medicinal products;
9. Council Directive 89/342/EEC of 3 May 1989 on immunologicals (vaccines, toxins or serums and allergens);
10. Council Directive 89/343/EEC of 3 May 1989 on radiopharmaceuticals;
11. Council Directive 89/341/EEC of 3 May 1989 amending Directives 65/65/EEC, 75/318/EEC and 75/319/EEC on the approximation of provisions laid down by law, Regulation or administrative action relating to proprietary medicinal products;
12. Council Directive 89/381/EEC of 14 June 1989 on products derived from human blood or human plasma;
13. Council Directive 91/356/EEC of 13 June 1991 on Good Manufacturing Practice (GMP);
14. Council Directive 92/25/EEC of 31 March 1992 on wholesale distribution;
15. Council Directive 92/26/EEC of 31 March 1992 on classification for supply;
16. Council Directive 92/27/EEC of 31 March 1992 on labelling and package leaflets;
17. Council Directive 92/28/EEC of 31 March 1992 on advertising;
18. Regulation (EEC) No 1768/92 of 18 June 1992 concerns the creation of a supplementary protection certificate for medicinal products, which thereby extended the patent protection for a medicinal product;
19. Council Directive 92/73/EEC of 22 September 1992 on homeopathic medicinal products;
20. Council Directive 93/39/EEC of 14 June 1993 on pharmacovigilance and which also provided that in the event of a disagreement between Member States about the quality, safety or efficacy of a medicinal product that is the subject of the decentralised Community authorisation procedure, the matter should be resolved by a binding Community Decision following a scientific evaluation of the issues involved within a European medicinal product evaluation agency.

A number of these Directives had been frequently amended subsequent to their initial adoption. Therefore, in the interests of clarity and rationality, they were assembled in a single text, Directive 2001/83/EC of 6 November 2001, codifying the latest versions of 11 of these Directives, including 65/65/EEC, 75/318/EEC and 75/319/EEC – the three key legislations.

18.3.2 Legislation during the period January 1995 to April 2004

In order to achieve wider and deeper harmonisation within the Member States, steps were taken in early 1990s to introduce more sweeping pharmaceutical legislation and procedures ('Future Systems') that became effective on 1 January 1995.

Council Regulation (EEC) 2309/93 of 22 July 1993 laid down Community procedures for the authorisation and supervision of medicinal products for human and veterinary use. Article 1 established a European Agency for the Evaluation of Medicinal Products (EMEA) and Article 5 established a 'new' CPMP to replace the 'old' CPMP which was established by Article 8 of Directive 75/319/EEC.

The EMEA began its activities on 1 February 1995 and was the administrative and scientific secretariat, working in close liaison with national authorities of the Member States. With its headquarters in London, it provided a forum and stimulus for further discussions of the safety and efficacy of drugs to determine a pan-European approach. The EMEA functioned as a secretariat to four scientific advisory committees of the EU on human as well as veterinary pharmaceuticals:

1. Committee for Proprietary Medicinal Products (CPMP);
2. Committee for Orphan Medicinal Products (COMP);
3. Committee for Herbal Medicinal Products (HMPC) (to be established under the then new Directive 2004/24/EC of 31 March 2004 and was a Working Party);
4. Committee for Medicinal Products for Veterinary Use (CVMP).

The activities of the EMEA were supported by fees payable to the EMEA, which were mandated by Council Regulation (EC) No 297/95 of 10 February 1995.

18.3.2.1 Committee for Proprietary Medicinal Products

The 'new' CPMP took over the functions of 'old' CPMP and met for the first time in January 1995 at which Professor J-M. Alexandre (France) was elected as its first chairman. It was also constituted of two members from each of the 15 Member States and was legally empowered and was responsible for formulating Opinions to the EC on any question concerning the admissibility of the files submitted in accordance with the centralised procedure, the granting, variation, suspension or withdrawal of an authorisation to place a medicinal product for human use on the market arising in accordance with the provisions of the Regulation, and pharmacovigilance. The CPMP was also responsible for arbitration ('referral') on differences among the Member States on a whole range of issues. The CPMP consisted of two voting members, nominated by the national authority of

each Member State. For an Opinion to be adopted, it required an absolute majority (16 of the potential 30 votes). In addition, the CPMP also included members appointed by each of the EEA-EFTA States as of 2000. These members had previously participated in the discussions but were excluded from the voting process, although their positions were recorded separately in the CPMP Opinion and the minutes of the meeting.

On completion of his two terms in December 2000, Professor Alexandre retired and was succeeded in January 2001 by Dr Daniel Brasseur (Belgium). The last meeting of this 'new' CPMP took place on 20–22 April 2004 and the May 2004 meeting was postponed to 1–3 June 2004. Following a further review of the legislation, the functions of the CPMP were transferred to the Committee for Medicinal Products for Human Use (CHMP) (see section 18.4.2) effective from 1 June 2004. The pharmaceutical legislation in the EU was further strengthened during the period January 1995 to April 2004.

Commission Regulation (EC) No 540/95 of 10 March 1995 laid down the arrangements for reporting suspected unexpected adverse reactions that are not serious to medicinal products for human or veterinary use authorised in accordance with the provisions of Council Regulation (EEC) No 2309/93, whether these reactions occurred in the Community or in a third country.

Commission Regulation (EC) No 541/95 of 10 March 1995 harmonised the examination of variations to the terms of a marketing authorisation granted by a competent authority of a Member State, whereas Commission Regulation (EC) No 542/95 of 10 March 1995 similarly harmonised the examination of variations to the terms of a marketing authorisation falling within the scope of Council Regulation (EEC) No 2309/93.

Commission Regulation (EC) No 1662/95 of 7 July 1995 laid down certain detailed arrangements for implementing the Community decision-making procedures in respect of marketing authorisations for products for human or veterinary use, establishing the Standing Committee on Medicinal Products for Human Use and the Standing Committee on Veterinary Medicinal Products.

Directive 2001/83/EC was also subsequently amended by:

1. Directive 2002/98/EC of 27 January 2003, setting standards of quality and safety for the collection, testing, processing, storage and distribution of human blood and blood components;

2. Commission Directive 2003/63/EC of 25 June 2003, replacing Annex 1 of Directive 2001/83/EC (detailing scientific and technical requirements) with a new Annex (requirements for the dossier to be submitted in Common Technical Document (CTD) format);

3. Directive 2004/24/EC of 31 March 2004 as regards traditional herbal medicinal products;

Council Directive 2003/63/EC of 25 June 2003 amending Directive 2001/83/EC, introduced the CTD in compliance of ICH, replacing the previous format of the dossier which consisted of Parts I–IV. The broad overview of CTD format of the dossier is shown in Box 18.1. Module 1 of the CTD is region-specific and varies in different ICH regions. The non-clinical and clinical overviews and summaries are equivalent to the Expert Report required under the earlier requirements. Annex 1 of Directive 2001/82/EC specifies the details and the structure of what is expected and required under each heading. The objectives behind the CTD are to reduce the time and resources needed to compile applications, to facilitate electronic submissions, regulatory reviews and communications, and facilitate exchange of information between regulatory authorities. The CTD is not intended to indicate what studies are required – these are essentially the same as before – but merely to indicate an appropriate internationally harmonised format for the presentation of the data that have been generated.

Starting as an ad hoc Working Group on Herbal Medicinal Products in May 1997, there evolved a Herbal Medicinal Products Working Party (HMPWP) which had been operational as regards traditional herbal medicinal products until August 2004. Article 16h of Directive 2004/24/EC of 31 March 2004 formally established the Committee for Herbal Medicinal Products (HMPC) (see section 18.4.4), which was to replace the HMPWP.

Later, the EC also introduced two implementing Regulations dealing with examination of variations:

1. Commission Regulation (EC) No 1084/2003 of 3 June 2003 concerning the examination of variations to the terms of a marketing authorisation for medicinal products for human use and veterinary medicinal products granted by a competent authority of a Member State;

2. Commission Regulation (EC) No 1085/2003 of 3 June 2003 concerning the examination of variations to the terms of a marketing authorisation for medicinal products for human use and veterinary medicinal products falling within the scope of Council Regulation (EEC) No 2309/93.

BOX 18.1 Summary of the contents of the modules of the Common Technical Document (CTD)

Module 1: EU-specific requirements
1.1 Module 1 comprehensive table of contents (Modules 1–5)
1.2 Application form
1.3 Product literature
    1.3.1 Summary of product characteristics (SPC)
    1.3.2 Labelling and package leaflet
    1.3.3 Mock-ups and specimen
    1.3.5 SPCs already approved in the Member States
1.4 Information about experts
1.5 Specific regional requirements for different types of applications
1.6 Environmental risk assessment

Module 2: CTD Summaries
2.1 CTD table of contents (Modules 2–5)
2.2 CTD introduction
2.3 Quality overall summary
2.4 Non-clinical overview
2.5 Clinical overview
2.6 Non-clinical summaries
    Introduction
    Pharmacology – written and tabulated
    Pharmacokinetics – written and tabulated
    Toxicology – written and tabulated
2.7 Clinical summary
    Biopharmaceutics and associated analytical methods
    Clinical pharmacology studies
    Clinical efficacy
    Clinical safety
    Synopsis of individual studies

Module 3: Quality
3.1 Format and presentation
3.2 Content: basic principles and requirements

Module 4: Non-clinical study reports
4.1 Format and presentation
4.2 Content: basic principles and requirements
    4.2.1 Pharmacology
    4.2.2 Pharmacokinetics
    4.2.3 Toxicology

Module 5: Clinical study reports
5.1 Format and presentation
5.2 Content: basic principles and requirements
    5.2.1 Reports of bio-pharmaceutics studies
    5.2.2 Reports of studies pertinent to pharmacokinetics using human bio-materials
    5.2.3 Reports of human pharmacokinetic studies
    5.2.4 Reports of human pharmacodynamic studies
    5.2.5 Reports of efficacy and safety studies
    5.2.6 Reports of post-marketing experience
    5.2.7 Case reports forms and individual patient listings

18.3.2.2 Orphan drug legislation

Following the success of the US orphan drug legislation passed in 1983, a number of countries introduced similar legislation (Japan in 1993 and Australia in 1998). Orphan diseases are those that are sufficiently rare that there are no commercial incentives to research these diseases and develop effective therapy. In 1999, the EU also passed legislation relating to this important area of drug development.

There are two primary pieces of orphan drug legislation in the EU. The first founding legislation is Regulation (EC) No 141/2000 of the European Parliament and the Council of 16 December 1999 on orphan medicinal products. This is concerned with the purpose, definitions, criteria for designation of a drug as orphan drug, establishing the COMP (see section 18.4.3), procedures, provision of protocol assistance, access to centralised procedure without further justification for Community marketing authorisation, market exclusivity and other incentives. The other is the Commission Regulation (EC) No 847/2000 of 27 April 2000 laying down the provisions for implementation of the criteria for designation and definitions of the concepts of 'similar medicinal product' and 'clinical superiority'. The COMP considers and gives Opinions on the applications for designation of drugs as orphan drugs (see section 18.7.6).

18.3.2.3 Clinical Trials Directive

It had long been evident that there were marked variations between the Member States in terms of the requirements for and conduct and approval of clinical trials. With a view to harmonising the conduct of clinical trials across the EU, Directive 2001/20/EEC was finally agreed on 14 December 2000 and was formally adopted in May 2001 with a 3-year transition period for its implementation.

The EU Clinical Trials Directive contains specific provisions regarding the conduct of clinical trials, including multicentre trials, on human subjects. It requires the introduction of procedures in the Community that will provide an environment where new medicines can be developed safely and rapidly (see section 18.7.11 and Appendices 2 and 3).

18.3.2.4 Good Manufacturing Practice

In 2003, the provisions of Commission Directive 91/356/EEC on GMP were extended to accommodate the Directive on clinical trials. Directive 91/356/EEC was replaced by Directive 2003/94/EC of 8 October 2003 laying down the principles and guidelines of GMP in respect of medicinal products for human use

and investigational medicinal products for human use. This new Directive lays down the principles and guidelines of GMP in respect of medicinal products for human use whose manufacture requires the authorisation referred to in Article 40 of Directive 2001/83/EC and in respect of investigational medicinal products for human use whose manufacture requires the authorisation referred to in Article 13 of Clinical Trials Directive 2001/20/EC. This new Directive on GMP deals with issues relating to inspections, compliance with marketing authorisation, conformity with GMP, quality assurance system, personnel, premises and equipment, documentation, production, quality control, work contracted out, complaints, product recall and emergency unblinding of the blinded product(s) in a clinical trial, self-inspection and labelling.

18.3.3 Current legislation after May 2004

Regarding all activities for the regulation of pharmaceuticals at the EU level, Article 71 of Regulation EEC/2309/93 (establishing the EMEA and the new CPMP) required that 'Within 6 years of the entry into force of this Regulation, the Commission shall publish a general report on the experience of the procedures laid down in this Regulation, in Chapter III of Directive 75/319/EEC and in Chapter IV of Directive 81/851/EEC'.

The tender for review was awarded to a consortium of Cameron McKenna and Arthur Anderson. The full report from Cameron McKenna, dated October 2000 and entitled 'Evaluation of the Operation of Community Procedures for the Authorisation of Medicinal Products', was a comprehensive and highly constructive document that made a large number of recommendations for the reform of EU pharmaceutical legislation (Review 2001).

Following extensive discussions among all interested parties, such as the national authorities, the EMEA and the European Federation of Pharmaceutical Industries and Associations (EFPIA), the EC proposed comprehensive reform of the EU pharmaceutical legislation in March 2004, which was adopted by the European Parliament and the Council. The introduction of the new legislation just preceded the accession to the EU of 10 new Member States on 1 May 2004, bringing the EU membership to 25 Member States (and referred to as EU25).

18.3.3.1 Review 2001

Regulation (EC) No 726/2004 of the European Parliament and of the Council of 31 March 2004 laid down

Community procedures for the authorisation and supervision of medicinal products for human and veterinary use and establishing a European Medicines Agency – thus replacing Regulation EEC/2309/93.

Article 5 of Regulation (EC) No 726/2004 created the CHMP, which is responsible for drawing up the Opinion of the EMEA on any matter concerning the admissibility of the files submitted in accordance with the centralised procedure, the granting, variation, suspension or revocation of an authorisation to place a medicinal product for human use on the market and pharmacovigilance. The CPMP therefore became the CHMP.

Article 55 of Regulation (EC) No 726/2004 created the European Medicines Agency, comprising of a management board, an Executive Director and a secretariat as well as six scientific advisory committees (CHMP, CVMP, COMP and HMPC with the subsequent addition of the Paediatric Committee (PDCO) and the Committee for Advanced Therapies (CAT)). Thus, the former EMEA became the European Medicines Agency. However, for technical reasons, it had to retain the acronym EMEA (the acronym EMA belongs to European Medical Association). The Agency may also give a scientific Opinion, in the context of cooperation with the World Health Organization (WHO), for the evaluation of certain medicinal products for human use intended exclusively for markets outside the Community. The Committee for Advanced Therapies (CAT) was set up in 2009 (see section 18.4.6).

Following the above-mentioned review of European pharmaceutical legislation, Directive 2001/83/EC was also further amended extensively by:

1. Directive 2004/27/EC of the European Parliament and of the Council of 31 March 2004, amending Directive 2001/83/EC, on the Community code relating to medicinal products for human use;
2. Regulations (EC) No 1901/2006 and 1902/2006 of 12 December 2006 concerning medicinal products for paediatric use;
3. Regulation (EC) No 1394/2007 of 13 November 2007 on advanced therapy medicinal products;
4. Directive 2008/29/EC of 11 March 2008 concerning Comitology procedures.

18.3.3.2 Directive 2004/27/EC

Directive 2004/27/EC of 31 March 2004 concerned a variety of matters and also included borderline substances and generic products. Some of the key features of Directive 2004/27/EC are described below.

It is evident from the above that a number of products were outside the scope of the original Directive 65/65/EEC, such as radiopharmaceuticals, homeopathic medicines and vaccines, and that these too were gradually brought within the scope of pharmaceutical legislation. Consequently, Directive 2004/27/EC also amended the definition of a medicinal product. The new definition states that to be a medicine, a product must be:

1. Any substance or combination of substances presented as having properties for treating or preventing disease in human beings; or
2. Any substance or combination of substances that may be used in or administered to human beings either with a view to restoring, correcting or modifying physiological functions by exerting a pharmacological, immunological or metabolic action, or to making a medical diagnosis.

A new provision was also added to remove any uncertainties, which states that: 'In cases of doubt, where, taking into account all its characteristics, a product may fall within the definition of a product covered by other Community legislation the provisions of this Directive shall apply.' Taken together, these provisions are intended to ensure that where doubt exists over whether a product – those on the 'borderline' between, for example, medicines and medical devices, medicines and cosmetics, medicines and food supplements – should be regulated under medicines legislation or a legislation enforced by another sector, the stricter medicines regulatory regime should apply.

Apart from changing the definition of a medicinal product, the definition of 'risks related to use of the medicinal product' was also changed. The definition includes four components – in addition to the prevailing definition which defined risk to public health in terms of the quality, safety and efficacy of the product, the revised legislation requires an assessment of any undesirable effects on the environment from use of the product. Under Article 26, the grounds for refusing a marketing authorisation have been amended under the review. The new provision allows a refusal if the risk–benefit balance of the product is not favourable, if the therapeutic efficacy is insufficiently substantiated or if its qualitative and quantitative composition is not as declared. The application may also be refused if the documents are not submitted in accordance with the requirements set out in the Directive. The marketing authorisation holder or the applicant is responsible for the accuracy of the data and documentation submitted. An unfavourable risk–benefit balance is also a ground for refusal (although in practice this principle has been applied previously).

Article 1(28)a of Directive 2004/27/EC defines the risk–benefit balance as an evaluation of the positive therapeutic effects of the product in relation to the risks to patients' or public health. The environmental component of the definition of risks is excluded from the risk–benefit balance. Under the new legislation, the risk–benefit balance is considered as part of Article 23, which enables the competent authority to continuously assess the risk–benefit balance by requesting relevant data from marketing authorisation holder.

The new EU legislation is regarded as helpful in stimulating the generics industry. The definition of a generic medicine, the concept of a European reference product, restrictions on strategic withdrawals, the decentralised procedure, the option to use the centralised procedure, a legal framework for biogenerics/biosimilars and the Bolar provisions are all regarded as stimulating the generics industry. Generic versions of centrally approved reference medicinal products may use the centralised procedure. To harmonise data protection, Article 10 of the revised legislation provides for 10 years' *market* exclusivity following initial authorisation of the reference (innovator) products that are authorised under Articles 6 and 8 of the amending Directive. Second applicants for generic product authorisations based on abridged dossiers may submit applications no earlier than 8 years (the *data* exclusivity period) from the date of initial authorisation of the innovative reference product and obtain a marketing authorisation. However, they may not place their products on the market until the 10-year period has elapsed. The 10-year period of *market* exclusivity for innovative products may be extended to a maximum of 11 years if, during the first 8 years from the date of initial authorisation, the marketing authorisation holder obtains an authorisation for one or more new therapeutic indications which are deemed to bring a significant clinical benefit in comparison with existing therapies. Presumably, significant clinical benefit would be expected to include new indications and/or new categories of patients. It is anticipated that whether a new indication represents a significant clinical benefit, and hence whether the product qualifies for an additional year of market exclusivity, will be evaluated as part of the product assessment and will be included in the assessment report. Where these reports are shared with EMEA and other Member States for purposes of centralised, decentralised or mutual recognition procedures for authorisation, there will be an opportunity for the Member States to establish an agreement on the significance, or otherwise, of the new indication.

There is a reordering of the information to be included in the SPC (see section 18.9.1). With regard to generic medicines, the final paragraph of Article 11

states that for authorisations under Article 10, those parts of the SPC of the reference product referring to indications or dosage forms that are still covered by patent law at the time when a generic medicine is marketed need not be included. However, for centrally approved reference product, this means that the EC will have to issue separate marketing authorisations for each Member State (depending on the local laws on data exclusivity). This provision will allow the authorisation of generic products with indications that vary between Member States to take account of usage patents in force on the innovative product in certain Member States. Under the current rules, some Member States would only accept an authorisation of the generic with those indications that did not have a usage patent anywhere in the EU. Some Member States, including the UK, have taken the view that while it may be acceptable to omit reference to certain indications and dosage forms, it may not be permissible to omit associated warnings or contraindications where those are important for the protection of public health. Therefore, the extent of modifications possible for a particular generic product SPC will be judged on a case-by-case basis.

Articles 21(3) and 21(4) oblige the competent authorities to make publicly available or accessible without delay the marketing authorisation, SPC, assessment report and reasons for the Opinion after deletion of commercially confidential information.

Under Article 23a, after a marketing authorisation has been granted, the holder of the authorisation must inform the competent authority of the authorising Member State of the date of actual marketing and also notify the competent authority if the product ceases to be placed on the market of the Member State, either temporarily or permanently. This notification typically should be made no less than 2 months before the interruption of the supply. The marketing authorisation holder may also be required to provide data on sales and any data in his possession relating to the volume of prescriptions.

Under Article 24 of the revised legislation, only a single renewal is required when the product has been authorised for 5 years. A second renewal may take place after a further 5 years if there are justified pharmacovigilance grounds. In addition, any authorisation that is not followed by placing on the market within 3 years (or that is not present on the market for 3 years) shall cease to be valid (see sections 18.7.2.6 and 18.7.5.6). Member States may grant exemptions from the 3-year rule, if justified on public health grounds.

Article 126a allows a Member State to authorise on public health grounds the marketing of a product on its territory even if the marketing authorisation holder has not made an application for an authorisation to that competent authority. It requires, nonetheless, that the authorising Member State ensures that the following requirements of the legislation can still be met: titles V (leaflets and labels), VI (classification), VIII (advertising), IX (pharmacovigilance) and XI (supervision and sanctions).

18.3.3.3 Micro, small and medium-sized enterprises office

Article 70.2 of Regulation (EC) No 726/2004 introduced a provision for financial and administrative assistance for micro, small and medium-sized enterprises (SMEs). Commission Regulation (EC) No 2049/2005 of 15 December 2005 is an implementing regulation laying down rules regarding the payment of fees to, and the receipt of administrative assistance from, the EMEA by SMEs. An SME Office was established on 15 December 2005 to provide a single interface between the SMEs and the EMEA. It has a dedicated structure within the Agency with its own secretariat.

The primary aim of the SME initiative is to promote innovation and the development of new medicinal products by smaller companies. As of 18 December 2008, 372 undertakings had been assigned SME status and a further 40 were under review. The large majority of companies are developing medicinal products for human use.

The incentives available to SMEs include:
1. Administrative and procedural assistance;
2. Fee exemptions for certain administrative services;
3. Fee reductions;
4. Deferral of fee for application for marketing authorisation or inspection;
5. Conditional fee exemption; and
6. Translation of product information.

Article 12 of the Regulation called for a user guide on the administrative and procedural aspects of medicines legislation that are of particular relevance to smaller companies. This user guide was published in 2006 and the final updated version appeared in October 2008 (http://www.emea.europa.eu/pdfs/SME/43039908en.pdf).

18.3.3.4 Paediatric medicines

The development of medicines for paediatric use had long attracted the attention of the EC since 1997 when the EC organised at the EMEA a round table conference of experts to discuss paediatric medicines. One of the conclusions at that time was that there was a need to strengthen the legislation, in particular by introducing a system of incentives.

In 1998, the Commission supported the need for international discussion on the performance of clinical trials in children in the context of the ICH and an ICH guideline was therefore agreed.

Aware of the unmet medical needs of the paediatric population, the CHMP took the initiative of creating an ad hoc Expert Group on Paediatrics (PEG). Dr Daniel Brasseur, chairman of the CHMP and a paediatrician himself, chaired this group. With the implementation of title IV of Regulation (EC) No 726/2004, the PEG was transformed into a temporary Paediatric Working Party, which was constituted in 2005 under a new mandate.

Regulation (EC) No 1901/2006 of 12 December 2006 on paediatric medicines amended Regulation (EEC) No 1768/92, Directive 2001/20/EC, Directive 2001/83/EC and Regulation (EC) No 726/2004. The Clinical Trials Directive 2001/20/EC had already taken into account some specific concerns about performing clinical trials in children, and in particular it laid down standards for their protection in clinical trials.

Regulation (EC) No 1901/2006 of the European Parliament and of the Council, as further amended by Regulation (EC) No 1902/2006 of 20 December 2006 of the European Parliament and of the Council, was adopted to facilitate the development and availability of medicinal products for use in the paediatric population, to ensure that medicinal products used to treat this group are subject to ethical research of high quality and are appropriately authorised for use in children, and to improve the information available on the use of medicinal products in various paediatric populations. These objectives should be achieved without subjecting the paediatric population to unnecessary clinical trials and without delaying the authorisation of medicinal products for populations of other age groups. The Regulation also established a scientific committee, the Paediatric Committee (PDCO) (see section 18.4.5). This Regulation creates a system of obligations and incentives or rewards for the development of medicines for paediatric use.

To encourage paediatric drug development, Regulation (EEC) No 1768/92 on supplementary protection certificate was amended to provide a reward in the form of a 6-month extension of the supplementary protection certificate. Because of frequent amendments to it, Directive 2001/83/EC was last consolidated in March 2008 and published in the *Official Journal* on 21 March 2008.

Volume 1 of the publications 'The rules governing medicinal products in the European Union' is a compilation of the EU legislation in the pharmaceutical sector for medicinal products for human use and can be accessed at http://ec.europa.eu/enterprise/pharmaceuticals/eudralex/vol1_en.htm. For further discussion on medicines for paediatric use, the reader is referred to Chapter 19.

18.4 EMEA and scientific advisory committees

As far as the medicinal products for human use are concerned, the EU is served by the above five advisory committees (CHMP, COMP, HMPC, PDCO and CAT) with representation from each Member State. These committees are a part of the EMEA which provides the secretariat and is a coordinating centre. All these committees have an advisory role.

The chairperson and vice-chairperson of these advisory committees are elected by and from amongst its members for a term of 3 years, which may be renewed once. The chairman loses the right to vote and is replaced by another member to represent his or her nominating Member State. The members appointed by the EEA-EFTA States may not be elected chairperson or vice-chairperson of the committee.

The quorum required for the adoption of Scientific Opinions or recommendations by the any of these committees shall be reached when two-thirds of the total members of the committee eligible to vote are present. The votes shall be positive or negative (unless the provision concerning the conflicts of interest is applied).

Whenever possible, Scientific Opinions or recommendations of the committee shall be taken by consensus. If such a consensus cannot be reached, the Scientific Opinion or recommendation will be adopted if supported by an absolute majority of the members of the committee (i.e. favourable votes by at least half of the total number of committee members eligible to vote plus one). The exception is the COMP which requires a majority of two-thirds for an Opinion to be adopted. The divergent positions of and the names of the members expressing the divergent positions in the scientific evaluation shall be mentioned in the Opinion of the committee and, where relevant, the minutes of the committee. Members having divergent positions shall provide them in writing, stating clearly the reasons on which they are based. They will be appended to the Opinion. The reasons for the divergent Opinions shall be publicly available together with the document made publicly available where appropriate. In the event of no absolute majority position, the committee's Opinion is deemed to be negative.

The members from the EEA-EFTA States may not vote but their positions shall be stated separately in the Opinion, where relevant, in the minutes of the committee and, in case of divergent Opinions, these positions shall be appended to the committee's Opinion. Their position is not counted in reaching the committee's Opinion.

18.4.1 European Medicines Agency

The European Medicines Agency (EMEA), being the secretariat, is responsible for coordinating the existing scientific resources of the Member States for the provision of scientific advice, evaluation of safety, quality and efficacy, supervision and pharmacovigilance of medicinal products for human and veterinary medicinal products, orphan designation and agreement on paediatric investigation plans (PIPs), and SME assignment. It has access to about 4300 European experts. It is a decentralised agency of the EU and not part of the EC, with offices at 7 Westferry Circus, Canary Wharf, London E14 4HB, UK.

The EMEA, in collaboration with its scientific advisory committees, adopts Opinions which are ratified into binding Decisions by the EC. The EC must justify its decisions should these be at variance with the Opinions of the EMEA. The only exception is with regard to PIPs for which the decision-making power is vested into the EMEA Executive Director .

The Executive Director, currently Dr Thomas Lönngren (Sweden), is the Agency's legal representative and is ultimately responsible for all decisions of the EMEA. His duties are set out in Regulation (EC) No 726/2004 and the Agency is supervised by a management board to whom he reports. The staffing of the EMEA has increased from 67 in 1995 to 441 in 2007 (in addition to 124 contract agents and national experts seconded to the Agency).

The Executive Director is supported by a legal team, a senior medical officer, executive support staff and integrated quality management and audit team and five unit heads report to him. These units, with the structures of the two concerned with evaluation of human medicines, are:

1. Pre-authorisation Evaluation of Medicines for Human Use:
- Scientific advice, paediatrics and orphan drugs;
- Quality of medicines;
- Safety and efficacy of medicines.
2. Post-authorisation Evaluation of Medicines for Human Use:
- Regulatory affairs and organisational support;
- Pharmacovigilance, risk management and post-authorisation safety and efficacy of medicines;
- Medical information.
3. Veterinary Medicines and Inspections.

4. Communications and Networking.

5. Administration.

The Agency's total budget was just over €163 million in 2007 compared with just over €14 million in 1995. Since it became fully functional in early 1996, the proportion of the budget represented by fees has been increasing progressively and in 2007 it was 67% of the EMEA income, the rest was the EU subsidy. About one-third of the EMEA budget is paid to the national authorities of the Member States, who provide expertise on a contract basis at the request of the EMEA. In 2007, this amounted to approximately €53 million.

18.4.2 Committee for Medicinal Products for Human Use

The Committee for Medicinal Products for Human Use (CHMP) consists of one member and one alternate appointed by each of the EU Member States, after consultation of the management board, for a term of 3 years, which may be renewed, and a chairperson. The alternates represent and may vote for the members in their absence and can also act as rapporteurs in their own right. In addition, the CHMP also includes one member and one alternate appointed by each of the EEA-EFTA States, for a term of 3 years, which may be renewed. As permitted by the Regulation, the committee, in order to complement its expertise, has appointed five co-opted members chosen on the basis of their specific scientific competence, from the experts nominated by Members States or the Agency. At present, the expertise of these co-opted members includes medical statistics, pharmacovigilance, pharmacoepidemiology and risk management, quality of non-biologic products and quality and safety of biologicals with expertise in advanced therapies. Co-opted members are also appointed for the term a term of 3 years, which may be renewed, and they do not have alternates.

The task of the CHMP is to prepare the Agency's Opinions on all questions concerning medicinal products for human use, in accordance with Regulation (EC) No 726/2004. The CHMP has a vital role in the marketing procedures for medicines in the EU:

• In the Community or centralised procedure, the CHMP is responsible for conducting the initial assessment of medicinal products for which a Community-wide marketing authorisation is sought. The CHMP is also responsible for several post-authorisation and maintenance activities, including the assessment of any modifications or extensions (variations) to the existing marketing authorisation.

• In the mutual recognition and the decentralised procedures, the CHMP arbitrates in cases where there is a disagreement between Member States concerning the marketing authorisation of a particular medicinal product (arbitration procedure). The CHMP also acts in referral cases, initiated when there are concerns relating to the protection of public health or where other Community interests are at stake (Community referral procedure).

The CHMP also has an important role in EU-wide pharmacovigilance activity by closely monitoring reports of potential safety concerns (adverse drug reaction reports) and, when necessary, making recommendations to the EC regarding changes to a product's marketing authorisation or the product's suspension or withdrawal from the market. In cases where there is an urgent requirement to modify the authorisation of a medicinal product because of safety concerns, the CHMP can issue an urgent safety restriction (USR) to inform health care professionals about changes as to how or in what circumstances the medication may be used.

The EMEA publishes a European Public Assessment Report (EPAR) for every centrally authorised product that is granted a marketing authorisation, setting out the scientific grounds for the committee's Opinion in favour of granting the authorisation, plus the SPC, labelling and packaging requirements for the product, and details of the procedural steps taken during the assessment process. EPARs are published on the website of EMEA, and are generally available in all official languages of the EU. Assessment reports are also available in case of negative outcomes including withdrawals of the marketing authorisation application.

Other important activities of the CHMP and its working parties include:

1. Provision of assistance to companies researching and developing new medicines;

2. Preparation of scientific and regulatory guidelines for the pharmaceuticals industry; and

3. Cooperation with international partners on the harmonisation of regulatory requirements for medicines.

Each national competent authority is expected to monitor the level and independence of the evaluation carried out and to facilitate the activities of nominated members and experts. Members States are expected to refrain from giving committee members and experts any instruction that is incompatible with their own individual tasks or with the tasks and responsibilities of the Agency.

The chairman of previous CPMP, Dr Daniel Brasseur, was elected chairman of CHMP during its inaugural meeting on 1–3 June 2004. On conclusion of his term, he was succeeded by Dr Eric Abadie (France) as chairman on 18 June 2007. Dr Abadie is a physician who specialises in internal medicine, diabetes and cardiology. He was a member of the CPMP from 1997 to 2004 and of CHMP from 2004 onwards. Details of the Rules of Procedure of CHMP can be found at http://www.emea.europa.eu/pdfs/human/regaffair/4511007en.pdf.

18.4.3 Committee for Orphan Medicinal Products

In order to encourage pharmaceutical companies to invest in orphan drug development, legislation provides for a number of incentives: market exclusivity, protocol assistance and reductions of fees for application and inspection. In the EU, there is waiver of the fee applicable to the provision of any scientific advice (i.e. protocol assistance) for designated orphan drugs. From 1 February 2009, the reductions applicable are full (100%) reduction for protocol assistance and follow-up advice, full (100%) reduction for pre-authorisation inspections, 50% reduction for new applications for marketing authorisation to applicants other than SMEs, full (100%) reduction for new applications for marketing authorisation only to SMEs and full (100%) reduction for post authorisation activities including annual fees only to SMEs in the first year after granting a marketing authorisation. The funds made available by the Community for fee exemptions for orphan medicinal products amounted to €4.77 million in 2008. This accounted for 79% of the total fund of €6 million.

The period of market exclusivity is 10 years from authorisation of the product. As a consequence of market exclusivity in the EU, a Member State must not accept another application for a marketing authorisation or grant a marketing authorisation or accept an application to extend an existing marketing authorisation for the same therapeutic indication in respect of a similar medicinal product. A 'similar medicinal product' means a medicinal product containing a similar active substance or substances as contained in a currently authorised orphan medicinal product, and which is intended for the same therapeutic indication. A 'similar active substance' means an identical active substance, or an active substance with the same principal molecular structural features (but not necessarily all of the same molecular features) and which acts via the same mechanism. An 'active substance'

means a substance with physiological or pharmacological activity. Two active substances may only be considered to have the same mechanism of action provided that both share the same pharmacological target and pharmacodynamic effect. However, exclusivity may be lost by the first applicant consenting to a second application from another applicant, if the first is unable to meet demand, if a similar product is found to be clinically superior, if the criteria are no longer met or if, at the end of 5 years, a Member State can show that the product is (excessively) profitable.

The members of the COMP are nominated by the Member States and are chosen on the basis of their qualifications and expertise with regard to the evaluation of medicinal products. They do not have alternates and serve on the committee for a renewable term of 3 years.

Until April 2004, the COMP was constituted of a member from each Member State, three nominated by the EC on a proposal from the EMEA and three from patient organisations, making a total of 21 representatives. Following the accession of new Member States, the voting membership has increased to 33 and the committee is currently composed of the following:
1. A (non-voting) chairman, elected by COMP members;
2. One (voting) member nominated by each of the 27 EU Member States;
3. Three (voting) members nominated by the EC to represent patients' organisations;
4. Three (voting) members nominated by the EC on recommendation from EMEA;
5. One (non-voting) member nominated by each of the EEA-EFTA states (Iceland, Liechtenstein and Norway); Representatives of the EC and the EMEA (all non-voting) can attend the meetings. In addition, there are general observers who do not enjoy any voting rights.

The COMP is responsible for reviewing applications from persons or companies seeking 'orphan medicinal product designation' for products they intend to develop for the diagnosis, prevention or treatment of life-threatening or very serious conditions that affect not more than 5 in 10,000 persons in the EU.

The COMP is also responsible for advising the EC on the establishment and development of a policy on orphan medicinal products in the EU, and assists the EC in drawing up detailed guidelines and liaising internationally on matters relating to orphan medicinal products. Although the determination of safety and efficacy of an orphan medicinal product at the stage of marketing authorisation application are the remit of CHMP, it is also the remit of COMP to evaluate that application to confirm that the criteria for designation are met before an orphan medicinal product is granted a marketing authorisation and enjoy the market exclusivity.

The COMP has access to the expertise of all the Expert Working Parties set up by CHMP (see section 18.5) and is highly proactive in promoting the development of orphan drugs and interacting with academia, industry and patient groups.

The committee may establish any working groups and, when necessary, the committee and its working groups may avail themselves of the services of experts in specific scientific or technical fields. Such experts shall be included in the European experts list.

The COMP held its inaugural meeting in April 2000 and its first chairman was Professor Josep Torrent-Farnell (Spain). On completion of his second term in April 2006, he was succeeded by Dr Kerstin Westermark (Sweden). Details of the Rules of Procedure of COMP can be found at http://www.emea.europa.eu/pdfs/human/comp/821200en.pdf.

18.4.4 Committee for Herbal Medicinal Products

The HMPC was established in September 2004, replacing the CPMP Working Party on Herbal Medicinal Products.

Herbal medicines of long tradition are in wide use in a number of Member States of the EU. A significant number of these medicinal products, despite their long tradition, do not fulfil the requirements of a well-established medicinal use with recognised efficacy and an acceptable level of safety and so are not eligible for a marketing authorisation. The long tradition of these medicinal products makes it possible to reduce the need for clinical trials, in so far as the efficacy of the medicinal product is plausible on the basis of long-standing use and experience. Preclinical tests do not seem necessary where the medicinal product, on the basis of the information on its traditional use, proves not to be harmful in specified conditions of use. However, even a long tradition does not exclude the possibility that there may be concerns with regard to the product's safety, and therefore the competent authorities are entitled to ask for all data necessary for assessing its safety. The quality aspect of the medicinal product is independent of its traditional use so that no derogation is made with regard to the necessary physicochemical, biological and microbiological tests. These products should comply with quality standards in relevant European Pharmacopoeia monographs or those in the pharmacopoeia of a Member State.

A herbal medicinal product is defined as any medicinal product exclusively containing as active ingredients one or more herbal substances or one or more herbal preparations, or one or more such herbal substances in combination with one or more such herbal preparations.

All herbal substances are defined as mainly whole, fragmented or cut plants, plant parts, algae, fungi, lichen in an unprocessed, usually dried form, but sometimes fresh. Certain exudates that have not been subjected to a specific treatment are also considered to be herbal substances. Herbal substances are precisely defined by the plant part used and the botanical name according to the binomial system (genus, species, variety and author).

Herbal preparations are defined as preparations obtained by subjecting herbal substances to treatments such as extraction, distillation, expression, fractionation, purification, concentration or fermentation. These include comminuted or powdered herbal substances, tinctures, extracts, essential oils, expressed juices and processed exudates.

The HMPC is composed of scientific experts in the field of herbal medicinal products. It has one member and one alternate member nominated by each of the 27 EU Member States and by each of the EEA-EFTA States Iceland and Norway. Up to five additional members (European experts nominated by the Member States or by the Agency) may be co-opted to contribute additional expertise to the HMPC. Currently, the committee has co-opted members with expertise in clinical pharmacology, experimental/non-clinical pharmacology, toxicology, paediatric medicine, and general and family medicine. The HMPC also has observers from the European Directorate for the Quality of Medicines (EDQM) and – as part of the EU Enlargement Programme 'Transition Instrument for Pre-accession Programme' – from Croatia, Turkey and the Former Yugoslav Republic of Macedonia.

The activities of the HMPC are aimed at assisting the harmonisation of procedures and provisions concerning herbal medicinal products laid down in EU Member States, and further integrating herbal medicinal products in the European regulatory framework. As part of these objectives, the HMPC provides EU Member States and European institutions its Scientific Opinion on questions relating to herbal medicinal products. Other core tasks include the establishment of a draft 'Community list of herbal substances, preparations and combinations thereof for use in traditional herbal medicinal products', as well as the establishment of Community herbal monographs.

The inaugural meeting of the HMPC took place on 23–24 September 2004 and the current chairman is Dr Konstantin Keller (Germany). Details of the Rules of Procedure of HMPC can be found at http://www.emea.europa.eu/pdfs/human/hmpc/13980004en.pdf.

18.4.5 Paediatric Committee

The Paediatric Committee (PDCO) is composed of five CHMP members with their alternates, appointed by the CHMP itself, one member and one alternate appointed by each Member State (except Member States already represented through the members appointed by the CHMP), three members and their alternates representing health professionals, and three members and their alternates representing patients' associations. Members of the PDCO are appointed by the EC for a renewable term of 3 years.

The main responsibility of the PDCO is to assess the content of PIPs and adopt Opinions on them in accordance with Regulation (EC) No 1901/2006 as amended. This includes the assessment of applications for a full or partial waiver and assessment of applications for deferrals (see section 18.7.9).

Other main tasks of the PDCO include assessing data generated in accordance with agreed PIPs and adopting Opinions on the quality, safety or efficacy of any medicine for use in the paediatric population (at the request of the CHMP or a competent authority), providing advice on any question relating to paediatric medicines (at the request of the EMEA Executive Director or the EC), establishing and regularly updating an inventory of paediatric medicinal product needs and advising the EMEA and the EC on the communication of arrangements available for conducting research into paediatric medicines.

The PDCO is not responsible for marketing authorisation applications for medicinal products for paediatric use. This remains fully within the remit of the CHMP. However, the CHMP or any other competent authority may request the PDCO to prepare an Opinion on the quality, safety and efficacy of a medicinal product for use in the paediatric population if these data have been generated in accordance with an agreed PIP.

The PDCO, replacing the previous Paediatric Working Party, held its inaugural meeting on 4–5 July 2007 and Dr Daniel Brasseur, who had chaired the Paediatric Working Party, was elected as its first chairman. Details of the Rules of Procedure of PDCO can be found at http://www.emea.europa.eu/pdfs/human/pdco/34844008en.pdf.

18.4.6 Committee for Advanced Therapies

In January 2009, CAT was established in accordance with Regulation (EC) No 1394/2007 on advanced-therapy medicinal products (ATMPs). It is a multidisciplinary committee, bringing together some of the best available experts in Europe to assess the quality, safety and efficacy of ATMPs, and to follow scientific developments in the field.

The main responsibility of the CAT is to prepare a draft opinion on each ATMP application submitted to the EMEA, before the CHMP adopts a final opinion on the granting, variation, suspension or revocation of a marketing authorisation for the medicine concerned. At the request of the Executive Director of the EMEA or of the EC, an Opinion is also drawn up on any scientific matter relating to ATMPs.

Other responsibilities of the CAT include:
• participating in EMEA procedures for the certification of quality and non-clinical data for small and medium-sized enterprises developing advanced-therapy medicinal products;
• participating in EMEA procedures for the provision of scientific recommendations on the classification of advanced-therapy medicinal products in accordance with Article 17 of Regulation (EC) No 1394/2007;
• contributing to the EMEA's provision of scientific advice, following relevant procedures established between the CAT and the Scientific Advice Working Party (SAWP);
• involvement in any procedure regarding the provision of advice for undertakings on the conduct of efficacy follow-up, pharmacovigilance and risk-management systems of ATMPs;
• advising, at the request of the CHMP, on any medicinal product which may require, for the evaluation of its quality, safety or efficacy, expertise in ATMPs;
• assisting scientifically in the elaboration of any documents related to the fulfilling the objectives of Regulation (EC) No 1394/2007;
• providing at the request of the European Commission, scientific expertise and advice for any Community initiative related to the development of innovative medicines and therapies that requires expertise on ATMPs;
• assisting, at the request of the CHMP, in the tasks identified in the work programmes of the CHMP working parties.

The Committee for Advanced Therapies is composed of:
• five members of the CHMP, with their alternates, appointed by the CHMP itself;

• one member and one alternate appointed by each EU Member State whose national competent authority is not represented among the members and alternates appointed by the CHMP;

• two members and two alternates appointed by the EC to represent clinicians;

• two members and two alternates appointed by the EC to represent patients associations.

Members of the CAT are appointed for a renewable period of 3 years. The Chairperson of the CAT is elected from its members for a term of 3 years, which may be renewed once. The inaugural meeting of CAT was held on 15 and 16 January 2009 at the EMEA and Dr Christian Schneider (Germany) was elected as its first Chairman on 12 February 2009. Details of the Rules of Procedure of CAT can be found at http://www.emea.europa.eu/pdfs/human/cat/45444608en.pdf.

18.5 Expert Working Parties

The CHMP has four levels of expertise available to it:

1. Individual experts consulted by the rapporteur/co-rapporteur or coordinators within the framework of centralised applications, referral and scientific advice;

2. Ad hoc groups such as that on drug-induced QT interval prolongation; and

3. Scientific advisory groups (SAGs).

In addition, there are also expert working parties established to provide advice in specific areas.

At present, there are 12 expert working parties:

1. Biologics Working Party (BWP);
2. Blood Products Working Party (BPWP);
3. Cell-based Products Working Party (CPWP);
4. Efficacy Working Party (EWP);
5. Gene Therapy Working Party (GTWP);
6. Joint CHMP/CVMP Quality Working Party (QWP);
7. Patients' and Consumers' Working Party (PCWP);
8. Pharmacogenomics Working Party (PGWP);
9. Pharmacovigilance Working Party (PhVWP);
10. Safety Working Party (SWP);
11. Scientific Advice Working Party (SAWP);
12. Vaccine Working Party (VWP)

These working parties have been established progressively over time as necessitated by advances in science. These Working Parties produce guidelines relevant to their areas of expertise and these guidelines as well as those produced by ICH can be accessed at http://www.emea.europa.eu/htms/human/humanguidelines/background.htm.

The following groups are also established by the CHMP to provide expertise in their respective areas:

• (Invented) Name Review Group (NRG); and
• Working Group on Quality Review of Documents (QRD).

Whenever required by a project of a temporary or ad hoc nature, the CHMP may establish a temporary working party to conduct it. Two examples are the ad hoc Group of Experts on QT interval and the Similar Biological (Biosimilar) Medicinal Products Working Party (BMWP).

The Healthcare Professionals Working Group has become an EMEA/CHMP Working Group with Healthcare Professionals' Organisation (HCPWG), and its meeting are held with the Patients' and Consumers' Working Party (PCWP) members attending.

Of the above Expert Working Parties, the workings and the procedures of three deserve particular description in view of their significance for most applicants.

18.5.1 Efficacy Working Party

The Efficacy Working Party (EWP) has been established to provide recommendations to the CHMP on all matters relating directly or indirectly to the clinical part of drug development and to prepare, review and update guidelines in specific therapeutic areas and on methodology and interpretation of clinical trials (this might include statistical issues, but also consideration of alternative methodology for specific situations, such as clinical trials in small populations). Some of the other tasks of EWP include:

1. At the request of the CHMP, support to dossier evaluation.

2. At the request of the CHMP, support to scientific advice on general and product specific matters related to the clinical part of drug development.

3. When requested, provide support to the CHMP in international cooperation on clinical and related matters (interaction with the FDA, and other regulatory Agencies and with the WHO).

4. Liaison and contribution with SAWP on general and specific matters related to clinical trials.

5. Where needed and agreed by the CHMP, interaction with the COMP.

6. Contribution to ICH efficacy issues.

The Efficacy Working Party agrees a work programme with CHMP and may also identify and propose topics for consideration by the CHMP. Any proposal for a guideline, in the form of a Concept Paper providing adequate justification, is transmitted to the CHMP for discussion and endorsement by the CHMP.

The EWP is composed of experts selected from the European experts list according to their specific expertise. All members of the committee are invited to nominate one expert to be member of the EWP (one member per Member State). When necessary, the EWP may avail itself of the services of experts in specific scientific or technical fields.

The Executive Director of the Agency, members of the EMEA secretariat, and representatives of the Commission, may attend all meetings of the working party. CHMP members are encouraged to take an active role in the activities of the EWP.

The chairperson and vice-chairperson of the EWP are elected by the members of the CHMP for a term of 3 years. The chairperson is invited to attend plenary CHMP meetings to report on the activities on the EWP and ensure liaison with the work of the CHMP.

The efficacy guidelines issued by EWP and/or ICH can be located at http://www.emea.europa.eu/htms/human/humanguidelines/efficacy.htm and http://www.emea.europa.eu/htms/human/ich/ichefficacy.htm.

18.5.2 Pharmacovigilance Working Party

The mission of the Pharmacovigilance Working Party (PhVWP) is to provide recommendations to the CHMP on all matters relating directly or indirectly to 'pharmacovigilance' – the constant monitoring of medicinal products on the market. This involves providing advice on the safety of medicinal products and on the investigation of adverse reactions associated with medicinal products authorised in the EU, enabling the CHMP to effectively identify, assess and manage risk at any phase in the lifecycle of a medicinal product (see section 18.10).

Some of the other responsibilities of PhVWP include evaluation of potential signals arising from spontaneous reporting, provision of advice on confirmation and quantification of risk and on regulatory options, risk management, monitoring regulatory action, setting standards for procedures and methodologies to promote good vigilance practice, promotion of communication and exchange of information between the EMEA and national competent authorities and international cooperation.

The PhVWP frequently holds teleconferences with the FDA in the margins of the PhVWP meetings. The frequency of such teleconferences is agreed between the PhVWP, the EMEA and the FDA.

The PhVWP is composed of experts selected from the European experts list according to their specific expertise. The PhVWP consists of one representative per Member State. The representatives are appointed by the national competent authorities. Additional experts may attend the meetings of the PhVWP. Representatives from Iceland, Liechtenstein and Norway are also invited to attend the meetings of the PhVWP but they may not be elected chairperson or vice-chairperson. When necessary, the PhVWP may avail itself of the services of experts in specific scientific or technical fields.

The PhVWP meets 11 times per year (excepting August). Meetings of the PhVWP are held in parallel with the meetings of the CHMP in order to allow interaction between PhVWP representatives and the CHMP. The Executive Director of the EMEA, members of the EMEA secretariat, members of the CHMP and representatives of the Commission may attend all meetings of the PhVWP.

The chairperson of the PhVWP is appointed by the CHMP for a renewable term of 3 years. The chairperson is invited to attend plenary CHMP meetings to report on the activities of the PhVWP and ensure liaison with the work of the CHMP.

Details of the Rules of Procedure of PhVWP can be found at http://www.emea.europa.eu/pdfs/human/phvwp/phvwpmandate.pdf.

18.5.3 Scientific Advice Working Party

In accordance with Council Regulation (EEC) 2309/93 the group responsible for advising applicants during drug development started its activities as a CPMP consultation group (1996), as a Scientific Advice Review Group (1999) and as a formal CPMP Working Party (Scientific Advice Working Party (SAWP)) in 2003. As of 2001, with the introduction of Regulation (EC) No 141/2000, the activities of the group extended to providing protocol assistance for orphan drugs. In order to deal with the increasing number of applications and improve dialogue with industry, the meetings were separated from CPMP meetings and extended to two full days. New procedures for scientific advice and protocol assistance were also put in place.

Article 56(3) of Regulation (EC) 726/2004 provides that:

The Executive Director, in close consultation with the Committee for Medicinal Products for Human Use and the Committee for Medicinal Products for Veterinary Use, shall set up the administrative structures and procedures allowing the development of advice for undertakings, as referred to in Article 57(1)(n), particularly regarding the development of new therapies.

Each committee shall establish a standing working party with the sole remit of providing scientific advice to undertakings.

Article 57(1) of Regulation (EC) 726/2004 provides that: 'the Agency, acting particularly through its committees, shall undertake the following tasks: (n) advising undertakings on the conduct of the various tests and trials necessary to demonstrate the quality, safety and efficacy of medicinal products.'

Therefore, as of May 2004, the CHMP and the COMP established the SAWP as a standing working party with the sole remit of providing scientific advice and protocol assistance to applicants.

The SAWP is a multidisciplinary expert group. The CHMP appoints 22 members for a renewable term of 3 years, upon proposals from CHMP members. These SAWP members may be CHMP members or European experts. The COMP nominates three of its members for a renewable term of 3 years. The SAWP includes at least the following expertise:

1. *Preclinical safety* – at least two representatives;
2. *Pharmacokinetics* – at least one representative;
3. *Methodology and statistics* – at least two representatives. Experience in small population methodology and pharmacoepidemiology are particularly important;
4. Therapeutic fields for which there are frequent requests and/or defined in the annex of the new Regulation (e.g. cardiology, oncology, diabetes, neurodegenerative disorders and infectious diseases including HIV infection).

The respective chairperson of the SWP and EWP as well as the chairperson and vice-chairperson of the CHMP are also invited to each SAWP meeting. In addition, the CHMP members are also encouraged to take an active role in the activities of the SAWP. The SAWP meets 11 times a year (excepting August) at the EMEA for a 3-day meeting, generally set 2 weeks before the CHMP.

The SAWP may consult relevant working parties or scientific advisory groups in relation to the evaluation of preclinical and/or clinical questions including safety, for a specific product within the agreed timelines. The SAWP also delegates the task of evaluating quality related issues to the Biotechnology Working Party (BWP) or Quality Working Party (QWP). The SAWP may also avail itself of additional expertise (including patients' representatives) when considering scientific advice or protocol assistance, which could involve any aspects of drug development (pharmaceutical, preclinical, clinical and significant benefit). Additional expertise is also consulted in particular for the provision of protocol assistance for orphan medicinal products.

The chairperson of the SAWP is elected by the members of the CHMP for a renewable term of 3 years. Where the chairperson does not belong to the CHMP, he or she is invited to attend plenary CHMP meetings to report on the activities on the SAWP and ensure liaison with the work of the CHMP. Details of the Rules of Procedure of SAWP can be found at http://www.emea.europa.eu/pdfs/human/sciadvice/sawpmandate.pdf.

18.6 Scientific Advisory Groups

The CPMP/CHMP has established a number of SAGs, each dedicated to a particular therapeutic area and consisting of independent academic experts, to assist them with the evaluation of specific types of medicinal products or treatments. So far, seven SAGs have been set up and the link to each of these is provided below:

1. Scientific Advisory Group on Cardiovascular Issues (SAG-CVS) http://www.emea.europa.eu/htms/general/contacts/CHMP/CHMP_SAG-CVS.html
2. Scientific Advisory Group on Anti-infectives (SAG-AI) http://www.emea.europa.eu/htms/general/contacts/CHMP/CHMP_SAG-AI.html
3. Scientific Advisory Group on Clinical Neuroscience (SAG-CNS) http://www.emea.europa.eu/htms/general/contacts/CHMP/CHMP_SAG-CNS.html
4. Scientific Advisory Group on Diabetes/Endocrinology (SAG-DE) http://www.emea.europa.eu/htms/general/contacts/CHMP/CHMP_SAG-DE.html
5. Scientific Advisory Group on Diagnostics (SAG-D) http://www.emea.europa.eu/htms/general/contacts/CHMP/CHMP_SAG-D.html
6. Scientific Advisory Group on HIV/Viral Diseases (SAG-HIV) http://www.emea.europa.eu/htms/general/contacts/CHMP/CHMP_SAG-HIV.html
7. Scientific Advisory Group on Oncology (SAG-O) http://www.emea.europa.eu/htms/general/contacts/CHMP/CHMP_SAG-O.html

SAGs are created by the CHMP to deliver answers, on a consultative basis, to specific questions addressed to them by the committee. SAGs could also be consulted on centralised applications, scientific advice and protocol assistance, referrals, guidelines or any other scientific issues. The SAG has the opportunity to identify scientific issues that may need further discussion within or outside the discipline of the SAG subject to the agreement of the CHMP.

SAGs are composed of experts selected from the European experts list according to their specific expertise. A SAG is comprised of both a core group and other individual experts who may be called upon to participate at a given meeting or series of meetings on a specific issue about which they have appropriate expertise. The core group would ensure continuity and consistency within the group. The other individual members would bring additional expertise in specific domains and on a case-by-case basis.

Core group members (typically 6–9 members) will be selected for their clinical expertise in the field of interest and the core group should reflect a balanced composition of scientific expertise. The composition of the core group reflects as far as is possible different 'schools of thinking' or EU therapeutic practices. The CHMP members and the EMEA propose experts to be the core group members of SAG. Core group members of SAG elect one of its core members to be proposed to the CHMP to act as chairperson for the SAG and one to act as vice-chairperson.

The CHMP rapporteur, the co-rapporteur, the working party rapporteur or the scientific advice coordinators are invited to attend the SAG meeting, to present the List of Questions for the SAG, and to provide any additional information requested by the SAG. Assessors from the application-specific team set up by the rapporteurs or the coordinators are also expected to attend the meeting when necessary. An applicant or a marketing authorisation holder or a third party may be invited to provide an oral explanation to the SAG following agreement of the CHMP.

SAG Answers and Comments to the CHMP will contain answers to the CHMP List of Questions for the SAG, and a justification for each answer. Where consensus cannot be reached on an answer to the CHMP List of Questions for the SAG, the conclusion reached by the majority, together with any divergent positions within the SAG, will be noted in the SAG Answers and Comments to the CHMP. The divergent positions shall be explained in that document and where relevant in the minutes of the meeting. Members having divergent positions shall convey these clearly stating the reasons on which they are based.

Once finalised, the part of the draft 'SAG Answer and Comments to the CHMP' that relates to the 'product' will be released to the concerned company. The other parts of the SAG answer document and the minutes of the SAG meeting remain confidential. The CHMP List of Questions for the SAG, and the SAG Answers and Comments to the CHMP shall be reflected in the CHMP assessment reports, as appropriate, and thus appended to the CHMP Opinion. If, on request by the applicant the committee has consulted with the SAG in connection with the re-examination of its Opinion, the views of the SAG should also be included in the CHMP assessment report adopted by the committee.

The chairperson of SAG is responsible for the conduct and running of the meetings. Whenever possible, the chairperson of the SAG shall be available during a CHMP meeting, to provide feedback from the SAG discussions including divergent views to the CHMP. Because members of SAG are independent experts, the CHMP, while taking into account the position expressed by the SAG, remains responsible for its final Opinion.

18.7 Procedures for applications

The EMEA as well as the national authorities of the Member States are under considerable pressure from a heavy workload. Therefore, these authorities require prior notice, preferably well ahead of the proposed dates for the meeting or the submission of an application. In addition, as far as the national authorities are concerned, the applicants should not expect to secure their desired time-slot when requesting these authorities to act as Reference Member State for an application to be submitted through the mutual recognition or the decentralised procedure or when requesting a meeting for national scientific advice if these requests are made without adequate prior notice to or discussions with them.

It is therefore recommended that for all and any of the applications for marketing authorisation when the applicants' regulatory strategy has been decided, unless requested otherwise by the EMEA, the applicants open a dialogue with the appropriate authority by a provisional letter of intent, giving the pertinent background information on the product, sent about 8–10 months ahead of the intended submission date. This can be followed by a more definitive letter of intent about 3–4 months ahead of the realistic submission date. It is also recommended that the applicants request one pre-submission meeting and this request should be made well ahead of the desired date of the meeting. One pre-submission meeting should take place approximately 6–7 months prior to the anticipated date of submission of the application. These pre-submission meetings are extremely helpful because they provide an opportunity to discuss the development programme, secure advice on the contents and the format of the application and obtain procedural, regulatory and legal advice as well as appoint the evaluation teams. This guidance information and successful pre-submission meetings should enable applicants to submit applications that are in conformity with the legal and regulatory requirements and which can be validated speedily. Pre-submission meetings will also enable applicants to establish contact with the EMEA or the national authority staff closely involved with the application as it proceeds. Above all, these pre-submission meetings should not be treated as pre-submission evaluation of the data by inappropriate questions, but rather as opportunity of discussing the strengths and deficiencies of the development programmes. This is particularly important when seeking scientific advice. Checking of compliance with the Paediatric Regulation obligations can also take place ahead of the validation of the application.

It is recommended that the applicants follow a similar approach when seeking meetings with national authorities when they desire to obtain the views of these authorities on their perspectives on regulatory requirements, interpretation of and conformity (or otherwise) with various guidelines and the availability of the desired time-slots for applications.

Each application requires a full marketing authorisation application dossier (Module 1–5 according to the EU-CTD format) in English, including the applicant's part of the Active Substance Master File, if any. The contents vary with the type of application (e.g. a new chemical entity or a biological product, generic product or a substance with well-established use) and the details are specified in Annex 1 of Directive 2001/83/EC. Besides the submission of paper copies of the dossier, the EMEA strongly encourages the submission of complete copies using electronic storage media following advance discussion with the EMEA. At a minimum, the applicant should submit an electronic (WORD) copy of Modules 1 and 2, including the English WORD version of SPC, labelling and package leaflet. Applicants wishing to use this option must sign a letter in which they commit themselves to supplying a full paper copy of the marketing authorisation application within 48 hours upon request and confirm that the data on the CD-ROM/DVD supplied is identical to that in any written submission. There are other technical initiatives adopted by the EMEA to maximise the efficiency of the assessment process. These include e-CTD and Product Information Management (PIM) standard. The applicant should liaise with the EMEA in this regard.

With regard to an application for marketing authorisation, the Community legislation provides for two primarily different procedures: a Community procedure involving all the Member States or a national procedure which can involve only the Member States that are of interest to the applicant.

The Community procedure is compulsory for certain types of drugs and therapeutic classes of products and is optional for others at the discretion of the CHMP. The types of product that fall within the scope of Council Regulation (EEC) No 2309/93 as amended, were set out in the Annex to that Regulation. For medicinal products falling within the scope of Part A of the Annex applicants were obliged to use the centralised procedure, whereas for products falling within the scope of Part B of the Annex the applicants may also use the centralised procedure. The scope of the medicinal products that must go through the centralised route has been further extended by the Annex to Regulation (EC) No 726/2004.

Article 3(1) of Regulation (EC) No 726/2004 defines the so-called 'mandatory' scope of the centralised procedure. Medicinal products intended for prevention or diagnosis of diseases (as opposed to their treatment) are not included (but recommended to be considered by the applicant) in the compulsory scope of the centralised procedure unless they fall under other indents of the Annex to the Regulation. Apart from the products originally covered by Part A, the products falling within the 'mandatory' scope included new active substances used to treat HIV/AIDS, cancer, neurodegenerative diseases and diabetes as well as orphan medicinal products (Box 18.2). In addition, human medicinal products used to treat auto-immune diseases and other immune dysfunctions and viral diseases have been added from 20 May 2008.

Article 3(2) of Regulation (EC) No 726/2004 defines the so-called 'optional' scope of the centralised procedure as follows:

Any medicinal product not appearing in the Annex may be granted a marketing authorisation by the Community in accordance with the provisions of this Regulation, if:
(a) the medicinal product contains a new active substance which on the date of entry into force of this Regulation, was not authorised in the Community;
or
(b) the applicant shows that the medicinal product constitutes a significant therapeutic, scientific or technical innovation or that the granting of authorisation in accordance with this Regulation is in the interests of patients or animal health at Community level.

BOX 18.2 Human medicinal products to be authorised by the Community

Mandatory

1. Medicinal products developed by means of one of the following biotechnological processes:
   - Recombinant DNA technology
   - Controlled expression of genes coding for biologically active proteins in prokaryotes and eukaryotes including transformed mammalian cells
   - Hybridoma and monoclonal antibody methods
2. Medicinal products for human use containing a new active substance which, on the date of entry into force of this Regulation, was not authorised in the Community, for which the therapeutic indication is the treatment of any of the following diseases:
   - AIDS
   - Cancer
   - Neurodegenerative disorder
   - Diabetes
   and with effect from 20 May 2008:
   - Auto-immune diseases and other immune dysfunctions
   - Viral diseases
   After 20 May 2008, the Commission, having consulted the Agency, may present any appropriate proposal modifying this point and the Council shall take a decision on that proposal by qualified majority
3. Medicinal products that are designated as orphan medicinal products pursuant to Regulation (EC) No 141/2000

Optional

Medicinal products that, although not belonging to the abovementioned categories, are nevertheless:

1. New active substances (this may include a new chemical or biological substance, a new radiopharmaceutical substance, a different salt, ester, ether, isomer, mixture of isomers, a complex or derivative of a chemical substance that differs significantly in properties with regard to safety and/or efficacy from a chemical substance of an authorised medicinal product, a biological substance that differs in molecular structure from that of a medicinal product previously authorised or a new fixed combination of active substances)
2. Of significant therapeutic, scientific or technical innovation
3. Of benefit to society or to patients (e.g. certain medicinal products that can be supplied without a medical prescription)
4. Generic medicinal products authorised by the Community, provided that this in no way undermines either the harmonisation achieved when the reference medicinal product was evaluated or the results of that evaluation

These new provisions, and in particular the second new provision, pave the way for the authorisation, through the centralised procedure, of certain medicinal products that can be supplied without a medical prescription. Indeed, in October 2008, the EMEA recommended the first switch from prescription only to non-prescription status for a centrally authorised medicine (orlistat).

For further guidance on the EMEA procedure for confirmation of eligibility, and for examples of medicinal products that may have access to the centralised procedure based on innovation or patient interest criteria, the applicant should consult the 'Guideline on Article 3(2) of Regulation (EC) No 726/2004 – Optional scope of the centralised procedure' published on the EC website in Volume 2C of the Notice to Applicants and accessed at http://pharmacos.eudra.org/F2/eudralex/vol-2/home.htm.

Even generic versions of centrally approved products may also use the centralised procedure. To this end, Article 10(2)a of Directive 2004/27/EC defines a reference medicinal product and Article 10(2)b goes on to define a generic medicinal product as 'a medicinal product which has the same qualitative and quantitative composition in active substances and the same pharmaceutical form as the reference medicinal product, and whose bioequivalence with the reference medicinal product has been demonstrated by appropriate bioavailability studies'. The different salts, esters, ethers, isomers, mixtures of isomers, complexes or derivatives of an active substance shall be considered to be the same active substance, unless they differ significantly in properties with regard to safety and/or efficacy. In theory therefore, a copy of a biological/biotechnology reference medicinal product may be regarded as a 'biogeneric' product but, for obvious reasons, different criteria will apply when it comes to defining these.

The national procedure applies to products not obliged to use Community procedure and can be a mutual recognition procedure or a decentralised procedure. No parallel evaluation of national authorisation can take place in the EU. Both the mutual recognition procedure and the decentralised procedure aim to facilitate access to a single market by relying upon the principle of mutual recognition. Thus, with the exception of those medicinal products that are subject to the centralised procedure, a marketing authorisation or the assessment in one Member State (the so-called Reference Member State (RMS)) ought in principle to be recognised by the competent authorities of the other Member States (the so-called

Concerned Member States (CMS)), unless there are grounds for supposing that the authorisation of the medicinal product concerned may present a potential serious risk to public health.

In the mutual recognition procedure, the application is first made to one Member State and the marketing authorisation already granted by that Member State can then be entered for mutual recognition by other Member States. In the decentralised procedure, an alternative to the mutual recognition procedure, the application is submitted to all the Member States of interest with the evaluation proceeding simultaneously in all the Member States but one of them (nominated by the applicant) acting as the RMS. Because of the complete Community *acquis*, Iceland and Norway are parties to these procedures, including the Community procedure.

Sections 18.7.2 and 18.7.5 summarise special provisions that apply to applications approvable by centralised and mutual recognition/decentralised procedures, respectively.

18.7.1 Applications through Community (centralised) procedure

A successful application under the centralised procedure delivers a single marketing authorisation (a single decision from the EC) for a medicinal product valid throughout the Community under a single trade name and a common SPC. The EMEA is required to ensure that the Opinion of CHMP is given within 210 days after the receipt of a valid application.

Conceptually, this procedure for Community authorisations resembles a hybrid of the national procedure and the mutual recognition procedure, with the differences that, first, the application is submitted to EMEA; secondly, the dossier supporting the application undergoes a detailed assessment by the CHMP; thirdly, the applicant is provided with an opportunity to clarify any issues raised by any of the CHMP members; fourthly, the procedure naturally has an extended time frame but still with predetermined deadlines; and finally but perhaps most importantly, the applicant ends up with an approval or a refusal to market the product in all or any Member States of the EU.

At least 7 months before submission, applicants should notify the EMEA of their intention to submit an application and give a realistic estimate of the month of submission. At the time of receipt of the letter of intent, the proposed invented (trade) name will be checked. However, review of the trade name more than 6 months in advance of the submission date only serves to detect objections that exist at that time and not later. In any case, the applicant should submit the proposed invented name(s) at the earliest 12 months and at the latest 4–6 months prior to the planned submission date of the marketing authorisation application. In order to identify, at an early stage, potential difficulties presented by the invented name(s) proposed by an applicant, a satellite group of the CHMP, the invented Name Review Group (NRG), has been set up. The NRG consists of representatives of Member States, the European Commission and the EMEA. This check is performed in order to determine whether the name proposed would raise any identifiable public health concern. In particular, the invented name: (a) should not convey misleading therapeutic or pharmaceutical connotations; (b) should not be misleading with respect to the composition of the product; and (c) should not be liable to cause confusion in print, handwriting or speech with the invented name of an existing medicinal product. If any public health concern emerges, these should be resolved as soon as possible.

If the proposed invented name cannot be accepted prior to submission, the marketing authorisation application can be submitted either under any of the proposed invented names, the common name or scientific name accompanied by a trade mark or the name of the marketing authorisation holder. At the latest 1 month prior to the adoption of the CHMP Opinion on the application concerned, the applicant will in such case have to inform the EMEA Product Team Leader (PTL) and the NRG secretariat on the acceptable invented name of their choice. If no suitable invented name has been identified at that stage, the Opinion will be adopted according to the common name or scientific name accompanied by the name of the marketing authorisation holder.

In certain cases, companies may wish to obtain more than one marketing authorisation for the same medicinal product, through either simultaneous or subsequent applications. A specific procedure has been agreed for this between the EMEA and the EC. Under this procedure, companies should inform both the EMEA and the EC Services, at the latest 4 months prior to submission of their intentions, in particular providing the EC with an explanation of the underlying motives for the multiple applications and their intentions regarding exploitation of any authorisations granted, which could be related to the availability of medicinal products or for co-marketing reasons.

For applications to be processed via the centralised procedure, the CHMP appoints one of its members to act as rapporteur for the coordination of the evaluation of an application for a marketing authorisation. The CHMP may, and usually does, also appoint a second member to act as co-rapporteur. For line extensions, the CHMP will decide on the need for appointment of a co-rapporteur on a case-by-case basis. All members have an equal opportunity to act as the rapporteur or co-rapporteur, and therefore the CHMP members are invited submit a description of their evaluation team in writing in advance of the meeting at which rapporteurs are appointed. Appointments of rapporteur and co-rapporteur are made on the basis of the expertise and availability of the evaluation team of CHMP members based on their expertise. The CHMP now no longer take into account preferences expressed by applicants in selecting rapporteurs. In addition, some CHMP members may be assigned to 'peer review' the (co)-rapporteurs' scientific evaluation, as well as the validity of the scientific/regulatory conclusions reached, and to improve the quality of the Day 120 List of Questions. The peer review is carried out in the period between the release of the initial assessment reports (day 80) by the rapporteur(s) and the adoption of the CHMP List of Questions (day 120).

An EMEA Product Team will be set up for each application intended to be submitted through the centralised procedure. The Product Team consists of a Product Team Leader (PTL) and Product Team Members nominated by the EMEA. The applicant will be notified of the appointed PTL. The PTL, in close cooperation with the rapporteur and co-rapporteur, will also ensure that the applicant is kept informed of all issues relating to the application. The PTL will serve as the main liaison person between the EMEA, the rapporteur, the co-rapporteur and the applicant. The Product Team is responsible for the handling of all procedural aspects of the application, both in the pre- and post-authorisation stages, including providing procedural and regulatory guidance during the pre-submission phase, coordinating the validation of the application submitted, monitoring compliance with the time-frame, preparing the CHMP assessment report and coordinating all the activities with regard to the progression and final determination of the application.

The EMEA requires from the applicant:

1. One full copy of the dossier (Modules 1–5 according to the EU-CTD format), including the applicant's part of the Active Substance Master File, if any. In those cases where an Active Substance Master File exists, the applicant should ensure that the Active Substance Master File is submitted by the active substance manufacturer to the EMEA, rapporteur and co-rapporteur at around the same time as the main application.

2. Two additional copies of Modules 1 and 2 including the draft SPC, labelling and package leaflet in English.

3. One electronic copy of module 1 and 2 (at least 2.1–2.5) in WORD.

Electronic-only applications are now mandatory and the reader is referred to the following website for details. http://www.emea.europe.eu/pdfs/human/regaffair/59688107en.pdf.

In addition, applicants must submit the dossier to both the rapporteur and the co-rapporteur in parallel with the EMEA.

Applicants must include evidence of establishment in the EEA, as well as documents showing their capacity to discharge all the responsibilities required of the marketing authorisation holder under Community pharmaceutical legislation, whether they do it themselves or via one or more persons designated to that effect. The centralised procedure is shown in Figure 18.1.

On receipt of a valid application via the EMEA, the rapporteur and the co-rapporteur prepare their separate detailed assessment reports, which are circulated to the EMEA and all other Member States by day 80 from the start of the procedure. By day 100, rapporteur, co-rapporteur, CHMP members and EMEA receive comments from all other members of the CHMP. A consolidated draft list of questions is prepared by the rapporteur and circulated to the members by day 115 and may undergo peer review. A final consolidated List of Questions is agreed by the CHMP on day 120 and communicated to the applicant, and the clock of the procedure is stopped (usually up to 3 months and possibly extended by a further 3 months maximum).

This consolidated List of Questions includes any major objections, points for clarification and changes to the SPC raised by the committee. The applicant is also provided with the overall conclusions and review of the scientific data. The applicant is entitled to seek clarification from the rapporteur if necessary before responding to these issues raised. These clarification meetings between the applicant and the rapporteurs are crucial. During the procedures in 2004, 61% of the applicants had requested such meetings and the vast majority found these very useful in terms of formulating their responses. After receipt of the responses, the clock starts (day 121) and the CHMP adopts a timetable for the evaluation of the responses.

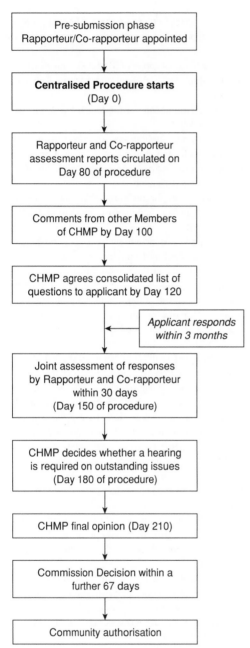

Figure 18.1 Centralised procedure. CHMP, Committee for Medicinal Products for Human Use.

The rapporteur and co-rapporteur prepare a joint assessment (of responses) report which is circulated by day 150 to all members of the CHMP. The deadline for comments from CHMP members to be sent to rapporteur and co-rapporteur, EMEA and other CHMP members is day 170. Any issue(s) still outstanding are discussed on day 180 of the procedure at the CHMP and a decision may be made on whether to issue a positive CHMP Opinion.

If there still are any outstanding issues identified, the CHMP will ask the applicant to address in writing and/or during an oral explanation. Applicants should normally respond (or prepare for an oral explanation that should normally last not more than 30–40 minutes) within 1 month. In exceptional circumstances, a 1 or maximum 2 months extension may be granted if the applicant provides appropriate justification and subject to a review of these justification and agreement by the CHMP.

Day 181 is the start of the clock when any further written response is assessed and oral explanation takes place. Days 181–210 of the procedure involves preparation of the final draft of English SPC, labelling and package leaflet sent by applicant to the rapporteur and co-rapporteur, EMEA and other CHMP members. On or before day 210, the CHMP adopts its Opinion in light of the final recommendation of the rapporteur and co-rapporteur and further evidence presented at the oral explanation. In case of an oral explanation and where the procedural timetable allows, the CHMP Opinion will be adopted at the following CHMP meeting, allowing applicant, (co)-rapporteur and CHMP members to finalise the product information and Assessment Report as appropriate. The deadline for adopting an Opinion and preparation of the CHMP Assessment Report is day 210 of the procedure with a timetable for the provision of final versions of product information translations.

If positive, the CHMP Opinion is communicated to the applicant and the EC for a binding Decision. Should the CHMP want to record any follow-up measures they will be included in the Assessment Report and referenced in a letter of undertaking signed by the applicant, which will be annexed to it. Once the medicinal product is authorised and in all cases *before* the medicinal product is placed on the market, specimens of the final outer and immediate packaging and the package leaflet must be submitted to the EMEA within a time-frame agreed between the EMEA and the applicant.

A CHMP Opinion, whether positive or negative, may be the subject of an appeal (called re-examination), a procedure that has its own time-frame. The EMEA immediately informs the applicant when the Opinion of the CHMP is that the application does not satisfy the criteria for authorisation set out in the Regulation. The following documents are annexed and/or appended to the Opinion: first, the CHMP Assessment Report stating the reasons for its negative conclusions, and secondly, when appropriate, the divergent positions of committee members, with their grounds.

The applicant may notify the EMEA/CHMP of their intention to appeal within 15 days of receipt of the Opinion (after which, if the applicant does not appeal, they are deemed to have agreed with the Opinion and it becomes the final Opinion). The grounds for appeal must be forwarded to the EMEA within the next 45 days (i.e. 60 days from receipt of the negative Opinion). The applicant may request consultation of a Scientific Advisory Group in the re-examination procedure. If the applicant wishes to appear before the CHMP for an oral explanation, this request should also be sent at this stage.

The EMEA will publish in the CHMP Press Release/'Monthly Report' a short statement on the re-examination request. Within 60 days from the receipt of the grounds for appeal, the CHMP will consider whether its Opinion should be revised. The CHMP will appoint a new rapporteur and where necessary (a) new co-rapporteur(s), different from those appointed for the initial Opinion, to co-assess the grounds for the re-examination of the Opinion. If considered necessary, an oral explanation can be held within this 60-day time-frame. The re-examination may deal only with the points of the Opinion initially identified by the applicant and may be based only on the scientific data available when the CHMP adopted the initial Opinion.

After adoption of a CHMP Opinion by day 210, the preparation of the annexes to the Commission Decision is carried out in accordance with a pre-determined timetable. For new Community author-isations, the overall duration from Opinion to Decision should not exceed 67 days. Article 10 of Regulation (EC) No 726/2004 prescribes the timelines for decision-making process by the EC. By day 215 at the latest, the applicant provides the EMEA with draft Annex A (pack sizes and pharmaceutical forms), Annex I (SPC), Annex II (legal status, manufacturer of the biological active substance and manufacturing authorisation holders responsible for batch release, conditions of the marketing authorisation, conditions or restrictions regarding supply and use imposed on the marketing authorisation holder, conditions or restrictions with regard to the safe and effective use of the medicinal product and specific obligations to be fulfilled by the marketing authorisation holder) and Annex III (labelling and package leaflet) in all the 24 languages (all official EU languages, plus Norwegian and Icelandic). EMEA circulates draft translations to Member States for review. Member States send their comments to the EMEA and final translations are agreed by day 232. By day 237 at the latest, the Opinion and the final translations of Annexes in all EU languages are transmitted to the Commission, Members of the Standing Committee, and Norway and Iceland and the applicant. The Standing Committee Consultation, that can last 22 days, begins on day 239 and this is followed by adoption of the EC Decision by day 277.

Once a product goes through the centralised procedure, all its post-approval activities are undertaken by the same rapporteur(s) and go through this procedure. Once granted a Community marketing authorisation based on Article 3(2) of the Regulation, a medicinal product can no longer be the subject of a subsequent (or previous) national marketing authorisation.

Where an applicant decides to withdraw the application before an Opinion has been adopted by the CHMP or during the appeal process, the applicant is required to communicate its reasons for doing so to the EMEA. The EMEA will make this information publicly accessible and publish the Assessment Report, if available, after deletion of all information of a commercially confidential nature (as justified by the applicant and according to the EMEA policy). Withdrawal of the application after adoption of the Opinion is treated similarly.

Chapter 4 of Volume 2A of Notice to Applicants (EudraLex) provides details of the centralised procedure and can be accessed at http://ec.europa.eu/enterprise/pharmaceuticals/eudralex/vol2_en.htm. Various guidelines concerning centralised applications and related procedures can be accessed at http://www.emea.europa.eu/htms/human/raguidelines/pre.htm.

18.7.2 Special provisions for centrally approvable products

The EU pharmaceutical legislation provides for special applications for unique medicinal products. These are applications that fall within the scope of Regulation (EC) No 726/2004 (covering Community marketing authorisations), which are categorised as applications that qualify for accelerated assessment, approval under exceptional circumstances or conditional marketing authorisation. If the applicant intends to benefit from these special provisions for their applications, this intention should be declared in the letter of intent but the final decision rests with the CHMP.

18.7.2.1 Accelerated assessment

Article 14(9) of Regulation (EC) No 726/2004, states that when an application is submitted for a marketing authorisation in respect of medicinal products for human use that are of major interest from the point of view of public health and in particular from the viewpoint of therapeutic innovation, the applicant may request an accelerated assessment procedure.

The accelerated assessment procedure is applicable to marketing authorisation applications for medicinal products for human use falling within the scope of Articles 3(1) and 3(2) of Regulation (EC) No 726/2004. This includes medicinal products intended for treatment, prevention or diagnosis.

Applicants requesting an accelerated assessment procedure should justify that the medicinal product is expected to be of major public health interest particularly from the point of view of therapeutic innovation. Based on the request, the justifications presented and the recommendations of the rapporteurs, the CHMP will formulate a decision on the request for accelerated assessment. At the time of the request, the CHMP assessment of the request is based on the justification presented in favour of a claim of major public health interest and not on the assessment of the marketing authorisation application. The CHMP will review the justifications and claims, and formulate a view on whether the request can be granted. Additionally, the CHMP can decide to shorten the time-frame of assessment on its own volition.

When an application is accepted for accelerated assessment, the time limit shall be reduced from 210 to 150 days. After a request has been granted, at any time during the marketing authorisation application evaluation, if the CHMP considers that it is no longer appropriate to conduct an accelerated assessment the CHMP may decide to continue the assessment under standard centralised procedure timelines according to Article 6(3) of Regulation (EC) No 726/2004. The duration of the assessment outside a formal request for accelerated assessment is part of the normal function of the CHMP and is outside the scope of the guideline on accelerated assessment available at http://www.emea.europa.eu/pdfs/human/euleg/41912705en.pdf.

18.7.2.2 Exceptional circumstances

In accordance with Article 14(8) of the Regulation, in exceptional circumstances, and following consultation with the applicant, an authorisation may be granted subject to a requirement for the applicant to introduce specific procedures, in particular concerning the safety of the product. Such authorisation must be based on one of the grounds set out in Directive 2001/83/EC, namely when, in respect of particular therapeutic indications, the applicant can show that he is unable to provide comprehensive data on the efficacy and safety under normal conditions of use, because:

1. The indications for which the product in question is intended are encountered so rarely that the applicant cannot reasonably be expected to provide comprehensive evidence;
2. In the present state of scientific knowledge, comprehensive information cannot be provided; or
3. It would be contrary to generally accepted principles of medical ethics to collect such information.

The applicant should include a statement on the appropriateness of the granting of a marketing authorisation under exceptional circumstances as part of the letter of intent to submit a centralised application. The applicant may request advice from the EMEA about the appropriateness of applying for a marketing authorisation under exceptional circumstances. This should preferably occur during the pre-submission meeting between the EMEA and applicant and occur at least 4–7 months before the submission of a marketing authorisation application.

Marketing authorisation may be granted under exceptional circumstances on the following conditions:

1. The applicant completes on identified programme of studies within a time period specified by the competent authority, the results of which shall form the basis of a reassessment of the benefit–risk profile;
2. The medicinal product in question may be supplied on medical prescription only and may in certain cases be administered only under strict medical supervision, possibly in a hospital, and for a radio pharmaceutical by an authorised person;
3. The package leaflet and any medical information shall draw the attention of the medical practitioner to the fact that the particulars available concerning the medicinal product in question are as yet inadequate in certain specified respects.

Continuation of the authorisation shall be linked to the annual reassessment of these conditions. Guideline on procedures for the granting of a marketing authorisation under exceptional circumstances can be accessed at http://www.emea.europa.eu/pdfs/human/euleg/35798105en.pdf.

18.7.2.3 Conditional marketing authorisation

The legal basis for conditional approval is Commission Regulation (EC) 507/2006 of 29 March 2006 on the conditional marketing authorisation for medicinal products for human use falling within the scope of Regulation (EC) No 726/2004 of the European Parliament and of the Council.

In the case of certain categories of medicinal products, in order to meet unmet medical needs of patients and in the interests of public health, it may be necessary to grant marketing authorisations on the basis of less complete data than is normally the case and subject to specific obligations, hereinafter referred to as 'conditional marketing authorisations'. However, the benefit–risk balance of the product should already be judged positive. The medicinal products that may qualify for conditional approval are those that are aimed at the treatment, prevention or medical diagnosis of seriously debilitating or life-threatening diseases, or medicinal products to be used in emergency situations in response to public health threats.

In accordance with Article 14(7) of the Regulation (EC) No 726/2004, following consultation with the applicant, the CHMP may adopt an Opinion recommending a marketing authorisation to be granted subject to certain specific obligations to be reviewed annually. The list of these obligations is made publicly accessible.

The granting of a conditional marketing authorisation will allow medicines to reach patients with unmet medical needs earlier than might otherwise be the case, and will ensure that additional data on a product are generated, submitted, assessed and acted upon. The applicant should notify the EMEA about its intention to request a conditional marketing authorisation as part of the letter of intent to submit a centralised application. Conditional marketing authorisations will be valid for 1 year, on a renewable basis. Before expiry, the marketing authorisation holder shall apply for the renewal of the marketing authorisation.

18.7.2.4 Compassionate use

By way of exemption from Article 6 of Directive 2001/83/EC, Member States may make available for compassionate use a medicinal product for human use belonging to the categories referred to in Article 3(1) and (2) of Regulation (EC) No 726/2004.

For the purposes of this Article, 'compassionate use' means making a medicinal product available for compassionate reasons to a group of patients with a chronically or seriously debilitating disease or whose disease is considered to be life-threatening, and who cannot be treated satisfactorily by an authorised medicinal product. The medicinal product concerned must either be the subject of an application for a marketing authorisation in accordance with Article 6 of this Regulation or must be undergoing clinical trials. The Member State permitting the compassionate use must inform the EMEA.

When compassionate use is envisaged, the CHMP, after consulting the manufacturer or the applicant, may adopt Opinions on the conditions for use, the conditions for distribution and the patients targeted. The Opinions shall be updated on a regular basis. These CHMP Opinions are forwarded to the Member States who shall take them into account. However, the CHMP Opinions do not affect the civil or criminal liability of the manufacturer or of the applicant for marketing authorisation.

Where a compassionate use programme has been set up, the applicant shall ensure that patients taking part also have access to the new medicinal product during the period between authorisation and placing on the market.

Guideline on compassionate use of medicinal products can be accessed at http://www.emea.europa.eu/pdfs/human/euleg/2717006enfin.pdf.

18.7.2.5 Enforcement and penalties

In June 2007, the EC adopted Commission Regulation (EC) 658/2007 concerning the imposition by the Commission of financial penalties on the holders of marketing authorisations in order to ensure the enforcement of certain obligations connected with marketing authorisations granted in accordance with the centralised procedure. This Regulation implements Article 84(3) of Regulation (EC) No 726/2004 and came into force in July 2007.

The Regulation lists the obligations linked to marketing authorisations and the conditions which may lead to Community enforcement, and provides for the maximum amount for penalties, the criteria for the imposition of penalties and the elements of the infringement procedure. Article 1 of this Regulation lists 17 types of infringements. Among others, this includes the completeness and the accuracy of the particulars and documents contained in an application for marketing authorisation, conditions or restrictions included in the market authorisation and concerning the supply or use of the medicinal product, conditions or restrictions included in the marketing authorisation with regard to the safe and effective use of the medicinal product, the introduction of any necessary variations to the terms of the marketing authorisation to take account of technical and scientific progress and enable the medicinal products to be manufactured and checked by means of generally accepted scientific methods, the supply of any new information that may entail a variation to the terms of the marketing authorisation, the notification of any prohibition or restriction imposed by the competent authorities of any country in which the medicinal product is marketed, or the supply of any information that may influence the evaluation of the risks and benefits of the product, the supply at the request of the Agency of any data demonstrating that the risk–benefit balance remains favourable, notification to the Agency of the dates of actual marketing and of the date when the product ceases to be on the market, recording and reporting of suspected serious adverse reactions, reporting of suspected serious unexpected adverse reactions and suspected transmission of infectious agents, communication of information relating to pharmacovigilance concerns to the general public and collation and assessment of specific pharmacovigilance data.

These new provisions are expected to contribute to the strategic goals of the Community framework for the authorisation and surveillance of medicinal products, thereby ensuring that public health is adequately protected across the Community, and supporting the achievement of the internal market for the pharmaceutical sector.

To that effect, the Regulation aims to strengthen the application of the Community pharmaceutical rules through a stronger involvement of the EMEA and the Commission in the area of marketing authorisations granted through the centralised procedure. The Regulation will raise the deterrent effect of the Community rules and will increase the efficiency of the enforcement system for marketing authorisations granted through the centralised procedure, by providing for a single mechanism for the enforcement of obligations linked to these authorisations where the infringement has a Community dimension or effect.

18.7.2.6 Sunset clause

The marketing authorisation remains valid if at least one presentation of the marketing authorisation is placed on the market in the Community (in at least one Member State) including Iceland, Norway and Liechtenstein. In accordance with Article 14(4) of Regulation (EC) No 726/2004, any marketing authorisation that is not followed by the actual marketing in the Community within 3 years after the granting of the authorisation shall cease to be valid. However, the start of the 3-year period should be the date when the medicinal product can be placed on the market by the marketing authorisation holder. For generic applications, this is as of the end of the 10- or 11-year

period of market exclusivity of the reference medicinal product and at the end of other protection rules which must be respected.

Article 14(5) of Regulation (EC) No 726/2004 makes a similar provision for any medicinal product previously placed on the market but no longer actually present on the market for 3 consecutive years.

This new provision applies prospectively to all centrally authorised medicinal products from the date of entry into force of the Regulation (i.e. 20 November 2005).

Therefore, for medicinal products which have been granted a marketing authorisation before 20 November 2005 and for which no more presentations are marketed in the Community at this date, the 3-year period which may lead to the marketing authorisation ceasing to be valid will start counting as of 20 November 2005.

The EMEA will monitor the application of the sunset clause provision via an electronic tool (so-called 'sunset timer') which will run and be updated based on the marketing status data reported by the marketing authorisation holder for a specific medicinal product.

According to the Articles 14(6) of Regulation (EC) No 726/2004, the Commission may grant exemptions from the application of the sunset clause on public health grounds and in exceptional circumstances. Exemptions can apply at any time of the marketing authorisation life cycle, depending on the type of exemptions. It is the responsibility of the marketing authorisation holder to provide an adequate justification for consideration by and decision of the Commission.

18.7.3 Applications through mutual recognition procedure

Once a medicinal product has been granted a marketing authorisation by one of the Member States, the marketing authorisation holder may request that the marketing authorisation be entered into this procedure for mutual recognition by other Member States. Within 90 days of the receipt of this request, the original competent authority (the RMS) transmits the assessment report (updated if necessary), together with the SPC approved by it, to each Member State (the CMS) from whom the applicant seeks a marketing authorisation. The applicant submits an identical application (with the dossier updated if necessary) to each Member State from whom the applicant seeks a marketing authorisation (CMS).

During this procedure, the original competent authority and the applicant act jointly. The role of the

RMS is to act as the scientific assessor of the dossier, regulatory advisor to the applicant, a moderator in facilitating discussions between the applicant and the CMSs, to arrange, chair and administer the face-to-face meeting (breakout session) between the applicant and the CMSs and to close the procedure appropriately.

On receipt of an application for mutual recognition, each CMS treats the application almost as a national application with the important differences that, first, they deal with the RMS (rather than the applicant) in respect of any concerns, queries or need for clarification and, secondly, the procedure is driven by predetermined immutable deadlines.

This procedure applies when a medicinal product has been granted a marketing authorisation by one of the Member States or when the same medicinal product is being examined by more than one Member States. Where a Member State is informed that another Member State has authorised a medicinal product which is the subject of a marketing authorisation or notes that an application for the same medicinal product is being examined in another Member State, the Member State concerned shall reject the application and shall advise the applicant accordingly.

The procedure has a finite immutable duration of 90 days. At the completion of the procedure, the applicant should anticipate receiving a number of essentially identical marketing authorisations, the only differences being in the authorisation number, product name, pack size or marketing authorisation holder.

The mutual recognition procedure is shown in Figure 18.2. The procedure begins on day 1 following validation of the application by all CMSs. For practical purposes, the exact date of day 1 is determined so that day 75 approximately would coincide with a meeting of the Coordination Group for Mutual Recognition and Decentralised Procedures for Human Medicinal Products (CMD(h)) (see section 18.7.5.3) and is normally within 14 days of validation. By day 50, all CMSs are required to have communicated their concerns to the RMS.

In response to the objections or questions communicated to the applicant by the CMSs, it is recommended that the applicant should provide a draft response document to the RMS well before day 60, so that the RMS can comment on the responses and support the applicant's response document, when considered as satisfactory, with a letter. By day 60, the applicant should respond to the CMSs, enclosing an RMS-approved revised SPC. Additional information from the applicant should always be sent to all the CMSs and to the RMS but it should be noted that the applicant does not have the possibility of addressing questions and/or objections by providing additional studies during the procedure.

The RMS should in all situations evaluate the response given by the applicant (to the issues raised by the CMSs) and communicate these in writing to all CMSs by day 68 at the latest.

By day 75, outstanding issues of serious risks to public health should be communicated by the CMSs to the applicant and the RMS and these are discussed in a face-to-face meeting, known as the Breakout Session. The 'Breakout Session' is organised under the responsibility of the RMS to discuss the applications and/or to resolve outstanding questions. Breakout sessions are arranged, where possible, to coincide with CMD(h) meetings. The RMS will inform the marketing authorisation holder if it is considered that representatives from the applicant should be available at the relevant meeting to aid in the resolution of these issues. Although applicants should be aware that they may not be required to participate in the session, they may be asked to agree amendments to the SPC, package leaflet and labelling or to answer questions from the CMSs. Applicants should therefore ensure that their representatives are able to take decisions on amendments to the SPC, package leaflet and labelling being proposed by Member States.

All CMSs should give their final Opinion at latest on day 85. On occasion, further discussion may be needed (either by telephone conference, videoconference or in a meeting) around day 85 to avoid a procedure in the CMD(h) or an arbitration by the CHMP. Any further changes in the SPC, package leaflet and labelling should be agreed on by the RMS and all other CMSs.

All CMSs notify the RMS and the applicant of their final position by day 90. If consensus is reached, the RMS closes the procedure with a final version of the SPC. In case of a negative position and the Member States are unable to reach a consensus, the CMS also notifies the secretariat of the CMD(h) at the EMEA. The application is referred to the CMD(h) (see section 18.7.5.3) with the RMS submitting to CMD(h) within 7 days the points of disagreement submitted by CMS(s) on day 90 of the procedure. (For withdrawal of applications during mutual recognition procedure see section 18.7.5.2.)

Once a product goes through the mutual recognition procedure, all its post-approval activities (variations and extensions) are undertaken by the original RMS and go through the same procedure. Specific

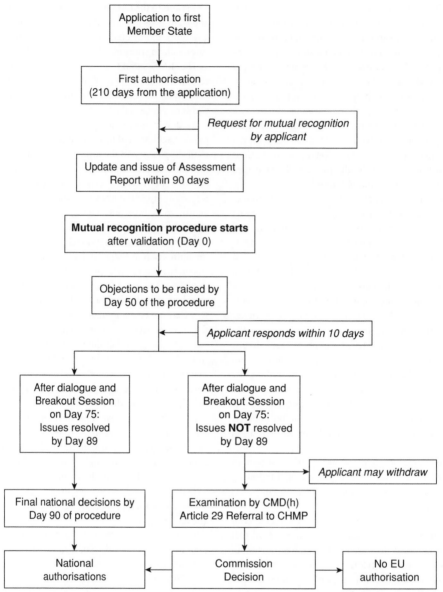

Figure 18.2 Mutual recognition procedure: CMD(h) Coordination Group for Mutual Recognition and Decentralised Procedures for Human Medicinal Products.

national requirements for labelling and package leaflet have to be presented in a so-called 'blue box' and these are listed in Section 10 of Chapter 7 of Volume 2A of Notice to Applicants (EudraLex).

Chapter 2 of Volume 2A of Notice to Applicants (EudraLex) provides details of the mutual recognition procedure and can be accessed at http://ec.europa.eu/enterprise/pharmaceuticals/eudralex/vol2_en.htm.

18.7.4 Applications through decentralised procedure

The decentralised procedure has proved to be very popular and some Member States have been inundated with requests to act as RMS. In 2007, five Member States accounted for 85% of all decentralised procedures (Germany with 273, the UK with 222, Denmark with 218, the Netherlands with 140 and

Sweden with 49 procedures). As a result, following discussions with a Member State well in advance of the proposed submission date, one Member State will be appointed by the applicant to act as RMS who will allocate a slot for submission and on receipt of a validated application, prepare a draft assessment report with a draft SPC and a draft of the labelling and package leaflet.

The decentralised procedure is to be used in order to obtain marketing authorisations in several Member States where the medicinal product in question has not yet received a marketing authorisation in any Member State at the time of application.

It is an alternative to mutual recognition procedure for new products. The procedure to be followed will depend upon whether it is a Member State or the marketing authorisation holder that initiates the decentralised procedure.

As set out in Directive 2001/83/EC, Member States have to approve during the decentralised procedure the assessment report, the SPC, the package leaflet and the label. Specific national requirements for labelling and package leaflet have to be presented in a so-called 'blue box' and these are listed in Section 10 of Chapter 7 of Volume 2A of Notice to Applicants (EudraLex). The assessment process during decentralised procedure takes place in two steps.

Step I is a 120-day procedure followed by step II procedure, which has duration of a further 90 days. If no agreement can be reached at the end of step II, the application then requires referral to the CMD(h) (see section 18.7.5.3). The decentralised procedure is shown in Figure 18.3.

Step I commences when the RMS starts the procedure on day 0 and forwards the preliminary assessment report (PrAR), SPC, patient information leaflet (PIL) and labelling to the CMSs on day 70. The CMSs have until day 100 to send their comments to the RMS. By day 105, there is consultation between the RMS, CMSs and applicant. If consensus not reached, the RMS stops the clock to allow the applicant to supplement the dossier and respond to the questions. The applicant sends the final response document to the RMS and CMSs within a recommended period of 3 months, which could be extended if justified. On receipt of the responses, the clock is restarted as day 106 and the RMS updates the PrAR to prepare a draft assessment report (DAR), draft SPC, draft labelling and draft PIL which are sent to CMSs by day 120. The RMS may close the procedure if consensus is reached.

If on day 120 of step I consensus is not reached, step II begins with the RMS sending the DAR, draft SPC, draft labelling and draft PIL to CMSs who have a further 25 days (day 145) in which to send their comments. The RMS may close procedure if consensus is reached (day 150) but if not, the RMS should communicate any outstanding issues to the applicant, receive any additional clarification and prepare a short report for discussion within the next 30 days (day 180). A Breakout Session involving the Member States should reach consensus on the matter within the next 25 days (day 205). Over the next 5 days (day 210), the procedure is closed with the CMSs approval of assessment report, SPC, labelling and PIL. If consensus is not reached by day 210, the application is referred to the CMD(h) with a view to resolving the points of disagreement (see section 18.7.5.3).

When consensus is reached at any time during steps I and II of the procedure or following resolution of the points of disagreement by CMD(h), the procedure is closed. This is followed by a 30-day period for national authorisations to be granted. To this end, the applicant has 5 days during which to send high quality national translations of SPC, labelling and PIL to the CMSs and RMS. The Member States then have a further 25 days in which to issue the marketing authorisations.

If the points of disagreement remain unresolved following the end of referral to CMD(h), the application is referred to the CHMP for arbitration.

Chapter 2 of Volume 2A of Notice to Applicants (EudraLex) provides details of the decentralised recognition procedure and can be accessed at http://ec.europa.eu/enterprise/pharmaceuticals/eudralex/vol2_en.htm.

18.7.5 Special provisions for mutual recognition and decentralised procedures

18.7.5.1 Definition of potential serious risk to public health

Following the reform of the legislation, in March 2006 the EC issued a guideline on the definition of a potential serious risk to public health. For the application of this guideline, a 'risk' is defined as the probability that an event will occur and a 'potential serious risk to public health' is defined as a situation where there is a significant probability that a serious hazard resulting from a human medicinal product in the context of its proposed use will affect public health. 'Serious' in this context means a hazard that could result in death, be life-threatening, result in patient hospitalisation or prolongation of existing hospitalisation, result in persistent or significant disability or incapacity, or be a congenital anomaly/birth defect or permanent or

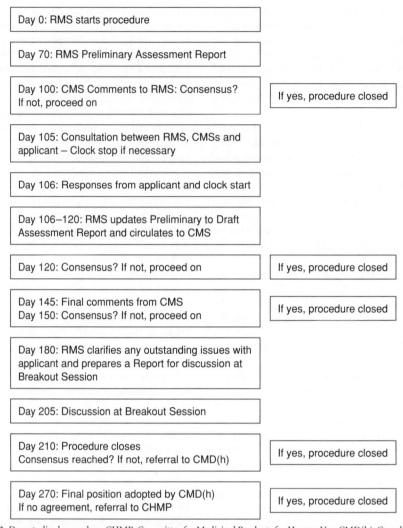

Figure 18.3 Decentralised procedure. CHMP, Committee for Medicinal Products for Human Use; CMD(h), Coordination Group for Mutual Recognition and Decentralised Procedures for Human Medicinal Products; CMS, Concerned Member State; RMS, Reference Member State.

prolonged signs in exposed humans. The assessment of a 'potential serious risk to public health' cannot be made in isolation but has to take into account the positive therapeutic effects of the medicinal product in question.

Therefore, a potential serious risk to public health in relation to a particular medicinal product can be considered to exist when:

1. The data submitted to support therapeutic efficacy in the proposed indication(s), target population(s) and proposed dosing regimen (as defined by the proposed labelling) do not provide sound scientific justification for the claims for efficacy or adequate proof of bioequivalence of the generic medicinal products to the reference medicinal product is lacking.

2. The evaluation of the preclinical toxicity and/or safety pharmacology, clinical safety data and post-marketing data does not provide adequate support for the conclusion that all potential safety issues for the target population have been appropriately and adequately addressed in the proposed labelling or the absolute level of risk from the medicinal product, in the context of its proposed use, is considered unacceptable.

3. The proposed production and quality control methods cannot guarantee that a major deficiency in the quality of the product will not occur.

4. The overall risk–benefit balance for the product is not considered to be favourable, taking into account the nature of the identified risk(s) and the potential benefit in the proposed indication(s) and target patient population(s).

5. The product information is misleading or incorrect for either the prescribers or patients to ensure the safe use of the medicinal product.

Any major objection must be scientifically justified, taking into account the nature and degree of any hazards, the magnitude of the risks involved, the benefits associated with the use of the product and the feasibility and practicality of the implementation of any measures to mitigate the risks. Any objection on the grounds of a potential serious risk to public health cannot be justified by differences in national administrative or national scientific requirements, or internal national policies, unless the conditions or Article 29(1) of Directive 2001/83/EC are fulfilled.

Although it will ultimately depend on the nature of each individual medicinal product, it is questionable whether major objections based on any of the following are sustainable:

1. The absence of an active comparator study versus a specific medicinal product.

2. The lack of clinical trials in a subgroup of patients who are not the target of the medicinal product. However, in this context, it is well to remember that regulatory authorities are now anxious that medicinal products are investigated in patient populations that are all inclusive of the society (in terms of age, gender and ethnicity).

3. The absence of evidence demonstrating added therapeutic value of the new medicine in comparison to existing medicines.

4. The length of the treatment varies according to national medical practices in the various Member States.

5. The targeted population is too narrow, and should include patients who are allergic or intolerant to medicinal products approved for the same indications.

6. A Member State requires a special interaction study with a medicinal product that is not usually prescribed or used together with the new medicinal product.

18.7.5.2 Withdrawal during the procedures

During the mutual recognition or the decentralised procedure, the applicant may withdraw the applications anytime before day 90 from those CMSs (on average one or two) that still have major public health concerns. If the applicant refuses to withdraw the application from a CMS that has major public health concerns, the CMS has no choice but to refer the application to the CMD(h) (see section 18.7.5.3). The RMS (but not the applicant) too is free to, and should, refer the application to the CMD(h) if it considers any major objection to be unreasonable. Although an application for a marketing authorisation may be withdrawn by the applicant at any time during the mutual recognition procedure, once a potential serious risk to public health has been raised to be dealt with by the CMD(h) and if not resolved successfully, by the CHMP in an arbitration procedure, the Opinion of the CMD(h) and of the CHMP will be given unless all applications and existing marketing authorisations for the product are withdrawn. In other words, withdrawing from a Member State is not sufficient to avoid arbitration. In the latter case, the CHMP may decide either to close or to continue the referral procedure if there still is a public health concern.

Member States that have approved the assessment report, the draft SPC and the labelling and package leaflet of the RMS may, at the request of the applicant, authorise the medicinal product without waiting for the outcome of the referral procedure. In that event, the authorisation granted is without prejudice to the outcome of that procedure.

18.7.5.3 Referral to the Coordination Group (CMD(h))

In contrast to the earlier legislation whereby a referral for arbitration was made directly to the CPMP, the new legislation requires that the arbitration by CHMP is preceded by an examination of any question relating to marketing authorisation by the CMD(h) set up in accordance with the legal procedures laid down.

The CMD(h) started its activities in November 2005 and replaced the former informal Mutual Recognition Facilitation Group, which was in operation for over 10 years, to coordinate and facilitate the operation of the mutual recognition procedure. In contrast, the CMD(h) is a legally empowered body which has been set up in compliance of the revised pharmaceutical legislation (Directive 2004/27/EC amending Directive 2001/83/EC) for the examination of any question relating to marketing authorisation of a medicinal product in two or more Member States in accordance with the mutual recognition procedure or the decentralised procedure. The CMD(h) holds monthly meetings at the EMEA and the meetings take place during the week of the CHMP meeting and have a duration of 2 to 3 days.

CMD(h) is composed of one representative per Member State (including Norway, Iceland and Liechtenstein) appointed for a renewal term of 3 years. Members of the CMD(h) may arrange to be accompanied by experts. Its responsibilities also include:

1. To consider the points of disagreement in case of disagreement between the Member States involved in a mutual recognition or decentralised procedure on the assessment report, the summary of product characteristics, labelling or the package leaflet on the grounds of 'potential serious risk to public health'.

2. To establish, yearly, a list of medicinal products for which a harmonised summary of product characteristics should be drawn up, to promote harmonisation of marketing authorisations across the Community.

Mrs Truus Janse-de Hoog (the Netherlands) was elected chairperson of the CMD(h) for a term of 3 years and re-elected in November 2008. The vice-chairperson of the CMD(h) is the member of the CMD(h) who is representing the Member State that holds the presidency of the Council of the European Union for the duration of the term of the presidency.

Where one or more of the CMSs cannot approve the assessment report, the SPC, labelling or the package leaflet of an application for a marketing authorisation, submitted through the mutual recognition or the decentralised route, the points of disagreement are referred to the CMD(h). The reasons for disagreement shall be on grounds of potential serious risk to public health. The Member State(s) that cannot approve the documents mentioned above shall notify the RMS, other CMSs, the CMD(h) secretariat at the EMEA and the applicant at day 90 for mutual recognition applications and at day 210 at the latest for decentralised applications. The notification should include a detailed exposition of the reasons for the negative position. It is the duty of the RMS to refer the matter to the CMD(h). In cases where the RMS is negative on the application but one or more CMSs are positive, it is likewise the duty of the RMS to refer the matter to CMD(h).

From the legislation it is clear that a referral to CMD(h) should be made if any Member State cannot approve the assessment report, SPC, labelling and the package leaflet within the time period laid down in Article 28(4). The time period in Article 28(4) is the 90-day procedure of the mutual recognition procedure and the 90-day period following the submission of the draft documents referred to in Article 28(3) (i.e. the end of the assessment step II in the decentralised procedure).

Within the CMD(h), all Member States are expected to use their best endeavours to reach agreement on the action to be taken. They should allow the applicant the opportunity to make their point of view known orally or in writing. If, within 60 days of the communication of the points of disagreement, the Member States reach an agreement, the RMS shall record the agreement, close the procedure and inform the applicant accordingly. Each Member State in which an application has been submitted shall adopt a decision in conformity with the approved assessment report, the SPC and labelling and package leaflet as approved and grant a marketing authorisation within 30 days after acknowledgement of the agreement.

The secretariat will propose a starting date for the 60-day procedure which should be no later than day 30 after day 90/210 of the procedure concerned and day 60 of the referral is recommended to be set at least 5–10 days after a CMD(h) meeting. The procedure does not include a clock stop.

This referral begins with day 0 when the RMS distributes a proposal for the list of questions to all Member States for agreement. On day 10, the CMD(h) secretariat sends the agreed list of questions to the applicant and inquires whether the applicant wishes to make his point of view known in writing only or have it presented orally at a CMD(h) meeting. Applicants are advised to discuss with the RMS the need for an oral explanation for all or specific questions. On about day 20 (corresponding to the meeting of CMD(h) and referred to as meeting 1), the list of questions is tabled for information. If needed, Member States can discuss the reasons for the referral and the positions of the RMS and CMSs. The CMD(h) will also consider taking advice from the CHMP, the HMPC or their working parties and other scientific advisory groups. On or before day 25, the applicant sends the responses to the list of questions to all CMD(h) members. Around day 35, the RMS should circulate an updated assessment report to all CMD(h) members and to the applicant. Seven days before the next meeting of the CMD(h), referred to as meeting 2, all members of CMD(h) should preferably state their view on the response document in writing to all other CMD(h) members. The comments from the CMSs on the response document will be shared by the RMS with the applicant. The main scientific discussion should take place at the following CMD(h) meeting (referred to as meeting 2). The members of CMD(h) can be accompanied by relevant national experts who should preferably be different from those taking the decisions in the advisory committees of the EMEA but it is up to the individual Member States to decide on participation. The views from the applicant, orally or in writing, should be taken into account.

In summary, CMD(h) is informed of the List of Questions at meetings 1 on or about day 20, and the full discussion among all the parties concerned on these issues takes place at meeting 2 on or about day 50, of the referral and the procedure is concluded on day 60. To ensure the efficiency of the procedure, the members of CMD(h) should have the proper mandate to make it possible to reach an agreement according the Article 29 of the Directive. In case no agreement could be reached at the meeting, the full 60 days, as foreseen in the legislation, should be used to obtain an agreement between the RMS, CMSs and the applicant. In this situation, the RMS should circulate the final proposal for agreement on the procedure on day 55 at the latest. The RMS should ensure that all CMSs have been provided the opportunity to state their final view until the end of the given timeline.

If the Member States reach an agreement within these 60 days, the RMS shall record the agreement, close the procedure and inform the applicant of the outcome. Subsequently the Member States shall adopt the decision in conformity with the agreed SPC, labelling and PIL within 30 days after reaching the agreement. To obtain an approval in the Member States where the application has been withdrawn, a repeat use procedure must be started.

If the Member States fail to reach an agreement during the 60-day period, the RMS should immediately inform the EMEA and the applicant and provide a detailed statement of the unresolved issues and the reasons for the disagreement, with a view to proceeding with the arbitration by CHMP (Article 29 referral, of Directive 2001/83/EC; see section 18.8). The EMEA shall be provided with a detailed statement of the matters on which the Member States have been unable to reach agreement and the reasons for their disagreement. A copy shall be forwarded to the applicant. As soon as the applicant is informed that the matter has been referred to the EMEA, the applicant shall forthwith forward to the EMEA a copy of relevant information and documents referred to in the first subparagraph of Article 28(1) of Directive 2001/83/EC.

18.7.5.4 Change of RMS

A change of RMS cannot take place during a pending procedure. In *exceptional* circumstances, the marketing authorisation holder may request a change of the RMS. The change may be needed for a variety of commercial reasons or when a medicinal product has more than one RMS for the different pharmaceutical forms of the medicinal product. These are examples and other reasons might be justified. However, a request for the change of RMS based on scientific disagreement between the marketing authorisation holder and the current RMS is not acceptable. The competent authority of a Member State may decide upon other reasons of non-acceptance.

18.7.5.5 Repeat use

It is possible to use the mutual recognition procedure more than once for subsequent applications to other Member States in relation to the same medicinal product (so-called repeat use). However, it is recommended that, wherever feasible, the marketing authorisation holder considers involving all Member States where the product is intended to be marketed in the first use of mutual recognition procedure or decentralised procedure.

In the case where the applicant withdraws his application for marketing authorisation during a mutual recognition or decentralised procedure, this does not prevent the marketing authorisation holder from initiating a second procedure of mutual recognition for that/those Member State(s) at a later stage. Each subsequent procedure will be treated as a new mutual recognition procedure including the possibility for the new CMSs to raise objections based on potential serious risk to public health.

In the case of such a repeat use procedure, the subsequent application for mutual recognition will have to comprise the original dossier updated by any variation or renewal that had been approved and/or amended after authorisation; if necessary, additional data accepted by all Member States involved in the previous procedure and a proposal for an SPC, package leaflet and labelling identical to that currently authorised. The RMS will send the original assessment report, including the assessment of the updated dossier and variations, as an Annex or as an updated assessment report to the CMSs.

In order to initiate a repeat use of a previous mutual recognition procedure after 30 October 2005, the applicant will have to obtain harmonisation of the package leaflet and labelling of the medicinal product concerned. Differences between the SPC, package leaflet and labelling approved in one Member State and the SPC, package leaflet and labelling submitted in another Member State do not automatically prevent the latter from a mutual recognition procedure. If these differences have no therapeutic implications (no difference in the efficacy and safety profile, i.e.

both products have the same qualitative and quantitative (strength) composition in active substance and the same pharmaceutical form), they have to be considered as being the same and a mutual recognition procedure has to be followed.

Member States concerned in any repeated mutual recognition procedure shall normally recognise the authorisation granted in the previous procedure. In exceptional circumstances, where a CMS considers that there are grounds for supposing that authorisation of the medicinal product concerned may present a potential serious risk to public health, the Member State shall refer the matter to the CMD(h). The applicant cannot stop this procedure by subsequently withdrawing the application in the referring Member State. If no agreement can be reached in this group the matter is referred for arbitration to the EMEA. Any matter dealt with by the CMD(h) in a previous mutual recognition procedure or decentralised procedure may not be raised again in any subsequent procedure except for justified reasons. Similarly, matters dealt with in arbitration in a previous mutual recognition procedure or decentralised procedure may also not be raised again in any subsequent procedure.

18.7.5.6 Sunset clause
The CMD(h) have recently given their interpretation of the legislation with regard to the fate of marketing authorisations that have been obtained through the mutual recognition or the decentralised procedure concerning the product(s) which are subsequently not marketed in the RMS or CMS. According to the CMD(h), the provisions of Article 24(4–6) of Directive 2001/83/EC should be applied individually to each separate marketing authorisation granted by a national competent authority even where those authorisations are duplicates. Therefore, it is not enough if the product approved by the 'original marketing authorisation' is marketed if the duplicate has not been marketed for 3 consecutive years. The marketing authorisation of the duplicate should then cease to be valid. The same principle applies if only the duplicate is marketed and not the 'original'. The change of ownership to a marketing authorisation does not change the application of the sunset clause.

18.7.6 Application for orphan drug designation
In order to benefit from the incentives available to them, sponsors of medicinal products intended for rare diseases can apply for orphan designation. Sponsors should notify the EMEA of their intention to submit an application at least 2 months prior to the planned submission date and are generally advised to have a pre-submission meeting with the EMEA secretariat.

A sponsor applying for designation of a medicinal product as an orphan medicinal product can apply for designation at any stage of the development of the medicinal product before the application for marketing authorisation is made. This means that if a marketing authorisation application for the same medicinal product has already been submitted by the same sponsor in any Member State within the Community or centrally through the EMEA, whether or not the marketing authorisation has been granted, then that medicinal product is no longer eligible for designation as an orphan drug in the indication that is the proposed therapeutic indication in the marketing authorisation application.

To meet the criteria for a successful orphan designation, the applicant should establish:

1. That the medicinal product is intended to treat, prevent or diagnose a disease or condition (medical plausibility);
2. The life-threatening or debilitating nature of the condition;
3. That the prevalence of the condition in the Community is not more than 5 in 10,000; or that it is unlikely that marketing the medicinal product in the Community, without incentives, would generate sufficient return to justify the necessary investment;
4. That no satisfactory method of diagnosis, prevention or treatment exists, or if such a method exists, that the medicinal product will be of significant benefit to those affected by the condition.

All four criteria must be satisfied and all claims require supporting data or should be adequately substantiated to the satisfaction of the COMP. A sponsor may apply for designation of a medicinal product as an orphan medicinal product for an already approved medicinal product provided the orphan designation concerns an unapproved therapeutic indication. In this case, at the time of application for a marketing authorisation, the marketing authorisation holder shall apply for a separate marketing authorisation (with a different trade name) which will cover only the orphan indication(s). If more than one orphan indication is applied for the same product, separate designation applications should be submitted for each such indication. In this regard, 'treatment' and 'prevention' of the same condition are considered as two separate indications.

In addition to all the required administrative information, the application should include detailed information concerning:

1. Description of the condition;
2. Prevalence of the condition;
3. Potential for return on investment (when this is the basis for the application);
4. Existence of other methods of diagnosis, prevention or treatment;
5. Description of the stage of development;
6. Bibliography.

The sponsor of a medicinal product for human use may desire to seek orphan designation of its medicinal product from the EC and from the US FDA. In such a case, the sponsor may apply for orphan designation of the same medicinal product for the same use in both jurisdictions by using the common application form which is then submitted to both the EMEA and the FDA.

On receipt of a valid application, the COMP appoints two or three coordinators (one or two COMP members, one EMEA staff member) for each application. The EMEA coordinator, in association with the COMP coordinator(s), will prepare a summary report on the application. The summary report will include data reported in the sponsor's application, a critical review and a conclusion. Where there is a need for written or oral explanation from the sponsor, this will be highlighted in the summary report. In this case, the report will identify the main issues to be addressed by the sponsor.

Following agreement between the EMEA coordinator and the COMP coordinator(s), the summary report will be circulated to the COMP members for comments. Members of COMP will forward comments to EMEA, with other COMP members on copy, in accordance with the adopted timetable. The summary report is discussed at the COMP meeting (day 60). If the COMP is satisfied that the criteria are met, a positive Opinion is issued. More often than not, there are issues that require clarification and a list of questions or issues to be addressed is sent to the applicant and an invitation to a hearing. The responses are assessed by the two coordinators and discussed at the next meeting (day 90). If there are outstanding issues, these can be dealt with during an oral hearing on day 90, following which the Opinion is issued. In case of a negative Opinion, the applicant has full appeal rights with the appeal procedure which has a 30-day time-frame. In practice, this time-frame is much shorter because the appeal is determined at the next COMP meeting. This re-examination is usually subject to a review by a different set of coordinators. It is worth stressing that in contrast to CHMP Opinions, only a negative Opinion from COMP can be the subject of an appeal.

Designation of a product as orphan is based on presumptions for significant benefit and is not an endorsement of its safety or efficacy in the indication proposed because the designated product has yet to be shown and assessed to be safe and effective.

Once final, the Opinion of COMP is forwarded to the EC who issue a binding Decision within 30 days and the designated product is placed on the Community Register of Orphan Medicinal Products. This is followed by publication of the Summary of COMP Opinion on the EMEA website.

As of 6 November 2008, a total of 569 medicines have been awarded orphan designation status by the EC, based on recommendations of the COMP. Of these, 50 have now been successful in obtaining a positive EMEA Opinion on marketing authorisation, with many more positive Opinions expected over the coming years. The list of these 50 products is available at http://www.emea.europa.eu/pdfs/human/comp/56357508en.pdf.

The Commission guideline on the format and content of applications for designation as orphan medicinal products and on the transfer of designations from one sponsor to another can be accessed at http://www.emea.europa.eu/pdfs/human/comp/628300en.pdf. A number of guidelines relevant to orphan drug designation are available at http://www.emea.europa.eu/htms/human/raguidelines/orphans.htm.

18.7.7 Application for scientific advice or protocol assistance

In order to optimise drug development, it is often necessary to obtain scientific views (scientific advice) from the authorities on issues that are not regulatory in nature and that are *not* covered by existing guidelines, or when the applicant is proposing to deviate from these guidelines. Scientific advice also facilitates the evaluation of the dossier, as there are no ambiguities or inconsistencies between Member States. It is particularly important to seek this advice before embarking on phase III studies. Protocol assistance is the term used for scientific advice for the development of orphan medicinal products.

Protocol assistance for orphan drugs is essential in view of the unique challenges associated with the development of these products (small sample sizes, widely distributed patient population, study designs, use of comparators versus placebo, the choice of endpoints and making sure that all criteria for designation are likely to be addressed, especially demonstrating significant benefit over authorised products).

Applicants are free to solicit advice from individual Member States and, according to various surveys conducted by the European Federation of Pharmaceutical Industries and Associations, they often do. Apart from the FDA, these surveys reveal the EU Member States most often consulted are Germany, France, the Netherlands, Sweden and the UK. However, it is often important to secure pan-European advice.

The SAWP currently faces a continuous increase in the number of procedures and meetings with applicants. A steep increase in the number of procedures was observed since 2001, nearly doubling in 4 years (109 procedures were finalised in 2004). Therefore, a new procedure was adopted by the CHMP in April 2005, providing for earlier and greater involvement of internal assessors and external experts from the pre-submission phase to final scientific advice. The objective has been to streamline the procedure to allow finalisation within 40 or maximally 70 days (compared with the 100-day procedure in the previous framework). This new framework will also consolidate the involvement of CHMP by formalising the peer review before final adoption of the letter to maximise the clarity and ensure consistency in the provision of scientific advice. The success of the new procedures is reflected by the fact that 288 procedures (including 73 for protocol assistance) were finalised in 2007. During 2008, this number had increased to 328 procedures, of which 65 were for protocol assistance.

Fees are chargeable for the scientific advice and the level depends not on the number of questions but on whether the advice is requested on all or any combination of safety, quality and efficacy and also on whether it is a follow-up request. Scientific advice is free for any paediatric question and protocol assistance for orphan drugs and fee reductions are in place for SMEs.

18.7.7.1 Scientific advice and protocol assistance from CHMP

A pre-submission meeting for scientific advice or for protocol assistance is highly recommended at the time of submission of the letter of intent (about 8 weeks in advance of the anticipated start of the procedure). A scientific advice team is created by the coordinators, the EMEA and additional experts nominated by SAWP members. Once a meeting date is agreed, companies will then be requested to send the relevant background information containing the draft scientific advice or protocol assistance request. These should be sent to the EMEA at least 10 working days before the anticipated meeting. Appointed SAWP coordinator(s), EMEA scientific advice administrators and, product team leaders/members may participate in these pre-submission meetings.

Once the request is validated by the EMEA, it is forwarded to SAWP and to other relevant working parties. The SAWP appoints two coordinators. For protocol assistance, if the request includes issues relating to demonstration of significant benefit, a third coordinator who is one of the COMP representatives to the SAWP will also be appointed as an additional coordinator.

On day 0, the coordinators introduce the company's request, highlighting the main issues (this meeting is referred to as SAWP 1). By day 20, the coordinators send their *first* reports to the EMEA secretariat. The reports are forwarded for comments to the SAWP, the relevant working parties and any additional experts and to the COMP (for protocol assistance). On day 30, SAWP (SAWP 2) discusses the first reports, focusing on controversial issues. The SAWP confirms at this stage whether the advice can be adopted at day 40 or whether it is necessary to invite the applicant for a discussion meeting.

If the SAWP decides at SAWP 2 that there is no need for a discussion meeting and that the procedure can be finalised in 40 days, the coordinators send their joint report to the EMEA secretariat. The joint coordinators' report and the draft advice letter to the company are adopted on day 33 by the SAWP through a *written procedure*. The CHMP/SAWP/EMEA peer review takes place to check content consistency and coherence. On day 40, the final advice letter is adopted by the CHMP (and by the COMP in case of question on significant benefit for protocol assistance) and sent to the company.

If the SAWP decides at SAWP 2 that it is necessary to invite the applicant for a discussion (at day 60 of the procedure), for example in cases of disagreement with the proposed development, a list of issues to be addressed by the company at the discussion meeting is adopted by the SAWP and sent to the company. The SAWP may request the applicant to address issues in writing only. In this case a list of issues to be addressed by the company in writing is adopted by the SAWP and sent to the company. In such an event, the coordinators send their joint report on day 50, highlighting the controversial issues from SAWP 2 discussion, to the EMEA secretariat. The applicant may also propose in writing to the EMEA additional points for discussion that are not part of the adopted list of issues and submit in writing an amended development programme ahead of the discussion meeting. The report is forwarded for comments to all the members of SAWP, the relevant working parties and any additional experts and to the COMP (for protocol assistance). On day 60 (SAWP 3), a discussion meeting takes place with the company. The coordinators present a preliminary conclusion at the end of the discussion meeting and also debrief SAWP by presenting the outcome of the discussion meeting.

On day 63, the coordinators send their revised joint report to the EMEA secretariat. The coordinators' joint report and the draft advice letter to the company are adopted by the SAWP through a *written procedure*. The CHMP/SAWP/EMEA peer review takes place to check content consistency and coherence. On day 70, the final advice letter is adopted by the CHMP (and by the COMP in case of question on significant benefit for protocol assistance) and sent to the company. If needed, the applicant may request a clarification after receipt of the final advice letter. This is *only* intended to provide the applicant with the opportunity to clarify the meaning of CHMP advice that is perceived as being not clear or precise enough.

The answer and the advice given are based on the question and the documentation submitted without prejudice to evolution and developments in the state-of-the-art. Furthermore, companies should note that the advice provided is without prejudice to applicable legislation relating to the particulars and documents, which must be submitted in support of a marketing authorisation application. It is also without prejudice to any intellectual property rights of third parties. When providing scientific advice or protocol assistance, the CHMP or COMP (for questions related to demonstration of significant benefit within the scope of protocol assistance) do not pre-empt the outcome of the evaluation of any subsequent marketing authorisation application.

Advice is given in good faith but circumstances can change, especially in the case of early advice or subsequent scientific developments. In some cases (e.g. as a result of scientific developments), an alternative approach to that advised may be more appropriate. In this case it is recommended that companies request a follow-up to the initial scientific advice or protocol assistance given. However, where companies choose not to apply the advice, they are requested to justify clearly their position in any subsequent marketing authorisation application. Likewise, the CHMP/COMP will provide argumentation during the evaluation of the marketing authorisation application when diverging from the advice it gave.

18.7.7.2 Parallel Scientific Advice from FDA/CHMP

Effective from 1 January 2005, there is a scheme for parallel scientific advice meetings between SAWP and FDA. The goal of this pilot is to provide a mechanism for EMEA and FDA assessors and sponsors to exchange their views on scientific issues during the development phase of new medicinal products. These parallel scientific advice meetings usually occur at the request of the sponsor but, in special circumstances, may also be initiated by either the EMEA or the FDA in cooperation with the sponsor.

Prime candidates for parallel scientific advice under this pilot should be important (e.g. products for orphan indications or paediatric populations) or breakthrough medicinal products, especially if the product is being developed for indications for which development guidelines do not exist or, if guidelines do exist, those from the EMEA and from the FDA differ significantly. Most parallel scientific advice meetings conducted under this scheme should be a single occurrence focused on the specific development issue raised. Each agency will provide their independent advice to the sponsor on the questions posed during the parallel scientific advice, according to their usual procedures. The advice of each agency may still differ after joint discussion.

Regulatory and procedural guidelines for scientific advice and protocol assistance can be accessed at http://www.emea.europa.eu/htms/human/raguidelines/sa_pa.htm.

18.7.8 Application for change in classification for supply

Legislation already existed in the USA (Durham–Humphrey Amendment of 1951) that defined the kinds of drugs that could not be used safely without medical supervision and restricted their sale to prescription by a licensed practitioner. In 1958, the FDA published the first list of substances generally recognised as safe (GRAS). Medicinal products containing these substances could be dispensed without a medical prescription.

In the EU, each Member State had its own national system for switching or reclassifying a prescription-only medicine to its availability over-the-counter without a prescription. Directive 92/26/EEC of 31 March 1992 concerning the classification for the supply of medicinal products for human use was adopted as an initial step towards harmonising the basic principles applicable to the classification for the supply of medicinal products in the Community or in the

Member States concerned. The relevant articles in Directive 2001/83/EC are Articles 70–75.

Recital 32 of Directive 2001/83/EC states: 'It is appropriate, as an initial step, to harmonise the basic principles applicable to the classification for the supply of medicinal products in the Community or in the Member States concerned.'

Article 70 of Directive 2001/83/EC provides two classifications for the supply of medicinal products for human use in the Community: medicinal products subject to medical prescription; and medicinal products not subject to medical prescription. Article 71 provides the criteria for classifying a medicinal product as subject to medical prescription. Thus, a medicinal product that meets these criteria is subject to a medical prescription and a medicinal product that does not meet these criteria is by default not subject to a medical prescription, as stated in Article 72. The legislation permits for subcategories of classifications which may be available for medicinal products not subject to a medical prescription at Member State level, such as those available in pharmacies only following initial medical diagnosis or available on general sale, as the case may be.

There are four criteria, any one of which may render a medicinal product subject to prescription control:
1. When they are likely to present a danger either directly or indirectly, even when used correctly, if utilised without medical supervision;
2. When they are frequently and to a very wide extent used incorrectly, and as a result are likely to present a direct or indirect danger to human health;
3. When they contain substances or preparations thereof the activity and/or side effects of which require further investigation;
4. When they are normally prescribed by a doctor to be administered parenterally (for injection).

Article 4(4) of the Directive 2001/83/EC does not affect the application of national legislation prohibiting or restricting the sale, supply or use of medicinal products as contraceptives or abortifacients. The Member States, however, shall communicate the national legislation concerned to the Commission.

According to Article 71(4) of Directive 2001/83/EC, a medicinal product that meets any of the criteria for supply subject to medical prescription may be classified for supply not subject to medical prescription if the maximum single dose, the maximum daily dose, the strength, the pharmaceutical form, certain types of packaging and/or other circumstances of use, can make supply without medical prescription appropriate.

An application for a change in classification status should be accompanied by data on safety and efficacy as well an expert report and the proposed product information.

In practice, the application of the prescription status is heterogeneous following Member States' national legislations; therefore, at European level, the decision only defines medicinal products that require prescription and those that do not.

18.7.8.1 Expert report or the clinical overview

In all cases, an expert report (or its CTD equivalent, the clinical overview), which is a critical analysis of the proposed availability of the product without a medical prescription with the dose and indications as stated in the application, must be provided. The expert is expected to take a clear position, defend the proposal in light of current scientific knowledge, and demonstrate why none of the criteria that determine classification for supply subject to a medical prescription applies to the product.

18.7.8.2 Safety

Safety data are vital in supporting any application for a change in the classification. Such data will cover a wide range of safety issues. A summary should be given of, or references to, animal studies or studies on humans that show low general toxicity and no relevant reproductive toxicity, genotoxic or carcinogenic properties relevant to the experience/exposure of the product. Experience in terms of patient exposure to the substance needs to be considerable and should be outlined. Normally, active substances which are suitable for supply without a medical prescription will have been in widespread use for 5 years in medicinal products subject to a medical prescription. However, provided enough data are available, this does not exclude the possibility of an authority accepting a shorter time. Adverse drug reactions to the pharmaceutical form and dose proposed for supply not subject to a medical prescription should in normal conditions be minor and should cease on discontinuing therapy. Information should be provided on adverse reactions, including experience of use without medical supervision (e.g. in another Member State or in a third country). Risks of drug interactions should be detailed. Consequences concerning misuse (e.g. use for longer periods than recommended), as well as accidental or intended overdose and the use of higher doses, should be discussed. Consequences of the use of the product by a patient who has incorrectly assessed his or her condition or symptoms should be considered. The application should consider the consequences of incorrect or delayed diagnosis of a patient's condition or symptoms resulting from self-medication with the product.

18.7.8.3 Efficacy

Evidence of the product's efficacy is not normally considered in the application for changing the classification for supply, unless this application also includes changes to the indications or posology. If other parts of the dossier are changed (e.g. indication, posology or strength), then supporting data should be provided. A suitable time period for treatment of the suggested indication(s) should be justified and given, together with a proposed pack size.

18.7.8.4 Product information

For a medicinal product classified for supply without a medical prescription, the proposed product label and leaflet are important elements of the application and will be closely examined for comprehensive information and effectiveness in protecting patients from any safety hazards.

18.7.8.5 Data exclusivity

Article 10 of Directive 2001/83 provides data exclusivity for 1 year to the applicant if the switch from prescription control to non-prescription use requires significant preclinical tests and/or clinical trials. Article 74a of Directive 2001/83/EC as amended by Directive 2004/27/EC requires that where a change of classification of a medicinal product has been authorised on the basis of significant preclinical tests or clinical trials, the competent authority shall not refer to the results of those tests or trials when examining an application by another applicant for or holder of marketing authorisation for a change of classification of the same substance for 1 year after the initial change was authorised.

Preclinical tests and/or clinical trials are significant if they are related to a new strength or posology, using a new route of administration, new pharmaceutical form or for a new indication particularly one not previously authorised for a medicinal product not subject to medical prescription or a subpopulations (e.g. the elderly, children, certain racial groups and those having certain medical conditions). Studies that concern a lower strength or posology are significant if it is necessary to confirm that the reduced strength or posology retains the efficacy. For a new indication, confirmatory clinical trial(s) are very likely to be necessary and significant. Similarly, if duration or

modalities of treatment are changed, new non-clinical and/or clinical studies may become necessary and would be subject to protection.

Where the safety or efficacy profile of a medicinal product requires confirmation, either within the prescription setting or within the envisioned non-prescription environment, resulting in the generation of new safety/efficacy data (e.g. actual use studies), such data are likely to be eligible for exclusivity.

18.7.8.6 Other provisions

For products that are subject to national or mutual recognition/decentralised procedure only, it is expected that data exclusivity would be applied by each competent authority, irrespective of whether the data were common to more than one application.

For marketing authorisations processed through the mutual recognition or decentralised procedures, each competent authority will take its own decision as to whether the 1-year data exclusivity period is to be granted. Nevertheless, in the interest of maintaining harmonisation already achieved previously during the original approval of the product, the Member States are encouraged to use their best endeavours to reach agreement on the legal status of a medicinal product and on the 1-year data exclusivity. The decision of each competent authority authorising the change will contain a clear statement of whether the change in classification is based on significant preclinical tests or clinical trials.

For centrally authorised products, where the change in classification is submitted within an existing marketing authorisation, the change requires the submission of a type 2 variation application, unless it introduces the need for an extension application (e.g. a new strength, pharmaceutical form, route of administration or any other significant change). Alternatively, a separate stand-alone application for marketing authorisation could be submitted. The CHMP will assess the preclinical or clinical trials and issue a single Opinion for the change of the classification. A Commission Decision will authorise the change in classification including a clear statement of whether the change in classification is based on significant preclinical tests or clinical trials.

The legislation also requires the competent authorities to draw up a list of the medicinal products subject, on their territory, to medical prescription, specifying, if necessary, the category of classification. The list should be updated annually. The Directive also requires that when new facts are brought to their notice, the competent authorities should examine and, as appropriate, amend the classification of a medicinal product. Each year, Member States have to communicate to the EC and to the other Member States the changes that have been made to the list referred to above.

A guideline on switch in classification for supply, published in January 2006, can be accessed at http://ec.europa.eu/enterprise/pharmaceuticals/eudralex/vol-2/c/switchguide_160106.pdf.

18.7.9 Application for paediatric investigation plan or a waiver

The Paediatric Regulation (EC) No 1901/2006 requires, where necessary, the early submission of a paediatric development plan for medicines – the Paediatric Investigation Plan (PIP). The normal development of a medicine requires that various studies be performed to ensure its quality, safety and efficacy. The development plan can be modified with increasing knowledge about the medicine.

A PIP is a development plan aimed at ensuring that the necessary data are obtained through studies in children, when it is safe to do so, to support the authorisation of the medicine for children. The plan should be submitted by pharmaceutical companies to the Paediatric Committee, which is responsible for agreement or refusal of the plan.

The PIP includes a description of the studies and of the measures to adapt the way the medicine is presented (formulation) to make its use more acceptable in children (supporting a full indication in all age groups of children). For example, children cannot swallow large tablets so the availability of liquid formulation may be more appropriate. The PIP should cover the needs of all age groups of children, from birth to adolescence. The PIP also defines the timing of studies in children compared to adults. In some cases, studies will be deferred until after the studies in adults have been conducted, to ensure that research with children is performed only when it is safe and ethical to do so.

18.7.9.1 Application for a paediatric investigation plan

This should include the following information in detail:

A. Administrative and product information:

A1: Name or corporate name and address of the applicant and contact person;

A2: Type of product;

A3: Name of the active substance;

A4: Details of the medicinal product;

A5: Regulatory information on clinical trials related to the condition and to the development in the paediatric population;

A6: Marketing authorisation status of the medicinal product;

A7: Advice from any regulatory authority relevant to the development in the paediatric population;

A8: Orphan drug status in the EEA;

A9: Planned application for marketing authorisation/line extensions/variation;

A10: Any annexed documentation where appropriate such as:

• A letter of authorisation for the person authorised to communicate on behalf of the applicant;

• A copy of any scientific advice given by the EMEA/CHMP or any other EEA national competent authority;

• A copy of US FDA written request and/or any advice, Opinion or decision relating to paediatric information given by a regulatory agency outside EEA;

• A copy of any Commission decision on orphan designation;

• A copy of any previous EMEA decision on a PIP or a negative Opinion of the Paediatric Committee on such plans;

• A copy of a representative SPC recently granted in the EEA.

A11: Table of translations of the EMEA decision.

B. Overall development of the medicinal product including information on the conditions:

B1: Discussion on similarities and differences of the disease/condition between populations;

B2: Discussion of anticipated similarities and differences of the effect of the product on the disease/condition;

B3: Prevalence and incidence in the paediatric population;

B4: Current methods of diagnosis, prevention or treatment in paediatric populations;

B5: Significant therapeutic benefit or fulfilment of therapeutic needs.

18.7.9.2 Applications for paediatric waivers

No product specific waiver may be necessary to satisfy the requirements of Articles 7 and 8 of the Paediatric Regulation if the therapeutic indication and the subset of the paediatric population are already covered by a class waiver. Where the requirements of Articles 7 and 8 of the Paediatric Regulation are partially covered by class waiver but a product specific waiver is necessary to satisfy the requirements, the class waivers should be referred to when specifying the scope of the product specific waiver.

Companies are encouraged to inform the Paediatric Committee when new information becomes available that suggests that a class or product specific waiver should be reviewed in accordance with Article 14(2) of the Paediatric Regulation.

As some diseases do not affect children (e.g. Parkinson's disease), the development of medicines for these diseases should not be performed in children, and so a PIP will not be required by the Paediatric Committee; the requirement for a PIP will therefore be waived in these cases.

The grounds for a waiver of the paediatric development are defined in Article 11 of the Paediatric Regulation. These include the lack of significant therapeutic benefit, the likelihood for the product to be ineffective or unsafe, and/or as in the example above, the fact that the disease only occurs in adults.

On 24 September 2008, the EC published the final version of the guideline entitled 'Guideline on the format and content of applications for agreement or modification of a PIP and requests for waivers or deferrals and concerning the operation of the compliance check and on criteria for assessing significant studies'. This guideline can be accessed at http://www.emea.europa.eu/pdfs/human/paediatrics/Guideline_2008_C243_01.pdf.

18.7.10 Application for registration of herbal medicinal product

In order to obtain traditional use registration, the applicant shall submit an application to the competent authority of the Member State concerned. The applicant and registration holder shall be established in the Community. The application shall be accompanied by the particulars and various documents, any authorisation or registration obtained by the applicant in another Member State, or in a third country, to place the medicinal product on the market, and details of any decision to refuse to grant an authorisation or registration, whether in the Community or a third country, and the reasons for any such decision, appropriate required expert evidence and bibliographic safety data.

Article 16a–c of Directive 2001/83/EC as amended by 2004/24/EC provides for a simplified registration procedure for herbal medicinal products that fulfil all of the following criteria:

1. They have indications exclusively appropriate to traditional herbal medicinal products which, by virtue of their composition and purpose, are intended and designed for use without the supervision of a medical practitioner for diagnostic purposes or for prescription or monitoring of treatment.

2. They are exclusively for administration in accordance with a specified strength and posology.

3. They are an oral, external and/or inhalation preparation.

4. The period of traditional use for the medicinal product in question, or a corresponding product in medicinal use throughout is a period of at least 30 years preceding the date of the application, including at least 15 years use within the Community.

5. The data on the traditional use of the medicinal product are sufficient; in particular, the product proves not to be harmful in the specified conditions of use and the pharmacological effects or efficacy of the medicinal product are plausible on the basis of long-standing use and experience.

The requirement to show medicinal use throughout the period of 30 years referred to above, is satisfied even where the marketing of the product has not been based on a specific authorisation. It is likewise satisfied if the number or quantity of ingredients of the medicinal product have been reduced during that period. However, this simplified procedure should be used only when no marketing authorisation can be obtained through procedures for typical medicinal products.

The simplified registration should be acceptable only where the herbal medicinal product may rely on a sufficiently long medicinal use in the Community. Medicinal use outside the Community should be taken into account only if the medicinal product has been used within the Community for a certain time. Where there is limited evidence of use within the Community, it is necessary to assess carefully the validity and relevance of use outside the Community.

In order to promote harmonisation, Member States are expected to recognise registrations of traditional herbal medicinal products granted by another Member State based on Community herbal monographs or consisting of substances, preparations or combinations thereof contained in any EU list that may have been established.

Where the product has been used in the Community for less than 15 years, but is otherwise eligible for simplified registration, the Member State where the application for traditional use registration has been submitted shall refer the product to the HMPC. The Member State shall submit relevant documentation supporting the referral. The HMPC shall consider whether the other criteria for a simplified registration as referred to above are fully complied with. If the HMPC considers it possible, it shall establish Community herbal monographs as referred to in Article 16h(3) which shall be taken into account by the Member State when taking its final decision.

When new Community herbal monographs are established, the registration holder shall consider whether it is necessary to modify the registration dossier accordingly. The registration holder shall notify any such modification to the competent authority of the Member State concerned.

18.7.11 Application for Clinical Trial Authorisation

Until harmonised in May 2004, the regulation of clinical trials within the EU was very heterogeneous. Although a recent survey in December 2007 showed that there are still some areas of different practices among the Member States, the conduct of clinical trials in the EU is now highly regulated by Directive 2001/20/EEC and there is much greater harmony than before. This Directive contains specific provisions regarding the conduct of clinical trials, including multicentre trials, on human subjects. It sets standards relating to the implementation of Good Clinical Practice and Good Manufacturing Practice, with a view to protecting clinical trial subjects. Commission Directive 2005/28/EC of 8 April 2005 lays down the principles and detailed guidelines for Good Clinical Practice and Commission Directive 2003/94/EC of 8 October 2003 lays down the principles and guidelines of Good Manufacturing Practice.

Directive 2001/20/EEC is very detailed and comprehensive, addressing ethical and scientific standards. It defines 'clinical trial' as any investigation in human subjects intended to discover or verify the clinical, pharmacological and/or other pharmacodynamic effects of one or more investigational medicinal product(s), and/or to identify any adverse reactions to one or more investigational medicinal product(s), and/or to study absorption, distribution, metabolism and excretion of one or more investigational medicinal product(s) with the object of ascertaining its (their) safety and/or efficacy, and defines the human 'subject' as an individual who participates in a clinical trial as a recipient of either the investigational medicinal product or a control. Thus, all healthy volunteer studies, including investigations of bioavailability and bioequivalence, are included and must comply with the requirements of the Directive.

Conversely, non-interventional studies are excluded where medicinal products are prescribed in the usual manner in accordance with the terms of the marketing authorisation.

The Directive defines the sponsor as an individual, a company, an institution or an organisation. The sponsor does not need to be located in an EU Member State but has to have a legal representative in the EU. The legal representative shall have the position of the sponsor with regard to civil and criminal liability in the Community. It is required to have one legal representative located in the EU for a non-EU sponsored trial taking place in EU. It is acceptable to use an established company as a legal representative. It is also acceptable to have one central legal representative in EU for all trials. The investigator and the sponsor may be the same person.

Clinical trials have to be entered in the EudraCT database. Before submitting an application to the competent authority, the sponsor should obtain a unique EudraCT number from the EudraCT database. An authorisation of a clinical trial by the competent authority of a Member State will be a Clinical Trial Authorisation and will only be valid for a clinical trial conducted in that Member State. Following changes to European legislation, the EMEA will soon be able to make public some of the information in EudraCT.

According to Article 9(2) of the Directive, the applicant must submit a valid request for authorisation to the competent authority and this should include:

1. Covering letter;
2. Allocation of the EudraCT number;
3. Application form;
4. Protocol;
5. Investigator's brochure; and
6. Data related to the investigational medicinal product.

A reduced information requirement may apply for the investigational medicinal products that are already known to the competent authority concerned. There are detailed provisions for notification of amendments, suspension of a trial by the competent authority and for declaration of the end of a clinical trial. In October 2005, the EC also issued a detailed guidance for the request for authorisation of a clinical trial on a medicinal product for human use to the competent authorities, notification of substantial amendments and declaration of the end of the trial. This guidance details the information required by each competent authority within the EU.

Each competent authority is responsible for determination of an application for clinical trials in the territory under its jurisdiction. Where an application for a clinical trial is submitted in more than one Member State, the sponsor/investigator can commence a clinical trial in the Member State concerned if the positive Opinion of the ethics committee in that Member State and the authorisation/statement of no grounds for non-acceptance of the competent authority in question have been received.

The Directive lays down specific obligations for the Member States. If the competent authority of the Member State notifies the sponsor of grounds for non-acceptance, the sponsor may, on one occasion only, amend the content of the request to take due account of the grounds given. There are specific measures before the commencement and end or early termination of a clinical trial, including a time limit not exceeding 60 days for Member States to consider a valid request. No further extension to this period is permissible except in the case of trials involving medicinal products for gene therapy or somatic cell therapy or medicinal products containing genetically modified organisms for which an extension of a maximum 30 days is permitted. For these products, this 90-day period may be extended by a further 90 days under certain circumstances. In the case of xenogenic cell therapy no time limit to the authorisation period is allowable. It is important to note that 'The Member States may lay down a shorter period than 60 days within their area of responsibility if that is in compliance with current practice', and that 'The competent authority can nevertheless notify the sponsor before the end of this period that it has no grounds for non-acceptance.'

The Directive contains detailed articles on the conduct of a clinical trial, exchange of information between Member States, EMEA and the EC, the reasons and procedures for suspension of the trial by a Member State, and notification of adverse events, including serious adverse reactions.

As required by the Directive, the EC has issued detailed guidance on several aspects including:
1. Application format and documentation to be submitted in an application for an ethics committee Opinion on the clinical trial on medicinal products for human use (February 2006);
2. European Clinical Trials (EudraCT) Database (April 2003);
3. European database of suspected unexpected serious adverse reactions in clinical trials (April 2004);
4. Collection, verification and presentation of adverse reaction reports arising from clinical trials on medicinal products for human use (April 2006); and

5. Requirements to the chemical and pharmaceutical quality documentation concerning investigational medicinal products in clinical trials (March 2006).

The EudraCT database created by Directive 2001/20/EC was confidential and accessible only to competent authorities of the Member States, the EC and the EMEA. Further to the Paediatric Regulation, modifications to the database are being implemented to give public access to part of the information regarding protocols and results of paediatric clinical trials performed within the EEA and those performed completely outside of the EEA when they are part of a PIP. The EudraCT database can be accessed at https://eudract.emea.europa.eu/index.html. Volume 10 of the 'The rules governing medicinal products in the European Union' contains guidance documents applicable to clinical trials and can be accessed at http://ec.europa.eu/enterprise/pharmaceuticals/eudralex/vol10_en.htm.

18.8 Community referrals to the CHMP

The EU has a highly structured legislative framework for resolution of referrals to its scientific advisory committees – for new applications as well as for products already authorised. Community pharmaceutical legislation has created a binding Community arbitration mechanism. The legal basis for referrals is provided in Directive 2001/83/EC (applications) and Regulation (EC) 1084/2003 (variations).

Depending on the specific procedure, a referral under Directive 2001/83/EC can be initiated by an applicant, a marketing authorisation holder, a Member State and/or the EC:
1. Article 29 referral procedures can be initiated, during a mutual recognition or decentralised procedure, by Member States concerned in the procedure on the grounds of potential serious risk to public health.
2. Article 30 referral procedures can be initiated by any Member State, the EC or the marketing authorisation holder of a particular medicinal product and concerns divergent decisions having been adopted by Member States concerning the authorisation, suspension or withdrawal of a particular medicinal product. For example, where such medicinal product has been nationally authorised in two or more Member States and the authorisations diverge (e.g. different indications, contraindications or posology). Once harmonised, the medicinal product in question will follow a mutual recognition procedure, avoiding future disharmony.
3. Article 31 referral procedures can be initiated by any Member State, the EC or the applicant or the

marketing authorisation holder and concerns specific cases where the interest of the Community is involved. The expression 'Community interest' has a broad meaning but it refers particularly to the interests of the public health in the Community, for example, following concerns related to the quality, efficacy and/or safety of a medicinal product, a range of products or several products of the same therapeutic class (e.g. when new pharmacovigilance information becomes available).

4. Article 36 referral procedures can be initiated by any Member State or the EC to resolve any post-harmonisation divergences that may arise between Member States. It may be triggered by a Member State when it is considered that a variation, suspension or withdrawal of a harmonised marketing authorisation is necessary for the protection of public health. Article 37 provides that Articles 35 and 36 shall apply by analogy to medicinal products authorised by Member States following an Opinion of the 'old' CPMP, given in accordance with Article 4 of Directive 87/22/EEC before 1 January 1995 (making centralised applications mandatory for high technology medicinal products, particularly those derived from biotechnology).

As far as the variations are concerned, the referrals are:

5. Referral under Article 5(11) of Regulation (EC) 1084/2003 which can be initiated by Member States concerned by a mutual recognition procedure or by the marketing authorisation holder (this concerns type 1b variations).

6. Referral under Article 6(12) of Regulation (EC) 1084/2003 which can be initiated by Member States concerned by a mutual recognition procedure (this concerns type 2 variations that are initiated by Member State(s)).

7. Referral under Article 6(13) of Regulation (EC) 1084/2003 which can be initiated by the marketing authorisation holder (this concerns type 2 variations that are initiated by the marketing authorisation holder or the applicant).

A fee is payable only for referral procedures under Articles 30 and 31 initiated by the applicant of a marketing authorisation or the holder of an existing marketing authorisation. This fee is independent of the number of marketing authorisations or applications held by a specific applicant or marketing authorisation holder and independent of the number of pharmaceutical forms, dosages or pack sizes.

The referral procedures for the CHMP Opinion and EC decision are laid down in Articles 32–34 of Directive 2001/83/EC. Article 32 describes the time-lines and the procedures to be followed following a referral. When reference is made to the procedure described in this Article, the CHMP has to consider the matter concerned and issue a reasoned Opinion within 90 days of the date on which the matter was referred to it. However, in cases submitted to the CHMP in accordance with Articles 30 and 31, this period may be extended by 90 days. When appropriate, the CHMP may suspend a timetable. Conversely, in case of urgency, on a proposal from its chairman, the CHMP may agree to a shorter deadline.

In order to consider the matter, the committee appoints one of its members to act as rapporteur. The committee may also appoint individual experts to advise it on specific questions. When appointing experts, the committee shall define their tasks and specify the time limit for the completion of these tasks. The applicant or the marketing authorisation holder is provided an opportunity to present written or oral explanations within a specified time limit. The Opinion of the committee is accompanied by a draft SPC for the product and a draft text of the labelling and package leaflet. If necessary, the committee may call upon any other person to provide information relating to the matter before it. The EMEA then notifies the applicant or the marketing authorisation holder forthwith where the Opinion of the committee is that:

1. The application does not satisfy the criteria for authorisation;

2. The SPC proposed by the applicant or the marketing authorisation holder should be amended;

3. The authorisation should be granted subject to certain conditions, in view of conditions considered essential for the safe and effective use of the medicinal product including pharmacovigilance; or

4. A marketing authorisation should be suspended, varied or revoked.

Within 15 days after receipt of the Opinion, the applicant or the marketing authorisation holder should notify the EMEA in writing of the intention (if any) to request a re-examination of the Opinion. In that case, the detailed grounds for the request should be forwarded to the EMEA within 60 days after receipt of the Opinion. Within 60 days following receipt of the grounds for the request, the CHMP is required to re-examine its Opinion in accordance with Article 62(1) of Regulation (EC) No 726/2004.

Chapter 3 of Volume 2A of Notice to Applicants (EudraLex) provides details of the Community referrals and can be accessed at http://ec.europa.eu/enterprise/pharmaceuticals/eudralex/vol2_en.htm. Various guidelines on referrals can be accessed at http://www.emea.

europa.eu/htms/human/raguidelines/referrals.htm. A question and answer document on referrals can be accessed at http://www.emea.europa.eu/pdfs/human/referral/q_a/Q&A.pdf.

18.9 Product literature, promotion and advertising

18.9.1 Summary of Product Characteristics (SPC)

For all practical purposes, the most important document is the Summary of Product Characteristics (SPC). Its terms are carefully scrutinised by the competent authority in light of the dossier accompanying the application. The approved SPC sets out the agreed position of the medicinal product as distilled during the course of the assessment process. It is the definitive statement between the competent authority and the marketing authorisation holder and it is the common basis of communication between the competent authorities of all Member States. As such, the content cannot be changed except with the approval of the originating competent authority. The agreed SPC forms the basis for subsequent marketing of the medicinal product and includes all information which may/should be made available to health professionals and the patients.

It is easy to see why an SPC coming out of all the EU procedures is a highly effective document in terms of the therapeutic claims allowed, a dose schedule that is carefully scrutinised, and detailed safety information and/or monitoring requirements. In rare instances, the SPC comes out too restricted or unbalanced because of the differences in medical practices and cultures among the Member States.

Article 11 of Directive 2001/83/EC prescribes the information, and the order in which this information is presented, to be included in the summary of the product characteristics (Box 18.3).

Involving as it does the scrutiny of pharmaceutical, preclinical and clinical assessors from each of the Member States, the unique Euro-SPC of a medicinal product is a highly effective document, doing full justice to the efficacy of the product and delineating precise indications and dose schedules for its clinical use while providing all information aimed at or necessary for safeguarding the public.

The marketing authorisation holder needs the approval of the competent authority should it wish to vary the terms of the SPC. Such variations require supporting data.

BOX 18.3 Contents of summary of product characteristics

1. Name of the medicinal product followed by the strength and the pharmaceutical form
2. Qualitative and quantitative composition in terms of the active substances and constituents of the excipient, knowledge of which is essential for proper administration of the medicinal product. The usual common name or chemical description should be used
3. Pharmaceutical form
4. Clinical particulars:
   4.1 Therapeutic indications
   4.2 Posology and method of administration for adults and, where necessary, for children
   4.3 Contraindications
   4.4 Special warnings and precautions for use and, in the case of immunological medicinal products, any special precautions to be taken by persons handling such products and administering them to patients, together with any precautions to be taken by the patient
   4.5 Interaction with other medicinal products and other forms of interactions
   4.6 Use during pregnancy and lactation
   4.7 Effects on ability to drive and to use machines
   4.8 Undesirable effects
   4.9 Overdose (symptoms, emergency procedures, antidotes)
5. Pharmacological properties:
   5.1 Pharmacodynamic properties
   5.2 Pharmacokinetic properties
   5.3 Preclinical safety data
6. Pharmaceutical particulars:
   6.1 List of excipients
   6.2 Major incompatibilities
   6.3 Shelf life, when necessary after reconstitution of the medicinal product or when the immediate packaging is opened for the first time
   6.4 Special precautions for storage
   6.5 Nature and contents of container
   6.6 Special precautions for disposal of a used medicinal product or waste materials derived from such medicinal product, if appropriate
7. Marketing authorisation holder
8. Marketing authorisation number(s)
9. Date of the first authorisation or renewal of the authorisation
10. Date of revision of the text
11. For radiopharmaceuticals, full details of internal radiation dosimetry
12. For radiopharmaceuticals, additional detailed instructions for extemporaneous preparation and quality control of such preparation and, where appropriate, maximum storage time during which any intermediate preparation such as an eluate or the ready-to-use pharmaceutical will conform with its specifications

18.9.2 Package leaflet

The package leaflets (or patient information leaflet (PIL)) and labels are now regulated by Articles 54–69 of Directive 2001/83/EC as amended by Directive 2004/27/EC. The package leaflet, intended for patient information, should be drawn up in lay language in accordance with the SPC and must contain the information in the order shown in Box 18.4.

BOX 18.4 Contents of package (patient information) leaflet

(a) Identification of the medicinal product:
  (i)   Name of the medicinal product followed by its strength and pharmaceutical form and, if appropriate, whether it is intended for babies, children or adults. The common name shall be included where the product contains only one active substance and if its name is an invented name
  (ii) Pharmacotherapeutic group or type of activity in terms easily comprehensible for the patient
(b) The therapeutic indications
(c) A list of information which is necessary before the medicinal product is taken, taking into account the particular condition of certain categories of users (children, pregnant or breastfeeding women, the elderly, persons with specific pathological conditions), possible effects on the ability to drive vehicles or to operate machinery and listing of those excipients knowledge of which is important for the safe and effective use of the medicinal product:
  (i)   Contraindications
  (ii)   Appropriate precautions for use
  (iii) Forms of interaction with other medicinal products and other forms of interaction (e.g. alcohol, tobacco, foodstuffs) which may affect the action of the medicinal product
  (iv)   Special warnings
(d) The necessary and usual instructions for proper use, and in particular:
  (i)   Dosage
  (ii)   Method and, if necessary, route of administration
  (iii) Frequency of administration, specifying if necessary the appropriate time at which the medicinal product may or must be administered and, as appropriate, depending on the nature of the product
  (iv)   Duration of treatment, where it should be limited
  (v)   Action to be taken in case of an overdose (such as symptoms, emergency procedures)
  (vi)   What to do when one or more doses have not been taken

---

BOX 18.4 continued

  (vii) Indication, if necessary, of the risk of withdrawal effects
  (viii) A specific recommendation to consult the doctor or the pharmacist, as appropriate, for any clarification on the use of the product
(e) A description of the adverse reactions that may occur under normal use of the medicinal product and, if necessary, the action to be taken in such a case; the patient should be expressly asked to communicate any adverse reaction that is not mentioned in the package leaflet to his or her doctor or pharmacist
(f) A reference to the expiry date indicated on the label, with:
  (i)   A warning against using the product after that date
  (ii)   Where appropriate, special storage precautions
  (iii) If necessary, a warning concerning certain visible signs of deterioration
  (iv)   Full qualitative composition (in active substances and excipients) and the quantitative composition in active substances, using common names, for each presentation of the medicinal product
  (v)   For each presentation of the product, the pharmaceutical form and content in weight, volume or units of dosage
  (vi)   Name and address of the marketing authorisation holder and, where applicable, the name of the appointed representatives in the Member States
  (vii) Name and address of the manufacturer
(g) Where the medicinal product is authorised under different names in the Member States concerned, a list of the names authorised in each Member State
(h) The date on which the package leaflet was last revised

Although Article 12.2 of Directive 92/27/EEC provided that the guidelines on legibility and readability should be adopted as a Commission Directive, the Pharmaceutical Committee considered it more appropriate to adopt these recommendations as a guideline. This guideline on legibility and readability, adopted in September 1998 to be effective from January 1999, described the format of the package leaflet (in terms of print and font size, use of colours, syntax and contents) and provided an example of a model leaflet in its Annex 1a together with further guidance on its content in Annex 1b. It was recommended that this example of a model leaflet and the guidance on its content should be followed in so far as the resulting leaflet complies with Directive 92/27/EEC and, upon testing (e.g. in accordance with Annex 2) by applicants for a marketing authorisation, is shown to be readable to the patient/consumer.

This guideline on legibility and readability was updated in September 2006 to include further details to improve legibility and readability of leaflets (e.g. headings, use of italics and underlining and their layout, quality of paper). Chapter 2 of this updated guideline includes specific recommendations regarding the need of the blind and partially sighted patients and requires the name of the product to be provided in Braille on the packaging. Chapter 3 provides further guidance concerning consultations with target patient groups for the package leaflet. Therefore, the package leaflet must reflect the results of consultations with target patient groups to ensure that it is legible, clear and easy to use.

The competent authority shall refuse the marketing authorisation if the labelling or the package leaflet does not comply with the provisions of this title or if they are not in accordance with the particulars listed in the SPC. However, Article 60 of Directive 2001/83/EC as amended requires that Member States may not prohibit or impede the placing on the market of medicinal products within their territory on grounds connected with labelling or the package leaflet where these comply with the requirements of this title.

All proposed changes to an aspect of the labelling or the package leaflet covered by this title and not connected with the SPC shall be submitted to the authorities competent for authorizing marketing. If the competent authorities have not opposed a proposed change within 90 days following the request, the applicant may put the change into effect.

18.9.3 Promotion and advertising

The requirements for regulating advertising, previously by Council Directive 92/28/EEC of 31 March 1992, are now codified as Articles 86–100 of Directive 2001/83/EC as amended by Directive 2004/27/EC.

Article 86 defines advertising of medicinal products as including any form of door-to-door information, canvassing activity or inducement designed to promote the prescription, supply, sale or consumption of medicinal products. It includes in particular the advertising of medicinal products to the general public, to persons qualified to prescribe or supply them, visits by medical sales representatives to persons qualified to prescribe medicinal products, the supply of samples, the provision of inducements to prescribe or supply medicinal products by the gift,

offer or promise of any benefit or bonus, whether in money or in kind, except when their intrinsic value is minimal, sponsorship of promotional meetings attended by persons qualified to prescribe or supply medicinal products, sponsorship of scientific congresses attended by persons qualified to prescribe or supply medicinal products, and in particular payment of their travelling and accommodation expenses in connection therewith.

Member States have an obligation to prohibit any advertising of a medicinal product in respect of which a marketing authorisation has not been granted in accordance with Community law. All parts of the advertising of a medicinal product must comply with the particulars listed in the SPC. The advertising of a medicinal product should encourage only the rational use of the medicinal product, by presenting it objectively and without exaggerating its properties, and not so as to be misleading.

There are special provisions for advertising to the general public as well as to the health professions. Member States must prohibit the advertising to the general public of medicinal products for therapeutic indications specified in the Directive. When permissible, all advertising to the general public of a medicinal product has to be set out in a prescribed manner. Article 90 of the Directive specifies the material or information that should not be contained in the advertising of a medicinal product to the general public.

In respect of advertising to health professionals, there are detailed requirements in respect of provision of information, free samples, and gifts and hospitality as well as the training and duties of medical sales representatives.

Member States have an obligation to monitor advertising and are required to ensure that there are adequate and effective methods to monitor the advertising of medicinal products. Such methods, which may be based on a system of prior vetting, must in any event include legal provisions under which persons or organisations regarded under national law as having a legitimate interest in prohibiting any advertisement inconsistent with the Directive may take legal action against such an advertisement, or bring such an advertisement before an administrative authority competent either to decide on complaints or to initiate appropriate legal proceedings.

Under the legal provisions, Member States must confer upon the courts or administrative authorities powers enabling them, in cases where they deem such measures to be necessary, taking into account all the interests involved and in particular the public interest, to order the cessation of, or to institute appropriate legal proceedings for an order for the cessation of, misleading advertising, or if misleading advertising has not yet been published but publication is imminent, to order the prohibition of, or to institute appropriate legal proceedings for an order for the prohibition of, such publication, even without proof of actual loss or damage or of intention or negligence on the part of the advertiser. Member States must also make provisions for the statutory measures that confer various powers upon the courts or administrative authorities.

The legislation, however, does not exclude voluntary control of advertising and promotion of medicinal products by self-regulatory bodies and recourse to such bodies, if proceedings before such bodies are possible in addition to the judicial or administrative proceedings referred to above. One example of such voluntary control is the Code of Practice established by the Association of British Pharmaceutical Industry (ABPI), which covers promotion in its widest aspects (see Chapter 12).

Article 98 lays down the obligations of the marketing authorisation holder, including particularly retention of samples of all advertising material, conformity of the advertisement with the provisions of the Directive, verification of the training of sales force, advertising title of the Directive, provision of information and assistance the regulatory authorities require to carry out their responsibilities for monitoring advertising of medicinal products and full and immediate compliance with their decisions.

18.10 Pharmacovigilance

Every Member State had local legislation and obligations for maintaining effective pharmacovigilance and there were criminal, civil and/or regulatory penalties for non-compliance by marketing authorisation holder. Directive 93/39/EEC introduced the concept of pharmacovigilance in the EU and the harmonisation of pharmacovigilance within the EU also gained momentum. The changes to the legislation following 'Review 2001' are intended to strengthen the protection of public health of EU citizens through the effective regulation of medicines for human use. Not surprisingly, pharmacovigilance in the EU, as elsewhere under other jurisdictions, has now moved to the top of regulatory agenda.

The legislative framework for pharmacovigilance across the EU is already provided in a number of Regulations, Directives and guidelines. These consist of Commission Regulation No 540/95, Regulation (EC) No 726/2004 and Commission Directive 2000/38/EC. Various legislations have been codified as Articles 101–108 of Directive 2001/83/EC as amended by Directive 2004/27/EC.

Article 102 of Directive 2004/27/EC includes a provision that requires Member States to share information collected through their pharmacovigilance system with other Member States and the EMEA. A central EudraVigilance, a data processing network and management system for reporting and evaluating individual case study reports (ICSR) and suspected unexpected serious adverse reactions during the development and following the marketing authorisation of medicinal products in the EEA, has been developed to allow Member States and the EMEA to share information on adverse drug reactions once all Member States have populated it. This database was created as part of the implementation of the Clinical Trials Directive 2001/20/EC. It can be accessed at http://eudravigilance.emea.europa.eu/highres.htm.

The text of Articles 104–107 includes a new requirement for the marketing authorisation holder to submit adverse drug reactions data in electronic format except in exceptional circumstances. Table 18.1 summarises the current legal requirements for expedited (within 15 calendar days from receipt) reporting of adverse drug reactions. This applies to initial as well as follow-up information (day 0 is defined as the day the marketing authorisation holder becomes aware of a case that fulfils minimum information). The role and responsibilities of the marketing authorisation holder include having a named Qualified Person responsible for pharmacovigilance at the EU level (whose rigorous duties are strictly specified), and there may be a need for an additional named person at the national level when this is required.

18.10.1 Periodic safety update reports

Two major advances in harmonisation of pharmacovigilance activities in the EU and elsewhere globally were the acceptance of MedDRA (ICH topic M1) as a common medical dictionary for regulatory work and the acceptance of Periodic Safety Update Reports (PSUR) (ICH topic E2C) for drugs marketed in the EU.

The frequency of PSURs has also been increased. Once a medicinal product is authorised in the EU, even if it is not marketed, the marketing authorisation holder is required to submit PSURs at 6-monthly intervals. When launch dates are planned, this information should be reflected in the upcoming

Table 18.1 Expedited (within 15 calendar days) reporting requirements

Authorisation type	ADR type	Destination
Reaction originating in the EU Member State		
Centralised	All serious adverse reactions,	Member State where the reaction occurred
Mutual recognition or decentralised	including any suspected	Member State where the reaction occurred
or subject to referral	transmission via a medicinal	and to the RMS
Purely national	product of an infectious agent	Member State where the reaction occurred
Reaction originating in non-EU country		
Centralised	All serious unexpected adverse	All Member States and to the EMEA
National mutual recognition or	reactions and any suspected	All Member States where the product is
decentralised or subject to referral	transmission via a medicinal	authorised and to the EMEA
	product of an infectious agent	

ADR, adverse drug reaction; EMEA, European Medicines Agency; RMS, Reference Member State.

PSUR. Once marketed, 6-monthly PSUR submissions should be continued following initial placing on the market in the EU and until 2 full years of marketing experience in the EU has been gained. Then, PSURs should be submitted once a year for the following 2 years and thereafter at 3-yearly intervals. PSURs should also be submitted upon request of a competent authority or the EMEA at any time after granting of the marketing authorisation. The increased frequency of PSURs is linked with the changes to the renewals procedure and will ensure regular examination of safety issues, undertaken in a coordinated manner across the EU.

However, there may be exceptions where the cycle may be restarted or an exemption to the requirement for 6-monthly and annual PSURs is granted. Circumstances where less frequent submissions may be appropriate include:
• Products authorised through line extensions to existing medicinal products;
• Newly authorised generic medicinal products.
Circumstances where more frequent submissions may be appropriate include:
• Variations introducing new indications, populations, dosage forms and routes of administration;
• An active substance that is a different salt/ester or derivative (with the same therapeutic moiety);
• The presence of an excipient without an established safety profile; and
• A risk management plan in place for a corresponding originator product requiring specific monitoring of a safety concern.

For medicinal products authorised under the centralised procedure, PSURs should be submitted to the competent authorities of all countries of the EEA and to the EMEA. It is recommended that information on all indications, dosage forms, routes of administration and regimens for a given active substance for medicinal products authorised to one marketing authorisation holder should be included in a single PSUR, with a single data lock point common for all aspects of product use. PSURs should be submitted within 60 days of the data lock point. If a time gap occurs between the data lock point of a regular PSUR and a request from a competent authority (e.g. renewal, review of risk–benefit, ad hoc PSUR request), a PSUR Addendum Report should also be submitted.

Where a product is authorised to more than one marketing authorisation holder, in the case of multiple applications, submission of common PSURs is acceptable provided that the products remain identical in all respects apart from their invented names and that the PSURs are submitted separately by each marketing authorisation holder. The data lock point should be based on the 'birth date' used for the first authorised product. When data received from any partner company might contribute meaningfully to the safety analysis and influence any proposed or effected changes in the product information of the reporting marketing authorisation holder, these data should be included, with source indicated, and discussed in the PSUR, even if it is known that they are included in the PSUR of another marketing authorisation holder.

After several years of preparatory work under the auspices of the Heads of Agencies (HMA), a large work-sharing scheme was successfully launched in 2007. This scheme does not, however, apply to centrally authorised products. For the rest of the products covered by this scheme, innovator companies were asked to propose dates for substances for which they considered their product to be the originator, and this was used as a basis for compiling a list of European harmonised birth dates (EU HBD) and data lock points (DLPs) for active substances.

The products have been distributed between the authorities, and the time limits for submitting PSURs have been set for products with an active substance authorised the first time after 1976. This list has now been adopted by all national agencies and is published on the HMA website. An additional list of EU HBD and DLPs has recently been published on the HMA website. Both these lists can be accessed at http://heads.medagencies.org and http://www.hma. eu/80html.

Under this scheme all products involving the same active substance will have the same EU HBD and DLP and therefore the same PSUR submission cycle. This will allow sharing of the PSUR assessment work load across the EU. Each active substance will be allocated a P-RMS (Reference Member State for the PSUR) who will take the lead in the assessment. For mutually authorised marketing authorisations, the P-RMS and RMS may not be the same EU Member State. Thus, companies are now encouraged to submit all PSURs with the same active substance in the same time period (i.e. to let the PSUR submission take place synchronously in all countries and for all companies). One authority is then in charge of assessing all PSURs with the same active substance and of communicating with the companies in question. The project has not been anchored in any legislation yet, but it is expected that the new PSUR procedures will be made statutory in connection with the development of the new pharmacovigilance legislation.

These PSURs are seemingly accessible to public. Recently, in three instances, the Danish Ministry of the Interior and Health has decided that access can be granted (in part) to PSURs on medicinal products under the Danish Act on Access to Public Records, subject to the exceptions listed in the Access to Public Administration Files Act.

18.10.2 Safety-related regulatory actions

Because Iceland, Liechtenstein and Norway have adopted the complete Community *acquis*, they are parties to the Community procedures. Consequently, the pharmacovigilance guidelines and procedures do not only apply with regard to the marketing authorisation holder's obligations towards competent authorities in Member States of the EU but also to those in Iceland, Liechtenstein and Norway. Likewise, the obligations that apply to the competent authorities of the Member States of the EU also apply to the competent authorities in these States.

18.10.2.1 Urgent safety restrictions

As provided for in Commission Regulations (EC) 1084/2003 and 1085/2003, provisional urgent safety restrictions may be taken in the event of a risk to public health. An urgent safety restriction may be taken by the marketing authorisation holder if the competent authority in the Member State or, for centrally authorised products, the EMEA does not raise any objection within 24 hours after the marketing authorisation holder's notification. The competent authority may also impose an urgent safety restriction.

In the case of a centrally authorised product, a Rapid Alert may be issued by the rapporteur, the Member State or the EMEA when a signal is identified that leads to concern about the risk–benefit balance of a centrally authorised product and that could lead to major changes for the status of the authorisation. If it is the marketing authorisation holder who first identifies a potentially urgent and serious issue, they needs to inform the EMEA without delay. The Rapid Alert is transmitted to the contact points of the Member States, the EMEA and the EC, and to the rapporteur of the centrally authorised product that is the subject of the Rapid Alert. The EMEA, in agreement with the rapporteur, promptly starts an inquiry and information exchange with the marketing authorisation holder(s). The EMEA coordinates the process. The rapporteur works closely with the originator of the concern to evaluate the issue. Agreement is reached in each case on the responsibility for the Assessment Report on the risk–benefit balance, by the rapporteur, the Member State where the signal originated from, or jointly. Following risk evaluation a discussion is held at the PhVWP and subsequently at the CHMP within a defined time-frame. Any resulting CHMP Opinion on the measures to ensure the safe and effective use of the centrally authorised product is transmitted by the EMEA to the EC, in order to issue a binding Decision.

Should this concern a product authorised through the mutual recognition or the decentralised procedure, the Rapid Alert system should be used to communicate information on safety concerns. The RMS should preferably take the lead, but in case the concern was raised in a CMS, agreement needs to be reached regarding who will transmit the Rapid Alert. The Rapid Alert should be transmitted to the designated contact points in all Member States, the EMEA and the EC. The RMS should inform the marketing authorisation holder at the same time. The RMS should work closely with the CMS where the concern was raised (if not the RMS) and responsibilities for management and assessment of the safety concern should be agreed between them. They should also decide what additional information should be requested from the marketing authorisation holder and other CMSs. Following risk evaluation, a discussion should be held at the PhVWP with the aim of finalising an agreed position. In cases of a particularly pressing safety issue, a special meeting of the PhVWP may need to be convened and the RMS should keep the CMD(h) informed.

An urgent safety restriction should be followed by submission by the marketing authorisation holder of a variation application immediately and in no case later than 15 days after the initiation of the urgent safety restriction.

18.10.2.2 Safety-related suspension, revocation or variation

When, as a result of the evaluation of pharmacovigilance data, a Member State considers that a marketing authorisation should be suspended, revoked or varied in accordance with Article 107 and the guidelines referred to in Article 106(1), it shall forthwith inform the EMEA, the other Member States and the marketing authorisation holder. Where urgent action to protect public health is necessary, the Member State concerned may suspend the marketing authorisation of a medicinal product, provided that the EMEA, the EC and the other Member States are informed no later than the following working day.

18.10.2.3 Safety-related referral to CHMP

Under the terms of Articles 31, 36 and 37 of Directive 2001/83/EC, a Member State, the EC or the marketing authorisation holder may refer a pharmacovigilance matter relating to a nationally authorised product, including those authorised through the mutual recognition or the decentralised procedure, to the CHMP whenever the interests of the Community are involved. These matters may be referred by the CHMP to the PhVWP for consideration. The EC Decision issued on the basis of the CHMP Opinion is binding on all Member States.

18.10.3 Compliance with obligations for pharmacovigilance

The Position Paper on Compliance with Pharmacovigilance Regulatory Obligations (CPMP/PhVWP/ 1618/01), adopted in November 2001, has now evolved into requirements for monitoring for compliance and inspection. Competent authorities should monitor marketing authorisation holders for compliance with pharmacovigilance regulatory obligations. Furthermore, competent authorities exchange information in cases of non-compliance and will take appropriate regulatory action as required. It should be noted that enforcement action is within the competency of individual Member States. Article 84 of Regulation (EC) 726/2004 sets out the roles of the Member States, the Agency and the Commission with respect to the imposition of penalties for infringement of that Regulation or regulations adopted pursuant to it.

Some national authorities such as the MHRA have established a Pharmacovigilance Inspectorate. In the UK MHRA, it is part of the Inspections and Standards Division of the agency. It assesses pharmaceutical companies' compliance with UK and EU legislation relating to the monitoring of the safety of medicines given to patients.

It is one of the five inspectorates at the MHRA. The other four being:

1. Good Clinical Practice (GCP) Inspectorate;
2. Good Distribution Practice (GDP) Inspectorate;
3. Good Laboratory Practice (GLP) Inspectorate;
4. Good Manufacturing Practice (GMP) Inspectorate.

The legal basis for the conduct of pharmacovigilance inspections is set out in Article 111 of Directive 2001/83/EC and in Article 19(1) of Regulation (EC) 726/2004. Documentation supporting the pharmacovigilance system (and its detailed description) may be required during the pre-authorisation period, or post-authorisation, for purposes such as assessment or inspection.

There are three types of inspections:

1. *Routine national inspections* – these are scheduled inspections which marketing authorisation holders undergo on a periodic basis. Marketing authorisation holders are notified of these inspections in advance. These inspections are generally systems-based, meaning that inspectors examine the systems and procedures used by a marketing authorisation holder to comply with existing EU and national pharmacovigilance Regulations and guidance.

2. *'For cause' national inspections* – these are ad hoc inspections which are triggered as a result of, for example, safety issues, suspected violations of legislation relating to the monitoring of the safety of medicines or referrals by other Member States. In rare circumstances, marketing authorisation holders may not be notified of these inspections in advance.

3. *CHMP requested inspections* – the CHMP may request inspections of marketing authorisation holders in association with specific centrally authorised products. These can either be routine or triggered.

The current focus is on risk management strategies and the EC have drawn up a number of guidelines in consultation with the EMEA, Member States and interested parties in accordance with Article 106 of Directive 2001/83/EC as amended and Article 26 of Council Regulation (EC) 726/2004.

Volume 9A of 'The rules governing medicinal products in the European Union' concerns pharmacovigilance for medicinal products for human use (version September 2008) and is a compilation of all the pharmacovigilance guidelines and can be accessed at http://ec.europa.eu/enterprise/pharmaceuticals/eudralex/vol-9/pdf/vol9a_09-2008.pdf. The pharmacovigilance guidelines issued by PhVWP and/or ICH can be located at http://www.emea.europa.eu/htms/human/phv/phvwp.htm; http://www.emea.europa.eu/htms/human/ich/ichefficacy.htm; and http://www.emea.europa.eu/htms/human/raguidelines/pharmacovigilance.htm.

18.11 Wholesale distribution, pricing and reimbursement

Directive 2004/27/EC extended the harmonisation process to cover many aspects of wholesale distribution enshrined in Directive 92/25/EEC and these are set out in Recitals 34–38 and Articles 76–85 of Directive 2001/83/EC.

The EC has in the past tried to achieve a harmonisation of prices but this could not be achieved and produced the Transparency Directive (89/105/EEC). Therefore, Article 4(3) of Directive 2001/83/EC specifies that its provisions shall not affect the powers of the Member States' authorities either as regards the setting of prices for medicinal products or their inclusion in the scope of national health insurance schemes, on the basis of health, economic and social conditions.

Each Member State of the EU operates its own policy regarding the pricing of pharmaceutical products. The contents of the Transparency Directive (89/105/EEC) can be summarised by its various Articles as follows:

Article 1 If the authorities fix prices of the medicinal products, they must comply with the rules of this Directive;

Article 2.1 Time limit to comply with rules is 90 days;

Article 2.2 Reasons must be given by authorities if the price is other than that sought by the person putting the product on the market;

Article 3 Deals with procedures where price increases are sought;

Article 4 Imposed price freezes;

Article 5 Deals with profit regulation schemes;

Article 6 Deals with limited lists (positive lists);

Article 7 Deals with limited lists (negative lists);

Article 8 Classification of products by therapeutic class for inclusion or exclusion;

Article 9 Report on the operation of the Directive to be made within 2 years of its adoption;

Article 10 A committee to be set up;

Article 11 Demand that all Member States conform.

Essentially, the Directive allowed Member States to operate whatever scheme they chose provided they operated to 'objective and verifiable criteria'. In the UK, the primary tool is the Pharmaceutical Price Regulation Scheme (PPRS), which is better described as a profit-regulating scheme. The PPRS is the method by which the UK government seeks to control the prices of branded medicines. It is a voluntary scheme negotiated every 5 years between the Department of Health and the ABPI. The current scheme runs from 2005 to 2010. The Office of Fair Trading in the UK recommended in February 2007 that the PPRS should be reformed, to deliver better value for money from NHS drug spend and to focus business investment on drugs that have the greatest benefits for patients. This has been dealt with in detail elsewhere in this book (see Chapter 29). Other Member States have created various but differing combinations of price fixing, profit or volume limiting and product listing (positive or negative) to control health care spending relating to medicinal products. Generic substitution is encouraged or even mandatory in many Member States.

18.12 International harmonisation and conclusions

It is evident that despite being a union of 27 sovereign Member States, much has been achieved in harmonisation of legislation and regulation of human medicinal products across the EU. The process of harmonisation is underpinned by a desire for transparency, promoting public health and protecting consumer safety, without impediments to scientific advance, free trade and competition. It has been highly successful in bringing safe and effective medicines to the market in a timely manner across the entire EU. If sovereign Member States can achieve such broad and deep harmonisation, the scope for much wider harmonisation was clearly appreciated in early 1980s.

In June 1984, the EC had decided that a meeting with the Japanese authorities, attended by M.F. Sauer (France) and the chairman and vice-chairman of the Safety Working Party, Dr J.P. Griffin (UK) and Professor R. Bass (Germany), respectively, and the chairman of the Efficacy Working Group, Professor J-M. Alexandre, should take place in Tokyo. These discussions provided an opportunity for initiating wider harmonisation. Subsequently, the US FDA and Pharmaceutical Research and Manufacturers of America (PhRMA) joined the dialogue. However, it was at the WHO Conference of Drug Regulatory Authorities (ICDRA), at Paris, in 1989, that specific plans for action began to materialise. Soon afterwards, the authorities approached the International Federation of Pharmaceutical Manufacturers Association in Geneva to discuss a joint regulatory–industry initiative on international harmonisation. These efforts culminated ultimately in the ICH process, where the WHO, Canadian Health Protection Branch and the EFTA countries enjoy an observer status. The EU has proved to be a highly proactive partner in the ICH process and has provided important leads to other regulatory authorities of the world, either indirectly or formally through the ICH. In fact, some of the toxicology guidelines produced by the Safety Working Party set up by the 'old' CPMP has formed the basis of a number of ICH guidelines.

However, it is interesting to note that harmonisation is extending well beyond the scope envisaged in the ICH initiatives. In order to increase transparency and to benefit from exchange of information, the EC has signed agreements of bilateral cooperation with the US FDA in September 2003. The agreement allowed the two to exchange confidential information as part of their regulatory processes, both pre-approval and post-approval, including scientific advice, orphan drug designation, paediatric development and inspection reports, marketing approvals and post-authorisation surveillance information. In May 2006, the agreement was extended to include joint FDA/EMEA briefing meetings with sponsors following voluntary submission of genomic data. The areas of cooperation were further extended in October 2008 to cover advanced therapy medicines and nanotechnology-derived medicinal products, as well as exchange of pharmacovigilance information. Following a visit of Dr Margaret Hamburg, the new FDA commissioner to Brussels in July 2009, the EU and the FDA agreed that both agencies will share more data and expertise. In addition, both have already agreed to post experts in each other's food and drug safety agencies to enhance further coordination of policies. In February 2007, the EU and the Japanese Ministry of Health, Labour and Welfare (MHLW) signed an agreement to enable the EMEA and Japanese Pharmaceuticals and Medical Devices Agency (PMDA) to exchange confidential information about the authorisation and safety of medicines. In December 2007, a similar agreement was signed with Health Products and Food Branch of Health Canada to enable the regulatory experts from the two sides to exchange confidential information about the authorisation and safety of medicines. A similar agreement is under discussion with the Australian Therapeutic Goods Administration.

19 Paediatric regulation

Heike Rabe

Brighton & Sussex University Hospitals, UK

19.1 Introduction

The development of paediatrics as a speciality in its own right has been established for over 100 years. Health care professionals working in this field are aware that children are not small adults. However, with regard to developing correct dosages of drugs for children, and especially neonates, the dose calculations have often been 'down' calculated from the adult dosage by body weight only. This has led to toxic over-dosing in the past. For example, in the 1950s, chloramphenicol was applied to newborn infants at 100–200 mg/kg/day, which led to cardiovascular collapse (Gray's syndrome). Following evidence regarding the physiologically immature activity of the glucuronyl-transferase of the liver, the dose was adjusted to 25 mg/kg/day.

With evolving techniques in paediatrics and neonatology, more neonates and children are surviving severe illnesses, yet up to 50–90% of prescribed drugs are not approved for use in these age groups.

19.2 Case study

To illustrate the problems faced daily by clinicians, imagine the case of Lucy (fictitious name and history; see Figure 19.1). Lucy was born prematurely at 26 weeks' gestation (thus 14 weeks too early). After birth a neonatal team took care of her. An immediate problem in those born preterm is immature lungs, for which an endotracheal tube was passed into her lungs through which surfactant could be applied to relieve her respiratory distress syndrome and improve

The Textbook of Pharmaceutical Medicine. Edited by John P. Griffin. © 2009, ISBN: 978-1-4051-8035-1.

oxygen delivery. Altogether she received 11 drugs on her first day of life. Of these only four are currently licensed for use in premature infants in the UK: vitamin K, surfactant, benzylpenicillin and gentamycin. Would such a situation be acceptable for adult patients?

19.3 Paediatric population in the European Union

The European Union (EU) currently consists of 28 Member States with more countries waiting to join in the future. About 20% of the EU population are less than 16 years of age which equates to 100 million children. These children need to be divided into groups by age and maturity: preterm neonate; term neonate; infant; child and adolescent. At each developmental stage their body system will react differently to administered drugs. Gender differences might also have a role, especially in puberty, but not much attention has been paid to this possibility in the past. A shift of early onset of pubertal stages, particularly in girls, will need to be taken into account in future studies of drug efficacy and safety.

19.3.1 Special paediatric physiology

With respect to normal and abnormal physiological processes, preterm and term infants, children and adolescents have a wide variation in bodily functions. For example, the percentage of total body water and extracellular fluid volume decreases significantly from a preterm infant to an adult, while the body fat content increases (Figure 19.2). After birth a great transition takes place as the body's organs begin to carry out functions that were previously supported by the placenta. In preterm infants renal function can be impaired as a result of immature function and fewer numbers of receptors leading to increased water

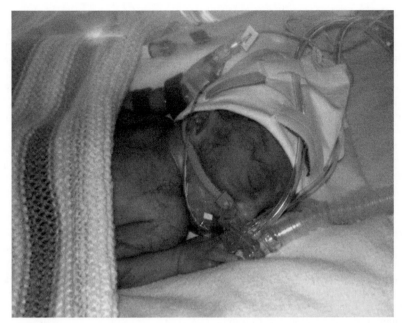

Figure 19.1 Preterm baby.

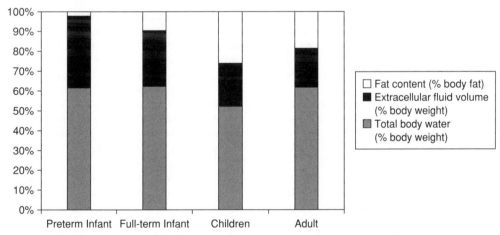

Figure 19.2 Comparison of body composition in premature infants, full term infants, children and adults.

and electrolyte losses. As the infant matures, renal function will mature, but will still be different from older children and adults. This is reflected in different normal values for different age groups. Similarly, gut absorption of metabolites varies according to age and maturity. Skin barrier is different, which can lead to increased absorption of drugs applied locally, which might offer an alternative route of application. Liver function can be immature even in full-term infants, which often leads to neonatal jaundice as a result of hyperbilirubinaemia from immature action of the uridine diphosphate-glucuronyl transferase in the endoplasmatic reticulum. All such functional variation will have an impact on any drug absorption and uptake into the body as well as metabolism and excretion pathways.

Pharmacogenetics, pharmacokinetics and pharma-codynamics according to age and maturity should be taken into account when designing studies on new and existing medicinal products for children. More information is needed in this area, in particular for preterm and term neonates, but also about gender differences, which might occur during pubertal stages. Meticulous attention is needed to all aspects of drug metabolism including possible side effects and inadvertent or unexpected reactions. All such reactions should be recorded, especially if unexpected. Quite often these will only occur once the drug is already marketed. A central reporting system is necessary to identify all such problems at an early stage.

19.3.2 Orphan diseases

An orphan disease in this context is a disease that has not been 'adopted' by the pharmaceutical industry because it provides little financial incentive for the private sector to make and market new medications to treat or prevent it. An orphan disease may be a rare disease by number of people affected in a population. According to US criteria, an orphan disease is one that affects fewer than 200,000 people. There are more than 5000 such rare disorders. For the paediatric population these are often inborn errors of metabolism, for which life-long treatment is necessary. Drugs for metabolic diseases are often difficult to develop and test and are therefore expensive to produce as the volume of demand is small compared to those for common diseases.

Another definition of orphan diseases might be a common disease that has been ignored (e.g. tuberculosis, cholera, typhoid and malaria) because it is far more prevalent in developing countries than in the industrialised world. Lattery, these diseases are recurring with the increased mobility of people and also with the increased spread of HIV and AIDS. The US Orphan Drug Act of 1983 offered tax incentives on clinical trials and 7 years of marketing exclusivity for drugs developed for conditions that occur only rarely in the USA. Since then, more than 200 orphan drugs have been approved by the US Food and Drug Administration (FDA) and have reached the market. Similar legislation has been adopted in Japan and Australia. In the year 2000, the European Union adopted 'orphan medicinal products' legislation modelled on the US law, but including tropical diseases and other disorders prevalent only in the developing world. The EU law provides for 10 years of marketing exclusivity, but no tax incentives as there is no centralized EU taxation system.

19.3.3 Long-term effects of drugs

One major difference for studies performed in children is the much longer life expectancy, not only of newly born generations of children but also in general compared to an adult who is enrolled in a trial at the age 50 or 60 years. There are currently no data available on long-term effects of drugs that have been studied in newborn infants. Limited data are emerging from studies in children with cancer or leukaemia who have been treated as young children and are now 20–30 years old.[1,2] The effect of drugs given in early infancy or childhood might be very difficult to study as individuals are exposed to environmental factors that might influence the development of illnesses in later life. However, for future studies, prospective long-term follow-up should be part of the paediatric investigation plan (PIP), so that confounding factors can be accounted for. In particular, in multicentre multinational trials with a large patient cohort, valuable evidence might emerge from such studies.

19.4 New paediatric drug regulation

19.4.1 History of legislative initiative

The new paediatric drug regulation came into force on 26 January 2007.[3] This was enabled by a 10-year process which started with a round table discussion of the European Commission (EC) and the European Medicines Agency (EMEA) in December 1997 following the Food and Drug Administration Modernization Act (FDAMA), which the US Congress passed in the same year. The latter encourages studies of certain therapies being used in paediatrics by providing an exclusivity incentive provision.

The round table meetings were followed by an EC Council Resolution in December 2000. A formal consultation with EU Member States was performed between November 2001 and January 2004. In parallel, an extended impact assessment for improving the provision of labelled and licensed drug use in children was initiated as part of 'Better regulation for Europe' in 2003–2004. From these activities a draft regulation was adopted by the EU Commissioners in September 2004. The First Reading by the EU Council of Ministers in November 2004 was followed by the First Reading in European Parliament in April 2005, which was followed by a vote in September 2005. The Second Readings took place in the Council in the first quarter of 2006 and in the Parliament in the second quarter of 2006. The adopted regulation was published in December 2006, from which the Entry into force resulted in January 2007.

19.4.2 Aims and objectives of the regulation

The major aims of the new regulation are the reduction of unlicensed or off-label use of medicines in children and especially in neonates. In order to achieve this goal there needs to be a coordinated effort on a European and international level. This aims at avoiding repeating studies for approval of medicines by different drug regulatory bodies such as FDA and EMEA. The necessary studies should be performed according to the principles laid out in the Good Clinical Practice (GCP) guidelines. The legal framework for these have been laid in the Clinical Trials Directive (2001/20/EC)[4] and the International Conference on Harmonisation (ICH) guidelines E11 and E6 (GCP).[5] The ethical framework already exists through the Declaration of Helsinki and its updates and recently was defined in more detail by EU recommendations on ethics of clinical trials in children.[6]

The legislation will improve the health of children by increasing the volume of high quality ethical research into medicines for use in children. Through this it will increase the availability of authorized medicines for children and the information about them. All the above goals need to be achieved without delaying the authorization of new drugs to the adult population.

19.4.3 Changes applying to industry

In the future, investigation plans for the study of new drugs will only be approved if they incorporate a PIP.

This applies to all drugs, which might be relevant for the treatment in children as well as in adults. The PIPs will be thoroughly reviewed by the Paediatric Board, in order to avoid any unnecessary studies in children. At the same time, the approval of drugs for use in adults should not be delayed by studying the drugs in children as well. The study of drugs in children will increase the cost of new drug development. As an incentive, the industry will be offered an extension of the protective patent by 6 months. The standard length of patent protection is 17 years with an average effective patent duration of 10 years when development time is taken into account (under certain circumstances a Supplementary Patent Certificate may be awarded). The increase of costs will be well compensated by large innovative pharmacology industry but for smaller companies and for generic drugs this might be more difficult. It will need to be closely observed whether the new legislation will have negative effects for such smaller enterprises.

19.4.4 New regulatory bodies

19.4.4.1 Paediatric Board

The previously established Paediatric Expert Group (PEG) housed by the EMEA has been replaced by the new Paediatric Board (PB). This consists of experts from national competent authorities, representatives of patient and parent groups, health care professionals and members of the Committee for Medicinal Products for Human Use (CHMP) from the EMEA. All EU Member States should have one representative through the above composition, which makes it a large committee to work within (Figure 19.3). The work of the PB will be overseen by the EMEA. The PB

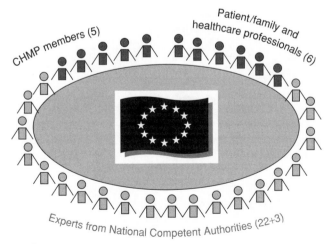

Figure 19.3 Paediatric Board.

will have a key role in approving PIPs for new drugs. For currently used drugs its members will review available knowledge and grant waivers and deferrals. New PIPs for existing drugs, which will focus on specific questions and new applications, will also be considered and approved.

19.4.4.2 Paediatric Use Marketing Authorization

A new type of marketing authorization related to paediatrics, the Paediatric Use Marketing Authorization (PUMA), will have a key role in the approval of existing drugs already used in children. Through this task it can concentrate on paediatric drugs only. The information from the literature on existing drugs already used off-label in children will be reviewed in order to grant waivers and deferrals as appropriate. This will support the aim of the new regulation of avoiding unnecessary studies and doubling up of efforts. PUMA will be involved in approving PIPs for new drugs. It will oversee the post-marketing requirements and surveillance, especially with regard to safety aspects and inadvertent side effects. This is particularly important for drugs used in orphan diseases, where not many children are affected in each country.

19.4.5 Role of the European Medicines Agency

The EMEA has a key role in the implementation of the new regulation. The Medicines for Children branch coordinates the work of the PB, communicates with other official government bodies such as the European Commission Directorate General Research, Brussels, the US Food and Drug Administration, the National Institute of Health, Washington DC, pharmaceutical industry, national and international paediatric expert societies and parent and patient representatives associations. The goal of this coordination is to work towards acknowledging each other's drug authorization, thus avoiding repeating studies in children in the USA and Europe for example.

Details about the framework, regulations and ongoing activities can be found on the EMEA's website.[7] Together with the expert societies the paediatric branch of the EMEA has been drawing up concept papers about specialist aspects on drug trials in children with regard to organ function and disease areas. Specific attention needs to be given to variations in pharmacogenetics, pharmacodynamics and therapeutic range in different age groups.

More recently, the stakeholders have issued priority lists of off-label use drugs which should be studied urgently (Figure 19.4). As the patent on these drugs has often expired, extra government funding is available in the European Union and the USA to fund such studies.[8]

A thorough review of the available literature and surveys on the use of existing paediatric medicines are ongoing in order to provide evidence for the priority lists.

An online database of all existing and future paediatric drug trials is essential for avoiding doubling up studies. This database should contain the basic

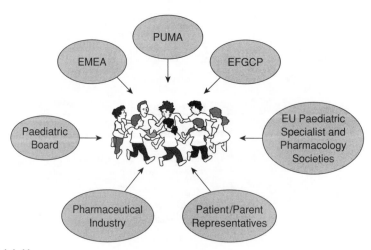

Figure 19.4 Stakeholders.

data on study: title, contact details, participating centre/countries, disease studied, age and sex of study patients, aim of study, inclusion and exclusion criteria, name of study drug and type of trial (e.g. therapeutic efficacy, pharmacokinetics, dose finding, safety, toxicity). A sample of a database can be found at www.dec-net.org.[9] Currently, a number of databases exist.[10–12] In addition, a number of states have national study databases where all ongoing trials are registered. In the UK trials are automatically entered on the appropriate database by the supervising research and development department of the host institution. There is clearly a need for a European trial database or even an international one. Most journals have now implemented a policy that they will only consider a manuscript on a drug trial for review if this trial had been registered on one of the databases.

It is anticipated that a number of studies can only be performed successfully with recruitment rates over a reasonable time period if they are performed within national or international study networks and consortia. The European and US paediatric expert societies have a major role in initiating and coordinating study networks in their expert field (e.g. neonatology or paediatric oncology). Specific emphasis lies in incorporating new EU Member States and associated countries into the expert networks. The networks can then apply for funding to study drugs from the EMEA/FDA priority lists.

Some EU member states already had well-functioning paediatric networks, such as PAED-NET in Germany[13] which has expanded its role in order to cover the new regulation. Others have initiated the foundation of a national agency, such as the Medicine for Children Research Network (MCRN) in the UK, which has been divided into regional subnetworks by geographical area or by speciality (e.g. neonatology).[14] These networks are supporting the EMEA in its role (e.g. by conducting surveys on the use of drugs in children). They also support the aims of the regulation by informing the public, and especially children, about the purpose and need of studying new and existing drugs. This can be achieved by visiting school programmes, children's focus groups and workshops or other public meetings, which are currently tested in Germany and England, for example. The regulation will only be successful if studies are initiated and recruited into. This requires the enthusiasm and engagement of health professionals, who are prepared to take up the extra work, quite often without no or very little remuneration.

19.5 Ethical aspects of studies in children

The new regulation takes into account that children are not small adults. In the past, drug trials in children have been approached with caution as they are more difficult to perform than in adults, they might take longer to recruit to and bear extra cost during the drug approval process. It was said that trials might even be unethical. Thus, most studies of medicinal products have been performed by industry in young adults rather than children or even neonates.

However, recent publications demonstrate that studies are not impossible in children. Parents give consent for their child to participate even in the very young age groups. Certainly, the experience from the USA shows that a positive motivation from industry is paramount. This can be achieved by extending the patent protection and has therefore been implemented into the European regulation. Instead of excluding children from research as a means of false protection, including them will provide sound evidence about the safety and efficacy of medicinal products. Therefore, obtaining proper scientific evidence is ethically justified.

Special attention has been given to the question how informed consent should be obtained. It is generally accepted that even young children can learn and understand the purpose of a drug study if this is explained in an age-appropriate way. Children often gain more knowledge and understanding as they go through the process of treatment and other therapy for their illness. Information should be given by an experienced health professional with a paediatric background. Information can be supported by pictures, simple drawings, videos and other means of communication such as written information leaflets in simple language. Children have the right to be informed about their treatment, especially as certain drugs might have life-long consequences, which are currently unknown.

The EMEA has issued guidance on ethical aspects with regard to drug trials.[6] It specifically outlines the rights of children and the ages at which assent should be sought. Adolescents might even be eligible for giving legally valid consent for themselves, depending on their cognitive maturity rather than simply age. This needs attention in particular in cases of conflict, where for example the parents or legal guardian of a child would give consent but the child does not agree to participate in a trial. National legal regulations might vary in such case in different EU countries.

19.5.1 Ethics committees in the European Union

The new drug regulation can only be put into practice if all required institutions and committees are set up and are functioning. All studies of medicinal products have to be reviewed and passed through either a national or local ethics committee. In case of multicentre and multinational studies this can be a lengthy process. Therefore guidance documents have been produced to speed up this process and also to make it safe and transparent.

The ethics working group of the European Forum for Good Clinical Practice (EFGCP) have published a structured report on 'The Procedure for the Ethical review of Protocols for Clinical Research Projects in the European Union'.[15] There is quite a variation in how ethics committees are set up, their membership structure and their code of practice. Interestingly, new EU member states, who did not have formal ethical review processes in the past, have been able to implement the European guidelines more easily as they have not had to deal with the sometimes slow to adjust historic ways of workings in ethics committees. The report still revealed a number of areas where further work will be needed (e.g. the training of research ethics committees, their quality assurance, the recruitment of vulnerable subjects and the handling of safety reports, specifically suspected unexpected serious adverse reactions (SUSARs)).

Several workshops are being held throughout Europe in order to bring ethics committees and stakeholders together. The work will feed back into any possible amendments of the Clinical Trial Directive 2001/20/EC.

Streamlining the ethics review process will certainly help to encourage the studies on medicinal products in children, if possible with removing any unnecessary international hurdles.

19.6 Conclusions

The new regulation on the use of medicinal products in children provides the unique opportunity for the products to be licensed for the use in children and adults at the same time. In the future this will provide sound evidence for the health care professional who is prescribing the drug, as well as the patients and their carers about the safety and efficacy of the new drug. For the currently off-label or unlicensed drugs used in the children, extra government or central European funding will be needed in order for these drugs to be licensed. There are still many questions to be answered with regard to funding, ethical reviews of studies, quality assurance, training for health care professionals involved in trials and adequate rapid distribution of knowledge. A key area will be multinational cooperation with countries outside the European Union so that unnecessary repetition of studies can be avoided and drugs can be approved quickly. It is very important that all stakeholders, including industry, work closely together to achieve these goals. The information on the topic is constantly changing and being updated. Therefore it is recommended that the interested reader has a regular look at the websites provided in the reference list.

References

1 von der Weid NX. Adult life after surviving lymphoma in childhood. *Support Care Cancer* 2008;16:339–45.
2 Schellong G, Pötter R, Brämswig J et al. High cure rates and reduced long-term toxicity in pediatric Hodgkin's disease: the German–Austrian multicenter trial DAL-HD-90. The German–Austrian Pediatric Hodgkin's Disease Study Group. *J Clin Oncol* 1999;17:3736–44.
3 Regulation (EC) No 1901/2006 of the European Parliament and of the Council of 12 December 2006 on medicinal products for paediatric use. *Official Journal* 2007; 26 Jan.
4 Directive 2001/83/EC of the European Parliament and of the Council of 6 November 2001 on the Community code relating to medicinal products for human use. *Official Journal L* 2001;311:67–128.
5 http://www.ich.org/cache/compo/475-272-1.html
6 http://ec.europa.eu/enterprise/pharmaceuticals/paediatrics/docs/paeds_ethics_consultation20060929.pdf
7 www.emea.europa.eu/htms/human/paediatrics/introduction.htm
8 www.nih.gov
9 www.dec-net.org
10 www.trialscentral.org
11 www.clinicaltrials.gov
12 www.fda.gov
13 www.paed-net.org
14 www.mcrn.org.uk
15 www.efgcp.org

20 European regulation of medical devices

Christopher J.S. Hodges

University of Oxford, Oxford, UK

20.1 Introduction

The regulatory system for medical devices is quite different from that for pharmaceuticals. It does not involve the assessment of a product by a medicines agency or the grant of a marketing authorisation. Instead, the onus of ensuring and declaring that a product conforms to the legal essential requirements is placed on the manufacturer, but in many instances this is subject to approval by an independent technical organisation (known as a notified body).

A manufacturer must apply an appropriate conformity assessment procedure to their device in order to ensure that it complies with the essential requirements, after which they must certify this fact by completing a declaration of conformity. There is usually a choice of conformity assessment procedures open to a manufacturer, depending on a risk-based classification of the class into which the device falls. The two main approaches to conformity assessment are based either on an approved total quality management system audited to ISO 9000 series standard, as customised for medical devices with EN 46000 series standard, or individual product assessment.

The essential requirements relate to the safety in use of the device, including labelling requirements, but are principally expressed in terms of scientific and technical performance characteristics. Efficacy, as such, is not a criterion. Confirmation of conformity must include evaluation of clinical data for many devices, generated from either a compilation of scientific literature or the results of clinical investigations on the product, for which prior ethical and regulatory approval is required. Conformity of a device with the essential requirements is denoted by affixing a CE marking to the device. CE marking, which must be marked on the device, acts in effect as the passport that authorises the device to be placed on the market and to circulate freely within the European Economic Area (EEA).

The legal obligation is that a product must comply with the relevant essential requirements, but where the manufacturer chooses to apply a national standard that adopts a European harmonised standard (EN series) to an aspect of the product, conformity will be prima facie presumed in respect of the aspects of the essential requirements covered by that standard. Other national or international standards do not have this regulatory benefit. Compliance with the essential requirements at the time of placing the device on the market, or declaration of this fact, should mean that the device is safe but it may later transpire that this is not the case. Manufacturers therefore have some post-marketing vigilance requirements. If a marketed device is unsafe, the competent authority of a Member State has power under a safeguard clause in each Directive to take regulatory action to effect the withdrawal of the product from the market in its jurisdiction: the matter is then referred to the Commission and all Member States who then coordinate their actions.

European pharmaceutical regulation has been in existence since the mid-1960s and over four decades has successively extended from control of the requirements for placing a product on the market and the data necessary to justify this, coupled with control on manufacture, to virtually all aspects of dealing with a medicine, including wholesale dealing, advertising and clinical research. In contrast, systematic regulation of medical devices is more recent and dates from the 1990s. It essentially covers the requirements for placing a product on the market, coupled with aspects

The Textbook of Pharmaceutical Medicine. Edited by John P. Griffin. © 2009, ISBN: 978-1-4051-8035-1.

of manufacture, labelling and clinical investigation. Aspects such as distribution may be regulated soon under amendments to the medical devices legislation and/or the 'new approach' legislation, and are regulated in general terms for consumer products. Generic controls cover advertising and trade practices [1]. The central difference is that many activities with pharmaceuticals require prior competent authority approval, which is not the case with devices.

Before the medical devices Directives came into being, most medical devices were unregulated in most European states. In some states some were regulated (illogically, but this was the only available mechanism) as if they were medicines. Examples of products formerly regulated as medicines in the UK include: contact lens products; intrauterine contraceptives; certain medicated dressings, surgical ligatures and sutures; absorbent or protective materials; and dental filling substances.

20.2 Law on specific devices

The EEA law on the marketing of medical devices is governed by three principal Directives, each of which adopt the Community's matrix scheme for product regulation known as the 'new approach'.[1] The new approach applies to many product sectors, such as machinery, personal protective equipment, low voltage equipment and electromagnetic compatibility (EMC) requirements but not to pharmaceuticals or cosmetics. Both the 'new approach' and medical devices models were reviewed in the first decade of the twenty-first century and extensions and reforms are anticipated. There are three device Directives:

1. Directive 90/385/EEC on active implantable medical devices (AIMDs) came into force on 1 January 1993 and is mandatory from 1 January 1995. This covers all powered implants or partial implants that are left in the human body, such as a heart pacemaker.

2. Directive 93/42/EEC on medical devices came into force on 1 January 1995 and became mandatory on 14 June 1998. This covers a wide range of devices ranging from first aid bandages, tongue depressors and blood collection bags to hip prostheses and active (powered) devices.

3. Directive 98/79/EC on *in vitro* diagnostics (IVDs) came into force on 7 June 2000 and is mandatory from 7 December 2003. This covers products such as pregnancy tests, blood glucose monitoring and tests for transmissible diseases.

A transitional period is provided under each of these Directives so that during the period from the coming into force of the Directive until it is mandatory, manufacturers may choose whether to apply the Directive to their device or the national rules that were in force immediately prior to the date on which the Directive came into force. From the date a Directive becomes mandatory, a device that is covered by national law implementing that Directive must comply with it.

Under Community law, a Directive is binding on each Member State, which is obliged under the EC Treaty to implement the Directive into its national law. A Member State has the discretion to choose the manner in which the Directive may be implemented so long as the effect of the Directive is achieved under its national legal order. Most Member States transpose Directives into their national law by enacting domestic legislation that follows the text of the Directives closely, if not verbatim. However, differences between implementing laws can arise, particularly in relation to enforcement and sanctions for non-compliance, which are aspects only governed by Directives in broad terms so are in any event matters for the national authorities. It is the national law that is directly binding on people, companies and operations within a particular state, not the Directive. However, because the Directive ultimately governs the national law, people often colloquially refer to the Directive rather than the national law and this approach will be adopted in this chapter. Nevertheless, in any given situation, one must always check the relevant national law and consider, first, what its provisions are; secondly, to what extent they differ from the Directive; and, thirdly, whether any difference constitutes a breach of Community law by the Member State and what consequences might follow, such that the national provision might be unenforceable.

The UK legislation is the Medical Devices Regulations 2002/618.

The basic structure, concepts and terminology of the three Directives on AIMDs, medical devices and IVDs are identical; the differences that exist among them arise out of the different nature of these products. The following discussion will therefore focus on the medical devices Directive (MDD), because this

---

[1] Directive 2005/29/EC on unfair business-to-consumer commercial practices, implemented by the Consumer Protection from Unfair Trading Regulations 2008, SI 2008/1277.

is the central Directive and covers most products. Short sections follow on AIMDs and IVDs. Detailed analysis of the relevant provisions would fill a large book: what is intended here is to highlight the important aspects which should be considered.

The basic purpose of the MDDs, as with all product Directives based on Article 95 (formerly 100a) of the EC Treaty, is to ensure that devices placed on the EEA market ensure *a high level for the protection of safety and health* of patients, users and others, when properly maintained and used in accordance with their intended purpose.[2] The reference to a 'high level' of protection should be noted: the standard of safety and protection required by the legislation is significant. Strictly speaking, this high level only applies where a device is properly maintained and used in accordance with its intended purpose. In practice, however, danger arising where a device has not been properly maintained or as a result of misuse would be highly likely to lead to action by the authorities.

Despite the emphasis of the legislation on safety, an equally important basic purpose of the legislation relates to the EEA's commerce and the economy. All Directives have as a basic purpose the creation of a European internal market without internal barriers to trade and with a single harmonised set of laws governing the placing of a product on the market and its free movement within the market.[3]

The intention behind the legislative scheme is that a product should essentially be regulated under a single product-specific regime as a medicinal product,[4] AIMD, medical device, IVD, cosmetic,[5] blood or blood product,[6] or personal protective equipment.[8] However, certain other Directives might apply to particular medical devices, including:

1. Directive 89/336/EEC on electromagnetic compatibility (the EMC Directive): EMC requirements are included within the essential requirements of the MDDs so the EMC Directive only applies to medical devices before the relevant MDD is applicable.

2. Directive 2001/95/EC on general product safety (GPS): this applies to all consumer products, some of its obligations apply to medical devices used by consumers.

20.3 Resolution of uncertainties

Because this legislation is extensive, complex, frequently written in generalised terms and seeks to create an entirely new regulatory system for products that were formerly largely unregulated, difficulties of interpretation or application are bound to arise. As the Directives constitute a legal system, ultimate authority for interpretation rests with the courts, fundamentally with the Court of Justice of the European Communities in Luxembourg, to which questions of interpretation of Community law may be referred by national courts. A mechanism exists, however, under the MDDs by which measures and interpretations may be formally adopted: in the case of the MDD this is the Article 7 Committee, which is a committee of representatives of Member States chaired by the Commission. Under the Article 7 procedure, the Commission may submit to the Committee a draft of measures to be taken, on which the Committee delivers its opinion based on a weighted majority of representatives. The Commission will adopt the measures envisaged if they are in accordance with the opinion of the Committee. If there is divergence, the Commission then permits a proposal to the Council of Members, which acts by a qualified majority of votes.

Less formal, non-binding procedures also exist. There are frequent meetings between representatives of the Commission, Member States and notified bodies. The Commission is also assisted by a Working Group of Experts. A sequence of guidance notes have been issued by the Commission (MEDDEV series), by certain competent authorities (such as the UK Agency's Bulletins) arising out of the meeting of notified bodies, by trade associations and others.

20.4 Competent authorities and notified bodies

Each Member State has designated a competent authority, which is the governmental authority responsible for implementing the Directive in that Member State. In the case of the UK, the competent authority is the Medicines and Healthcare products Regulatory Agency (MHRA). The principal function of a competent authority in practice is to ensure the safety and health of patients and users of medical devices.

A competent authority is not involved in the assessment or authorisation for placing a medical device on the market. As stated above, the legal responsibility in each case rests with the individual manufacturer. However, in many cases the manufacturer is required to obtain independent certification from a third-party testing house, called a notified body. Such testing houses are private commercial enterprises that may apply for, and be approved for, the purposes of the legislation by the competent authority in their Member State and are then notified within the Community by their approval being published in the *Official Journal*. Notified bodies may be approved for all devices or only for specific classes of devices. Criteria that they must satisfy in order to be approved are set out in an Annex to the relevant Directive (Annex XI for the MDD). In effect, therefore, notified bodies, although private entities, perform certain delegated regulatory functions. A manufacturer who is required by law to utilise the services of a notified body may choose any notified body within the Community who has the appropriate certification, irrespective of where either of them is located. The relationship between manufacturer and notified body is based on contract even though certain actions of the notified body have regulatory authority.

20.5 What is a medical device?

A medical device is defined as any instrument, apparatus, appliance, material or other article, whether used alone or in combination, including the software necessary for its proper application intended by the manufacturer to be used for human beings, for the purpose of:

1. Diagnosis, prevention, monitoring, treatment or alleviation of disease;
2. Diagnosis, monitoring, treatment, alleviation or compensation for an injury or handicap;
3. Investigation, replacement or modification of the anatomy or of a physiological process; or
4. Control of conception, and which does not achieve its principal intended action in or on the human body by pharmacological, immunological or metabolic means, but which may be assisted in its function by such means.[8]

An accessory is also considered to be a medical device. An accessory is defined as: an article that, while not being a device, is intended specifically by its manufacturer to be used together with a device to enable it to be used in accordance with the use of the device intended by the manufacturer of the device.[9]

20.6 The drug–device borderline

Difficult borderline questions arise in relation to a significant number of products, particularly whether they are to be classified as medicinal products or as medical devices. As a general rule, a relevant product is regulated either under the MDDs or by the medicinal products Directives (MPDs). Normally, the procedures of both Directives do not apply cumulatively. The Commission has issued guidelines on this drug–device borderline issue[10] and also on what constitutes medical devices, AIMDs and accessories. In order to decide which regime applies, the relevant criteria are:

1. The intended purpose of the product, taking into account the way the product is presented (this is likely to establish if either the MDD or MPD apply, rather than distinguish between the two regimes).
2. The method by which the principal intended action is achieved. This is crucial in the definition of a medical device. Typically, the medical device function is fulfilled by physical means (including mechanical action, physical barrier, replacement of, or support to, organs or body functions). The action of a medicinal product is achieved by pharmacological or immunological means or by metabolism.

The principal intended action of a product may be deduced from:

- The manufacturer's labelling and claims;
- Scientific data regarding mechanism of action.

Although the manufacturer's claims are important, it is not possible to place the product in one or other category in contradiction with current scientific data. Manufacturers may be required to justify scientifically their rationale for classification of borderline products.

Medical devices may be assisted in their function by pharmacological, immunological or metabolic means, but as soon as these means are not any more ancillary with respect to the principal purpose of a product, the product becomes a medicinal product. The claims made for a product, in accordance with its method of action may, in this context, represent an important factor for its classification as medical device or medicinal product. Examples of medical devices incorporating a medicinal substance with ancillary action include catheters coated with heparin or an antibiotic, bone cements containing antibiotic, and blood bags containing anticoagulant.[11]

20.7 Drug–device combinations

The MDD specifies the following approaches:[12]

1. A device that is intended to administer a medicinal product (e.g. an unfilled syringe) is a medical device. The medicinal product itself remains regulated as a medicine.

2. If the device and the medicinal product form a single integral product which is intended exclusively for use in the given combination and which is not reusable (e.g. a pre-filled syringe), that single product is regulated as a medicine. An application for a marketing authorisation must be made under Directive 2001/83/EC. However, the safety and performance of the device features of the integral product are assessed in accordance with the essential requirements of Annex I of the MDD.

3. Where a device incorporates, as an integral part, a substance that, if used separately, may be considered to be a medicinal product and that is liable to act upon the body with action ancillary to that of the device (e.g. a heparin-coated catheter), the product is classed as a medical device. However, the medicinal product is to be assessed in accordance with the requirements of Directive 75/318/EEC (replaced by 2001/83/EC and updated by 2003/63/EC). A notified body undertaking conformity assessment on a medical device that incorporates a medicinal substance having ancillary action has a responsibility to consult a national medicines agency about the medicinal substance, to verify its safety, quality and usefulness by analogy with the appropriate methods specified in Directive 75/318/EEC.

20.8 Classification of devices

The purpose of classification of devices is simply so as to provide options for conformity assessment methods. Under the MDD, medical devices are categorised into four classes, generally according to the degree of risk that they represent. In summary, Class I covers those that do not enter or interact with the body; Classes IIa and IIb are invasive or implantable devices or those that do interact with the body; Class III is for devices that affect the functions of vital organs. Implantables with an energy source are covered by the AIMD Directive (AIMDD). The detailed classification rules are lengthy and are set out in Annex IX of Directive 93/42/EEC. A sequence of rules must be worked through: charts and software are available to assist this.

The classification system uses three basic criteria, in various combinations: duration of contact with the body, degree of invasiveness and the anatomy affected by the use of the device.

Duration is based on continuous use (i.e. uninterrupted actual use) and categorised as transient (<60 min), short term (±30 days) or long term (>30 days). Invasive devices penetrate wholly or partly inside the body by way of an orifice or via the surface of the body. A body orifice is a natural opening in the body and includes the external surface of the eyeball and any permanent artificial opening, such as a stoma. Surgically invasive devices penetrate via the surface to the inside of the body by surgical intervention. Implantable devices are surgically invasive devices intended to be totally introduced to the body, to replace an epithelial surface or the surface of the eye and intended to remain in place after the procedure, and also includes those partially introduced surgically invasive devices remaining in place for at least 30 days. The central circulatory system is defined by the following vessels: arteriae pulmonales, aorta ascendens, arteriae coronarieae, arteria carotis communis, arteria carotis externa, arteria carotis interna, arteriae cerebrales, truncus brachicephalicus, venae cordis, venae pulmonales, vena cava superior, vena cava inferior. The central nervous system consists of the brain, meninges and spinal cord. Active medical devices depend on a power source, such as electricity, for its operation, but not sources of power generated by the human body or gravity.

Non-invasive devices are covered by rules 1–4 and include the following classes:

1. Class I, for example, ostomy pouches, wheelchairs, eye glasses, incontinence pads, cups and spoons for administering medicines, wound dressings, such as cotton wool and wound strips.

2. Class IIa, for example, transfusion equipment, storage and transport of donor organs, polymer film dressings, hydrogel dressings.

3. Class IIb, for example, haemodialysers, dressings for chronic extensive ulcerated wounds.

Invasive devices are covered by rules 5–8 and include the following classes:

1. Class I, for example, dressings for nose bleeds, hand-held dentistry mirrors, enema devices, reusable surgical instruments.

2. Class IIa, for example, contact lenses, urinary catheters, tracheal tubes connected to a ventilator, needles used for suturing, infusion cannulae, dental bridges and crowns.

3. Class IIb, for example, urethral stents, insulin pens, devices supplying ionising radiation, intraocular lenses, maxillofacial implants.

4. Class III, for example, prosthetic heart valves, rechargeable non-active drug delivery systems, absorbable sutures, spinal stents, neurological catheters, temporary pacemaker leads. Hip, knee and shoulder joint replacements were reclassified from Class IIb to Class III [2].

Active devices, while covered under the above rules, are largely covered by rules 9–12 and include the following classes:

1. Class I, for example, examination lights, surgical microscopes, wheelchairs, thermography devices, recording, processing or viewing of diagnostic images.

2. Class IIa, for example, suction equipment, feeding pumps, anaesthesia machines, ventilators, hearing aids.

3. Class IIb, for example, lung ventilators, incubators for babies, surgical lasers, X-ray sources.

Special rules 13–18 govern several hazardous characteristics that may be found in certain devices and require a certain level of control and conformity assessment. Rule 13 deals with devices incorporating a medicinal substance whose action is ancillary to that of the device – Class III, for example, antibiotic bone cements, condoms with spermicides, heparin-coated catheters.

Rule 14 deals with devices used for contraception or the prevention of transmission of sexually transmitted diseases – Class IIb, for example, condoms, contraceptive diaphragms and if they are implantable or long-term invasive; Class III, for example, intrauterine devices.

Rule 15 deals with devices for specific disinfecting, cleaning and rinsing and includes contact lens disinfecting, cleaning, rinsing and hydrating – Class IIb, for example, contact lens solutions, comfort solutions, and devices specifically intended for disinfecting medical devices; Class IIa, for example, disinfectants for use with endoscopes.

Rule 16 classifies non-active devices specifically intended for recording X-ray diagnostic images as Class IIa, for example, X-ray films.

Rule 17 classifies all devices utilising animal tissues or derivatives rendered non-viable and coming into contact with breached skin as Class III, for example, biological heart valves, porcine xenograft dressings, catgut sutures, collagen implants and dressings.

Rule 18 puts blood bags into Class IIb.

If several rules apply to a device, the strictest rule resulting in the higher classification applies. It must be reiterated that classification is based on the manufacturer's intended use and thus the listing of devices into classes must be taken as guidance only. No classification system can be perfect and thus the

aim is to capture the majority of products while recognising that there will always be products that are borderline either between classes or with other product types, such as drugs and cosmetics, and also new innovative products that do not fit the criteria laid down.

20.9 Conformity assessment procedures and CE marking

Depending on the class of the device, a manufacturer may be able to choose between a number of alternative conformity assessment procedures in the assessment of whether a medical device conforms to the essential requirements. Although the rules should be considered in detail in each case,[13] the basic options might be summarised as follows:

1. For all products in Classes IIa, IIb and III, and AIMDs, a full quality assurance system, audited periodically by a notified body (Annex II of the MDD), which includes examination and certification by the notified body of the design dossier of each product covered. The manufacturer must keep documentation on the quality system and the design dossier of each product plus other documentation. The quality system obligations include post-marketing and vigilance aspects. Compliance with Annex II may be achieved (this is not mandatory but is invariably adopted voluntarily) by compliance with the EN 29000 and 46000 series standards, which apply the ISO 9000 series.

2. For products in Classes IIa, IIb and III, and AIMDs, examination and certification by a notified body of a specimen product (type examination: Annex III of the MDD) coupled with a varying degree (partially restricted by product class) of product or production quality assurance (MDD Annexes IV, V and VI), which ensures that the manufacturing process produces products that conform to the certified type and might involve a quality system for manufacture and final inspection (Annex V), or a quality system for final inspection and testing (Annex VI).

3. For products in Class I, the manufacturer must have specified technical documentation on the design of the product showing that it conforms to the essential requirements: manufacturing aspects are not covered and a notified body is not involved unless there is a measuring function and/or the product is sterilised. (Annex VII: EC declaration of conformity.)

In all cases, the specified documentation must be kept for 5 years after the last product has been

[2] Commission Directive 2005/50/EC, implemented by the Medical Devices (Amendment) regulations 2007, SI 2007/400.

manufactured. The Annex VII procedure is also available for Class IIa devices if coupled with the Annex IV or V or VI procedure.

20.10 Registration

The manufacturer of a Class I device or of a custom-made device, or a person who markets a system or procedure pack, must inform the competent authority of the manufacturer's registered place of business and the description of the devices concerned.[14] Such manufacturers who are located outside the EEA must designate persons established within the Community who are responsible for such registration.

20.11 Harmonised standards

Manufacturers may voluntarily decide to apply any standard to their product or business. Devices that are in conformity with a national standard adopted pursuant to a harmonised EC standard published in the *Official Journal of the European Communities* are presumed by Member States to comply with those aspects of the essential requirements that are covered by the standard. Harmonised standards are those adopted by the EC standards bodies pursuant to a mandate issued by the Commission, in this case the European Committee for Standardisation (CEN) and the European Committee for Electrotechnical Standardisation (CENELEC). A large number of standards are contemplated but may take time to be written and adopted. Standards may be horizontal (covering aspects common to all or a number of product types) or vertical (dealing only with a specific aspect or specific product type). Important harmonised standards exist on the following:

• EN 13485 Medical devices – Quality management systems – Requirements for regulatory purposes;
• EN 1041 information and labelling for medical devices;
• EN 980 graphical symbols;
• EN 10993 series biological evaluation of medical devices;
• EN 14155-1 Clinical investigation of medical devices for human subjects – Part 1: General requirements; EN 14155-2 Clinical investigation of medical devices for human subjects – Part 2: Clinical investigation plans;
• EN 60601 series medical electrical equipment;
• EN 14971 – Medical devices – Application of risk management to medical devices.

20.12 Custom-made devices

A new device that is specifically made in accordance with a duly qualified medical practitioner's written prescription and which gives, under the practitioner's responsibility, specific design characteristics, and is intended for the sole use of a particular patient is permitted to be marketed without CE marking under provisions referring to custom-made devices.[15] The prescription may be made by any person authorised by virtue of their professional qualifications to do so. Mass produced devices that need to be adapted to meet the specific requirements of the medical practitioner or any other professional user are not considered to be custom-made devices.

The manufacturer must undertake to keep available for the competent authorities documentation on the design, manufacture and performance of the product so as to allow assessment of conformity with the essential requirements. The manufacturer must also draw up a statement containing the following information:
1. Data allowing identification of the device in question.
2. A statement that the device is intended for exclusive use by a particular patient, together with the name of the patient.
3. The name of the medical practitioner or other authorised person who made out the prescription and, where applicable, the name of the clinic concerned.
4. The particular features of the device as specified in the relevant medical prescription.
5. A statement that the device in question conforms to the essential requirements set out in Annex I of the Directive and, where applicable, indicating which essential requirements have not been fully met, together with the grounds.
Manufacturers must inform the competent authorities of their registered place of business and the description of the devices concerned.

20.13 Systems and procedure packs

A number of items are sometimes assembled and marketed together as a particular system or to be used with a particular medical procedure. The individual items might or might not already bear CE marking. Where all the devices bear CE marking and are put together within the intended purposes specified by their manufacturers, a person or manufacturer who puts them together must draw up a declaration stating the following:

1. They have verified the mutual compatibility of the devices in accordance with the manufacturers' instructions and have carried out their operations in accordance with these instructions.

2. They have packaged the system or procedure pack and supplied relevant information to users incorporating relevant instructions from the original manufacturers.

3. The whole activity is subjected to appropriate methods of internal control and inspection.

The system or procedure pack must not bear additional CE marking and must be accompanied by the original manufacturers' information. The declaration must be kept for 5 years.

Where the above conditions are not met, as in cases where the system or procedure pack incorporates devices that do not bear CE marking or where the chosen combination of devices is not compatible in view of their original intended use, the system or procedure pack must be treated as a device in its own right and the appropriate conformity assessment procedure must be followed.

20.14 Essential requirements

The essential requirements contained in Annex I of each new approach Directive specify the aspects of safety and performance that must be satisfied at the time at which a relevant product is placed on the market. Essential requirements are stated as principles or as generalised aspects and exclude detailed technical requirements. The scheme of the Community's new approach is that detailed technical aspects are not required as legal obligations but, if they are generally accepted, may be applied voluntarily by manufacturers through being included in official standards.[16] The essential requirements are intended to be comprehensive and all must be satisfied save for those requirements that do not apply to a particular product as a matter of common sense.

The essential requirements in the MDD fall under two headings: general requirements and requirements regarding design and construction. The general requirements include the following provisions:

1. The devices must be designed and manufactured in such a way that when used under the conditions and for the purposes intended, they will not compromise the clinical condition or the safety of patients, or the safety and health of users or, where applicable, other persons, provided that any risks that may be associated with their use constitute acceptable risks when weighed against the benefits to the patient and are compatible with a high level of protection of health and safety.

2. The solutions adopted by the manufacturer for the design and construction of the devices must conform to safety principles, taking account of the generally acknowledged state of the art. In selecting the most appropriate solutions, the manufacturer must apply the following principles in the following order:

(a) Eliminate or reduce risks as far as possible (inherently safe design and construction);

(b) Where appropriate, take adequate protection measures including alarms if necessary, in relation to risks that cannot be eliminated;

(c) Inform users of the residual risks due to any shortcomings of the protection measures adopted.

3. The devices must achieve the performances intended by the manufacturer and be designed, manufactured and packaged in such a way that they are suitable for one or more of the functions as specified by the manufacturer.

4. The characteristics and performances referred to in sections 1–3 above must not be adversely affected to such a degree that the clinical conditions and safety of the patients and, where applicable, of other persons are compromised during the lifetime of the device as indicated by the manufacturer, when the device is subjected to the stresses that can occur during normal conditions of use.

5. The devices must be designed, manufactured and packed in such a way that their characteristics and performances during their intended use will not be adversely affected during transport and storage, taking account of the instructions and information provided by the manufacturer.

6. Any undesirable adverse effect must constitute an acceptable risk when weighed against the performances intended.

Section 2 above implies that a manufacturer must carry out a risk analysis. A harmonised standard is available on this topic, EN 14971, which amplifies the methodology for risk analysis, elimination or reduction required by section 2.

The essential requirements regarding design and construction are too extensive to be summarised here. They cover the following headings:

- Clinical, physical and biological properties;
- Infection and microbial contamination;
- Construction and environmental properties;
- Devices with a measuring function;
- Protection against radiation;
- Requirements for medical devices connected to, or equipped with, an energy source; and

• Information supplied by the manufacturer (see below).

20.15 Information supplied by the manufacturer

The general principle is that each device must be accompanied by the information needed to use it safely and to identify the manufacturer, taking account of the training and knowledge of the potential users. This information comprises the details on the label and the data in the instructions for use. A series of 13 particular requirements are specified for inclusion in the label and the same 13 requirements plus a further 15 categories of information must be included in the instructions for use.

As far as practicable and appropriate, the information needed to use the device safely must be set out on the device itself and/or on the packaging for each unit or, where appropriate, on the sales packaging. If individual packaging of each unit is not practicable, the information must be set out in the leaflet supplied with one or more devices. Instructions for use must be included in the packaging for every device. By way of exception, no such instructions for use are needed for devices in Class I or IIa if they can be used safely without any such instructions.

Where appropriate, this information should take the form of symbols. Any symbol or identification colour used must conform to the harmonised standards. In areas for which no standards exist, the symbols and colours must be described in the documentation supplied with the device.

It will be noted that in the above three paragraphs, which are quoted verbatim from Annex I, certain flexibility is permitted through use of the words 'where appropriate': this is a feature of many of the other essential requirements. The manufacturer is permitted some discretion over compliance with the essential requirements, based on an application of common sense to the circumstances of his particular product.

20.16 Who is a manufacturer?

A manufacturer is defined as the natural or legal person with responsibility for the design, manufacture, packaging and labelling of a device before it is placed on the EU market under that manufacturer's own name, regardless of whether these operations are carried out by that manufacturer or on their behalf by a third party. The Directives also apply to those who assemble, package, process, fully refurbish or label a product and in certain other situations.

The intention is that the person (more normally, the company) who assumes the legal responsibility of 'manufacturer' need not be the person who assembles the product. One or more of the activities of design, manufacture, packaging or labelling may be subcontracted by the legal manufacturer. The name or tradename and address of the legal manufacturer must appear on the label and instructions for use.[17] In addition, for devices imported into the Community, the label, or the outer packaging, or instructions for use, must contain the name and address of either the authorised representative of the manufacturer established within the Community, or of the importer established in the Community (this is in effect for devices whose importation is not authorised by the manufacturer), or for the person who has the responsibility to register with the competent authorities in the case of Class I or custom-made devices.

20.17 Manufacturers outside the EEA

A non-EEA manufacturer may place a Class I or custom-made medical device or a system or procedure pack on the EU market under their own name provided it has undergone a relevant conformity assessment procedure and bears CE marking, and the competent authorities in the relevant Member State have been informed of either:

1. The manufacturer's registered place of business in that Member State, if they have one, and the description of the device; or

2. The registered place of business in that Member State of a person designated by the manufacturer as responsible for marketing the device in the European Union, and the category of the device.[18]

In relation to devices in Classes II, IIa and IIb, a manufacturer must certify conformity personally under the Annex II procedure, but an authorised representative established in the European Union may do this in place of the manufacturer under the Annex III and IV procedures.

The functions of an authorised representative are not precisely defined in the Directives except for the IVDD, but such a person is explicitly designated by the manufacturer, and acts and may be addressed by authorities and bodies in the Community instead of the manufacturer with regard to the latter's obligations.[19] It would be good practice for the manufacturer to have a written contract recording their relationship.

20.18 'Placing on the market' and 'putting into service'

The Directives provide that devices may be placed on the market and put into service only if they comply with the requirements laid down in the Directive when duly supplied and properly installed, maintained and used in accordance with their intended purpose.[20] Devices, other than devices that are custommade or intended for clinical investigations, that are considered to meet the essential requirements set out in Annex I of the relevant Directive must bear the CE marking of conformity when they are placed on the market.[21]

The CE marking of conformity, as specified in MDD Annex XII, must appear in a visible, legible and indelible form on the device or its sterile pack, where practicable and appropriate, and on the instructions for use. Where applicable, the CE marking must also appear on the sales packaging. It must be accompanied by the identification number of the notified body responsible for implementation of the relevant conformity assessment procedure. It is prohibited to affix marks or inscriptions that are likely to mislead third parties with regard to the meaning or the graphics of the CE marking. Any other mark may be affixed to the device, to the packaging or to the instruction leaflet accompanying the device provided that the visibility and legibility of the CE marking is not thereby reduced.

The concepts of 'placing on the market' and 'putting into service' are standard in Community 'new approach' Directives. For the purposes of the MDD, they are defined as follows:

1. *Placing on the market* means the stage of first making available in return for payment or free of charge a device other than a device intended for clinical investigation, with a view to distribution and/or use on the Community market, regardless of whether it is new or fully refurbished.

2. *Putting into service* means the stage at which a device has been made available to the final user as being ready for use on the Community market for the first time for its intended purpose.[22]

The European Commission has issued guidance on these concepts in the context of all 'new approach Directives'.[23] In essence, a device is placed on the market when it is first put into the stream of distribution or commerce by its manufacturer. A device that is fully refurbished is treated as if it were a new device and must be subject afresh to the requirements of the Directive. Difficulties arise over the definition of what constitutes refurbishment (simple servicing is clearly not included) and aspects, such as upgrading.

20.19 Clinical investigation

Confirmation of conformity with the essential requirements must be based on clinical data in the case of:
• (As a general rule) implantable and long-term invasive devices falling within Classes IIa and IIb, and all Class III devices under the MDD;[24]
• All active implantable devices under the AIMDD.[25]

The adequacy of such clinical data must be based on either:
• A compilation of the relevant scientific literature and, 'if appropriate', a written report containing a critical evaluation; or
• The results of all clinical investigations made.

Thus, evaluation of the clinical safety and performance is required for all devices, whereas a clinical investigation of each device may or may not be necessary (the term 'clinical trial' is not used in relation to devices). The Directives give some latitude over the circumstances in which a clinical investigation of a non-CE marked device is required. Guidance issued by the MHRA[26] states that an investigation would be required where:

1. There is the introduction of a completely new concept of device into clinical practice where components, features and/or methods of action, are previously unknown.

2. An existing device is modified in such a way that it contains a novel feature, particularly if such a feature has an important physiological effect; or where the modification might significantly affect the clinical performance and/or safety of the device.

3. A device incorporates materials previously untested in humans, coming into contact with the human body or where existing materials are applied to a new location in the human body, in which case compatibility and biological safety will need to be considered.

4. A device, either CE marked or non-CE marked, is proposed for a new purpose or function. Clinical investigation will also be required where a CE marked device is to be used for a new purpose.

The regime of the Directives is that if clinical evaluation is required, it must be subject to ethical approval in accordance with the principles of the Declaration of Helsinki.[27] The Directives specify[28] that the purpose of a clinical investigation is to:

1. Verify that, under normal conditions of use, the performance of the devices conform to (those intended by the manufacturer, viz. the device should be designed and manufactured in such a way that it is suitable for the functions specified by the manufacturer).
2. Determine any undesirable side effects, under normal conditions of use, and assess whether they are acceptable risks with regard to the intended performance of the device.

The Directives also specify the methodology to be adopted in clinical investigations. Adverse incidents occurring in the investigation must be reported to the competent authority. A general requirement in the MDD is:

'Clinical investigations must be performed on the basis of an appropriate plan of investigation reflecting the latest scientific and technical knowledge and defined in such a way as to confirm or refute the manufacturer's claims for the device; these investigations must include an adequate number of observations to guarantee the scientific validity of the conclusions.'[29]

The primary consideration of a clinical investigation of a device is assessment verification of the manufacturer's claims for the technical performance of the device. Safety considerations are, nevertheless, relevant in that the clinical investigation should determine and assess any undesirable adverse effects, but the main thrust of the clinical evaluation, and in particular of the conformity assessment by a notified body or the manufacturer to permit marketing, is on technical performance rather than a complete evaluation of safety. It is an essential requirement for marketed devices that '[A]ny undesirable side-effect must constitute an acceptable risk when weighed against the performances intended'.[30]

Both the AIMDD[31] and the MDD[32] specify that a manufacturer must submit a statement [in the specified form (MDD Annex VIII) containing information as detailed as design drawings, manufacturing methods, descriptions and explanations and the results of calculations and technical tests] to the competent authority of the Member State in which the investigation is to be conducted. For Class II devices and implantable and long-term devices in Classes IIa and IIb the investigation may commence either after 60 days unless the authority has objected, or earlier if the authority so authorises, provided a favourable ethics committee opinion is available. For devices

other than those just specified, the Member State may authorise immediate commencement after receipt of notification, provided a favourable ethics committee opinion has been issued. A device that is intended for clinical investigation must not bear CE marking. Compliance with the requirements relating to clinical investigations (AIMDD Annex VII; MDD Annex X) is assisted by adoption of standards EN 14155-1 – Clinical investigation of medical devices for human subjects – Part 1: General requirements; EN 14155-2 – Clinical investigation of medical devices for human subjects – Part 2: Clinical investigation plans. These are very similar to pharmaceutical Good Clinical Practice.

Clinical investigation is not required for IVDs.

20.20 *In vitro* diagnostics

An IVD medical device is defined as any medical device that is a reagent, reagent product, calibrator, control material, kit, instrument, apparatus, equipment or system, whether used alone or in combination, intended by the manufacturer to be used *in vitro* for the examination of specimens, including blood and tissue donations derived from the human body, solely or principally for the purpose of providing information:

1. Concerning a physiological or pathological state or congenital abnormality;
2. To determine the safety and compatibility with potential recipients; or
3. To monitor therapeutic measures.

For the purpose of this Directive, a specimen receptacle, whether evacuated or not, specifically intended by its manufacturer to contain a specimen for the urposes of an IVD examination, is considered to be a device. Products for general laboratory use are not devices unless such products, in view of their characteristics, are specifically intended by their manufacturer to be used for IVD examination.[33]

The IVD Directive follows the same general 'new approach' scheme as the other MDDs with the following major differences. IVDs are divided into two classes: Annex II devices and everything else. Annex II devices are themselves divided into List A (high risk) and List B which include the following (each case also including calibrators and control materials):

1. List A:
(a) Reagents and reagent products for determining the following blood groups: ABO system, Rhesus (C, c, D, E, e) anti-Kell;
(b) Reagents and reagent products for the detection, confirmation and quantification in human specimens

of markers of HIV infection (HIV 1 and 2), human T-cell lymphocytotrophic virus (HTLV) I and II, and hepatitis B, C and D.

2. List B:

(a) Reagents and reagent products for determining the following blood groups: anti-Duffy and anti-Kidd;

(b) Reagents and reagent products for determining irregular anti-erythrocytic antibodies;

(c) Reagents and reagent products for the detection and quantification in human samples of the following congential infections: rubella, toxoplasmosis;

(d) Reagents and reagent products for diagnosing the following hereditary disease: phenylketonuria;

(e) Reagents and reagent products for determining the following human infections: cytomegalovirus, *Chlamydia*;

(f) Reagents and reagent products for determining the following human leucocyte antigen (HLA) tissue groups: DR, A, B;

(g) Reagents and reagent products for determining the following turmoral marker: PSA;

(h) Reagents and reagent products, including software, designed specifically for evaluating the risk of trisomy 21;

(i) The following device for self-diagnosis: device for the measurement of blood sugar.

One of the following two conformity assessment procedures may be followed for devices covered by Annex II:

1. The EC Declaration of Conformity procedure (full quality assurance: Annex IV); or

2. the EC type examination procedure (Annex V) coupled with either the EC verification procedure (Annex VI) or the EC Declaration of Conformity (production quality assurance: Annex VII).

All devices other than those covered by Annex II are subject to the EC Declaration of Conformity procedure (Annex III), which does not involve the intervention of a notified body, but which includes supplementary requirements for devices for self-testing, which does involve a notified body (Annex III).

Common technical specifications (CTS) are to be adopted by the Article 7.2 Committee (a working group of scientific experts appointed by the Member States) which will apply to devices in Annex II List A and, when required, devices in Annex II List B. There is some uncertainty about the circumstances in which the requirement might apply to List B devices. CTS establish appropriate performance evaluation and re-evaluation criteria, batch release criteria, reference methods and reference materials. If, for duly justified reasons, manufacturers do not comply with the CTS,

they must adopt other solutions that are at least equivalent to these specifications. CTS are intended mainly for the evaluation of the safety of the blood supply and organ donations.

Manufacturers shall notify competent authorities:

1. For reagents, reagent products, reference and control materials, of information concerning common technological characteristics and/or analytes, as well as any important and subsequent modification, including suspension of marketing authorisation.

2. For other IVDs, appropriate indications.

3. For devices in Annex II and devices for self-testing, all data allowing identification and the analytical parameters and, where applicable, for diagnostic products in Annex 1.3, results of evaluation of performance in accordance with Annex VIII and certificates of notified bodies.

Clinical evaluation is not appropriate for IVDs but a procedure is specified for performance evaluation studies in clinical laboratories or in other appropriate environments outside the manufacturer's premises (Annex VIII). Manufacturers who place devices on the market under their own name must notify the competent authorities of the Member State in which they have their registered place of business of the address of that registered place of business, the categories of devices as defined in terms of common characteristics of technology and/or analytes, and of any significant change thereto.

20.21 Advanced therapy medicinal products

Tissue engineered products are to be subject to the special regulatory regime for advanced therapy medicinal products (ATMPs) [3]. The rules may apply to tissue engineered products from January 2009 and become mandatory from January 2013. A tissue engineered product is one that contains or consists of engineered cells or tissues, and is presented as having properties for, or is used in or administered to human beings with a view to regenerating, repairing or replacing a human tissue [4]. Products containing or consisting exclusively of non-viable human or animal cells and/or tissues, which do not contain any viable cells or tissues and which do not act principally by

---

[3] Regulation (EC) 1394/2007.
[4] Regulation (EC) 1394/2007, Article 2.1.

pharmacological, immunological or metabolic action, are excluded from this definition [5].

ATMPs are regulated under the Community's centralized procedure for medicinal products, subject to certain extra requirements, including on traceability, labelling, post-authorisation follow-up of efficacy and adverse reactions, and risk management [6]. The donation, procurement and testing of human cells or tissues is regulated by Directive 2004/23/EC, discussed above. A medical device that forms part of a combined ATMP shall also meet the essential requirements for medical devices [7].

20.22 Adverse event reporting: vigilance

All adverse events with medical devices of which the manufacturer becomes aware must be recorded. The detailed legal requirements in relation to recording and reporting are, curiously, more onerous in relation to medical devices than AIMDs. However, the Commission's guidance is that they should be treated the same in practice. In general, a manufacturer of general medical devices should report, and a Member State record and evaluate:

1. Any malfunction or deterioration in the characteristics and performance of a device, or inadequacy in the labelling, that might lead to, or have led to, the death of a patient or user or to a serious deterioration in their state of health.

2. Any technical or medical reason in relation to the characteristics or performance of a device for the reasons referred to above, leading to systematic recall of devices of the same type by the manufacturer.

Guidance is issued by the European Commission on medical device vigilance[34] which includes an explanation of the difficult concept of when a deterioration in state of health should be considered serious:

• Life-threatening illness or injury;

• Permanent impairment of a body function or permanent damage to a body structure;

• A condition necessitating medical or surgical intervention to prevent permanent impairment of a body function or permanent damage to a body structure.

Regulatory data is (to be) stored on a European Database on medical devices accessible only to competent authorities. This will include data on registration, certificates issued or withdrawn and vigilance.[35]

20.23 General Product Safety Directive

Directive 2001/95/EEC [8] imposes GPS obligations on producers and distributors (as defined) of products 'intended for consumers or likely to be used by consumers'.

The obligations on producers are that they must:

1. Place only safe products on the market.

2. Provide consumers with the relevant information to enable them to assess the risks inherent in the product throughout the normal or reasonable foreseeable period of its use, where such risks are not immediately obvious without adequate warnings, and to take precautions against those risks.

3. Adopt measures commensurate with the characteristics of the products which they supply, to enable them to be informed of risks which these products might present.

4. Take appropriate action to avoid these risks including, if necessary, withdrawing the product in question from the market or recalling it.

5. Batch-mark products.

6. Immediately notify the competent authorities in each Member State in which the product is in circulation if a product placed on the market no longer complies with the definition of a safe product.

7. Inform the competent authorities of actions taken, or intended, to prevent risks.

8. Collaborate with the authorities on action taken to avoid risks.

Other obligations apply to distributors of consumer products. The GPS obligations apply in the absence of other specific rules of Community law governing the safety of such products. It is clear that the obligations under the MDDs cover most, if not all, producers' obligations which arise under the GPS Directive as set out above. Manufacturers are obliged, for example, under MDD Annex II, to undertake their notified body that they will institute and keep up to date a systematic procedure to review experience

---

[5] Regulation (EC) 1394/2007, Article 2.1.

[6] Regulation (EC) 1394/2007, Articles 4–15.

[7] Regulation (EC) 1394/2007, Article 6; see Directive 93/42/EEC or for active implantable medical devices Directive 90/385/EEC below.

---

[8] Implemented by the General Product Safety Regulations 2005, SI 2005/1803.

gained from devices in the post-production phase and to implement appropriate means to apply any necessary corrective action. This undertaking includes an obligation to notify the authorities of reportable adverse events. Whatever the strict legal position on whether GPS obligations do or do not apply to medical device manufacturers, their general principles should be followed as a matter of prudence and for product liability reasons.

20.24 Recall

A manufacturer may have a number of post-marketing obligations arising under either the medical devices legislation and/or the GPS legislation, and under product liability or negligence law. The precise legal provisions constitute a somewhat incomplete matrix, although the UK MHRA has issued guidance on the subject of recall (defined to include the return, modification, exchange, destruction or retrofit of a device) which covers in general terms the circumstances in which a recall might be appropriate and how it should best be implemented.[36]

20.25 Enforcement and sanctions

The MDDs authorise Member States to take enforcement action against medical devices that prove to be unsafe. The specific powers, offences, sanctions and penalties are subject to the discretion of Member States. Accordingly, these matters are provided for under national legislation and practice. It must be remembered that relevant national provisions may be found not only within national legislation implementing the relevant MDD, but also in other provisions such as general consumer protection, trade descriptions or criminal legislation. Where a Member State invokes the 'safeguard clause' under a MDD, removing a product from the market on grounds of safety, a mechanism must be followed under which the Commission and other Member States are notified, the position discussed, and a unified approach taken by the authorities.

Enforcement provisions are generally of two types: first, powers to investigate and take action against a product and, secondly, offences that may be committed by individuals for breach of which they may be prosecuted by the authorities and subject to criminal sanctions. In the UK, for example, the first category of provisions arise under the product-specific regula-

tions and Part II of the Consumer Protection Act 1987. The offences are as specified in the product-specific regulations. There is a considerable variation between Member States in the number and wording of criminal offences that may be committed and in the penalties that might be imposed.

Different national agencies have different practices on what action they may take when faced with dangerous products. The UK MHRA, for example, operates a practice of issuing a sequence of three advisory notices to UK health services, for which the criteria for the various safety warning categories are as follows.[37]
• Hazard notices are issued:
(a) In cases of actual death or serious injury, or where death or serious injury would have occurred but for the fortuitous circumstances or the timely intervention of health care personnel (or a carer);
(b) Where the medical device is clearly implicated;
(c) Where immediate action is necessary to prevent recurrence.
• Device alerts are issued:
(a) In cases where there is the potential for death or serious injury, or there may be implications arising from the long-term use of the medical device;
(b) Where the medical device is likely to be implicated;
(c) Where the recipient is expected to take immediate action on the advice.
• Safety notices are used to recommend or inform:
(a) Where action by the recipient will improve safety;
(b) Where it is necessary to repeat warnings on long-standing problems;
(c) To support or follow-up manufacturers' field modifications.

References

1 Council resolution of 7 May 1985 on a new approach to technical harmonisation and standards, OJ 1985 No. C 136/1, 4.6.85. [A Regulation and Directive were adopted in 2008 (reference unavailable at time of writing) to extend the 'new approach' matrix in relation to obligations on distributors, on post-marketing surveillance, information and recall of products, strengthening the accreditation system for conformity assessment bodies and strengthening the Community market surveillance system. Some of these aspects are already covered in the medical devices legislation.]
2 Directive 93/42/EEC, recitals 2, 3 and 5 and Article 2.
3 For example, Directive 93/42/EEC, recital 1.
4 Directive 65/65/EEC as amended and related Directives.
5 Directive 76/768/EEC as amended.
6 A Directive or Directives will be forthcoming on these products.

7 Directive 89/686/EEC as amended.

8 Directive 93/42/EEC, Article 1.2(a); Directive 90/385/EEC, Article 1.2(a).

9 Directive 93/42/EEC, Article 1.2(b).

10 Guidelines, European Commission, MEDDEV 2.1/3 rev. July 2001.

11 Draft Commission Guidelines, MEDDEV 14/93 rev. 2.

12 Directive 93/42/EEC, Recital 6 and Article 1.3 and 1.4.

13 Directive 93/42/EEC, Article 11.

14 Directive 93/42/EEC, Article 14.

15 Directive 93/42/EEC, Articles 1.2(d), 12.6 and Annex VIII.

16 Council Resolution of 21 December 1989 on a global approach to conformity assessment, OJ 1989 No. C10/1, 16.1.90.

17 Directive 93/42/EEC, Annex 1, paragraph 13.1.

18 Directive 93/42/EEC, Article 14.

19 Directive 98/79/EC, Article 1.2(g).

20 For example, Directive 93/42/EEC, Article 2.

21 For example, Directive 93/42/EEC, Articles 17 and 3.

22 Directive 93/42/EEC, Article 1.2(h) and (i) as amended by Article 21 of Directive 98/79/EC.

23 *Guide to the Implementation of Directives Based on the New Approach and the Global Approach*, European Commission 2000.

24 Directive 93/42/EEC, Annex X and Article 15.

25 Directive 93/42/EEC, Article 9, Annex 2 paragraph 4.1 and Annex 3 paragraph 3.

26 *Guidance Notes for Manufacturers on Clinical Investigations to be carried out in the UK*, MHRA, July 2008.

27 Directive 93/42/EEC, Annex 7, paragraph 2.2 and Directive 93/42/EEC, Annex X, paragraph 2.2.

28 Directive 93/42/EEC, Annex 7 and Directive 93/42/EEC, Annex X.

29 Directive 93/42/EEC, Annex X, Requirement 2.3.1.

30 Directive 93/42/EEC, Annex l, Requirement 6.

31 Directive 93/42/EEC, Article 10.

32 Directive 93/42/EEC, Article 15. 33. Directive 98/79/EC, Article 1.2(b).

33 Directive 98/79/EC, Article 1.2(b).

34 *Guidelines on a Medical Devices Vigilance System*, European Commission, MEDDEV 2.12-1 rev 5, April 2007.

35 Directive 93/42/EEC, Article 14a.

36 *Guidance on the Recall of Medical Devices*, Medical Devices Agency, 2000.

37 Medical Devices Agency, Safety Notices, 2001.

21 Technical requirements for registration of pharmaceuticals for human use: the ICH process

Dean W.G. Harron

School of Pharmacy, Medical Biology Centre, Belfast, Northern Ireland, UK

21.1 Introduction

The International Conference on Harmonisation of Technical Requirements for Registration of Pharmaceuticals for Human Use (ICH) is a unique project that has brought together the regulatory authorities of Europe, Japan and the USA and experts from the pharmaceutical industry in the three regions to discuss scientific and technical aspects of product registration. The purpose is to make recommendations on ways to achieve greater harmonisation in the interpretation and application of technical guidelines and requirements for product registration in order to reduce or obviate the need to duplicate the testing carried out during the research and development of new medicines. The objective of such harmonisation is a more economical use of human, animal and material resources, and the elimination of unnecessary delay in the global development and availability of new medicines while maintaining safeguards on quality, safety and efficacy, and regulatory obligations to protect public health.

21.2 ICH organisation

21.2.1 Members

Harmonisation, under ICH, involves the European Union, Japan and the USA, with the assistance initially of observers from the World Health Organization (WHO), the European Free Trade Association (EFTA) and Canada. The six co-sponsors of the Conference are:

1. European Commission – European Union (EU);
2. European Federation of Pharmaceutical Industries and Associations (EFPIA);
3. Ministry of Health and Welfare, Japan (MHW);
4. Japan Pharmaceutical Manufacturers Association (JPMA);
5. US Food and Drug Administration (FDA); and
6. Pharmaceutical Research and Manufacturers of America (PhRMA).

In addition, the International Federation of Pharmaceutical Manufacturers and Associations (IFPMA) participates as an umbrella organisation for the pharmaceutical industry, and provides the ICH secretariat.

21.2.2 The Steering Committee

The ICH Steering Committee oversees the preparations for ICH conferences, and the harmonisation initiatives that are undertaken under the ICH Process. The Committee normally meets two or three times a year.

21.2.3 Expert Working Groups

The Steering Committee is advised on technical issues concerned with harmonisation topics by Expert Working Groups.

These are joint regulatory–industry Working Groups for which experts are nominated from the six co-sponsors of the conference. The Working Groups deal with individual harmonisation topics under general headings: Safety (pre-clinical toxicity and related tests); Quality (pharmaceutical development and specifications); Efficacy (clinical testing programmes and safety monitoring); and Multidisciplinary (cross-cutting topics including regulatory communications and timing of toxicity studies in relation to clinical studies).

In October 1994, the ICH Steering Committee announced a 'new direction' in the harmonisation work coming within the review of ICH. In response to

The Textbook of Pharmaceutical Medicine. Edited by John P. Griffin. © 2009, ISBN: 978-1-4051-8035-1.

developments in communications technology and the need to avoid divergence in the three regions, which could affect the efficiency of the regulatory process, it was agreed that two aspects on Regulatory Communications should be included in the ICH programme; these are the development of an international Medical Terminology and agreement on Electronic Standards for the Transfer of Information and Data.

21.3 The ICH process

On the basis of experience to date, the Steering Committee has outlined a step-wise ICH Process (Figure 21.1) for monitoring the progress of the harmonisation work and identifying the action that is needed in order to reach a defined endpoint.

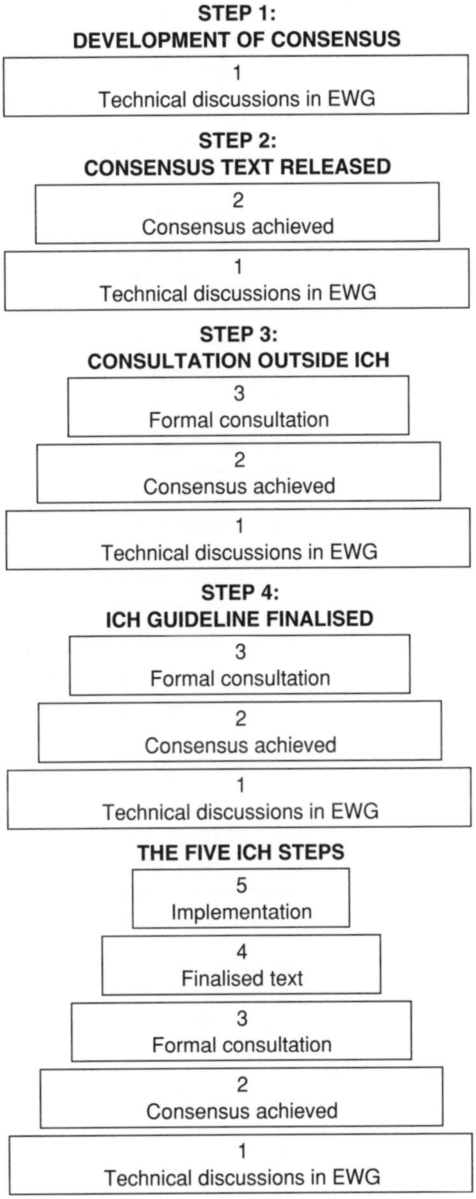

21.3.1 ICH Meetings and Conferences

It was agreed, from the start, that the focus for discussions of tripartite harmonisation should be an international conference or series of conferences. The Steering Committee recognised the importance of ensuring that the process of harmonisation is carried out in an open and transparent manner and that ICH discussions and recommendations are presented in open forums.[1-4]

• First International Conference on Harmonisation (ICH 1) Brussels, November 1991, hosted by the European Commission and EFPIA.
• Second International Conference on Harmonisation (ICH 2) Orlando, Florida, 27–29 October 1993.
• Third International Conference on Harmonisation (ICH 3) Yokohama, Japan, 29 November to 1 December 1995.
• Fourth International Conference on Harmonisation (ICH 4) Brussels, 16–18 July 1997.
• Fifth International Conference on Harmonisation (ICH 5) San Diego, USA, 9–11 November 2000.
• Sixth International Conference on Harmonization (ICH 6) Osaka, 12–15 November 2003.

21.3.2 Status of ICH Harmonisation Initiatives

It was generally assumed that following the ICH 4 meeting in 1997 that International Harmonisation had reached an interim conclusion and that the future would focus on developing a Common Technical Document (CTD) to improve efficiency in documenting new medicines for regulatory purposes. However, the ICH Process has continued not only for developing the CTD, but also ICH 5 and ICH 6 conferences

STEP 1:
DEVELOPMENT OF CONSENSUS

1
Technical discussions in EWG

STEP 2:
CONSENSUS TEXT RELEASED

2
Consensus achieved

1
Technical discussions in EWG

STEP 3:
CONSULTATION OUTSIDE ICH

3
Formal consultation

2
Consensus achieved

1
Technical discussions in EWG

STEP 4:
ICH GUIDELINE FINALISED

3
Formal consultation

2
Consensus achieved

1
Technical discussions in EWG

THE FIVE ICH STEPS

5
Implementation

4
Finalised text

3
Formal consultation

2
Consensus achieved

1
Technical discussions in EWG

Figure 21.1 The ICH process.

have been convened; the total number of finalised tripartite guidelines has now reached 59[5-11] (20 Quality, 13 Safety, 17 Efficacy, 7 Multidisciplinary, 2 eCTD), for examples see Tables 21.1–21.5. Full details are available on www.ich.org.

21.3.3 Common Technical Document

The adoption of the CTD was a major event that required a global level conference (ICH 5), both to

Table 21.1 ICH: guidelines (quality examples)

Topic	Guidelines	Step
Stability		
ICH Q1A(R2)	Stability testing of new drugs and products (revised guideline)	Step 5 (2003)
ICH Q1B	Photostability testing of new drug substances and products	Step 5 (1996)
ICH Q1C	Stability testing for new dosage forms	Step 5 (1996)
ICH Q1D	Bracketing and matrixing designs for stability testing of drug substances and drug products	Step 5 (2002)
ICH Q1E	Evaluation of stability data	Step 5 (2003)
ICH Q1F	Stability data package for registration in Climatic zones III and IV	Step 5 (2003)

Table 21.2 ICH: guidelines (safety examples)

Topic	Guidelines	Step
Safety		
ICH S1A	Guideline on the need for carcinogenicity studies of pharmaceuticals	Step 5 (1995)
ICH S1B	Testing for carcinogenicity of pharmaceuticals	Step 5 (1997)
ICH S1C	Dose selection for carcinogenicity studies of pharmaceuticals	Step 5 (1994)
ICH S1C(R)	Addendum to SIC: addition of a limit dose and related notes	Step 5 (1997)
Genotoxicity studies		
ICH S2A	Genotoxicity: guidance on specific aspects of regulatory tests for pharmaceuticals	Step 5 (1997)
ICH S2B	Genotoxicity: a standard battery for genotoxicity testing for pharmaceuticals	Step 5 (1997)

Table 21.3 CH: guidelines (efficacy examples)

Topic	Guidelines	Step
Good Clinical Practice		
ICH E6	Good Clinical Practice consolidated guideline	Step 5 (1996)
Clinical Trials		
ICH E7	Studies in support of special populations geriatrics	Step 5 (1993)
ICH E8	General considerations for clinical trials	Step 5 (1997)
ICH E9	Statistical principles for clinical trials	Step 5 (1998)
ICH E10	Choice of control group in clinical trials	Step 5 (2000)
ICH E11	Clinical investigation of medicinal products in the pediatric population	Step 5 (2000)
Guidelines for Clinical Evaluation by Therapeutic Category		
ICH E12A	Principles for clinical evaluation of new antihypertensive drugs (ICH principle document)	Step 5 (2000)
ICH E14	Clinical evaluation of QT/QTc interval prolongation and pro-arrhythmic potential for non-antiarrhythmic drugs	Step 2 (2003)

Table 21.4 ICH: guidelines multidisciplinary topics

Topic	Guidelines	Step
ICH M1	Medical terminology (MedDRA)	
ICH M2	Electronic standards for transmission of regulatory information (ESTRI)	
ICH M3	Timing of Pre-clinical studies in relation to clinical trials	
ICH M4	Organisation including the granularity documents that provides guidance on document location and paginations (common technical document)	Step 5
	(Revised annex: granularity document, November 2003) CTD: Q&As (updated November 2003)	Step 5 (2003)
ICH M4Q	Quality: the section of the application covering chemical and pharmaceutical data including data for biological/ biotechnological products (re-edited) CTD quality; Q&As	Step 5 (2002) Step 5 (2003)

Table 21.5 ICH: guidelines multidisciplinary/eCTD

Topic	Guidelines	Step
ICH M4S	The non-clinical section of the application (re-edited) CTD safety: Q&As (updated November 2003)	Step 5 (2002) Step 5 (2003)
ICH M4E	The clinical section of the Application (re-edited) CTD efficacy: Q&As (updated November 2003)	Step 5 (2002) Step 5 (2003)
eCTD	The electronic CTD eCTD: Q&As (updated November 2003)	Step 5 (2002) Step 5 (2003)
ICH M5	Data elements and standards for drug dictionaries	Step 1 (2003)

present the final document and consider implementation issues.

The arguments in favour of a CTD have been forcefully presented. Having harmonised the technical requirements for the demonstration of quality, safety and efficacy of a new medicinal product under the first phase of the ICH process, it seemed reasonable that the three regions should now agree on the way in which this information should be presented for the purpose of obtaining authorisation to place the medicinal product on the therapeutic market. This would obviously save unnecessary duplication and reworking and would decrease the time and resources required for submission of the regulatory documents, ultimately benefiting patients in the three regions and in the rest of the world.

The industrialists performed a feasibility study in Europe and the USA to determine some of the resource requirements for producing a CTD. They evaluated the time and resources required to convert a New Drug Application (NDA) to an EU application and vice versa. For eight international companies, it took an average of 3–4 months to convert one submission to the other; obviously a costly operation in terms of time and resources. However, the report showed the feasibility of developing the CTD and this was presented to regulators in advance of an ICH Steering Group Meeting. The feasibility report revealed slight differences between the three regions in the proposed format of technical dossiers. Agreed harmonisation of format was considered to be relatively easy to achieve, but harmonising content was considered to be harder as differences were greatest between the three regions with regard to the detail required in reports submitted to the regulatory authorities.

Thus, the CTD is feasible, but it is a formidable challenge. ICH has already demonstrated its ability to deliver and enforce consensus decisions based upon good science and mutual trust. There is therefore an opportunity to develop in common a more logical, more efficient, more user-friendly way of compiling the technical requirements for registration purposes, taking into account the most recent advances of regulatory science and the extraordinary potentials of new information technologies. The ICH Steering Committee agreed to a 2-year schedule to produce a document. It was also considered, and this is an important development, that the CTD would apply to generics and over-the-counter products and that their manufacturers should also be involved in discussions as to content. Up to this point, generic manufacturers and over-the-counter producers had been largely ignored by the ICH.

21.4 ICH 5 Meeting Report

21.4.1 Common Technical Document

Prior to the Conference, during which the ICH Expert Working Group and Steering Committee met, the ultimate objective of ICH 5 was achieved. The CTD was agreed, setting out a harmonised format for regulatory submissions (Table 21.6).

• *Module 1 – Administrative Information and Prescribing Information*. This contains documents specific to each region including, for example, application forms or the proposed label for use in the region; the content and format of this module will be specified by the relevant regulatory authorities.

• *Module 2 – Summaries*. In addition to a table of contents and a one-page introduction, this module contains the quality overall summary, the non-clinical overview and the clinical overview; these are followed by the non-clinical written summaries, the non-clinical tabulated summaries and the clinical summary [separate documents (M4Q, M4S, and M4E) give guidance on the format and content of the summaries].

• *Module 3 – Quality*. This covers information on manufacture, specifications, quality control and stability, which must be presented in the structured format described in Guideline M4Q.

• *Module 4 – Non-clinical Study Reports*. This covers reports on animal and *in vitro* tests, which must be presented in the order described in Guideline M4S.

• *Module 5 – Clinical Study Reports*. This covers human study reports and related information presented in the order described in Guideline M4F.

Table 21.6 Organisation of the common technical document (CTD) for the registration of pharmaceuticals for human use

---

Module 1: Administrative information and prescribing information
A. Table of contents
B. Documents specific to each region (e.g. application forms, prescribing information)

Module 2: Common technical document summaries
A. Overall common technical document table of contents
B. Introduction
C. Quality overall summary
D. Non-clinical overview
E. Clinical overview
F. Non-clinical summary
  1. Pharmacology
    a. Written summary
    b. Tabulated summary
  2. Pharmacokinetics
    a. Written summary
    b. Tabulated summary
  3. Toxicology
    a. Written summary
    b. Tabulated summary
A. Clinical summary
  1. Summary of biopharmaceutics and associated analytical methods
  2. Summary of clinical pharmacology studies
  3. Summary of clinical efficacy
  4. Summary of clinical safety
  5. Synopses of individual studies

Module 3: Quality
A. Table of contents
B. Body of data
C. Key literature references

Module 4: Non-clinical study reports
A. Table of contents
B. Study reports
C. Literature references

Module 5: Clinical study reports
A. Table of contents of clinical study reports and related information
B. Tabular listing of all clinical studies
C. Clinical study reports
D. Literature references

21.4.2 Implementation of the CTD

All three of the ICH regulatory parties: the European Commission, FDA and MHW, made firm commitments to implement the CTD, when their representatives spoke in a panel on *What the CTD will mean to Regulators* in the Closing Plenary.

By common agreement, at the ICH Steering Committee meeting, all three parties would accept applications in the CTD format from 1 July 2001. This will be on a so-called voluntary basis, as the time required before implementation can become mandatory will vary according to the formal steps needed in the three regions. It was apparent that a question in the minds of many in the audience was whether the new format would really replace current requirements. At several points in the CTD there is provision for authorities to ask for additional information according to 'regional requirements'.

Background
Each region has its own requirements for the organisation of the technical reports in the submission and for the preparation of the summaries and tables. In Japan, the applicants must prepare the GAIYO, which organises and presents a summary of the technical information. In Europe, Expert Reports and tabulated summaries are required, and written summaries are recommended. The US FDA has guidance regarding the format and content of the New Drug Application. To avoid the need to generate and compile different registration dossiers, this guideline describes a format for the Common Technical Document that will be acceptable in all three regions. (Organisation of the Common Technical Document M4.)

Harmonisation of the requirements for summaries (Module 2) has been the most challenging task for the CTD Working Groups. A background note in the CTD text (see extract above) identifies the current requirements that will be changed by CTD, but there was concern, for example, that FDA would still retain an additional 'regional' requirement for the Integrated Safety Summary (ISS) and Integrated Efficacy Summary (IES).

Dr Janet Woodcock, Director of the FDA Centre for Drug Evaluation and Research (CDER) confirmed that implementation of the CTD would require changes in the Code of Federal Regulations (CFR) and hoped that it would be possible to 'rewrite a more flexible and less specific CFR'. She cautioned, however, that this would take time and that the full consultations required under FDA's Good Guidance Practices must be followed. In response to questions about the ISS she indicated that this was still regarded as a 'crucial document' in assessment of safety but that FDA recognised the need to address the subject further in order to achieve the goal of a single clinical summary.

Ms Emer Cooke, Principal Administrator in the Pharmaceuticals and Cosmetics Unit of the European Commission Enterprise Directorate-General, presented a timetable under which the CTD could be fully implemented in the EU by July 2002:
• Revision of *Notice to Applicants*, Vol IIB, first quarter of 2001;
• Acceptance of applications in the new format, July 2001;
• Proposal for revision to Directive 75/318/EEC (technical directive), mid- to end-2001;
• Date for CTD to become mandatory, provisionally July 2002.

Dr Yoshinobu Hirayama, Director, Evaluation Division 1, of the MHW Pharmaceuticals and Medical Devices Evaluation Centre confirmed that 'the current GAIYO will be replaced by CTD Module II documents'. He cautioned, however, that although the CTD provides a common content and format, there will be cases where differences would necessarily occur in dossiers for the three regions (e.g. there may be different dosage recommendations and different quality requirements). He sympathised with the impact on industry who would feel 'the burden of transition more than regulators' and indicated that the transition time before the CTD became mandatory might depend on how much preparatory work needs to be done by industry. Progress on the electronic version of the CTD was discussed. It was anticipated that the eCTD specification would reach draft consensus (or Step 2 of the ICH Process) in May 2001 and be finalised (Step 4) by the end of 2001.

The Steering Committee for ICH 5 issued a statement on the future of ICH which emphasises the intentions of ICH to focus its activities on: implementing and maintaining existing guidelines, preventing disharmony, encouraging scientific dialogue and harmonisation in new areas (e.g. new technologies or therapies), and undertaking efforts towards global cooperation with non-ICH regions and countries. At its May 2001 meeting, the Steering Committee discussed practical aspects, including the possibility of harmonisation efforts in the area of the post-marketing activities.

21.5 The CTD post-ICH 5

21.5.1 Organisation of the CTD
The common format of the CTD has been changed slightly compared with the Step 2 version agreed in July 2000 (e.g. the 'Overall Summary' is now called 'Overview'). The new version of the organisation is shown in Table 21.6 (www.ich.org).

21.5.2 Benefits for authorities and applicants

A common format is of value to both applicants and reviewers as the order of documents is logical, more user-friendly, shortens review time, saves resources and facilitates the exchange of information and discussions. Janet Woodcock, Director of FDA's CDER, speaking at ICH 5, expects more 'reviewable' applications, more complete, well-organised submissions, a format that is more predictable and, as a consequence, more consistent reviews.

21.5.3 Hurdles for harmonisation of the content of Module 3

21.5.3.1 Quality

Unfortunately, up to now it was not possible to harmonise either the content of the quality dossier or the format. One of the major reasons for this is that there are some areas where there has never been an ICH guideline developed (e.g. for synthesis of drug substances, manufacturing of drug products, process validation and packaging material). These points were also highlighted by Cone.[12] That means that national guidelines apply. Also, it seems to be of high priority for FDA to develop new national guidelines and regulations incorporating ICH guidelines where they

exist. In consequence, applicants may be able to submit common dossiers but should not expect identical query letters or common decisions issued by the various regulatory agencies concerned.

The other reason for disharmony of the content is the fact that the three major pharmacopoeias are different in terms of monographs and methods required, with the consequence that industry is forced to duplicate testing and generate different specifications, analytical testing, validation of methods, stability testing and summaries. In order to harmonise General Methods of Analysis and Excipient Monographs, the *Pharmeuropa* (*Ph. Eur*), the *Japanese Pharmacopoeia* (*JP*) and the *United States Pharmacopeia* (*USP*) formed a pharmacopoeial discussion group (PDG) in 1989. At the time of ICH 5, only four of 11 general chapters defined as essential in Q6A have reached stage 6 of the PDG procedure, six are still in stage 4, and one in stage 3. Only one excipient monograph out of 50 reached stage 6, 31 are in stage 5, and nine in stage 4 (Table 21.7), only three general monographs moved forward between ICH 5 and ICH 6.[13] These were bacterial endotoxins, residue on ignition and sterility.

In addition to these regulatory issues there are some homemade limitations to common quality documentation (e.g. normally, pharmaceutical companies

Table 21.7 The pharmacopoeial discussion group (PDG) process

PDG Stage No.	Status
Stage 1	Selection of subjects to be harmonised and nomination of a coordinating pharmacopoeia for each subject
Stage 2	Investigation on the existing specifications, on the grade of products marketed and on the potential analytical methods Preparation of a first draft text (Stage 3 draft)
Stage 3	Publication of the draft text in the forum of each pharmacopoeia: *Pharmeuropa* (*Ph Eur*), *Japanese Pharmacopoeial Forum* (*Japanese Pharmacopoeia*) and *Pharmacopoeial Forum* (*United States Pharmacopoeia*) Comments received and consolidated Preparation of a second draft text (Stage 3 draft)
Stage 4	Publication of the Stage 4 draft Comments received and consolidated Preparation of a revised version (Stage 5A draft)
Stage 5A	Stage 5A draft reviewed and commented on Revised provisional harmonised document prepared and reviewed until consensus is reached by all three pharmacopoeias (Stage 5B draft)
Stage 5B	Consensus document is signed off by the three pharmacopoeias
Stage 6	Adoption of the signed-off document by the organisation responsible for each pharmacopoeia Publication of the adopted document by the three pharmacopoeias in supplements or new editions
Stage 7	Implementation of published document in each region

prefer to market tablets in polyethylene bottles in the USA, in contrast to blister packs for the European market and different trade names, colours or pack sizes are also unavoidable in certain cases). The consequence of these differences is the fact that a common Module 3 (Quality) and therefore a common Quality Summary in Module 2 cannot be compiled.

21.5.3.2 Safety
Safety CTD is causing the fewest problems.[12]

21.5.3.3 Efficacy
The efficacy CTD discussions are dominated by the debate on the need for, and positioning of, the ISS and the ISE that are required for FDA applications.[12,14]

21.5.4 Other problems facing regulatory agencies and the pharmaceutical industry
In addition and in parallel to the legal changes to be made, several internal aspects have to be faced by the regulatory agencies concerned, for example:
• The impact of the new format on the current review process has to be checked;
• Current good review practices need to be adapted;
• New templates and technical guidelines are to be set up;
• Internal training of reviewers and document staff will be required; and
• A feedback mechanism for applicants based on experience in the voluntary phase will have to be created.

Internationally operating pharmaceutical companies as well as contract research organisations (CROs) are busy these days with similar activities in order to gain first-hand experience with the new format, and to take part in the voluntary phase by filing applications simultaneously as soon as possible.

Sooner rather than later, CTD-formatted dossiers should also be made acceptable for other types of products (e.g. generics, line extensions, herbals, radiopharmaceuticals and blood products). Also applications for clinical trials [e.g. CTX in the UK, Investigational New Drug Application (IND) in the USA], as well as applications for variations, and Drug Master Files could be formatted according to the CTD guideline. However, before this becomes reality, national regulations and guidelines need to be adapted accordingly.

21.5.5 Impact on non-ICH countries
In addition to the ICH regions USA, EU and Japan that agreed to accept a CTD-formatted dossier as of July 2001, other authorities in non-ICH countries announced they will also accept this, in particular the ICH observers, Canada and Switzerland.

The Swiss authorities intend to make the CTD format mandatory as of 1 July 2002 for new chemical entities (NCEs), as of 1 January 2003 for generics, and as of 1 July 2003 for over-the-counter products and herbals. The same applies to the other EFTA countries (i.e. Iceland, Norway and Liechtenstein).

Mike Ward, representing the Canadian authorities' point of view in San Diego, supported a simultaneous filing of applications, and therefore expected an early acceptance of CTD formatted dossiers. He also mentioned, however, some challenges linked to the implementation of the CTD in Canada (e.g. defining and adopting requirements, systems and procedure for CTD-based NDS is a complex task; also, the electronic submissions will need to be adjusted to the CTD format). An implementation master plan has been drafted and just needs to be completed. The Canadian authorities seem to be committed to ICH and the CTD. Health Canada will continue with their templates used since 1996 for the comprehensive summaries and evaluation reports, adapted to the CTD guideline accordingly.

South Africa, Australia, New Zealand, and countries in Latin America, the Middle East and South-East Asia are expected to adopt the CTD guideline, or at least will hopefully not insist in any particular national format. That means, in consequence, that applicants would just need to compile one common dossier in a modular approach following the CTD format, and would be able to submit this to the authorities concerned in all their target countries at the same time.

21.5.6 Developments: Brussels, February 2002
The ICH process is continuous, with the Steering Committee meeting in Brussels on February 2002 reporting on the CTD, eCTD, and MedDRA (Medical Dictionary for Regulatory Activity) terminology, the setting up of the Global Cooperation Group, and the status of the technical guidelines. This information can be obtained from the website (www.ifpma.org). As has been stated, the success of the ICH process and full implementation of the CTD is fraught with difficulties, not only from current regional reporting differences, but also from the impact of local factors such as disease prevalence, ethnicity and local medical practice. The integration of these disparate views will be encouraged with the eCTD, which will provide a medium to transfer data through the world

instantaneously. These changes will require companies to develop their own technical and human resources to meet the 'e' demand.

With the adoption of the ICH CTD from July 2002 and mandatory use in the EU and Japan from July 2003 (and its use strongly encouraged by the US FDA), 'aids' to finding our way round the CTD are beginning to appear. One of these is produced by Quintiles Regulatory Affairs Europe as a teaching aid and is reproduced in the *Regulatory Affairs Journal.*[8]

21.5.7 Developments: Washington, September 2002

• Electronic version of Common Technical Document (eCTD) was adopted and would move forward for adoption in the three ICH regions.
• Paper version of CTD upgraded/clarification on Quoting References in the Scientific Literature.
• ICH has published a list of frequently asked questions (FAQs) on its website.
• ICH guidelines on pharmacovigilance have been further developed.
• Open workshop on gene therapy convened and recommended amongst other topics; the need to review the safety issue relating to germ-line integration following administration of either viral or non-viral based vectors.
• The steering committee agreed to establish an Expert Working Group to develop harmonised Guidelines on bioequivalence of biotech products (Q5).
• Implementation Working Group set up to develop recommendations and clarifications for the E5 Guideline on ethnic factors in acceptability of foreign clinical data.
• Other guidelines being further developed include:
Residual solvents (Q3C(M));
Impurities in new drug products (Q3B);
Safety pharmacology studies for assessing the potential for delayed ventricular repolarisation (QT interval prolongation) by human pharmaceuticals (S7B); and MedDRA Version 5.1 released.

21.6 ICH 6: November 2003, Osaka

The issues discussed at this conference included:[10]
1. *Harmonization with countries outside the ICH remit.* This enlargement process was mediated through an expanded ICH Global Cooperation Group (GCG). The new members included representatives from:
(a) Asia-Pacific Economic group (APEC);
(b) Association of Southeast Asian Nations (ASEAN);
(c) Southern African Development Community (SADC);
(d) Pan American Health Organization (PAHO).
WHO and the PAN American Network for Drug Regulatory Harmonization (PANDRH) were also included.
2. *MedDRA.* The global standard medical terminology for regulatory activities (MedDRA) continued to evolve. Version 6.1 was released in September 2003, Version 7.0 and 7.1 in March 2004 and September 2004, respectively. A Spanish Version 6.1 was issued in December 2003.
3. *Gene therapy.* This is a relatively new ICH initiative (September 2002); the current issues include:
• The safety and design of lentiviral vectors;
• The charactisation and use of adenoviral reference material and other reference materials;
• Detection of replication competent adenovirus and adenovirus by infectivity polymerase chain reaction;
• Cytoplasmic gene therapy using Sendai virus vectors;
• Current requirements on inadvertent germline integration; and
• Insertional mutagenesis/oncogenesis.
4. *Common Technical Document.* The meeting discussed the implementation of both the paper and electronic versions of the CTD with particular relevance to biotech products and new chemical entities.
5. *Assessment of innovative therapies.* Discussions focused on the new ICH initiative about risk-based approach to drug product quality and Good Manufacturing Practice. Talks also focused on new technologies to enhance drug development, challenges in the area of biotechnology, and pharmacogenetics and targeted medicines.
6. *Quality.* Guidelines discussed included:
• Comparability of biotechnological and biological products subject to changes in their manufacturing processes (ICH Q5E);
• Bracketing and matrixing designs for stability testing of new drug substances and drug products (ICH Q1D);
• Evaluation of stability data (ICH Q1E);
• Stability data package for registration in climatic zones III and IV (ICH Q1F);
• Impurities in new drug substances [ICH Q3A(R)];
• Impurities in new drug products [ICH Q3B(R)];
• Impurities: Residual solvents (Maintenance) [ICH Q3C(M)];
• Specifications for new drug substances and products: chemical substances (ICH Q6A and ICH Q4).
7. *Safety and efficacy.* It was announced that concerted discussions would continue on the following:

Table 21.8 What's new on the ICH website?

M3 (R2): Guidance on non-clinical safety studies for the conduct of human clinical trials and marketing authorization for pharmaceuticals
Released for public consultation on 15 July 2008-09-26
July 2008

All Step 2 guidelines open for public consultation are available here
July 2008

New ICH Concept Paper for the revision of S6 guideline: preclinical safety evaluation of biotechnology-derived pharmaceuticals
S6 (R1) Concept Paper, June 2008
June 2008

NEWLY RELEASED GUIDELINES:
The Guidelines that were signed in Portland, Oregan, May 31–June 5, 2008 are now available on the ICH website:

Step 4 Tripartite Harmonised ICH Guidelines recommended for implementation:

Q4B Annex 2	Evaluation and recommendation of pharmacopoeial texts for use in the ich regions on test for extractable volume of parenteral preparations general chapter
Q4B Annex 3	Evaluation and recommendation of pharmacopoeial texts for use in the ich regions on test for particulate contamination: sub-visible particles general chapter
Q10	Pharmaceutical quality system
E14 Q&As	Q&As document for the E14 guideline on the clinical evaluation of qt/qtc interval prolongation and proarrythmic potential for non-antiarrythemic drugs

---

Step 2 Consensus Draft Guidelines released for open consultation:

Q4B Annex 4A	Evaluation and recommendation of pharmacopoeial texts for use in the ICH regions on microbiological examination of non-sterile products: microbial enumeration tests general chapter
Q4B Annex 4B	Evaluation and recommendation of pharmacopoeial texts for use in the ICH regions on microbiological examination of non-sterile products: tests for specified micro-organisms general chapter
Q4B Annex 4C	Evaluation and recommendation of pharmacopoeial texts for use in the ICH regions on microbiological examination of non-sterile products: acceptance criteria for pharmaceutical preparations and substances for pharmaceutical use general chapter
Q4B Annex 5	Evaluation and recommendation for pharmacopoeial texts for use in the ICH regions on disintegration tests general chapter
E2F	Development safety update report
June 2008	

PRESS RELEASE: Portland, Oregan, May 31–June 5, 2008

'Monitoring and Protecting the Global Public Health'
The international Conference on Harmonisation (ICH) Steering Committee and its expert working groups met in Portland, Oregan from 31 May to 5 June 2008. The main achievements are outlined below.
June 2008

Continued

PRESS RELEASE: Portland, Oregan, USA, MedDRA® Management Board Meeting

Portland, 1 June 2008 – MedDRA Management Board Endorses Free MedDRA Training
The Board authorized the MSSO to offer free training on coding and data analysis at various locations throughout the EU and USA for all MSSO subscribers, with immediate effect. This action extends the Board's policy to reduce barriers to MedDRA's use, such as the recent elimination of subscription fees for small business, not-for-profit, and academic organizations.
June 2008

The *Global Cooperation Group (GCG) Reports* of the previous meetings (May 2007 and October 2007) are available now from the GCG/Reports section.
May 2008

Step 2 Guideline for public consultation by end of May 2008:
S2 (R1): Guidance on Genotoxicity Testing and Data Interpretation for Pharmaceuticals Intended for Human Use

Second revision of SIC(R1) directly under Step 4, without further public consultation:
SIC (R2): Dose Selection for Carcinogenicity Studies of Pharmaceuticals
April 2008

New topic: Q11
Development and Manufacture of Drug Substances (chemical entities and biotechnological/biological entities)
The Concept Paper and Business Plan are available here
April 2008

The UMC and ICH MedDRA Management Board Announce:
MedDRA's Implementation in Vigibase
Uppsala, March 18, 2008

The Proceeding of the ICH Tokoyo Symposium : Hot Topics and Influence on Asia, Tokyo,
2 November 2007

• Clinical evaluation of QT/QTc interval prolongation and proarrhythmic potential for non-antiarrhythmic drugs (ICH E14);
• Safety pharmacology studies for assessing the potential for delayed ventricular repolarisation (QT interval prolongation) by human pharmaceuticals (ICH S7B); and
• Ethnic factors in the acceptability of foreign clinical data (ICH E5).
8. *Pharmacovigilance.* The implementation issues concerning the standard of electronic reporting: data elements fo the transmission of individual base safety reports [ICH E2B(M)] were adopted as was post-approval safety data management: definitions and standards for expedited reporting (ICH E2D). Pharmacovigilance planning (ICH E2E) reached Step 2 in

November 2003. Also discussed were Addendum to E2C: perodic safety update reports for marketed drugs (ICH E2 Cadd), ICH E2D and ICH E2E.

21.7 Future formats of meetings

The meeting of ICH 6 at Osaka, Japan, 2003 was the last meeting in the current format. It was recommended that the conferences should be held every 18 months in each ICH region as a 1-day additional meeting at the end of ICH Steering Committee and Expert Working Group/Implementation Working Group meetings. This culminating in the ICH Tokyo Symposium entitled 'Hot Topics and Influence on Asia' in November 2007. All updates up to and including this meeting are available from kishi@jpma.or.jp.

Between ICH 6 in Osaka in 2003 and November 2007 there took place seven Global Cooperation Group Meetings: Yokohama, 2004 (GCG 15F); Brussels, 2005 (GCG 19F); Chicago, 2005; Yokohama, 2006 (GCG 41F); Chicago, 2006 (GCG 50F); Brussels, 2007 (GCG 65F); and Yokohama, 2007 (GCG 78F). A final report of each of these meetings is available on the ICH website (http://www.ich.org).

21.7.1 Web updates

Fot web updates see Table 21.8.[15]

21.8 Conclusions to date

The whole ICH process is continually changing – the concept is universally accepted but it is a dynamic process that has to be m+odified to suit new technologies and the aspirations of all the participants.

References

1 Cone M, D'Arcy PF, Harron DWG. ICH international conference on harmonisation of technical requirements for registration of pharmaceuticals for human use. *Int Pharm J* 1996;10:104–6.

2 D'Arcy PF. ICH 3: a report and background. *Adverse Drug React Toxicol Rev* 1996;15:125–7.

3 D'Arcy PF. ICH 4: a report and background. *Adverse Drug React Toxicol Rev* 1997;16:199–206.

4 D'Arcy PF, Harron DWG. Proceedings of the Fourth International Conference on Harmonisation, Brussels 1997. Published at the Queen's University of Belfast, 1998.

5 Cone M. Meeting Report: Fifth International Conference on Harmonisation. *Regul Affairs J* 2000;11:954–5.

6 Zahn M. The Common Technical Document (CTD) Post-ICH 5. *Regul Affairs J* 2001;12:113–7.

7 Nick C. The CTD and beyond: surviving the impact. *Regul Affairs J* 2002;13:373–4.

8 Winzenrieth A. CTD roadmap. *Regul Affairs J* 2002; 13:463–8.

9 Cone M. ICH Update. *Regul Affairs J* 2002;13:814–6.

10 Anon. Worldwide update; ICH 6. *Regul Affairs J* 2004; 15:30–2.

11 Anon. Worldwide update: ICH Guidelines. *Regul Affairs J* 2004;15:63–8.

12 Cone M. Reflections on the International Conference on Harmonization. *Regul Affairs J Pharma* 2004;15:87–92.

13 Potter C. Pharmacopoeial harmonization revisited. *Regul Affairs J Pharma* 2004;15:97–9.

14 De Crémiers. ICH 6 CTD Efficacy. *Regul Affairs J Pharma* 2004;15:174.

15 What's new on the ICH website? http://www.ich.org (Accessed 18 August 2008).

22 The regulation of drug products by the US Food and Drug Administration

Peter Barton Hutt

Covington & Burling LLP, Washington, DC, USA

22.1 Introduction

The regulation of drug products by the Food and Drug Administration (FDA) in the USA is extraordinarily detailed and complex, and has enormous public costs as well as public benefits.[1] This chapter provides only a broad overview of this subject. Entire books,[2] and thousands of articles, have been devoted both to a comprehensive review of the area and to specific aspects. Anyone who wishes to understand it in greater detail must consult the governing statutes, regulations and guidance, as well as the experience of experts who have spent their entire careers working in the field. This chapter therefore presents a bare outline, permitting a glimpse into this extremely important and fascinating area but not a definitive analysis of any of its myriad aspects.

22.2 Regulatory framework

22.2.1 Federal regulatory requirements

In the USA, regulatory policies are established by statutes enacted by Congress and signed by the President. These laws govern all regulatory requirements imposed by the FDA upon drug products. No additional or different requirements can be imposed by any administrative official, but the statutory requirements are continually subject to reinterpretation and thus expansion as they are implemented by administrative action.

Laws are usually written by Congress in relatively general terms. They are intended to be implemented and enforced by administrative officials, in this instance

located in the FDA. Under the Federal Food, Drug, and Cosmetic Act (FD&C Act) of 1938,[3] the FDA is empowered to promulgate regulations implementing the statute, in accordance with the procedural requirements established by the Administrative Procedure Act.[4] These procedural requirements require that most regulations initially be published as proposals in the Federal Register, accompanied by a lengthy preamble explaining the purpose and meaning of the proposed regulations.[5] Time is then given for public comment. After the public comment has been received, the FDA reviews the comment, makes a final decision on the regulations and promulgates the final regulations, together with a preamble explaining the decision with respect to each comment received and the reasons for the final version of the regulation. The regulations are then codified in the Code of Federal Regulations, without the explanatory preambles.

Following the promulgation of a federal regulation, any interested person may challenge the legality of the regulation in the courts.[6] The primary grounds for any such legal challenge are that the regulation exceeds the FDA statutory authority or that it is arbitrary or capricious. Any person who challenges an FDA regulation in this way has a heavy burden to demonstrate that the regulation is illegal, and in most instances the FDA regulations are upheld by the courts.

Even though the FDA regulations are more detailed than the governing statute, they are nonetheless still often worded in general terms, and thus it becomes important to have more specific and detailed documents to guide daily decision-making in the agency. Such detailed policy comes in many forms, including the preambles to the regulations, written guidance, letters, speeches and a host of other documents, as well as unwritten tradition and practice. It is this area that largely governs daily FDA action. Because the vast bulk of FDA policy is not set forth either in the statute

---

The Textbook of Pharmaceutical Medicine. Edited by John P. Griffin. © 2009, ISBN: 978-1-4051-8035-1.

or in the regulations, it is uniquely a field where experience and judgement have a very large role.

22.2.2 State regulatory requirements

Decades ago, the individual states played an important part in the regulation of pharmaceutical products. However, as pharmaceutical science has become more complex and as the FDA regulation of the pharmaceutical industry has become more intense and pervasive, the states have shifted their traditional regulatory responsibilities to concentrate more heavily on food products and other items that are more appropriate for local control. Thus, state regulation of drug products is a relatively insignificant aspect of drug regulation in the USA today.

The individual states have retained their statutes governing both non-prescription and prescription drugs, and on occasion will exercise their authority to regulate in these areas. In recent years, this regulation has largely been limited to non-prescription drugs. For example, California has guidelines for slack fill in the packaging of non-prescription drugs.[7] On some occasions, states have also switched a non-prescription drug to prescription status in order to address a local abuse problem – usually only for a short duration. State regulation of drugs is not considered further in this chapter.

22.2.3 Product liability

The one aspect of state 'regulation' of pharmaceutical products that has increased is that of product liability. Drawing upon common law precedent extending back to medieval English origins, an individual harmed by a pharmaceutical product may bring a civil tort action under state law against the manufacturer or distributor of the drug for damages sustained. This can be a potent form of regulation. If a pharmaceutical product causes widespread damage to patients, the resulting tort liability could endanger the future of the manufacturer. One example is the Dalkon Shield, the damage actions from which resulted in the bankruptcy of AH Robbins. Further discussion of the field of product liability is beyond the scope of this chapter.

22.3 FDA history

The US Patent Office began its interest in agricultural matters in the 1830s. Eventually, an Agricultural Division was established in the Patent Office, and a chemical laboratory was funded in that division.[8]

When Congress created the US Department of Agriculture (USDA) by statute in 1862,[9] the Agricultural Division of the Patent Office, and its chemical laboratory, were transferred to form the nucleus of the new department. A Chemical Division was immediately formed within USDA. This became the Division of Chemistry in 1890,[10] the Bureau of Chemistry in 1901,[11] the Food, Drug and Insecticide Administration in 1927[12] and the FDA in 1930.[13]

The FDA remained a part of USDA until it was transferred to the new Federal Security Agency in 1940.[14] When the Department of Health, Education and Welfare (HEW) was established in 1953, as the successor to the Federal Security Agency, FDA became a part of HEW.[15] HEW was renamed the Department of Health and Human Services (HHS) in 1979.[16]

Throughout this period, the FDA (and its predecessor agencies) were created by administrative action, not by Congress. The governing statutes were all officially delegated for implementation and enforcement to the Secretary of Agriculture/HEW/HHS, not to the Commissioner of Food and Drugs. It was not until the Food and Drug Administration Act of 1988[17] that Congress officially established the FDA as a government agency. To this day, however, the governing statutes delegate responsibility for implementation and enforcement to the Secretary of HHS.

Throughout this history, the Commissioner of Food and Drugs and his or her predecessors have also occupied a position that was created solely by administrative action, not by Congress. The Food and Drug Administration Act of 1988 also officially created the position of the Commissioner of Food and Drugs, and required that the Commissioner be appointed by the President with the advice and consent of the Senate.

The Secretary of HHS is a Cabinet position, appointed by the President with the advice and consent of the Senate. The Commissioner of Food and Drugs reports to the Secretary of HHS.

Within the FDA, there is an Office of the Commissioner and five product-oriented centres (for food, drugs, biologics, medical devices and veterinary medicine) located in the Washington DC area.[18] The Center for Drug Evaluation and Research and the Center for Biologics Evaluation and Research are responsible for regulation of drug products. Outside Washington DC, FDA has an extensive field force located in regions and districts throughout the USA, where FDA employees inspect drug establishments and conduct enforcement activities. The FDA field force is also responsible for the inspection of foreign drug establishments located throughout the world.

The FDA is funded through annual congressional appropriations. When it became clear that Congress would not appropriate sufficient funds to support FDA drug review programs, in 1992 the regulated industry agreed to the enactment of user fees dedicated to FDA evaluation of new drugs (see section 22.4.17). Even then, congressional appropriations were insufficient to support all of the FDA's drug regulatory responsibilities. A major report issued by a subcommittee of the FDA Science Board in November 2007 exposed the weakened condition of the agency,[19] resulting in agreement by Congress to increase FDA appropriations substantially.

22.4 Historical overview of drug regulation statutes

Government concern about the adulteration and misbranding of pharmaceutical products extends back to ancient times.[20] Pliny the Elder, for example, in the first century AD, criticised 'the fashionable druggists' shops which spoil everything with fraudulent adulterations'.[21] As a result, various forms of government control to prevent the adulteration and misbranding of food and drugs can be found in virtually every recorded civilisation. These regulatory controls were brought to the American colonies by early settlers, were enacted into state law following the American Revolution and eventually were adopted by Congress as nationwide requirements in a series of federal statutes.

During most of the nineteenth century, regulation of food and drug products was thought to be a matter of state and local concern, not appropriate for federal legislation, under the US Constitution. During this period, most federal laws governing food and drugs therefore related to foreign commerce rather than to domestic commerce. It is only since 1900 that regulation of food and drugs in the USA has been concluded to be a matter of national concern that justifies the enactment of federal statutes. The following paragraphs present a brief chronology of the major federal regulatory statutes governing non-prescription and prescription drug products in the USA.

22.4.1 Vaccine Act of 1813
Following Edward Jenner's discovery of a smallpox vaccine in 1798, and the demonstration by Benjamin Waterhouse in the USA in 1800 that the vaccine was effective, fraudulent versions of the vaccine were marketed throughout the country. A Baltimore physician, John Smith, initially convinced the Maryland legislature to enact a statute designed to ensure the availability of an effective smallpox vaccine supply, and then persuaded Congress to enact the Vaccine Act of 1813[22] for the same purpose. This statute authorised the President to appoint a federal agent to 'preserve the genuine vaccine matter and to furnish the same to any citizen' who requested it.

The President promptly appointed Dr Smith as the first and, as it turned out, only federal vaccine agent. Following an outbreak of smallpox in North Carolina in 1821, which was thought to be caused by a contaminated lot of vaccine supplied by Dr Smith under the 1813 statute, the matter was investigated by two committees of the House of Representatives. The second committee concluded that regulation of smallpox vaccine should be undertaken by state and local officials rather than by the federal government, and as a result the 1813 Act was repealed in 1822.[23] As discussed below, 80 years later another drug tragedy led to the enactment of a new statute in 1902 under which vaccines are currently regulated by the FDA.

22.4.2 Import Drug Act of 1848
A congressional investigation in 1848 discovered that a wide variety of drugs imported into the USA for use by US troops in Mexico were adulterated. Congress therefore enacted a statute dealing solely with imported drugs. The 1848 Act[24] required that all imported drugs be labelled with the name of the manufacturer and the place of preparation, and be examined and appraised by the US Customs Service for 'quality, purity and fitness for medical purposes'. The Customs Service was directed to deny entry into the USA of any drug determined to be so adulterated or deteriorated as to be 'improper, unsafe or dangerous to be used for medical purposes'. This law remained in effect until it was repealed in 1922.[25]

22.4.3 Biologics Act of 1902
As the result of a series of problems with biological drugs during the late 1890s, culminating in the death of several children in St Louis from a tetanus-infected diphtheria antitoxin, Congress enacted the Biologics Act of 1902.[26] This statute is the first known regulatory law in any country that required premarket approval. It required approval of both a product licence application (PLA) and an establishment licence application (ELA) before any biological product could be marketed. Although it was recodified in 1944[27] and 1997,[28] it has remained in effect without significant change since 1902. It was initially implemented by the

Public Health Service, but was transferred to the FDA in 1972.[29] Today it is implemented partly by the Center for Biologics Evaluation and Research (CBER) within the FDA, which is located in buildings on the campus of the National Institutes of Health (NIH), where it had been located prior to the 1972 transfer to the FDA, and partly by the Center for Drug Evaluation and Research (CDER).

22.4.4 Federal Food and Drugs Act of 1906

The first legislation to establish comprehensive nation-wide regulation of all food and drugs was introduced in Congress in 1879. Largely because regulation of food and drugs was at that time thought to be a matter for state and local control, Congress debated this legislation for 27 years, ultimately enacting the Federal Food and Drugs Act in 1906.[30] This law broadly prohibited any adulteration or misbranding of drugs marketed in interstate commerce. Although it was quite short, and very broad and general in nature, it was extremely progressive for its time and included sufficient authority to permit the FDA to take strong enforcement action against the unsafe, ineffective and mislabelled products that flooded the US market in the late 1800s. Unlike the Biologics Act of 1902, it contained no provisions requiring premarket testing or approval for new drug products. An attempt by the FDA to obtain this type of authority in 1912 was unsuccessful. Thus, Congress initially provided premarket approval authority for biological drugs but not for other drugs.

22.4.5 Federal Food, Drug, and Cosmetic Act of 1938

Shortly after President Franklin D Roosevelt took office in 1933, the Commissioner of Food and Drugs persuaded the new administration to propose legislation to modernise the Federal Food and Drugs Act of 1906. The legislation was introduced in 1933, debated by Congress for 5 years, and ultimately enacted as the Federal Food, Drug, and Cosmetic Act of 1938 (the FD&C Act).[31] Initially, it was intended to add cosmetics and medical devices to the 1906 Act and to require additional affirmative labelling for food and drug products. In September 1937, however, more than 100 people died of diethylene glycol poisoning following use of Elixir Sulfanilamide, which used this chemical as the solvent without any form of safety testing. As a result, Congress added a premarket notification requirement for new drugs to the pending legislation and enacted the new law in June 1938.

Under this statute, a 'new drug' was defined as a drug that was not generally recognised as safe for its intended use. Before a new drug could be marketed, it was required to be tested on humans in accordance with investigational new drug (IND) regulations promulgated by the FDA. When sufficient data were obtained under the IND to demonstrate the safety of the drug, the manufacturer was required to submit a new drug application (NDA) for the drug to the FDA. If the FDA did not disapprove the NDA within 60 days after filing, the NDA became effective and the drug could be marketed. The FD&C Act has been amended more than 200 times since 1938, and is now a very lengthy, detailed and complex law. The more important amendments relating to drugs are summarised below.

22.4.6 Insulin and Antibiotics Amendments

Following enactment of the FD&C Act in 1938, insulin, penicillin and other antibiotic drugs were developed and marketed. Because of the unique production processes for these new pharmaceutical products, Congress enacted special provisions in the law requiring both that the FDA approve each of them as safe and have the authority to require that each batch be certified by the FDA as conforming to standards established for them by the agency. Thus, insulin and antibiotics were regulated by the FDA under provisions that were similar to, but nonetheless different from, those established both for biologics and for chemical drugs.[32]

22.4.7 Durham–Humphrey Amendments of 1951

The FD&C Act made no distinction between non-prescription and prescription drugs. A company could label a drug either way, depending upon marketing strategy. However, in 1939, the FDA promulgated regulations declaring that any drug for which adequate directions for lay use could not be prepared must be sold only on prescription, thereby for the first time creating a mandatory prescription class of drugs. In order to make certain that the same drug, at the same dosage and for the same indication, could not be marketed both as a non-prescription and a prescription drug, in 1951 Congress codified the FDA regulations into law by enacting the Durham–Humphrey Amendments.[33]

22.4.8 Drug Amendments of 1962

Although thalidomide was marketed throughout Europe, the NDA for this drug was not allowed to become effective and thus thalidomide was not marketed in the USA. When it was learned in mid-1962 that thalidomide was a potent human teratogen, Congress immediately enacted the Drug Amendments of 1962 to strengthen the new drug regulatory system to make certain that the FDA had adequate statutory authority to ensure that no such drug could be marketed in the future.[34]

The 1962 Amendments made a number of important changes. First, and most important, the amended law requires the FDA explicitly to approve an NDA, rather than simply allowing the NDA to become effective through FDA inaction. Thus, the new drug provisions of the law were converted in 1962 from premarket notification to premarket approval, making them parallel with the Biologics Act of 1902. Secondly, a new drug was required to be shown to be effective as well as safe. Thirdly, the FDA was given additional authority to require compliance with current Good Manufacturing Practices (GMP), to control the advertising of prescription drugs, to register drug establishments and to implement other regulatory requirements. Finally, the FDA was required to review all NDAs that had become effective during 1938–1962, to determine whether these drugs were effective as well as safe.

22.4.9 Controlled Substances Act of 1970

Beginning in the early 1900s, Congress enacted a series of laws to control narcotic drugs and other drugs subject to abuse. All of these laws were repealed in 1970 and replaced by the Controlled Substances Act.[35] Responsibility for enforcement rests with the Drug Enforcement Administration (DEA) of the Department of Justice. The FDA may approve an NDA for any controlled substance that has a legitimate medical use, but the DEA may impose upon any new drug that is also a controlled substance additional regulatory requirements to prevent abuse and misuse by classifying it into one of four categories: schedules II (most restrictive) to schedule V (least restrictive).

22.4.10 Poison Prevention Packaging Act of 1970

In response to concern about household poisoning of children with hazardous household products, Congress enacted the Poison Prevention Packaging Act[36] to require the use of special child-resistant packaging. In accordance with regulations established by the Consumer Product Safety Commission, this type of packaging is now common for virtually all prescription drugs and for most non-prescription drugs.[37]

22.4.11 Drug Listing Act of 1972

The Drug Amendments of 1962 included a requirement that every owner of a US drug establishment register that establishment with the FDA. Congress enacted the Drug Listing Act of 1972[38] to add the requirement that every person who registers an establishment shall include a list of all drugs manufactured at that establishment.[39]

22.4.12 Orphan Drug Act of 1983

An orphan drug is one that is intended for use in rare diseases and thus for which there is not a sufficient market to justify the investment needed to demonstrate safety and effectiveness in order to obtain approval of an NDA. For more than 20 years the FDA had permitted orphan drugs to be distributed through a permanent IND, with little or no thought that it would ever progress to an approved NDA.

In 1983, Congress enacted the Orphan Drug Act[40] to provide economic incentives for the industry to make the investment necessary to develop this category of drugs. When that proved insufficient, the Act was amended in 1984 to expand its coverage substantially, by providing that any drug with a use that has a target patient population of fewer than 200,000 people in the USA is automatically classified as an orphan drug.[41] Although the Orphan Drug Act does not provide for any different regulatory requirements from those applied to non-orphan drugs, the tax incentives and, in particular, a 7-year period of market exclusivity during which no competing NDA may be approved by the FDA, combined with the extraordinary expansion in 1984 of the number of drugs covered by this statute, has had a major impact on drug development in the USA.

22.4.13 Drug Price Competition and Patent Term Restoration Act of 1984

Under the new drug provisions as initially enacted in 1938 and as amended in 1962, all information in an IND and NDA was regarded as confidential proprietary business information that could not be revealed by the FDA to the public or any competitor, and could not be used as the basis for any subsequent approval of a generic version of the pioneer new drug. Even after the patent for a pioneer new drug expired, competitors were unable to obtain an approved NDA for a generic version without duplicating all the animal and human testing needed to demonstrate safety and effectiveness. Congress therefore enacted the Drug Price Competition and Patent Term Restoration Act of 1984,[42] which authorised the FDA to approve an abbreviated NDA for a generic version of a pioneer new drug after the patent and the statutory period of market exclusivity for the pioneer drug had expired. The result has been a substantial increase in the number of generic drugs available in the USA.

At the same time, Congress recognised that the effective patent term of pioneer drugs was dramatically reduced because of the time required for drug development by the FDA IND/NDA requirements prior to marketing. On average, the effective patent life for a pioneer drug was less than half the 17-year period then specified by Congress under the patent law, as of the time of NDA approval. For some drugs, no patent could be obtained. As part of the 1984 legislation, Congress therefore directed the Patent Office to extend the patent for a pioneer drug for up to 5 years in order to compensate for the lost patent life resulting from FDA regulatory review requirements. Congress also specified a minimum period of 3 or 5 years of market exclusivity during which no generic version could be approved by the FDA even if there was no patent protection.

22.4.14 Drug Export Amendments Act of 1986

Under the FD&C Act as enacted in 1938, adulterated and misbranded drugs may lawfully be exported but an unapproved new drug could not. This was a drafting error, but it was nonetheless enforced by the FDA. Congress therefore enacted the Drug Export Amendments Act of 1986,[43] which authorised the limited export of unapproved new human drugs and biological products after the FDA had approved an export application. An export application could be approved only if:

- There was an active IND;
- Approval of an NDA was actively being pursued in the USA;
- The product was for export to one or more of 21 listed countries with sophisticated regulatory systems;
- The product was currently approved and marketed in the receiving country;
- The FDA had not disapproved the product;
- The product was manufactured in conformity with GMP and was not adulterated;
- The product's labelling listed the countries to which the FDA permitted it to be exported;
- The FDA had not determined that domestic manufacture of the drug for export was contrary to the public health and safety of the USA;
- The product was properly labelled for export.

Not surprisingly, these restrictions were so tight that most US companies preferred to move their manufacturing facilities overseas, and thus to source a drug from abroad, rather than to make it in the USA and attempt to obtain FDA approval for an export application. As a result, in 1996 the 1986 Amendments were repealed and replaced with substantially more flexible provisions.[44]

22.4.15 Prescription Drug Marketing Act of 1987

Congressional investigations in the mid-1980s demonstrated that pharmaceutical products were being exported from the USA and later imported back into the country without adequate assurance that they had not become adulterated or misbranded while abroad. Congress responded by enacting the Prescription Drug Marketing Act of 1987,[45] which makes the reimportation of US drugs by anyone other than the manufacturer illegal. It also prohibits the sale of drug samples and the resale of drug products initially sold to health care institutions. Distribution of drug samples by pharmaceutical manufacturers is permitted only in response to a written request, for which a receipt is obtained. The provisions requiring state licensure of wholesale distributors of prescription drugs were subsequently clarified in the Prescription Drug Amendments of 1992.[46]

22.4.16 Generic Drug Enforcement Act of 1992

Following enactment of the Drug Price Competition and Patent Term Restoration Act of 1984, the FDA embarked upon a major campaign to expedite approval of abbreviated NDAs for generic versions of important pioneer drugs for which the patents had expired. Because of the enormous economic profit that could be made by the generic drug company that marketed the first generic version of an important pioneer drug, a number of generic drug manufacturers submitted fraudulent data to the FDA as part of abbreviated NDAs, and even paid illegal bribes to FDA officials in an attempt to obtain preferential handling of their applications. When this scandal came to light, in addition to the criminal prosecution of the individuals and companies involved, Congress enacted the Generic Drug Enforcement Act of 1992[47] to increase the penalties for such illegal behaviour. These new penalties include mandatory and permissive debarment of corporations and individuals, suspension and withdrawal of approval of abbreviated NDAs, and civil money penalties. Although the 1992

Act applies primarily to generic drugs, it also provides mandatory and permissive debarment for individuals who engage in wrongdoing with respect to any drug, whether generic or pioneer. All of the provisions of the Act apply to both non-prescription and prescription drugs.

22.4.17 Prescription Drug User Fee Act of 1992

Following enactment of the Drug Amendments of 1962, the time needed to develop the data and information to demonstrate the safety and effectiveness of a new drug, and to obtain FDA approval of an NDA, escalated. As a result, a 'drug lag' developed between the pharmaceutical products available in the rest of the world and those available in the USA. The FDA on many occasions pointed out that the time needed for FDA review of an IND or an NDA was at least in part a function of the resources available to the agency. Although both the FDA and the pharmaceutical industry initially opposed the imposition on the industry of 'user fees' that would generate additional revenue to permit the FDA to hire additional people to review INDs and NDAs, both abruptly reversed their earlier positions and agreed to enactment of the Prescription Drug User Fee Act (PDUFA) of 1992.[48]

Under this statute, the FDA was authorised to collect user fees for 5 years based on annual fees levied for each pioneer prescription drug and each pioneer prescription drug establishment, as well as a one-time fee for each NDA for a pioneer new drug. The fees do not apply to generic drugs or to pioneer drugs after they become subject to generic competition. All of the revenue from these user fees is required to be in addition to the existing FDA budget and must be used solely for the IND/NDA review system. User fees were extended for another 5 years under the Food and Drug Modernization Act of 1997,[49] and for another 5 years each under the Prescription Drug User Fee Amendment of 2002[50] and the Prescription Drug User Fee Amendments of 2007.[51]

22.4.18 FDA Export Reform and Enhancement Act of 1996

Following the November 1994 elections, in which the Republican Party won control of both the House of Representatives and the Senate for the first time in 40 years, Congress began to consider statutory reform of the FDA in earnest. When the reform legislation became stalled in 1996, the provisions dealing with the export requirements of the FD&C Act were separated out and enacted.[52] The 1996 Act repealed the

Drug Export Amendments Act of 1986[53] and adopted a much more liberal and expansive approach. A drug that is not approved in the USA may now be exported to any country in the world if it complies with the laws of that country and has valid marketing authorisation by the appropriate authority in any country included in a new list of 25 countries with sophisticated regulatory systems. A drug that is not approved in the USA may be exported for investigational use in any listed country. FDA approval of the export of a drug that is not approved in the USA is required only if it is exported for investigational use in a non-listed country. Although the 1996 Act is a major improvement over the 1986 Act, the export provisions of the FD&C Act continue to be the most stringent in the world, and thus many US companies continue to manufacture products abroad in order to avoid its cumbersome requirements.

22.4.19 Food and Drug Administration Modernization Act of 1997

One year after the drug export provisions of the FD&C Act were reformed, Congress enacted the remainder of the reform legislation that it had been considering. The Food and Drug Administration Modernization Act of 1997[54] is a lengthy, comprehensive and complex statute. Although the impact of this statute has been modest at best, it is the first statute since the FD&C Act was enacted in 1938 that has attempted significant reform. The following brief summary of the major provisions in the 1997 Act is sufficient to convey the broad scope of this legislation:
- Reauthorises prescription drug user fees for another 5 years;
- Establishes for a period of 5 years an additional 6 months of market exclusivity for paediatric studies of new drugs;
- Establishes a fast-track system for the study and approval of new drugs that address unmet medical needs related to serious or life-threatening conditions;
- Establishes a data bank in the NIH to provide information on research relating to new drugs for serious or life-threatening diseases, for use by the general public;
- Establishes new criteria for permitting health care economic information relating to new drugs in labelling and advertising;
- Clarifies the requirements for NDA approval to say that data from one adequate and well-controlled study, together with confirmatory evidence, may, with the discretion of the FDA, constitute substantial evidence of effectiveness of a new drug;

- Requires the FDA to consult with the NIH and representatives of the pharmaceutical industry to review and develop guidance on the inclusion of women and minorities in clinical trials;
- Adds a provision that is intended to reduce the number of post-market manufacturing changes requiring FDA approval and otherwise to make it easier to implement manufacturing changes for approved new drugs;
- Reduces the amount of information required to be submitted to the FDA as part of an IND application;
- Clarifies the power of the FDA to prevent or halt a clinical investigation of a new drug through use of a clinical hold;
- Requires the FDA to issue guidance describing when abbreviated reports may be submitted in lieu of full reports for clinical and non-clinical studies required to be included in an NDA;
- Requires the FDA to issue guidance for NDA reviewers relating to promptness in conducting the review, technical excellence, lack of bias and conflict of interest, and knowledge of regulatory and scientific standards;
- Requires the FDA to meet with a sponsor upon reasonable written request for the purpose of reaching agreement on the design of pivotal trials, and provides that, after testing begins, the agreement cannot be changed unilaterally by the FDA unless the director of the reviewing division issues a written decision that the change must be made because of a safety or effectiveness issue identified after the testing has begun;
- Provides that a decision by the reviewing division is binding on the FDA field and compliance personnel unless the reviewing division agrees to change its decision;
- States that no action of the reviewing division may be delayed based on a delay in action by field personnel;
- Provides for the use of scientific advisory committees to provide expert advice and recommendations to the FDA regarding clinical investigation and approval of new drugs;
- Requires the FDA to promulgate separate regulations governing the approval of radiopharmaceuticals;
- Amends the Public Health Service Act to eliminate the requirement of separate product and establishment licences and directs the FDA to harmonise the review and approval requirements for biological products and new drugs to the extent possible;
- Provides that a drug manufactured in a pilot or other small-scale facility can be used to establish safety and effectiveness and to obtain marketing approval

prior to scale-up unless the FDA determines that a full-scale facility is necessary to ensure safety or effectiveness;
- Eliminates the separate regulatory requirements for insulin and antibiotics, and makes these drugs subject to the IND and NDA requirements;
- For prescription drugs replaces the old label statement 'Caution: Federal Law prohibits dispensing without a prescription' with a new 'Rx Only' designation;
- Deletes the obsolete statutory provisions relating to labelling of 17 listed 'habit-forming' drugs;
- Establishes an entire new programme to control pharmacy compounding;
- Reauthorises a clinical pharmacology programme in the FDA;
- Establishes new requirements for phase IV studies that the manufacturer has agreed to conduct as a condition for NDA approval;
- Requires notice to the FDA from the sole manufacturer of a life-supporting product 6 months before the manufacturer discontinues production;
- Establishes national uniformity in the regulation of non-prescription drugs;
- Requires the label of a non-prescription drug to bear the quantity or the proportion of each active ingredient;
- Requires the label of a non-prescription drug to bear the name of each inactive ingredient, listed in alphabetical order;
- Authorises manufacturers of new drugs to disseminate information on unapproved (off-label) uses of approved products under very limited conditions;
- Authorises expanded access to drugs that are still undergoing investigation for serious diseases and conditions;
- Attempts to reduce the disincentives to the submission of supplemental NDAs by reducing the cost and increasing the efficiency of handling them within the FDA;
- Establishes dispute resolution mechanisms for the resolution of scientific controversies relating to new drugs;
- Requires the FDA to promulgate a regulation regarding the development, issuance and use of guidance documents, and requires the FDA to ensure that employees do not deviate from guidance without appropriate justification and supervisory concurrence;
- Establishes a statutory mission statement for the FDA, which includes both the promotion of public health by taking appropriate action on the marketing of regulated products in a timely manner and the

protection of public health by ensuring that regulated products are safe, effective and properly labelled;
• Requires the FDA to publish a plan to bring the agency into compliance with each of the obligations established under the FD&C Act, and to review and revise the plan biennially;
• Requires the FDA to publish an annual report in the Federal Register on its performance under the agency plan;
• Requires the FDA to establish an information system regarding all submissions to the agency requesting agency action;
• Requires the FDA to provide training and education programmes for employees relating to their regulatory responsibilities;
• Requires the FDA to support the office of the US Trade Representative to reduce the burden of regulation and harmonise international regulatory requirements consistent with the purposes of the FD&C Act;
• Requires FDA support of efforts to move towards the acceptance of mutual recognition agreements between the European Union and the USA;
• Requires the FDA to participate in meetings with foreign governments to discuss and reach agreement on methods and approaches to harmonise regulatory requirements;
• Provides that an environmental impact statement prepared in accordance with FDA regulations shall be considered to meet the requirements of the National Environmental Policy Act, notwithstanding any other provision of law;
• Requires the FDA to implement programmes and policies that will foster collaboration between FDA, NIH and other science-based federal agencies in order to enhance the scientific and technical expertise available to the FDA in discharging its duties with respect to regulating drugs;
• Authorises the FDA to enter into contracts with any organisation or individual with relevant expertise to review and evaluate any application or submission for the approval or classification of an article, for the purpose of making recommendations to the agency on the matter;
• Provides that a person who submits an application or other submission under the FD&C Act may ask the FDA for a determination respecting the proper regulatory classification of the product and the organisation within the FDA that will regulate the product;
• Requires registration of foreign drug establishments;
• Establishes a rebuttable presumption of interstate commerce for drugs;

• Provides that any report or information relating to the safety of a drug that is submitted to the FDA shall not be construed to reflect necessarily a conclusion that the report constitutes an admission that the product caused or contributed to an adverse experience;
• Repeals the former provision in the FD&C Act that prohibited any representation in labelling or advertising that the FDA had approved an application for a new drug.
Only some of these provisions have been implemented by the FDA, and the full impact of most of them remains to be determined.

22.4.20 Medicine Equity and Drug Safety Act of 2000

The Prescription Drug Marketing Act of 1987 prohibited the reimportation into the USA of any prescription drug that had been exported. In response to public concern about the high cost of prescription drugs in the USA, Congress passed the Medicine Equity and Drug Safety Act of 2000[55] to authorise the reimportation of prescription drugs if the Secretary of HHS certifies to Congress that its implementation would impose no risk to the public health and safety and that it would result in a significant reduction of the cost of covered products to the US consumer. The Secretary of HHS under both the Clinton and the Bush administrations determined that these certifications could not be made and this law has therefore never been implemented.

22.4.21 Best Pharmaceuticals for Children Act

The paediatric drug testing provisions in the FDA Modernization Act of 1997 had an automatic 5-year sunset limitation. In January 2002, Congress enacted the Best Pharmaceuticals for Children Act[56] reauthorising these provisions, with changes, for another 5 years. The 2002 Act, like the 1997 provisions, relies upon incentives for voluntary industry testing of drugs used for children. It was similarly revised and extended for another 5 years in 2007.[57]

22.4.22 Public Health Security and Bioterrorism Preparedness and Response Act of 2002

Congress passed the Public Health Security and Bioterrorism Preparedness and Response Act of 2002[58] as part of the Homeland Security Act, in response to the terrorism attacks of 11 September 2001. The new law contains several provisions that are designed to strengthen the public health system generally, and the availability of drugs, biological products and medical devices for countering bioterrorism in particular.

22.4.23 Pediatric Research Equity Act of 2003

Following enactment of the Best Pharmaceuticals for Children Act in 2002, a court ruled that the FDA regulation requiring mandatory paediatric testing of new drugs is not authorised under the FD&C Act and is thus illegal.[59] Congress responded by enacting the Pediatric Research Equity Act of 2003,[60] providing specific authorisation for the FDA to require mandatory paediatric testing for new drugs. The statute was reauthorised in 2007 for another 5 years.[61]

22.4.24 Food and Drug Administration Amendments Act of 2007

When the Republicans retook the House and Senate in 1994, they enacted the FDA Modernization Act of 1997 in an attempt to reform the IND/NDA system in order to expedite the approval of new drugs. When the Democrats retook the House and Senate in 2004, they enacted the FDA Amendments Act of 2007[62] in an attempt to reform the IND/NDA system in order to slow down the approval of new drugs. Because both largely enacted provisions that followed existing FDA policy and practice, it is primarily the discretionary action of individual FDA employees that has determined how the IND/NDA provisions are implemented. As in 1997, however, the 155-page statute (the longest amendment of the FD&C Act in history) contains an impressive array of new powers:

- Reauthorises prescription drug user fees for another 5 years;
- Authorises user fees to support FDA review of direct-to-consumer advertising of prescription drugs;
- Reauthorizes the Pediatric Research Equity Act for another 5 years;
- Reauthorizes the Best Pharmaceuticals for Children Act for another 5 years;
- Established the Reagan–Udall Foundation for the Food and Drug Administration as a private–public partnership to modernise medical product development, accelerate innovation and enhance product safety;
- Tightens conflict of interest requirements for FDA advisory committee members;
- Expands and makes mandatory the registration of all clinical trials except phase I on ClinicalTrials.gov;
- Requires the disclosure of the results of clinical trials for approved drugs in a new database;
- Authorises the FDA to require drug labelling changes;
- Authorises the FDA to require phase IV testing relating to drug safety;
- Establishes a public–private partnership for a system of active post-market surveillance of drug safety;
- Establishes civil money penalties as an enforcement tool for specified violations;
- Authorises the FDA to require a risk evaluation and mitigation strategy (REMS) to assure that a drug's benefits outweigh its risks;
- Increases the security of the drug supply;
- Prevents the abuse of citizen petitions to delay approval of generic drugs;
- Requires the FDA to make publicly available FDA documents supporting approval of an NDA;
- Requires a new internet website that will consolidate drug safety information about all approved products;
- Requires the FDA to post on the internet the approved physician labelling within 21 days after approval or any change;
- Requires the FDA to screen adverse events biweekly and post new safety information quarterly;
- Requires the FDA to review all phase IV testing commitments each year to determine whether any should be revised or eliminated;
- Requires the FDA to establish an Advisory Committee on Risk Communication;
- Requires the FDA to issue guidance on clinical trials for antibiotic drugs;
- Requires the FDA to issue a priority review voucher, which can be sold to another company, to any firm that obtains an approval of a new drug to treat a neglected or tropical disease.

The impact of these provisions will not be known for several years.

22.5 Other pharmaceutical products

In addition to biological and chemical drugs, two other categories of pharmaceutical products deserve brief mention: animal drugs and human medical devices. Both are beyond the scope of the present chapter.

22.5.1 Animal drugs

Under the Federal Food and Drugs Act of 1906 and the FD&C Act of 1938, animal feed and drugs were regulated under the same provisions as human food and drugs. A separate statute, the Animal Virus, Serum and Toxin Act of 1913[63] was enacted by Congress to authorise the USDA to regulate biological drugs intended for use in animals, and the USDA retains jurisdiction over that statute to this day. To simplify

FDA regulation of animal feed and drugs, Congress enacted the Animal Drug Amendments of 1968.[64] Following the approach of the 1984 statute authorising FDA approval of generic versions of human new drugs, Congress also enacted the Generic Animal Drug and Patent Term Restoration Act of 1988,[65] the Animal Drug Availability Act of 1996,[66] the Animal Drug User Fee Act of 2003[67] and the Minor Use and Minor Species Animal Health Act of 2004.[68]

22.5.2 Medical devices

Medical devices were first made subject to FDA regulation under the FD&C Act of 1938. At that time, the statute included no requirement for premarket testing or approval. Congress enacted the Medical Device Amendments of 1976[69] to require premarket notification for all medical devices, and premarket approval for some old and new devices for which there was no adequate assurance of safety and effectiveness. The 1976 Amendments established a broad new array of statutory requirements and enforcement provisions. This new regulatory approach was supplemented by the Safe Medical Devices Act of 1990[70] and further refined by the Medical Device Amendments of 1992,[71] the Food and Drug Administration Modernization Act of 1997,[72] the Medical Device User Fee and Modernization Act of 2002,[73] the Medical Devices Technical Corrections Act of 2004[74] and the FDA Amendments Act of 2007.[75]

22.6 Two classes of drug products

There are two classes of drugs under the FD&C Act in the USA: non-prescription and prescription. Neither the Federal Food and Drugs Act of 1906 nor the FD&C Act of 1938 distinguished between non-prescription and prescription drugs or established a class of mandatory prescription drugs. Shortly after the FD&C Act was enacted in 1938, however, the FDA promulgated regulations establishing criteria for a class of drugs that could only lawfully be sold by prescription.[76] Those regulations were later codified into law by Congress in the Durham–Humphrey Amendments of 1951.[77] Under this statute, prescription status is mandatory for drugs that are not safe for use except under a practitioner's supervision, and drugs limited to prescription sale under an NDA. The statutory criteria for determining prescription status are toxicity, other potential for harmful effect, and the method of use and collateral measures necessary to use the drug. In all instances today, the prescription or

non-prescription status of a new drug is determined by the NDA.

A drug may be switched by the FDA from prescription to non-prescription status.[78] Prior to 1970 this was most often accomplished by FDA promulgation of a regulation. During 1970–1990, a switch from prescription to non-prescription was most frequently accomplished as part of the FDA OTC Drug Review, discussed in detail below. Now that the OTC Drug Review is substantially complete, and with the availability of market exclusivity under the Drug Price Competition and Patent Term Restoration Act of 1984, a switch from prescription to non-prescription status is accomplished primarily through a supplemental NDA.

Non-prescription drugs may be sold at any kind of retail store in the USA, ranging from a pharmacy to a grocery store or a gasoline filling station. There are no criteria or limitations on their method of distribution and sale. Pharmacy groups have contended that the FDA should establish a 'third class' of drugs that would be available only through a pharmacy, and have used those prescription drugs that are in the process of being switched to non-prescription status as one example of the need for such a new class. The FDA has declined to establish such a third class, on both policy and legal grounds.[79] First, the FDA has stated that any drug switched by the agency from prescription to non-prescription status is sufficiently safe for sale in any retail establishment, and that a requirement limiting sale to a pharmacy would provide an unjustified monopoly to pharmacists. Secondly, the FDA has stated that the FD&C Act provides no authority for the FDA to restrict distribution of a non-prescription drug to pharmacies. In a number of instances, however, drug companies have voluntarily placed non-prescription drugs behind the counter, either for safety or for marketing reasons.

22.7 Regulation of non-prescription drugs

22.7.1 Adulteration and misbranding

Since 1906, the adulteration or misbranding of a non-prescription drug has been illegal in the USA.[80] Both 'adulteration' and 'misbranding' are terms of art, defined in the FD&C Act. Adulteration includes such acts as the failure to comply with Good Manufacturing Practices; the use of a container that may render the contents injurious to health; the use of an illegal colour additive; failure to comply with United States

Pharmacopeia requirements; failure to meet labelled strength or purity; and related prohibited acts. Misbranding includes such labelling violations as any false or misleading labelling and:

- The failure to contain mandatory information relating to the name and address of the manufacturer and the net quantity of contents;
- The failure to bear adequate directions for use and warnings against unsafe use;
- The failure to meet packaging and labelling requirements established by the United States Pharmacopeia;
- The failure to use packaging and labelling to reduce product deterioration;
- Danger to health when used as recommended in the labelling;
- The failure to obtain batch certification for an antibiotic for which such certification is required;
- The failure to comply with a large number of other statutory requirements, including drug establishment registration and product listing, and poison prevention and tamper-resistant packaging.

The adulteration and misbranding provisions of the statute itself are continually expanded by FDA regulations that impose additional requirements either for all non-prescription drugs or for specific categories. Accordingly, current requirements can be determined only by consulting FDA regulations and other policy statements, as well as the statute itself.

22.7.2 IND/NDA system

Since 1938, non-prescription drugs have been subject to the new drug provisions of the Act as well as the adulteration and misbranding provisions. As a practical matter, however, the new drug provisions cover only those non-prescription drugs that have been switched from prescription status through a supplemental NDA. Almost all new chemical entity drugs are initially restricted by the FDA to prescription status. Only a handful of new chemical entity drugs that require an NDA – perhaps one per decade – are marketed initially with non-prescription status. For those non-prescription drugs that do go through the IND/NDA system, the requirements are no different than for a prescription drug. These requirements are discussed in detail below.

22.7.3 OTC Drug Review

During the period beginning with enactment of the new drug provisions in the FD&C Act in 1938 and ending with enactment of the Drug Amendments of 1962, there were approximately 420 NDAs that became effective for non-prescription drugs. Many of these NDAs were for long-established ingredients for which no NDA was actually required, but it was so simple to obtain an effective NDA during that time that many were submitted simply to obtain a perceived marketing advantage. As part of the Drug Amendments of 1962, the FDA was required to review these 420 NDAs and to determine whether the drugs were effective as well as safe. Rather than limit its inquiry to these 420 specific non-prescription drug products, the FDA decided instead to broaden the scope of its review to all active ingredients used in all non-prescription drugs on the market at that time. The agency also decided to review the safety and labelling as well as the effectiveness of the active ingredients in these products.

In 1972, the FDA announced the beginning of its massive OTC Drug Review – the largest and most extensive review of the safety, effectiveness and labelling of non-prescription drugs ever undertaken.[81] The FDA established panels of experts to review individual categories of non-prescription drugs and to prepare reports on their conclusions and recommendations. Those reports were published as proposed monographs establishing the conditions for safe, effective and properly labelled non-prescription drugs within each category. Following public comment, the FDA published a tentative final monograph. Following additional public comment and a public hearing before the Commissioner, the FDA established the final monograph. The documents that comprise these public proceedings represent an extremely important record of the status of non-prescription drug active ingredients and finished products in the USA.

By the early 1980s, all of the FDA panels had completed their deliberations and issued their reports. Because the industry largely followed the conclusions and recommendations of these reports, most of the impact of the OTC Drug Review has already been reflected in the marketplace. Nonetheless, a number of monographs remain to be completed and it will be some years before the OTC Drug Review is fully finished.

An OTC drug monograph establishes those conditions under which a non-prescription drug is generally recognised as safe, effective and properly labelled, and thus may be lawfully marketed in the USA without the need for an NDA or any other type of FDA approval. Any person may market a non-prescription drug in the USA in compliance with one of these monographs (or, where no final monograph has been issued, in accordance with a tentative final monograph). One of the major purposes behind the OTC Drug Review was to establish, by regulations, the criteria under which an NDA is not required. Where a product is marketed with any deviation from an OTC drug monograph, however, some form of NDA is required in order to justify that deviation before marketing will be permitted.[82] In short, complete compliance with an OTC drug monograph guarantees immediate marketing without any form of premarket approval. Of course, all non-prescription drugs must comply with the general adulteration and misbranding provisions of the law, including GMP, establishment registration and drug listing.

22.7.4 Tamper-resistant packaging

In September 1982, it was discovered that several people living in Chicago had died from cyanide poisoning after taking Extra-Strength Tylenol capsules. The FDA promptly promulgated regulations requiring tamper-resistant packaging for most non-prescription drug products.[83] Congress followed by enacting the Federal Anti-Tampering Act of 1983,[84] which makes it a crime to tamper with a consumer product with reckless disregard for the risk of persons or with intent to cause injury to a business. A number of individuals have been prosecuted for illegal tampering under this statute.

22.7.5 Non-prescription drug labelling

Based on an extensive rule-making, the FDA promulgated regulations in March 1999 establishing completely new labelling requirements for all non-prescription drug products.[85] The new regulations require the use of a 'Drug Facts' box using a standardised format and type size. The new labelling requirements are being phased in, in coordination with the development of final monographs for non-prescription drugs. Industry has petitioned the FDA for modification of some of the new requirements, and changes may be adopted through revision of the new labelling regulations, revisions of individual monographs or the issuance of guidance.

22.7.6 Non-prescription drug advertising

In 1914, Congress enacted a statute to prohibit unfair methods of competition and created the Federal Trade Commission (FTC) to implement this new law.[86] The FTC and the courts interpreted unfair methods of competition to include false or misleading labelling and advertising of non-prescription drugs and other consumer products. In 1933, when the legislation that became the FD&C Act was first introduced, it proposed to transfer the jurisdiction over food and drug advertising from the FTC to the FDA. Not surprisingly, the FTC objected. Congress ultimately resolved this controversy in 1938, by enacting both the Wheeler–Lea Amendments to the FTC Act[87] and the FD&C Act. Congress gave the FTC jurisdiction over advertising and FDA jurisdiction over labelling. However, because the FTC was also given jurisdiction over all unfair or deceptive acts or practices, it has jurisdiction over labelling as well as advertising. And because the courts have agreed with the FDA that the agency may refer to advertising to determine the proper regulatory classification and requirements for a product under the FD&C Act, the FDA to some extent indirectly regulates advertising. To clarify the situation, in September 1971 the FTC and FDA entered into a Memorandum of Understanding.[88] Under this agreement, the FTC has primary jurisdiction over advertising and the FDA has primary jurisdiction over labelling of non-prescription drugs and other FDA-regulated products.

22.7.7 Industry self-regulation

The Consumer Healthcare Products Association (CHPA), the US trade association representing the non-prescription drug industry, has established a number of voluntary codes and guidelines to supplement FDA regulation of non-prescription drugs. Among these are recommended package sizes for non-prescription drug categories, label 'flags' to bring the attention of consumers to significant product changes, bulk mail sampling of non-prescription drugs, expiry dating of non-prescription drugs, product identification of solid dosage non-prescription drugs and label readability for non-prescription drugs. Although these are not legal requirements, they are widely followed in the non-prescription drug industry.

22.8 Regulation of prescription drugs

It is particularly difficult to summarise FDA regulation of prescription drugs. The statutory provisions are long and complex, the regulations consume hundreds of pages in the Code of Federal Regulations, the preambles cover thousands of pages in the Federal Register, and the guidelines and policy directives are numerous and diverse. The discussion will therefore begin with a historical overview of the development of FDA regulation of prescription drugs. This is followed by a brief analysis of how the current system works.

This section is limited to drugs regulated under the FD&C Act. Biological drugs are considered in the next section.

22.8.1 Historical overview

As enacted in 1938, the FD&C Act defined a 'new drug' as any drug that was not generally recognised as safe.[89,90] Section 505 of the 1938 Act provided that an NDA must be submitted for every new drug, and authorised the FDA to permit an NDA to become effective or to disapprove it, but not affirmatively to approve an NDA. If the FDA took no action within 60 days after the filing of an NDA, the NDA automatically became effective and the drug could lawfully be marketed.

During the first few years after 1938, the pharmaceutical industry submitted thousands of NDAs. Because the FDA was unprepared to deal with this large number, it advised drug manufacturers that NDAs were not required for 'old drugs' that were generally recognised as safe (GRAS), and in fact refused to accept NDAs for these drugs. This substantially reduced the numbers of NDAs that were submitted to, and accepted by, the FDA. For example, more than 4000 NDAs had been submitted by 1941 but by 1962 NDAs for only 9457 individual drug products had become effective. Most prescription drugs were marketed on the conclusion of the FDA or the manufacturer that they were GRAS, and hence old drugs that did not require an NDA.

Following enactment of the Drug Amendments of 1962, the FDA immediately encountered two problems. First, the pharmaceutical industry submitted a substantially increased number of INDs and NDAs, which again overwhelmed the resources of the FDA to deal with them. Secondly, the 1962 Amendments required the FDA to review all of the NDAs that had become effective between 1938 and 1962 on the basis of a demonstration of safety, and to determine whether these drugs were also effective. Because of the overwhelming number of current INDs and NDAs for new products, the FDA had no resources to devote to this requirement. Accordingly, in June 1966 the FDA contracted with the National Academy of Sciences (NAS) to conduct the review of 1938–1962 NDAs.

The NAS review was conducted by panels of experts in specific drug categories. Drugs were rated in one or other of the following six categories:

1. Effective;
2. Probably effective;
3. Possibly effective;
4. Ineffective;
5. Effective but other drugs are preferable; or
6. Ineffective as a fixed combination.

Because roughly half of the drugs were no longer marketed, the NAS ultimately reviewed approximately 4000 different drug formulations. Brief reports, many consisting only of a single sentence, were transmitted to the FDA by the NAS in 1967–1968. The FDA then undertook to implement these reports in the form of notices published in the Federal Register as part of what the agency called the Drug Efficacy Study Implementation (DESI) programme.

In order to implement the NAS reports, the FDA found that it must first address a number of important policy issues. First, the FDA was required to determine whether the NAS findings would apply only to the pioneer drug for which the NDA was submitted or would also apply to all subsequently marketed generic versions of the drug. The FDA determined that the latter approach was required, which led to extensive litigation. FDA policy on this matter was ultimately upheld by the Supreme Court in June 1973.[91]

Secondly, the FDA had to confront the fact that prior to the 1962 Amendments it had issued hundreds of 'old drug' opinion letters for generic versions of pioneer new drugs. It therefore issued a statement of policy in May 1968 revoking all of those opinions.[92]

Thirdly, the FDA was confronted with potentially thousands of requests for formal trial-type administrative hearings before it could remove from the market pre-1962 new drugs that were found to be less than effective. The requirement of formal administrative hearings would have effectively precluded implementation of the 1962 Amendments. The FDA resolved this by publishing in the Federal Register regulations defining the new statutory requirement of adequate and well-controlled clinical investigations,[93] and issuing summary judgement notices withdrawing approval of new drugs that failed to submit clinical studies which met the requirements of the new regulations. The regulations defining adequate and well-controlled clinical investigations were upheld in the courts, and the summary judgement procedure was also upheld.[94] Thus, the number of drugs for which formal administrative hearings were required was substantially reduced.

Fourthly, the FDA established a new procedure for regulating generic versions of pre-1962 pioneer drugs that were found under the DESI programme to be safe and effective. The FDA established the 'abbreviated' NDA, which required the submission of information to the FDA on bioequivalence and manufacturing controls only, and not on basic safety and effectiveness.[95] Any manufacturer who wished to market a generic version of a pre-1962 pioneer drug found to be safe and effective under the NAS review could obtain FDA approval through an abbreviated NDA.

In 1972, 10 years after the 1962 Amendments were enacted, three lower court rulings threatened to destroy the FDA approach to these matters. The agency successfully took all three cases, as well as a fourth in which the FDA had prevailed, to the US Supreme Court, and in June 1973 the Supreme Court sustained the FDA on all of the legal issues involved.[96] From then on, the basic approach to FDA implementation of the 1962 Amendments was established and strengthened.

The FDA pace of implementation of the 1962 Amendments was, however, necessarily slow. The American Public Health Association therefore brought a lawsuit to require the FDA to complete its DESI programme for pre-1962 new drugs, and the federal district court entered an order requiring completion within 4 years.[97] Although the FDA to this day has still not completed this programme, the court order did impose a greater sense of urgency and led the FDA to devote greater resources to the matter.

Throughout this time, the FDA was groping for a consistent approach to the handling of generic drugs. Initially, it revoked all 'old drug' opinion letters. Later, it proposed a procedure for determining old drug status for products.[98] Following that, it concluded that an abbreviated NDA should be submitted for all generic versions of pre-1962 new drugs.[99] In 1975, it again reversed itself and decided to develop old drug monographs, similar to the non-prescription drug monographs, for which an NDA would not be required.[100] Still later, it abandoned that approach and again stated that an abbreviated NDA would be required for all generic versions of pre-1962 new drugs.[101] That position was challenged in the courts, but was upheld by the Supreme Court.[102]

An attempt was made during 1977–80 to resolve all of these issues through a comprehensive revision of the new drug provisions of the FD&C Act. The legislation passed the Senate in 1979[103] but did not reach the floor of the House and, because the legislation was so detailed and complex, it was never again seriously considered.

By 1980, a new problem had emerged. The FDA had administratively created the concept of an abbreviated NDA to handle generic versions of pre-1962 pioneer new drugs, but there was no similar mechanism for the approval of generic versions of post-1962 new drugs. As time went by, more and more post-1962 pioneer new drugs lost patent protection, but retained an equivalent protection under the FD&C Act because the FDA had no authority to approve any form of an abbreviated NDA for generic versions of

these drugs. The FDA therefore began to search for a solution to this problem. In 1978, the FDA announced it would approve a 'paper' NDA for a generic copy of a post-1962 pioneer new drug based on the published scientific data for the drug. This policy was upheld in the courts,[104] but it had relatively little impact because there were insufficient published animal and human data to approve generic versions of most post-1962 new drugs. Thus, relatively few paper NDAs were approved by the FDA.

Another drug tragedy in early 1984 focused the FDA on yet another aspect of regulating prescription new drugs. An intravenous vitamin E product marketed without an NDA produced serious adverse reactions that required a nationwide recall.[105] The FDA concluded that there were approximately 5000 prescription drugs marketed without an approved NDA of any kind. Some 1800 would eventually be subject to the requirement for an abbreviated NDA when the DESI programme was fully implemented, but another 3200 were never subject to the NAS review because they were on the market prior to the FD&C Act of 1938, or were otherwise grandfathered. In a September 1984 Compliance Policy Guide, the FDA was forced to concede that these products could remain on the market until the agency could find the resources to review them and consider appropriate regulation.[106] Indeed, new versions of these products can still be marketed as long as they are identical to the previously marketed versions. The FDA did promulgate a regulation requiring adverse drug reaction reports for all prescription drugs marketed without an approved NDA, in order to track any potential public health problem,[107] but because the FDA has failed to take action against the vast majority of these unapproved drugs, it is now estimated that they have increased to some 16,000 in number and represent about 2% of annual prescriptions.[108]

In the past three decades, the FDA has proceeded slowly but surely with the DESI programme implementing the NAS review of pre-1962 new drugs. Where drugs have been found ineffective, most have been taken off the market using the summary judgement procedure. A few manufacturers have succeeded in requiring an administrative hearing, but none has prevailed before an administrative law judge, the Commissioner, or the courts.

In a surprisingly large number of instances, manufacturers decided to market new drugs without any NDA, and outside the 1984 FDA policy that permits such products if they are identical to old products that never had an NDA, solely on the basis that they were old drugs because they were generally recognised as safe and effective (GRAS and GRAE) and therefore did not require an approved NDA. The FDA brought enforcement actions against dozens of these products and, because the agency prevailed in every case, this approach is rarely tried today. As indicated above, the status of generic versions of both pre-1962 and post-1962 new drugs was settled by Congress in the Drug Price Competition and Patent Term Restoration Act of 1984.[109] That statute will be discussed in greater detail below.

Accordingly, the large conceptual issues that confronted the FDA following enactment of the Drug Amendments of 1962 have now been resolved, and most (but not all) of the large categories of DESI prescription drug products on the market have been brought under regulatory control. The major category of products that remains without any form of NDA approval are the pre-1962 new drugs that were never the subject of an NDA and for which the FDA has not yet conducted some form of regulatory review.

22.8.2 Regulatory categories of prescription drugs

There are two primary categories of prescription drugs: those not currently subject to any form of NDA approval, and those subject to some form of NDA approval.

22.8.2.1 No NDA

Those not subject to any form of NDA approval consist largely of products for which an NDA has never been required or obtained, and which thus were not subject to the NAS review of 1938–1962 new drugs. This is a narrow category but it encompasses about 16,000 drug products and represents about 2% of all US prescriptions.

In its September 1984 policy statement,[110] the FDA stated that until some form of regulatory control was instituted, new versions of these drugs could be marketed only if the new version was in all significant respects identical to the old version. The life of one of these products is, of course, uncertain. The FDA could at any time decide to regulate any or all of these products in a more comprehensive way. The FDA announced a new Compliance Policy Guide in June 2006 that confirmed and strengthened the September 1984 FDA policy.[111] The precise status of any of these drugs can be determined only by a detailed review of all of the facts available for the specific product involved.

22.8.2.2 Three forms of NDA

The vast bulk of prescription drugs on the market today are subject to the requirement for some form of an approved NDA. Following enactment of the Drug Price Competition and Patent Term Restoration Act of 1984,[112] there are now three clearly established types of NDA: a full NDA, a paper NDA [now called a Section 505(b)(2) NDA, after the provision in the FD&C Act that created it] and an abbreviated NDA. Each of these is discussed in the sections that follow.

22.8.2.2.1 The full NDA For any new chemical entity drug, whether or not it has been first marketed abroad, and whether or not it is chemically related to some other approved new drug, the FDA requires compliance with the full IND/NDA process.

The IND. Before submitting an NDA to FDA, the sponsor of a drug must conduct, or arrange to be conducted, various types of non-clinical (*in vitro* and animal) tests and clinical (human) studies designed to demonstrate that the drug is safe and effective for its intended use.[113]

For non-human studies no IND is required. Companies may perform *in vitro* testing, for example, to obtain chemical information necessary to set exact specifications for the active ingredient or to obtain stability data. The company may also conduct animal toxicology tests to establish an adequate margin of human safety. Animal toxicology testing must be conducted in accordance with the FDA Good Laboratory Practice (GLP) regulations,[114] but no IND or any other type of notice to FDA is required for any type of non-human studies. The FDA also has both formal and informal guidelines to govern animal toxicity testing.

After adequate preclinical testing has been completed, an IND must be submitted to the FDA to justify clinical investigation in humans. The content and format of an IND are set out in detail in the FDA regulations, and therefore need not be repeated here. The IND must contain all relevant information about the safety and effectiveness of the new drug, the protocols intended to be used in the investigations, the chemistry, manufacturing and control information, pharmacology and toxicology information, previous human experience and other pertinent information. In all respects, the FDA IND regulations must be followed in detail.

After submission, the FDA has 30 days within which to evaluate the IND. By the end of 30 days, one of several things will have occurred. First, the FDA may approve the IND, in which case testing can begin. Secondly, the FDA may place the IND on formal clinical hold, in which case testing cannot begin.[115] Thirdly, the FDA may say nothing, may raise questions, may offer suggestions or may say virtually anything in response to the IND. The sponsor must then determine whether to proceed in light of these developments or to delay testing until the matter is clarified. Many sponsors conclude that the only reasonable thing to do is to delay testing until all issues are fully resolved, but others proceed in the face of open questions.

Once the initial 30-day period has expired, the IND may be amended and updated periodically. For example, additional protocols may be added. There is no 30-day delay for any subsequent amendment. Once again, however, sponsors must determine whether to delay testing until the FDA is consulted and any issues are fully resolved.

An essential element of the IND is approval of the investigation by an institutional review board (IRB), either constituted by the institution in which the drug will be tested or established as a for-profit private IRB.[116] The IRB is charged with reviewing the ethical and moral dimensions of the study as well as the scientific merit. IRB approval does not guarantee FDA approval, nor does FDA approval guarantee IRB approval. They are separate and independent requirements, and both must be fulfilled before testing may begin under an IND.

Adherence to the IND by the sponsor is essential. Deviations from any aspect of it are not permitted. Before there can be any change in any aspect of the IND – including the specifications of the drug, the nature of the manufacturing process, the protocol for the investigation and the identity of the investigators, to name just a few – the IND must be amended.

No investigational new drug may be promoted or otherwise commercialised. No charge may be made for an investigational new drug without the prior approval of the FDA.

The FDA IND regulations contain requirements for various types of records and reports, which must be adhered to without exception.[117] Immediate reports to the FDA are required for any serious and unexpected adverse experience associated with the drug. Annual reports are required for every IND. Records must be kept to document all aspects of the IND.

Clinical testing under an IND is usually regarded as proceeding through three phases. Phase I includes the initial introduction of an investigational new drug into humans under closely monitored conditions, usually in a teaching hospital. This phase involves a relatively small number of subjects and is intended to obtain basic information on the pharmacology of the drug. Phase II includes controlled clinical studies conducted to evaluate the effectiveness and optimum dosage of the drug, and to determine common side effects and other risks. It involves a greater number of subjects, but is not a large-scale trial. Phase III involves expanded controlled and uncontrolled trials to gather additional information about safety and effectiveness that is needed to evaluate the overall benefit–risk relationship, and may involve up to several thousand subjects. In recent years, these three phases have tended to overlap substantially, and approval has been obtained on the basis of phase II or II/III studies for a number of important drugs.

Three types of unusual IND situations deserve special mention. First, the regulations contain a provision governing emergency use of an investigational new drug, where the FDA will permit such use by telephone or other rapid communication means.[118] In these situations, the IND must subsequently be amended to reflect the new situation. Secondly, the FDA will approve specific treatment protocols for compassionate use of an investigational new drug, where the drug is intended to treat a serious or immediately life-threatening disease, there is no satisfactory alternative, the drug is under clinical investigation pursuant to an IND and marketing approval is actively being pursued with due diligence.[119] After a treatment IND has been approved, the sponsor may provide the drug to any patient who meets the criteria in the treatment IND, and may charge in order to recoup the cost of the drug. Thirdly, the FDA will approve 'parallel track' protocols for AIDS where there is no therapeutic alternative and individuals cannot participate in the controlled clinical trials, in order to assure widespread use of the most promising drugs at the earliest possible stage.[120] As a practical matter, it is difficult, if not impossible, to distinguish between a parallel track IND and a treatment IND.

Compassionate use of investigational new drugs has been permitted by the FDA since the 1950s in order to assure that individual patients who have no other alternative are not denied promising treatment. The more recent terminology of 'treatment IND' and 'parallel track' is therefore simply a continuation of this long-standing policy, with no significant substantive change. In addition to these new forms of compassionate use INDs, the pharmaceutical industry continues to use the traditional form of compassionate use protocol as well.

The results of clinical trials conducted under an IND have traditionally been regarded as confidential business information that the FDA was prohibited from releasing to the public under the Freedom of Information Act and that the publication of which was determined solely by the drug sponsor. The Food and Drug Administration Modernization Act of 1997 established a clinical trial data bank for drugs for serious or life-threatening disease and required the inclusion of information on all effectiveness trials for these drugs. As a result of widespread concern about the lack of public availability of information about all clinical trials and their results, individual companies and the Pharmaceutical Research and Manufacturers of America announced programmes to make this information public and the editors of important scientific and medical journals have determined that they will not publish studies unless this information is made public.[121] The NIH has also announced that such information from NIH trials will be made public. To provide a single comprehensive data bank for this information, Congress included in the FDA Amendments Act of 2007 an expansion of the website established by the NIH, ClinicalTrials.gov, under the FDA Modernization Act of 1997.[122] The expanded website will include both a registry of clinical trials and the results of each trial.[123]

The NDA. After the sponsor has completed all non-clinical and clinical testing necessary to demonstrate the safety and effectiveness of the drug, the test results must be compiled in an NDA for submission to the FDA.[124] As with the IND, the content and format of the NDA are set forth in the FDA regulations and must be followed in detail. The NDA must begin with a summary, to be followed by technical sections relating to:

1. Chemistry, manufacturing and controls;
2. Non-clinical pharmacology and toxicology;
3. Human pharmacokinetics and bioavailability;
4. Microbiology;
5. Clinical data; and
6. Statistics.

Proposed labelling must also be included. The typical NDA comprises tens of thousands or even hundreds of thousands of pages.

The FD&C Act requires that a new drug must be shown to be both safe and effective. Because no drug has ever been shown to be completely safe or effective, in all cases this has been interpreted to mean that the benefits of the drug outweigh its risks under the labelled conditions of use for a significant identified patient population. The statute is very broadly worded with respect to the required proof for safety and effectiveness, and the FDA has exercised substantial discretion in applying these requirements. New drugs have been approved on the basis of only one study, on the basis of phase II studies that have never progressed to phase III, on the basis of foreign studies alone and with results that could not be regarded as definitive from a scientific standpoint.

In most instances, the FDA requires more than one adequate and well-controlled clinical trial. However, in the FDA Modernization Act of 1997, Congress clarified the law by providing that the FDA may base the approval of an NDA on data from one adequate and well-controlled clinical investigation and confirmatory evidence.[125] The FDA has in practice implemented this provision only when the single adequate and well-controlled clinical investigation has statistical significance that is an order of magnitude greater than is normally required (i.e. 0.005 rather than the customary convention of 0.05).

Under the FD&C Act, the FDA has always been required to evaluate the NDA and approve or disapprove it within 180 days. Until 1992, this almost never occurred. The average time for approval of an NDA was 2–3 years. This time remained largely unchanged for the years between 1962 and 1994, in spite of repeated promises and attempts by the FDA to speed up the process. The FDA was able to avoid the 180-day statutory time deadline in several ways. First, the agency started the clock when it accepted the NDA for filing, not when it was submitted. Secondly, the FDA stopped the clock, and restarted it, whenever new submissions were made. Thirdly, the FDA requested an extension of time from the applicant, who had no choice but to agree. Fourthly, the FDA simply ignored the 180-day deadline, and there was nothing that the applicant could do about it.

For many years it was proposed that user fees should be assessed on NDAs and that the proceeds should be used to hire sufficient FDA personnel to process applications more expeditiously. In 1992, the regulated industry and the FDA finally agreed on this approach and Congress enacted the PDUFA of 1992.[126] The PDUFA was initially authorised for 5 years, and was reauthorised for another 5 years each under the FDA Modernization Act of 1997,[127] the Prescription Drug User Fee Amendments of 2002[128] and the FDA Amendments Act of 2007.[129] The legislation provides for three types of user fee: drug applications, drug products and drug establishments. These fees have allowed the FDA to more than double the number of personnel reviewing NDAs. As a result, the time for NDA approval was initially halved. In 1999 and 2000, however, this trend has reversed and the time for approval has begun to increase significantly. Reflecting this increase in approval time, the FDA began to issue 'approvable' or 'complete response' letters within the user fee time guidelines, and then to take a substantial additional period to negotiate remaining issues (often including labelling) before a final approval letter was sent. In July 2000, the FDA abandoned the use of 'approveable' and similarly designated letters and now issues either a 'complete response' or an 'approval' letter.[130]

In response to criticism that the agency was not moving quickly enough to approve new drugs for AIDS and other serious or life-threatening illnesses, in 1992 the FDA established regulations to establish an accelerated approval process.[131] This is commonly referred to as the subpart H process, after the designation in the FDA regulations. The regulations describe two subpart H procedures. Under the first, the FDA is authorised to approve a new drug based on a surrogate endpoint that has not yet been validated but that is 'reasonably likely . . . to predict clinical benefit', if the sponsor agrees to conduct and submit data from post-marketing studies. Under the second procedure, the FDA may grant accelerated approval to beneficial but highly toxic drugs if the sponsor agrees to post-approval distribution restrictions. Under the regulations, both of these procedures are voluntary.

Subsequent to the establishment of subpart H, Congress enacted separate 'fast-track' procedures for new drugs to treat a serious or life-threatening condition that had the potential to address unmet medical needs under the FDA Modernization Act of 1997.[132] The FDA is required to respond to requests for designation of new drugs as fast-track products within 60 days, and must expedite the development and review of a fast-track NDA. Approval may be based on a determination that the product has an effect on a clinical endpoint or on a surrogate endpoint. If it is based on a surrogate endpoint, post-approval studies can be required to confirm the effect on the clinical endpoint. The NDA sponsor must submit copies of all promotional materials prior to NDA approval and subsequently. Approval of a fast-track product may be withdrawn using expedited procedures. FDA has issued a guidance, but no regulations, to implement this provision.

Following market withdrawal of several new drugs because of toxicity that had not been uncovered in the non-clinical or IND studies, in 1998 the FDA established a Task Force on Risk Management to evaluate the FDA system for managing the risks of FDA-approved medical products. The task force con-cluded that the rates of drug withdrawals and adverse events remain consistently low, but recommended a new risk management approach in order to better identify and control these risks as early as possible in the NDA process.[133] Implementation of this report had a substantial impact on the IND/NDA process. FDA reviewers required more patients in clinical trials, more dosage levels, longer follow-up and more trials. A number of NDAs that had been expected to obtain FDA approval were disapproved and required additional evidence of safety and effectiveness. As already noted, the time for NDA approval increased significantly following the release of the report. The release in late 1999 of the widely publicised Institute of Medicine report on the number of deaths caused by medication errors undoubtedly contributed to the new FDA wave of conservatism.[134] Patients have com-plained that their interests are not being considered, as drugs have been withdrawn or withheld because of concern about toxicity to a few individuals, and the benefits to large numbers of patients are not being taken into account.

The widespread publicity about the potential risk from COX-2 inhibitor drugs, and the withdrawal of Vioxx from the market, propelled the FDA and Congress into another wave of conservatism. The FDA Amendments Act of 2007 included several pro-visions confirming FDA authority to impose stringent safety requirements for new drugs. These include the authority to require drug labelling changes, phase IV testing and REMS programmes.

The FDA divides NDAs into two categories for the purpose of review: priority drugs and all other drugs. For priority drugs, the FDA sets a target of NDA review within 6 months. For all other drugs, the target is 10 months. These targets are subject to periodic adjustment when the PDUFA is renegotiated every 5 years, but it is unlikely that they will be substantially reduced.

During the NDA evaluation there are no guidelines or rules that require open communication between FDA and the applicant. It is impossible to generalise about the relationship between drug applicants and FDA reviewers. The CDER review divisions have quite varied reputations for openness, promptness and cordiality. Thus, discussion between an FDA review division and the applicant varies all the way from virtually no communication to constant discussion. Relations range from friendliness to near hostility. The NDA review process is, in short, entirely an ad hoc and informal process of negotiation that may go very well or very poorly, and over which the applicant has virtually no control. Attempts to obtain resolution of disputes through the FDA ombudsman or by appealing issues to higher officials are almost never successful, and often worsen relations with the NDA reviewers. Pharmaceutical companies uniformly fear retaliation unless they cooperate fully with every request from the NDA reviewers.

For every NDA, some clinical study is almost certain to remain in progress at the time when the NDA is submitted. Safety update reports are therefore required to be submitted to the FDA by the applicant while the NDA is pending, and particularly following receipt of a complete response letter.[135] Detailed systems and procedures are required to ensure that the data in the NDA and the safety updates are accurate and complete, and failure to meet these requirements is regarded by the FDA as a serious deficiency.

It is customary for the FDA to submit one or more letters of disapproval as part of the NDA review process. These frequently lead to the submission of new information, a revision of labelling and further negotiation. In a relatively small number of cases, the FDA will issue a definitive disapproval letter determining that there is no additional information on the basis of which the drug could be approved. There are then various administrative and judicial appeals that the applicant can make. In no instance since 1938, however, has any applicant successfully challenged FDA denial of approval of an NDA.[136] For this reason, it is generally understood that there is no practical way to challenge whatever the FDA requires during the NDA process, and that the only realistic alternative is to negotiate the best possible approach with the FDA in a cooperative spirit.

Confidentiality of information. Under the Freedom of Information Act, all information in government files is subject to public disclosure unless it falls within a specified exemption.[137] Both the FD&C Act[138] and the Federal Trade Secrets Act[139] prohibit the public disclosure of confidential commercial information and trade secrets. The FDA has promulgated detailed regulations governing the status of general categories of data and information in its files,[140] and particularly data and information submitted as part of an IND or NDA.[141] In general, no data or information submitted to the FDA as part of an IND or NDA will be made public prior to FDA approval or disapproval of the NDA. Even the existence of an IND or NDA was once kept confidential by the FDA if it was not disclosed by the sponsor, although all clinical trials must now be disclosed by the sponsor through the registry established by NIH at ClinicalTrials.gov. Upon approval,

the FDA issues a summary of the basis for the agency approval of the product, which describes the safety and effectiveness data on which the agency relied.[142] The FDA Amendments Act of 2007 requires the FDA to publish on its website the action package for approval of a new chemical entity new drug within 30 days of NDA approval.[143] Whether the FDA will also release the reports and data relating to the testing for safety and effectiveness will depend upon whether the company can convince the agency that these data retain value as 'confidential commercial information'.[144] In general, the FDA will release the full data and information on safety and effectiveness after a drug becomes subject to generic competition, but not before. Agency regulations spell out the FDA's confidentiality policies in great detail, but there are still often disputes about their application to any particular set of facts.

Advisory committees. There is no statutory requirement that the FDA review the approval of an NDA with an advisory committee before final action is taken. Since the 1970s, however, this has been the customary practice, particularly with important new drugs. This prompted Congress to enact a specific provision dealing with the establishment of drug advisory committees under the FDA Modernization Act of 1997.[145] The FDA Amendments Act of 2007 carried this one step further by requiring for every new chemical entity new drug either advisory committee review or a statement by the FDA why such review is unnecessary.[146]

The review of an NDA by an advisory committee is an extremely important step in the approval process. It represents the best opportunity that the applicant has to address the agency and the public about the evidence of safety and effectiveness and the importance of the drug to public health. In the majority of cases, the FDA accepts the recommendation of the advisory committee for approval, further testing or outright disapproval. Where the advisory committee recommends approval and the FDA disagrees, however, the agency will almost always take a long time to implement the advisory committee recommendations, or may even add additional testing requirements before approval is eventually obtained. The importance of advisory committee review is widely recognised in the pharmaceutical industry, and it is common for a company to engage in extensive preparation for the company presentation and to seek supportive statements from independent outside experts and patients as well.

The FDA has long been faced with the dilemma that the most respected medical experts in the country are almost always retained as consultants by the regulated industry, which raises the issue of a conflict of interest when considered for service on an FDA advisory committee. In the FDA Amendments Act of 2007, Congress ordered the FDA to reduce the number of conflict of interest waivers granted to advisory committee members by 5% per year from 2007 through 2012.[147]

Post-approval requirements. Following approval of an NDA, the FDA requires the submission of three different types of reports by the owner of the NDA.[148] First, serious and unexpected adverse drug experiences must be immediately reported to the FDA regardless of whether or not the company believes they are causally related to the drug. Secondly, all adverse drug experiences, as well as other safety and effectiveness information, must be reported periodically to the FDA, at intervals specified in the FDA regulations. Thirdly, information relating to all other aspects of the drug must be reported immediately to the FDA if they represent a potential problem, but otherwise may be included in an annual report. Foreign as well as domestic adverse experiences and other information must be included in these reports.

Changes in the NDA after approval. Any significant change from the detailed terms and conditions specified in the approved NDA must be the subject of a supplemental NDA and cannot be put into effect until the supplemental NDA has been approved by the FDA.[149] The only changes in an approved NDA that may be made without approval of a supplemental NDA are set forth in the FDA regulations, and those exceptions must be reflected in the annual report submitted to the FDA. Where the FDA finds that changes have been made from an approved NDA, beyond those permitted without a supplemental NDA, very stringent regulatory action can be taken, including recall of the product and the inability to manufacture any more product until the unapproved changes are eliminated or approved. Accordingly, it is essential that all aspects of an approved NDA be followed in detail unless a clear exception is created in the FDA regulations. In close cases, the FDA should be consulted.

Summary suspension of approval. The statute provides that the Secretary of HHS may summarily suspend approval of an NDA upon a finding that the drug represents an imminent hazard to the public health.[150] This authority is delegated to the Secretary of HHS alone, and cannot be exercised by the FDA or anyone else. It has been used only once, and its use was upheld in the courts.[151]

Antibiotic drugs. New antibiotic drugs are subject to the same IND and NDA requirements contained in the FDA regulations as other new drugs. Although the FD&C Act initially provided that the FDA could require batch certification for antibiotics, in 1982 the FDA exempted all classes of antibiotic drugs from this requirement because of the high level of manufacturer compliance with antibiotic standards. Because the FDA Modernization Act of 1997 repealed the old antibiotic provisions of the FD&C Act,[152] antibiotics today are regulated in the same way as all other new drugs.

User fees. Under the PDUFA of 1992, as extended 5 years each by the FDA Modernization Act of 1997, the Prescription Drug User Fee Amendments of 2002, and the FDA Amendments Act of 2007, the FDA has the authority to collect user fees for pioneer drugs until such time as generic competition is approved.[153] The fees include:

1. A one-time NDA fee;
2. An annual product fee; and
3. An annual establishment fee.

The precise amount of each fee escalates each year and is subject to modification according to detailed provisions in the statute. The funds obtained from these fees must be in addition to the existing congressionally appropriated resources for the IND/NDA system as adjusted for cost-of-living increases, and must be used solely for the IND/NDA process. In return for receiving user fees, the FDA has committed to specific goals for improving the drug review process, by reducing the backlog of applications, meeting specified time deadlines and making improvements in the process. The extent to which these commitments are kept becomes apparent only in subsequent years.

22.8.2.2.2 Section 505(b)(2) NDA When Congress enacted the Drug Price Competition and Patent Term Restoration Act of 1984, it included a provision based on the concept of a paper NDA but which in fact expanded that concept significantly. The former paper NDA is therefore now called a Section 505(b)(2) NDA, after the statutory provision that creates it.[154] It applies to those situations where a pioneer drug is no longer protected by patents or market exclusivity but where an applicant is unable to submit an abbreviated NDA because the modified drug differs in some substantial way from the pioneer drug. A Section 505(b)(2) NDA relies upon the pioneer NDA for all information except the data needed to support the element of substantial difference. Thus, the Section 505(b)(2) NDA need not include any data relating to the basic safety and effectiveness of the drug, except in so far as the difference between the pioneer drug and the applicant's modification of that drug bears upon safety or effectiveness.

Minor differences between a pioneer drug and a generic version of that drug may be approved by the FDA as appropriate for an abbreviated NDA pursuant to a 'suitability petition'. Where those differences become substantial, however, the FDA will deny the suitability petition and will require the approval of a more complete NDA. In these circumstances, the Section 505(b)(2) paper NDA will be sufficient, and a full NDA will not be required. Thus, the Section 505(b)(2) NDA is midway between a full NDA and an abbreviated NDA. The same regulations and requirements apply to a Section 505(b) (2) paper NDA under the 1984 Act as apply to a full NDA. The FDA interprets Section 505(b)(2) to authorise the agency to rely on confidential commercial information in a pioneer NDA in order to approve a generic competitor's version of the drug. The regulated industry takes the position that this would be illegal under the FD&C Act. This disagreement must ultimately be resolved in the courts.

22.8.2.2.3 Abbreviated NDA All of the regulations and requirements for an abbreviated NDA developed by the FDA in the late 1960s as part of the implementation of the Drug Amendments of 1962, and all of the proposed changes that the FDA considered to adapt those requirements to post-1962 new drugs, were eliminated when Congress enacted the Drug Price Competition and Patent Term Restoration Act of 1984. The 1984 Act established detailed requirements that supersede everything that went before.[155]

Under the 1984 Act, an abbreviated NDA may be approved by the FDA for a generic version of a pioneer new drug after: (1) all relevant product and use patents have expired for the pioneer drug; and (2) all relevant periods of market exclusivity for the pioneer drug have also expired. The statute contains detailed and complex rules for determining precisely how this system works. No attempt will be made here to discuss the specific provisions, but they are extremely important in determining the commercial value of a pioneer new drug because they govern when the drug will become subject to generic competition. Of particular importance, Congress expanded the length of protection granted under the 1984 Act in the FDA Modernization Act of 1997, as extended by the Best Pharmaceuticals for Children Act in 2002 and 2007, by providing an extra 6 months of market exclusivity

at the end of the extended patent term (or market exclusivity term, if the patent has already expired) when the sponsor conducts paediatric testing requested and approved by the FDA.[156]

There are basically two types of situation where an abbreviated NDA may be submitted. The first situation is where the generic version is the same as the pioneer version in all material respects. Where this is true, the applicant for the generic product simply submits the abbreviated NDA and the FDA may approve it without further consideration about the basic safety and effectiveness of the drug. The second circumstance is where the generic version is different from the pioneer drug in any significant respect (e.g. a different route of administration, dosage form or strength). In these circumstances, the generic applicant must first submit to the FDA a 'suitability petition' demonstrating that the difference between the drugs is not sufficient to preclude an abbreviated NDA, and that additional studies to show safety and effectiveness are not needed. If the FDA grants the suitability petition, an abbreviated NDA may be submitted. If the suitability petition is denied, the applicant must submit either a Section 505(b)(2) paper NDA or a full NDA. In all other respects, the regulations and requirements for an abbreviated NDA are the same as those for a full NDA.

22.8.3 Applications integrity (fraud) policy

As a result of the generic drug scandal described above, where generic drug manufacturers submitted fraudulent data and bribed FDA officials, the FDA adopted a 'fraud policy' in September 1991, which was later called the 'applications integrity policy,' to cover situations where the FDA concluded that an applicant who had engaged in a wrongful act would need to take corrective action to establish the reliability of data submitted to the FDA in support of pending applications and to support the integrity of products already on the market.[157] Under this policy, the FDA issues a formal letter invoking the policy and requiring the applicant to cooperate fully with the FDA investigation. The applicant is required to identify all individuals associated with the wrongful act and to ensure that they are removed from any substantive authority on matters under FDA jurisdiction. A credible internal review must be conducted to identify all instances of wrongful acts, to supplement the FDA's own investigation. The internal review should involve an outside consultant or team qualified by training and experience to conduct such a review. Finally, the applicant must commit in writing to developing and implementing a corrective action operating plan. Although this fraud policy was developed in response to the generic drug scandal, it also applies to pioneer drug companies and to data in full NDAs. Because the FDA has invoked the fraud policy against innocent companies whose rogue employees have acted illegally, and who have voluntarily reported the illegal activity to the agency, companies are reluctant to disclose such incidents where such disclosure is not otherwise required under the law.

22.8.4 Labelling and advertising

The labelling for a new drug must be included as part of the NDA and must be explicitly approved by the FDA. FDA regulations establish detailed requirements for the format and content of the physician labelling (often called the 'package insert') for a prescription drug. When the FDA revised these requirements in January 2006, it included in the preamble a highly controversial determination that the FDA decisions reflected in the physician labelling are intended to pre-empt any contrary decision by a federal or state court.[158] No significant change may be made in the labelling without prior FDA approval through a supplemental NDA. Because this rule is so clear and so stringent, the pharmaceutical industry seldom takes chances with deviations in product labelling that could result in FDA enforcement action. The FDA has long permitted the use of 'changes being effected' supplemental NDAs to allow new safety information to be added to a drug's labelling. In August 2008, the FDA revised this regulation to clarify that this procedure can be used only if there is 'sufficient evidence of a causal relationship' to justify the labelling change.[159]

At one time the FDA promulgated regulations to require mandatory patient package inserts for prescription drugs, but these regulations were revoked and replaced with a voluntary patient information programme.[160] The FDA then promulgated regulations requiring mandatory medication guides, called 'medguides' for short, for a limited number of drugs with a narrow therapeutic index or other potential for serious harm.[161] Under the FDA Amendments Act of 2007, the FDA now has the statutory authority to require either a medication guide or a patient package insert as part of a REMS programme for any prescription drug.[162]

The Drug Amendments of 1962 gave the FDA the authority to regulate advertising for prescription drugs, as well as labelling.[163] However, the FD&C Act was not amended to give the FDA premarket approval over advertising, similar to its premarket approval over labelling. Accordingly, the FDA must rely upon general policing of prescription drug advertising to determine whether it is false or misleading. Under FDA regulations, however, advertising must be submitted to the FDA promptly after it is first disseminated.[164]

In accordance with its statutory authority, the FDA has promulgated regulations that illustrate ways in which prescription drug advertising may be false, lacking in fair balance or otherwise misleading.[165] As the pharmaceutical industry has expanded its promotional activities, the FDA has also issued a variety of policy statements on various types of advertising practice that do not fall within the existing regulations. These policy statements deal with such issues as press conferences, medical seminars, journal supplements, TV and radio talk shows and a wide variety of other means of communication.[166] It is essential that anyone engaging in prescription drug marketing be fully familiar with the latest FDA policy in these areas.

A recent innovation has been direct-to-consumer (DTC) prescription drug promotion in the broadcast media. Because FDA regulations require a summary of the entire approved package insert to appear with any prescription drug advertisement, it was extremely difficult to use radio or television advertising for this purpose. Most consumer advertising for prescription drugs was therefore limited to the print media. However, beginning in July 1997, the FDA has issued guidance that allows the package insert requirement to be satisfied with more flexible ways to provide the same information to consumers.[167] This has resulted in an explosion of DTC prescription drug advertising on television. The FDA reviews these advertisements very carefully, and thus caution must be used in preparing them. It is sound practice to review proposed advertising of this type with the FDA prior to its use. Because of criticism that DTC prescription drug advertising may contribute to unwarranted use of prescription drugs and to higher drug prices, the FDA is conducting a thorough review of the current requirements for this category of advertising. It is likely that the agency will require greater emphasis on the potential risk of prescription drugs in future DTC prescription drug advertising. Under the FDA Amendments Act of 2007, the FDA is authorized to require submission of DTC advertising for a drug at least 45 days before dissemination of the advertisement. The FDA may make recommendations about the advertisement but may not require that changes be made, except for a serious risk.[168]

22.8.5 Good Manufacturing Practices

One of the most important parts of an NDA is the description of the chemistry, manufacturing and controls (CMC).[169] The FDA has traditionally placed substantial reliance upon this part of the NDA in ensuring the safety and effectiveness of the drug. One study conducted two decades ago found that more questions were raised by FDA reviewers about this section of the NDA than about the safety and effectiveness of the drug itself.

Beginning in 1991, moreover, the FDA announced a new enforcement technique designed to assure adequate GMP compliance before an NDA is approved.[170] Prior to FDA approval of the NDA, the FDA field force now conducts a pre-approval inspection (PAI) of the establishment where the new drug is to be manufactured. If the manufacturing facility deviates in any way from either the description in the NDA or the general requirements for GMP in the FDA regulations,[171] the NDA will be held hostage and will not be approved until full compliance is achieved. Pursuant to this policy, the approval of numerous NDAs has been substantially delayed. Compliance with GMP is therefore essential to any NDA approval. Because of widespread concern about this practice, Congress included in the FDA Modernization Act of 1997 a specific provision stating that an NDA approval may not be delayed because of unavailability of information from, or action by, the FDA field personnel unless the reviewing division determines that a delay is necessary to assure the marketing of a safe and effective drug.[172] In spite of this provision, the FDA has continued to hold drugs hostage as a result of a PAI without a finding that this is necessary to ensure the marketing of a safe and effective drug.

After approval of an NDA, the FDA periodically inspects a drug establishment for two purposes. First, the FDA determines whether any unapproved changes have been made in the manufacturing process from those set forth in the approved NDA. If any such changes are made beyond those permitted without a supplemental NDA, the FDA may well bring stringent enforcement action. Secondly, the FDA routinely inspects all establishments to determine compliance with GMP. Although the FDA has not changed its GMP regulations, the interpretation and application of those regulations by FDA inspectors are thought by the pharmaceutical industry to have been substantially tightened and made more strict in the past few decades.

Where the FDA determines any deviation from GMP, the inspector leaves a form FDA-483, specifying the manufacturing deficiencies. It is essential in these circumstances that the company immediately make all corrections and respond to the FDA in writing about them. It can be expected that the FDA will reinspect the establishment and look both for what has been done to correct the prior deficiencies and for any new deficiencies that can be found. The pharmaceutical industry believes that the FDA often lists insignificant matters, that establishments that have passed without observed deficiencies in the past suddenly will be the subject of major deficiencies because of a change of inspectors or of interpretation, and that the requirements vary widely from individual inspector to individual inspector and from FDA district to FDA district. However, the industry has found that its complaints fall on deaf ears, and thus that it must comply with whatever is required by the individual inspector or face the threat of serious regulatory action.

Realising that the agency had not reviewed its drug GMP regulations and requirements since 1979, the FDA announced in 2002 an initiative to conduct a thorough evaluation of all aspects of its implementation of drug GMP requirements. In 2004, the FDA issued a final report announcing a number of reforms relating to drug GMP.[173] Of primary importance, drug GMP decisions in the future are to be based upon scientific principles of risk analysis and risk management. The FDA also established a technical dispute resolution process for GMP disputes between FDA inspectors and the regulated industry. Five years after the FDA announced these GMP reforms, however, there has been no discernable impact on daily FDA GMP compliance decisions.

22.8.6 Pharmacy compounding

Prior to 1997, there was no provision in the FD&C Act that explicitly authorised pharmacy compounding. FDA policy recognised the practice of pharmacy compounding, but the agency brought action against compounding pharmacists when they began to advertise specific drugs or to stockpile substantial quantities of drugs.[174]

Under the FDA Modernization Act of 1997, Congress for the first time addressed the requirements and limitations of pharmacy compounding. To take advantage of the authority to compound, a pharmacy would have been precluded from advertising that specific compounded drugs were available from that pharmacy. In 2002, the Supreme Court held that this restriction was unconstitutional, in violation of the right of free speech under the First Amendment to the US Constitution.[175] Because a US Court of Appeals had ruled that the advertising restriction could not be separated from the other pharmacy compounding provisions, the result was that none of these provisions remained effective. Accordingly, pharmacy compounding was now back to where it was before the 1997 Act. The FDA reiterated its views regarding when pharmacy compounding becomes illegal manufacture.[176] In 2008, however, a second US Court of Appeals ruled that the advertising restriction could in fact be separated from the other pharmacy compounding provisions of the FDA Modernization Act of 1997 and thus that those other provisions remain effective.[177] This direct conflict between the two courts can be resolved only by Congress or the Supreme Court.

22.8.7 Distribution controls

On one occasion, the FDA sought to limit the distribution of a new drug to hospital-based pharmacies and to prohibit it through community pharmacies. Upon challenge by the pharmacy profession, the courts ruled that this was an illegal restriction that was not authorised by the FD&C Act.[178] Since then, the FDA has approved labelling for new drugs under which sponsors have voluntarily included restrictions on distribution, including under subpart H,[179] but the agency has not itself imposed distribution controls on any new drug. Under the FDA Amendments Act of 2007, however, the agency has been authorized to impose distribution controls as part of a mandatory REMS programme to assure the safety of a drug.[180]

22.8.8 Import and export
22.8.8.1 Import

In general, a prescription drug may lawfully be imported into the USA only in full compliance with all the laws and regulations applicable to domestic drugs. However, there is one exception. Since 1977, the FDA has stated that the agency will not detain unapproved new drugs imported for personal use.[181] This became important when patients with AIDS began to import drugs not available in the USA. Subsequently, AIDS organisations established buying clubs to import drugs for all of their members. The FDA has not sought to prohibit this activity except where it is done for commercial profit or involves unsafe or fraudulent products for which the agency has issued an import alert (such as RU-486). Where the FDA has considered cracking down on such imports, public pressure has forced the agency to back off from enforcement action.

The USA is the only country in the world that does not fix the prices for prescription drugs. Patented prescription drug costs in the USA are therefore higher than in any other country, and the cost of generic drugs in the USA are lower than in any other country. Because of the large price differential between the USA and other countries for patented prescription drugs, internet pharmacies and other organisations ship prescription drugs illegally into the USA, without an approved NDA or in violation of the prohibition against reimportation under the Prescription Drug Marketing Act of 1987. The FDA has vigorously opposed these illegal imports as well as any legislation designed to change the current statutory requirements for imported new drugs. Under both the Clinton and the Bush administrations, the Secretary of HHS has declined to certify that importation of unapproved drugs from abroad could be undertaken safely and would result in significant cost savings to the US consumer. Accordingly, the provisions of the Medicine Equity and Drug Safety Act of 2000 that would have provided for prescription drug imports have never been put into effect. The FDA continues to enforce the FD&C Act against illegal drug imports, many of which are counterfeit products.[182]

22.8.8.2 Export

The FD&C Act of 1938, and even the Drug Export Amendments Act of 1986, placed such stringent limitations on the export of unapproved drugs from the USA that they raised enormous commercial potential for foreign countries. Many US pharmaceutical companies reasonably anticipated that their drugs would receive approval for use outside the USA before they were approved by the FDA, and could not take the risk that they would be able to obtain and maintain FDA approval of an export application. Under these circumstances, they had no option other than to build their manufacturing facilities abroad rather than in the USA. For that reason, foreign countries competed in attempting to attract these pharmaceutical factories.

The FDA Export Reform and Enhancement Act of 1996 eliminated many, but far from all, of the restrictions on FDA export of unapproved new drugs. For example, although unapproved new drugs may be exported to any of the 25 listed countries for investigational use, these drugs may not be shipped to any other country for the same purpose without FDA approval – which can take a year or more. No other country in the world controls exports in the same way as the USA, and thus a pharmaceutical establishment may be located anywhere other than the USA without fear of unreasonable limitations on international trade. Accordingly, it is essential for any US or foreign company to be able to source its drugs abroad, rather than in the USA, if it is to be assured of the ability to investigate and market its new drugs throughout the world.

22.8.9 Orphan drugs

Under the Orphan Drug Act of 1983[183] and its amendments, an orphan drug is eligible for two types of benefit. The first, which is often of minor significance, consists of tax credits. The second type, which has proved to be of enormous importance, is the market exclusivity provided by the prohibition against any form of FDA approval of the same drug for another company for 7 years. The company that obtains FDA approval of an NDA for an orphan drug is thus assured of greater protection under the Orphan Drug Act than under any other statute, including the patent laws. The 7-year orphan drug market exclusivity can be broken if the FDA determines that a subsequent version of the same drug is clinically superior.[184]

As enacted in 1983, the Orphan Drug Act had relatively little impact because the scope of the term 'orphan drug' was considered by the FDA to be relatively narrow. When Congress amended the law in 1984[185] to define an orphan drug as any drug, or any single indication for a drug, for a condition afflicting fewer than 200,000 patients in the USA, the impact of the law changed dramatically. Some orphan drugs became blockbusters on which entire companies have been founded. Although Congress has considered legislation to cut back some of the provisions of the Orphan Drug Act, one such bill was vetoed by the President[186] and no other has since come close to enactment. Even if the benefits available from the Orphan Drug Act are changed, they are likely to remain important to drug companies for the foreseeable future.

22.8.10 Physician prescribing

The FD&C Act has been interpreted by the FDA as applying only to the labelling, advertising and marketing of a new drug, not to the practice of medicine as reflected in the physician's prescription of the drug for a particular patient. In a policy first published in 1972,[187] and reiterated many times,[188] the FDA has stated that the physician may, within the practice of medicine, lawfully prescribe an approved drug for an unapproved use. Because the Drug Price Competition and Patent Term Restoration Act of 1984 provides no significant market protection for companies that obtain FDA approval of new uses for previously

approved new drugs, companies rarely submit supplemental NDAs to request FDA approval of an unapproved use for an approved drug. As unapproved uses expand, the prescription drug package insert approved by the FDA has become substantially outdated. In many areas, the unapproved uses of a new drug overwhelm the approved uses. Although the FDA has deplored this fact, it has thus far done nothing to find an adequate resolution.

Although the FDA has stated since 1938 that the agency has no authority to require an NDA sponsor to conduct testing for uses that the sponsor has not included in the proposed labelling, the FDA nonetheless promulgated regulations in late 1998 to require paediatric testing of new drugs in most situations in order to reduce unapproved use of new drugs in infants and children.[189] The FDA regulation on paediatric testing was determined to be illegal by a court in 2002, but was restored by Congress in the Pediatric Research Equity Act of 2003. In the FDA Modernization Act of 1997, as extended for 5 years each by the Best Pharmaceutical for Children Act in 2002 and by the FDA Amendments Act of 2007, Congress included not only 6 months of marketing exclusivity for paediatric testing,[190] but also a provision to allow dissemination of information on unapproved uses of approved new drugs under specific limited conditions.[191]

While the 1997 Act was being considered by Congress, the FDA policy prohibiting dissemination of information on unapproved uses of approved new drugs was being challenged in the courts. The US District Court held that the FDA policy violated the First Amendment to the US Constitution, even taking into consideration the new statutory provision added by the 1997 Act, and issued an injunction that permitted a drug manufacturer to disseminate to physicians and other medical professionals information on unapproved uses of approved new drugs from a peer-reviewed professional journal or a reference textbook, or to suggest content or speakers to an independent programme adviser for a continuing medical education programme. The injunction permitted the FDA to require the drug manufacturer to disclose the company's interest in the drug and the fact that the use of the drug had not been approved by the FDA.[192] The FDA then changed its legal position and argued on appeal that its policy merely constituted a 'safe harbour', and that a violation would not necessarily bring an enforcement proceeding. As a result, the US Court of Appeals reversed the District Court's decision on procedural grounds, without in any way disagreeing with it.[193] The District Court then revoked its injunction, although indicating that it had not changed its opinion on the matter.[194] The FDA subsequently published a notice stating its continued intent to enforce its policy,[195] and the Washington Legal Foundation has raised serious legal objections. It is extremely unlikely that the FDA will enforce its unapproved use policy under the circumstances permitted by the now-dissolved District Court injunction, regardless of the outcome of this case, and FDA officials have so stated.

In February 2008, the FDA released a draft guidance essentially incorporating the dissolved District Court injunction.[196] Thus, the First Amendment right of free speech in the USA makes it even more difficult for the FDA to attempt to force NDA sponsors to submit supplemental NDAs for unapproved uses, absent unequivocal statutory authority to require that drugs be tested for these uses and that applications be submitted for including them in approved labelling. When a drug loses its patent status, the problem of requiring the generic and the pioneer sponsors to conduct such testing is overwhelming.

22.8.11 Patient freedom of choice

Beginning with enactment of the Drug Amendments of 1962, organised patient groups have argued strenuously that they should have the freedom to purchase whatever drugs they may wish to use, regardless of their FDA status, particularly where individuals have life-threatening diseases. Cancer patients argued for the use of Krebiozen and Laetrile, but the FDA sought to prohibit those drugs by every means available, and the courts ultimately supported the agency.[197] More recently, a US Court of Appeals, sitting en banc, determined that a terminal patient does not have the right under the US Constitution to access to an unapproved drug that has progressed to phase II testing.[198]

With the dramatic rise in AIDS, however, a larger, more vocal and more politically active interest group challenged the authority of the FDA to deny experimental and unapproved drugs to any patient who wishes to use them. This time, the activists had a greater impact.[199] The FDA has declined to take enforcement action in many instances where it would have done so in the past. The agency has also expedited the approval of AIDS drugs on the basis of scientific information that would not have been accepted as sufficient for any other disease area. Thus, the FDA has bent its rules for putative AIDS treatments but has refused to expand its flexibility to include other disease areas. The result is an inconsistent series of decisions approving drugs for one disease on the basis

of preliminary information and withholding approval of more extensively tested drugs for other diseases.

22.8.12 Costs and benefits of the IND/NDA system

There have been hundreds of investigations and reports on the IND/NDA system.[200] Numerous analyses have been carried out of the costs and benefits, and hundreds of recommendations have been made about ways to improve the system. Feelings run deep on these subjects, and the philosophical and emotional element often dwarfs the factual and analytical element.

A 1991 study demonstrated that the average NDA requires an investment of about $231 million.[201] In the last year of NDA approval, the average carrying cost (cost of capital) alone was $31 million. Today, these figures have escalated to an estimated $1.7 billion[202] or more. Critics argue that this is largely the result of unrealistic regulatory requirements that cause higher drug prices, that the delay in drugs reaching the market substantially harms the public health and that the high cost of drug development discourages drug research and development and directly hinders the development of life-saving drugs for the future. Supporters of the system point to drug tragedies of the past, argue that any relaxation of regulatory controls will dramatically increase drug risks and reduce drug effectiveness and state that the only sound way to protect the public health is to continue and indeed to strengthen the present system. Supporters of biotechnology charge that the present system is destroying the opportunity presented by this new technology, and critics of biotechnology applaud that result.

22.9 Biological drugs

For a full century, biological drugs have been regulated under the Biologics Act of 1902, in accordance with statutory requirements that have not significantly changed.[203] When the FDA was delegated the responsibility for regulating biologics in 1972, however, the agency promulgated regulations adding a number of the drug regulatory provisions under the FD&C Act to those already available under the Biologics Act. Current regulation of biologics therefore incorporates requirements from both statutes.

22.9.1 Biologics licence application

Prior to 1996, the FDA required the submission and approval of both an ELA and a PLA. This bifurcated submission and approval process was widely criticised as inefficient. Following the November 1994 elections and the realisation that the FDA would be a major target for legislative reform, the agency revised its regulations to eliminate the requirement for a separate ELA and to substitute a single biologics licence application (BLA) for four categories of well-characterised biological products.[204] In the FDA Modernization Act of 1997, however, Congress eliminated the ELA and PLA for all biological products and substituted the single BLA.[205] Congress also ordered the FDA to take measures to minimise differences in the review and approval of biological products under Section 351 of the Public Health Service Act and new drugs under Section 505(b)(1) of the FD&C Act. The FDA promptly amended the regulations governing biologics licences to implement this requirement.[206]

Before a company may manufacture any biological product, a BLA must be submitted to and approved by the FDA for the product involved. Under Section 351 of the Public Health Service Act as it is now revised, the product approval system for a biological drug is the same as for a new drug. Non-clinical studies may be conducted without FDA knowledge or approval. Clinical investigation in humans must be preceded by the submission of an IND, and all the IND regulations discussed above for chemical drugs apply equally to a biological drug. It is only the BLA that has a different name and a somewhat different focus.

A basic premise of the regulation of biological drugs is that, because they come from natural sources, they cannot adequately be characterised by chemical specifications and must instead be regulated very rigidly by rigorous adherence to detailed manufacturing procedures. For this reason, approval of a BLA depends upon the specific establishment specified and approved in that BLA. If the owner of an approved BLA wishes to manufacture all or part of the biological drug in a new establishment, it has long been standard policy under the Biologics Act to require not just that the new product be shown to be the same as the old, but also that new clinical studies independently demonstrate the safety and effectiveness of the new product as manufactured in the new establishment. This goes beyond the requirements that the FDA has applied to new drugs.

This FDA policy has important ramifications for the generic drug industry. When Congress enacted the Drug Price Competition and Patent Term Restoration Act of 1984, it included only new drugs and it excluded biological drugs. Nonetheless, a small number of biological products were handled under NDAs rather than BLAs, the most prominent of which is human growth hormone. Generic drug manufacturers have in fact submitted abbreviated NDAs or Section 505(b)(2) NDAs for human growth hormone. Thus, the FDA must decide whether generic versions of this biological product may be approved without the requirement of the same type of clinical testing that was required for the pioneer product. For all other biological products that have been licensed through BLAs under the Biologics Act of 1902, however, the advent of generic versions must await a revision of the statute by Congress.

With the advent of biotechnology, work in the CBER has changed dramatically. For decades, the only biological products regulated under the Biologics Act of 1902 were vaccines, blood, allergenic extracts and other related products that did not pose the difficult problems of balancing benefits against risks which were daily faced by the CDER. As a result, the CBER was able to review and approve ELAs and PLAs rapidly, in a fraction of the time that it took the CDER to do the same job. Now, the two are indistinguishable. The time required for review and approval of a BLA became even longer than that for an NDA. The backlog at the CBER rose dramatically. Critics suggested that review and approval of new pharmaceutical products by the CBER was slower and more difficult than by the CDER. The FDA therefore announced in 2002 that the handling of most biological drugs would be transferred from the CBER to the CDER, but that regulation of traditional biological products, such as vaccines and blood, will remain with the CBER. Approximately one-third of the CBER resources were transferred to the CDER as part of this reorganisation.

22.9.2 Biologics Review

When implementation of the Biologics Act was transferred to the FDA in 1972, a process was just being formulated by the Division of Biologics Standards in the NIH to review the safety, effectiveness and labelling of the biological products that had been licensed during the past 70 years under the 1902 Act. The FDA promptly established written procedures and undertook the Biologics Review.[207] The Biologics Review was patterned after the OTC Drug Review and is similarly not yet completed.

22.10 Enforcement

The FDA has available to it a wide variety of formal and informal enforcement authorities under the FD&C Act. They apply equally to all products regulated by the FDA. For generic drugs, the FDA also can rely upon the provisions of the Generic Drug Enforcement Act of 1992. The following sections summarise some of the more important enforcement provisions used by the FDA to regulate all pharmaceutical products.

22.10.1 Formal enforcement authority

22.10.1.1 Factory inspection

For purposes of enforcing the law, FDA inspectors may at any time inspect any factory manufacturing a non-prescription or prescription drug.[208] For both, FDA inspectors may see all records and documents except those that relate to financial data, sales data other than shipment data, pricing data, personnel data and research data.[209] An FDA inspector may spend whatever amount of time is necessary to complete such an inspection – even weeks or months. Where significant enforcement issues have been found, FDA inspectors have been known to spend more than a year at a single establishment.

22.10.1.2 Seizure

The FDA has statutory authority to request the Department of Justice to 'seize' any illegal product.[210] If the FDA asserts that the drug is dangerous to health or the labelling is fraudulent or misleading in a material respect, the statute authorises multiple seizures throughout the country. Prior to 1997, the FDA was required to prove the requisite shipment in interstate commerce in order to establish the agency's jurisdiction. Under the FDA Modernization Act of 1997, Congress established a rebuttable presumption of interstate commerce for purposes of FDA enforcement jurisdiction, thereby making all FDA enforcement action substantially simpler.[211]

22.10.1.3 Injunction

The FDA also has statutory authority to request the Department of Justice to seek a court injunction against continued violations of the law by a drug manufacturer or distributor.[212] The FDA has had mixed results in attempting to obtain injunctions from the courts, who realise that an injunction can shut down a company entirely or subject it to arbitrary demands by the FDA. The FDA has therefore sought to obtain the equivalent in the form of stipulated agreements with companies that are filed in court as consent decrees and thus are fully enforceable as a requirement of law.

22.10.1.4 Criminal penalties

All violations of the FD&C Act are automatically criminal violations of law.[213] On two occasions the US Supreme Court has held that any person standing in a responsible relationship to a violation of the FD&C Act is criminally liable, regardless of the lack of knowledge or intent.[214] The nature of the offence is the failure of an individual to take action to prevent a violation and to ensure compliance with the law.

This is an extremely harsh statute. As a practical matter, the FDA exercises its prosecutorial discretion only to bring cases for continuing violations of law, violations of an obvious and flagrant nature and intentionally false or fraudulent violations. Although there have been attempts to change the criminal liability standard under the FD&C Act by legislation, none has been successful.

22.10.1.5 Section 305 hearing

The FD&C Act provides that, before any violation is reported by the FDA for institution of a criminal proceeding, the person against whom the proceeding is contemplated shall be given appropriate notice and an opportunity to present views.[215] In accordance with this provision, it is the custom of the FDA to provide an informal hearing to individuals, to show cause why they should not be prosecuted. When a grand jury is convened, however, the FDA usually does not provide this type of hearing. Where such a hearing is given, it is obviously important for the individual to demonstrate a good faith attempt to comply with the law and an intent to correct and prevent any deficiencies in the future.

22.10.1.6 Other criminal statutes

The US Code contains a number of criminal provisions related to enforcement of the FD&C Act. These laws prohibit any criminal conspiracy,[216] false reports to the government,[217] mail fraud,[218] bribery,[219] perjury[220] and other similar illegal activity. The FDA has used these provisions on a number of occasions to bring criminal prosecution against individuals and companies who have violated the FD&C Act.

22.10.1.7 Civil money penalties

The Prescription Drug Marketing Act of 1987 includes civil penalties for violation of the drug sample provisions of the FD&C Act.[221] The law provides that a manufacturer or distributor who violates these provisions is subject to a civil penalty of not more than $50,000 for each of the first two violations resulting in a conviction in any 10-year period, and for not more than $1 million for each violation resulting in a conviction after the second conviction in any 10-year period. These penalties may be imposed only by a

Federal District Court. The FDA has no administrative authority to impose any civil penalties under these provisions. Under the FDA Amendments Act of 2007, Congress expanded the authority to impose civil money penalties to include violations of the new labelling, REMS, phase IV testing, and clinical trial registry and results database provisions.[222]

22.10.1.8 Restitution

One court interpreted the FD&C Act in the 1950s as not authorising the FDA to require restitution by a manufacturer to purchasers of a product that has been found to violate the FD&C Act,[223] but two more recent court decisions have upheld restitution.[224] The Medical Device Amendments of 1976 explicitly provide such authority for medical devices.[225]

22.10.2 Informal compliance authority

22.10.2.1 Recall

For decades, the FDA has worked with product manufacturers to request, and to help carry out, the recall of illegal products from the market. Courts have disagreed on whether the FD&C Act authorises an injunction that includes a requirement for product recall.[226] As a practical matter, however, the precise legal authority of the FDA on this matter is irrelevant. Manufacturers routinely cooperate with the FDA on the recall of any dangerous product. The FDA has established detailed administrative policy governing recall procedures.[227]

22.10.2.2 Warning letters

The FD&C Act authorises the FDA to decline to institute formal enforcement proceedings for minor violations whenever the FDA believes that the public interest will be adequately served by a suitable written notice or warning. In accordance with this provision, in the early 1970s the FDA began to issue a 'regulatory letter' in lieu of bringing formal court enforcement action. This permitted more rapid, less costly and more efficient compliance with the law. In the early 1990s, regulatory letters were renamed 'warning letters', and lost their impact because they were no longer approved by FDA top management and the Chief Counsel. Nonetheless, any warning letter must be given immediate attention in order to avoid more serious formal enforcement action in the courts.

22.10.2.3 Publicity

The FDA has explicit statutory authority to issue information to the public.[228] The courts have upheld the right of the FDA to publicise illegal activity and to issue publicity about products and practices that it concludes to be harmful to the public health.[229] This is regarded by many as the most potent compliance tool available to the FDA. Instead of using the formal enforcement authority established in the FD&C Act, for example, the FDA issued strong negative publicity about the dangers of phenylpropanolamine and ephedra and destroyed the market for both of these products overnight.

22.10.3 Enforcement statistics

In the first few decades of the 1900s, the FDA brought hundreds of seizure and criminal actions to enforce the FD&C Act. Beginning in the 1970s, the formal court enforcement actions have been replaced in two ways. First, the FDA has promulgated hundreds of regulations and guidance that establish the precise requirements of the law, thus reducing the need for many court enforcement actions. Secondly, formal court enforcement actions have been replaced by informal administrative compliance actions such as recalls and warning letters. FDA statistics initially demonstrated that the increase in administrative compliance actions was greater than the decrease in formal court enforcement actions, and thus that overall FDA enforcement activity continued to increase, but more recent statistics show a significant decrease in enforcement.[230]

22.11 Conclusions

This brief survey of the FDA regulation of pharmaceutical products demonstrates the breadth and depth of FDA activity in this field. Although there are repeated calls for reform of the IND/NDA system, it appears unlikely that any substantial change will occur in the near future. It is therefore important that any person who enters the prescription drug industry in the USA be fully informed about the requirements, understand the regulatory risks involved and comply adequately with all of the FDA requirements.

References

1 An earlier version of this chapter was published in Burley DM, Binns TB, Clarke J, Lasagna L, eds. *Pharmaceutical Medicine*, 2nd edn. Hodder Arnold, 1993, Chapter 9.
2 For example, Hutt PB, Merrill RA, Grossman LA. *Food and Drug Law: Cases and Materials*, 3rd edn. 2007.

3 52 Stat. 1040 (1938), 21 U.S.C. 301, *et seq.* FDA's internet website contains a large amount of information about the agency, the statutes it implements, its regulations and guidances, and other pertinent documents: www.fda.gov.

4 5 U.S.C. 551 *et seq.*

5 21 C.F.R. 10.40.

6 21 C.F.R. 10.45.

7 Section 12606 of the California Business and Professions Code.

8 Hutt PB. A historical introduction. *Food Drug Cosmet Law J* 1990;**45**:17; The transformation of United States Food and Drug Law. *J Assoc Food Drug Off* 1996;**60**:1.

9 12 Stat. 387 (1862).

10 26 Stat. 282, 283 (1890).

11 31 Stat. 922, 930 (1901).

12 44 Stat. 976, 1002 (1927).

13 46 Stat. 392, 422 (1930).

14 54 Stat. 1234, 1237 (1940).

15 67 Stat. 631, 632 (1953).

16 93 Stat. 668, 695 (1979).

17 102 Stat. 3048, 3120 (1988).

18 21 C.F.R. 5.200.

19 Report of the Subcommittee on Science and Technology for the FDA Science Board. *FDA Science and Mission at Risk*, 2007; Hutt PB. The state of science at the Food and Drug Administration. *Adm Law Rev* 2008;**60**:431.

20 Hutt PB, Hutt PB II. A history of government regulation of adulteration and misbranding of food. *Food Drug Cosmet Law J* 1984;**39**:2.

21 Pliny. *Natural History* 207 (Rackham H, ed. 1949).

22 2 Stat. 806 (1813).

23 3 Stat. 677 (1822).

24 9 Stat. 237 (1848).

25 42 Stat. 858, 989 (1922).

26 32 Stat. 728 (1902).

27 58 Stat. 682, 702 (1944).

28 111 Stat. 2296, 2323 (1997), 42 U.S.C. 262.

29 37 Fed. Reg. 12865 (June 29, 1972).

30 34 Stat. 768 (1906).

31 Note 3 supra.

32 55 Stat. 851 (1941); 59 Stat. 463 (1945); 61 Stat. 11 (1947); 63 Stat. 409 (1949).

33 65 Stat. 648 (1951).

34 76 Stat. 780 (1962).

35 84 Stat. 1236, 1242 (1970), 21 U.S.C. 801.

36 84 Stat. 1670 (1970).

37 16 C.F.R. part 1700.

38 86 Stat. 559 (1972).

39 21 C.F.R. part 207.

40 96 Stat. 2049 (1983).

41 98 Stat. 2815, 2817 (1984); section 526 (a)(2) of the FD&C Act, 21 U.S.C. 360bb(a)(2).

42 98 Stat. 1585 (1984).

43 100 Stat. 3743 (1986).

44 110 Stat. 1321, 1321–313 (1996), as amended, 110 Stat. 1569, 1594 (1996); section 802 of the FD&C Act, 21 U.S.C. 382.

45 102 Stat. 95 (1988).

46 106 Stat. 941 (1992).

47 106 Stat. 149 (1992).

48 106 Stat. 4491 (1992); Kuhlik BN. Industry funding of improvements in the FDA's new drug approval process: the Prescription Drug User Fee Act of 1992. *Food Drug Law J* 1992;**47**:483.

49 111 Stat. 2296, 2298 (1997).

50 116 Stat. 594, 687 (2002).

51 121 Stat. 823, 825 (2007).

52 Note 44 supra; Hutt PB, Kuhlik BN. *Export Expertise: Understanding Export Law for Drugs, Devices and Biologics*, 1998.

53 Note 43 supra.

54 111 Stat. 2296 (1997).

55 114 Stat. 1549A–35 (2000).

56 115 Stat. 1408 (2002).

57 121 Stat. 823, 876 (2007).

58 116 Stat. 594 (2002).

59 *Association of American Physicians and Surgeons, Inc. v. FDA*, 226 F Supp. 2d 204 (D.D.C. 2002).

60 117 Stat. 1936 (2003).

61 121 Stat. 823, 866 (2007).

62 121 Stat. 823 (2007).

63 37 Stat. 822 (1913), 21 U.S.C. 151.

64 82 Stat. 342 (1968), section 512 of the FD&C Act, 21 U.S.C. 360b.

65 102 Stat. 3971 (1988).

66 110 Stat. 3151 (1996).

67 117 Stat. 1361 (2003).

68 118 Stat. 891 (2004).

69 90 Stat. 540 (1976); Hutt PB. A history of government regulation of adulteration and misbranding of medical devices. *Food Drug Cosmet Law J* 1989;**44**:99–117.

70 104 Stat. 4511 (1990); Flannery EJ. The Safe Medical Devices Act of 1990: an overview. *Food Drug Cosmet Law J* 1991;**46**:129.

71 106 Stat. 238 (1992).

72 Title III of 111 Stat. 2296, 2332 (1997).

73 116 Stat. 1588 (2002).

74 118 Stat. 572 (2004).

75 121 Stat. 823, 852 (2007).

76 Hutt PB. A legal framework for future decisions on transferring drugs from prescription to non-prescription status. *Food Drug Cosmet Law J* 1982;**37**:427–40.

77 Note 33 supra.

78 Note 76 supra.

79 For example, 39 Fed. Reg. 19880, 19881 (June 4, 1974).

80 Sections 7 and 8 of the 1906 Act, 34 Stat. 768, 76971 (1906), sections and 502 of the FD&C Act, 21 U.S.C. 351 and 352.

81 37 Fed. Reg. 85 (January 5, 1972); 37 Fed. Reg. 9464 (May 11, 1972), 21 C.F.R. part 330.

82 21 C.F.R. 330.11.

83 47 Fed. Reg. 50442 (November 5, 1982); 21 C.F.R. 211.132.

84 97 Stat. 831 (1983), 18 U.S.C. 1365.

85 62 Fed. Reg. 9024 (February 27, 1997); 64 Fed. Reg. 131254 (March 17, 1999); 21 C.F.R. 201.66.

86 38 Stat. 717 (1914).

87 52 Stat. 111 (1938), 15 U.S.C. 41 *et seq.*

88 36 Fed. Reg. 18539 (September 16, 1971).

89 Note 2 supra at 477–487.

90 52 Stat. 1040–1042 (1938).

91 *USV Pharmaceutical Corp. v. Weinberger*, 412 U.S. 655 (1973).

92 33 Fed. Reg. 7758 (May 28, 1968); 21 C.F.R. 310.100.

93 34 Fed. Reg. 14596 (September 19, 1969); 35 Fed. Reg. 3073 (February 17, 1970); 35 Fed. Reg. 7250 (May 8, 1970); 21 C.F.R. 314.126.

94 *Upjohn v. Finch*, 422 F.2d 944 (6th Cir. 1970); *Pharmaceutical Manufacturers Ass'n v. Richardson*, 318 F Supp. 301 (D. Del. 1970).

95 34 Fed. Reg. 2673 (February 27, 1969); 35 Fed. Reg. 6574 (April 24, 1970).

96 *USV Pharmaceutical Corp. v. Weinberger*, 412 U.S. 655 (1973); *Weinberger v. Bentex Pharmaceuticals, Inc.*, 412 U.S. 645 (1973); *Ciba Corp. v. Weinberger*, 412 U.S. 640 (1973); *Weinberger v. Hynson, Westcott & Dunning, Inc.*, 412 U.S. 609 (1973).

97 *American Public Health Ass'n v. Veneman*, 349 F. Supp. 1311 (D.D.C. 1972).

98 33 Fed. Reg. 7762 (May 28, 1968).

99 Note 95 supra.

100 40 Fed. Reg. 26142 (June 20, 1975).

101 41 Fed. Reg. 41770 (September 23, 1976); FDA, *Compliance Policy Guide* 440.100.

102 *United States v. Generix Drug Corp.*, 460 U.S. 453 (1983).

103 S. Rep. No. 96–321, 95th Cong. 1st Sess. (1979); 125 Cong. Rec. 2244–75 (September 26, 1979).

104 *Burroughs Wellcome Co. v. Schweiker*, 649 F.2d 221 (4th Cir. 1981); *Upjohn Manufacturing Co. v. Schweiker*, 681 F. 2d 480 (6th Cir. 1982).

105 Deficiencies in FDA's Regulation of the Marketing of Unapproved New Drugs: The Case of E-Ferol, H.R. Rep. No. 98–1168, 98th Cong., 2d Sess. (1984).

106 49 Fed. Reg. 38190 (September 27, 1984); FDA, *Compliance Policy Guide* 440.100.

107 50 Fed. Reg. 11478 (March 21, 1985); 51 Fed. Reg. 24476 (July 3, 1986); 21 C.F.R. 310.305.

108 Note 2 supra at 616.

109 Note 42 supra.

110 Note 106 supra.

111 68 Fed. Reg. 60703 (October 23, 2003); 71 Fed. Reg. 33466 (June 9, 2006).

112 Note 42 supra.

113 21 C.F.R. part 312.

114 21 C.F.R. part 58.

115 Section 505(i)(3) of the FD&C Act, 21 U.S.C. 355(i)(3).

116 21 C.F.R. parts 50 and 56.

117 21 C.F.R. 312.32 and 312.33.

118 21 C.F.R. 312.36.

119 21 C.F.R. 312.34 and 312.35.

120 55 Fed. Reg. 20856 (May 21, 1990).

121 DeAngelis C, Drazen JM, Frizelle FA, et al. Clinical trial registration. *JAMA* 2004;**292**:1363–4.

122 42 U.S.C. 282(j).

123 Zarin DA, Tse T. Moving toward transparency of clinical trials. *Science* 2008; **319**:1340–2.

124 21 C.F.R. part 314.

125 Section 505(d) of the FD&C Act, 21 U.S.C. 355(d).

126 Note 48 supra.

127 Note 54 supra.

128 Note 50 supra.

129 Note 62 supra.

130 73 Fed. Reg. 39588 (July 10, 2008).

131 57 Fed. Reg. 13234 (April 15, 1992); 57 Fed. Reg. 58942 (December 11, 1992); 21 C.F.R. part 314, subpart H.

132 Section 506 of the FD&C Act, 21 U.S.C. 356.

133 FDA. *Managing the Risks from Medical Product Use: Creating a Risk Management Framework*, 1999.

134 Institute of Medicine. *To Err is Human: Building a Safer Health System*, 1999.

135 21 C.F.R. 314.50(d)(5)(vi)(b).

136 For example, *Ubiotica Corp. v. FDA*, 427 F.2d 376 (6th Cir. 1970); *Edison Pharmaceutical Co., Inc. v. FDA*, 600 F.2d 831 (D.C. Cir. 1979).

137 80 Stat. 250 (1966), 5 U.S.C. 552.

138 Section 301 (j) of the FD&C Act, 21 U.S.C. 331(j).

139 18 U.S.C. 1905.

140 37 Fed. Reg. 9128 (5 May 1972); 39 Fed. Reg. 44602 (December 24, 1974); 21 C.F.R. part 20.

141 21 C.F.R. 312.130 and 314.430.

142 21 C.F.R. 314.430(e)(2)(i).

143 Section 505(l)(2) of the FD&C Act, 21 U.S.C. 355(l)(2).

144 21 C.F.R. 314.430(f); 130 Cong. Rec. 24977–24978 (September 12, 1984).

145 Section 505(n) of the FD&C Act, 21 U.S.C. 355(n); 21 C.F.R. 14.160.

146 Section 505(s) of the FD&C Act, 21 U.S.C. 355(s).

147 Section 712 of the FD&C Act, 21 U.S.C. 379d-1.

148 Section 505(k) of the FD&C Act, 21 U.S.C. 355(k); 21 C.F.R. 314.80 and 314.81.

149 21 C.F.R. 314.70.

150 Section 505(e) of the FD&C Act, 21 U.S.C. 355(e); 21 C.F.R. 2.5.

151 *Forsham v. Califano*, 442 F. Supp. 203 (D.D.C.1977).

152 111 Stat. 2296, 2325 (1997).

153 Section 735 of the FD&C Act, 21 U.S.C. 379g.

154 Section 505(b)(2) of the FD&C Act, 21 U.S.C. 355(b)(2); 21 C.F.R. 314.50.

155 Section 505(j) of the FD&C Act, 21 U.S.C. 355(j); Flannery EJ, Hutt PB. Balancing competition and patent protection in the drug industry. *Food Drug Cosmet Law J* 1985;**40**:269–309.

156 Section 505A of the FD&C Act, 21 U.S.C. 355a.

157 55 Fed. Reg. 52323 (December 21, 1990); 56 Fed. Reg. 46191 (September 10, 1991); FDA, *Compliance Policy Guide* 120.100.

158 65 Fed. Reg. 81082 (December 22, 2000); 71 Fed. Reg. 3922 (January 24, 2006); 21 C.F.R. 201.56 and .57.

159 73 Fed. Reg. 2848 (January 16, 2008); 73 Fed. Reg. 49603 (August 22, 2008); 21 C.F.R. 314.70(c)(6)(iii).

160 Note 2 *supra* at 511–520.

161 21 C.F.R. part 208.

162 Section 505–1(e)(2) of the FD&C Act, 21 U.S.C. 355-1(e)(2).

163 Section 502(n)(2) of the FD&C Act, 21 U.S.C. 352(n).

164 21 C.F.R. 314.81(b)(3)(i).

165 21 C.F.R. part 202.

166 62 Fed. Reg. 14912 (March 28, 1997).

167 FDA. *Guidance for Industry: Consumer-Directed Broadcast Advertisements*. Draft July 1997 and Final August 1999.

168 Section 503B of the FD&C Act, 21 U.S.C. 353b.

169 Section 505(b)(1)(D) of the FD&C Act, 21 U.S.C. 355 (b)(1)(D); 21 C.F.R. 314.50(d)(1).

170 58 Fed. Reg. 47340 (January 28, 1991); 56 Fed. Reg. 3180 (September 8, 1993).

171 21 C.F.R. parts 210 and 211.

172 Section 505(b)(4)(F) of the FD&C Act, 21 U.S.C. 355(b)(4)(F).

173 FDA. *Pharmaceutical CGMPs for the 21st Century: A Risk-Based Approach,* 2004.

174 For example, *Cedars North Towers Pharmacy, Inc. v. United States*, 1978–80 FDLI Judicial Record 668 (S.D. Fla. 1978).

175 *Thompson v. Western States Medical Center*, 535 U.S. 357 (2002).

176 FDA. *Compliance Policy Guide* Section 460.200.

177 *Medical Center Pharmacy v. Mukasey* (5th Cir. 2008).

178 *American Pharmaceutical Ass'n v. Weinberger*, 377 F. Supp. 824 (D.D.C.1974), affirmed per curiam, 530 F .2d 1054 (D.C. Cir. 1976).

179 Note 131 supra.

180 Section 505-1(f)(3) of the FD&C Act, 21 U.S.C. 355-1(f)(3).

181 Note 2 supra at 563–565.

182 Note 2 supra at 1383–1388.

183 Note 40 supra.

184 21 C.F.R. 316.25(a)(3).

185 Note 41 supra.

186 26 Weekly Compilation of Presidential Documents 1796 (October 9, 1990).

187 37 Fed. Reg. 16503 (August 15, 1972).

188 For example, 21 C.F.R. 312.2(d).

189 62 Fed. Reg. 43900 (August 15, 1997); 63 Fed. Reg. 66632 (December 2, 1998); 21 C.F.R. 314.55.

190 Note 156 supra.

191 Section 551 of the FD&C Act, 21 U.S.C. 360aaa.

192 *Washington Legal Foundation v. Friedman*, 13 F. Supp. 2d 51 (D.D.C. 1998), 36 F. Supp. 2d 16 (D.D.C. 1999), and 56 F. Supp. 2d 81 (D.D.C. 1999).

193 *Washington Legal Foundation v. Henney*, 202 F.3d 331 (D.C. Cir. 2000).

194 *Washington Legal Foundation v. Henney,*128 F. Supp. 2d 11 (D.D.C. 2000).

195 65 Fed. Reg. 14286 (March 16, 2000).

196 73 Fed. Reg. 9342 (February 20, 2008).

197 *United States v. Rutherford*, 442 U.S. 544 (1979); *Rutherford v. United States*, 806 F.2d 1455 (10th Cir. 1986).

198 *Abigail Alliance v. Eschenbach*, 495 F.3d 695 (D.C. Cir. 2007) (en banc).

199 Note 2 supra at 552–566.

200 Hutt PB. Investigation and reports respecting FDA regulation of new drugs: parts I and II. *Clin Pharmacol Ther* 1983;**33**:537–48,674–87.

201 DiMasi JA, Hansen RW, Grabowski HG, Lasagna L. Cost of innovation in the pharmaceutical industry. *J Health Econ* 1991;**10**:107–42.

202 Gilbert J, Henske P, Singh A. Rebuilding big pharma's business model. *In Vivo: Business Med Rep* 2003;**21**:73.

203 Notes 26–28 supra.

204 61 Fed. Reg. 2733 (January 29, 1996); 61 Fed. Reg. 24227 (May 14, 1996).

205 Section 123 of the FDA Modernization Act of 1997, 111 Stat. 2296, 2323 (1997), Section 351(a) of the Public Health Service Act, 42 U.S.C. 262(a).

206 63 Fed. Reg. 40858 (July 31, 1998); 64 Fed. Reg. 56441 (October 20, 1999); 21 C.F.R. 601.2.

207 37 Fed. Reg. 16679 (August 18, 1972); 38 Fed. Reg. 4319 (February 13, 1973); 21 C.F.R. 601.25.

208 Section 704 of the FD&C Act, 21 U.S.C. 374.

209 The non-prescription drug industry traded records inspection for national uniformity under the FDA Modernization Act of 1997, 111 Stat. 2296, 2374, 2375 (1997).

210 Section 304 of the FD&C Act, 21 U.S.C. 334.

211 Section 709 of the FD&C Act, 21 U.S.C. 379a.

212 Section 302 of the FD&C Act, 21 U.S.C. 332.

213 Section 303(a) of the FD&C Act, 21 U.S.C. 333(a).

214 *United States v. Dotterweich*, 320 U.S. 277 (1943); *United States v. Park*, 421 U.S. 658 (1975).

215 Section 305 of the FD&C Act, 21 U.S.C. 335.

216 18 U.S.C. 371.

217 18 U.S.C. 1001.

218 18 U.S.C. 1341.

219 21 U.S.C. 209.

220 21 U.S.C. 1623.

221 Section 303(b) of the FD&C Act, 21 U.S.C. 333(b).

222 Section 303(f) of the FD&C Act, 21 U.S.C. 333(f).

223 *United States v. Parkinson*, 240 F.2d 918 (9th Cir. 1956).

224 *United States v. Universal Management Systems, Inc.*, 191 F. 3d 750 (6th Cir. 1999).

225 Section 518 of the FD&C Act, 21 U.S.C. 360h.

226 For example, *United States v. Superpharm Corp.*, 530 F. Supp. 408 (E.D.N.Y 1981); *United States v. Barr Laboratories, Inc.*, 812 F. Supp. 458 (D.N.J. 1993).

227 21 C.F. R. 7.40.

228 Section 705 of the FD&C Act, 21 U.S.C. 375.

229 *Hoxsey Cancer Clinic v. Folsom*, 155 F. Supp. 376 (D.D.C. 1957); *Ajay Nutrition Foods, Inc. v. FDA*, 378 F. Supp. 210 (D.N.J. 1974), affirmed, 513 F.2d 625 (3rd Cir. 1975).

230 Hutt, Note 19 supra, at 466.

23 The US FDA in the drug development, evaluation and approval process

Richard N. Spivey[1], Judith K. Jones[2], William Wardell[3] and William Vodra[4]

[1] Meda Group, Somerset, New Jersey, USA
[2] Georgetown University, Washington, DC, USA
[3] Wardell Associates International LLC, Ponte Vedra, FL, USA
[4] Arnold & Porter, Washington, DC, USA

23.1 Introduction

23.1.1 Background

The Food and Drug Administration (FDA) is one of the largest and most complex agencies dealing with drug development, evaluation and approval. Separate centres handle drugs and therapeutic biologics, vaccines and blood products, devices and food. At the same time, personnel within the agency are accessible and a wealth of information is readily available to help guide novice and experienced pharmaceutical personnel alike through the process. The FDA has a website (http//:www.fda.gov) which gives ready access to food and drug law, official guidelines and unofficial guidance documents for drugs, biologics, devices and foods. Also, one can find FDA press releases and 'talk papers' on a variety of topics of current interest as well as information concerning the FDA advisory committees. Chapter 21 of the Code of Federal Regulations (21 CFR) contains the official regulations for the FDA. A printed version is available through the US Superintendent of Documents. The Public Health Service Act governs biologics. Regulation of biologics and drug development has been largely harmonised and regulatory responsibilities for drugs and therapeutic biologics has been consolidated within the Centre for Drug Evaluation and Review (CDER) (see section 23.1.2.2).

The FDA, like all drug regulatory agencies worldwide, is in the midst of rapid change in response to the pressures of consumers and health care professionals for more rapid approval of life-saving drugs and from the push for international harmonisation of review and approval procedures. At the same time,

the frequent occurrence of safety problems, some of which reach political proportions, acts as a restraining force on too-rapid change. The FDA Modernization Act (FDAMA) of 1997 represents congressional response to some of these pressures. The FDAMA, until recently, was the most extensive legislative changes made to the Food, Drug and Cosmetic Act (FD&C Act) since the landmark 1962 Kefauver–Harris Amendments, which added the explicit requirement that drugs demonstrate efficacy in addition to being safe. For the most part, however, the FDAMA merely codified current FDA practice rather than making substantial reforms. Specific references will be made to the FDAMA changes in this chapter, plus the recent 2007 Food and Drug Administration Amendments Act (FDAAA), but it is important always to check the implementing regulations.

Of late, there has been increasing pressure on the FDA from a new front. Access to medication from ex-US sources (parallel importing) is being demanded by consumers, and the FDA is being asked to ensure a safe high-quality supply chain. How this issue is resolved could have significant implications on FDA resources, especially for field inspection staff. In addition, there have surfaced many topics that consume FDA resources, ranging from risk management programs for newly marketed products to identifying drug development impediments and offering advice to the industry on ways to expedite development (for the 'Critical Path' Initiative of 2004 see Chapter 24), as well as very recent renewed concerns on how the FDA assures the safety of drugs.

In addition, there continues to be great concern by consumers and Congress about various industry practices: promotional activity, interactions with health care professionals, disclosure of clinical trial information and safety of new and existing products. The FDAAA addresses some of these issues and,

The Textbook of Pharmaceutical Medicine. Edited by
John P. Griffin. © 2009, ISBN: 978-1-4051-8035-1.

importantly, gives the FDA wider enforcement powers than previously existed. More details regarding the FDAAA can be found in Chapters 22 and 24.

23.1.2 Evolution of the FDA's approach to drug effectiveness

23.1.2.1 The 1962 Act and the Drug Effectiveness Study Implementation project

Before 1962, the FDA was legally empowered to evaluate evidence on safety of a proposed new pharmaceutical, but not evidence on effectiveness. However, in practice, the agency did consider efficacy, at least in the case of drugs with major side effects. It reasoned that the decision to approve a drug for marketing had necessarily to involve both safety and efficacy, because the amount of risk allowed had to take into account each drug's efficacy. Nevertheless, this approach was the exception, not the rule, and the agency rarely acknowledged any formal evaluation of effectiveness. By 1962, at least 13,000 new drug applications (NDAs), covering approximately 4000 unique formulations of active ingredients and over 16,000 distinct therapeutic claims, became effective under the 1938 statute.

The 1962 legislation changed this situation in several respects. First, it required affirmative agency approval of the NDA. Under the old law, if the FDA failed to object in the first 60 days after an NDA was submitted, the drug could enter the market. Thus, Congress delayed marketing until the FDA had acted. Secondly, it insisted that a drug be effective for its declared use. Thirdly, the legislation required that effectiveness be proved by adequate and well-controlled investigations, including clinical investigations. Finally, Congress directed the FDA to reassess all drugs that had entered the market under the prior law, to ensure their effectiveness.

This last provision had, in many respects, the most significant impact on the agency and the pharmaceutical industry over the next 15 years. Initially, the agency contracted with the National Academy of Sciences – National Research Council (NAS-NRC) to conduct a review of the marketed products. The NAS-NRC in turn hired teams of physicians, pharmacologists and clinical researchers to perform the actual reviews. At the end of 1968, the NAS-NRC reported back that, for almost 15% of the claims, the products did not work; for another 24%, the claims were supported, but there were superior products treating these conditions; and for another 42%, the evidence supporting efficacy was equivocal. In short, less than 20% of the efficacy claims were found to be supported without qualification. Moreover, the NAS-NRC found a large number of products ineffective as fixed combinations in that there was no substantial reason to believe that each ingredient added to the effectiveness of the combination.

The NAS-NRC report set the FDA and the pharmaceutical industry on a collision course. The agency was under orders from Congress to remove the ineffective products. The industry faced the choice of giving up products (and revenues) or investing in new research for old products. The Drug Effectiveness Study Implementation (DESI) program resulted in protracted litigation and painful disputes between drug companies and the FDA over prescription drugs. In the process, both parties learned much more about the nuances and complexities of 'adequate and well-controlled' clinical investigations in many diverse and previously inadequately studied diseases. The agency promulgated the first regulations defining the elements of such investigations and then, after much litigation, applied them to deny formal hearings to NDA holders in order to complete the DESI effort. Companies, physicians and regulators grappled with how to design and interpret clinical trials in virtually all areas of pharmacotherapy. By the time DESI was over (1984), and partly in response to it, the science of drug development had taken an enormous leap forward. Moreover, academia, industry and the FDA had largely replaced disputes over the drug effectiveness requirement with a common understanding and acceptance of the methods and value of adequate well-controlled studies. In sum, there had been a complete paradigm shift.

The intensity and focus of the DESI program influenced the process of evaluating new NDAs. After 1962, the agency had greatly increased the number of physicians, pharmacologists, toxicologists, statisticians and pharmacists to carry out both DESI and the review of pending NDAs. Many of these technical experts started their careers with scepticism about the merits of manufacturers' claims for drugs (vindicated by the DESI findings) and with an intense course in the meaning of 'adequate and well-controlled' studies needed to carry out the DESI project. The subsequent adverse effects on products in the pipeline gave rise to the drug lag and patient access debates (see below).

Another collateral effect of the DESI project was the development of the abbreviated NDA (ANDA), by which a generic version of the innovator product could satisfy the statutory preconditions for entering the market, without repeating the preclinical and clinical studies of the innovator. This administrative creation, designed to assure that generics were both pharmaceutically equivalent and bioequivalent to the pioneer product, was endorsed by Congress in 1984. As will be seen, this development had a staggering impact on the business model of the pharmaceutical industry.

23.1.2.2 FDA organisation and attitudes toward industry

Implementation of the 1962 amendments, and subsequent challenges, led to a series of organisational changes within the agency. In the 1960s, the FDA was organised along disciplinary lines (e.g. Bureaus of Medicine, Science and Compliance). In 1970, it was reorganised along product lines (e.g. Bureau of Drugs, Bureau of Foods). Within the new Bureau of Drugs, the old separation between 'new' drugs (NDA evaluation) and 'marketed' drugs (evaluation of supplements and safety information) was eliminated by the creation of the Office of New Drugs. In 1972, a departmental reorganisation resulted in the transfer of the Division of Biologic Standards from the National Institutes of Health (NIH) to the FDA, which renamed it the Bureau of Biologics. For a brief period in the 1980s, the Bureau of Drugs was consolidated with that for Biologics into the National Centre for Drugs and Biologics. The marriage failed, and by the late 1980s the agency created the Centre for Drug Evaluation and Research (CDER) and the Centre for Biologics Evaluation and Research (CBER). In 2002, jurisdiction for many therapeutic biologicals was reassigned from CBER to CDER.

Throughout this period, the agency has undergone a series of reorientations regarding its relationship with the regulated industry. In the 1960s and early 1970s, the attitude was frankly adversarial. The drug industry was characterised as unscrupulous seekers of profits. In *Pills, Profits, and Politics*, Philip Lee (Assistant Secretary for Health in the Lyndon Johnson Administration) and Milton Silverman attacked the pharmaceutical industry. Even in the early to mid-1970s, Senators Ted Kennedy (Democrat – MA), Gaylord Nelson (Democrat – WI) and congressman LH Fountain (Democrat – NC) conducted hearings that regularly sought to expose problems with drug safety and alleged misconduct by the pharmaceutical industry or the FDA (or often both). While ignoring the obvious slowdown in new drug approvals, these well-publicised congressional investigations attempted to embarrass the FDA for failing to regulate the industry adequately. Among the outcomes of these investigations were greater agency attentions both to post-approval adverse event monitoring

and to rigorous enforcement of rules to assure the integrity of research data.

By the mid-1970s, however, attitudes within the agency were changing. While some still viewed their role as finding industry errors, a new professional ethic emerged in which the FDA was to judge objectively the evidence presented. By the mid-1980s, the orientation shifted further, in light of the AIDS crisis. The picture changed to one where new drug approval was no longer deemed to be a zero-sum game in which benefit for some was possible only at the expense of harm to others. Drug development was understood to be a process wherein approval could be speeded by efficient and timely review of relevant animal and human data so that every sector could benefit – the sick obviously, but also the medical profession, the FDA and the industry. In the 1990s, the terminology became one of 'stakeholders' in which the agency viewed itself as a neutral party mediating between divergent interests and serving all constituent groups, including industry. This 'customer' focus itself became a target of criticism by those who felt the FDA could not serve both industry and the public at the same time.

23.1.2.3 Investigational new drug

Prior to 1962, the agency had played no part until the NDA was submitted. After learning, however, that pregnant woman were given thalidomide (to prevent morning sickness) without being told what the drug was or that it was experimental, Congress demanded federal oversight and informed consent from all research subjects. The result was the investigational new drug (IND) application, and a new series of FDA regulations governing informed consent, protections of the rights and safety of human subjects and Good Clinical research Practices (GCPs).

In response to demands to accelerate the drug review process, however, the FDA perceived opportunities to use the IND process to improve the chances that the subsequent NDA would answer the essential regulatory questions, or eliminate them by answering these questions before the NDA was submitted. Gradually, the chemistry, manufacturing and controls segments of the IND application moved from merely being adequate to assure the safety and consistency of the investigational product, to being complete and acceptable for NDA purposes. Clinical reviewers provided more guidance on study design, to avoid fundamental flaws that would render the final results scientifically invalid. Pharmacologists and toxicologists urged completion of all preclinical studies early in the IND process, so that issues could be flagged in advance of the NDA filing. Overall, the IND became burdened with regulatory requests that were unnecessary for subject protection but might shorten NDA review times and increase the chances for ultimate drug approval.

23.1.2.4 The drug lag debate and its consequences

By the early 1970s, many observers were questioning the impact and value of FDA review of NDAs for effectiveness. In particular, cardiologists could point to the fact that in a period of almost 5 full years, the FDA had not approved a single new molecular entity (NME) in their field. The pharmaceutical industry was keenly aware of the decline in approvals of NMEs via the NDA process, despite the fact that many new products were available in Europe. William Wardell identified a 'drug lag', showing that the USA had fallen behind other pharmaceutically advanced countries (e.g. the UK) in terms of the number of new drugs approved and the overall capabilities of the therapeutic armamentarium available. Work on the drug lag and the wider issues of pharmaceutical policy in government and industry led in 1974 to the founding of the Centre for the Study of Drug Development (CSDD) by Louis Lasagna and William Wardell at the University of Rochester Medical Centre. The CSDD moved to Tufts University in the 1980s.

A few personal touches emerged to underline the drug lag issue, such as an FDA commissioner taking propranolol for hypertension at a time when it was not approved by the FDA for that purpose. Meanwhile, the more cautious parties cited the dangers of the perceived rapid and less stringent approvals in Europe and the example of practolol, a beta-blocker that was found to cause a severe 'mucocutaneous syndrome' with sclerosis of eyes and internal organs which was severely debilitating and sometimes fatal. Its prodrome, 'itchy eyes', had been noted and discounted in the clinical trials.

Although the charges of drug lag were greeted with hostility from Congress, the FDA and the anti-drug lobby, they were welcomed by the drug industry. In the end, the proponents had tremendous influence over the future of drug regulation in the USA.

Interestingly, the debate went beyond the regulated parties. Economists and libertarians commenced a campaign to let the marketplace determine which drugs were effective. Advocates of laetrile (a purported cancer cure) fought in court for an exception to the effectiveness requirements for drugs intended for per-

sons with terminal illnesses that could not be treated by any approved or recognised methods.

No one was officially declared the winner in the drug lag debate. The FDA, fearing for the survival of the effectiveness requirement, refused to admit that a lag existed, but pledged to eliminate it anyway. At the same time, the agency presented to Congress a legislative proposal that put the efficacy standard on the table, for ratification or repeal. Leaders in both Houses made clear that repeal was out of the question. At about the same time, the Supreme Court rejected the arguments of the laetrile proponents, observing that the effectiveness requirement also protected patients with incurable diseases from quackery. Industry, moving past DESI and getting more and faster approvals of important new products, lost interest in attacking the efficacy provision and focused its attention on two new objectives. First, it sought restoration of patent life for time lost in the development and review process; this law was enacted in 1984. Secondly, it agreed to fund the FDA directly to provide more resources to shorten review times. The Prescription Drug User Fee Act (PDUFA) was enacted in 1992, and renewed in 1997, 2002 and 2007. Under PDUFA, each manufacturer of innovator prescription drugs pays an annual assessment fee based on the number of establishments it operates. In addition, for each original NDA or supplement that requires review of clinical data, the applicant pays a fee. The revenues are earmarked for drug review activities and may not be used by the agency to offset the funding it receives for these activities from the federal treasury.

By the mid-1990s, after two decades of attention, the drug lag had been eliminated; indeed, the pendulum had swung clearly in favour of the FDA. Whether because of the PDUFA resources, the advent of more bureaucracy overseas (e.g. the formation of the European Union's central drug approval authority) or criticism of delays at the agency, today the USA is often the first country to approve new drugs.

23.1.2.5 The patient access debate and its consequences

While the drug lag debate was waning, a new challenge emerged to the FDA standards for drug effectiveness. This time, it was patient advocates who led the charge.

Orphan diseases are those that affect such a small number of patients that the market cannot sustain the cost of research to find treatments. For some time, the agency, the industry and patient support groups had recognised the problem; indeed, the FDA worked with various drug firms to find 'homes' for potentially valuable orphan products. Nevertheless, the economics worked against those with rare diseases.

In 1979, Dr Louis Lasagna wrote a seminal article, 'Who will adopt the therapeutic orphans?' which helped Abby Meyers, the founder of the National Organisation for Rare Disorders (NORD), to obtain enough congressional attention to start the move towards supportive legislation.[1] Beginning in 1983, Congress responded to this situation by enacting (and in 1985 and 1986 strengthening) the Orphan Drug Act. This legislation allowed sponsors to seek FDA designation of pipeline products as 'orphan drugs' for specific indications. Once designated, the sponsors could seek funding grants and could receive tax credits for research costs. Most significantly, if a sponsor was the first to obtain a particular product approved for an orphan indication, no other company could obtain FDA approval of an identical product for the same use for 7 years. This exclusivity incentive proved powerful and as a result many new drugs have reached the market.

In the mid-1980s, the AIDS crisis exploded. Activists behaved in ways no patient advocacy group had ever done, including picketing the agency's offices. Initially, they demanded immediate access to any drug that might help the disease, and they objected to placebo-controlled trials as unethical. Libertarian and politically conservative (including White House) voices were also heard, calling for a broader suspension of the effectiveness standard. In its first response, the agency rushed through the approval of the first diagnostics for HIV and the first therapies for AIDS and related opportunistic infections. It also adopted regulations (just before the 1988 Presidential elections) to expedite the development, evaluation and marketing of new treatments for life-threatening diseases. These so-called Subpart E rules allowed for early consultations between sponsors and the agency on study requirements, treatment protocols, active FDA monitoring of ongoing studies, phase IV studies to delineate additional information after approval and a risk–benefit analysis that explicitly recognised the severity of the disease and the absence of alternative therapies as factors to be considered.

The political pressures to expand early access for patients did not abate. Other policy changes occurred, such as the encouragement of community-based simple studies, and the initiation of fast-track review procedures (giving priority for important new drugs over those offering smaller contributions to patient health). In 1992, the agency adopted another set of regulations to provide for the accelerated approval of new drugs for life-threatening illnesses. These rules, called Subpart H, were similar to the Subpart E policies (which remained in place) but now authorised the FDA to approve drugs based on surrogate endpoints rather than mortality effects, to restrict the distribution of drugs so approved to special settings, to preclearance of advertising copy and to expeditious withdrawal of approval if phase IV trials failed to demonstrate a clinical benefit.

It is important to note that the majority of AIDS activists, after initially opposing controlled investigations, came around to recognise that improvements in HIV therapy could only be identified through such studies.

In 1997, Congress stepped in once again to tinker with the federal FD&C Act. With regard to drug effectiveness, it directed the agency to develop guidelines on those situations in which a single adequate and well-controlled study would be adequate for approval of a new drug or a new indication for an approved product. The FDA issued guidance the following year. To some observers, it offered little meaningful change from past practice.

Thus, by the end of the 20th century, the effectiveness requirement, requiring proof through more than one adequate and well-controlled clinical investigation, remained the standard to which most new drugs were held. Important therapeutic breakthroughs, however, could reach patients earlier or faster through one or more administrative mechanisms created by the agency. As a result of the resources provided by PDUFA, the FDA has become the largest and best-staffed drug regulatory agency in the world, setting standards that influence all other countries.

Criticisms of slowness, rigidity and authoritarianism are still heard from industry, but with less frequency. One can debate whether the decline is because of improvements within the agency, or because industry now contains a large number of employees whose careers depend largely on satisfying the FDA's demands or the reluctance of industry to express concerns publicly. The FDA has become a significant 'sponsor' or 'patron' of many diverse elements within the industry; its laws provide economic benefits to the industry (such as limiting parallel imports and generic competition); it has the power to cripple or destroy individual companies. Thus, for many reasons, regulatory decisions may be less vigorously challenged or resisted by industry today than 40 years ago, at the height of DESI.

In 2003, then-Commissioner Mark McClellan, both a physician and an economist, recognised the high

and increasing cost of drug development and proposed, as part of a strategic plan, that the agency
should consider ways to reduce it. The following year,
the agency announced its 'Critical Path' initiative, to
identify (and, one hopes, ultimately to solve) problems in drug development science that increase costs
and add time to the process. A mutual commitment
on the part of industry and the FDA to boosting
efficiency and output represents a critical opportunity
for drug developers.

23.1.3 Evolution of the FDA's approach to drug safety

In 1938 the concept of drug safety focused on premarket testing and post-approval adulteration. Adverse
events emerging after a drug entered the marketplace
were not really considered part of the FDA's responsibility. When, in the early 1950s, chloramphenicol
was discovered to cause aplastic anaemia, the alarm
was sounded by the American Medical Association
(AMA). The AMA joined with hospital and pharmacy
organisations to create a registry for reporting these
cases, and later, adverse events associated with other
drugs, thus forming the origins of what would ultimately be the FDA's adverse reaction system. The
registry was transferred to the FDA in 1969 after a
further flurry of drug safety concerns in the wake of
the thalidomide tragedy with the placement of new
authority for monitoring drug safety into regulations
in the late 1960s.

The agency developed these specific regulations
for mandatory reporting of adverse events by holders
of NDAs, but not by health care professionals who,
instead, were encouraged to report voluntarily. Also,
uniquely in the world, the agency accepted reports
directly from consumers; although attempts are
made to obtain medical verification of such reports,
this is one feature that has created skepticism over the
value of the FDA adverse events data. This structure
remains in place today. Voluntary reporting for all
drugs tends to spike in the wake of publicity about
safety issues requiring withdrawal of a product [e.g.
phenformin (1977), benoxaprofen and ticrynafen
(1982), nomifensine (1987) and fenfluramine (1997)].

In the USA in the late 1960s and early 1970s, there
was widespread concern over the wide use of illicit
drugs (e.g. marijuana) as well as the new psychoactive
benzodiazepine drugs such as chlordiazepoxide and
diazepam. There also existed widespread concern over
drug interactions and the need for 'drug utilization
review' that had been incorporated into the management of the newer government health insurance

plans for the indigent and elderly (Medicaid and
Medicare), mandated in the mid-1960s. Both of these
activities underlined the lack of information about the
utilization and effects of drugs in the USA. Senator
Ted Kennedy, acting in the wake of these movements
as well as the concerns raised in *Pills, Profits and
Politics*, formed a commission, the National Commission on Prescription Drug Use, in the mid-1970s.

Deliberating for over 2 years, the discussions of
this Commission, chaired by Ken Melmon, MD, professor at the University of California, San Francisco
and later Stanford, and in their 8-volume report
laid some of the groundwork for formalising the
FDA's post-marketing surveillance system, and proposed methods that went beyond spontaneous reports
for formal surveillance of drugs after marketing.[2]
Dating from the time of this Commission, there
was increased regulatory focus on recurring areas of
drug toxicity, ranging from birth defects (allegedly
associated with the anti-emetic drug Bendectin in
1980, and clearly demonstrated for the anti-acne drug
isotretinoin in 1984) to hepatic or renal injury and
blood dyscrasias.

In the early 1990s, with the advent of the discovery
of sudden cardiac death from torsades de pointes
associated with the very widely used antihistamine
terfenadine and the gastrointestinal drug cisapride,
drug safety entered a newer era with the root cause
of such reactions becoming incorporated into pre-
approval decision-making. In the case of these two
drugs, it was found that both drug problems were
usually associated with drug interactions, specifically
at the 3A4 cytochrome p450 metabolising site. Thus,
requirements for premarket testing for these and
analogous interactions that might increase toxicity
gradually became routine parts of the NDA requirements. Secondly, for these drugs and several others
introduced in the 1990s, the discovery of preventable
risks was rapidly followed by labelling changes and
'Dear health care professional' letters, as had been the
agency's routine practice for decades. However, careful studies demonstrated that these warnings had little
or no impact on physicians' prescribing behaviour;
the life-threatening risks brought about by drug
interactions were still occurring. The FDA concluded
that label changes had little or no impact. Thirdly,
an analysis of drug surveillance studies estimated that
adverse events associated with drugs accounted for
approximately 100,000 deaths per year, making this
event a major public health problem, approximating
the burden of major diseases such as chronic obstructive pulmonary disease.

In response, in 1999 the FDA unveiled a new initiative, one identifying and preventing risks from medical products and, in May 2004, the agency produced several specific proposed guidances on risk management, covering premarketing risk assessment, risk management programs and pharmacovigilance programs, as well as a proposal for regulations that represent the most comprehensive overhaul of the adverse event reporting regulations ever undertaken. Although this extensive set of proposed safety regulations has not been finalized, many features of the proposed guidances that are being implemented greatly extend the focus on drug safety from phase I clinical studies right through the commercial life of a product. The FDA now expects detailed collection and analyses of clinical safety data in the NDA, plus comprehensive pharmacovigilance programs that encompass not only passive spontaneous report surveillance but also proactive programs.

The rigor of this examination is most recently reflected in extensive guidelines for the NDA safety review in February 2005. For drugs identified as posing significant risks, the FDA now requires plans in the NDA, originally called risk management action plans [RiskMAPs; now renamed as risk evaluation and mitigation strategy (REMS)] that must go beyond the usual education programs to efforts to modify behaviour of the prescriber, pharmacist and/or patient to optimize utilization of the drug and reduce risk. Further, there is the expectation that these efforts and outcomes are evaluable and measurable. In general, it is anticipated that these programs extend over the life cycle of the drug.

The FDA has also formed a Drug Safety and Risk Management Advisory Committee during this time, provided specific training for the members and has subsequently placed selected members on advisory committee panels to consider various risks or to review existing risk management programs.

The focus on safety has continued to accelerate, driven in part by what many consider as a watershed event in September 2004. The manufacturer of rofecoxib, a COX-2 inhibitor non-steroidal anti-inflammatory drug (NSAID) for arthritis, suspended marketing worldwide because of cardiovascular risks under discussion at an advisory committee. In another case, in August 2004, the agency determined that at least some selective serotonin reuptake inhibitors (SSRIs) for depression may increase the risk of suicide in some patients, particularly children. In both cases, the risks were identified (and only identifiable) through randomised controlled clinical trials, which tradition-

ally have focused only on drug effectiveness. Some experts began suggesting the expanded use of such trials to assess safety. Meanwhile, congressional hearings unearthed scientific dissent within the agency and called for more effective safety monitoring. In February 2005, the agency announced a new Safety Oversight Board, comprising of experts from the FDA, other government agencies and academia, to provide oversight to the drug safety assessment process.

The FDA's approach to drug safety since this time has been the topic of constant scrutiny and study. The Institute of Medicine took on the themes sounded in 1999, and convened panels and published reports on medication errors and on the FDA's drug safety process (in part at the request of the FDA).[3,4] Congress went on to develop and pass major legislation that addressed a number of recommendations, particularly in the latter report. This legislation, a congressional endorsement and rewrite of the FDA's recent policy initiatives, incorporates major requirements for expanded function of safety responsibility, and requires a number of reports to Congress. Further, it authorized considerably more resources for this part of the agency and mandated the establishment of a national Sentinal System to proactively collect data on all FDA-regulated products through various networks of electronic data in the health care system. These activities also have the oversight of at least two relatively independent bodies, the Regan–Udall Commission and the Health Information Technology Board formed by the Department of Health and Human Services to coordinate use of electronic data.

In the wake of all these activities, there is a growing concern that the FDA is becoming more risk-averse, resulting in more requirements for pre-approval safety testing, more delays in drug approvals and more restrictions on post-approval use of drugs. Recent figures on drug approvals show a considerable decline, although not all of the FDA's refusals to approve were related to safety.[5] In fact, any actual demonstration of risk averseness is difficult, in part because many drugs reviewed are being used to extend mortality in patients with life-threatening conditions (e.g. cancer, AIDS) where the benefit–risk balance is clearly unusual.

23.1.4 Phases of drug development

As described in more detail in section 23.2, initiation of clinical testing must be preceded by submission of an IND application to the FDA for review, prior to introduction in humans. Investigations may proceed if a review of the preclinical data provides no basis for the agency to place a clinical hold on testing. Clinical drug development leading to product approval is often described in three phases. In the US regulations phase I is described as the initial introduction into humans. Studies conducted in this phase of development are intended to determine the tolerance (dose range), metabolism and pharmacological actions of the drug in humans and to characterise the adverse experiences associated with increasing doses. Studies in phase I are usually closely monitored and may be conducted in patients as well as healthy subjects, depending on the nature of the drug as well as the type of information being sought. Drug interaction studies are also likely to be conducted.

In phase II studies are conducted to prove the therapeutic concept, and evaluate efficacy and assure that measures of efficacy are adequate. Importantly, dose–response studies are conducted to determine the therapeutically useful dose range and to establish doses to be used in full-scale clinical trials. These studies are closely monitored and well controlled in a small to moderate numbers of patients with the condition of interest. Study results may also give some idea of common dose-related adverse events following short-term therapy.

Phase III studies are usually large and parallel-controlled in design. They provide expanded information concerning the efficacy and safety of the drug in the intended patient population. For the FDA, these studies have traditionally been to provide information on benefit–risk, as well as prescribing information for physicians. Historically, two adequate and well-controlled studies (usually phase III) were required for drug approval, often including the use of placebo. In addition, for chronic use drugs, longer term experience is required (i.e. beyond 6–12 months of treatment). International Conference on Harmonization (ICH) guidelines now describes recommended durations and numbers for chronic testing (see FDA website). For oncology and AIDS drugs, phase II studies have been accepted in support of approval, and in some cases only a single adequate and well-controlled study was considered sufficient. To clarify the requirement for the number of studies, FDAMA specifically stated that a single 'adequate and well-controlled' study is sufficient provided that 'confirmatory evidence' is obtained before or after the trial. Any sponsor considering relying on a single study should discuss the acceptability of the proposed single trial with the FDA early in the development process.

It is important to note that the phases described above are not mutually exclusive and are not necessarily performed in strict linear order. These definitions

have become increasingly blurred with the accelerated development plans seen with drugs for the treatment of serious and life-threatening disorders. It is becoming more important to ask of each study, what will be learned and what the study contributes to proof of either efficacy or safety, or ultimately to the product label. The evidence required for approval increases inexorably year by year. For example, increasing emphasis has been placed on exploring drug use in special populations, such as the elderly, the young and patients with hepatic or renal impairment, and to characterise possible major drug interactions. The most recent major addition has been studies to address cardiovascular safety (e.g. QTc prolongation) which may alone add a cost of one to several million dollars to each development program.

23.1.5 Working with the FDA

The FDA is open to meaningful and productive communication. Meetings can be by tele-conference, video-conference or face to face. The FDA procedure refers to a 'centre [FDA] component', which in most cases will be the FDA division responsible for the IND, and eventually for the NDA [or in the case of biologics, the biologics licence application (BLA)]. The meeting request must be in writing, usually preceded by a telephone call to the consumer safety officer (CSO) or project manager responsible for the drug to discuss the need for the meeting and to make preliminary arrangements. The written request for the meeting should specify the purpose of the meeting, a list of specific objectives that the sponsor has for the meeting, a proposed agenda, a list of sponsor attendees, a request for FDA attendees and the timing of submission of a background document for the meeting.[6]

The director of the FDA component, usually the division director, will determine whether the meeting is appropriate. Normally, the background document must be sent to the FDA at least 4 weeks prior to the meeting. Once the division director has agreed to a meeting, the reviewing division has 14 days to set a date with the sponsor (the earliest date when FDA participants can be available) within 30–75 days, depending on the type of meeting.

The FDA is usually quite accommodating about meetings, but meetings should not be requested frivolously or prematurely. In preparing for an FDA meeting the sponsor should prepare and submit an agenda and background document to the FDA reviewing division. This should not be too lengthy, and large documents should be submitted as appendices to the background document. The sponsor should submit specific questions for the FDA to address. Any presentation should conform to the written material submitted and should be succinct and focused. It is rare to obtain more than 1 hour and time must be allotted for dialogue. Rehearsal is important to avoid unclear presentations and to focus clearly on key questions and meeting objectives. Because the agency usually has an internal meeting to discuss the questions prior to the meeting with a sponsor, at the sponsor meeting the agency often decides to dispense with the formal presentation and go straight to the sponsor's questions and discussion. When the FDA requests that presentations be omitted, the sponsor should follow the agency's lead and listen and respond to the comments. If, during the discussion, there are areas that require clarification, there may be parts of the planned presentation that can be used. The timing of the meeting may have some importance in terms of confidentiality; for example, there are regulations protecting the confidentiality of an existing IND, but they may not apply to a meeting held before an IND has been submitted.

It is very important for the sponsor and the FDA to keep complete and accurate minutes of official meetings, and in some cases these are taken at the meeting with both parties agreeing to the wording. Often, the FDA provides draft responses to questions posed by the sponsor prior to or at the time of the actual meeting. This greatly facilitates communication of issues and possible pathways to address data requirements. The FDA procedure for meetings outlines distribution within the agency. The minutes of the meeting should be exchanged between agency and sponsor to minimise misunderstandings. These minutes provide a record of agreements reached and they may be very important as development proceeds and at the time of NDA submission. Sponsors may request assessment of specific protocols [special protocol assessments (SPA)] to determine if they are adequate to meet scientific and regulatory requirements:

1. Animal carcinogenicity protocols;
2. Final product stability protocols; and
3. Clinical protocols for phase III trials.

These assessments, if agreed to by sponsor and the FDA, are produced in writing.[7]

23.2 The investigational new drug application

23.2.1 General considerations

An IND is required before clinical testing of a new drug can begin in the USA. The information require-

ments for the IND are found in chapter 21, part 312 of the Code of Federal Regulations (21 CFR 312). The purpose of the IND is to provide a scientific rationale for studying the drug in humans and sufficient information from preclinical studies to warrant the risk of exposure in humans. Although the information to be submitted is specified in the regulations, there is flexibility as to the amount and type of information needed, based on the design of the first trials to be performed under the IND. For example, if all that is needed initially is to test the bioavailability of a drug in humans, the requirements for data may be less than for a more extensive phase I programme. Although there are exceptions, the FDA generally requires a separate IND for each dosage form and research target (e.g. heart failure and asthma). Cross-referencing to information contained in an existing IND is permitted and reduces the need for duplicate paperwork.

The FDA has clarified the minimum requirements for an IND submission in three areas: chemistry, toxicology reports (draft) and size (2–3 volumes, each 3 inches thick) in an attempt to relax current practices somewhat, to the level required for a UK clinical trial exemption (CTX). However, full reports are to be provided within a short time after the initial drafts.[8] Conversely, information needed to conduct human studies in the European Union has increased recently, with the implementation of the Clinical Trial Directive.

An individual (rather than an industrial sponsor) may also submit an IND for the purpose of conducting clinical investigations. Such an individual is referred to as an investigator-sponsor. If the investigator plans to study a drug already subject to an IND held by an industrial or other sponsor, he or she can request that the sponsor allow them to cross-reference the existing IND. A letter from the IND sponsor allowing cross-referencing by the investigator-sponsor is usually all that is needed. These situations usually occur when an investigator wishes to pursue a research target not of interest to the industrial sponsor. The request for cross-referencing may be denied if the planned investigation is felt not to be consonant with the development of the drug. An investigator-sponsor may, however, proceed if he or she supplies information independent of the industrial sponsor to support the investigator-sponsor application and thus meet FDA data requirements. This is usually beyond the individual capabilities of the investigator-sponsor, especially for drugs not yet approved for any indication.

The question of the benefits and risks of investigator-sponsored INDs is often raised by small pharmaceutical companies, who are attracted to the independence, and often the lower initial cost, that this entails. Investigators are responsible for all the administrative support of their own INDs and maintain responsibility for meeting all IND reporting and performance obligations. Usually, the initial costs are indeed less to the small company, as the investigator is often willing to handle the IND requirement because he or she may have independent funding for the conduct of the study. The risk to the company is the lack of control over the study (and the drug) that this independence entails. The investigator may not perform the study to the standards needed, or may fail to report safety data in an appropriate and timely manner. Any of these failures could raise issues for the development of the drug and could have an adverse impact on the drug, the programme and the company.

Similar issues of control and development priorities are raised when studies are conducted under the auspices of any organisation not contractually bound to the company. Examples include NIH entities such as the National Cancer Institute or any of the cancer cooperative study groups, or the AIDS Cooperative Trials Group. The company is at the mercy of the priorities, sense of urgency, objectives, standard operating procedures, auditing standards, case report forms, coding dictionaries and databases of these groups when the latter are the sponsors independent of the company. At the same time, these groups may well be the most cost-efficient and expeditious way of developing a new drug, and they may control access to specialised resources (e.g. specialised clinical laboratories). These factors (in addition to ownership issues) must be carefully weighed before a decision is taken to rely on any outside sponsorship for drug development.

23.2.2 IND submission and review

An IND is submitted to the appropriate reviewing division within CDER (see 21 CFR 312.23 for IND content and format). If there is uncertainty as to the appropriate reviewing divisions, one should check with the division considered most likely and obtain guidance. For both drugs and biologics, one may also consult the office of the deputy director. Once an IND is submitted the reviewing division will acknowledge receipt, and the date of receipt becomes the official date for review purposes. Once an IND is submitted, the FDA reviewing division has 30 days from the official submission date in the acknowledgment letter in which to evaluate the information contained in the IND and to decide whether the information supports proceeding with the initial human study protocol. There is no official 'approval' of an IND; rather, it is 'allowed'.

If the FDA raises no 'hold' issues during the 30-day evaluation period, the sponsor is free to proceed. However, it is generally good practice to contact the agency prior to study initiation to confirm that there are no concerns related to starting the planned study.

The FDA may respond to the IND with questions and concerns in writing. These may be requests for clarification or issues that need to be addressed during the drug development process. If the FDA feels that the planned study poses a significant safety risk to human subjects they may inform the sponsor that the study cannot proceed. This act is referred to as placing a 'clinical hold' on the IND. A clinical hold may be complete or partial. In the latter case, the FDA may place a hold on certain aspects of the planned development while permitting the sponsor to proceed with other aspects. For example, the planned study may be a dose-escalation trial and the FDA may only permit a single dose level based on the information provided in the IND. The FDAMA has codified FDA obligations to a sponsor whose IND is placed on clinical hold (Section 117). The FDA is obliged to explain its concern and make clear to the sponsor what is needed to respond. Guidance documents adopted before the legislative changes require the reviewing division to communicate its concerns by telephone and with a written communication within 5 working days. The sponsor then responds and the FDA must reply within 30 days as to the adequacy of the response.[9] If the hold is not lifted, formal appeal to the office level may be needed to resolve differences of opinion.

23.2.3 IND meetings (see 21 CFR 312.47)

23.2.3.1 Early IND meetings

One of the decisions that a sponsor should make regarding the time immediately before or after filing an IND is whether to request a meeting with FDA to discuss the submission. The FDA has become more receptive in recent years to offering early advice and counsel. As a result, meetings during early development are much more common than they were a decade ago. Reasons for requesting a meeting in the early phases of an IND are varied. The sponsor may have concerns regarding some element of the IND; for example, they may wish to have as a first study relatively long exposure, and there may be problems with the adequacy of the animal toxicological data to support the exposure planned. The sponsor may wish to introduce the FDA to what they feel is a very interesting and promising development project. Another reason for requesting a meeting might be to determine whether the early development programme is adequate to achieve the stated objectives. If the latter is the primary purpose of the meeting, it is highly recommended that the sponsor present a plan to the FDA for comment and discussion, rather than asking the agency how to proceed. This latter approach can lead to less productive dialogue and perhaps a less than focused or less commercially feasible development programme.

23.2.3.2 End of phase II meeting

For most drugs, one of the most important meetings with the FDA in the new drug development process is the end of phase II meeting. This was initially directed at drugs of specific interest because of either medical need or possible toxicity. This meeting is now standard at the FDA for development planning. Its purpose is to present to the FDA the results of studies conducted during phases I and II to gain the agency's concurrence that it is safe and reasonable to proceed to phase III. More importantly, assuming there is concurrence to proceed, the meeting serves to review plans for phase III development. Under the FDAMA, written agreements on the adequacy of design of the key efficacy trials can be obtained (Section 119). Because phase III can be very expensive for the sponsor and critical to the ultimate approval of the drug, it is vital to obtain FDA commitment at this juncture.

The timing of the end of phase II meeting is important. The meeting should be scheduled when sufficient information from earlier phases of development is available, yet early enough to permit planning and preparation for phase III. The information available must be in a condition to permit adequate summary and analysis. The background package of information presented to the FDA is critical to achieving the objectives of the meeting. At this stage, one should have ready a 'target package insert' with clearly stated desired claims and careful annotation showing the existing or planned studies that are intended to support these claims. This is pivotal for obtaining detailed advice and opinion from the agency. A clinical development plan has little meaning unless related to the precise language of a package insert 'Indications' section. Also, if any specific safety statements are desired or anticipated these should be highlighted and the data supporting them referenced in the background material. This meeting needs intense preparation. In order to achieve the objectives in the limited time available, any presentations must be concise and focused. If the FDA has reviewed the background material the agency may wish to omit the sponsor's presentations, but the sponsor must still be prepared.

After the meeting, at the sponsor's discretion, an SPA request may be submitted to the FDA for review and agreement.

Another important aspect is that the FDA is required to 'provide its best judgement, at that time, of the paediatric studies required for the drug product and whether their submission will be deferred until after approval' [21 CFR 312.47(b)(v)]. This is crucial to understand early, and to be able to develop an appropriate program. Minutes of the meeting are developed and provided by the FDA to the sponsor.

23.2.3.3 IND amendments

The IND evolves with the development programme. It is amended with each new protocol and with each meaningful change in an existing protocol. It is particularly important to remember to amend a protocol when there is a change in design or in the scope of the study. The sponsor may begin a new study or implement a change in protocol when the protocol or protocol amendment has been submitted to the FDA for review and approval obtained from the institutional review board responsible for the study.

There are also information amendments submitted to the IND that incorporate new information concerning the drug under study. Examples include new toxicology data or new information concerning chemistry, manufacturing or controls of the drug. These amendments are essential to support new clinical protocols or amendments. There are proposals currently being discussed to determine the feasibility and desirability of submitting the original IND and subsequent amendments electronically. If this is done well, the body of information can be more accessible to the FDA reviewers and lead to a more comprehensive knowledge base in anticipation of a future NDA submission. This concept has been referred to as a 'cumulative' IND.

The IND safety report is another important type of IND amendment. Any serious unexpected adverse experience associated with the use of the drug occurring in clinical trials or in animal studies must be submitted to FDA; the regulations define 'serious' and 'unexpected' (21 CFR 312.32). 'Associated with' is somewhat more subjectively defined as an event for 'which there is a reasonable possibility that the event might have been caused by the drug'. The sponsor must report to the FDA and notify all participating investigators in writing within 15 calendar days following the initial receipt of the report. It does not matter whether or not the source of the event was a study conducted under the IND for it to be reportable. If the safety report concerns a fatal or life-threatening event of the type described, the FDA is to be notified by telephone within 7 calendar days. This is to be followed by the written report within 15 calendar days of the initial receipt of the report. It is critical that the regulations concerning IND safety reports be reviewed in detail as there are several nuances of interpretation, and strict compliance is essential.

23.2.3.4 IND annual reports

Within 60 days of the anniversary date on which the IND went into effect, the sponsor must submit an annual report. Regulations (21 CFR 312.33) outline the requirements for this report. It should include a brief summary of the status of each study completed or in progress. If a study is complete, a brief description of the findings should be presented, and if in progress any interim results available should be summarised. A summary of all IND safety reports submitted during the year must be included, along with tabulations of the most frequent and serious adverse experiences observed. Listings of all patients who died or who discontinued from the study because of adverse events (regardless of causality) must also be included. All preclinical studies completed or in progress during the year should be listed and any new findings summarised. New manufacturing information should also be presented. There is flexibility in the format of the report but it is important to submit it in a timely manner. Extensions may be granted upon request to the agency.

23.2.3.5 IND issues for drugs that treat serious or life-threatening conditions

The FDAMA widened and codified 'fast-track' procedures that had previously been addressed in part by 21 CFR 312 Subpart E, for drugs intended to treat 'life-threatening and severely debilitating illnesses'. The act refers to drugs 'intended for the treatment of a serious or life-threatening condition and it demonstrates the potential to address unmet medical needs for such a condition' (Section 112). Sponsors apply for 'fast-track' status and, if this is granted, receive expedited review of the application based on clinical or surrogate measures 'reasonably likely to predict clinical benefit'. The FDAMA also codifies the process of a 'rolling review', whereby an incomplete application can be reviewed, while results from ongoing studies are added as the review progresses. Both the FDAMA and existing Subpart E regulations place several conditions and limitations on drugs approved under 'fast track'. These include commitments to carry out

definitive studies post-approval, pre-clearance of promotional material by FDA and a procedure for accelerated withdrawal of the drug from the market in cases where clinical benefit is not confirmed. Because development is accelerated under this procedure, sponsor and agency interactions are more frequent and intense than for other applications. For example, the enhanced interactions allow for an end of phase I meeting, where guidance might be offered that would allow an adequate and well-controlled phase II study or studies to be used as the basis of approval.

Another set of regulations (21 CFR 312.34) governs the availability of a treatment IND or protocol. A treatment IND or protocol allows a drug to be made available to patients not otherwise eligible to participate in clinical studies that are part of the drug development programme. A treatment protocol may be filed when the drug provides a possible treatment for a serious or life-threatening disorder where no alternative therapy is available. A treatment protocol may be filed during phase III, or when all clinical studies have been completed. When the drug is clearly valuable, a treatment IND can be filed as early as phase II. The regulations spell out the information that must be provided when submitting a treatment protocol. The FDA must determine that there is sufficient information to suggest that the drug may offer the prospect of efficacy and that the risks for use are acceptable. The sponsor must also give assurances that they are continuing the development of a drug with due diligence. The sponsor should be aware that there is a risk that making the drug available under a treatment protocol may reduce the ability of the sponsor to recruit patients into the controlled trials, thereby delaying ultimate approval of the NDA.

23.3 The new drug application (NDA or BLA)

23.3.1 General considerations

The NDA is an organised presentation of all the information collected during the drug development process assembled into a format allowing FDA review. Despite the voluminous nature of a full NDA, the essence of the product is captured in the proposed labelling. The labelling essentially summarizes important aspects of the development program. More importantly, the labelling provides information about the product and how to use it, what patient population might benefit from treatment and what important considerations should drive the safe use of the product. The FDA focuses on the intended use of the product, and their review is always considered in that context.

The regulations governing the NDA are found in 21 CFR 314. In addition, the FDA has issued detailed guidelines on the content and format of the NDA, which can be accessed on the FDA website. It is important to note, however, that the reviewing division may have specific format or organisational needs for the data to ensure speedy review (see pre-NDA meeting). Commonly, case report forms and data tabulations have been submitted in electronic portable document file (PDF) format, greatly reducing the volume of paper that needs to be submitted to the FDA. It is now possible – and soon to be mandatory – that NDAs be submitted entirely in electronic form. Several guidelines have been issued which outline the requirements for such submissions, including the need for electronic signatures.

Recently, the FDA has promulgated specific proposed guidances on the structure and activities for pre-marketing risk assessment, and final guidances have been issued.[10] This guidance is in the context of an overall initiative by the FDA to promote 'risk management' planning as part of the NDA process. (There are two additional companion guidances on RiskMAPs and pharmacovigilance which relate more to post-marketing activities). The expectation implicit in these proposed guidances and other actions by the FDA is that each NDA may need to consider whether a RiskMAP is needed for a particular risk. It is also implied that if this is the case, the NDA should include descriptions of this plan and how it will be evaluated, which may include pre-market testing of the RiskMAP as part of the NDA clinical trials. This testing may include evaluation of communications or other interventions to be used in the post-marketing period.

The NDA is a 'layered' document. There are summary documents, individual study reports and actual data tabulations. It differs in two main ways from the dossier submitted in the European Union:

1. In the amount of raw data contained in the NDA submission; and

2. In the presence of expert reports in the European dossier, compared with well-defined integrated summaries in the NDA.

This resulted from historical, cultural and structural differences between US and European regulatory bodies. In general, Europeans have relied more heavily on outside experts to review applications. The ICH Conferences have made considerable progress in harmonising the content of many sections of the US NDA and the EU dossier. The ICH has now agreed on the common technical document (CTD) that will, as the name implies, be a common approach to dossiers in the three participating regions of the world: the USA, the European Union and Japan. In addition, work has begun on elaborating the requirements for the electronic version, the eCTD. If companies are interested in submitting via eCTD, they must contact the FDA well in advance in order to make sure that submissions will meet the requirements and that appropriate testing of the eCTD system can occur.

23.3.2 The pre-NDA meeting

As preparations for the submission of an NDA begin, there needs to be a pre-NDA meeting with the FDA reviewing division. This meeting focuses on format, not content, and is important to eliminate delays that can occur when an NDA does not meet the specific needs of the assigned reviewers at the FDA (21 CFR 312.47). The sponsor should provide to the FDA an idea of the types and volume of information to be submitted, as well as the plan for data summary, presentation and analysis. The FDA should provide to the sponsor any specific requests for the display and analysis of data. Electronic formats and requests have become more routine, and a good understanding of what is planned and needed can help improve efficiency and minimise later difficulties.

23.3.3 NDA submission

The sponsor submits the NDA along with an appropriate application fee (currently in the range of $1.3 million), and the FDA reviews the application for completeness, that is to determine whether all parts of the NDA are present, in particular the information critical for their review. If the NDA is complete enough for review it is 'filed' (accepted) by the FDA. The agency has 60 days in which to perform this 'completeness' review, and communicates the status of the review in a '74-day' letter (i.e. 2 weeks after the 60-day period expires). The completeness review is important under user fee legislation, as the review clock starts with the FDA's receipt of an NDA for review. If the FDA finds that some critical information is missing, the agency will notify the sponsor that the NDA is not filed (i.e. not complete). In that case the agency must state the nature of the deficiency so the sponsor can resubmit with the needed information. The sponsor forfeits half of the application fee if the NDA is not accepted for filing. For drugs reviewed under fast-track procedures, an incomplete NDA can be filed for review and additional data submitted during the review process (the 'rolling review' referred to earlier).

The official filing date is 60 days after receipt of the submission, if no significant deficiencies in the application have been found. The PDUFA set specific performance targets for the agency and in general sponsors can anticipate a complete review within 10 months of submission. In the past, FDA review times were highly variable, but performance has improved considerably since the passage of this Act. There is a 'sunset' clause in the PDUFA that requires reapproval every 5 years. It was last renewed in 2007.

23.3.4 NDA classification

The PDUFA provides for the classification of NDA submissions as being subject to either standard or priority review. Priority applications are targeted for, and tracked to, an action at 6 months. The standard applications are targeted for action at 10 months. The sponsor may request the priority review status to be applied. This request is usually contained in the covering letter, along with the rationale for the request. Although there are general guidelines that address the basis for ascribing priority review status, decisions are not always clear-cut and arguments provided by the sponsor may help guide the agency. Nevertheless, the FDA considers for priority review classification a drug product that would be a significant improvement compared to marketed products, demonstrated by:

1. Evidence of increased effectiveness in treatment, prevention or diagnosis of disease;
2. Elimination or substantial reduction of a treatment-limiting drug reaction;
3. Documented enhancement of patient compliance; or
4. Evidence of safety and effectiveness in a new subpopulation.[11]

23.3.5 Monitoring the review of the NDA

Once the NDA has been filed, the sponsor should monitor the progress of the NDA review in order to detect problems or concerns at the earliest possible moment. This monitoring or tracking must be carried out with great sensitivity. If contacts are too frequent or poorly timed they can quickly become an annoyance, which can hamper further communications. The FDA project manager is the usual point of contact. If there is difficulty with a particular review, then the reviewer should be contacted (with consideration, obviously, for the reviewer's time), but the project manger should always be informed of any such contacts.

One must consider the reviewer's style and preferred method of communication. Most reviewers prefer requests to go through the project manager. One reviewer might be very responsive to e-mail, whereas another might prefer a telephone call. The contacts during an NDA review can be numerous – the exact number will vary with the application and the reviewing division. The purpose of contacts should not only be to track or monitor, but whenever possible to assist the reviewer in resolving quickly minor issues which can sometimes cause the reviewer to slow or even halt a review.

All substantial requests, whether received informally or through official notification, must be addressed as promptly and completely as possible. An attempt to gloss over an issue usually leads to further delay. Issues raised by the reviewer represent significant concerns and should be treated as such. The amount and type of any new information needed to answer a request must be carefully considered. Under user fee guidelines, the FDA likes to keep the review moving without the need to review large amounts of new data which, if too large, may cause the FDA to 'reset the clock' (i.e. extend the review time-frame). The effect of such a submission on the review should be discussed with the agency and balanced against the need for the information.

Some new drug applications may contain particularly innovative or controversial approaches to therapeutic interventions. In some cases, the FDA seeks advice from an external panel of experts, deemed an advisory committee (21 CFR 14). Individual participants on these panels must be recognized for their particular expertise and satisfy various conditions, including an evaluation as to any conflict of interest. These panels provide advisory input to FDA questions and issues; however, the actual final decision remains with the FDA.[12]

23.3.6 FDA actions

Until quite recently the actions of the FDA concerning an NDA were expressed in an approval letter, an approvable letter or a non-approval letter. In the case of a non-approval letter, the deficiencies were noted that were felt by the agency to require substantial action by the sponsor because a positive action by the agency in the present review cycle was not possible. Where the issues could be solved promptly by the sponsor, a non-approval letter was not necessarily a bad result because it officially clarified the remaining issues.

An approvable letter usually stated some minor area of concern that needed to be resolved prior to final approval. The letter usually stated that if these concerns were resolved approval would be granted shortly.

In contrast, an approval letter meant that the submitted information justified approval. The only action usually requested for this type of letter was the submission of final printed labelling and advertising. In some cases, an approval letter could spell out other conditions for approval, such as post-approval studies, or restrictions on distribution or promotion. These conditions were generally discussed with the sponsor and agreed to prior to issuance of the letter.

The FDA has now implemented a two-tier approach to action letters: approval and complete response. The latter replaces non-approval and approvable letters with a letter that lists all the deficiencies the sponsor will need to correct to obtain approval. If deficiencies are substantial, the letter will read more like the old non-approval letter; if the deficiencies are minor, the letter would read more like an approvable letter.

The sponsor will usually be made aware of the deficiencies prior to the action letter, and this allows a more rapid response. If post-approval studies are to be performed as a condition of approval, the agency now has clear authority to require the sponsor to report on those studies under Section 130 of the FDAMA. Under the previous law, the FDA's authority in this regard was never clear, and post-approval studies had been conducted under a 'gentleman's agreement' without a firm legal basis.

23.3.7 Post-approval reporting

Following the approval of an NDA, the sponsor has ongoing reporting responsibilities. The most important of these is the monitoring of clinical safety once the drug is on the market, to ensure that the product's benefits outweigh any risks identified when it is introduced to larger, more diverse populations. Clinical safety regulations for drugs are found at 21 CFR 314.80, and for biologics at 21 CFR 600.80 and basically require that all reports of safety concerns, whether or not thought to be causally associated with the product, received by the sponsor are captured and reported to the FDA. These regulations describe specific and rigidly enforced requirements, regarding the timing of submissions of individual spontaneous reports of suspected adverse events, determined by the type of report (e.g. serious and unlabelled events are reported in 15 calendar days, whereas most other events are submitted in periodic reports). The information required is described on a standard form (3500A), which closely corresponds to the international Council

for International Organizations of Medical Sciences form for event reporting which is accepted in most countries.

In the past decade, there has been increased emphasis on drug safety, and more public visibility of safety problems. The volume of reports now approaches 500,000 spontaneous reports per year, and the FDA has just initiated its public reports of suspect adverse events that are currently under examination. These are highlighted in the medical press and also in the general media. In 2003, the FDA released extensive proposed new regulations for post-approval reporting, in part to harmonise requirements with ICH recommendations for periodic safety update reports in use in many other countries, and use of standardised terminology (MedDRA) and standards for electronic reporting of adverse events. These proposed regulations also include broader definitions for reporting serious events, as well as actual and potential medication errors. As of this time of writing these proposed regulations have not been finalized, but their publication served to alert the regulated industry to possible forthcoming final regulations. Most needed, and likely to emerge in the final new regulations, are activities that relate to harmonization in terminology (MedDRA, already used by the FDA) and periodic reporting requirements.

In parallel, the FDA has focused much more intently on safety, in both NDA reviews and in the post-marketing period. This has been prompted by the need to withdraw a number of products, such as cisapride, phenylpropanolamine, terfenadine, troglitazone, cerivastatin and rofecoxib. Also, there is increased scrutiny of products associated with particular adverse events, such as cardiac arrhythmias (torsades de pointes) and hepatic necrosis, because many of the safety problems have involved these particular events. In the case of many of these drugs, initial attempts to improve the safe use of the products through additions to the product label (e.g. bolded warnings, black boxes) were found not to be heeded either by prescribers or by the pharmacies dispensing the products.

In part because of this lack of impact, the agency generally concluded that label changes are insufficient for preventing significant risks. Further concern was raised by the publication, in the *Journal of the American Medical Association*, of a combined analysis of several studies of adverse effects resulting in or occurring in hospital.[13] This study concluded that adverse events were a major health problem (approximately the fifth most common cause of morbidity), and the topic was rapidly reviewed by both the Institute of Medicine and the FDA, who published a lengthy monograph on the importance of drug safety and set about to define guidances to address this. The result has been a growing emphasis on the concept of 'risk management' of a product.

This risk management concept evolved, after open hearings in 2004 and feedback, into the concept of RiskMAPs, described in FDA's Final Guidance released in May 2004.[14] The Risk Management Guidance identified the need to:

1. Identify potential risks in the indication population;
2. Determine which tools (information as in labels, active interventions such as patient consent or restricted distribution) can be best applied to prevent them;
3. Develop methods to determine whether the interventions are effective or need to be further optimised; and
4. Describe methods to evaluate the effectiveness of the interventions.

Several risk management efforts are already in place (e.g. thalidomide, alosetron, isotretinoin, and more recently, natalizumab) and are regularly being evaluated by the FDA, as the guidances are starting to be implemented on a broader scale. These may involve formation of registries of all or some exposed patients, with follow-up after exposure to the drug.

With finalization of the guidances, there is a general trend for sponsors to develop at least some general plans for RiskMAPs as part of the NDA. Very recently, the concept of RiskMAPs has evolved into the concept of REMS which in part reflect the recently passed FDAAA legislation (see Chapter 24).

In addition to the required reporting of spontaneously reported and literature-based adverse events, there is a requirement for an NDA annual report that contains other information relevant to the NDA. Again, the requirements are detailed in 21 CFR 314. Annual reports must contain a brief summary of new information that might bear on the safety, efficacy or labelling of the drug. This summary should also include any regulatory actions taken or planned (anywhere in the world) as a result of the new information. The report also contains product distribution data (domestic and international), current labelling with any changes highlighted, as well as new information from preclinical and clinical studies. Updates are also needed for any ongoing studies.

Sponsors are required to submit copies of promotional materials (e.g. journal advertisements, detail pieces such as file cards) to the FDA at the time of initial dissemination. This means that the sponsor is to submit them to the FDA simultaneously with the use of that piece or program. It is also possible for companies to engage the FDA in review of proposed programs or advertisements, in order to gain feedback on acceptability. This is particularly important for broadcast advertisements aimed at consumers, such as those viewed on television. If promotional materials are deemed to be violative by the FDA (e.g. if they are false and misleading), a sponsor must withdraw the advertisements and in some cases undertake new campaigns to correct the objectionable statements.

The NDA is a living document for as long as a drug is marketed. It is also a 'contract' that cannot be modified without notice to (and in most cases approval by) the FDA of changes in its terms through the submission of a 'supplement' to the NDA. For example, supplements must be approved for labelling modifications such as new indications, patient populations, dosing instructions or cautionary advice. Similarly, most changes in the chemistry, manufacturing and controls provisions must be approved in advance of implementation, although some can be implemented at the time of notification to the FDA (and subject to FDA disapproval); other, minor changes need only be reported in the annual report to the NDA.

The maintenance of an NDA is nearly as important as the approval, because any neglect in this activity can place the product in jeopardy.

23.3.8 Post-approval labelling changes and REMSA

23.3.8.1 FDA's control of labelling after approval

The labelling of a new drug usually needs to evolve during its life on the market. The primary changes that occur in the labelling relate to new indications, new dose forms and augmented safety information.

23.3.8.2 Prior approval of new indications and/or new dose forms

Typically, clinical trials for additional indications for a drug will be ongoing or planned at the time of NDA approval. For example, it is common for companies to be evaluating their product for use in selected paediatric or other special populations at the time of NDA approval. It is also common to evaluate the product for related conditions not specifically tested in the original NDA clinical trials; thus, an antidepressant may be further evaluated in clinical trials for panic disorder. When adequate clinical trial information on the new indication (or dose form) is assembled and sufficient to warrant an efficacy and safety review, the sponsor will assemble a supplement to the NDA (SNDA). This dossier will be carefully reviewed, as for an NDA, including in particular the proposed labelling; this will need to be updated to reflect the new indication and probably the new population indicated to take the drug. In addition, the change may require new information in the adverse effects and dosing sections. Any supplemental submission relying on new clinical data is subject to a user fee (half of a full NDA fee, or approximately $650,000).

23.3.8.3 Power to order new safety disclosures

A second and equally common activity that results in changes to the label relates to new safety findings. Because a typical NDA only evaluates a drug in 3000–10,000 individuals, it is not surprising that new rarer effects will be seen when a drug is used in the broader population. In part this relates to use in populations not normally tested in clinical trials (e.g. pregnant women, children, frail elderly and those on many medications for several chronic diseases) where there may be special safety risks. In the USA, with its large population, these risks are often identified in the first 1–2 years of marketing through spontaneous reports and are incorporated into the label.

Occasionally, a newly introduced drug will be associated with a new adverse event that might be related to the product, or to another drug also commonly used in the indication population. This may require further research into the possibilities, and usually also a label change. Because events of special concern, such as serious liver events, are often not detected early, reports of these events associated with the drug will be carefully evaluated, and may be judged to warrant a special label warning, or 'black box' to warn physicians of this rare but life-threatening condition.

Congress heard concerns about the FDA's authority to order changes in labelling over the objections of the drug sponsor, and responded in the FDAAA by explicitly empowering the FDA to direct changes in labelling if discussion with the sponsor failed to resolve differences. Thus, the label, and an up-to-date edition of the *Physician's Desk Reference* of approved labels, has the latest regulatory (FDA) approved label summarizing the most recent information on the safety of a drug. The most recent FDA-approved labelling can also be obtained on the FDA website.

23.3.8.4 Ongoing REMS and RiskMAPs

Over the past decade, the FDA has required various sponsors to conduct enhanced surveillance of a par-

ticular product and to provide reports to the agency on the effectiveness of that surveillance. Indeed, in 1988 the product isotretinoin was subject to such enhanced surveillance long before today's formal requirements for surveillance, and serves as an early example of today's approach.

In the case of isotretenoin, although the risk of birth defects was discovered rapidly just after marketing, it was not until the late 1990s that a formal program was created to assure appropriate use of this anti-acne drug and in particular to prevent its use in pregnancy. Through monitoring of a segment of the population using the drug, as well as monitoring all pregnancies as the program evolved in the late 1980s and early 1990s, the company was able to track its relevant safety experience with the drug. Later, this evolved into formal registry, which has evolved several times; the FDA has continued to monitor isotretenoin and has found that the current program is effective in assuring appropriate use most of the time, but not in all cases.

With the evolution of drug safety still a major focus, the value of surveillance both before marketing (as a proactive activity drawing upon increasing knowledge of drug-associated conditions) and after marketing, has come under further scrutiny, in particular by the oversight parties that have developed concerns about the focus and regulation of drug safety.

1. For example, one oversight body that extends from Congress [the Government Accounting Office (GAO)] has repeatedly noted that new effects are discovered after marketing and require label changes. The GAO interprets this as suggesting a failure in the approval process. However, unexpected adverse events have always been expected with new drugs under both the older and present drug laws, simply because of the relatively small populations exposed before approval.

2. Another troublesome foray into drug safety interpretations has developed recently, based upon contentions made about the analysis of safety events in large clinical trials. This has been particularly problematic, because many of the trials were conducted with a priori efficacy endpoints, but not predefined safety endpoints, although these latter data were collected. When retrospective analyses of these non-predefined safety endpoints were conducted, some signals of possible problems arose. Because some of these large trials were published, this retrospective analysis inappropriately became an issue for the publishers of the clinical trials, drawing the

journal editors into a misplaced vortex of post hoc analysis and safety judgements based upon ill-defined data.

Overall, such types of publicised editorial activities, which extend well beyond the regulatory decision-making process, have altered the perception of drug approval and inevitably biased the decision-making process to one of assuring a high level of safety with less concern for efficacy. Unfortunately, in the absence of sufficient clinical trial data on the limited number of patients tested, quantitative data on the efficacy and practical effectiveness of a drug in the population is often harder to find than the quantitative data on safety.

The FDA has recognized this dilemma, and has advocated the development of quantitative benefit–risk models and data. Thus far, although some examples, such as the 'number needed to treat' vs. 'number needed to harm' have emerged, the appropriate use of such models and their application to the regulatory process is in its infancy, and remains to be defined.

23.4 Conclusions

The roles of the pharmaceutical industry and the FDA, and the relationships between them, have evolved to an enormous extent since the 1962 effectiveness amendments to the FD&C Act, and today the two parties are engaged in a close, complex and generally supportive – if sometimes fractious – relationship. There is no doubt that the achievements of these two parties, both individually and together, have been spectacular – even historic – as their effectiveness and safety standards have been embraced by the whole world. Indeed, these standards are now recognised as a landmark in post-enlightenment science, as well as a forerunner and example of the current philosophy of evidence-based medicine.

Now, however, there are growing worries in a new direction: that the drug development effort has become bogged down in exaggerated regulatory process and compliance activities. The resulting fear is that drug development is slowing down, failing more often than it should and could eventually grind to a halt because of the increasing weight of regulatory demands. In Chapter 24 these concerns are considered, together with other aspects of the future of the drug development and approval process.

References

1 Lasagna L. Who will adopt the orphan drugs? *Regulation* 1979;3:27–32.

2 *Final Report: Joint Commission on Prescription Drug Use, January 1980.* Department of Health, Education and Welfare (DHEW). US Government Printing Office, January 1980.

3 Aspden P, Wolcott JA, Bootman JL, Cronenwett LR, eds. *Preventing Medication Errors.* Quality Chasm Series. Institute of Medicine. Washington DC: National Academies Press, 2006.

4 Baciu A, Stratton K, Burke SP, eds. *The Future of Drug Safety: Promoting and Protecting the Health of the Public.* Institute of Medicine. Washington DC: National Academies Press, 2007.

5 CDER Drug and Biologic Approvals for Calendar Year 2007, http://www.fda.gov/cder/rdmt/InternetNDA07.htm

6 *Guidance for Industry: Formal Meetings with Sponsors and Applicants for PDUFA Products.* February 2000.

7 *Guidance for Industry: Special Protocol Assessment.* May 2002.

8 *Guidance for Industry: Content and Format of Investigational New Drug Applications (INDs) for Phase 1 Studies of New Drugs, including Well-Characterised, Therapeutic, Biotechnology-derived Products.* November 1995.

9 *Guidance for Industry: Submitting and Reviewing Complete Responses to Clinical Holds.* April 1998.

10 *Guidance for Industry: Pre-marketing Risk Assessment.* March 2005.

11 *Manual of Policies and Procedures (MAPP 6020.3) Review Management Priority Review Policy.*

12 *Guidance for Industry: Advisory Committees: Implementing Section 120 of the Food and Drug Administration Modernization Act of 1997.*

13 Lamareaux J, Pomeranz BH, Corey PN. Incidence of adverse reactions in hospitalized patients. *JAMA* 1998; 279:1200–5.

14 *Guidance for Industry: Development and Use of Risk Minimization Action Plans.* March 2005.

Further reading

Temple R. Special study designs: early escape, enrichment, studies in non-responders. *Commun Stat Theory Methods* 1994;23:499–531.

Temple R. Are surrogate markers adequate to assess cardiovascular disease drugs? *JAMA* 1999;282:790–5.

Temple R. Policy developments in regulatory approval. *Stat Med* 2002;21:2939–48.

Temple R, Ellenberg S. Placebo-controlled trials and active-control trials in the evaluation of new treatments. *Ann Intern Med* 2000;133:455–63.

24 Future prospects of the pharmaceutical industry and its regulation in the USA

William Wardell[1], Judith K. Jones[2], Richard N. Spivey[3] and William Vodra[4]

[1] Wardell Associates International LLC, Ponte Vedra, FL, USA
[2] The Degg Group, USA
[3] Corporate Technology Policy Pharmacia, Peapack, NJ, USA
[4] Arnold & Porter, Washington, DC, USA

24.1 Introduction

In the previous chapter (Chapter 23) we described how the adoption in 1962, and subsequent implementation, of the key standards of effectiveness and safety has revolutionized drug development and therapeutics, and how the details and interpretation of these standards have evolved to the present day. We also described how the pharmaceutical industry and the Food and Drug Administration (FDA) work together, respectively, to discover and develop and to evaluate and approve new drugs, and to ensure their effective and safe use in the marketplace.

This chapter considers the wider aspects of these achievements, including how this history has shaped the current state of the industry and its regulation, and what changes may await us in the future.

Now is an opportune time to make these observations. Both the pharmaceutical industry and the FDA are under unprecedented stresses. Analysts are projecting that the industry may, in 2010, suffer its first drop in revenues (11%) of modern times. Given the bleak and declining output of drug discovery efforts and the extraordinary costs of drug research and development (R&D) today, there is understandably much hand-wringing over the industry's future prospects and even its survival. Surprisingly, there is no overall high-level plan to remedy the declining situation. (One intriguing suggestion for responding to this need is described in section 24.3.2.)

These pressures are having negative effects on the discovery and evaluation of new drugs and on their availability to physicians and patients. To start, we review the evolution of the US drug development and regulatory system, including the extensive changes since the 1962 Drug Amendments, in order to understand what may (or should) happen in the future.

The USA began regulating drugs to any significant degree in 1906, focusing mainly on the adulteration and misbranding of patent medicines. (Biologics regulations began in 1902.) In 1938, Congress, prompted by drug safety concerns, adopted a comprehensive overhaul of the Federal Food, Drug and Cosmetic Act. Frequently since then, the national legislature has found new issues and problems warranting additions to the 1938 Act, notably with the major 1962 Amendments and most recently with important changes in the FDA Amendments Act of 2007 (FDAAA). The full practical implications of the FDAAA are only now being understood, and one FDA official has opined that it may take 30 years to implement the FDAAA fully. The key Acts are discussed in Chapter 23, but there are many others, such as the Bioterrorism Act (2003) and the addition of prescription drug coverage to the Medicare programme (2004).

For purposes of drug research, development and marketing, the Drug Amendments of 1962 constituted the most significant single piece of legislation, creating for the first time a legal requirement for evidence of drug effectiveness and defining how it should be obtained. Specifically, Congress mandated that drugs be proven effective for their intended uses through 'adequate and well-controlled' clinical investigations. This deceptively simple requirement profoundly changed the pharmaceutical industry's, the FDA's and the USA's – indeed, the whole world's – standards and expectations for therapeutic agents. The Drug Amendments also directed the FDA to become involved in clinical research through the investigational new drug (IND) process, required companies to adhere to current Good Manufacturing Practices in making pharmaceuticals, allowed the

The Textbook of Pharmaceutical Medicine. Edited by John P. Griffin. © 2009, ISBN: 978-1-4051-8035-1.

FDA greater access to corporate records, and transferred regulatory control over the advertising of prescription drugs from the Federal Trade Commission to the FDA.

The innovative standards of the 1962 Drug Amendments have affected the entire spectrum of therapeutic interventions. The methods of approaching, analysing and implementing the steps needed to prove the effectiveness and safety of therapeutic drugs, and to guide their proper use in patient care, have enabled the broad field of evidence-based medicine and created its most extensive and well-defined example. The influence of drug regulation has also extended to FDA-regulated biological therapies and medical devices, as well as to all other therapeutic and diagnostic interventions – including surgical procedures, diet and watchful waiting – and established a new paradigm which continues to percolate through other branches of medicine and related sciences. These conceptual and operational advances in ensuring effectiveness and safety may arguably be among the most significant made in the field of therapeutic interventions since the Enlightenment. Those privileged to work in this field have a ringside seat (and a role) in the intellectual, scientific, medical and business struggles that it takes to develop a new product up to the present high standards of this era, and bring it to the market.

This chapter considers the changing environment in which drug development and marketing is occurring, how the economics of industry are being affected by these changes, how public attitudes toward industry and drug safety are evolving, and how the FDA is adapting to demands for greater oversight of drug safety. Finally, suggestions are offered on how public policy and FDA regulation might help sustain drug development in the future.

24.2 Wider aspects of the evolution of the FDA and the pharmaceutical industry from 1962 to 2008

24.2.1 Changing economic environment affecting the pharmaceutical industry

The business model for the pharmaceutical industry has undergone considerable changes, especially in the last 15–20 years. Moreover, the pace of change is accelerating, challenging the managers who must guide their companies forward. While many factors are at play, some that are unique to the pharmaceutical industry merit special recognition.

24.2.1.1 Impact of generic drug competition

Generic drugs have always been available in the US market. When the Drug Efficacy Study Implementation (DESI) programme assessed the effectiveness of drugs subject to new drug applications (NDAs) under the 1938 Act (prior to the 1962 Amendments), the FDA estimated that there were between 5 and 13 products without NDAs that were identical, similar or related to each of the 13,000 products under NDAs. These products might contain the same active ingredient in the same quantity and dosage form; often, though, they claimed some unique characteristic – a different salt or ester, a different quantity of drug, a different dosage form or an 'extra-added active ingredient'.

As part of the DESI project, the FDA sought to introduce uniformity and control over these products. First, the agency required any generic copy to be identical to the NDA product in the precise active ingredient (e.g. salt), the amount of that ingredient, the dosage form and the route of administration, unless the proponent obtained FDA permission to vary from the innovator. Secondly, the manufacturer had to obtain an 'abbreviated' NDA (ANDA) showing that the product was identical and could be made consistently. In essence, it was an application that contained all of the chemistry, manufacturing and control information of a full NDA, but omitted any preclinical or clinical data. A number of generic firms initially opposed even these requirements, and significant litigation followed before the FDA prevailed.

While the ANDA process was evolving, a new problem arose. Physicians reported that patients with congestive heart failure who had been titrated carefully to a specific dose of digoxin had uncontrolled concentrations upon getting prescriptions refilled. Investigation revealed that digoxin, a pre-1938 drug that was never subject to an NDA, varied from manufacturer to manufacturer, and even lot to lot from the same manufacturer. The variations were not in quantity of actual drug per tablet, but in the amount of drug released from the tablet into the body. The consequences could be life-threatening. The agency ordered that each manufacturer submit bioavailability studies showing the rate and extent of absorption into the body of each lot of digoxin, until standards could be set. Thus was born the idea of 'bioequivalence,' that generic products must be not only pharmaceutically identical to an approved reference product, but also show no significant difference in the rate or extent of absorption in studies comparing the proposed and reference products.

The ANDA process and bioequivalence rules permitted the agency for the first time to declare individual generic products to be 'therapeutically equivalent' to approved brand name versions, in that the generics could be fully expected to produce the same clinical effect and safety profile as the brand name product. The FDA began making such declarations on a limited basis around 1975; by 1979, the agency began to publish them in the *Approved Drug Products with Therapeutic Equivalence Evaluations* (Orange Book). This step was critically important to the evolution of generic success. Before this point, generics did not pose a great competitive threat, because pharmacy laws in the different US states did not permit the substitution of a generic for the innovator drug that had been prescribed. The premise of these laws was that pharmacists were not in a position to assure that generic products would perform like the innovators. However, once the FDA gave its imprimatur of equivalency, the rationale for non-substitution disappeared. In 1979, the Federal Trade Commission unveiled a model drug product selection law, which guided state legislatures on how to amend pharmacy laws to permit pharmacists to substitute equivalent generics, without the permission of the prescribing physician. Within a few years, all US states had adopted a version of this law.

Even this step had a limited effect, because the ANDA mechanism was only available to generic copies of drugs first approved before 1962. In 1984, as part of the compromise to obtain restoration of patent life that was being lost during the drug development and review process, the pharmaceutical industry agreed to extension of the ANDA requirement to copies of any previously approved product, once the patent for the product had expired or was declared invalid (and at least 5 years had passed since the reference product was first approved, to assure a minimum period of data exclusivity). The impact of this change was first felt in the late 1980s, when important innovator products went off patent. Prior to the ANDA process and drug product substitution laws, an innovation could rely on retaining over 80% of its market share for years after generic entry; now, companies found themselves losing 90% of the market in just 3–6 months.

The effect of these developments on the pharmaceutical business model has been profound. Henceforth, the only period during which a research-based drug sponsor could expect to profit from the sales of a new product was the time window from approval and launch to the date of expiration of patents and data exclusivity.

Within the 1984 law were seeds of further troubles for the pharmaceutical industry. One provision rewarded a generic manufacturer who challenged an innovator patent: if the patent were found to be invalid or not infringed, the challenger would be rewarded with 6 months of exclusive marketing of the generic. During this window, not only would the innovator lose its market share, but the generic could charge a premium price and make substantial profits. Experience began to reveal that, after three or four generics entered the market, their prices fell to pure competitive or 'commodity' levels, with very low profit margins. The generic firm, to survive and prosper, would have to become aggressive in finding other innovator patents to 'break'. By the end of the 1990s, it was increasingly common for generics to contest patents rather than wait for this expiration.

This foreshortening of the commercial life of a pharmaceutical would necessarily affect the projected return on investment for a pipeline product. The incentives were skewed in favour of 'blockbuster' developments that would command both high prices (so-called 'value-based prices') and high demand despite the high prices.

24.2.1.2 Accelerating rate of innovator competition

The pharmaceutical marketplace is indeed crowded, especially in the more traditional therapeutic areas. Further, the time lag between when the first member of a class enters the market and a 'me-too' follow-on product is approved is lessening. As a result, the ability of a company to maintain high prices even before the entry of generic competition is compromised.

24.2.1.3 Emerging demand for cost-effectiveness

Health care costs in the USA have become a major issue for governments (which subsidise health care for the poor, disabled and elderly), businesses (which subsidise health care for employees), labour unions (which are increasingly fighting to preserve benefits and jobs, rather than to increase wages) and politicians (who recognise that a huge proportion of the population has no health insurance whatsoever). Historically, drug costs were a trivial part of the health care budget. Indeed, in 1964, when Congress enacted the original Medicare programme, prescription drugs were not covered. The political perception was that the products were inexpensive, not necessarily effective and certainly drug subsidies were not critical to patient care.

Beginning in the 1990s, prescription drug expenditures accelerated as a percentage of total health care costs. This shift should be viewed as a positive development, reflecting the discovery and introduction of agents to address a population whose life expectancy has been extended, thanks to drugs and other medical advances. Unfortunately, but realistically, there are limits to the proportion of the economy that can be allocated to health. As a result, third-party payers started searching for ways to reduce the total cost. At the same time, for the reasons just discussed, manufacturers introduced 'value-based' pricing for new pharmaceuticals. The first drug to cost more than $10,000 per year for a single patient was AZT, the first AIDS drug. After initial complaints, the high price was accepted, and now products are launched at annual per person costs that are much higher (in the case of biotech drugs, some exceeding $100,000 per year, and one at approximately $300,000 per year). Thus, it is no surprise that payers have focused on prescription drugs as a way to control overall costs.

'Newer' does not automatically mean 'better', and today payers are insisting that innovations be more cost-effective than competitor products, in particular low-price generic competitors. It was once possible to launch profitably an eighth or twelfth beta-blocker or NSAID. Now, so-called 'me-too' products must at least offer some cost–benefit advantage over the innovator. The prizes go to the first-in-class product (because it will have the greatest volume of use to support safety) and to the best-in-class (because it would have been shown to be superior in some way to the others). The rest fight over the crumbs left by patients who do not respond to the first- or best-in-class products.

Furthermore, some therapeutic areas have relatively inelastic demand. For example, in the case of migraine, the market shows no sign of growth, despite the fact that there are now at least seven triptans available for patients, including four distinct dosage forms. New entrants employ large sales forces to launch new products, but results are often meagre, until continued investment proves prohibitive to do even that. Meanwhile, managed care organisations decide that only one or two representatives of a class will be reimbursable, thus placing additional pressure on marketing organisations.

The economic implications should be clear. Today's drug development decisions must be made with a careful regard to the drug's place in the queue of likely competitors, and to the sponsor's ability to demonstrate therapeutic advantages. In the case of some drugs, such as proton pump inhibitors, the very mechanism of action limits the potential for significant improve-

ments by later generations. In other areas, such as the calcium channel blockers diltiazem and verapamil, the chemistry may not permit a second generation molecule.

24.2.1.4 Declining productivity of research and development

The productivity of R&D efforts within the pharmaceutical industry has declined significantly in the past decade. While large numbers of INDs are submitted each year, only a small proportion in the pipeline emerges as NDA submissions or approvals. NDA approvals for new molecular entities (NMEs) have fallen from a high of 53 in calendar year 1996, to 18 and 16 in 2006 and 2007, respectively. No clear reasons exist for this decline, especially in the face of record high levels of R&D investment. Speculation suggests that the 'easy' targets have already been exploited; that profit potential for pipeline products cannot meet ever-increasing financial targets, causing their abandonment; and that safety concerns require inordinately clean risk profiles for new products even to be submitted to the FDA.

Research technology has advanced particularly rapidly over the past two decades, and techniques such as robotics, high throughput screening and computer-aided design and simulations have been instituted in discovery and early development labs. Given the declining level of NME NDA submissions and the industry's continuing ordeal of consolidations and layoffs, it appears that there has not yet been a high degree of payoff for these technological innovations, despite some significant successes such as trastuzumab. However, biotechnology product approvals are increasing and represent a bright spot in an otherwise gloomy picture.

24.2.1.5 Pharmacogenomics and 'personalized therapeutics'

One of the most popular therapeutic ideas over the past 10 years is the claim that pharmacogenomic (PGx) diagnostics will open up an era of 'personalized therapeutics' and thereby revolutionize medical treatment. In the area of cancer chemotherapy, PGx diagnostics have indeed started to deliver advances in selecting the most appropriate drug(s) for a particular patient's cancer; areas outside cancer are also steadily acquiring helpful genomic information.

The FDA now publishes on its website a very useful *Reference Table of Valid Genomic Biomarkers in the Context of Approved Drug Labels*. About 10% of labels for drugs approved by the FDA now contain genomic information that can be relevant to prescribers in identifying responders and non-responders, avoiding toxicity and adjusting the dosage of drugs to optimize their effectiveness and safety. In drug labels, these genomic biomarkers are classified on the basis of their specific use: clinical response and differentiation, risk identification, dose selection guidance, susceptibility and resistance, differential disease diagnosis and polymorphic drug targets.

The FDA's table (nine pages long) lists valid genomic biomarkers in the context of FDA-approved drug labels, and links to relevant pharmacogenomic data. Most drug labels listed in this table provide pharmacogenomic information with no immediate recommendation for a specific action (e.g. genetic testing). However, a few of these labels now recommend or require genetic testing, thereby specifying the use of these markers for reaching a therapeutic decision. Currently, there are 28 drugs in the table, plus reference to 40 additional drugs that share one or others of the relevant biomarkers. This site is worth visiting (http://www.fda.gov/cder/genomics/genomic_biomarkers_table.htm).

In some therapeutic areas, PGx is still mostly a promise that has yet to achieve its extremely broad claims, but the amount of relevant genomic information is steadily accumulating, along with its relevance and impact. In the case of drug safety, two recent examples show that safety may be improved through genomic diagnostic testing. First, it has been shown to provide improved accuracy in selecting the initial dosing of the anticoagulant warfarin. [It is only the initial (loading) dose that is being predicted, because thereafter maintenance dosing must be controlled by regular international normalised ratio (INR) testing.] Genotypes of two genes (*CYP2C9* and *VKORC1*), plus certain clinical characteristics of each patient, can account for approximately half the variance in a population's response to warfarin. In mid-2007, the FDA relabelled warfarin to inform physicians that lower initial doses of the drug should be considered for patients with certain genetic variations in *CYP2C9* and *VKORC1*, in what may be considered one of the first steps the agency has taken to put 'personalised medicine' in a drug product label. Later in 2007, the FDA also approved a change in labelling for carbamazepine. Asian patients may have an allele (*HLSB*1502*) that hugely increases the risk of incurring the Stevens–Johnson syndrome when they take carbamazepine. Simply testing for this allele, and avoiding carbamazepine, will exclude those at increased risk for this devastating reaction.

The warfarin example is particularly interesting because the traditional phenotypic marker used for decades (the INR) is also the actual surrogate endpoint, and is easily measured in 2 minutes after a finger-stick test. Thus, the cost and effectiveness hurdles for showing improvement in anticoagulation by adding the genomic test are quite high in this case.

The task of developing a genomic test to predict drug effectiveness during a drug's clinical development phases will be much more complex, and will greatly impact the drug's development process. To meet the 'substantial evidence' standard for efficacy, the sponsor will presumably first have to show that the genomic diagnostic is appropriately sensitive and specific, accurate and reproducible; that the test can discriminate between those who will respond (therapeutically) to the drug and those who will not; and that the drug is clinically more effective or safe within the group of patients selected using the PGx diagnostic, compared with a control group of patients without genomic testing. In practical terms, this policy will probably require studying the drug–diagnostic combination in both phase II and III – a significant challenge of time and cost in the drug's pre-approval programme.

Thus, in phase II and earlier, the development programme will presumably need to define the relationship between genetic variation and response to the drug in defined populations, along with development of valid tests to measure the variations. The phase III controlled studies will need to demonstrate that the addition of PGx testing actually improves health outcomes for patients. The benefit added by the diagnostic testing will influence the pricing of the test (i.e. whether the test – and the test procedure – is cost-effective compared with usual care). In addition to its impact on patients, this set of questions is typically of great relevance to clinicians and third-party payers who will be the ultimate gatekeepers for the clinical integration of pharmacogenetics.

To date, nearly all of the research efforts and funding for PGx have been focused on the science – basic and clinical. Now PGx must face the regulatory standards for safety and effectiveness, to prove its value for both clinical and economic decision-making. Although it has been estimated that some 1700 potential PGx tests currently exist (nearly 300 of which have received some degree of recognition as commercial diagnostics), very few have yet been recognized for the ultimate PGx application (i.e. selecting a specific drug for an individual patient's therapy) which has been demonstrated to be more likely to improve therapeutic outcome in that patient.

24.2.1.6 Increasing costs of drug development

The costs of bringing a new drug to the market keep rising exponentially. This fact compounds the problems of persistently long development time (now averaging 12 years) and a remarkably high failure rate (75% or more) in the clinical research phase. The latest estimate from the Tufts Center for the Study of Drug Development puts large pharmaceutical companies' average out-of-pocket cost, including failures, of developing a new chemical entity to the point of NDA approval, at $403 million ($121 million preclinical plus $282 million clinical). When the cost of the capital, expended over the 12-year average time of product development, is included, this figure rises to $802 million ($336 million preclinical plus $466 million clinical). Development speed and failure rates have a large effect on the cost of development: if development time could be cut in half, the $802 million would drop to $568 million. If the failure rate were reduced from 75% to 67%, total costs would be lowered by $217 million.

Other estimates are even higher, in the $1–2 billion range with a success rate as low as 8%, but much depends on the methodology of the estimate.

Some of the more potent causes of these increasing costs include the following:

1. Chronic and complex indications demand longer, larger and more complex studies.

2. Comparative trials (comparing two active drugs), needed for regulatory approval when placebo trials are unacceptable, and often merely to compete in the marketplace, require larger populations and longer durations to have sufficient power to determine equivalency, non-inferiority or superiority.

3. Special pre-approval studies are now expected, or required, to explore safety and effectiveness in special subpopulations. These groups include the elderly; children (four subsets: neonates and infants, toddlers, and preschoolers, prepubescent school-aged children, and postpuberty adolescents); women of child-bearing potential; persons with renal or hepatic impairment; and persons using foreseeable concomitant medications (looking for dangers such as QTc interval prolongation, a signal for possible torsades de pointes).

4. More trials, with greater numbers of subjects, necessitate a larger infrastructure to manage sites, collect and verify data, assure protocol compliance plus adherence to Good Clinical Practice (GCP) regulations. This need has led to the need for outside consultants and contract research organisations (CROs). The number of outside companies who now draw their livelihood from the growing size and complexity of the drug development process is an ominous portent because it signifies that there is no end in sight, nor means of containing, the inexorable ratcheting-up of details, standards, employment and costs.

5. Competition for a limited pool of patients has caused study recruitment and retention problems and the need for direct payments to subjects for their participation. It has also encouraged efforts to perform clinical trials in countries with less-developed health care systems, in which large numbers of treatment-naïve patients may be found. Undertaking controlled studies in these countries may be difficult. Between 2003 and 2007, according to the FDA, the percentage of clinical trials filed with the agency that were performed in countries in Central or Eastern Europe, the Middle East, Africa, South America, Asia or the Pacific rose from 9% to 18%, with Russia, India, Brazil and China being major players. The time and cost savings from locating trials in these areas may be reduced if new infrastructures have to be created to train and monitor investigators.

6. Increased use of information technology, such as remote electronic data entry and electronic diaries, creates the further need for additional data integrity controls and audit trail.

7. More rigorous demands for the format of regulatory submissions. The FDA initiatives to eliminate unnecessary paperwork through electronic filings can lead to expensive technology investments which have yet to show economy and efficiency.

8. Greater and broader concern over safety of the product. As the number of allegedly 'missed' safety problems (e.g. troglitazone and rofecoxib) has emerged as an issue of public and political concern, FDA reviewers have tended to request more data and/or studies to elaborate on the safety profiles of pending drugs.

9. New fields of expertise are emerging as necessary or desirable to interact with regulatory authorities. Whenever regulators express a general interest in, or concern about, a new type of scientific issue, sponsors naturally commit resources to anticipate how this issue might affect their pipeline products. Thus, the R&D organisation may have to acquire and manage persons with skills that do not directly advance drug development itself. For example, the current regulatory interest in pharmacogenomics has led to the establishment of PGx departments in drug firms, well before the value of PGx to drug development has been proven.

In summary, the compounding effect of so many added burdens from all directions has itself produced new dimensions of complexity and costs not readily apparent to those outside – or even inside – the system. There is a real danger that the system will collapse of its own weight. The growth of burdens at this pace cannot continue for ever, and the currently pessimistic business climate for the pharmaceutical industry reflects – and compounds – the problem.

24.2.2 Economic consequences of this changing environment on the pharmaceutical industry

24.2.2.1 Consolidation within the industry

The steeply rising costs (not only in R&D but also in marketing and supply operations), combined with a foreshortened period of generic-free competition, initially drove the industry into maintaining large marketing and sales operations and an efficient supply chain. Its business model evolved to focus on blockbuster drugs, ones that generated at least $1 billion per year in order to make a profitable return on investment before generics or 'me-too' products enter the market. However, the declining productivity of R&D has forced the industry to cast a wider net to discover compounds and take them through the initial phases of development. Despite this, the lack of sufficient blockbuster products has forced other changes in the business model. A recent change has been a shift from the blockbuster strategy to finding profitable niche products in specialised areas, such as oncology.

The most common response to the declining pipeline, however, has been consolidation of the industry, in order to support the sales and manufacturing operations and ongoing R&D. Unprecedented consolidation has taken place over the last 10–15 years because of these economic pressures, and the pace of consolidation has sharply increased in the past 2 years, with large-scale layoffs and consolidations.

While these mergers may yield efficiencies in marketing and production, it is doubtful whether the same efficiencies hold in drug development. The search for blockbuster and high-value niche drugs has compelled research organisations to be driven more by the market than by science. One result of consolidation had been the creation of mega-R&D organisations, some of which had 15,000–20,000 staff or more, with multiple research sites on several continents. The very size of these organisations has produced the further challenge of managing these resources. Paradoxically, there is as yet no evidence that the consolidation improved innovation, or that huge R&D organisations have useful economies of scale or efficiencies in discovery or development. It is conceivable that the consolidation has actually achieved the opposite of its intent in R&D, and that discovery and innovation have declined as a result.

24.2.2.2 Rise of the biotechnology industry

A new drug discovery industry has emerged in parallel with the consolidation of the pharmaceutical industry. Beginning in the 1970s, boosted by the Bayh–Dole Act of 1980 (encouraging outlicensing of university-based discoveries made with National Institutes of Health funds), and funded by venture capital, start-up biotechnology ('biotech') companies, proliferated. The term 'biotech' originally applied to the tools offered by recombinant DNA and monoclonal antibody technologies, but now loosely embraces start-up and small companies in general, including small molecule design and discovery, genomics and proteomics, bioinformatics, therapeutic vaccines, novel drug delivery systems, combinations of a medical device with a drug or biologic, nanotechnology and other cutting edge biomedical research ideas and tools. Unfortunately, the great potential of these new technologies has not yet been fully realised. A staggering number of products and the start-up companies that spawned them have failed. Other great promises, such as interferon, endorphins and gene therapy, have proved so far to have limited clinical applications or unsuspected toxicity. The translation of new technologies to the hospital, pharmacy and bedside is taking longer, and costing more, than was expected in the enthusiasm of the 1990s. Part of the reason for the disappointment to date may lie in the excessive exuberance for its potential that was intrinsic to raising venture capital to create new companies and fund novel research.

Nevertheless, biotechnology has made a substantial and growing contribution to the pharmaceutical pipeline and the therapeutic armamentarium, with approximately 6–8 NME products reaching the market each year. The largest biotech companies (e.g. Amgen and Genentech) are now indistinguishable, in the business sense, from traditional pharmaceutical companies. The vibrant biotech small company sector, particularly at the discovery and early development level, is supplying drug candidates for licensing or acquisition by pharmaceutical companies that need to supplement their own internal research operations. The relationship has proven mutually beneficial. Pharmaceutical companies cannot afford to finance the scale of drug discovery operations needed to maintain a pipeline; companies funded by venture capital and stock offerings assume much of the risk of early failures; and both parties share the rewards of success. As a result, every major pharmaceutical company scouts for new opportunities, and the most promising drug candidates become the subjects of intensive bidding competitions.

If pharmaceutical companies cannot increase their traditional internal R&D productivity, then the rate of biotech discoveries reaching the market must increase rapidly to sustain the overall pharmaceutical pipeline. At the very least, the advent of the biotech industry has greatly changed the face of pharmaceuticals worldwide, and is now being seen as the creative force that may be saving the pharmaceutical industry – at least for the present.

24.2.2.3 Outsourcing

The steady rise of outsourcing since the 1960s has greatly expanded the operating capacity and expertise base of the pharmaceutical industry. It began with the clinical CROs which handled the logistics of clinical trials and with animal testing laboratories compliant with the FDA's Good Laboratory Practice (GLP) regulations. Subsequently, the field expanded to include firms in all areas of drug development: production of active pharmaceutical ingredients, design of pharmaceutical formulations, stability programmes, pharmacokinetic studies, biostatistics, data management, clinical site management, auditing for compliance with GLP/GCP requirements and preparation of regulatory submissions. Even the duties of institutional review boards (IRBs) are often undertaken for multicentre trials by free-standing for-profit companies.

A recent event may foreshadow even greater levels of outsourcing in the future. In 2008, Eli Lilly sold the entire campus of one of its preclinical facilities to the CRO Covance, a move that has precedents in the manufacturing area but not previously in R&D. The Lilly–Covance deal is one of the first large-scale examples of this type of facility sale in early stage drug development (a function that until recently was contained within the big pharmaceutical companies). Under the terms of the agreement, 260 Lilly employees who work in toxicology, pharmacology and imaging services will work for Covance, which plans to upgrade the site and double or triple the workforce.

The future of outsourcing is clearly strong, but it also reveals a growing pressure for cheaper ways to satisfy the requirements for evidence of effectiveness and safety. One recent and growing solution is to move clinical research activities out of the USA and other high-cost countries to Eastern Europe, India and China. One CRO, for example, recently relocated its entire electrocardiography (ECG) monitoring services to India and promises 1-hour 24/7 turnaround, in the same way that some US hospitals have outsourced the reading of radiographs. Other specific functions such as data management, analysis and information technology can also be performed offshore. Recently, it was reported that India, which performed about 1% of all clinical trials around the world in 2007, would seek to expand its market share to 15% by 2011. While these trends may appear to reduce costs, there are caveats to consider, in that not all offshore countries, or contractors, may be of the high standards that are essential for regulatory submissions. Expansion of the infrastructure to support a growth in the volume of clinical trials in India, for instance, could be very expensive upfront, and even more expensive later, if the studies prove not to meet GCP standards and cannot support regulatory approvals. Thorough evaluation and caveat emptor are the watchwords. In addition, the shift of GLP and GCP trials from the USA and Western Europe could have long-term adverse effects on the scientific capacity of those countries to sustain pharmaceutical R&D generally.

24.2.2.4 Frontloading the drug development process

Advances in the sciences of drug discovery and early development, such as computer modelling and simulation ('in silico' testing), offer the possibility that candidate drugs can be screened earlier in the development process for potential problems, thereby reducing the failure rate at later stages. The results to date have been disappointing, however, and the very low success rate of compounds that enter development has not been raised. The FDA's Critical Path initiative is another attempt to address the development failure problem. These approaches also create a new challenge: by investing more in the numerous technologies available at the early stage of a drug's development, one 'frontloads' each compound's early development costs. Thus, if the compound still ultimately fails, the economic savings may be less than initially hoped for. The value of frontloading strategies needs ultimately to be judged by its effect on the late-stage pipeline and on the volume of new drug approvals and corporate profitability.

In general, the frontloading of the development process by further use of any of the numerous modern available technologies would be attractive if one had a reasonable and data-supported basis for believing that it would work. To date, it has not produced enough successful results to determine whether it is a superior strategy. Nevertheless, investments are proceeding to frontload R&D without this evidence.

24.2.3 Changing public attitudes toward the pharmaceutical industry

In recent years, the drug industry has come under increasing criticism on a wide variety of fronts within the USA. The cumulative impact makes the industry look bad and lose public support. A short catalogue of the public concerns and perceptions illustrates the complexity of the public relations challenge facing drug firms:

• *High prices for prescription drugs.* Americans know that they are paying more for drugs than residents outside the USA, because of price controls elsewhere. Polls indicate that Americans feel they are paying more than their fair share for the cost of drug development. Moreover, those individuals not covered by health insurance covering prescription drugs may have to choose between food and medical care. In 2004, Congress enacted a prescription drug benefit programme for Medicare patients, but the uninsured are still estimated to be in the 45–50 million range, out of 300 million US residents. The importation of brand name drugs purchased more cheaply abroad is a perennial political issue.

• *Excessive total costs for prescription drugs.* Insurers and other third-party payers see drugs as the fastest rising component in total health care spending. For them, it is not merely the question of price per pill, but the aggregate utilisation of drugs. With the advent of 'lifestyle' drugs, and later-generation medicines that may offer no convincing advantages over those that are available as generics, there are real concerns about the diversion of limited resources to unnecessary products, plus the soaring costs for employee benefits that must be built into cost of goods sold.

• *Dubious practices in promoting prescription drugs.* Americans have long had a love–hate relationship with advertising, but the reported excesses and misconduct linked to prescription drug marketing has produced intense public outrage. Gifts, luxury trips and six-figure consulting contracts for physicians smack of bribes. The ratio of sales representatives to prescribing physicians is stunning. The introduction of direct-to-consumer (DTC) advertising has led to charges that the public is being seduced to believe that pills are a solution for any ailment, as well as being lulled into ignoring the risks associated with prescription drugs. At the same time, the total amount spent on DTC advertising has reached levels that inevitably are linked to the high prices for and total costs of prescription drugs. Finally, stories about the marketing of drugs for indications or populations in which they have not been tested or approved (so-called 'off-label'

promotion) have shocked prosecutors, politicians and the media.

• *Disconnection between high industry profits and R&D spending.* For years, the industry's justification for its prices and profits was the need to have sufficient money to carry out new research, as well as to reward the inherently high risks of drug discovery. Revelations that many companies spend more on promotion than on R&D, combined with the decline in the introduction of major new therapies coming to market, have made people sceptical of this claim. Sir Thomas McKillop, while CEO of AstraZeneca, publicly acknowledged that this argument was no longer credible.

• *Fundamental distrust of the industry's ethics.* Repeated revelations that adverse research studies have been withheld from public view, or released in partial and misleading form, have created new statutory requirements (and corresponding medical journal demands) for sponsors to disclose publicly, in government registries, all phase II and III clinical trials before patients are enrolled. More seriously, apparent delays in removing or issuing warnings about products, coupled with the precipitous withdrawal of widely marketed drugs and the suspicion that safety risks could have been identified before approval gives support to the anti-industry charge that 'companies put profits before people.' It does not help the pharmaceutical industry's image that in the last decade a large number of major companies have been successfully prosecuted by the federal government for violations of a myriad of different laws. Taken together, these events seem to underscore the appearance of deficiencies in basic ethical standards within the industry.

The net result of the changing public attitudes toward the industry is an increasing reluctance of US voters and consumers to accept the need to pay for the high costs of new drug development and other medical advances that improve the quality of life and the savings of health care money.

24.2.4 Changing public perceptions of drug safety and FDA responses

Over the years, the amount of knowledge available about a candidate drug has increased tremendously by the time of NDA submission. The size of NDAs has grown to a point that it is not uncommon for an NDA to contain data generated from scores of trials involving more than 10,000 patients. Much of this growth is in response to regulatory demands for a clearer delineation of the safety profile of a drug before approval.

Despite this record level of premarket risk information, new problems are invariably identified after approval. Over the past decades, roughly 2–3% of the drugs approved by the FDA and by the major European regulatory agencies each year, have ultimately been removed from the market for safety reasons. This situation is understandable and expected; in fact, recognition that the post-market experience inevitably reveals new adverse effects forms the basis for the requirement for post-marketing pharmacovigilance. The initial approval of an NDA has always involved a trade-off between known benefits and known and unknown risks, because the clinical trials cannot have realistically evaluated a drug in all the populations who may ultimately use it. Spontaneous reports from the entire population, plus phase IV studies, have usually provided the first signals of new adverse events. No matter how large the number of patients studied prior to marketing, discovery of new adverse events will always occur. Because of the very large size of the US market, relatively rare events may have a better opportunity to be discovered there earlier, and thus lead to changes in warnings or removals from the market.

These realities are frequently misunderstood or ignored, especially by sensationalist media, plaintiffs' lawyers and political opportunists, whose public posturing on drug safety issues might be summarised as follows:

1. Unless a drug is live-saving, it should generally not have any serious or life-threatening risks. Drugs for symptomatic relief or for lifestyle choices, especially for which there are alternatives, simply do not justify any chance of causing permanent injury or death.

2. The risks we are familiar with are 'safer' (i.e. more acceptable) than the one we have just heard about. In the debate surrounding the withdrawal of rofecoxib, for example, the media rarely attempted to discuss the risks of life-threatening gastrointestinal bleeds caused by first generation NSAIDs but avoided by rofecoxib. Instead, the discussion focused entirely on the newly identified cardiovascular risks of the COX-2 inhibitor.

3. Good well-conducted science should be able to reveal all side effects during drug development. The failure to do so suggests concealment and/or incompetence by industry and/or the FDA.

4. Safety is a clear-cut issue, with an easy answer. Discussions of conflicting and inadequate data, problems of background noise or study bias, and the differing values placed on specific benefits and risks (as well as individual freedom to accept risks) merely confuse the public.

Whenever a drug is withdrawn for toxicity therefore, one can expect to hear arguments that the standards for drug approval should be increased. Often, the FDA is accused of being lax in enforcing current requirements for safety, or urged to adopt more rigorous ones. In contrast, FDA officials have contended that the agency is more willing to admit (and leave) drugs on the market than other national authorities. They assert that the FDA can do so because it has been proactive in developing programmes to manage the known risks for a drug with a narrow benefit–risk ratio.

In fact, over the past decade, the FDA has greatly enhanced its approach to risk management (after studies of the effects of new warnings and labelling changes demonstrated that they had done little to affect prescribing behaviour). The agency recognised that it needed new tools to minimise preventable risks and to inform physicians and patients about risks. Accordingly, it developed an approach called a risk minimisation action plan (RiskMAP) consisting of more aggressive physician and patient education programmes, and in extreme cases, actual limitations on access to high-risk products. Congress endorsed and strengthened this approach, and renamed it 'risk evaluation and mitigation strategies' (REMS) in the FDA Amendments of 2007. Internal organizational changes at the FDA have also increased the agency's resources and sought to integrate better decision-making on drug risk–benefit issues.

If risk management activities are used to permit the marketing of drugs that otherwise would be kept off the market because of serious safety concerns, and the activities are effective, the public will be better served. On the other hand, if REMS are routinely applied to drugs that could be marketed safely without them, they may unnecessarily inhibit deny access of physicians and patients to, or appropriate use of, valuable and acceptably safe medicines. How the FDA will strike this important balance remains to be seen.

24.3 Improvements needed for the future

From our discussion in this chapter, it is obvious that the economic pressures on the industry pose significant challenges for the discovery, development and introduction of novel drugs. Unless new products can be found to replace the revenue provided by those going off patent and becoming available as generics, the ability of the industry to continue funding R&D

will be impaired. If, in turn, this process leads to a long-term decline in finding new drugs to treat diseases and conditions that currently do not have adequate therapies, all of us will suffer.

Clearly, having better drug candidates and better ways of choosing which of them should enter into development would be an important step forward. Although the enormous increase in power of the biological and pharmaceutical sciences has increased the range and quality of development candidates over recent years, prediction of consistently successful ones is still elusive. Equally critical is improving the success rate of the overall process, which has changed little over the last few decades. Estimates of the overall success rate of a drug from the point of IND allowance range as low as 8% today. It has been estimated that increasing the success rate by 10% across a portfolio of drugs at all stages of clinical development would have the same effect on development costs as reducing the development time by more than 20%. But changes in regulatory policy would seem unlikely to have much immediate and direct effect – other than through raising time and costs – on either the quantity or quality of candidates to take into development or the ultimate success rate among these candidates.

Regulators, of course, might facilitate research to permit candidates to fail earlier in the process and thus be eliminated at lower cost. Despite numerous attempts in the past to streamline it, the drug development and approval process still takes too long and is too expensive. The FDA recognized this reality a few years ago, and launched its Critical Path Initiative, in an effort to identify new strategies and tools to assess safety and effectiveness at lower cost, in less time. We applaud this effort. Some of our recommendations fit within the Critical Path Initiative.

For 35 years it has been recognised that fundamental reforms are needed. The answer, we believe, is to work within the legal and regulatory framework of the current system, and to implement some of the best reforms that have already been proposed. It is the difficulty of implementation, rather than the lack of ideas, that has prevented progress and allowed the system itself to become an ever-larger impediment.

Our main proposals are as follow:
1. Lessen the regulatory requirements for IND filing and phase I and II studies, to facilitate new products' exploratory development and proof-of-concept in patients. Safety requirements should not be raised unnecessarily at this stage.
2. At the NDA stage, make more use of the NDA's existing conditional approval mechanisms, so that in a wider range of circumstances a drug may be approved for the market for limited indications considerably earlier than it would be at present, on condition that the development programme continues and that the conditions of initial approval are enforced. In this way, the law's ultimate effectiveness and safety standards for a full approval are safeguarded, not compromised. While this avenue exists and is used, it has not generally been commercially attractive for wide-scale use. (It is used to good effect, however, in orphan drug INDs and NDAs.)
3. In addition, we have a number of smaller proposals that, taken together, would further facilitate the process. At present, the FDA expends considerable resources and has too many requirements for formulation changes, new dose forms, extended release preparations and combinations, treating them almost like NCEs. This is an example of an opportunity to streamline the agency, saving resources on both sides.

24.3.1 Simplify the IND submission, and the phase I–II clinical programme, through proof-of-concept

The FDA has differentiated between the regulatory purposes in reviewing phase I IND submissions versus phase II and III protocols. Overall requirements for an IND have continued to rise in complexity and size. We recommend simplifying the IND requirements further through the proof-of-concept stage, so that key safety and basic efficacy studies can be performed easily in humans with similar protections, but at less time and cost than they are at present.

The administrative burdens (including the amount of data required) that go into managing IND submissions and amendments, in both large pharmaceutical companies and small start-ups, is excessive. The cost of impediments at this early stage is greater than might appear at first sight because they contribute greatly to the frontloading of the clinical development time and costs that we have described.

The filing of a full IND, with a formal coordinated write-up of all the supporting data (in effect, a mini-NDA), while perhaps necessary 45 years ago, is now an excessive requirement in the early stage clinical programmes of most large pharmaceutical firms and CROs that carry out this work. It is a barrier to the easy access to human studies that is needed for proof-of-concept studies (phases I and IIa). Very little risk to public health and safety has been seen in the past 20 years with early work under INDs filed by experienced and responsible individuals, corporations and institutions; the FIAU experience and the Gelsinger gene therapy tragedy stand out in their isolation, and neither were prevented by the IND process. The system can now be safely adjusted to recognise this fact, by scaling back the IND requirements for responsible entities, based on what has been learned in the past 45 years.

Our proposal goes considerably beyond the FDA's 'phase 0' stage for first-in-man pharmacokinetic and similar activities, and beyond the FDA's 'exploratory IND' guidance of 2006. Our proposal would cover all early human studies through clinical proof-of-concept (phase IIa). Only in the large pivotal studies (phases IIb–III), when there is more assurance that the drug candidate has a solid chance of getting to an NDA submission, and where larger numbers of patients are treated at full doses, would the full formal IND filing be necessary. (These proposals are the opposite of what has been introduced by the EC Clinical Trial Directive.)

The streamlined system would work like this:
• Experienced pharmaceutical companies, CROs and medical research institutions would be qualified by the FDA as 'responsible' to conduct early clinical trials without full IND review by the FDA. These qualified bodies would still have to comply with IND requirements for reporting safety events, obtaining independent ethical review and informed consent, and recordkeeping. The FDA could establish standards and procedures for qualifying these organisations, and for revoking 'responsible' status if misconduct occurred.
• For sponsors that qualify for this new status, the IND and all phase I and IIa studies under it would be allowed by simple notification to the FDA – rather than by the FDA's scrutiny and formal allowance in each case. This system would be similar, in some respects, to the former German *Hinterlegungsstelle* ('deposition'), whereby the sponsor made a simple deposition of the supporting data that the sponsor deemed sufficient, with no review or attention needed by the agency unless a problem arose. If a problem did arise, the data deposition package would be opened and reviewed by the agency, and the sponsor held liable (and, among other penalties, would lose its 'responsible' status) if safety or other key deficiencies were found.

The rationale for this proposal is that phases I and II (first-in-man and early efficacy studies) are of small size and are relatively safe when performed by experienced investigators; and that entities and individuals with a good track record and a reputation to lose have

a powerful incentive to keep their record spotlessly clean and so retain their 'responsible' status privileges.

For investigators and institutions that have not been qualified as 'responsible', the present IND system would apply unchanged, with the expectation that a process would be developed for evaluating and qualifying candidate 'responsible entities'.

24.3.2 Reform the NDA by extending the option of provisional approval

While the standards of ultimate NDA approval, based on effectiveness and safety, should be carefully maintained, existing regulations already provide for attaining full approval in multiple stages. Our proposal is that these options should be made available in a wider range of circumstances, including at the request of the sponsor. The model would be similar to that developed by the FDA and sponsors so successfully over the past several decades for handling drugs for accelerated approval, and would be tailored to the case of each particular drug. That is, the sponsor would have the option of requesting earlier approval under, for example, a restricted range of uses or increased post-market controls and obligations.

This proposal reflects the reality of many approvals today, plus the fact – not yet fully recognised in the context of the approval process – that in the past few decades there has arisen, outside the core FDA drug regulatory system, an expanding set of additional utilisation controls of considerable power that can further shape drug use in many ways. Over the past 40 years, the marketplace has developed its own powerful expanding set of utilisation controls (based on payment, marketing, managed care and information feedback) which already function as a *de facto* add-on utilisation control system, and this can – and in some cases already does – act as an additional safeguard for the use of new drugs in the early post-marketing situation.

In summary, a conditional approval step could be integrated with the existing system of marketplace utilisation controls, and thus be used as an option to expedite approvals for earlier access to promising therapies. It would be important, however, not to burden new drugs unnecessarily with conditional approval status if there is not a real reason to do so.

24.3.2.1 'Economic Darwinism'

A thoughtful and more detailed way of implementing and providing incentives for provisional approval has been proposed by Wood.[1] Wood suggests modifying and focusing on particular key details of the regulatory

Table 24.1 Improving the drug approval process through 'economic Darwinism'. From Wood (2006)[1] with permission

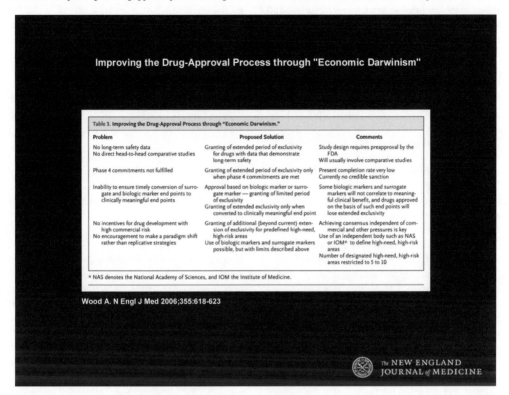

approval process: to create greater incentives for industry to develop drug candidates of high scientific risk, and to carry out long-term safety studies.

Wood identified six fundamental problems (Table 24.1) and proposes to address them through a radical 'carrot and stick' approach that he terms 'economic Darwinism', designed to induce sponsors to perform such useful tasks as undertaking high commercial risk projects; completing long-term safety data commitments; performing head-to-head comparative studies; fulfilling phase IV commitments; and converting surrogate or biomarker endpoints promptly to meaningful clinical endpoints.

Sponsors who undertake and fulfil the relevant tasks would be rewarded with the 'carrot' of easier approval (on surrogate endpoints, including biomarkers) and/or increased exclusivity. Sponsors who choose not to participate would endure the 'stick' of having to cope with the present system.

A novel central element of Wood's proposal is the use of varying periods of market exclusivity, depending on the amount of clinical work the sponsor has carried out. At the present time, US law assures the sponsor of any new chemical entity at least 5 years of data exclusivity, plus any additional period provided by a valid and enforceable patent. Congress has also provided a special incentive to perform pediatric studies, by extending any existing exclusivity by one or two additional 6-month periods. This special incentive has proven enormously successful. Wood offers the idea of adding other exclusivity rewards in exchange for further work to develop the drug after initial approval. Failure to do so would invite early generic competition.

This approach should be given serious consideration, because it does not require a major philosophical change in the present system, but instead uses relatively minor legislative adjustments that actually produce powerful changes in the incentives to sponsors.

The agency's ability to grant a sponsor's request for earlier approval, with conditions such as these, would especially help those small companies and products for which approval in some form, even with extensive restrictions, is an increasingly necessary step to finance further work. These powers would be particularly useful, for example, for patients who might benefit from orphan-type drugs, and for drugs developed by the growing number of small pharmaceutical and biotechnology companies that have products in development for limited or special indications.

24.3.2.2 Provisional approval and off-label marketing of drugs

In the USA, a physician is generally permitted to prescribe or administer an approved drug product for any bona fide medical use, even if the drug is not approved for that particular use. Exceptions exist for drugs subject to RiskMAP and REMS programmes, as well as controlled substances. Otherwise, the decision to use a drug 'off-label' is up to the physician, subject to any utilisation controls imposed under formulary or reimbursement schemes (and, of course, malpractice liability).

Drug companies are not legally permitted to promote their products for off-label (unapproved) uses. At the same time, they face an abrupt loss of market revenues when generic competition begins (discussed above). The incentive to maximise sales during the period of product exclusivity is strong – and has led companies to violate the prohibition against off-label marketing.

The issue goes to the safety and effectiveness of the drugs for the unapproved applications. Senator Charles Grassley recently asked the Government Accounting Office (GAO), the investigative arm of Congress, to review the FDA's effectiveness in monitoring drug companies' efforts to promote off-label uses, because of concerns about the possible effects of such promotion on doctors' prescribing practices and on patients' safety. The GAO responded that concerns about off-label use had grown in recent years, citing a 2006 study that found more than 20% of prescriptions for 100 of the 500 most commonly used prescription drugs to be for off-label uses. The GAO went on to conclude that the FDA does a poor job of policing off-label promotion and that its systems were disorganized and slow.

Nevertheless, the government – acting through the FDA but also through the Department of Justice, the Office of Inspector General of Health and Human Services and the Attorneys General of the various states – and aided by whistleblowers who can obtain substantial rewards for turning in violators – has engaged in a major campaign over the last decade-plus against promotion of drugs for unapproved uses. Numerous companies have reached settlements involving payments of millions of dollars, including Pfizer (for gabapentin), Lilly (for raloxifene) and

Cephalon (for tiagabine, modafinil and oral transmucosal fentanyl).

The very fact that major pharmaceutical firms have been charged with off-label marketing demonstrates that the risks these practices might incur under a plan of provisional approval for limited purposes are real. We are not making any recommendations to address this risk, but recognize that it is an issue to be resolved if our proposal for greater use of earlier qualified approvals is adopted.

24.3.4 Other opportunities for improving drug discovery and development

Finally, we discuss here a further set of potential areas for improvement across a wide area of the drug development process.

24.3.4.1 The FDA's skills

Using the increased skills and talents of the greater number of qualified staff now at the FDA (made possible in particular by the budget expansions of the Prescription Drug User Fee Act (PDUFA) and other appropriations, and now in more concrete form in the agency's critical path initiative) is another avenue. DiMasi and Manocchia[2] have shown that early and continuing discussions between the regulators and the regulated, in the form of FDA–sponsor conferences, facilitate drug approval. This is what one would expect if, by the time of filing an NDA, all the important questions had been asked and answered. The FDA's Critical Path Initiative is an obvious way in which the agency's skills and resources can be brought to bear, and the results of this effort will be followed with particular interest. Again, the amount and effect of frontloading of the process needs to be carefully compared against the results when they become available.

24.3.4.2 Avoid premature requirements for experimental drug development tools, and eliminate quickly requirements that are obsolete

The possibility that new tools of drug development can shorten timelines, reduce costs and improve success rates is exciting, and has attracted the interest of the FDA, industry and academia. We applaud the efforts to discover, test and validate such things as surrogate endpoints, biomarkers, pharmacogenomics, *in silico* testing and new laboratory and animal models for specific toxicity risks. At the same time, care should be taken to prevent enthusiasm from becoming routine expectations. For example, much faith is currently held for the potential effects of biomarkers, including genomic and other molecular markers, in improving the quality of targets and drug candidates, their progression through early development, and their tailoring to specific types of patients. Apart from examples in cancer therapeutics and a few such as those mentioned above, these promises are still somewhat hypothetical. It is probably too early to suggest that pharmacogenomics be integrated into every drug development programme.

We recommend that efforts be directed instead into government and industry efforts to assess and validate the tools in specific (and clinically important) situations. The FDA's Critical Path Initiative has focused on this process already, and is to be encouraged.

At the same time, industry and regulators should be vigilant for opportunities to get rid of testing requirements that have proven useless, redundant or outdated. When identified, they should be removed quickly. We should not repeat the extended period of time that it took to free industry from routine LD_{50} toxicity tests in laboratory animals, even when the precision sought in such studies was unnecessary for product development.

24.3.4.3 Observational and 'naturalistic' studies

The inclusion–exclusion criteria needed in formal clinical trials inevitably produce experimental populations that are not typical of patient populations in routine medical practice. More attention therefore needs to be paid to the 'naturalistic' study of drugs, after marketing, in general clinical practice. Such studies could lead to an increased understanding of both effectiveness and risk in the intended patient population. Benefits will almost certainly accrue by identifying, for example, empiric relations between genomic make-up and drug response, with the possibility of increasing benefit or decreasing harm. Progress in this area is unfortunately predicted too optimistically at present by scientists who should be aware of the length of time that will be required to achieve these goals, but nevertheless ultimate progress will be made if we apply ourselves to the task.

24.3.4.4 Incentives for obtaining new indications for older drugs

We have already discussed using incentives based on wider use of provisional approval.

Because some additional uses may only be discovered late in a drug's patent life (or even after the patent has expired), a company may be reluctant to spend the time and money to obtain formal FDA approval of new uses primarily to benefit generic manufacturers. Optimal medical practice, however, calls for access to sound and persuasive data on new indications for older drugs. Some method needs to be found to encourage sponsors to seek new indications during more of a product's patent life and – if possible – beyond.

The success of the various special-case incentives for drug development, such as for orphan drugs, for cancer, antibiotic, tropical disease and AIDS drugs, and for paediatric studies, could be a guide to how to approach – and what to avoid – in facilitating larger approaches to the development of new indications in the future.

24.4 Conclusions

After a difficult decade following the 1962 Amendments, the pharmaceutical industry and the FDA have in general worked well together, and the four decades from 1970 to 2008 mark an era of unparalleled achievement in the modernisation of drug development and approval. The present system has achieved much in its near half-century of operation. Nevertheless, it is becoming in part a victim of its own successes, as the once finely balanced processes are now paradoxically coming closer to bogging down under the weight of continually increasing requirements from many directions – particularly regulatory – in both the pharmaceutical industry and the FDA.

In the last 15 years, bigger cracks have become obvious in the system, just when it should be getting more efficient and faster. The pharmaceutical industry's output of new drugs has slowed despite unprecedented investment in discovery and development; and at the same time the industry, and the drug development and marketing process itself, has acquired the most negative public image ever, mainly because of pricing, marketing and safety issues. The FDA, too, has come under criticism over drug safety questions, in part because of communication problems.

The causes of this unfortunate state of affairs are numerous, and require a variety of solutions as we have described. Defining the roles of the industry and government in the pursuit of effective new therapies and their appropriate use is one of the areas where attention is needed in the future.

The pharmaceutical industry itself may be partially responsible for the increasing burdens in drug development. For example, its well-honed coping skills – evolved to respond to the tendency for society to pile on regulatory requirements and for the industry to cope with almost any challenge thrust upon it – have hindered the confrontations necessary to identify the problems and construct reforms. Thus, the system has accreted ever more obligations for the industry and for the FDA, without positive challenges to simplify the system.

International harmonisation may also risk becoming an effort that goes beyond its original aims, extending to create new regulations and – worse still – to become a self-perpetuating bureaucracy in itself. Some international safety consortia have developed similar expansionist activities. A key element in harmonization was the reservation of the right of each party to add requirements to those set by the multinational process. Unfortunately, domestic politics and national bureaucracies present a risk that divergent supplemental rules will be developed, which not only defeats the original purpose of the harmonisation efforts, but could easily result in new problems. Overall, the regulatory bodies have made considerable efforts to support the spirit of harmonisation; but in practice they continue to devolve interpretations of some of the policies to the individual countries. For example, the FDA proposed safety reporting regulations containing definitions for periodic safety update reports that deviate from the generally expected formats already adopted in many other countries under the International Conference on Harmonization (ICH) process.

More aggressive reforms are needed if pharmaceutical and regulatory agencies are to serve the public optimally. In this chapter we have considered how some of these hindrances – in particular, regulation of early drug development and also at the approval stage – could be addressed. As we have shown, there are:

1. Large parts of early IND research (phases I and IIa) that have become routine and could be safely deregulated, under appropriate controls, with beneficial effects; and

2. Considerable benefits that could be achieved at the NDA approval stage, simply by combining approval earlier in the development process with the existing available safeguards in drug utilisation controls necessary to guarantee safe use, until enough experience is obtained to relax the initial marketing restrictions.

There are many other areas that need to be addressed in addition to the ones we have considered here.

In summary, the main reforms we have suggested – involving both the IND and NDA, are a start, but much more is needed to adjust the pharmaceutical industry's productivity to the needs of society, while preserving the safety and effectiveness standards. Drug development and regulation will continue to be an interesting ride through the twenty-first century.

Acknowledgements

The authors wish to acknowledge the contributions of their friend and colleague Dr Louis Lasagna to the field of clinical pharmacology and to its wider applications in regulation, drug development and pharmaceutical medicine. Dr Lasagna contributed to previous editions of this chapter, and much of his writing is still in this edition. He died in August 2003.

References

1 Wood A. A proposal for radical changes in the drug-approval process. *N Engl J Med* 2006;355:618–23.
2 DiMasi JA, Manocchia M. Initiatives to speed new drug development and regulatory review: the impact of FDA-sponsor conferences. *Drug Info J* 1997;31:771–8.

Further reading

Center for the Study of Drug Development, Tufts University: *Outlook 2004* and other publications.
DiMasi JA. Risks in new drug development: approval success rates for investigational drugs. *Clin Pharmacol Ther* 2001;69:297–307.
DiMasi JA. The value of improving the productivity of the drug development process: faster times and better decisions. *PharmacoEcon* 2002;20:1–10.
DiMasi JA, Grabowski HG, Vernon J. R&D costs and returns by therapeutic category. *Drug Info J* 2004;38:211–23.
DiMasi JA, Hansen RW, Grabowski HG. The price of innovation: new estimates of drug development costs. *J Health Econ* 2003;22:151–85.
DiMasi JA, Paquette C. The economics of follow on drug development: trends in entry rates and the timing of development. *PharmacoEcon* 2004;22:1–14.
Food and Drug Administration. *Innovation, Stagnation: Challenge and Opportunity on the Critical Path to New Medical Products.* March 2004.
Food and Drug Administration Modernization Act of 1997 (FDAMA).
Food and Drug Administration Amendments Act of 2007 (FDAAA).
Jones JK. Joint Commission on prescription drug use. In: Velo G, Wardell W, eds. *Drug Development, Regulatory Assessment and Post Marketing Surveillance.* New York/London: Plenum Press, 1981;191–200.
Jones JK. Broader uses of post-marketing surveillance. In: Velo G, Wardell W, eds. *Drug Development, Regulatory Assessment and Post Marketing Surveillance.* New York/London: Plenum Press, 1981;203–16.
Jones JK. National/international systems for post marketing surveillance. In: Velo G, Wardell W, eds. *Drug*

Development, Regulatory Assessment and Post Marketing Surveillance. New York/London: Plenum Press, 1981;233–40.

Jones JK. Regulatory use of adverse reactions. In: *Detection and Prevention of Adverse Drug Reactions.* 1983 International Symposium, Stockholm, Skandia International Symposia, Almquist and Wiksall International, Stockholm, 1984;203–14.

Jones JK, Faich GA, Anello C. Post-marketing surveillance in the general population – the USA. In: Inman WH, ed. *Monitoring for Drug Safety,* 2nd edn. Lancaster, UK: MTP Press, 1985;153–63.

Jones JK, Idanpaan-Heikkila JE. Adverse reactions, post-marketing surveillance and pharmacoepidemiology. In: Burley DM, Clarke JM, Lasagna L, Edward Arnold, eds. *Pharmaceutical Medicine.* Hodder & Stoughton, 1993; 145–80.

Kaitin K, Cairns C. The new drug approvals of 1999, 2000, and 2001: drug development trends a decade after passage of the prescription Drug User Fee Act of 1992. *Drug Info J* 2003;4:357–71.

Lasagna L. Who will adopt the orphan drugs? *Regulation* 1979;3:27–32.

McMahon Commission Report. Commission on the Federal Drug Approval Process. Final Report 1982.

Normile D. The promise and pitfalls of clinical trials overseas. *Science* 2008;322:214–6.

Reichart J. Biopharmaceutical approvals in the US increase. *Regul Aff J Pharma* 2004;15:1–7.

Temple R. Special study designs: early escape, enrichment, studies in non-responders. *Commun Stat Theory Methods* 1994;23:499–531.

Temple R. Are surrogate markers adequate to assess cardiovascular disease drugs? *JAMA* 1999;282:790–5.

Temple R. Policy developments in regulatory approval. *Stat Med* 2002;21:2939–48.

Temple R, Ellenberg S. Placebo-controlled trials and active-control trials in the evaluation of new treatments. *Ann Intern Med* 2000;133:455–63.

Wardell W. The Drug Lag and American therapeutics: an international comparison. 22nd International Congress of Pharmacology, San Francisco, 1972.

Wardell W. Therapeutic implications of the drug lag. *Clin Pharmacol Ther* 1973;14:1022–34.

Wardell W, ed. *Controlling the Use of Therapeutic Drugs: An International Comparison,* Washington, DC: American Enterprise Institute for Public Policy Research, 1978.

Wardell W, Lasagna L. *Regulation and Drug Development.* Washington, DC: American Enterprise Institute for Public Policy Research, 1975.

Wood A. Improving the drug development process through 'economic Darwinism'. *N Engl J Med* 2008;355:618–23.

www.FDA.gov (The history section of the FDA's website is particularly informative.)

25 Regulatory and clinical trial systems in Japan

Yuichi Kubo[*]

Traslational Medicine and Clinical Pharmacology, Daiichi Sankyo Co. Ltd, Tokyo, Japan

25.1 Introduction

Japan is the second largest country in terms of pharmaceutical market, with a population exceeding 120 million. The importance of this market has long been recognised, but many pharmaceutical companies have excluded this particular area from their global development strategy. One reason for such an omission is Japan's unique marketing and distributing rules which handicap newcomers. Another obstacle was the Japanese notion that they were unique and different in every aspect from the rest of world, and therefore clinical data obtained in other countries were not applicable to the Japanese population.

The marketing and distributing rules in Japan have become almost identical to those in the West, and Good Clinical Practice (GCP) is updated in line with the International Conference on Harmonisation (ICH) GCP. ICH discussion on ethnic factors established a concept that foreign clinical data are accepted for a new drug application (NDA) if there are no concerns about ethnic differences in the effects or adverse effects of the product. In addition, the Japanese authorities compiled their concept towards involvement of Japanese clinical sites into global clinical trials.[1]

Because of these changes, many multinational pharmaceutical companies now include the Japanese market in their global development and marketing strategies. It is important to understand, however, that there are still some peculiarities for conducting clinical trials in Japan. These are because of the differences in medical practice and/or attitude of the Japanese people towards effects and side effects of medicinal products, which may not harmonise with the West in a short period of time. Therefore, it is important to conduct a careful feasibility study before commencing clinical trials in Japan if global development is planned.

25.2 Regulatory systems

25.2.1 Introduction

The procedures described below are essentially those that apply to the approval of ethical pharmaceutical products containing new chemical entities. Procedures for approval of drugs containing agents already listed in the Japanese pharmacopoeia, or modified drug formulations of already approved ones, or are *in vitro* diagnostic agents, are all subject to slightly different procedures. For a full description of these variations the reader is referred to *Drug Approval and Licensing Procedures in Japan*.[2]

The basis of the regulatory review and the clinical trial system was established in 1977 after significant amendment of the Pharmaceutical Affairs Law. Also, the revised GCP based on ICH has become a legal requirement, effective from 1 April 1997. A clinical trial review procedure has been instigated with a 30-day review period before trial initiation. Although clinical trial applications were previously sent to the Ministry of Health, Labour and Welfare (MHLW), the hospital and in-house institutional review boards (IRBs) also undertook active review.

Responsibility for regulatory review has been passed to an incorporated administrative agency, the Pharmaceutical and Medical Devices Agency (PMDA). The PMDA also intensively checks applications for GCP and reliability compliance. Another important

---

[*] The views expressed in this chapter are those of the author and not necessarily those of Daiichi Sankyo Co. Ltd.

The Textbook of Pharmaceutical Medicine. Edited by John P. Griffin. © 2009, ISBN: 978-1-4051-8035-1.

role of the PMDA is providing advice to sponsors on clinical trials and on which data should be submitted at the time of an NDA.

25.2.2 Type of approvals

Until March 2005, approvals fell into three categories: manufacturing approvals, import approvals and foreign manufacturing approvals. This has been changed from April 2005. Approval is no longer granted for manufacturing, import or foreign manufacturing, but for marketing, in line with the approval system of Western countries. This change of the approval system has no direct effect on the clinical trial system, but may provide opportunities for a foreign manufacturer seeking marketing opportunities in Japan.

25.2.3 Review process

The procedure by which applications are reviewed is described below and for all new drugs is shown schematically in Figure 25.1.

Applications for marketing should be sent to the MHLW. The application then passes to the PMDA, where the application splits into two different routes:

1. Good Laboratory Practice (GLP), GCP and reliability compliance check by the Office of Conformity Audit; and

2. Application review by the Offices of New Drugs or Office of Biologics.

First, the Office of Conformity Audit will conduct a compliance review to ensure that the dossier meets the standards of GCP, GLP and reliability. The GCP

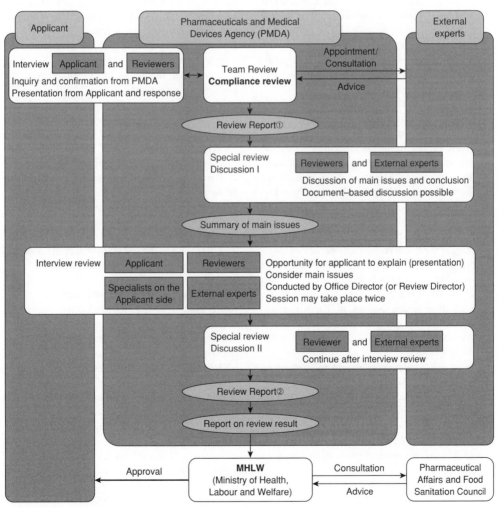

Figure 25.1 Review process for pharmaceuticals and medical devices.

compliance check is based on the inspection of both study sites and sponsor. For the submission of new active substance usually four study sites are inspected. If the pivotal studies are conducted overseas, the inspection may be conducted by the MHLW instead of the PMDA.

As well as GCP site inspections, an examination is undertaken of the raw or source data and records of Chemistry Manufacturing and Control (CMC), non-clinical and clinical reports that form the basis of the application. This is to ensure that the application dossier accurately reflects the source data. The procedure issued by the PMDA details that list of raw data and records must be provided. The applicant is required to bring the data and records to the PMDA on the specified days and when the examination finishes they should be retrieved. Therefore, the raw data and records stored at overseas sites are usually categorised as 'documents not to be submitted' and not subject to reliability review by the PMDA. Instead, the MHLW may investigate the data from non-Japanese studies at the site of storage because submission of a photocopy of the data is not permitted.

Review of the submission dossier will begin simultaneously with this compliance check. Review is undertaken by one of the four evaluation office teams, which comprised experts from medicine, pharmaceutical sciences, veterinary sciences and statistics. The team also includes external experts. Evaluation meetings are held at which questions are raised by the reviewing team and the applicant has the opportunity to discuss issues with the reviewers. The reviewer in charge will prepare a report of the application for the next stage of the special review and interview.

Once the PDMA review is completed, the result is reported to the Evaluation and Licensing Division of the MHLW. The report is then submitted to the Pharmaceutical Affairs Section of Pharmaceutical Affairs and Food Sanitation Council (PAFSC). Upon positive advice from the PAFSC, the minister of the MHLW grants approval.

The period required from receipt to approval of the application is treated as that for handling of the standard clerical service, except for replying to PAFSC enquiries and for correcting incomplete applications. The period for handling by the standard clerical service is 12 months. The applicant also has another 12 months to respond to queries and requests from the agency.

25.2.4 Effort to diminish 'drug lag'

Several surveys have showed that many drugs that contain new chemical entities are not available in Japan whereas they are elsewhere in the world. This non-availability is often called 'drug lag' and attributed mainly to the long period required for conducting clinical trials and for review after submission, and partly to the limited number of Japanese patients with the indication (therefore pharmaceutical companies may consider that the drug is not commercially feasible). The MHLW and PMDA are struggling to increase the number of reviewers to minimize the drug lag owing to the long review period, in addition to the implementation of the following review mechanisms.

25.2.4.1 Priority review

The priority review is applicable for orphan drugs, orphan medical devices and 'innovative drugs or medical devices that have been authorised to be highly necessary from a medical standpoint'. The standards to define orphan drugs are as follow:

1. Patient numbers with the disease indicated for the drug concerned is less than 50,000;
2. Exceptional usefulness of the drug from the medical standpoint; and
3. The development and the future use of the drug is fairly feasible.

The criteria for 'innovative drugs' other than the orphan drugs are that:

1. The indicated diseases are serious; and
2. The drug is clinically significantly superior to existing product.

The priority review system places the product in front of the review product queue and by this means expedites approval. It is important to note that there is no intention in the system to reduce the scientific standard or quality of the application data.

25.2.4.2 Approval of new indication without clinical trials

In the case in which a drug has been approved and marketed in Japan but lacks some indications approved elsewhere, a supplemental new drug application (sNDA) may be accepted without conducting clinical trials in Japan. Such sNDA are permitted when the drug meets the either of the following criteria:

1. The indications are approved by a foreign regulatory authority and the drug has been administered to a considerable number of patients with the relevant indication, and the submission dossier (or reliable scientific literature) is available for review; or
2. Efficacy and safety of the drug are supported with the results of clinical trials conducted by reliable academic or official organisation(s).

25.2.5 Data requirements for marketing approval in Japan

The data requirements for the application of new drugs were defined in the Pharmaceutical Affairs, Law and its Enforcement Regulations. Practical guidelines were issued in Pharmaceutical and Medicine Safety Bureau (PMSB) Director General Notification No. 481 dated 8 April 1999, *On Application for Drug Approval* and PMSB/ELD Notification No. 666 dated 8 April 1999, *On Requirements for Application for Drug Approval*, followed by ICH Common Technical Document (CTD) guidelines, PMSB Director General Notification No. 481 dated 21 June 2001, *On Application for Drug Approval* and PMSB Notification No. 899 dated 21 June 2001, *On Requirements for Application for Drug Approval.*

The various data, which must be submitted with applications for approval to manufacture ethical drugs, were specified in these notifications.

The application should be in the format of common technical document (CTD), which became mandatory from July 2003. The regional specific requirements are in the Modules 1 and 5 of CTD, which are described below.

25.2.5.1 Module 1

• NDA application form (format based on Pharmaceutical Affairs Law Enforcement Regulations);
• Certificates (including statement by a responsible person supervising collection and preparation of application data, documents related to GLP and GCP, copy of a written contract of co-development);
• Patent status information;
• Origin, background of the discovery and research and development (R&D) history (formerly in the first part of Gaiyo. This can be described in Module 2 instead of in Module 1);
• Status of use in foreign countries;
• List of other pharmaceuticals with similar pharmacological effect(s) and/or indications(s);
• Draft package insert (labelling);
• Documentation of non-proprietary name;
• Format for designation of poisonous/deleterious pharmaceutical ingredients;
• Draft for post-marketing surveillance including pharmacovigilance planning; and
• List of information/documents complied in the dossier.

In addition to Section 5.3.7 of Module 5, *Case Report Forms and Individual Patients Listing*, the following tabulations and charts are required:

• List of patients enrolled in the pivotal clinical trials including dose ranging studies and randomised controlled studies;
• List of patients who reported adverse reactions in all the submitted clinical trials;
• List of patients with serious adverse events in all the submitted clinical trials;
• List of patients in whom laboratory abnormal changes were observed in all the submitted clinical trials; and
• The charts that illustrate the change of laboratory tests in all the submitted clinical trials.

If any consultation with the PMDA (or formerly Drug Organisation) took place, the official records should be incorporated into Module 5.4.

Module 2 is termed Gaiyo (which means 'summary' in Japanese) as before and should be prepared in Japanese except for the figures and tables, if they are accompanied with translation of titles, legends and keywords. The original English reports are accepted in Modules 3–5 and a Japanese summary is no longer required.

After the approval of the product, the sponsor is requested to disclose Gaiyo to the public except for the parts containing trade secrets and private information. The electronic version of Gaiyo for disclosure can be obtained from: http://www.info.pmda.go.jp/info/syounin_index.html. (Please note that the homepage is written in Japanese.)

25.2.7 Clinical trial consultation

The PMDA consults with the sponsors on the protocol and the issues relating to drug development. There are a number of categories of consultations for drug development stages, starting from pre-phase I to pre-NDA and other consultations (Table 25.1). These consultations should be based on the scientific knowledge of the product obtained within the consultation time and should answer the queries of sponsors either on the design of study protocol, concepts

Table 25.1 List of major consultation meetings offered by the Pharmaceutical and Medical Devices Agency (PMDA), as of April 2008

Category	Fee (in Japanese Yen)
Pre-phase I meeting	4,239,400
Pre-early phase II meeting	1,623,000
Pre-late phase II meeting	3,028,400
End of phase II meeting	6,011,500
Pre-NDA meeting	6,011,400

of development or rationale for submission. The consultations provide the merits of both the Food and Drug Administration (FDA) meetings and the European Medicines Agency (EMEA) scientific advice. The consultation is chargeable and the fee is shown in the Table 25.1. The PMDA prepares the official records of the consultation, which is attached to the new drug application and will be considered by the reviewers.

25.3 Clinical trial systems

25.3.1 Introduction

Based on Step 4 of the ICH GCP guideline of May 1996, the Japanese authority issued *MHLW Ordinance of the Standards for Good Clinical Practice* on 27 March 1997 and the current version was recently revised on 29 February 2008. In Japan, GCP is based on the revised Pharmaceutical Affairs Law of June 1996, which requires that the data for new drug applications are obtained according to the standards set by the ministry, and therefore it is legally obligatory to adhere to the GCP in conducting clinical trials in Japan.

GCP follows the ICH GCP guideline but some unique aspects are added in order to cope with Japanese medical and clinical practices. Although some modifications have been made, the concept of the ICH guidelines is maintained, and this caused substantial change in clinical trial practice in Japan. The unique aspects of Japanese GCP and clinical trial practice are explained in the sections below.

25.3.2 Sponsor

GCP requires the sponsor to be fully responsible for all aspects of the clinical trial. This responsibility includes preparation of the clinical trial protocol, selection of investigators and study centres, monitoring and auditing, and writing the clinical trial reports. Previously, most of the responsibility for conduct of the clinical trial fell upon the chief investigator and, in a sense, the sponsoring company was immune from such responsibility. This mechanism deprived Japanese pharmaceutical companies of incentives to build medical and other expertise within the company. As many Japanese pharmaceutical companies have little expertise in the clinical area, the GCP guidelines require the sponsor to organise a study team consisting of specialists for a variety of aspects.

25.3.3 Medical adviser

There is serious shortage of medically qualified personnel including physicians in Japanese pharmaceutical companies; worse is the fact that they do not recognise the importance of such expertise in-house. GCP requires sponsoring companies to either employ or contract medical professionals in order to obtain medical advice in preparing protocols and conducting clinical trials.

25.3.4 Other specialists

Other specialists include biostatisticians, regulatory affairs personnel, pharmacokineticists, medical writers and so on, but GCP does not specify those specialists. If the sponsoring company does not possess such expertise, the sponsor can give it on contract.

25.3.5 Sponsor's in-house clinical trial review board

The government had required that the sponsors should have their own in-house clinical trial review board to review the ethical aspects of clinical trial protocols. Such a requirement was based on the former Japanese GCP (effective until 1996), which stipulated that the company should organise an internal formal body or mechanism that reviews and authorises its planned studies before submitting to either study centres or the MHLW for clinical trial plan notification.

The new Japanese GCP no longer contains a clause to this effect, but it seems that the authorities favour the sponsor maintaining the procedures for an in-house clinical trial review board and determining the appropriateness of the planned studies.

25.3.6 Contract research organisations

Contract research organisations (CROs) are formally recognised in Japanese GCP regulations, as it explicitly stipulates that the sponsor may contract all or some parts of clinical trial activity to contract bodies, and in such a case the contract between the sponsor and the study site should be executed between the sponsor, the study site and the CRO. Many CROs have been established because of heavy demand of trial monitors and data management specialists by sponsoring companies; further growth of CROs in terms of number and size is expected.

25.3.7 Protocol development

For confirmation studies, a single objective, clinically meaningful endpoint should be identified. Where an objective endpoint cannot be found, subjective endpoints can be used instead. If the endpoint is not well established or subjective, it must be validated. Study investigators or others who are involved in evaluation should be well trained, and their variation of evaluation results should be within an acceptable range.

Surrogate endpoints should be carefully chosen, if they are required. Some surrogate endpoints, such as blood pressure in hypertension, low-density lipoprotein cholesterol in hyperlipidaemia, forced expiratory volume in 1 minute in asthma or haemoglobin A1c in diabetes mellitus, are well established and can be used in the confirmatory studies. Conducting a true endpoint study is difficult if it is not incorporated into the global study because patient recruitment is still slow in Japan and hence relatively small numbers of study participants will be achieved within a reasonable time-frame.

25.3.8 Guidelines

It is always advised to check whether there is a specific guideline for evaluating a given medicinal product in the area of interest. Most of the study guidelines have not been updated for a long time in spite of authority's effort to revise them, and caution should be exercised to confirm that the contents therein are already obsolete and therefore invalid.

The agency had requested sponsors to adhere strictly to the guidelines, but now it explicitly warns sponsors that the guidelines were the guidelines at the time of their issue and the latest scientific standard will be applied when the agency reviews an NDA.

25.3.9 Study design

A double-blind randomised controlled study is recommended for the confirmatory study unless there are appropriate scientific reasons not to do so. In many cases, an active comparator is preferred to an inactive placebo as a control, as evidence of similar efficacy to the premium priced product will be an advantage for obtaining a favourable reimbursement price. Nevertheless, choice of the placebo has been increasing to demonstrate absolute efficacy of the drug and has been accepted by many study sites.

If conducting multinational studies in Japan, choice of an active comparator may be a difficult issue. There are many products that are not available, or their indication, dose and dosage or conditions of use are different from other countries.

25.3.10 Selection of study centres and investigators

25.3.10.1 Study site

GCP requires clinical trial sites to have adequate facilities to conduct clinical trials and be able to handle any clinical emergency. Adequately trained staff

should be available. The sites must prepare standard operating procedures (SOPs) for accepting, reviewing and operating the clinical trial. These requirements have been defined as the minimum requirements for any clinical trial to be conducted, in hospitals equipped with ample resources to manage many SOPs and office staff for clinical trials.

However, GCP also stipulates requirements when clinical sites contract out the above activities. By this means the trial-related offices can be established among a collection of study sites if the sites are those of general practitioners or small clinics. The contractors are called site management organisations (SMOs), which establish a network of clinical trial sites and provide faster patient recruitment capability in therapeutic areas for general practitioners or small clinics.

25.3.10.2 Number of patients at each site

An adequate number of patients per centre (e.g. 10 patients) is needed to confirm treatment-by-centre interaction in a multicentre clinical trial; however, some centres find it difficult to accommodate this number. This finding is supported by recent statistics which showed the number of patients recruited per centre is relatively small in Japan compared with other countries in global clinical trials.

If the number of patients at each centre is small, doctors cannot gain experience in the study and they cannot compare the responses of patients to the study medications. Study monitors have to cover a wide geographical area and a large number of study-related personnel in order to monitor a relatively small number of patients.

Rigorous efforts are being made to initiate and maintain clinical trial site networks in order to recruit ample numbers of patients by a variety of medical profession bodies and the private sector. It is always advisable to consider such networks when conducting clinical trials in Japan.

25.3.10.3 Institutional review board

GCP guidelines have expanded the IRB constitution and its role in the clinical trial. The IRB must consist of more than five members and must include non-medical personnel and someone not employed by the study centre. There are no requirements regarding gender balance. The head of the institute can attend the IRB meetings but cannot be a member nor discuss or vote at the meeting.

The IRB is responsible for reviewing protocols, the informed consent sheet, the investigator's brochure and other materials relating to the conduct of clinical trials. The IRB is also responsible for monitoring whether the clinical trials are conducted in compliance with both GCP and the IRBs requirements, if any. When the study period of a clinical trial exceeds 1 year the IRB should review the study every year. As GCP allows the study sponsor to pay a reasonable amount of money to the study subjects, the IRB is expected to review whether the amount and method of payment is reasonable and does not infringe upon the ethical aspects of the study. Also, the advertisement of a trial for patient recruitment is allowed, but the IRB's approval to implement this at the study centre is required.

By the recent amendment of GCP in February 2008, requirement for establishing an in-house IRB has been abolished and the head of institution can request a clinical trial review to any IRB that he or she considers appropriate. An IRB can be established in-house by the head of the institution, or more than two heads of different medical institutions with collaboration, or other medical organizations that are stipulated by the amended GCP.

IRBs are required to publish their operating procedures, names of review board members and the summary of review meetings.

25.3.10.4 Investigators
GCP clarifies the role of investigators. They are expected to take an active part in the study from the planning stage. Previously, the number of patients and the study protocols were allotted to each centre by the chief investigator, but now it is the responsibility of investigators as to whether they accept the protocol and the number of patients to be recruited, and then take part in the study.

Preparation of the patient informed consent sheet is the responsibility of each investigator, although support of the sponsor is requested. The investigator can nominate sub-investigators and other supportive staff for the study and establish a study team. The member list of the study team should be submitted to, and confirmed by, the head of the institute. The investigator should endorse the study protocol and the study contract, and must comply with them. Any deviations from the protocol should be recorded and reported to both the head of the institute and the sponsor.

Selection of study investigators is difficult and involves many factors. Among the factors, possible patient recruitment is the most important. It is not easy to predict patient recruitment at the time of protocol discussion, because the attitude of patients

towards clinical trials may not be entirely in favour of participation. Whether the study site is acceptable in the light of GCP is another important issue for the investigators. Although many centres are 'GCP compliant', close monitoring is required to confirm that such status is maintained during the conduct of the clinical trial. GCP system in hospitals is maintained by a small number of competent staff, mostly by pharmacy staff, and therefore the retirement or movement of the main staff may change the situation.

25.3.11 Clinical trial plan notification
An outline of the data from non-clinical studies must be submitted to the PMDA with the protocol for the proposed clinical trial before it is commenced. A notification is required for each protocol. The list of items required for clinical trial plan notification is shown in Box 25.1. Furthermore, supplementary data must be added on entry to subsequent clinical development phases. Such data are reviewed by the PMDA, and for this purpose the sponsor must wait for 30 days after submitting the initial notification before executing a contract with the medical institute. For a subsequent notification, the review period is reduced to 14 days. The notification also requires the names of all investigators, whether investigators or sub-investigators, and this list of investigators must be kept updated throughout the study period.

25.3.12 Contracts and funding
25.3.12.1 Head of study centre
Japanese GCP requires that the head of the medical institute and the sponsor execute a study contract, and does not allow the investigator to directly contract with the sponsor. Historically, a clinical trial is considered as an activity of the hospital as a whole, not

---

BOX 25.1 List of items required for clinical trial plan notification

- Description of trial drug
- Manufacturing method
- Anticipated indications, dose and dosage
- Purpose of trial
- Trial details including study period
- Name and address of each study centre
- Names of all investigators
- Name and address of establishing body of each institutional review board
- Amount of clinical supply for each centre
- Reasons if the supply is free of charge
- (Name and address of local clinical trial manager)

of an individual investigator. The reason behind this is that the investigator cannot conduct any study without the full support of hospital staff and access to hospital facilities. The head of the medical institute is responsible for selecting an IRB where the clinical trial documents are reviewed. Once the sponsoring company submits the clinical trial plan to the hospital, the head of the medical institute should submit the study document to the IRB for their opinion. The head cannot be a member of the IRB, is not allowed to discuss or vote on the clinical trial, but nevertheless attendance to the IRB is not prohibited.

The head of the medical institute should sign the study contract after receiving a favourable opinion from the IRB. The head cannot accept the study if the IRB decision is not favourable.

GCP stipulates essential clauses of the contract (Box 25.2).

BOX 25.2 Essential clauses of the contract between study sponsor and medical institution

- Date of contract
- Name and address of person sponsoring the clinical trial
- In the case where part of the work is entrusted to a contract research organisation (CRO), name and address of CRO, and range of the work entrusted
- Name and address of medical institution
- Name and title of persons responsible for contract
- Names and titles of investigators and others
- Period of clinical trial
- Target number of subjects
- Matters related to control of clinical trial drugs
- Matters related to preservation of records (including data)
- Matters related to report by sponsor and persons engaged at medical institution pursuant to Good Clinical Practice (GCP)
- Matters related to conservation of subjects' privacy
- Matters related to costs of clinical trials
- Statement that medical institution conduct the clinical trial in conformity with the protocol
- Statement that medical institution allow access to records (including documents) specified by GCP at the request of the sponsor
- In the case where it is evident that the medical institution adversely interfered with the proper clinical trial by violating GCP, protocol or the contract, the sponsor can cancel the contract
- Matters related to compensation to health damage to subjects
- Other matters necessary for ensuring that the clinical trial can be conducted properly and smoothly

---

The head of the institute must appoint a study drug manager, a document archiving manager and administration staff for clinical trials. In order to handle clinical trials in such a complex structure, SOPs for conducting clinical trials must be prepared at the hospital.

All serious adverse events, deviations from the protocol, extensions of study period or increase in patient numbers should be reported to the head of the institute by the investigator.

25.3.12.2 Clinical trial funding

The regulations on clinical trial funding differ among hospitals based on their background. For example, in the National Hospitals Organization there is a standard table which categorises clinical trial activities. To calculate the study budget, the activities are added up for each protocol and some hospital overheads, which cover general management costs, are also added. The entire study points are then multiplied by the index to change the points into actual currency. Private university hospitals set a similar rule but with higher overheads.

25.3.13 Ethical issues

25.3.13.1 Informed consent

Based on the ICH guidelines, written fully informed consent is required for all participating patients. If the patient cannot consent as a result of his or her health condition, a responsible caretaker is allowed to give consent in lieu of the patient.

The investigator should prepare an informed consent form for every study to be performed at the institute and should obtain an approval by the IRB that covers the institute. GCP lists a dozen points to be covered by the informed consent form (Box 25.3). GCP allows a reasonable amount of payment to the patient, such as transport costs. Patients should allow clinical trial monitors, auditors, IRB members and inspectors from the regulatory authority to verify the source documents. This requirement of obligatory written informed consent was regarded as a major challenge to the conduct of clinical trials in Japan, because Japanese patients were usually not informed of their medications and were unaware of possible outcomes or side effects. As this had been the normal practice in Japan for many years, patients did not expect any detailed explanation of their conditions, or to participate in decision-making of treatment choices. Also, it must be borne in mind that in Japan verbal agreements or contracts had been widely accepted, not only in the clinical setting, but also in

BOX 25.3 Items required in the informed consent form

- The fact that the clinical trial is conducted as a test
- Purpose of the clinical trial
- Name and title of the investigator, and contact site
- Methods of the clinical trial
- Anticipated efficacy of the clinical trial drugs and anticipated disadvantage to the subject
- Matters on other therapeutic methods
- Duration of participation in the clinical trial
- The fact that participation in the clinical trial can be withdrawn at any time
- The fact that the subject is never placed at any disadvantage by refusing to participate or withdrawal of participation
- The fact that monitor, auditor and the institutional review board can have access to source data on condition that the confidentiality of the subjects is kept
- The fact that confidentiality related to the subject is kept
- Contact site of the medical institution in case of health damage
- The fact that necessary treatment will be provided in the case of health damage
- Matters on compensation to health damage
- Type of institutional review board that reviews the study protocol, matters reviewed by the board and any other related matters on the board

society in general. It is easily imaginable in such an environment that patients might be frightened by a very detailed explanation of the disease, possible options of treatment including study drug, possible side effects (sometimes including fatalities) and compensation policy.

More recently, informed consent has become much more popular, not only for clinical trials, but also for everyday medical practice, and patients are now much more accustomed to giving their consent. Clinical trials have become more visible to the general public and the media reports studies with potential therapeutic benefit in a favourable manner.

25.3.13.2 Patient recruitment

Pharmaceutical Affairs Law prohibits advertisement of non-approved drugs (i.e. clinical trial drugs). However, if the study drug is not identified, the sponsor can advertise the clinical trial in order to recruit patients.

Similarly, hospitals were not able to advertise their involvement in clinical trials. There are detailed regu-

lations as to what hospitals can advertise, and these were amended in April 2001 so that hospitals can recruit patients by means of mass media.

Patient recruitment advertisements often appear in major newspapers or leaflets, which are delivered with newspapers, as most households subscribe one or more major newspapers. Some CROs established call centres to handle patient or volunteer applications or queries regarding the clinical trial and introduction of participating hospitals.

25.3.13.3 Payment to the participating patients

Participation in a clinical trial should be voluntary and there will be no payment unless the study provides no therapeutic benefit, such as tolerability and/or pharmacokinetic studies in healthy volunteers. When GCP was introduced, there was substantial discussion whether, in patients required to visit study sites more often than usual – for example, to attend additional examinations or treatments – it would be fair to put all financial burden on the patient.

In Japan, when patients receive medical services they pay 30% of the actual medical cost and the insurer pays the rest. There are ceilings of patient payment, if the patient's own payment exceeds predefined monthly limits or the patient falls into a certain category, such as the elderly or those with diseases designated as 'difficult to treat' by the government. The body of insurers and sponsoring companies agreed that the sponsoring company of the trial must pay:

1. All laboratory costs including radiological imaging during the study period;
2. Concomitant medication costs if such medication is used for the disease of concern in the study.

For this purpose, the study period is defined as 'between the first day of dosing and the last day of dosing'.

In addition, many study sites set rules that patients should be paid for their attendance at clinical examination or treatment during the study. It is roughly considered as the reimbursement of travel costs. There are no statistics on the amount of these payments, but the majority of hospitals set a standard of the equivalent to about £40 for each visit based on the protocol requirements.

25.3.14 Monitoring

GCP requires monitoring and on-site audit including source data verification (SDV) as in the ICH GCP guidelines. The difficulty in circumventing violation of privacy laws (medical law, criminal law and other related regulations) was resolved by obtaining informed consent from the patient that allows sponsor's monitors, auditors, IRB members and inspectors from regulatory authorities to access the source record, provided that the subject's privacy is respected. Furthermore, in most cases, the patient's name and other identifications are masked in order to avoid infringement of the patient's privacy.

The monitors put much emphasis on the SDV, as it is a new concept in Japanese clinical trials. The way case record forms (CRFs) are prepared causes difficult problems in monitoring. Most of the CRFs used in Japan are in the format of booklets with 8–12 pages. Investigators fill them in after completion of each case, or sometimes after completion of all cases. Therefore, there was a vague understanding that the SDV is a *post hoc* confirmation of CRF against the source data. This view is changing and more emphasis is placed on the initiation and ongoing monitoring to confirm that investigators adhere to the study protocol. Visit-type CRFs and electronic CRFs are being introduced in this connection and this becomes possible as sponsors enforce their data management capabilities and study sites and/or investigators introduce clinical trial coordinators.

Once many sponsors started monitoring based on GCP, they found that they were heavily understaffed. In previous times, a monitor was able to take care of 15–20 centres all over Japan. Now, most sponsoring companies consider that the appropriate number of centres per monitor should be around five. This number reflects not only the workload of study site monitoring, but also the complicated study initiation procedures required by GCP and serious adverse reaction reporting procedures as some major hospitals require the personal presence of the monitor to report such events. Sponsors are also aware that there is mismatch in monitors' qualifications, as most of monitors in major pharmaceutical companies are graduates, postgraduates or sometimes doctors in pharmaceutical or biosciences but they are not trained in the bedside setting. Their responsibilities are not limited to monitoring but include study planning, administration and medical writing. Sponsors recognise this is not an ideal situation, and they are introducing more medically trained monitors and separating other activities from them. Also they are increasing the contracting of monitoring activities to CROs.

25.3.15 Clinical research coordinator

It is agreed in Japan that the key person for the successful conduct of clinical trials is the clinical research coordinator (CRC), equivalent to the study nurse or study coordinator. Recently, the role of CRC in clinical trials has become well established and the number of CRCs is gradually increasing.

The role of the CRC is identical to that of European or US counterparts, but perhaps of a more complex nature because of the complicated Japanese GCP and medical system. Many professional bodies, some backed up by regulatory bodies and academia, provide training courses for CRCs and recent statistics showed the number of trainees has exceeded 4500 and activities of these graduates have enhanced the quality and productivity of clinical trials in Japan.

25.3.16 Audit

The new GCP requires that: 'sponsors shall compile plan and operating procedures on auditing and implement auditing in conformity with the plan and the procedures', thus auditors audit not only the sponsor's in-house process, but also processes at study sites. Within the sponsoring company, usually all CRFs and study reports are subject to the audit. Study sites are selected for audit based on auditors' SOP, usually based on sampling methodology. An audit certificate for each clinical trial is required to be incorporated into the new drug submission dossier. The typical sponsor's in-house audit is rigorous and the auditors require strict adherence to GCP clauses.

25.3.17 Serious adverse event reporting

All unexpected, serious and drug-related adverse events should be reported to the MHLW, the investigators and study sites. The requirement to report to the MHLW is identical to ICH guidelines with an additional definition that adverse events include any suspicious infection related to a study drug. This addition reflects the bitter experience of the spread of AIDS among haemophilia patients as a rsult of HIV-contaminated non-heat-treated human plasma products.

The agency reinforces the serious adverse event (SAE) reporting system rigorously during the clinical trial and this is reiterated at the time of GCP inspection. Some hospitals require the chief investigator to acknowledge the report before submitting it to the hospital study office. As the number of study centres for each protocol is rather large in Japan, such a requirement is resource consuming for the sponsoring companies.

The occurrences of study suspension or obtaining additional written informed consent from participating patients based on new SAEs vary from one ethics committee to another. There is no clear rule for this, and the decision of different sponsors whether they would suspend an entire study or not may differ. It is worthwhile to note that the SAE described here is not only life-threatening or of potential harm for the entire study population, but moderate or sometime mild adverse conditions, but, nevertheless, falls within the definition of serious.

25.4 Conclusions

The introduction of GCP and other study practices is aimed at bringing Japanese clinical trials to be accepted by regulatory bodies worldwide. Hospitals, regulatory authorities and pharmaceutical industries have worked to change many aspects of clinical trials, and they are establishing the new clinical trial system. There are considerable improvements in the quality and reliability of clinical trials and the objectives of the GCP are achieved in many ways. As the difference in medical practice or ethnic factors will, nevertheless, still remain, sponsors should consider incorporating such differences into their global development plan.

Acknowledgements

The author thanks Mr Kenichi Hayashi, Alamedic Co. Ltd., for his detailed review and advice. Also Drs Shunichi Sasaki and Hirofumi Nanjo, Clinical Development, Daiichi Sankyo Pharma Development, for their useful suggestions.

References

1 Basic principles on Global Clinical Trials, 2007. Available at http://www.pmda.go.jp/topics/h200110kohyo.html. (Accessed on 1 September 2008.)
2 *Drug Approval and Licensing Procedures in Japan*. Tokyo: Jiho, 2006.
3 Japan Pharmaceutical Manufacturers Association. *Pharmaceutical Administration and Regulation in Japan*. 2008. Available at http://www.jpma.or.jp/english/parj/0803.html.

Further reading

More information on regulatory affairs of Japan in English can be found at the following websites:

http://www.pmda.go.jp/index-e.html
http://www.mhlw.go.jp/english/index.html

26 The regulation of therapeutic products in Australia

Janice Hirshorn[1] and Deborah Monk[2]

1 Consultant, Rose Bay, NSW, Australia
2 Innovation and Industry Policy, Medicines Australia, Deakin, ACT, Australia

26.1 Introduction

The Commonwealth Therapeutic Goods Act 1989 sets out the legal requirements for the import, export, manufacture and supply of therapeutic goods in Australia. It is supported by the Therapeutic Goods Regulations 1990, the Therapeutic Goods (Medical Devices) Regulations 2002 and various orders and determinations. The aim of this legislation is to provide a national framework for the regulation of therapeutic goods in Australia, so as to ensure their quality, safety, efficacy and timely availability.

The Therapeutic Goods Administration (TGA), as part of the Commonwealth Department of Health and Ageing, has the responsibility for administering the Therapeutic Goods Act. It applies a risk management approach to therapeutic goods regulation, which is intended to ensure public health and safety while minimising the regulatory burden and associated costs. The TGA carries out a range of assessment and monitoring activities to ensure that all therapeutic goods available in Australia are of an acceptable standard:

• Pre-market quality, safety and efficacy evaluation of registered medicines, and quality and safety assurance of listed medicines intended for supply in Australia;
• Classification of medical devices based on level of risk and assessing compliance with a set of essential principles for their quality, safety and performance;
• Licensing of manufacturers in accordance with international standards under Good Manufacturing Practice (GMP);
• Post-marketing monitoring, through sampling, adverse event reporting, surveillance activities and response to public inquiries;

• The listing of medicines for export;
• Development, maintenance and monitoring of the systems for the regulation of therapeutic goods.

The term 'therapeutic goods' includes prescription medicines, non-prescription medicines, complementary medicines, medical devices and 'other therapeutic goods', including *in vitro* diagnostic devices (IVDs). The TGA also develops and implements national policies and controls for chemicals, gene technology, blood, tissue and cellular products.

A product's 'risk' is determined by a number of factors, including whether:

• The medicine contains a substance (drug) scheduled in the Standard for the Uniform Scheduling of Drugs and Poisons (SUSDP);
• The medicine's use can result in significant side effects;
• The medicine is used to treat life-threatening or very serious illnesses;
• There may be any adverse effects from prolonged use or inappropriate self-medication.

The scheduling of drugs is regulated under State and Territory (henceforth referred to as State) legislation controlling access to medicines, but is coordinated at a national level to ensure uniformity except in exceptional circumstances. All therapeutic goods must be included as either 'registered' or 'listed' medicines, medical devices or 'other therapeutic goods' in the Australian Register of Therapeutic Goods (ARTG) before they may be supplied in, or exported from, Australia unless they are exempt under the legislation.

Prescription medicines are medicines considered as having a higher level of risk. They must be registered on the ARTG, and the degree of assessment and regulation they undergo is rigorous and detailed, with sponsors being required to provide comprehensive safety, quality and efficacy data. They contain ingredients included in Schedule 4 (prescription) or

The Textbook of Pharmaceutical Medicine. Edited by John P. Griffin. © 2009, ISBN: 978-1-4051-8035-1.

Schedule 8 (controlled drugs) of the SUSDP, or are specified products such as sterile injectables. Biologics fall into the same overall approach – they are not handled separately.

Non-prescription medicines are medicines considered as having a lower level of risk than prescription medicines. They still must be registered on the ARTG, but undergo a lesser degree of evaluation. They contain ingredients included in Schedule 2 (pharmacy-only) or Schedule 3 (pharmacist-supervised supply) of the SUSDP. Non-prescription medicines have frequently been termed over-the-counter (OTC) medicines, and include analgesics, cough and cold products, and sunscreens.

Complementary medicines (also known as 'traditional' or 'alternative' medicines) include vitamin, mineral, herbal, aromatherapy and homeopathic products. They may be registered or listed on the ARTG, depending on their ingredients and the claims made. Most complementary medicines are listed.

All medicines supplied solely for export are listed (not registered) in the ARTG.

Medical devices also are required to be included if not exempt. Medical devices are classified based on intended use, level of risk and the degree of invasiveness in the human body, and classification determines the conformity assessment procedure used for conformity assessment. Certification by the TGA or an overseas notified body is required for higher risk devices.

For a new medicine to obtain public subsidy for patients in the community, the sponsor must successfully apply for the product to be included in the Pharmaceutical Benefits Scheme (PBS). Data are required on relative cost and effectiveness, and the scrutiny of this information according to prescribed criteria is described as the 'fourth hurdle', that is, in addition to quality, safety and efficacy requirements that medicines must overcome to be readily available to the Australian public.

The Commonwealth Government had agreed to establish a joint therapeutic products regulatory agency with the New Zealand Government, but in July 2007 this initiative was postponed indefinitely.

26.2 History of prescription medicine regulation

26.2.1 Quality, safety and efficacy

The Commonwealth Department of Health was established in 1921, but most health-related activities at that time remained the responsibility of the States.

The current title is the Department of Health and Ageing but its description frequently changes, so throughout this chapter the Department will be called the Department of Health, and the relevant Commonwealth Government minister will be called the Minister for Health.

The Therapeutic Substances Act 1937 gave the Minister for Health power to control the import and export of substances declared to be therapeutic substances in the *Commonwealth Gazette*. The Therapeutic Substances Act 1953 repealed the 1937 Act and gave the Commonwealth control of the import into Australia and interstate trading of therapeutic substances and controlled therapeutic substances (drugs of addiction).

In 1959, the National Biological Standards Laboratory (NBSL) was established, to test therapeutic products imported into Australia or supplied under the PBS for compliance with quality and manufacturing standards, largely based on the British Pharmacopoeia.

In the wake of the thalidomide tragedy, the Australian Drug Evaluation Committee (ADEC) was established in 1963 as a statutory committee to advise the government on the regulation of drugs intended for marketing in Australia. The adverse drug reaction (ADR) reporting scheme and the Adverse Drug Reactions Advisory Committee (ADRAC) were also introduced.

Furthermore, Commonwealth legislation was reviewed to give the Commonwealth powers to require companies to submit specified data to establish the quality, safety and efficacy of imported therapeutic goods. The resultant Therapeutic Goods Act 1966 provided the basis for the regulation of pharmaceuticals in Australia for over 20 years.

The Guidelines for Preparing Applications for General Marketing or Clinical Investigational Use of a Therapeutic Substance outlined information requirements for applications. Provision was also made for special Australian standards to apply where appropriate. Some States had separate arrangements that covered the few locally manufactured products sourced from local active ingredients, as the Commonwealth's jurisdiction was limited to imports, exports and goods crossing State borders (although the last power was thought unlikely to sustain a prosecution if taken to court).

A code of GMP was introduced in the late 1960s, covering principles and practices to be followed in the manufacture of therapeutic goods in Australia, but still relied upon State legislation and personnel for its enforcement.

The Customs (Prohibited Imports) Regulations were amended in 1970 to enable the Department of Health to further control importation through import permits for drug products.

The drug evaluation guidelines (known from 1976 as the NDF4 Guidelines) gradually became more detailed and were supplemented by appendices on specific issues such as bioavailability studies and bioequivalence. Rules were also introduced to address agency concerns that companies might manipulate the system; for example, by seeking review of data contained in a clinical trial application for a product that was already the subject of a general marketing application, thereby achieving speedier evaluation.

A revised clinical trial application evaluation scheme introduced in 1983 aimed for a response time of 45 working days for phase I and early phase II trials, and 80 working days for phase II and III trials, but in practice it took an average of 10–11 months from submission of data to receipt of written approval.

A Clinical Trial Exemption (CTX) scheme was introduced in Australia in 1987, with the intention of encouraging clinical trial activity. However, in addition to the aforementioned TGA restrictions, which required all clinical trials of an active substance underway in Australia to be completed before the review of a general marketing application relating to that substance, the specified data package included requirements unique to Australia, and the 60 working day review period compared with a 35 calendar day review under the UK CTX scheme.

Australia's drug evaluation system was increasingly criticised because of the 'drug lag' in availability of new and improved products in Australia, compared with other countries with well-regarded regulatory systems. Several government inquiries recommended streamlining and making better use of overseas experience. The pharmaceutical industry repeatedly expressed concern about the unique requirements that had led to significant delays in both the submission of applications and obtaining marketing approval; for example, requiring individual patient data (required in the USA but not in Europe) to be presented by parameter (uniquely to Australia) instead of by subject (as required in the USA).

By the late 1980s, it had also become clear that reliance on a combination of Commonwealth and State legislation was not the best way to ensure that desired standards were met. There were many complaints about loopholes and lack of uniformity. The way forward came from an unexpected source, a court case that confirmed that the Commonwealth

Government has powers over all corporations, and thus these powers could be used in relation to therapeutic goods matters even if they occurred within one State.

The Therapeutic Goods Act 1989 and Regulations came into effect on 15 February 1991, giving the Commonwealth more clearly defined regulatory authority. It changed the focus of control over therapeutic goods from the point of importation to the point of supply of the goods.

The Act applies to:

• All corporations who supply or manufacture medicines for supply (regardless of where) in Australia;
• Unincorporated parties who supply or manufacture medicines for supply in Australia outside their own state or territory;
• All parties (whether incorporated or unincorporated) who supply medicines under the PBS;
• All parties (whether incorporated or unincorporated) who import or export medicines.

Supportive State legislation is required only to cover activities of persons within one State, and specified areas (such as some aspects of labelling, packaging, distribution and fair trade) that are the responsibility of State governments.

Fees and charges were also introduced – through the Therapeutic Goods Act 1989 and Therapeutic Goods (Charges) Act 1989, respectively, and associated Regulations.

Pressure increased for the TGA to 'free up' the regulatory system for prescription medicines. In particular, the 1990 report by the Australian National Council on AIDS Working Party on the Availability of HIV/AIDS Treatments recommended that a notification scheme be introduced for clinical trials of unapproved products that had already been approved by respected agencies overseas.

In March 1991, the Commonwealth Government announced the introduction of an alternative clinical trial system. The Clinical Trial Notification (CTN) scheme was introduced in May 1991, following recognition of the negative effects of discouraging trials of investigational drugs – on patients (who were unable to access possible treatments for potentially life-threatening illnesses) and on pharmaceutical industry investment in research and development (R&D) in Australia. The government also announced a major review of drug evaluation processes in Australia.

Professor Peter Baume's report, *A Question of Balance: Report on the Future of Drug Evaluation in Australia*,[1] was released in July 1991, with a commitment from the Commonwealth Government to

speedily implement all 164 recommendations in the stated time-frames. Key aspects were:
• The retention of Australian sovereignty in deciding which drugs might be marketed in Australia;
• Recognition that considerable streamlining of drug evaluation procedures could be achieved;
• Acceptance that international harmonisation was a concept whose 'time had come', and that considerable benefit could flow from improved cooperation with other comparable developed countries;
• Recognition that no drugs were totally risk free, and that the need for a system of controls relating to the quality, safety and efficacy of therapeutic goods must be balanced against the more recently highlighted need for timely availability;
• Recommendations for reorganisation of the TGA and its advisory committees, with a new management plan and increased emphasis on performance;
• Provision of a timeline for Australia to bring about the reform of its drug evaluation processes within the next 2 years.

Recommendations were also made to streamline the CTX scheme for clinical trials and continue the CTN scheme, with further assessment in the future. Professor Baume noted that, in 1990, the TGA process of evaluation of new chemical entities (NCEs) was taking approximately twice as long as its target time of 16.5 months.

Following the Baume Report, changes were made to the Therapeutic Goods Act and Regulations to introduce specific target evaluation times, together with a fee penalty of 25% if a decision on an application was not made within the specified period.

The statutory time-frames led to a major reorganisation of TGA processes to focus on meeting them and complex measuring arrangements were introduced to ensure that only 'TGA working days' were included in the calculations. The clock is stopped whenever questions are raised with the product sponsor, and only restarted when no queries are outstanding.

New data requirements came into force from 1993 that closely aligned Australian marketing applications with those in the European Community (EC). The Australian Guidelines for the Registration of Drugs – Volume 1: Prescription and Other Specified Drug Products (AGRD1) specified that the document to support a prescription drug registration application should be compiled in accordance with the current version of *The Rules Governing Medicinal Products in the European Community*, Volumes II and III with Addenda and supplementary *Notes for Guidance* published by the Committee for Proprietary and Medicinal Products (CPMP), and also described specific

administrative requirements for registration applications in Australia.

Information about the overseas status of the product was also now sought as part of an application. The list of countries mentioned in this context in the AGRD1 included members of the Pharmaceutical Evaluation Report (PER) scheme, other EC countries and the USA. Expert reports also began to be utilised in the evaluation of applications.

In June 2004, the Australian Regulatory Guidelines for Prescription Medicines (ARGPM) were issued by the TGA to replace the AGRD1. Under the ARGPM the format for registration applications in Australia is the Common Technical Document (CTD) developed through the International Conference on Harmonisation (ICH).

On 31 March 2008, the ARTG included 10,994 registered medicines (8556 of which were Schedule 4 and Schedule 8 medicines), 1939 listed medicines and 3266 export-listed medicines – a total of 26,970 medicines. It should be noted that this number reflects the separate inclusion of each strength, dosage form and brand as a distinct therapeutic item. There are also 28,221 medical devices on the Register, some of which are 'grouped', and some of which would be termed diagnostic products in other countries.

It is a requirement under the Therapeutic Goods Act that a sponsor takes responsibility for each therapeutic item that is imported, exported, manufactured or supplied in or from Australia. The sponsor must be a corporation or person within Australia. Sponsors must be able to substantiate all claims made by them about their therapeutic products. On 31 March 2008, there were 2790 sponsors of therapeutic goods on the ARTG.

In the 2005–2006 federal budget the government announced that it would commence consultation with industry with the intention of introducing cost recovery for the administration of the Pharmaceutical Benefits Advisory Committee (PBAC) and the process of listing a medicine on the PBS from 2007–2008. In May 2008 the new Labor government confirmed that it intended to introduce cost recovery for evaluation for PBS listing and listing a vaccine on the National Immunisation Schedule. It introduced the National Health Amendment (Pharmaceutical and Other Benefits – Cost Recovery) Bill 2008 to Parliament in May 2008. The Bill was subsequently referred to the Senate Community Affairs Committee to report on the impact of cost recovery and how cost recovery will improve the timeliness and effectiveness of the current PBS process for listing new medicines. Following the Committee's report in mid-August 2008 the

Bill was defeated in the Senate. There will be a delay of at least 3 months before a revised Bill may be reintroduced.

26.2.2 Availability to the community

The authority for the Commonwealth Government to provide pharmaceutical benefits was introduced in the 1940s. Prior to that, except for the federal scheme covering war veterans, health care was the province of the States.

The Commonwealth National Health Act 1953 (National Health Act), together with the National Health (Pharmaceutical Benefits) Regulations, introduced the current framework for the operation of the PBS.

The PBAC was established under Section 101 of the National Health Act, to give advice to the Minister for Health about products to be made available as pharmaceutical benefits. The minister is required to consider the PBAC's advice but is not required to follow its recommendations. The initial criteria for inclusion of new products on the PBS were comparative safety and efficacy.

Initially, 139 'lifesaving and disease preventing drugs' were provided under the scheme without charge to pension recipients and their dependants. By 1960, the scheme had expanded to include a wider range of drugs, and supply to the general public with some co-payment. PBS listing continued to be based primarily on medical considerations.

A non-statutory body called the Pharmaceutical Benefits Pricing Bureau (PBPB) was established in 1963 to make recommendations to government on the pricing of PBS-listed medicines.

Escalation of costs led to multiple measures to limit the increase in PBS expenditure, including the introduction of an authority system for new drugs from 1988. Co-payments were eventually also introduced for concessional patients – for disadvantaged patients in 1989 and for pensioners in 1990. Details of the early history of the PBS and the myriad of subsequent changes can be found in *A History of the Pharmaceutical Benefits Scheme 1947–1992*.[2]

Amendments to the National Health Act in 1987 introduced the additional requirement for the PBAC to consider cost and effectiveness. Sponsors were encouraged to provide cost-effectiveness substantiation from 1991, and from 1 January 1993 it became mandatory to include pharmaco-economic analyses in listing applications – the 'fourth hurdle'.

In 1988, the PBPB was replaced by the (also non-statutory) Pharmaceutical Benefits Pricing Authority (PBPA). The PBPA was required to review the prices

of items on the PBS and consider items recommended by the PBAC for listing, taking eight factors in account. Factor (f) – the level of activity being undertaken by the company in Australia – was not to be considered in the price determination of each item, but through a separate allocation of funds to the companies that were successful in their proposals under the Pharmaceutical Industry Development Programme [the factor (f) programme].

When the factor (f) programme concluded in 1999, it was followed by the Pharmaceutical Industry Investment Programme (PIIP). Both schemes were intended to partially compensate participating companies for the price suppression imposed by the government in exercising its monopsony purchasing powers under the PBS. The PIIP funds of A\$300 million over 5 years were awarded to nine companies who successfully applied for funding in return for increased R&D and/or production value-adding activity in Australia. The PIIP concluded in early 2004.

This programme was followed by the Pharmaceuticals Partnerships Programme (P3), which provided A\$150 million over 5 years from 1 July 2004 for successful applicants, who received (initially) 30 cents (later 50 cents) for each additional dollar spent on eligible R&D activities. A review of the P3 in 2008 recommended that the programme should not be renewed in its current form when it ends in June 2009 and any decision on a successor programme should be informed by the Review of the National Innovation System, which was announced by the Minister for Innovation Industry, Science and Research in January 2008.

The minister also established a Pharmaceuticals Industry Strategy Group to examine the drivers and barriers to attracting new internationally competitive and sustainable manufacturing, R&D and clinical trials investment in the pharmaceuticals sector. It will present a directions paper by the end of September 2008 and a final report by the end of the year. The Strategy Group and Review of the National Innovation Systems will be the primary determinants of any future pharmaceuticals industry development programme.

The overwhelming importance of gaining PBS listing in order to achieve widespread availability and use of a prescription medicine in Australia is evident from information published by the Australian Institute of Health and Welfare (AIHW).[3] Government expenditure on pharmaceutical benefits in 2006–2007 amounted to 82.6% of the total cost of PBS prescriptions. The remainder was patient contributions which amounted to A\$1151.3 million. The majority of government expenditure on PBS prescriptions was directed towards concessional cardholders (A$4401.4 million, 80.4% of the total). Government pharmaceutical benefits expenditure totalled A$6428.3 million.

The AIHW estimated that total expenditure on prescription pharmaceuticals in 2005–2006 was A$10,551 million. This included A$2014 million on drugs used by hospitals, comprising A$1658 million in public hospitals and A$356 million in private hospitals. During 2006 there were 168 million community PBS prescriptions – 142 million (84.5%) to concessional patients (pensioners, seniors, repatriation health beneficiaries) and 26 million to general patients. In addition, about 54 million prescriptions did not attract a subsidy – 34.6 million below the co-payment threshold and 19.3 million 'private' prescriptions (i.e. prescriptions for drugs not listed on the PBS or RPBS), for which the consumer pays the full cost of the medicine. Thus, 76.0% of prescriptions were for items subsidised through the PBS.

Eligibility for PBS is restricted to Australian residents and visitors from those countries with which Australia has a reciprocal health care agreement – currently, the UK (including the Republic of Ireland), Ireland, New Zealand, Malta, Italy, Sweden, the Netherlands and Finland. Proof of eligibility by means of a Medicare card or passport is an absolute requirement for the subsidy to be applied.

The government introduced a series of programmes aimed at 'preventing the unnecessary use of PBS subsidised medicines' and 'reinforcing the commitment to evidence-based medicine'. These included 'a more detailed consideration process' for new PBS listings, ensuring greater compliance by doctors with PBS prescribing requirements, and the enhancement of PBS restrictions to reduce prescriptions supplied to individuals in breach of PBS conditions. The government also strengthened measures to reduce pharmacy fraud and further encourage the use of generics.

Major PBS reforms were introduced by legislative amendment in August 2007, to substantially reduce government expenditure on out of patent PBS listed drugs, while offering patented drugs some protection from price reductions. These reforms are discussed in more detail in section 26.4.

In December 2007, the Schedule of Pharmaceutical Benefits included 819 drug substances in 2749 forms and strengths (items) supplied as 3481 different drug products (brands).

26.2.3 National Medicines Policy

The Australian National Medicines Policy aims to establish an appropriate balance between health,

economic and industry objectives. It has four central elements:

1. Timely access to the medicines that Australians need, at a cost individuals and the community can afford;
2. Medicines meeting appropriate standards of quality, safety and efficacy;
3. Quality use of medicines; and
4. Maintaining a responsible and viable medicines industry.

Although these goals are not enshrined in legislation, they have become increasingly accepted by successive governments as a sound basis for informed policy decisions.

26.2.4 Fees and charges

The Therapeutic Goods Act 1989 and Therapeutic Goods (Charges) Act 1989, respectively, and associated regulations stipulate the fees and charges payable to TGA for processing applications, GMP inspections and annual licences. When fees and charges were first introduced in 1991 they were intended to cover 50% of the costs attributable to the TGA's responsibilities under the Therapeutic Goods Act, including those deemed to be 'for the public good'. It took some time to reach those levels – in 1992–1993 only 28% of the TGA's relevant costs were covered.

By July 1996 the 50% target was reached, and the Commonwealth Government announced that fees and charges would increase over the following 3 years to raise industry's contribution to the government's therapeutic goods programme from 50% to 75%. In 1997 the government announced that the TGA would be required to recover 100% of its operating costs from 1998–1999.

In 2006–2007 the overall revenue raised by the TGA from fees and charges was A$78.6 million, of which the prescription medicines sector contributes approximately 60%. Fees apply to almost all evaluation activities undertaken by TGA – not only to the review of general marketing applications but also to minor marketing-related matters, clinical trial applications and notifications, and GMP evaluations and inspections in Australia or overseas, but not to ADR assessments.

In 2003 there was a major revision of the fees and charges structure for prescription medicines to simplify the structure and to rebalance revenue by reducing fees obtained from pre-market evaluations and increasing revenue from post-market activities to more closely reflect the actual costs. Under the new structure, the evaluation fees are no longer based on the number of pages of data submitted. Instead, a single evaluation fee is now charged for each type of application (e.g. NCE, extension of indications, new generic product).

The evaluation fee for an NCE decreased from A$235,720 (before 1 July 2003) to A$176,300 from 1 July 2008. The restructuring of fees and charges is now complete, although there will continue to be an annual reassessment of fees and charges, adjusted (as a minimum) in line with inflation, to ensure that 100% cost recovery is maintained. Sponsors are required to pay 75% of the evaluation fee at the time of submitting their application. The balance of 25% of the evaluation fee is payable when the TGA completes the evaluation within the legislated time-frame.

There is no application fee, but if an application is withdrawn before it is accepted for evaluation, a screening fee of 20% of the evaluation fee up to a maximum of A$7130 currently applies.

Annual charges apply to maintaining each product on the ARTG. The annual charge for continuing registration of a prescription medicine increased over the 5-year transition period to A$5250 for a biological product and A$3140 for a non-biological from 1 July 2008.

26.2.5 Marketing applications for prescription medicines

Prescription medicines and certain other high-risk medicines, such as injections, are evaluated for inclusion on the ARTG by the Office of Prescription Medicines (OPM) of the TGA. The types of medicines that are evaluated by the OPM are described in Schedule 10 of the Therapeutic Goods Regulations. Usually, medicines containing new active substances are evaluated by the OPM for inclusion on the register as registrable goods. However, a sponsor can submit a justification for an alternative route of evaluation of a new active substance by another branch of the TGA as a non-prescription medicine; for example, where there is experience with the active ingredient in non-prescription medicines in other countries. Guidelines for providing such a justification are available at the TGA website (www.tga.gov.au).

26.3 TGA registration

26.3.1 Applications for registration

The sponsor of a therapeutic product is responsible for submitting an application to the TGA for registration of the goods and, once the goods are registered,

for compliance with conditions of registration such as reporting any adverse drug reactions.

Australia has closely aligned its data requirements for the registration of prescription medicines with those of the European Union. The ARGPM describes certain administrative requirements and provides technical guidance complementary to EU technical guidance, relevant to applications for registration in Australia. Under the ARGPM, if a sponsor prepares a dossier in the CTD format for submission in the European Union, this will be also accepted in Australia.

Where registration is being sought for a new drug to treat a life-threatening illness or to treat a condition for which no satisfactory alternative therapy exists, the TGA will accept the application in either US or EU format.

The TGA will accept dossiers in an electronic format, in addition to hard copy, following discussion with the sponsor. The TGA has been monitoring international developments in relation to applications in electronic formats and is expected to adopt any agreed international standard arising from the ICH process.

There is a formal process for consultation with the pharmaceutical industry on the adoption of each EU guideline in Australia. Australia has adopted the majority of guidelines published by the CPMP without amendment. Guidelines that have not been adopted usually concern labelling or the content of the Australian Product Information (PI) document. All of the EU guidelines that have been adopted or not adopted in Australia are listed on the TGA website. Any changes or additional comments on an EU guideline agreed between the industry and TGA are also published on the TGA website.

26.3.2 Categories of application

There are three categories of applications relating to prescription medicines:

1. Category 1 applications are defined as being those that do not meet the requirements of Category 2 or 3 applications. Essentially, Category 1 applications are those that include clinical, preclinical or bioequivalence data, such as applications to register goods containing a new active ingredient, a new generic product, a new strength, dosage form or route of administration.

2. Category 2 applications are defined as those that include clinical, preclinical or bioequivalence data for which there are two evaluation reports from 'acceptable countries', where the submission is already approved. The evaluation reports must be independent (not based on each other) and the product must

be identical in Australia and the 'acceptable countries', in respect to formulation, directions for use and indications. The countries identified as 'acceptable' for the purposes of providing evaluation reports are currently Canada, Sweden, the Netherlands, the UK and the USA. As the availability of evaluation reports would assist the TGA to evaluate an application, Category 2 applications are subject to shorter legislated evaluation times. However, as most sponsors submit applications for registration in Australia at the same time, or shortly after, they are submitted in the 'acceptable countries', it is rare for two evaluation reports to be available to qualify for a Category 2 application. Hence, almost no Category 2 applications are submitted.

3. Category 3 applications seek changes to the pharmaceutical data of goods already included on the ARTG, which do not need to be supported by clinical, preclinical or bioequivalence data. Examples of Category 3 applications include changes to the specifications of the active ingredient, change of shelf life or storage conditions, and change of trade name.

It is a condition of registration that, with limited exceptions, no changes may be made to registered goods without prior approval from the TGA. An exception is that some narrowly specified changes to pharmaceutical and manufacturing aspects may be made without prior approval, as outlined in Appendices 12 and 13 (for biological products) of ARGPM. A number of general and specific conditions must be complied with under the 'self-assessable' changes provisions. These are primarily the proper validation of any change and the notification of the change to the TGA.

26.3.3 Evaluation time-frames
The Therapeutic Goods Regulations specify time-frames for completion of the evaluation of Category 1, 2 and 3 applications in 'working days', which excludes weekends and public holidays.

Category 1 applications are required to be:
• Accepted for evaluation, or rejected, in 40 working days from receipt of the application and the application fee; and
• Evaluated in 255 working days from the date of acceptance.

Category 2 applications are required to be:
• Accepted for evaluation, or rejected, in 20 working days from receipt of the application and the application fee; and
• Evaluated in 175 working days from the date of acceptance.

Category 3 applications are required to be approved or rejected or to have an objection raised within 45 working days of receipt of the application, or payment of the evaluation fee, whichever is the later day. There is no application acceptance period. If an objection to the application is raised, the applicant may respond and provide further information or data. A further 30 working days from receipt of this response is then allowed for consideration of the response before the application must be approved or rejected.

Under Section 31 of the Therapeutic Goods Act, the TGA may request a sponsor to provide additional information or seek clarification of information provided in a submission. Fee penalties apply only if the statutory evaluation period is not met. The evaluation times do not include the time-frames for initial acceptance or rejection of an application or the time taken by the sponsor to respond to TGA Section 31 requests. They apply to each application as an absolute criterion, not as an average performance target. The TGA has almost invariably met the legislated time-frames.

In addition, in 2000 the TGA undertook to target the following mean evaluation times for different sub-types of Category 1 applications:
• New chemical entities – 150 working days;
• New generics, except 'own generics' – 100 working days;
• New indications – 160 working days;
• Product information changes – 90 working days;
• Other Category 1 applications – 130 working days.
For applications finalised in the second quarter of calendar year 2007 the average elapsed time from submission of an application to registration, for an NCE, was approximately 52 weeks/12 months.

26.3.4 Confidentiality of submissions
Sponsors routinely require that data contained in their applications remain confidential. If another party requests access to such data under the provisions of the Commonwealth Freedom of Information Act 1982, the Department of Health will consult with the sponsor to establish whether release of the information is possible, and enable the sponsor to request a review by the Administrative Appeals Tribunal (AAT) of any decision made by the TGA to release the information.

The TGA will not comply with demands for undertakings of confidentiality that seek to limit the lawful use or release of information by the TGA. The TGA will not accept confidentiality statements from sponsors that seek to prohibit the evaluator's access to departmental records of prior applications, and the accumulated knowledge and experience gained from the evaluation of previous applications. Examples of acceptable confidentiality statements are provided in ARGPM.

26.3.5 Data protection
In 1998 an amendment to the Act was enacted introducing data exclusivity provisions. Under Section 25A, the TGA must not use 'protected information' about other therapeutic goods when evaluating therapeutic goods for registration. Protected information is information about a new active ingredient that is not available to the public, that is lodged with an application to register goods containing the new active ingredient, where that application has led to registration of the goods. A new active ingredient is defined as one that is not currently, and has never been, contained in goods included in the ARTG. Such information is protected for 5 years from the date of registration of the goods containing the new active ingredient. Thus, products containing new actives are given 5 years data exclusivity.

At the time the data exclusivity amendments were being discussed, the pharmaceutical industry sought to extend the provisions to protect data relating to new indications, new dosage forms or routes of administration, but was unsuccessful. The industry association, Medicines Australia, has reactivated its request to the government to increase the term of data protection and extend the range of data protected, in light of new initiatives to encourage innovation in Australia. However, at this point no changes have been foreshadowed. Indeed, a recent Federal Court ruling has emphasised that data protection does not automatically apply to the entire registration package – the information claimed to be subject to the protection has to be adequately identified and justified as confidential.

A sponsor of a generic unpatented product may avoid the need for TGA to refer to protected information by submitting a full Category 1 application for registration, including preclinical and clinical data.

26.3.6 Orphan Drug Program
The Australian Orphan Drug Program was introduced in 1998. Through a cooperative arrangement with the US Food and Drug Administration (FDA), it intended to improve access to treatments for rare diseases in Australia by utilising US orphan drug evaluations as the basis for Australian approvals where possible. It also waived evaluation fees for new medicines or indications designated as 'orphan'.

In order to be designated as an orphan drug in Australia, the prevalence of the disease to be treated is required to be equal to or less than 2000 affected individuals or, if the drug is a vaccine or *in vivo* diagnostic agent, the persons to whom the drug will be administered in Australia are equal to or less than 2000 per year. The prevalence limit in Australia is considerably lower than other countries' orphan drug programmes, both in absolute terms and as a proportion of the population.

Also, whereas the US Orphan Drug Program offers several incentives to sponsors to bring drugs to treat rare diseases to market, such as a period of market exclusivity, tax credits for clinical research costs, clinical research grants and waiver of FDA evaluation fees, the Australian program offers a 100% reduction of the evaluation fee for a designated orphan drug but no research incentives. The TGA guideline does state that an orphan drug will be granted 5 years market exclusivity, which can be shared by a clinically superior product, but this exclusivity is not supported by any legislation.

Since the Australian program commenced, 134 drugs have been designated as orphan drugs (as at 17 July 2008). In December 2001, a review of the Orphan Drug Program found that sponsors had lodged applications for marketing approval for 33 of the 42 drugs designated as orphan at the time, and 17 of 20 that had reached their conclusion were approved. Seven of these had been successful in obtaining government funding, as highly specialised drugs or under the life-saving drugs programme. Three drugs had been considered and rejected by the PBAC on the grounds of unacceptable cost-effectiveness.

The 2001 review found that there have been few opportunities for the TGA to utilise a review by the FDA. Of 215 orphan drugs granted marketing approval in the USA, only 63 had not already been approved for marketing in Australia or did not have an equivalent in Australia. Of these, the review stated that not more than a dozen would represent a significant gap in what has been approved for marketing in Australia, and most of these would fall into the category of 'like to have' rather than 'need to have because there is no alternative'. The review recommended a number of changes to the Australian Orphan Drug Program, primarily focusing on increasing the incentives for sponsors to bring orphan drugs to market by offering greater surety of obtaining public subsidy under the PBS. As at August 2008, the review recommendations have still not been implemented.

26.3.7 Priority evaluations

The OPM may allocate priority evaluation to applications for registration of important new medicines. The current criteria for priority evaluation are:
• The active ingredient is a new chemical entity;
• The drug is indicated for the treatment or diagnosis of a serious, life-threatening or severely debilitating disease or condition; or
• There is clinical evidence that the drug may provide an important therapeutic gain.

Priority evaluation status does not give a definite, shorter evaluation period. Rather, the application is simply moved ahead in the queue of applications under evaluation.

26.3.8 Good Manufacturing Practice

It is a requirement of the Therapeutic Goods Act that all steps in the manufacture of a prescription medicine, including the manufacture of bulk active drugs and finished pharmaceutical products, are performed in manufacturing facilities of acceptable standards. An updated list of manufacturing principles established under the Therapeutic Goods Act is available from the TGA website.

Manufacturing sites within Australia must comply with the Australian Code of GMP for Medicinal Products – August 2002, which is based entirely on the international standard Guide to Good Manufacturing Practices for Medicinal Products, Version PH1/97 (Rev 3), 15 January 2002, published by the Pharmaceutical Inspection Cooperation Scheme (PIC/S). The ICH GMP Guide for Active Pharmaceutical Ingredients has also been adopted.

The TGA conducts regular inspections of Australian manufacturing operations to ensure compliance with the code of GMP. Scrutiny has increased, including unannounced inspections, since the major recall of a contract manufacturer's wide range of products in 2003 (see section 26.3.20).

The standard of any steps of manufacture and quality control conducted outside Australia must also be shown to be acceptable for the inclusion of therapeutic goods on the ARTG. The TGA will accept certificates of GMP compliance issued under the provisions of a Mutual Recognition Agreement (MRA) where the manufacturer is located in the same country as a regulator that is a recognised participant in the MRA. Audits and GMP certification for manufacturers in third countries are no longer automatically accepted because they may not include all aspects of the manufacture of medicines for supply to Australia. The countries currently included through an MRA are EC and European Free Trade Association (EFTA) countries, Canada (except for complementary medicines), Singapore and Switzerland, as specified in the in the TGA document *Guidance on the GMP Clearance of Overseas Medicine Manufacturers*, 16th edition, March 2008.

The TGA does not automatically accept GMP Certification from PIC/S member countries or the FDA, although there is an agreement in place with the FDA that provides for the exchange of information in relation to manufacturers for regulatory purposes.

26.3.9 The evaluation process

Details of requirements for the registration of prescription medicines are contained in the ARGPM, which is available from the TGA website. Submissions to register new prescription medicines in Australia undergo a two-stage process of evaluation by the OPM: application acceptance and evaluation.

Prior to submitting an application for registration there is an opportunity for a sponsor to have a presubmission meeting with TGA delegates to discuss the application. Pre-submission meetings are strongly recommended for complex applications, where there is some uncertainty as to whether the data package to be submitted will meet all Australian regulatory requirements, and for orphan drugs and literature-based submissions.

An application is screened for acceptance by the Application Entry Team of the OPM. Although primarily intended to be an administrative check that the application is in the required format, the three main modules (quality data, non-clinical data and clinical data) are also briefly reviewed by the relevant evaluation sections to ensure that there are no major omissions of data.

Once an application has been accepted for evaluation, the Pharmaceutical Chemistry Evaluation Section, Toxicology Section and Clinical Evaluation Units evaluate the Module 3, 4 and 5 data, respectively. For applications relating to products of biological origin, a second copy of the Module 3 data is also evaluated by the Office of Laboratories and Scientific Services, which evaluates aspects such as laboratory methodology, method validation and shelf-life.

There are currently five clinical evaluation units within OPM, each headed by a senior medical officer and supported by pharmacists. Applications are distributed among the five evaluation units based on the therapeutic area of the drug under evaluation. The OPM contracts a number of external clinical evaluators who are specialist medical practitioners in the medical condition that the proposed new drug is intended to treat. External evaluators may also be contracted to evaluate the Module 4 data. The head of the clinical evaluation unit coordinates the evaluation and makes the final decision on marketing approval as a delegate under the Therapeutic Goods Act.

From receipt of an application until a final decision on an application, a OPM evaluator may request additional information or clarification from the sponsor under Section 31 of the Therapeutic Goods Act. During the period from issuing a Section 31 letter and receipt of responses to all questions, the clock is stopped and the elapsed time is not counted towards the TGA's statutory evaluation time frames. If several Section 31 requests overlap, the periods are not additive but the clock remains stopped until the final question is answered. A sponsor is given a time-frame in which a Section 31 request should be answered. Justification for an extension of time may be discussed with the evaluator. If a sponsor considers that a Section 31 request is unreasonable they can discuss this with the delegate who issued the request. If the sponsor is unable to resolve the matter with the delegate, it may seek review under an additional, non-statutory appeal mechanism by a three-member Standing Arbitration Committee or Pharmaceutical Sub-Committee.

At the conclusion of evaluation of the Module 3, 4 and 5 data the evaluators prepare an evaluation report for each module. The evaluation reports are sent to the sponsor as they are received to allow comments to the delegate. Once the three evaluation reports are finalised, the delegate evaluates the reports and prepares an overview of the evaluation and a proposed decision for consideration by ADEC, which are also provided to the sponsor. The sponsor is given 10 working days from receipt of the overview and proposed decision to provide a response and submit any additional comment on the application to ADEC. This 'pre-ADEC response' is limited to six A4 pages in 12-point font.

26.3.10 Submission of new data

Two classes of new data may be submitted after an application has been accepted: additional data and supplementary data. Additional data are data identified at a pre-submission meeting that the TGA agrees to accept during the course of an evaluation at a predetermined date, such as the results from an ongoing clinical study.

Supplementary data are clinical or preclinical data submitted at the initiation of the sponsor, after it has received either or both of the Module 4 and Module 5 evaluation reports. The sponsor must notify its intention to submit supplementary data within 5 working days of receipt of the last evaluation report. Only one submission of supplementary data is permitted for each of Modules 4 and 5, unless otherwise agreed by the TGA in writing. Supplementary data will not be accepted after commencement of the pre-ADEC process, which is signified by the issuing of the delegates overview and recommendation. Acceptance of supplementary data is at the discretion of the TGA and is dependent upon mutual agreement to a 'clock stop'.

Up to 60 working days is allowed for all additional data and fees to be presented to the TGA following the sponsor's notification of intent; and up to 135 days may be taken for evaluation of the supplementary data after all data and fees have been received by the TGA.

26.3.11 Australian Drug Evaluation Committee

The Australian Drug Evaluation Committee (ADEC) makes medical and scientific evaluations of drugs referred to it by the minister or the secretary, and gives advice to the minister or secretary in relation to the import, export, manufacture and distribution of therapeutic goods. It is important to note that the ADEC has an advisory function and is not the final decision-maker. The TGA delegate is guided by ADEC's advice but may make a decision contrary to ADEC's recommendations.

The ADEC comprises six or seven 'core' members – eminent practising physicians, pharmaceutical scientists and pharmacologists who attend each meeting. There are up to 20 'associate' members whose expertise is drawn on as appropriate to the applications under consideration at a particular meeting. ADEC members adhere to strict guidelines on competing interests, which effectively exclude a member from proceedings if they have any pecuniary interest in a pharmaceutical company whose product is under consideration or in any competitor company. Participation in company-sponsored clinical trials must also be declared, but does not necessarily exclude the member from proceedings. The ADEC Competing Interest Guidelines are available from the TGA website. ADEC is supported by specialist subcommittees, which currently include the Pharmaceutical Sub-Committee and ADRAC.

The ADEC meets six times a year in February, April, June, August, October and December. For each application it receives the sponsor's covering letter, all evaluation reports, the delegate's overview and proposed decision, and the sponsor's pre-ADEC response. The ADEC makes recommendations on applications referred to it for advice. This recommendation, termed an ADEC resolution, is sent to the sponsor 5 working days after the ADEC meeting. Ratified minutes of the meeting in which the resolution is made are available only after the next ADEC meeting, whereafter all positive recommendations relating to applications for registration are published in the *Commonwealth Gazette* and are posted on the TGA website. Occasionally, significant recommendations relating to a class of drugs or the content of the PI document are also published. The ADEC minutes are also provided to a number of overseas regulatory agencies.

Not all prescription medicine applications are referred to the ADEC. Category 3 applications and Category 1 applications other than new medicines may be dealt with entirely by the OPM. A process has been implemented whereby applications to extend the use of a registered product for which all the evaluators and the delegate recommend approval are considered by the Peer Review Committee within the OPM. The Peer Review Committee is a group of senior medical officers from all areas of OPM. They consider non-contentious applications, other than for new medicines. ADEC is advised of the delegate's decision following the peer review process.

In 2005, the TGA conducted a review to examine whether workflow practices within the Drug Safety and Evaluation Branch (now called the OPM) could be improved, with the intention to align with best practice and international standards, including greater transparency of prescription medicine evaluation. The review report is available from the TGA website.

The recommendations from the review were under consideration as part of the establishment of the Australia New Zealand Therapeutic Products Authority (see section 26.3.23) and are now being implemented by the OPM. One recommendation from the review was for consideration be given to enabling sponsors to respond to questions that might arise about an application during ADEC's consideration. It is proposed that sponsors will have the opportunity to make a short presentation to ADEC about key issues and directly respond to ADEC questions. This would be limited to applications where there are clearly contentious issues or the recommendation for rejection or approval is borderline. It is not intended that sponsors would appear before the ADEC for applications where the evaluation reports and delegate's recommendation are clearly in favour of approval.

26.3.12 Post-ADEC and the delegate's decision

Following consideration by ADEC or the Peer Review Committee, if the delegate proposes to approve the application, he or she will communicate with the sponsor to address any outstanding issues, and the final PI will be negotiated. Once all outstanding matters are resolved, a marketing approval letter is issued by the delegate, which states the conditions of registration, together with the approved PI. A certificate of registration is also issued detailing the information included on the ARTG. The annual registration charge is payable following the registration.

If the delegate proposes to reject the application, a letter is sent to the sponsor advising of this intent, giving the reasons for the decision. A sponsor may appeal the initial decision of the delegate.

26.3.13 Australian Public Assessment Report

The workflow practices review also recommended improved transparency through the publication of a summary of the TGA delegate's decision and the rationale for the decision, excluding any reference to confidential commercial information. An Australian Public Assessment Report (AusPAR), modelled on the European Public Assessment Report (EPAR), will be prepared for each product derived from the evaluation reports. The AusPAR would be drafted immediately prior to the ADEC meeting at which the product will be considered. The AusPAR will not be reviewed by ADEC. The AusPAR will be finalised post-ADEC, incorporating the delegate's decision and reasons, and will be agreed between TGA and the sponsor. The final AusPAR will be published on the TGA website within 1 month of registration. The introduction of the AusPAR is expected to occur in 2009.

26.3.14 Appeals against marketing application decisions

Under Section 60 of the Therapeutic Goods Act, appeal mechanisms are available to sponsor companies to challenge decisions made by officers of the TGA. Eligible appeals are defined in the Therapeutic Goods Act.

The decision of the secretary or delegate is called an initial decision. If the sponsor wishes to appeal an initial decision, it must do so within 90 calendar days of receiving advice of that decision. The appeal of the initial decision is directed to the minister, who generally appoints the TGA principal medical adviser to act as a delegate in considering that appeal, and the decision on the appeal must be issued within 60 days. The outcome of this stage is called a reviewable decision.

Reviewable decisions are so-called because they may be appealed through the AAT within 28 calendar days of receiving advice on the minister's decision.

Restrictions have been added over the years that strictly delineate the information that may be considered and the grounds for a successful appeal by this route. Although this process has led to a tribunal hearing only a few times since 1991, it has been successfully used by sponsors on a more regular basis to challenge TGA decisions and negotiate a satisfactory outcome.

26.3.15 Product information

The PI is the summary of the outcomes of the evaluation for registration, in the same way as the Summary of Product Characteristics (SPC) forms the basis for prescribing in the European Union. It is intended to provide appropriate information to health professionals for the safe and effective use of the product, and is negotiated between the delegate and sponsor following the ADEC meeting, taking into account ADEC's recommendations. Once approved by the delegate, the sponsor may not change any aspect of the PI without prior approval from the TGA, except in specific circumstances such as safety-related changes. Unlike the SPC, the PI is not subject to 5-yearly review, although this has been proposed.

Safety-related changes to the PI that may be made by the sponsor without prior approval are those that reduce the patient population or add a warning, precaution, contraindication or adverse event. They must be notified to the TGA within 5 days of implementation and the date of each safety-related change must be listed in the PI in addition to the TGA approval date.

Non-safety-related changes to the PI may only be made by the sponsor without approval if they are minor editorial matters such as changes to headings or relocation of text or a change consequent to self-assessable change made in accordance with ARGPM. These changes must also be notified to TGA within 5 working days.

For PI changes that require approval, OPM accepts three main types of submission:
1. Conventional submissions, containing full study reports of clinical trials;
2. Literature-based submissions; or
3. Hybrid submissions, comprising a mix of conventional and literature-based data.

The type of submission considered by OPM to be appropriate for a PI update depends on the regulatory and clinical history of the drug in Australia and over-seas, with special reference to the UK, USA, Sweden, Canada and the Netherlands. Submissions based on company-sponsored clinical trials are usually required for drugs marketed for less than 5 years, whereas any of the three types of submission can be used for drugs marketed for more than 10 years. Drugs marketed between 5 and 10 years will be considered on a case by case basis, but it is generally expected that either a conventional or hybrid submission will be submitted.

Published non-clinical (Module 4) and clinical (Module 5) data may be used for either a literature-based submission or as the literature-based component of a hybrid submission. However, published reports rarely include sufficient validation information for pharmaceutical chemistry (Module 3) data to be accepted in the form of published literature. Conventional Module 3 data may accompany literature-based Module 4 and/or Module 5 data. Full guidelines on the preparation of literature-based submissions are available from the TGA website.

26.3.16 Paediatric indications

It is recognised internationally that there is a lack of information from proper investigations of the use of drugs in children, and a problem with the availability of paediatric-specific formulations, leading to drugs being used outside their approved indications and, at times, being reformulated by pharmacists to make them more suitable for use by children.

The TGA has endeavoured to encourage the submission of paediatric data packages by offering fee reductions for products that are not commercially viable or whose supply is in the public interest, waiving fees for orphan drugs and indications, and by accepting literature-based submissions. The TGA has also adopted internationally recognised ICH/EU guidelines dealing with paediatric data generation and facilitating the extrapolation of data from one patient population to another.

26.3.17 Consumer medicine information

Since 1993, all new prescription products (including changes to existing products that lead to a 'new' entry on the ARTG) have been required to also have a consumer medicine information (CMI) document, referred to in the Therapeutic Goods Regulations as a patient information document. From 1 January 2003, all prescription medicines have been required to have a CMI. The content of the CMI must be consistent with the PI and contain the information described in Schedule 12 to the regulations. CMI is also required for pharmacist-only (Schedule 3) medicines approved for registration since mid-1995, in accordance with Schedule 13 to the regulations.

Enormous effort has been invested in CMI development in Australia, with the aim of producing highly useful and usable information for consumers. *Writing About Medicines for People* (the usability guidelines) are in their third edition, providing guidance to sponsors on how to prepare CMIs with highly consistent usability. Unlike the European Union, Australian sponsors are not required to provide the CMI as a pack insert but may distribute the documents in a form that enables the CMI to be given to a person to whom a product is administered or dispensed. A system has been developed for electronic distribution of CMIs, so that they may be printed by doctors or pharmacists from their computer software.

26.3.18　Post-marketing responsibilities

The standard conditions of registration require the sponsor to inform the TGA of any adverse drug reactions and safety alerts related to their product of which they become aware. The requirements for reporting adverse drug reactions to prescription medicines occurring in Australia or overseas are described in the Australian Pharmacovigilance Guideline, which is available at the TGA website.

For spontaneous reports of reactions occurring in Australia, serious reactions (whether expected or unexpected) should be reported immediately and in no case later than 15 calendar days of receipt of the report. Other reactions occurring in Australia should be reported on request or as line listings in a Periodic Safety Update Report (PSUR). Reports of reactions occurring in other countries are not required to be routinely submitted to TGA. However, any significant safety issue or action that has arisen from an analysis of foreign reports, or has been taken by a foreign regulatory agency, must be reported to the TGA within 72 hours.

Australia has harmonised its requirements for post-marketing reports with those of the CPMP/ICH Guideline on Periodic Safety Update Reports (CPMP/ICH/228/95). The timing and frequency of provision of PSURs has also been harmonised with the CPMP/ICH requirements. Thus, an Australian sponsor may submit PSURs prepared to meet international regulatory requirements to the TGA. Post-marketing reports must be provided annually until the period covered by such reports is not less than 3 years from the date of the Australian marketing approval letter. No fewer than three annual reports are required: if a PSUR is not available, the Australian sponsor must prepare a post-marketing report.

Another condition of registration is that a product recall (or similar regulatory action) in any other country, which has relevance to the quality, safety and efficacy of the goods to be distributed in Australia, must be notified to the TGA immediately. Other conditions of registration include conditions related to the sampling and testing of products and manufacturing premises.

26.3.19　Products of gene technology

The Commonwealth Gene Technology Act 2000 came into force in 2001, introducing a national scheme for the regulation of genetically modified (GM) organisms in Australia. The legislation regulates some GM products, but only where the products are not regulated by an existing agency. Thus, therapeutic goods that contain GM organisms or are products of GM organisms continue to be regulated by the TGA.

The Gene Technology Act requires the gene technology regulator to be notified by other regulators such as the TGA about GM products approved for sale in Australia. For example, if the TGA approves a GM medicine for sale in Australia, this must be entered in the centralised, publicly available database of all GM organisms and GM products.

26.3.20　Products manufactured or tested using human embryos or human embryonic stem cells

In late 2003 an amendment to the Therapeutic Goods Regulations introduced new requirements for products registered on or after 1 July 2004 that are manufactured or tested using a human embryo or human embryonic stem cells (HESC). For products manufactured using a human embryo or HESC, or any material sourced from these materials, including any testing associated with the manufacture of the product, there must be a statement included in the PI and CMI disclosing this use.

In addition, where information is provided to the TGA as part of an application for registration of a prescription medicine that refers to use of human embryos, HESC or materials derived from human embryos or HESC in research undertaken in the development of the medicine, the PI and CMI must also include a statement to that effect.

The sponsor must provide a declaration on these matters in Module 1 of the application for registration.

26.3.21　Recalls

Recalls are handled by the Australian recall coordinator within the TGA according to the voluntary uniform recall procedures for therapeutic goods, in conjunction with the States. The Australian recall coordinator also liaises with the Commonwealth minister responsible for consumer affairs in relation to safety-related recalls of therapeutic goods, which must be notified within 48 hours, in accordance with the Trade Practices Act 1974. A mandatory recall of faulty goods may be enforced where safety is involved.

In April–May 2003 the TGA forced the recall of approximately 1600 complementary medicines at retail level throughout Australia, because of concerns about the quality of their manufacture. The recalled products were manufactured in Australia by Pan Pharmaceuticals, principally as a contract manufacturer for other companies. As a consequence of the regulatory action, amendments were made to the Therapeutic Goods Act to increase maximum penalties for a range of existing offences; create new offences such as falsifying documents relating to therapeutic goods regulation; expand compulsory public notification and recall provisions; insert a 'fit and proper person' test in relation to granting manufacturing licences and conformity assessment certificates; insert new conditions of licence to ensure compliance with manufacturing principles; require sponsors to maintain records of all manufacturers involved in manufacture of each batch of a product and have these records available for inspection at any time; require better identification of therapeutic goods in the event of a recall; and improve adverse event reporting for listed goods. The Therapeutic Goods Amendment Act (No. 1) 2003 took effect on 27 May 2003.

26.3.22 Counterfeit goods and tampering

The Therapeutic Goods Act was amended in 2000 to make it a specific offence to supply counterfeit therapeutic goods in Australia. Offences were also introduced under the Therapeutic Goods Act for tampering with therapeutic goods or continuing to supply goods that may have been tampered with, and for failing to notify the TGA of any knowledge of actual tampering or threats associated with tampering.

26.3.23 Trans-Tasman Mutual Recognition arrangement

The Trans-Tasman Mutual Recognition Act 1997, developed under the policy of closer economic relations between Australia and New Zealand, came into force in 1998. The Act is intended to enhance Trans-Tasman trade by allowing goods available in one country to be acceptable in the other (and also recognise professional qualifications in both countries). A special exemption for therapeutic goods was immediately granted in recognition of the differences between the Australian and New Zealand regulatory systems. Special exemptions are required to be reviewed annually and may be extended for a further 12 months to 30 April the following year.

The two countries' therapeutic goods agencies had been working towards resolving the special exemption in consultation with the industry, consumers, medical and pharmacy professions. The health ministers in Australia and New Zealand had agreed that harmonisation of regulatory requirements for therapeutic goods was the best option and, in December 2003, the two governments signed a treaty committing them to establishing a 'single world-class agency' and a 'regulatory regime consistent with international best practice for the regulation of quality, safety and efficacy or performance of therapeutic products.' The Australia New Zealand Therapeutic Products Authority, responsible for implementing regulatory controls over the import, manufacture and supply of therapeutic products in both countries, was scheduled to begin operation on 1 July 2006.

Legislation establishing the new agency was presented to both parliaments in 2007. On 16 July 2007, the New Zealand Government announced that it did not have sufficient parliamentary support to ensure passage of the legislation, and negotiations on the joint authority were suspended indefinitely. The Australian Government is now considering how it can utilise the work done in developing the legislation and rules for the joint agency to progress regulatory developments in Australia. Consultations commenced in July 2008 on reforms for therapeutic goods regulation in Australia.

26.4 Listing on the Pharmaceutical Benefits Scheme – the 'fourth hurdle'

Applications for listing a product on the PBS are generally submitted by the pharmaceutical company sponsor, which has the data required to support the application, to the Pharmaceutical Benefits section of the Department of Health. However, submissions from medical bodies, health professionals or members of the public may also be considered.

A product may not be listed on the PBS until marketing approval is granted. However, a sponsor may apply for PBS listing once the TGA delegate has recommended to ADEC that the product be granted marketing approval. Thus, consideration of a listing application can to some extent overlap with the final stages of evaluation of an application for marketing approval.

Products may not be subsidised under the PBS for unapproved indications, and some approved indications may not be subsidised. Details of the medicines approved for subsidy are available from the Schedule of Pharmaceutical Benefits website (www.pbs.gov.au).

26.4.1 The PBAC process

The PBAC assesses applications for listing on the PBS for reimbursement against criteria specified in the National Health Act. These criteria include safety and efficacy compared with other available treatments including non-drug therapies, and comparative cost-effectiveness.

The current Guidelines for Preparing Submissions to the Pharmaceutical Benefits Advisory Committee (PBAC) (Version 4.2) December 2007 (PBAC submission guidelines) are available through www.aodgp.gov.au/internet/main/publishing.nsf/Content/pbacguidelines-index.

The guidelines must be followed for major submissions to the PBAC to:
• List a new drug on the schedule of pharmaceutical benefits;
• Request a significant change to the listing of a currently restricted drug (including a new indication or a de-restriction);
• Enable a review of the comparative cost-effectiveness of a currently listed drug in order to change a PBAC recommendation to the PBPA or its therapeutic relativity or price premium; or
• List a new formulation or strength of a currently listed drug for which a price premium is requested.

The guidelines are interpreted in a very prescriptive manner, and have been the subject of ongoing discussion. Improved health outcomes that are difficult to quantify, such as 'indirect' benefits, are accorded a low weighting. Also large head-to-head comparative studies with adequate power to yield significant differences may be required before superior outcomes are regarded as proven.

On receipt of a major application for listing, the PBAC secretariat forwards the application to the Pharmaceutical Evaluation Branch (PEB). The PEB evaluates these applications together with three external groups from academic institutions contracted for this work. The PEB provides an evaluation report to the Economic Sub-Committee (ESC) of the PBAC.

The ESC reviews and interprets the economic analyses and advises the PBAC on these analyses. The PBAC also receives advice from the Drug Utilisation Sub-Committee (DUSC).

The sponsor receives the PEB evaluation and DUSC report approximately 2.5 weeks prior to the PBAC meeting at which the application will be considered. The sponsor's response to the overview and commentary must be sent to the PBAC secretariat within 1 week and are provided to the PBAC along with the ESC advice and the PEB overview and commentary.

As with ADEC, conflict of interest guidelines are strictly applied to PBAC and its sub-committees. The membership of the PBAC was revised in 2001, allowing for a greater range of expertise to be included, and introducing restrictions on the length of term that members may serve. Amid some controversy, a member with pharmaceutical industry experience was included, in addition to medical practitioners and members with pharmacy and consumerist backgrounds. Following the untimely death of the pharmaceutical industry member, and the appointment of a new Minister for Health, the industry member was not replaced. In April 2004, the National Health Act was amended to increase the number of members of the PBAC to a maximum of 15.

The PBAC meets three times per annum, in March, July and November, as the culmination of the 17 week pre-meeting application cycle (see section 26.4.8). Positive PBAC recommendations are published by the Department of Health on the PBS section of its website (www.health.gov.au/internet/main/publishing.nsf/Content/Pharmaceutical+Benefits+Scheme+%28PBS%29-1) approximately 6 weeks after the PBAC meeting. If an application for listing is successful, the PBAC recommends the maximum quantity to be dispensed on each prescription and the number of repeat prescriptions. The PBAC may also recommend prescribing restrictions – an authority required item requires the prescriber to obtain prior approval from Medicare Australia, by telephone or post, unless it has been designated as being eligible for the streamlined authority process, and restricted benefit items may only be prescribed for specified therapeutic uses.

Only 55% of first time major submissions in 2007 led to recommendations for new PBS listings, compared with 92% of first time minor submissions. Of the first time major submissions, 41% of cost-effectiveness submissions were successful and 59% of cost-minimisation submissions. For major resubmissions, the figures were 75% and 25%, respectively.

26.4.2 Appeals against recommendations on PBS listing applications

The National Health Act does not include the option for PBAC recommendations to be appealed to the AAT. Generally, the only avenue is for the applicant to appeal to the PBAC. Following a review of the listing process in 2002, the opportunity for meetings between the PBAC and stakeholders was established. These meetings are not intended as an appeals mechanism but as a 'without prejudice' non-adversarial process to facilitate a resubmission by the sponsor. A stakeholder meeting may be sought where the drug is indicated for a serious disabling or life-threatening condition for which there is no other realistic management option. The Guidelines for Stakeholder Meetings are available from the PBS website.

PBAC rejections, and the lack of available appeal mechanisms, have been increasingly challenged in recent years. One available route is to pursue a legal challenge to the Federal Court of Australia for a review of the decision. Most recently, as an outcome of the Australia United States Free Trade Agreement (AUSFTA), an Independent Review Mechanism (IRM) was introduced for negative PBAC recommendations. The IRM has only been used once – unsuccessfully – and offers little other than a second opinion on the PBAC's assessment.

26.4.3 Free Trade Agreement

The AUSFTA came into force on 1 January 2005. The full text of the agreement is available from the Department of Foreign Affairs and Trade website (www.dfat.govau/trade/negotiations/us_fta/final-text/index.html). Annex 2C and the side letter outline that the following changes (in summary) would be made to enhance the processes for listing medicines on the PBS:

1. Annex 2C
- Greater transparency of the listing process for applicants and the public;
- A medicines working group to be established comprising officials from each government to promote discussion and understanding of the Annex;
- Enhanced dialogue between the TGA and the FDA with the view to expedite availability of innovative medicines;
- Companies to be permitted to provide truthful and not misleading information on their websites about medicines approved for sale.

2. Side letter
- Applicants will have the opportunity to consult with officials prior to submission, to respond fully to all

reports or evaluations, and to have a hearing before the PBAC, and will receive information on the reasons for the PBAC's determination;
- There will be an independent review process for PBAC determinations of listing applications where there is a negative recommendation;
- The listing process will be streamlined and expedited, with more frequent revisions of the schedule of pharmaceutical benefits;
- Applicants will be allowed to apply for an adjustment to a reimbursement amount.

An initiative arising from the AUSFTA transparency principles is the availability of Public Summary Documents (PSDs), which provide summary information concerning the rationale for the PBAC recommendation to include a medicine on the PBS. The PBAC is required by legislation to take into account the cost-effectiveness of medicines proposed for subsidy compared with other therapies, therefore the PSD includes information on the economic analysis presented by the sponsor company and the PBACs evaluation of the cost effectiveness claims. PSDs are published on the Health Department website approximately 4 months after the relevant PBAC meeting. PSDs are published for positive listing decisions and first time rejections, the latter are published approximately 2 weeks later than PSDs for positive outcomes.

26.4.4 Pricing of products on the PBS

The PBPA makes recommendations to the Department of Health on the prices for new items that have been recommended for PBS listing by the PBAC. It also reviews the prices for all items listed on the Schedule of Pharmaceutical Benefits at least once per annum. The PBAC provides advice to the PBPA regarding comparison with other treatments and comparative cost-effectiveness.

The Commonwealth Government negotiates an agreed wholesale price with the pharmaceutical company sponsor, through a senior officer in the pharmaceutical benefits branch. This process applies to all products subsidised as PBS-listed items under Section 85 of the National Health Act, including products that are priced below the general patient co-payment.

A wholesaler margin is then set on the supplier's price, a pharmacist margin is applied to the wholesaler's price, and a pharmacist dispensing fee is also added, determined by the Pharmaceutical Benefits Remuneration Tribunal. Patients pay the co-payment (and any premiums) to the pharmacist when the PBS-listed medicine is dispensed, with the balance of the cost of the product being paid to the pharmacist by the government.

Consumers' contributions to the cost of their medicines are limited by safety net thresholds, which are adjusted annually in relation to the consumer price index. Under the PBS the maximum cost for a listed item on 1 July 2008 was A$5.00 for concessional patients and A$31.30 for general patients, except where a brand premium, therapeutic group premium (TGP) or special patient contribution applied. There are two safety net thresholds. For general patients, once a patient has spent A$1141.80 on PBS medicines, the patient co-payment decreases to the concessional level of A$5.00 for the rest of the calendar year. For concessional patients the safety net threshold is A$290.00. Once concessional patients reach this level they receive PBS items free of charge for the rest of the calendar year. From 1 August 2003 information about the full cost of each item has been included on the label of the medicine, so that consumers will be better informed.

Determination of the agreed price for a product to be listed on the PBS is understandably one of the most contentious areas between the pharmaceutical industry and government. The pricing procedure and methods used by the PBPA in recommending prices for new items and in its annual review of prices of all items listed on the PBS, including Reference Pricing and Weighted Average Monthly Treatment Cost, are explained in a document that is available from the PBS website.

The PBPA sometimes recommends the use of price/volume arrangements, particularly where unit prices are reasonably high and there is the potential for significant volumes or where there is uncertainty about future volumes.

If the predicted annual cost to the government is greater than A$5 million in 1 year, including consideration of the potential for prescribing outside of the agreed restrictions, the Department of Health must obtain the Department of Finance's agreement to the estimated costs. If the predicted annual cost to government is greater than A$10 million, the listing must be approved by the Prime Minister and the Minister for Finance, in addition to the Minister for Health.

The PBAC and PBPA also consider the prices of pharmaceuticals listed under Section 100 of the National Health Act, which allows for an alternative means of providing an adequate pharmaceutical service in circumstances where pharmaceutical benefits cannot be conveniently and efficiently supplied in the usual manner under the PBS. The current Section 100

programmes are Highly Specialised Drugs (HSDs), human growth hormone, IVF/GIFT, opiate dependence treatment and the special authority programme. HSDs, such as medicines for HIV/AIDS, are reviewed by the Highly Specialised Drugs Working Party and are generally supplied through different dispensing arrangements in public hospitals under agreements with the States, without wholesaler involvement.

26.4.5 Brand premiums

Where there are two or more brands of the same form and strength of a drug listed on the PBS that are bioequivalent and hence interchangeable, the PBPA recommends the benchmark price for that drug, being the price of the lowest priced brand. Sponsors of the other brands may charge a premium above the benchmark price. Brands that are considered interchangeable are indicated in the schedule by alphabetic superscripts. The cost of the brand premium must be paid by the consumer in addition to any co-payment. A pharmacist may substitute brands to avoid a consumer paying a premium, provided the prescriber does not specifically prohibit this and the consumer agrees.

26.4.6 Special patient contribution arrangements

A sponsor may not seek to charge a product premium above the agreed listing price unless there is an alternative brand of the drug in the same form and strength listed on the PBS. If the sponsor and government cannot agree on a listing price for a new product, and there is no alternative listed on the PBS, the product cannot be listed with a brand premium. However, on rare occasions a special patient contribution can apply. This currently applies to only six PBS items.

26.4.7 Reference pricing and therapeutic group premiums

In 1998, the Commonwealth Government introduced TGPs, a form of reference pricing, to certain therapeutic groups listed on the PBS. The current therapeutic groups are H2 receptor antagonists, angiotensin-converting enzyme (ACE) inhibitors, proton pump inhibitors, angiotensin II inhibitors, HMG-CoA reductase inhibitors (statins) and calcium-channel blockers. Under this policy, the government will subsidise all drug products in the therapeutic group up to the price of the lowest priced product in the group – the benchmark. Different substances in a therapeutic group are deemed to be equivalent for the purpose of pricing, including patented and off-patent products.

If a sponsor chooses to charge a premium above the benchmark price, that premium must be paid by the consumer in addition to the co-payment, and does not count towards the PBS safety net threshold.

A prescriber may apply to the Medicare Australia for a TGP exemption for an individual patient for a particular product, if adverse effects or reactions are expected to occur with all of the benchmark priced products or the transfer to a benchmark priced product would cause patient confusion leading to problems with compliance. Pharmacists may not substitute between different substances in a therapeutic group.

When the policy was introduced it was thought that some sponsors would maintain significant premiums for their products over the benchmark price. However, over time, many reduced their price to the benchmark price or charged a reduced premium compared with the price prior to introduction of the TGP policy. At August 2008 the premiums ranged from A$4.02 to A$1.52 in four groups, with no premium charged on any of the HMG-CoA reductase inhibitors or ACE inhibitors.

Since 1 August 2005, the first new generic brand of a medicine listed on the PBS has been required to be listed at 12.5% below the current benchmark price. As a result of reference pricing arrangements this price reduction also flows to all products in the same reference pricing group. This price reduction applies once only for each medicine (and for the medicines in the reference pricing group).

26.4.8 PBS reforms 2007

In November 2006, the government announced major reforms to the PBS. It forecast savings of around A$500 million in the first 4 years, increasing to A$3 billion over 10 years, by introducing greater competition in the off-patent drug market, with the aim of ensuring that the PBS remained economically sustainable, while allowing for the inclusion of new innovative medicines on the PBS. The main features of the reforms were the creation of two drug formularies and changes to pricing mechanisms.

From 1 August 2007, PBS medicines were divided into two separate formularies:

• Formulary 1 (F1) for single brand medicines, except for single brand medicines that are interchangeable at the patient level with multiple brand medicines; and
• Formulary 2 (F2) for multiple brand medicines and any single brand medicines that are interchangeable with multiple brand medicines at the patient level. F2 was further divided into two sub-formularies: F2T comprising medicines that attracted significant

trading terms to pharmacy at 1 October 2006 (i.e. discounts of 25% or more), and F2A comprising medicines that did not attract significant trading terms.

A medicine is classified into only one formulary. If one formulation or strength of a medicine has multiple brands, then the substance is listed on the F2 formulary, even if multiple brands are not available in other formulations or strengths of that medicine. Combination products are placed on a list outside the two formularies.

Reference pricing continues to apply between F1 medicines that are linked within reference pricing groups, within TGPs, and across different brands of the same substance listed on F2, but there will be no ongoing price links between medicines listed on F1 and those listed on F2.

The 12.5% price reduction policy for the first new generic brand (see section 26.4.7) became a legislated requirement under the reforms, instead of being only a matter of policy, and introduction of the first generic brand of a substance now also causes the medicine to move from the F1 formulary to F2A.

Other mandated price reductions were introduced as follows:

• Price reductions of 2% per year for 3 years for all products containing F2A substances, commencing on 1 August 2008; and
• A one-off 25% price reduction on 1 August 2008, for all products containing F2T substances, except for a few F2T substances specified in the legislation, for which the 25% price reduction is to be phased.

F1 substances are protected from these statutory price reductions, so long as they remain in the F1 formulary. Some substances in specified forms and with specified routes of administration for use in special populations are also exempt from the statutory price reductions.

Finally, medicines listed in F2 will move to a system of price disclosure, with associated price reductions, so that the price that the government pays for a PBS medicine will more closely reflect the actual price at which the medicine is being sold. Suppliers listing a new brand containing an F2A substance on or after 1 August 2007 must agree to ongoing disclosure of the actual market price on a regular basis, as a condition of listing, with mandatory flow-on price reductions if the weighted average discount (based on a complex formula) is found to be more than 10%. From 1 January 2011, F2A and F2T will merge and suppliers listing a new product containing any F2 substance must agree to disclose the actual market price as a condition of listing, with subsequent price reductions if applicable.

To compensate for the reduced income resulting from these reforms, pharmacy mark-ups and dispensing fees were increased, pharmacists are being paid A$1.50 per prescription to dispense a 'premium free' medicine (this applies to both originator and generic brands of a medicine), and additional funding was provided to pharmaceutical wholesalers. Full details are available from the PBS reforms website (http://www.health.gov.au/pbsreform).

In November 2006, the Access to Medicines Working Group (AMWG) was formed to enable the Department of Health and Medicines Australia to work together more effectively and consider issues regarding timely and appropriate access to new medicines for the PBS. The group is jointly chaired by a Deputy Secretary of the Department and the Chairman of Medicines Australia, and comprises senior representatives of each organisation. It meets 3–4 times a year.

The terms of reference for the AMWG are as follow:
1. Providing strategic oversight of ongoing joint activities undertaken by the Department and Medicines Australia to enhance the PBS processes; and
2. As a result of reforms to the PBS announced in 2006, considering issues relating to timely and appropriate access to effective new medicines on the PBS, including:
• The capacity to further streamline and coordinate processes to reduce the time it takes to list a medicine on the PBS;
• Possible impacts on the listing process of mandatory price reductions from 1 August 2008 for medicines on the new F2 formulary;
• The potential for improving clinical trial, economic and financial data to inform PBAC and PBPA decision-making processes;
• In collaboration with the PBAC, developing and articulating a set of principles for assessing evidence and information relating to new medicines and for improving the transparency of the decision-making process;
• The practical limitations to the evidence available to the PBAC to facilitate decision-making around access to new medicines and the development of options to manage uncertainty in such situations; and
• Opportunities for informing and learning from the broader international debate about evidentiary requirements and trends in drug development to support the economic evaluation of new medicines.

26.4.9 Time-frames

It currently takes a minimum of 35 weeks from submission of an application for PBS listing to the time it may be prescribed as a PBS item if the application is successful the first time it is considered, although some of this process may overlap the final stages of registration approval (Table 26.1). Products are frequently not launched in Australia until PBS listing is achieved.

26.5 Access to medicines not registered or listed on the ARTG

Four avenues are available for access to medicines not registered or listed on the ARTG are available:
1. Clinical trials;
2. Special access scheme;
3. Authorised prescriber;
4. Personal importation.
Further details are available through the TGA website.

26.5.1 Clinical trials

There are two schemes under which clinical trials involving therapeutic goods may be conducted in Australia: the CTN and the CTX schemes. These schemes are used for clinical trials involving any product not entered on the ARTG, or use of a registered or listed product in a clinical trial beyond the conditions of its marketing approval.

Clinical trials in which registered or listed medicines (or medical devices) are used within the conditions of their marketing approval are not subject to CTN or CTX requirements but still need to be approved by a human research ethics committee (HREC) before the trial may commence.

All CTN and CTX trials must have an Australian sponsor. The sponsor is that person, body, organisation or institution that takes overall responsibility for the conduct of the trial. It need not be a pharmaceutical company. The sponsor usually initiates, organises and supports a clinical study and carries the medicolegal responsibility associated with the conduct of the trial.

In 2006–2007 there were 3182 CTN scheme notifications. It should be noted, however, that this does not indicate the number of different clinical trial protocols, which was approximately 782 in 2006–2007. This contrasts with six CTX 50 working day applications in the same period and zero 30 working day applications.

26.5.1.1 The CTN scheme

Under the CTN scheme the sponsor of the clinical trial provides detailed information about the proposed trial to the principal investigator who submits an

Table 26.1 Time-frame for Pharmaceutical Benefits Scheme (PBS) listing

Action	Weeks
Prior to PBAC meeting	
Cut-off date for major submissions	17
PBS evaluation and DUSC commentary sent to sponsor	7.5
Cut-off date for minor submissions	6–7
Pre-ESC and pre-DUSC responses provided by sponsors	6.5
DUSC meeting	5
ESC meeting	4.5
RWG meeting	4
ESC, DUSC and RWG advice sent to sponsors	2
Pre-PBAC comments provided by sponsor	1
ESC report and sponsor comments sent to PBAC	1
PBAC meeting	0
Post-PBAC meeting	
Verbal advice of recommendation given to sponsor	0.5
Written advice of recommendation sent to sponsor	3
Unratified minutes sent to sponsor	4–5
PBPA meeting	6
Approval by Minister for Health/Parliamentary Secretary	10–12
Closing date to amend Schedule of Pharmaceutical Benefits	14
Listing in the Schedule of Pharmaceutical Benefits	18

Drug Utilisation Sub-Committee (DUSC); Economic Sub-Committee (ESC); Pharmaceutical Benefits Advisory Committee (PBAC); Pharmaceutical Benefits Pricing Authority (PBPA); Restrictions Working Group (RWG).

application to conduct the clinical trial to the HREC at the institution or other site at which the trial is proposed to be conducted. The clinical trial application generally includes the protocol, the investigator's brochure, related patient information, supporting data and the CTN form. HRECs usually have their own standard format for applications to conduct a CTN trial at their institution. The HREC evaluates the scientific and ethical validity of the proposed clinical trial and the safety and efficacy of the medicine in the context of its stage of development. The TGA does not evaluate any information about the clinical trial.

If the HREC approves the conduct of the clinical trial, the chairman of the HREC signs the CTN form. The institution or organisation at which the trial will be conducted, referred to as the approving authority, gives the final approval for the conduct of the trial at the site, having due regard to advice from the HREC and also must sign the CTN form. In some cases, the HREC can also be the approving authority for a particular trial site.

In signing the CTN form the signatories agree that they will comply with all legislative and regulatory requirements, that the trial will be conducted in accordance with the Note for Guidance on Good Clinical Practice (GCP Guidelines) (CPMP/ICH/135/ 95), and the National Health and Medical Research Council (NHMRC) National Statement on Ethical Conduct in Human Research 2007 (National Statement), and that they will agree to release information to the TGA about the conduct of the trial in the event of an inquiry or audit of the trial.

The form is then submitted by the sponsor of the trial to the TGA, along with the appropriate notification fee. The current notification fee is A$260 for each notification, which can comprise a single site conducting a clinical trial, or multiple sites conducting the same trial notified together. Once the CTN form has been submitted to the TGA along with the relevant fee, the clinical trial may commence. The TGA acknowledges receipt of the CTN form and fee, which takes 2–3 days. Some sponsors choose to wait for receipt of this acknowledgement before commencing a trial, although this is not strictly necessary.

There is one CTN form for each site conducting the same clinical trial, such as multicentre trials. In some cases a composite site can be notified where a single HREC and approving authority have responsibility for all sites conducting the trial, such as a general practice network.

To assist the TGA to maintain a record of each CTN trial, the sponsor must subsequently notify the TGA of the date the trial was completed, the reason the trial ceased (e.g. concluded normally; insufficient recruits) and any changes to the trial with respect of information previously submitted.

26.5.1.2 The CTX scheme

Under the CTX scheme, a sponsor submits an application to conduct clinical trials to both the TGA and the HREC at each institution or site at which it is proposed to conduct the clinical trial. The TGA reviews the information about the product provided by the sponsor, including whether the medicine is under investigation or approved for marketing in other countries, proposed usage guidelines, a pharmaceutical data sheet and a summary of the preclinical data and clinical data.

There are two levels of evaluation of applications for clinical trials of medicines under the CTX scheme. A 30 working day period for evaluation of a CTX application applies when the supporting data relate only to chemical, pharmaceutical and biological issues. A 50 working day period applies for applications supported by chemical, pharmaceutical and biological, preclinical and clinical data. These evaluation times commence from the date of acceptance of the application or receipt of the appropriate fee. The fee for a 30-day CTX application as at 1 July 2008 is A\$1280 and for a 50-day application A\$15,900.

If the TGA delegate raises an objection, trials may not proceed until the objection has been addressed to the delegate's satisfaction. Even if no objection is raised, the delegate usually provides comments on the accuracy or interpretation of the summary information supplied by the sponsor. The sponsor must forward these comments to the HREC(s) at sites at which the sponsor intends to conduct the trial.

As with the CTN scheme, the sponsor prepares information for submission by the principal investigator to the HREC at the institution or other site at which the trial is proposed to be conducted. The HREC in each host institution and/or organisation is responsible for approving the proposed trial protocol after reviewing the summary information received from the sponsor and any additional comments from the TGA delegate. The approving authority gives the final approval for the conduct of the trial at the site, having due regard to advice from the HREC.

A sponsor may not commence a CTX trial until written advice has been received from the TGA regarding the application, and approval has been obtained from the HREC and the institution at which the trial will be conducted.

The sponsor may conduct any number of clinical trials under the CTX application without further assessment by the TGA, provided use of the product in the trials falls within the original approved usage guidelines. However, HREC approval of each protocol and approval from the institution or organisation for the conduct of each trial are still required.

26.5.1.3 Reporting adverse events and adverse drug reactions during clinical trials

Australia has largely harmonised its reporting requirements for adverse events and ADRs occurring during clinical trials with international requirements and has adopted, in principle, the Note for Guidance on Clinical Safety Data Management: Definitions and Standards for Expedited Reporting (CPMP/ICH/377/95) – in particular the definitions and reporting time-frames.

Despite the TGA's adoption of these international requirements, the local interpretation of these guidelines in relation to reporting serious and unexpected adverse reactions must be adhered to. Sponsors of clinical trials are required to report to TGA single cases of serious and unexpected adverse reactions. Fatal or life-threatening ADRs should be reported within 7 calendar days of the reaction first being notified to the sponsor. This should be followed by as complete a report as possible within 8 additional calendar days. All other serious and unexpected ADRs should be reported to TGA within 15 calendar days of first knowledge of the sponsor.

Information should be provided in the form of a detailed summary in the ADRAC 'Blue Card' format. Even if initial information is scanty, these details should be forwarded to the TGA pending receipt and provision of further data. This procedure should be followed even when the medicine in question is the subject of an application for registration and under evaluation by the TGA.

Sponsors are not required, as a matter of routine, to submit individual patient reports to the TGA of suspected adverse drug reactions occurring with use of the same product in another country, even if a trial is ongoing at Australian sites. However, the TGA requires that sponsors advise the Experimental Drugs Section of OPM within 72 hours of any significant safety issue that has arisen from an analysis of overseas reports or action with respect to safety taken by another country's regulatory agency. This advice must include the basis for such action.

26.5.1.4 Good Clinical Practice and ethical conduct of clinical trials

The TGA's regulation of clinical trials involving new medicines requires adherence to international standards of ethical conduct and Good Clinical Practice (GCP). A TGA authorised person may enter a site at which a clinical trial is being conducted and examine anything at the site relating to the clinical trial, including any documents or records relating to the trial.

In 2000, the TGA Guidelines on Good Clinical Research Practice 1991 were replaced by the CPMP/ICH GCP guidelines (see section 26.5.1.1), with some amendments to reflect Australian regulatory requirements.

Furthermore, Australia has a strong framework in place to support the ethical conduct of clinical trials, provided by the NHMRC, its principal committees and HRECs. In August 2008, there were 208 registered HRECs in Australia – 106 hospital (public and private), 55 university, 25 government and 22 associated with professional and other bodies.

The strategic intent of the NHMRC is to provide leadership and work with other relevant organisations to improve the health of all Australians by:

• Fostering and supporting a high quality and internationally recognised research base;
• Providing evidence-based advice;
• Applying research evidence to health issues thus translating research into better health practice and outcomes; and
• Promoting informed debate on health and medical research, health ethics and related issues.

A principal committee of the NHMRC, the Australian Health Ethics Committee (AHEC), provides guidance and support for HRECs in Australia, and is responsible for developing and publishing the National Statement on Ethical Conduct in Human Research 2007.

Compliance with the national statement is a requirement for all clinical trials conducted in Australia under the CTX and CTN schemes. The chairman of the HREC certifies that the HREC is constituted in accordance with guidelines issued by the NHMRC, has registered with the AHEC, and has approved the clinical trial in accordance with the guidance provided by the national statement.

The increased awareness of ethical issues relating to human research led to the release in 2002 of the *Human Research Ethics Handbook*, including detailed commentary on the national statement and discussion of ethical and legal issues, to further assist HRECs to assess and facilitate the ethical conduct of research involving human participants, and resolve the challenges encountered during this process. Both the national statement and the associated handbook are available at the NHMRC website (www.nhmrc.gov au).

AHEC has developed the National Ethics Application Form (NEAF), which is a web-based application form for submission to HRECs. The NEAF is intended to assist sponsors and investigators, who can now prepare applications in a single format rather than according to individual HREC requirements, which delays submission of applications in Australia and adds to workload. There have been some user difficulties with the first NEAF version. The updated NEAF2 is expected to be available in August 2008.

Another initiative to streamline clinical trial start up is the implementation in May 2007 of a standard format for the Clinical Trial Research Agreement (CTRA) for trials sponsored by a pharmaceutical company. The CTRA was developed collaboratively between Medicines Australia and the State health authorities in New South Wales, Victoria and Queensland. An additional standard contract format for clinical research organisations (CROs) acting as the trial sponsor is also near finalisation, as is a standard format for collaborative research groups.

The NHMRC has received funding from the government to implement national streamlined ethical review for multicentre health and medical research in humans. It is anticipated that within 2 years Australia will move to a national system of ethical and scientific review whereby an ethical and scientific review conducted by an appropriately competent human research ethics committee will be accepted by all other centres participating in the research. There is considerable development and negotiation required to bring about this significant change in approach, but overall stakeholders recognise the necessity to implement a more efficient and timely ethical review process.

26.5.1.5 Status of the Declaration of Helsinki

The AHEC has advised HRECs to regard the National Statement as the definitive guideline for the review and conduct of research in Australia. The World Medical Association Declaration of Helsinki is mentioned in the preamble to the National Statement. AHEC has also advised HRECs that wherever there is doubt regarding the interpretation and application of various ethical guidelines, the National Statement takes precedence.

The clinical trial guidelines published by the TGA specify that all clinical trials must be conducted in accordance with the Declaration of Helsinki.

26.5.1.6 Clinical trial compensation guidelines and indemnity

In order to promote a uniform approach to offering compensation to subjects and indemnity to investigators and institutions conducting clinical trials, Medicines Australia published a Form of Indemnity for Clinical Trials and Guidelines for Compensation for Injury Resulting from Participation in a Company-Sponsored Clinical Trial. These documents are based on those published by the Association of the British Pharmaceutical Industry and are available from the Medicines Australia website (www.medicinesaustralia.com.au).

Medicines Australia has also developed a Form of Indemnity for Clinical Trials for HREC Review Only, for use where the indemnified party is providing HREC review only of the study.

26.5.2 Special Access Scheme

The Special Access Scheme (SAS) allows for the import and supply of an unapproved therapeutic good to an individual patient on a case-by-case basis. The scheme envisages two categories of patients – Category A patients, who are defined in the Regulations as 'persons who are seriously ill with a condition from which death is reasonably likely to occur within a matter of months, or from which premature death is reasonably likely to occur in the absence of early treatment', and Category B, all other patients. A medical practitioner can supply an unapproved product to a Category A patient without the approval of the TGA, but must inform the TGA within 4 weeks following supply. Thus, no prior approval is required from the TGA.

For Category B patients, individual approval for each patient must be obtained from a TGA delegate or a delegate outside the TGA referred to as an external delegate. Classification of a patient as Category A or B lies with the medical practitioner. However, the TGA may review, seek clarification and request information regarding the classification of patients under Category A.

A medical practitioner can supply any unapproved medicine to a Category A patient, except medicines listed in Schedule 9 of the SUSDP, which are primarily drugs of abuse such as heroin or cannabis.

Adverse event and ADR reporting requirements are similar to those for clinical trials, with greater emphasis on the prescriber being responsible for reporting any ADR to the TGA, the sponsor and HREC.

26.5.3 Authorised prescribers

Another avenue for limited access to an unapproved medicine is through the authorised prescriber provisions of the Therapeutic Goods Act. A few specified medical practitioners are authorised by the TGA to prescribe a specific unapproved therapeutic good or class of unapproved therapeutic goods, to specified recipients or classes of recipients (identified by their medical condition) in their immediate care, without further approval from the TGA. The authorised prescriber must also have the endorsement of an appropriate HREC to supply the product.

A pharmaceutical company is not obliged to supply an unapproved product under the authorised prescriber provisions. If it does supply the specified product, the company must provide reports every 6 months of the amount of product supplied to authorised prescribers.

Adverse event and ADR reporting requirements are similar to those for clinical trials, with greater emphasis on the authorised prescriber being responsible for reporting any ADR to the TGA, the sponsor and HREC as the sponsor will not normally be actively monitoring the use of the product.

26.5.4 Personal importation

Individuals may personally import an unapproved therapeutic good by either bringing the goods with them as they enter Australia or arranging for someone outside Australia to send the goods to them. Personal importation may only be used for that person or their immediate family (i.e. the goods may not be given or sold to another person). Furthermore, the quantity that may be imported is restricted to 3 months' supply at one time and a total of 15 months' supply in a 12-month period at the manufacturer's recommended maximum dosage.

If a prescription medicine is to be imported in this way, the importer must have a prescription from a medical practitioner, unless the goods are being carried with the person. Certain medicines may not be imported under the personal importation provisions, including drugs of abuse, such as narcotics, amphetamines and psychotropic substances, and anabolic substances, androgenic steroids and treatments for alcohol and drug addiction. There are also controls over certain other medicines including erythropoietin, growth hormones and gonadotrophins.

An individual cannot import injections that contain substances of human or animal origin (except insulin) without an SAS approval. The TGA considers that these injections represent a high risk from inadequately or improperly prepared materials (including a lack of sterility) and, therefore, approvals will only be granted to the supervising physician.

26.6 Presentation

Under the Therapeutic Goods Act, presentation means the way in which the goods are presented for supply, and includes matters relating to the name of the goods, the labelling and packaging of the goods, and any advertising or other informational material associated with the goods. The term label refers to the display of printed information on, or supplied with, the goods and their packaging, rather than the broader meaning applied in the USA, which includes approved uses of the product. Labels fall within the definition of advertising.

26.6.1 Standard for the Uniform Scheduling of Drugs and Poisons

The SUSDP lists drugs and poisons according to the recommended restrictions on their availability to the public. The categories of the SUSDP most relevant to medicines on the ARTG are as follow:

• *Schedule 8* – controlled drugs (e.g. strong analgesics, such as morphine);
• *Schedule 4* – prescription only medicines;
• *Schedule 3* – non-prescription medicines for supply by pharmacists only;
• *Schedule 2* – non-prescription medicines the safe use of which may require advice from a pharmacist.

Schedules 5 and 6 of the SUSDP also include some therapeutic products, such as head lice preparations and some essential oils.

The National Drugs and Poisons Schedule Committee, established under the Therapeutic Goods Act, is responsible for the SUSDP, which includes requirements for signal headings, warning statements and safety directions to be included on the labels of medicines containing scheduled substances, and exemptions from scheduling gained by placement of specified warnings on labels.

Access to the substances listed in the SUSDP is usually restricted for a number of reasons, including toxicity, safety and the risks and benefits associated with the use of the product.

The SUSDP has recently been formally declared to be a legislative instrument under Commonwealth law, but it still relies on State legislation that refers to or reflects the SUSDP (occasionally with some differences in some States) for its implementation.

Medicines that are not scheduled in the SUSDP can be sold through any distribution outlet, such as a supermarket or health food store. Examples of medicines that are unscheduled include small packs of simple pain relievers, and most vitamins and minerals.

26.6.2 Labels and packaging

The labels of medicines are required to conform to Therapeutic Goods Order (TGO) 69: General Requirements for Labels for Medicines, except for goods solely for export or for use in clinical trials. The requirements include names and quantities of active ingredients, dosage form, batch number, expiry date, the registration or listing number (AUSTR or AUSTL number, respectively), identification of inactive ingredients, what labelling is adequate for special packs and small containers, and letter size and additional requirements in particular circumstances.

In addition, labels for medicines must conform to requirements for labelling described in the SUSDP the Required Advisory Statements for Medicine Labels (RASML) document has been established to enable the transfer of all mandatory label advisory statements from the SUSDP and the Therapeutic Goods Regulations to a new document, separate from, but linked to, TGO 69.

Non-prescription medicines must, in addition, comply with TGO 69A, which introduced performance-based labelling from 1 July 2004. Products with labels that have been designed in accordance with the industry code of practice, Labelling Code of Practice: Designing Usable Non-prescription Medicine Labels for Consumers, should achieve this aim. TGO 69, TGO 69A and RASML are available on the TGA website.

Certain medicines considered to have a high risk of poisoning children must be packaged in child-resistant packaging. The specified medicines and acceptable types of packaging are described in TGO 65: Child-Resistant Packaging for Therapeutic Goods.

Evaluation areas within the TGA responsible for the different categories of registered medicines make recommendations on the labelling of individual products as part of the registration process. Listed medicines are entered into the ARTG with a declaration from the sponsor that they meet the relevant standards and advertising requirements, and have acceptable presentations. Labels are not examined at the time of listing, but may be assessed following listing either as a result of a random review or if a problem arises.

26.6.3 Country of origin

Country of origin is generally not indicated on the labels of therapeutic goods marketed in Australia. As prescription medicines are prescribed by a medical practitioner rather than purchased 'off the shelf' by the consumer, there is generally little incentive to convey origin information. Where manufacturers choose to do so, they must comply with State Fair Trading Acts, and the Commonwealth Trade Practices Act 1974.

Prior to December 1994, an 'essential character' test, was used to determine the validity of country of origin claims, in the context of Sections 52 and 53(eb) of the Trade Practices Act 1974 in relation to false or misleading statements. However, in 1994 the Federal Court handed down a decision that effectively rejected the essential character test and created uncertainty about outcomes of future cases in this area.

In 1998, the Trade Practices Amendment (Country of Origin Representations) Act 1998 came into force. Manufacturers making unqualified statements about country of origin, such as 'Made in . . .' must be able to demonstrate substantial transformation and exceed a 50% production costs threshold. They therefore tend to use qualified claims, such as 'Made in Australia from local and imported ingredients', to ensure that labels are not misleading or deceptive.

26.6.4 Advertising

The Therapeutic Goods Act and Regulations, Trade Practices Act, and State legislation all contain sections relating to the promotion of therapeutic goods. In particular, the Therapeutic Goods Act specifies that advertising of a therapeutic good can only refer to the approved indications for that good.

Prescription medicines may only be advertised to health care professionals – they may not be advertised to consumers. Advertisements of prescription medicines directed at health care professionals are regulated under a self-regulatory code of conduct administered by Medicines Australia. First published in 1960, it includes standards for appropriate advertising, the behaviour of medical representatives, and relationships with health care professionals. The current edition (15th) of the *Medicines Australia Code of Conduct* is available from the Medicines Australia website.

Since July 2007, members of Medicines Australia have been required, under the code of conduct, to provide 6-monthly reports detailing prescribed information about all educational events conducted or sponsored by member companies. This information is published on the Medicines Australia website. Medicines Australia commissioned an independent analysis of the first round of reports, which led to 52 complaints for further consideration arising from 14,633 educational events, with only 21 eventually found to be in breach of the code of conduct – a compliance rate of 99.8%. The annual report of the outcome of all complaints considered by the code of conduct committee is also published on the website.

The Therapeutic Goods Advertising Code currently forms the basis for determining the acceptability of advertisements for therapeutic goods directed to consumers. All advertisements for therapeutic goods directed to consumers, published or broadcast in mainstream (designated) media, must be approved before publication or broadcast. The Minister for Health has delegated this responsibility to the Australian Self-Medication Industry (ASMI) and the Complementary Healthcare Council (CHC). Complaints about advertisements in specified media, such as broadcast media and magazines, may be subject to complaints under the Therapeutic Goods Advertising Code, even if they have been approved before publication.

The non-prescription, complementary medicines and medical devices industry are also subject to broader industry-specific codes of practice, including relations with health care professionals, under codes administered by ASMI, CHC and the Medical Technology Association of Australia, respectively.

26.7 Patents

The Patents Act 1990 conveys a 20-year standard term of patent protection. From July 1999, holders of patents for a pharmaceutical substance have been permitted to apply for an extension beyond the standard term, as long as the application is made within 6 months of the first marketing approval (inclusion in the ARTG) of a pharmaceutical product containing the substance. The extension granted may be for no more than 5 years and will permit a maximum of 15 years protection after marketing approval. Sponsors of generic products containing that substance are permitted to undertake certain preparatory activities, known as 'springboarding', within the patent period. Recent Federal Court decisions have clarified the limitations of patent extension, to strictly interpret what is meant by first inclusion of a product containing the substance in the ARTG to include inclusion in the export-only section of the ARTG and what is meant by the phrase 'containing the substance'.

The AUSFTA required amendment of the Therapeutic Goods Act to ensure that a generic manufacturer is not able to enter the market with a generic version of a medicine before a patent covering that product has expired. Applicants registering a generic medicine are required to provide a certificate to the Secretary of the Department of Health (effectively the TGA) stating either that they believe that the generic medicine would not infringe a valid patent or that they have given notice to the patent holder that they propose to market the generic medicine before the end of the patent term. These amendments commenced when the AUSFTA came into force on 1 January 2005.

Prior to passing the Implementation Bill, the federal opposition successfully argued for certain further amendments to the Therapeutic Goods Act that impose significant penalties on patent holders (up to A$10 million) if they commence proceedings under the Patents Act 1990 against a generic manufacturer unless they are to be commenced in good faith, have reasonable prospects of success and will be commenced without reasonable delay.

26.8 Non-prescription medicines and complementary medicines

Non-prescription or OTC medicines are considered to be 'low risk' in comparison with prescription medicines. They are evaluated for quality, safety and efficacy by the TGA and the Medicines Evaluation Committee, in accordance with the Australian Regulatory Guidelines for OTC Medicines, 1 July 2003 before they may be registered on the ARTG. The OTC Products Application Lodgement system enables electronic lodgement of applications for inclusion of OTC products in the ARTG, although a hard copy data package is also still required to be submitted. Further details are available from the TGA website.

Complementary medicines are most frequently listed rather than registered, but this depends on the ingredients and claims made. The Guidelines for Levels and Kinds of Evidence to Support Indications and Claims was developed to assist sponsors in determining the appropriate evidence to support indications and claims made in relation to complementary medicines, sunscreens and other listable medicines, and is available from the TGA website. The Australian Regulatory Guidelines for Complementary Medicines contain further advice. The Complementary Medicines Evaluation Committee provides scientific and policy advice relating to controls on the supply and use of complementary medicines, with particular reference to the quality and safety of products and, where appropriate, efficacy relating to the claims made. Approximately 25% of medicines listed in the ARTG via the electronic listing facility – without the need for pre-market evaluation of substantiating evidence – are randomly selected by the TGA for a review of their labels, product specifications and

the summary of supporting evidence held by the sponsor.

The appropriateness of the current risk-based approach to the regulation of medicines is under increased scrutiny – especially that claims may be made for listable therapeutic goods without prior evaluation of substantiating evidence. A product's principal use and the claims made are also key determinants of whether it is deemed to be a medicine or a food, or a medicine or a cosmetic. Guidance on these distinctions is available from the TGA website.

26.9 Medical devices

The Therapeutic Device Programme was established in 1984. In 1987, the Customs (Prohibited Imports) Regulations were amended to require the Department of Health's approval before devices in five 'designated' categories could be imported, and the Therapeutic Device Evaluation Committee (TDEC) was established.

The Commonwealth Government gradually introduced regulatory requirements for devices akin to those for medicines, especially where higher risks were associated to their use. These include formal guidelines for marketing and clinical trial applications, GMP requirements and an adverse event reporting scheme. However, TDEC was not as involved as ADEC in considering individual marketing applications.

When the Therapeutic Goods Act came into effect, most therapeutic devices were classified as listable goods. Registrable devices include implantable devices, biomaterials, intraocular lenses and fluids, intrauterine and other contraceptive devices, and drug infusion systems.

An MRA on standards and conformity assessment between Australia and the EC came into effect from 1999, covering eight industry sectors including GMP inspection and batch certification of medicinal products, and conformity assessment of medical devices.

The ECMRA applied to medical devices manufactured in the EC, Australia and New Zealand. It recognised the competence of designated conformity assessment bodies in the EC to undertake conformity assessment of medical devices to Australian regulatory requirements, and the competence of the TGA to undertake assessment of medical devices for compliance with the requirements for certification (CE marking) for entry onto the EC market.

Devices incorporating animal-derived tissues, radioactive materials, *in vitro* diagnostics and devices manufactured in other countries, such as the USA (even those devices that have CE marking) were excluded.

New procedures came into effect in October 2002. The Commonwealth Therapeutic Goods Amendment (Medical Devices) Act 2002 and the Therapeutic Goods (Medical Devices) Regulations 2002 introduced new harmonised requirements, which classified medical devices as falling into one of five classes – I, IIa, IIb, III and active implantable medical devices, based on intended use, level of risk and the degree of invasiveness in the human body. All medical devices already included in the ARTG as registered or listed devices had until October 2007 to comply with the new requirements. If a product was required to be transitioned and its sponsor did not lodge an effective application for inclusion in the ARTG or for TGA Conformity Assessment certification by 3 October 2007, the product was taken to have been cancelled from the ARTG on 4 October 2007 for the purposes of determining the legality of supply of that product.

The TGA is developing a consolidated reference document detailing the Australian regulatory requirements for medical devices – the Australian Regulatory Guidelines for Medical Devices. Current details of the regulation of medical devices and diagnostics in Australia may be obtained through the TGA website.

The TGA also initiated the development of new regulatory frameworks for IVDs and human tissues and cellular therapies, to be harmonised with international best practice. The information contained in the old DR4 guidelines applies to IVDs, devices incorporating human materials, disinfectants and tampons. In relation to the manufacture of medical devices, the TGA accepts its own conformity assessment certificate, certificates of conformity issued under the MRA with the EC, and EC certificates issued by a EU Notified Body under the EU Medical Devices Directive 93/42/EEC or EU Active Implantable Medical Devices Directive 90/385/EEC, but does not accept an International Standards Organisation 13485 compliance certificate (because it does not provide assurance that the Australian requirements have been taken into consideration) or a certificate from the FDA (because it has been issued against different auditing criteria to that required by the Australian legislation).

References

1 Baume PE. *A Question of Balance: Report on the Future of Drug Evaluation in Australia*. Canberra: Australian Government Publishing Service, 1991.

2 Sloan C. *A History of the Pharmaceutical Benefits Scheme 1947–1992*. Canberra: Australian Government Publishing Service, 1995.

3 Australian Institute of Health and Welfare. *Australia's Health 2008: The Eleventh Biennial Health Report of the Australian Institute of Health and Welfare*. Canberra: Australian Institute of Health and Welfare, 2008 (http://www.aihw. gov.au/publications/index.cfm/title/10585).

27 Pharmaceutical medicine in the emerging markets

Nadarajah Sreeharan[1] and Jennie A. Sykes[2]

[1] Transcrip LLP
[2] Asia Pacific, Japan and Emerging Markets, GlaxoSmithKline

27.1 Introduction

The pharmaceutical industry and its activities in pharmaceutical medicine (i.e. investments in drug discovery, development and commercialisation of medicines) have been primarily focused on the developed world over several decades until the mid to late 1990s. This has primarily been driven by the size and growth of the pharmaceutical market in the developed world, the impact and influence of the regulatory agencies in the USA, Western Europe and to a lesser extent Japan, and the investment strategy of the industry's research and development (R&D) departments. In addition to the mainstream pharmaceutical companies, the biotechnology industry has also seen its focus and investment primarily confined to North America and Western Europe. During this period the role of the medical departments in less developed markets was primarily confined to the provision of medical support to the commercialisation of products with only a minimal contribution to core R&D activities, including global clinical trials. Indeed, in many companies these departments functioned outside the mainstream R&D organisation.

However, over the last decade of the twentieth and the beginning of the twenty-first century, a paradigm shift has begun to shape the industry, leading to the increasing impact of, and the resultant investments in, the 'emerging markets' in the core capabilities of the pharmaceutical industry. Several factors have been responsible for this paradigm shift and include both 'pull' and 'push' factors:

• *Changes in the dynamics of the pharmaceutical market.* Sales growth in mature pharmaceutical markets like the US and Western Europe has been in decline over the last decade. In contrast, growth in the emerging markets has been an impressive 12–14%, with growth in the seven most prominent countries (Brazil, Russia, India, China, Mexico, Turkey and South Korea) averaging even higher at 15–20% over the last 5 years.[1]

The rising population of middle classes, combined with a strengthening of intellectual property protection, have enhanced the commercial attractiveness of these markets. Importantly, growth in the emerging markets can occur even if low pipeline productivity persists as many mature brands continue to demonstrate growth. In addition, governments are increasing their level of spending on health care, with China, Mexico and Turkey committing to coverage for all their citizens by the end of the decade.

• *Decline in R&D productivity.* The innovative pharmaceutical industry has seen a considerable decline in its productivity since the early 1990s. This has primarily been caused by the decline in output of new chemical entities and the soaring costs of drug discovery and development, including the cost of clinical trials. The industry began to shift clinical trials and other R&D activities to the emerging markets in an attempt to reduce the cost of drug discovery and development. Furthermore, this shift also gave the opportunity for the companies to make radical changes to their globalisation strategies. In the past, the focus of this strategy has been the US and European markets with initial regulatory submissions followed by a sequence of clinical development and regulatory activities in the other markets over a period of months and even years. The scheduling of clinical trials outside the traditional markets enabled a shift towards simultaneous regulatory submissions in many markets, thus enhancing market access globally.

• *Patient populations.* As many companies competed in crowded disease areas, the availability of patients

The Textbook of Pharmaceutical Medicine. Edited by John P. Griffin. © 2009, ISBN: 978-1-4051-8035-1.

for recruitment into global trials became a limiting factor in the developed world. Simultaneously, rising prosperity and changing lifestyles in the emerging markets have resulted in disease patterns in many instances resembling those found in the developed world. Additionally, the greater availability of treatment-naïve patients in these markets makes it easier to assess the treatment effect of novel agents in this setting.

• *R&D resources.* The increasing availability of highly trained and motivated staff to populate R&D departments and to act as clinical trial investigators in these emerging markets has become an attraction for investment. Furthermore, recognition of the quality of scientific research in many of these countries (e.g. South Korea, China and India) has been a driver to set up R&D centres and investments in the discovery process as well.

• *Changing regulatory and investment environment for research.* Many governments in the emerging markets have begun to take actions to improve not only the regulatory environment, but also to offer financial incentives for investments in research. Although the regulatory climates in these markets have been a disincentive and a bottleneck for both clinical trials and product approvals for a number of years, rapid and positive changes are being encountered, especially in North East Asia and Japan, where greater acceptance by the regulators of foreign Asian data has opened the way for more pan-Asian registration trials. However, the long approval time lines for clinical trials in some emerging markets (e.g. 10–12 months in China and 6 months or longer in Brazil) mean that involvement of these countries in global trials remains challenging, unless the studies have long recruitment windows.

• *Diseases of the developing world.* There has been increasing pressure on, and ongoing criticism of, the pharmaceutical industry for the lack of investment in medicines to treat diseases of the developing world. To their credit many companies have responded positively to enhance investment in preventative and therapeutic remedies for the 'neglected diseases' (e.g. tuberculosis, malaria) leading to the increased scheduling of clinical trials for these diseases in many less developed markets, including sub-Saharan Africa.

The incorporation of emerging markets into the core global strategy of R&D has been accompanied by a new set of issues and challenges for R&D and medical departments. These complex markets could not be approached with the same strategic and operational imperatives and with the comfort factor of conducting an 'R&D business as usual'. It required an understanding of the issues and the offering of innovative solutions to maximise the impact of being in the emerging markets. Some of these complex issues include:

1. The need to train and educate core staff based in North America and Western Europe on the cultural, medical and ethical issues of practising pharmaceutical medicine in the emerging markets. It is impractical and illogical to transfer unchanged the R&D strategies and operational models that have driven a successful pharmaceutical industry in the developed world for several decades.

2. Developing the competencies and capabilities of R&D departments in the newer markets. Although there has been an expansion in the output of qualified scientific and medical talent in these markets, the specialised nature of the competencies essential for a successful R&D-based industry requires a strong focus on appropriate training and development of local staff.

3. Ensuring the optimal link between the needs of the sponsor and the needs of these markets. The success of R&D strategies in developing economies is intricately linked to their degree of alignment with the healthcare priorities of the relevant countries.

4. Addressing many of the complex ethical issues such as the adequacy of informed consent, access to medications both post-trial and post-approval. Given the educational and cultural diversity in the emerging markets, special care needs to be taken in addressing many aspects of Good Clinical Practice (GCP) when involving these markets in global clinical trials.

5. Understanding the complex regulatory requirements for both clinical trials and product registrations across a broad range of markets. Unlike the regulatory environment of the developed world which has evolved over several decades into a relatively integrated and harmonised set of agencies [US Food and Drug Administration (FDA), European Medicines Evaluation Agency (EMEA), Ministry of Health, Labour and Welfare (MHLW)], the regulatory environment in the emerging markets remains as complex and varied as the markets themselves.

6. Developing strategies for market access, pricing and reimbursement. The affordability and access of medicines to these markets still remains a contentious issue. Novel pricing and reimbursement strategies are being developed by many companies. In addition, the past few years have seen multinationals diversifying their portfolios through the addition of generics.

Although considerable progress has been made in many of the issues related to the practice of pharmaceutical medicine in the emerging markets, it is an ever-changing and complex environment and even more focus is required by all stakeholders in the future to make this exciting venture a successful one.

27.2 What are 'emerging markets'?

The term 'emerging markets' has to be used with caution as it had traditionally included a wide array of markets outside the developed world of North America, Western Europe and Japan (and a few other countries such as Australia and South Africa). The characteristics that defined these emerging markets were a gross national product (GNP) per capita that was below that of the developed economies, the potential for market growth and an environment with continued economic and political instability. However, as many of these emerging markets have grown at differential rates and have economic and other drivers that are very different and disparate, definitions of this sector have become more fragmented. Terminologies used to cover these markets include 'BRIC' (Brazil, Russia, India and China),[2] the 'emerging and developing economies',[3] 'economies in transition from central planning'[4] and 'least developed countries' (LDCs)[5] (Appendix 27.1). However, for the purpose of this chapter, in defining the impact of pharmaceutical medicine in emerging markets, it is perhaps best to cluster these markets into groups as follows:

1. Central and Eastern Europe: many of these markets have over the last decade or so been actively involved in activities related to pharmaceutical medicine and have experienced a growth in investment especially in clinical trials. With the accession and impending accession of many of these markets into the European Union, they have now been integrated or are in the process of integration into the European model by the pharmaceutical industry. Hence, many aspects discussed in this chapter have only limited relevance to many markets in this region.

2. The BRIC markets have economies that are developing rapidly and are predicted to eclipse the economies of the developed world by the middle of the twenty-first century. The BRIC markets form an important focus of this chapter.

3. Other rapidly developing markets, particularly in Asia and Latin America, which have many of the characteristics of the BRIC markets apart from size, will continue to see an increasing level of investment in activities related to pharmaceutical medicine. The most important of these in terms of contribution to market growth are Mexico, Turkey and South Korea.

4. Markets in Africa, particularly sub-Saharan Africa, which could be called the 'frontier markets' for the pharmaceutical industry. These markets, which include many of the LDCs, do not have the necessary health care infrastructure and capabilities and are therefore unlikely to be the focus of substantial R&D investment or be included in many of the global trials targeting the traditional disease areas. However, the industry has been criticised in the past for an insufficient focus and investment in many of the specific diseases applicable to these markets such as malaria, tuberculosis and other tropical diseases. More recently, there has been a significant increase in R&D investments towards these 'diseases of the developing world' and a consequent increase in investment in clinical trials.

27.3 The pharmaceutical market

The global pharmaceutical market[1] has been growing around 5% per annum, slowing to 2.5–3.5% in 2009 to reach $750 billion. Whilst the market is expected to rebound as the global economy recovers, an unprecedented level of patent expirations in 2011–12 is expected to curb sales growth through 2013. In contrast, growth in the most prominent seven emerging markets has been averaging 15–20% for the last 5 years, and revenues are forecast to double by 2013. Brazil, Russia, India, China, Mexico, Turkey and South Korea together will contribute more than half of global market growth in 2009 and sustain an average 40% contribution through 2013. China, which is currently the sixth largest pharmaceutical market, is forecast to become the third largest by 2011. It is predicted that future global growth will be driven by growth in the biotechnology sector, vaccines, generics and by oncology products. Furthermore, chronic disorders including 'Western diseases' will continue to play an important part in the growth of emerging markets and this has particular relevance to the future scheduling of clinical trials. For example, the diabetic population will grow from 19.4 and 16 million in 1995 to 57.2 and 37.6 million by 2025 in India and China, respectively.

The pharmaceutical industry in many of the emerging markets remains fragmented with varying contributions between local and multinationals and this has an important bearing on pharmaceutical medicine related activities. For example, China is currently dominated by local companies with considerable lobbying power on pricing and reimbursement negotiations and on formulary listings. Furthermore, some well-publicised issues related to product quality have resulted in an increasing focus on compliance and medical governance activities. India has over 500 companies although the top players, again dominated by local generic companies, have approximately 40% of the market.

27.3.1 Epidemiology and disease burden

Planning for the various activities related to pharmaceutical medicine in the emerging markets requires a knowledge and understanding of the changing epidemiology and burden of disease. Data can be accessed via an ongoing programme on disease burden by the World Health Organization (WHO).[6]

Disease burden data in the low–mid income markets across the various WHO regions in comparison to the high income developed nations are shown as mortality rates (Figure 27.1) and disability adjusted life years or DALYs (Figure 27.2). It is seen that although Group 1 diseases (including communicable diseases) still cause a significant burden in Africa and some of the other emerging markets, Group II diseases including cardiovascular diseases and cancer (Figure 27.3) contribute in no small measure to the burden of disease. As the emerging markets transform their economic status from low and middle income countries towards high income and developed status,

the pattern of disease burden also undergoes a corresponding shift as illustrated in Figure 27.4.

27.4 Changing patterns of pharmaceutical medicine

The old paradigm in the emerging markets was an industry that was dominated by local companies with a major focus on generics, not only in supplying the home markets but increasingly as a major supplier of generics to the developed world. In many of these markets, the commercial strategy of the multinational pharmaceutical companies was restricted to having their own subsidiaries or in establishing alliances with local companies. The medical departments were small in size and limited to the provision of medical affairs support to the companies' own portfolio of products or to products that were licensed locally.

The paradigm shift started to emerge in the 1990s and was initially driven by outsourcing of low cost and high volume activities, primarily in the area of manufacturing and data management. The availability of a low cost but highly skilled labour force, especially in India and China, was the initial catalyst for this shift.

By the turn of the century, the success of this initial experiment ('pull' factor) and the rapidly developing pressures in the developed world as a result of

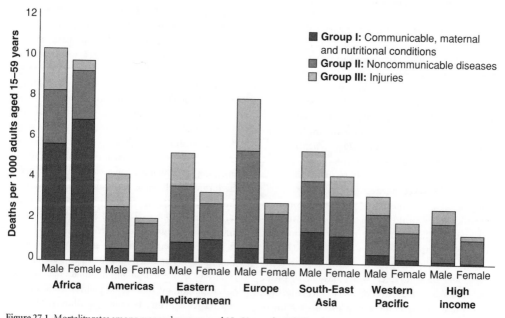

Figure 27.1 Mortality rates among men and women aged 15–59 years by WHO region.

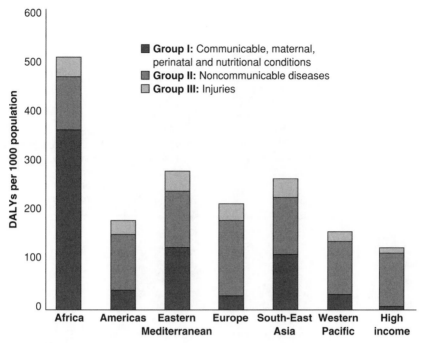

Figure 27.2 (DALYs) by WHO region.

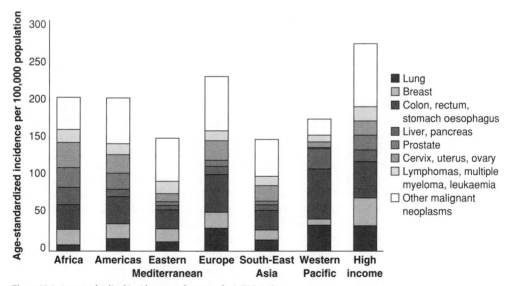

Figure 27.3 Age standardised incident rates for cancer by WHO region.

declining R&D productivity and an environment of cost containment ('push' factors) have contributed to an even more dramatic shift in R&D strategy and investments towards the emerging markets. This dramatic shift moved gradually up the value chain as a result of the increased scheduling of global clinical trials. More recently, moves towards investments in early clinical development, non-clinical development and discovery medicine have begun to emerge with the creation of R&D centres by many multinational

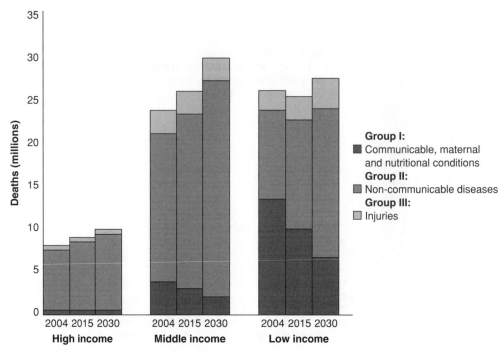

Figure 27.4 Projected deaths by cause for high, middle and low income countries.

companies. Analysts have predicted a future where independent and self-contained R&D activities, based in countries such as India and China, will be delivered across the entire value chain, from targets and molecules to medicines.

27.4.1 Intellectual property

One of the factors that impeded for decades the involvement of many of the emerging markets in the R&D activities of the global pharmaceutical industry had been the lack or perceived lack of political will to comply with different aspects of the trade-related aspects of intellectual property rights (TRIPS), which came into force in 1995.[7] Under TRIPs, World Trade Organisation (WTO) members were obliged to provide patent protection for any new product or process although some key exemptions were allowed as follows:

1. Developing countries and economies in transition from central planning were exempted from applying the TRIPs provisions until 1 January 2000. However, some developing countries delayed the approval of patents until January 2005, based on the provision to allow countries that did not have patent protection in a particular technology at the time of introduction of TRIPs up to 10 years to introduce the protection.

However, countries that followed this course had two obligations. First, they had to allow inventors to file applications, although decisions on the patent may not be taken until the end of the 10-year period. This process was called the 'mail-box' provision (literally a 'mail-box' is created to receive and date applications). Secondly, if the medicine was allowed to be marketed during this interim period, the government had to allow the applicant exclusive marketing rights for a 5-year period or until a decision on the patent application was made, whichever was shorter.

2. LDCs were exempted from TRIPs initially until 1 January 2006 and this was later extended to 2013 and subsequently under the Doha Declaration on the TRIPs[8] to 2016.

Compliance with TRIPs varied across many of the emerging markets for a number of years. Although China has, on paper, a satisfactory set of intellectual property related laws and regulations, deficiencies in implementation and enforcement continues to cause concern. Pharmaceutical counterfeiting is also still rampant in China and the government is conscious of the need to take stern action to facilitate China's emerging role in the global pharmaceutical arena.

India had, for years, delayed the implementation of TRIPs primarily as a result of lobbying power and the need to protect the productive generics industry. However, in 2005, in keeping with India's emergence as a global economic power, the government passed an amendment to the Patent Act to provide for pharmaceutical patents. However, a number of subsequent amendments to the Act, primarily resulting from local lobbying, have left the Act short of many of the provisions of TRIPs including some tight provisions on what is patentable.

In Brazil, 'pipeline patents' were introduced in 1996, as part of the various legal changes to comply with TRIPs, which allowed the granting of pharmaceutical patents for products in development that have received patent protection elsewhere. However, the involvement of an additional review process of pharmaceutical patents by the Agencia National de Vigilancia Sanitaria (ANVISA), the Brazilian Health Agency in addition to the Brazilian Patent Office (INPI) has resulted in an average time of 8 years from the submission to grant of patents, although steps are being taken to reduce this.

The intellectual property obligations of Russia are delivered as a signatory to the Paris Convention, a member of the World Intellectual Property Organisation (WIPO) although Russia is still not a member of the WTO. The legal framework of the intellectual property regulations in Russia is generally considered to be acceptable, although there are concerns with both the enforcement of these laws as well as in the considerable illegal market in counterfeit medicines.

Another major area of contention applicable to intellectual property and the emerging markets is the provision in the TRIPs for compulsory licensing. This is a provision under Article 31 of TRIPs (under 'other uses without authorisation of the patent holder') where a government allows an alternative source to produce the patented product without the consent of the patent holder. Certain conditions need to be met to comply with Article 31:

- The licensee must have made reasonable and unsuccessful prior attempts to obtain the license voluntarily from the patent holder (this provision could be waived in case of national emergencies or in the case of public non-commercial use);
- The licensee must pay adequate remuneration to the patent holder;
- The patent holder must still be allowed to continue to produce and commercialise the product;
- The license must primarily be given to supply the domestic market of the licensee. However, at the Doha Declaration in 2001, provisions were made to give extra flexibility so that countries that do not

have the capabilities locally could import supplies of patented drugs under compulsory licensing from other countries. This is termed the 'Paragraph 6' issue as it comes under that paragraph in the Doha Declaration.

In spite of the improvements in the intellectual property environment, significant issues still remain. For example, in India there have been some recent high profile refusals of patents on the grounds of prior known use or incremental innovation. Imatinib (Glivec) and gefitinib (Iressa) are notable examples. On the positive side, maraviroc (Celzentry) became the first HIV/AIDS drug to obtain a patent in India.

27.5 Late clinical development

The last decade has seen a major expansion in the conduct of global clinical trials outside the traditional countries in Western Europe and North America. The foray into Central and Eastern Europe in the 1990s has been well documented and the venture has had a satisfactory outcome with this region currently being the major contributor of clinical trials in Europe for many sponsors. The turn of the century has seen a similar expansion in global clinical trials to the emerging markets, particularly in Asia and Latin America. Although the recent growth in volume of patients enrolled into global clinical trials in the emerging markets has been clearly documented (Figure 27.5),[9] the 'core' Western countries still contribute the major share in absolute numbers of patients enrolled into these trials (Figure 27.6). Future trends in the globalisation of clinical trials (Table 27.1)[10] also demonstrate not only increased average relative annual growth rates in the emerging markets, but also a huge potential for future growth as shown by a low index of 'trial density' (number of recruiting sites divided by the country population in millions). The drivers for future growth in these markets are well documented and include both 'push' and 'pull' factors:

1. *Access to patient populations.* With the expansion of a plethora of novel targets and molecules resulting from the technological advances in genomics and combinatorial chemistry in the latter part of the twentieth century, more and more molecules are currently being evaluated in clinical trials across a wide range of diseases by a number of pharmaceutical companies. Many of the new agents are for chronic diseases and therefore involve lifelong therapy. The stringent regulatory environment increasingly mandates the assessment of risk–benefit in greater number of

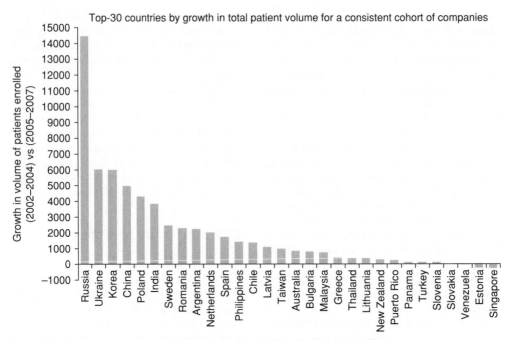

Figure 27.5 Growth in patient volume in global clinical trials in Traditional and Emerging Markets.

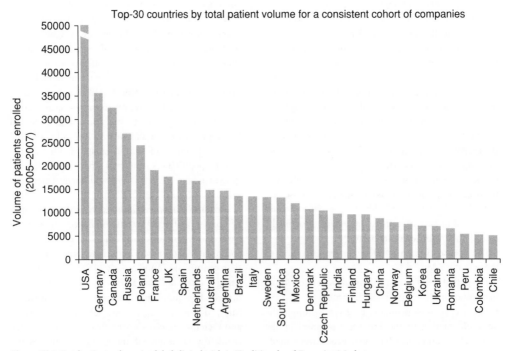

Figure 27.6 Total patient volume in global clinical trials in Traditional and Emerging Markets.

Table 27.1 Country trends in participation in biopharmaceutical clinical trials

Rank	Country	Number of sites	Share (%)	ARAGR (%)	Trial capacity	Trial density
1	USA	36,281	48.7	−6.5 ↓	43.7	120.3
2	Germany	4214	5.7	11.7 ↑	10.9	51.2
3	France	3226	4.3	−4.0 ↓	9.6	50.3
4	Canada	3032	4.1	−12.0 ↓	8.6	92.2
5	Spain	2076	2.8	14.9 ↑	6.8	46.4
6	Italy	2039	2.7	8.1 ↑	6.7	34.6
7	Japan	2002	2.7	10.3 ↑	33.4	15.7
8	UK	1753	2.4	−9.9 ↓	7.6	29.1
9	Netherlands	1394	1.9	2.1 ↑	6.8	85.0
10	Poland*	1176	1.6	17.2 ↑	5.3	30.9
11	Australia	1131	1.5	8.1 ↑	5.4	54.4
12	Russia*	1084	1.5	33.0 ↑	5.8	7.7
13	Belgium	986	1.3	−9.4 ↓	5.2	94.8
14	Czech Republic*	799	1.1	24.6 ↑	4.5	77.6
15	Argentina*	757	1.0	26.9 ↑	4.8	19.0
16	India*	757	1.0	19.6 ↑	5.8	0.7
17	Brazil*	754	1.0	16.0 ↑	5.1	4.0
18	Sweden	739	1.0	−8.6 ↓	5.1	81.0
19	Mexico*	683	0.9	22.1 ↑	4.0	6.2
20	Hungary*	622	0.8	22.2 ↑	4.1	62.5
21	South Africa*	553	0.7	5.5 ↑	4.3	11.9
22	Austria	540	0.7	9.6 ↑	3.8	65.1
23	China*	533	0.7	47.0 ↑	5.3	0.4
24	Denmark	492	0.7	9.2 ↑	4.4	90.3
25	South Korea*	466	0.6	17.9 ↑	3.4	9.5

Trial capacity is the number of sites in the country involved in large trials (20 or more sites) divided by the number of large trials in the country. Trial density is the number of recruiting sites on 12 April 2007 divided by the country population in millions. ARAGR, average relative annual growth rate (reproduced with permission from [10]).
* Countries in emerging regions.

patients and for longer periods. These factors have contributed to the saturation and shortage of patients and investigators for trials in Western Europe and North America and hence the need to look at alternative clinical trial sites in the emerging markets. The increase in prevalence of 'Western diseases' such as cardiovascular disorders and diabetes in many emerging economies makes it logistically feasible to include these countries in global trials.

The trials in non-traditional markets also offer other benefits in terms of access to patient populations. Because the trials will include patients with a wider ethnic variation, it allows the assessment of risk–benefit in subgroup of patients using pharmacogenetic technologies. Also in countries where currently available therapies are not routinely used, treatment-naïve patients can be recruited into appropriately designed protocols.

2. *Economics.* The cost of conducting trials in the emerging markets is considerably less than the developed world. However, the experience from Central and Eastern Europe has shown that this differential is often exaggerated as additional costs for infrastructure development have to be borne by the sponsor, at least in the early stages. Furthermore, as economies advance and earnings of the population rise, there is further erosion of the difference.

3. *Capabilities.* In many emerging markets, institutions and hospitals have standards of medical practice comparable to the developed world. These institutions are manned by academics and practitioners who are highly skilled and trained, many indeed having undergone the entirety or part of their training in the developed world, and are able to provide leadership to the clinical trials sites of global trials. Furthermore, these countries are continuing to produce high

> **BOX 27.1** (a) Prerequisite for local clinical trials for product registration in emerging markets
>
> *Markets that require local bridging studies*
> Korea*, Taiwan
>
> *Markets that require a pre-registration clinical trial†*
> China, India, Nigeria, Korea
>
> (b) Countries requiring information beyond investigator brochure and protocol for local trial.
>
> Argentina, Brazil, China, Costa Rica, Hong Kong, India, Indonesia, Korea, Malaysia, Singapore, South Africa, Taiwan, Thailand, Turkey, Vietnam
>
> * Either bridging study or local trial required.
> † Local trial may be waived, if sufficient patients are included in global trials.

quality science and medical graduates who are able to function as study monitors and clinical trial associates for the sponsors.

4. *Needs of the emerging markets.* There are several advantages to the emerging markets themselves in attracting this increase in high quality clinical trials:

• The trials will provide local clinical trial data to meet the prerequisite requirements of some of the national regulatory agencies, such as in China and India (Box 27.1 for list of countries that need local clinical trial data as a prerequisite for product registration);

• In some disease areas such as oncology, the clinical trial will provide the opportunity for these patients to have access to investigational compounds and/or approved therapies;

• The scheduling of global trials will enhance the capability of trial sites in these markets and train investigators and monitors;

• Increasing the capabilities in these markets will further facilitate the conduct of high quality trials in diseases of the developing world and neglected diseases.

The expansion in the scheduling of clinical trials in these newer markets also requires a good understanding of the complexities of these markets and the need to address some of the specific issues that are quite different to the developed world. Some of these factors are summarised below:

• The medical and scientific staff in the home R&D markets of the sponsor companies should be educated and trained in the varying cultural, ethical, medical and regulatory issues of these markets. They should also note that these issues vary enormously across the different markets and the region as a whole is less homogeneous than Western Europe or North America.

• The sponsors should proactively build local capacity and capabilities, particularly in some of the larger key markets (e.g. the BRIC markets). Employment of local staff and their ongoing training and development is a key contributory factor to success in these markets. However, it is also important not to dilute the clinical trial capabilities in a wide range of markets and each sponsor should strategically select the markets for investment.

• There needs to be recognition that all trials will be conducted to the same standard globally and in compliance with GCP of the International Conference on Harmonisation (GCP-ICH) and any specific national regulatory and legal requirements. This as a minimum should cover the use of scientifically and medically sound protocols, approval of the study by an independent ethics committee, selection and training of suitably qualified investigators and ensuring the rights, well-being and safety of the subjects.

There are some specific aspects of GCP and the Declaration of Helsinki that need special attention in the scheduling of clinical trials in the emerging markets:

• Obtaining informed consent can pose a particular challenge owing to local cultural factors and low literacy of some trial subjects. Extra precautions should be taken to ensure that all the key elements of the informed consent are in place and appropriate cultural nuances are included in the process of obtaining consent. This could involve the use of family members or local community leaders. Where consent cannot be in writing, the investigators need to work with independent witnesses to verify that the relevant information has been explained to and understood by the participants.

• Clinical trials should only be conducted in countries where the investigational medicine will be suitable, when available, for wider use in the community and where the trial programme fits into the health care strategy of the country. Clinical trials should not be conducted in countries where the sponsor has no prior intention to market the medicine.

• The protocol of the study should clearly address the provision of a locally relevant optimal standard of care on conclusion of the clinical trial. There should be a clear agreement between the sponsor and the institution conducting the trial that the health care system is responsible for and able to provide continued care, including the provision of nationally licensed medicines for trial participants. For life-threatening diseases, the sponsor should commit to the provision of the trial medication to those demonstrating meaningful benefit, even if the medicine has not been approved and licensed for use.

• Careful consideration should be given to the selection of the standard of care in the control groups of trials to determine whether the care should be the 'best current treatment available anywhere in the world' or reflect the 'treatment currently available in the participating country'. Selecting the latter option will be more relevant locally as it enables the comparison of the new treatment with the best available in the country and the data will be applicable to the care of patients in the community. However, in designing global trials, it may be scientifically and medically valid to select the 'best available treatment', particularly when there is widespread agreement. It is, of course, essential to ensure that the standard of care is never less than the locally acceptable standard. The criteria for using placebo in the control arm should be no different to that in the developed world.

• Compliance with the study treatment and maintaining regular follow-up could be problematic in trials in emerging markets. In many instances, the trial centres are in major cities while the participating patients may come from distant rural areas, often with very poor transport facilities. Additionally, other cultural factors such as variations in diets and the concomitant use of alternative therapies need to be factored into the design of the study and analysis of the data.

• The multitude of languages and dialects across many of these markets, let alone within a single country such as India, need to be taken into consideration prior to the selection of countries for participation in global trials. Although investigators and ethics committees in many countries are able to work with study documents in English, in other countries (e.g. China) documents need to be translated. Additionally, in most markets, patient-related documents including informed consent forms require translations. This becomes a particular issue with documents linked to study endpoints (e.g. quality of life questionnaires) as validation of the test material will be required.

27.6 Regulations

The regulatory environment in the emerging markets is extremely variable in terms of the requirements for both clinical trial applications and product registrations.

Two key requirements should be considered in the assessment of criteria for registration of products in the emerging markets. One is the provision of the Certificate of Pharmaceutical Product (CPP) by the applicant and the other is the need for local trials or the inclusion of local patients in global trials as a precondition for approval. The requirements for a CPP fall into five categories:[11]

1. A CPP is not required;
2. Submission can be made but a CPP is required prior to approval;
3. A CPP is required at submission, from a specified 'reference' agency (e.g. country of manufacture);
4. A CPP is required at submission from any suitable 'reference' agency;
5. Multiple CPPs are required at submission.

When the CPP is required to be from the country of manufacture, the sourcing strategy and anticipated labelling in that market become important components of overall strategic planning. The CPP should comply with the format specified by the WHO and gives details about a single named medicinal product, its manufacturing processes, its formulation and its manufacturing and packaging sites.

In some countries, there is a prerequisite to conduct efficacy clinical trial(s) or a bridging study in the country before a product can be approved for marketing. Furthermore, only a protocol and an investigator brochure needs to be provided for the approval of a clinical trial in some markets whereas others may request additional clinical and non-clinical technical information in a formal clinical trial application (Box 27.1).

Another issue is that the processes and regulations for the maintenance of licences are significantly underdeveloped with data requirements and timelines that are not aligned to ICH countries. This can result in delays in product supply (because of delays in approval of technical variations or source changes) and delays in label updates, including the provision of new safety information to health care professionals.

Some salient features of the regulatory processes for product approval in the BRIC countries are given below:

• The regulatory systems in Brazil are well established, under the national regulatory agency, ANVISA, and are understandably closely aligned to the FDA requirements and processes with approval times around 12 months. There is also a recent and welcome move to harmonise activities across some of the key Latin American regulatory agencies.

• Russian regulations are closely linked to the EU requirements for product registrations with average approval times ranging between 18 and 24 months. The Federal Ministry of Healthcare and Social Development provides executive oversight of policies and regulations with the Federal Service of Control and

Supervision (Roszdravnadzor) being responsible for review and approvals of products and the Federal State Establishment Scientific Centre of Expertise of Medicinal Products (FSE SC EMP) providing scientific advice.

• The regulatory environment in China is one of the most challenging amongst the BRIC countries. Although the Chinese Regulatory Authority, the State Food and Drug Administration, has recently been reorganised with the intention of shortening the regulatory processing time and a fast-tracking process has been introduced for medicines in AIDS, cancer and rare diseases, there are a number of areas that need to be improved. These include the implementation of the Regulatory Data Protection, a simplification of a currently complex categorisation system for review based on the phase of development of the medicine, restrictions in the export of tissue samples and a multitude of logistical and administrative issues. Currently, these combine to drive approvals for new products in China to time-lines generally 3–4 years after approval in ICH countries, with even longer time-lines for vaccines. Increasingly multinational companies are seeking to achieve the required patient numbers through inclusion of China in global or regional studies rather than conducting a local trial. This has the advantage of accelerating registration of products through the usual Class III route – a CPP being required prior to NDA submission rather than before a local study can be started.

Due to the increasing mutual acceptance of data between Japanese, Korean and Taiwanese authorities, these countries are increasingly being considered alongside China in pan-Asian registration strategies.

• The regulatory processes for product approvals in India generally follow international norms and approval times average 12–18 months. Although regulations require a local phase III study to be performed, this may be waived if sufficient Indian patients are included in global trials included in the dossier.

All the above issues are well recognised by industry and in the recent past much positive sharing of information and mutual challenges have taken place between the industry and the relevant agencies. Such discussions provide a much welcomed platform for the future rationalisation of regulatory requirements, the appropriate use of limited resources at the agencies and a more harmonised environment that encourages and facilitates true global development and registration. The next few years are likely to see development in the areas of classic R&D in the emerging markets (not simply local clinical studies for regulatory or commercial needs) and a higher degree of transparency – including more opportunity for meaningful pre-filing consultations with agencies, more technical transfer of value-added manufacturing operations and an increased level of information sharing between agencies.

27.7 Commercialisation of medicines

The emerging markets provide new challenges and dynamics in the commercialisation of medicines. Although the market was dominated by local companies and generics for several decades, there has been an increasing interest in launching branded products by multinational pharmaceutical companies, driven by the factors discussed earlier: the changes in the intellectual property environment, the cost containing environment in the traditional developed world markets and the growth of middle classes in the newer markets with increasing governmental and private investments in health care.

The marketing of medicines in the emerging markets has to take into consideration the price control mechanisms that operate in some countries (e.g. Brazil, Mexico, Taiwan, Turkey) either on a par with the developed world or, in others, such as South Korea, at an even more stringent level. Price controls operate in some private markets (e.g. Brazil, India) where there is little or no public drug provision. Other markets (e.g. China, South Korea, Taiwan) control prices for reimbursement of medicines in the public sector. There is an increasing trend for countries to develop their own Health Technology Assessment (HTA) programs, comparable to the UK's NICE program. The dilemma for the industry in the latter markets is whether to accept the price controls and retain the reimbursable status or to compete entirely in the private market. Interestingly, in many markets the rising middle classes demonstrate a preference for branded products, enabling these products to compete with generic products in some market segments. Nonetheless, health economic evaluations are becoming increasingly important for the public sector and managed care segments in many emerging markets (e.g. Brazil, Russia and South Korea).

Special strategies are needed to provide affordable medicines to the LDCs. For diseases that are confined to these countries (i.e. 'diseases of the developing world'/'neglected diseases'), innovative solutions including public–private partnerships (PPPs) and advanced market commitments (see section 27.8) and compulsory licensing (see section 27.4.1) could be considered. However, for diseases that are also relevant for high income markets (e.g. AIDS and 'Western diseases' such as diabetes and cardiovascular disorders), additional solutions are required to make these medicines affordable to the LDCs. The concept of differential pricing has been put forward and indeed implemented by many companies. This involves the supply of these essential medicines at lower (i.e. differential) prices to the LDCs while maintaining a market barrier for the reimporting of these medicines back into the high income markets by distributors.[12] This could be achieved by agreements with donor and host governments and purchasers to ensure market separation by using special markers for the products supplied to the LDCs. Another avenue open is the negotiation of confidential rebates with the LDCs without a difference in market price thereby making the products unattractive for reimportation.

It is also important to ensure the highest level of ethics and medical governance in the commercialisation of medicines in the emerging markets. Although BRIC and many other fast developing markets in Asia and Latin America have embarked on self-regulating codes of marketing practices modelled on the codes of the International Federation of the Associations of Pharmaceutical Physicians (IFAPP) and the International Federation of Pharmaceutical Manufacturers and Associations (IFPMA) and governmental laws and regulations are rapidly developing in these markets, it is the responsibility of pharmaceutical physicians to ensure compliance with the codes. Many pharmaceutical companies are increasingly developing corporate and R&D roles to oversee the global delivery of medical governance.

27.8 Development of medicines for the diseases of the developing world

The WHO data on burden of disease has highlighted the fact that although non-communicable chronic diseases such as cardiovascular disorders and diabetes are increasingly prevalent, particularly in the emerging economies of the BRIC countries, communicable diseases still continue to have a major impact, not only in sub-Saharan Africa and India but also in Russia, China and Brazil, where a three- to fourfold prevalence compared with the developed world is seen. HIV/AIDS, respiratory infections including tuberculosis, diarrhoeal disease and tropical diseases such as malaria are important contributors to mortality. Although indigenous factors such as poor education

and awareness of diseases together with a failure to use existing medications effectively impact on the disease burden, the paucity of new interventions to these diseases has remained a significant contributory factor. Additionally, a number of important, although relatively rare diseases, termed the 'neglected diseases', including African trypanosomiasis (sleeping sickness), South American trypanosomiasis (Chagas disease), leishmaniasis, schistosomiasis and filariasis have also suffered from the absence of new interventions. More recently, there has been a significant and positive change in the investments directed towards diseases of the developing world. Several factors have contributed to this change.

First, there is recognition that this complex issue can only be addressed by understanding the role and relative contributions of the various stakeholders: governments, non-governmental organisations and charities and the pharmaceutical industry. This has resulted in the establishment of several PPPs. Pharmaceutical companies have worked with or been part of PPPs to address and enhance investments towards searching for new therapies for the diseases of the developing world and the neglected diseases. Some examples of the PPPs are given below:[13]

1. Global Alliance for Vaccines and Immunization, which was launched in 2001. The primary objective is to increase the use and access of existing vaccines and to foster the development of new vaccines. The partnerships encompass a number of governmental and non governmental organisations (including the Gates Foundation, WHO, World Bank) and pharmaceutical companies.

2. Medicines for Malaria Venture, which was launched in 1999. The objective is to discover and develop new antimalarial drugs that are affordable and accessible. The Gates Foundation is a key contributor to the partnership.

3. Global Alliance for TB Drug Development (TB Alliance) with significant contributions from the Gates and Rockefeller Foundations has not only been exploring new interventions, but also looking at modifications to existing drugs and extending the use of existing antibiotics to the treatment of tuberculosis. One of the key initiative is to reduce cost and increasing compliance with existing therapies by simplifying treatment regimens.

4. Drugs for Neglected Diseases Initiative was set up in 2003 driven by Medecins Sans Frontieres partnering a number of research institutes and in close collaboration with the Special Programme for Research and Training of Tropical Diseases of the WHO.

Secondly, there is an increasing acceptance by the pharmaceutical industry of its social obligations and the development of the concept of a 'social contract' or 'corporate social responsibility'. This has now become an integral part of the strategy of many research-based pharmaceutical companies and includes a commitment to undertake activities related to health care in developing countries. These investments include activities encompassing a number of areas including the R&D of medicines for the developing world, improving affordability and access of medicines and investments in preventative and health education programmes.

Thirdly, there is recognition by governments that a private industry needs to be rewarded in terms of a reasonable return and that multiple stakeholders should share in the risks of investment in the R&D of medicines for these neglected diseases. The development of the concept of advanced market commitments, particularly for the development of vaccines, is an example of this approach. The primary principle of this concept is the commitment by governments of payments in advance at an agreed price dependent on the product meeting a pre-specified 'technical target product profile'. Such a commitment is espoused by several countries for the pneumococcal vaccine and by the UK and other European countries towards the development of a malarial vaccine.

27.9 The future: re-engineering R&D through emerging markets

Many analysts have predicted a dramatic expansion of core pharmaceutical R&D in the coming years, particularly in India and China and other BRIC markets. This will involve not only further expansions in both low cost and high volume ventures such as manufacturing and data management and in the globalisation of clinical trials, but also in investments further up the R&D value chain to discovery medicine, non-clinical development and early clinical development, including translational medicine. Various R&D models will develop to encompass this full spectrum of activities. These R&D models will range from alliances of multinational and local R&D-based companies, offshoring of components of drug discovery and development through contract research organisations and academic alliances to the full development of dedicated R&D centres based in some of these markets. However, these R&D centres, at least in the initial stages, are most likely to focus on specific areas,

functioning as R&D centres for the neglected diseases around the world, for locally prevalent diseases (e.g. hepatitis in China) or to a niche or a specified disease area dependent on the R&D strategy of the pharmaceutical company. Another area of possible involvement is the exploration of the untapped potential of indigenous therapies. However, it is also likely that the offshoring of research, unlike development activities, will take place at a slower pace and be confined to some key areas such as synthetic chemistry, animal and clinical pharmacokinetics and bioinformatics, driven by a shortage of skilled staff in the developed world and a comparable increase in talent in these areas in the newer markets.

Another factor contributing to the 'pull' of a broad R&D investment by multinationals is the change in strategy of the emerging markets themselves in increasing their own investment in pharmaceutical R&D in an attempt to transform themselves from generic manufacturers to global R&D-based companies. For example, six of India's top pharmaceutical companies increased their R&D investment by 20% between 2003 and 2005.[14] The regulatory environment in some of these markets is also more receptive to some of the more controversial areas such as stem cell research although the regulatory environment is more stringent for some other activities (e.g. animal experimentation in India and export of biological materials in China).

The eventual success of this venture is also dependent on the training and development of the staff in the emerging markets on all aspects of pharmaceutical medicine. This provides an opportunity for collaborative ventures on education and training between established institutes in the developed world, both university academic centres, R&D departments of pharmaceutical companies and accreditation bodies in pharmaceutical medicine such as the Faculty of Pharmaceutical Medicine of the Royal College of Physicians in the UK and similar institutes in the emerging markets. Recently, a number of programmes in pharmaceutical medicine have been launched in some of the emerging markets and it will be opportune to establish formal collaborations with many of the initiatives that are currently in place in Europe.

Acknowledgement

We are grateful to Alistair Davidson, Vice President, International Regulatory Affairs, GlaxoSmithKline for his contributions to section 27.6.

References

1 Global Pharmaceutical and Therapy Forecast, IMS Health. www.imshealth.com.

2 Global Economics Paper No 99. Goldman Sachs, 2003.

3 World Economic Outlook Database. International Monetary Fund, 2008.

4 Transition Report of the European Bank for Reconstruction and Development, 1994.

5 Report of UN-OHRLLS (UN Office of the High Representative for the Least developed countries, Landlocked developing countries and Small island developing states). www.unohrlls.org.

6 Global Burden of Disease 2008 report, WHO. http://www.who.int/topics/global_burden_of_disease/en.

7 *TRIPS and Pharmaceuticals Fact Sheet*. WTO, 2006. http://www.wto.org/english/tratop_e/TRIPS_e/factsheet_pharm00_e.htm.

8 Doha Development Round of the WTO.

9 *CMR R&D Factbook*, 2008.

10 Fabio AT, Anthony JS, Ernst RB. Trends in the globalisation of clinical trials. *Nat Rev Drug Discov* 2008;7:13–14.

11 TanLoh EA, Read KE, McAuslane JAN, Salek MS, Walker SR. New medicines in new markets: how long do patients have to wait and why? DIA Meeting, Boston, USA, June 22–26 2008.

12 Danzon PM, Towse A. Differential pricing for pharmaceutical: reconciling access, R&D and patents. *Int J Health Care Finance Econ* 2003;3:183–205.

13 *Fighting Diseases of Developing Countries*. Parliamentary Office of Science & Technology report, 2005. www.parliament.uk/documents.

14 IBM. *Pharma's new world view: transforming R&D through emerging markets*. IBM Institute for Business Value report, 2006.

APPENDIX 27.1 Classifications of emerging markets

(a) Emerging and developing economies:

Afghanistan
Albania
Algeria
Angola
Antigua and Barbuda
Argentina
Armenia
Azerbaijan
Bahamas
Bahrain
Bangladesh
Barbados
Belarus
Belize
Benin
Bhutan
Bolivia
Botswana
Bosnia and Herzegovina
Brazil*
Brunei Darussalam
Bulgaria
Burkina Faso
Burundi
Cambodia
Cameroon
Cape Verde
Chad
Chile
China*
Colombia
Comoros
Congo
Costa Rica
Côte d'Ivoire
Croatia
Czech Republic
Djibouti
Dominica
Dominican Republic
Ecuador
Egypt
El Salvador
Equatorial Guinea
Estonia
Eritrea
Ethiopia
Fiji
Gabon
Gambia
Georgia

Ghana
Grenada
Guatemala
Guinea
Guinea-Bissau
Guyana
Haiti
Honduras
Hungary
India*
Indonesia
Iran
Iraq
Jamaica
Jordan
Kazakhstan
Kenya
Kiribati
Kuwait
Kyrgyz Republic
Lao PDR
Latvia
Lebanon
Lesotho
Liberia
Libya
Lithuania
Macedonia
Madagascar
Malawi
Malaysia
Maldives
Mali
Mauritania
Mauritius
Mexico
Moldova
Mongolia
Montenegro
Morocco
Mozambique
Myanmar
Namibia
Nepal
Nicaragua
Niger
Nigeria
Oman
Pakistan
Panama
Papua New Guinea

Paraguay
Peru
Philippines
Poland
Qatar
Romania
Russia*
Rwanda
Samoa
São Tomé and
Príncipe
Saudi Arabia
Senegal
Serbia
Seychelles
Sierra Leone
Slovak Republic
Solomon Islands
Somalia
South Africa
Sri Lanka
St. Kitts and Nevis
St. Lucia
St. Vincent and the
Grenadines
Sudan
Suriname
Swaziland
Syria
Tajikistan
Tanzania
Thailand
Timor-Leste
Togo
Tonga
Trinidad and Tobago
Tunisia
Turkey
Turkmenistan
Uganda
Ukraine
United Arab Emirates
Uruguay
Uzbekistan
Vanuatu
Venezuela
Vietnam
Yemen
Zambia
Zimbabwe[2]

* BRIC (Brazil, Russia, India and China) markets.

APPENDIX 27.1 *Continued*

(b) Economies in transition from central planning.

Asia
Cambodia, China, Laos, Mongolia, Thailand, Vietnam

Central/Eastern Europe
Albania, Bosnia & Herzegovina, Croatia, Republic of Macedonia, Montenegro, Serbia

Commonwealth of Independent States
Armenia, Azerbaijan, Belarus, Georgia, Kazakhstan, Kyrgyz Republic, Moldova, Russia, Tajikistan, Turkmenistan, Ukraine, Uzbekistan

(c) Least developed countries.

Africa (33)

1 Angola	18 Madagascar
2 Benin	19 Malawi
3 Burkina Faso	20 Mali
4 Burundi[†]	21 Mauritania
5 Central African Republic	22 Mozambique
6 Chad	23 Niger
7 Comoros	24 Rwanda
8 Democratic Republic of the Congo	25 São Tomé and Príncipe
9 Djibouti	26 Senegal
10 Equatorial Guinea	27 Sierra Leone
11 Eritrea	28 Somalia
12 Ethiopia	29 Sudan
13 Gambia	30 Togo
14 Guinea	31 Uganda
15 Guinea-Bissau	32 United Republic of Tanzania
16 Lesotho	33 Zambia
17 Liberia	

Asia (15)

1 Afghanistan	9 Nepal
2 Bangladesh	10 Samoa
3 Bhutan	11 Solomon Islands
4 Cambodia	12 Timor-Leste
5 Kiribati	13 Tuvalu
6 Lao People's Democratic Republic	14 Vanuatu
7 Maldives	15 Yemen
8 Myanmar	

Latin America and the Caribbean (1)
1 Haiti

Part IV Pharmacoeconomic and other issues

28 Economics of health care

Carole A. Bradley[1] and Jane R. Griffin[2]

[1] Boehringer Ingelheim Canada Ltd, Burlington, ON, Canada
[2] Boehringer Ingelheim Ltd, Berks, UK

28.1 Introduction

Economics is about the allocation of resources to production and the distribution of the outputs that result. Economics exists as a discipline because the resources available globally, nationally, regionally or to any industry, organisation or individual are finite. At the same time, it would appear that no amount of output could ever satisfy all human wants and desires. Taken together, this means that choices about the level of resources to allocate to various sectors of the economy or to the production of specific outputs within those sectors are unavoidable. Equally, choices about distribution cannot be escaped. Thus, economics is the science of making choices.

Health economics is the application of the discipline of economics to the topic of health. When viewed in this light, health economics becomes first and foremost a way of thinking based on the principles of scarcity and the need for choice. Although the techniques of economic appraisal (discussed below) are the principal ways in which the discipline is applied, they are merely the 'toolkit'. The use of these tools without a proper understanding of the principles upon which they are based can be both ineffective and misleading.[1]

28.2 Economics of the National Health Service

28.2.1 Key principles of health economics: output, cost and efficiency
28.2.1.1 Output of health care
Health care services are not normally provided for their own sake. Few people receive any direct satisfac-

The Textbook of Pharmaceutical Medicine. Edited by
John P. Griffin. © 2009, ISBN: 978-1-4051-8035-1.

tion (utility) from consuming health care. Generally, these services are demanded because of an expectation that they will have a positive impact on present or future health. Consequently, the principal output of health care is 'health'. If health is viewed in the broadest sense of well-being then, if effective, interventions will make people better off than they would have been in the absence of the interventions. In other words, effective interventions will normally increase the length or improve the quality of life, or achieve some combination of the two.

The practical difficulties of viewing output in terms of health achieved is that health is notoriously difficult to define, measure and value. Broad definitions of health, such as a 'state of complete physical, mental and social well-being' given by the World Health Organization, are unhelpful when trying to compare the effectiveness of alternative therapies or to compare the health gain from either of these with that of some wholly unrelated area of health care.

Consequently, in practice, intermediate measures of output are often used as surrogate markers for final (health) outputs. This is generally considered to be acceptable, provided there is an established link between the surrogate marker and health. Thus, the evidence that a reduction in the number of exacerbations requiring hospitalisation is a strong indication of improved health in asthma patients means that 'number of exacerbations requiring hospitalisation' is an acceptable output measure. The less well established the link between the surrogate marker and health, the less useful the marker.

28.2.1.2 Cost of producing health
By definition, resources are those things that contribute to the production of output. In terms of health services, the output 'health' is produced using resources, such as doctors, nurses, hospital beds, operating

theatres, equipments and drugs. Money is needed in order to acquire these resources but, according to the above definition, money is not itself a resource as it only becomes productive if used to hire doctors, buy drugs, etc. Similarly, according to the above definition, resources can include the time of volunteers, informal caretakers or anything else that does not involve money payment but which, nevertheless, contributes to the production of health.[1]

A focus on resource use rather than money leads to a fundamental difference in how 'cost' is viewed in economics. Because resources are scarce, their commitment to any one use means sacrificing the benefits that could have been achieved if they had been used in an alternative way. In economics, cost is therefore equated to 'sacrifice', and the term 'opportunity cost' is used to emphasise the idea of an opportunity forgone. Money cost and opportunity cost may coincide – or they may not.

28.2.1.3 Basis on which resource allocation choices should be made – efficiency

Scarcity of resources means that it is not possible to do everything that we would like to do. Regardless of the level of resources currently being devoted to health care, it will always be possible to do more. This is partly because of the rapid development of new technologies, including pharmaceuticals, which allows more and more to be done each year, but also that resources devoted to health care incur opportunity costs elsewhere. The huge variety of human wants means that better health is not the only good thing that a society desires, and there are limits to how many other potential benefits society is willing to sacrifice in the pursuit of better health.

Scarcity means that resource allocation decisions cannot be avoided. If this is accepted, then it is clear that the basis on which these decisions are made should be explicit. Although economists do not claim to have the only – or even necessarily the best – answer for all choices that need to be made, at least economic criteria are explicit and hence open for criticism and debate.

The main criterion used in economic thinking is efficiency, which is about maximising the benefits from available resources. It concerns the relationship between inputs and outputs (i.e. the most benefit for the least cost). Being efficient means getting as much health as possible from the available resources; being inefficient means getting less. Viewed in this light, there is clearly an ethical justification for the pursuit of efficiency.

28.2.1.4 Acceptance of scarcity

A prerequisite to the use of health economics is an acceptance that no health care system can possibly do all things for all people. This means recognising explicitly that some form of prioritising is necessary and unavoidable. Such recognition has been slowly emerging over the past decade or so.

In the UK, annual expenditure on the National Health Service (NHS) is largely determined by government during public expenditure negotiations. Until recently, there has tended to be an implicit belief that this money (or the resources that this money could command) should be used to meet all health needs. Words such as rationing were avoided at all costs in official documents.

Whereas many in the UK would accept the need for rationing in the NHS, most would also wish to see additional resources made available. However, it is increasingly being recognised that although extra funding will ease the problem it cannot eliminate it. If need is believed to be the 'capacity to benefit from treatment', then clearly each new technological advance will increase need. Premature babies, born with low birthweights that were previously incompatible with life, only became 'in need' when the technology of neonatal intensive care allowed them to be saved. 'Need' is consequently a dynamic concept. As the pace of technological advance is unlikely to decrease, the gap between the need met (what is being achieved) and the total need (what could be achieved given infinite resources) will widen. Constantly increasing funding is therefore needed just to keep the gap from widening further, and as long as society has other needs (e.g. for education, defence, law and order, as well as private consumption needs) closing the health needs gap completely will not be possible.

28.2.1.5 Prioritisation in operation

As a result of this growing acceptance of scarcity, explicit prioritisation is becoming an increasingly common feature of the UK NHS. In the past decade, we have increasingly seen health authorities make clear choices about the kind of interventions that they will provide for their inhabitants. Many have gone so far as to remove certain procedures (e.g. tattoo removal, gender reorientation and fertility treatments) from the list of services that they will provide.

By the late 1990s, the issue of 'postcode prescribing' (patients being able to receive a particular treatment in one health authority but not if they resided in a neighbouring one) was a contributing factor in the election in Britain of the Labour government in 1997.

Table 28.1 Total health expenditure as a percentage of gross domestic product

	1975	1985	1995	1998	2002	2006
Australia	7.0	7.5	8.2	8.6	9.1	8.8
Canada	7.1	8.3	9.3	9.3	9.6	10.0
France	6.8	8.3	9.6	9.4	9.7	11.1
Germany	8.8	9.3	10.2	10.3	10.9	10.6
Italy	6.2	7.0	7.9	8.2	8.5	9.0
Japan	5.6	6.7	7.2	7.4	7.8	8.2
Spain	4.7	5.4	7.0	7.0	7.6	8.4
UK	5.5	5.9	6.9	6.8	7.8	8.4
USA	7.8	10.0	13.2	12.9	14.6	15.3

Source: OECD Health Database.

The Labour Party in their election manifesto promised to put an end to postcode prescribing, and since coming to power have endeavoured to establish measures to achieve this aim. One of these was the National Institute for Clinical Excellence (NICE; see section 28.4.2). NICE was created to rationalise the system of care rationing in the NHS by using the evidence base on the clinical and cost-effectiveness of new products to determine whether the NHS would reimburse them. The government believed that this 'fourth hurdle' would control costs and eradicate postcode prescribing. In the event they were wrong about both these issues.

First, NICE's recommendations are as likely to increase expenditure as to reduce it. The purpose of their evaluations has been clearly stated as being to identify 'value for money', not whether the NHS could afford the intervention. Secondly, postcode rationing exists because the exercise of clinical discretion locally results in treatments being available in one place and not in another. As new products are accepted by NICE, local decision-makers have to decide, given their finite resources, which 'old' products and procedures to eradicate and which efficient products and services to provide. Local choices will inevitably vary, and as a consequence one form of postcode rationing will simply replace another.[2]

28.2.2 Health service costs

The earliest developments in health economics concentrated on measuring the cost of health care. The work of Abel-Smith and Titmus[3] for the Guillebaud Committee in 1953 showed that rather than the NHS becoming too expensive, in reality the share that the NHS was taking up had fallen at a time when the population had grown. Since then the share of national income spent on the NHS has risen, but international

comparisons (Table 28.1) show that the UK remains a relatively low spender on health care services. This is partly explained by the strong positive correlation between total national income and the amount spent on health care (Figure 28.1). Clearly, richer countries can afford to spend more on health care services. However, as Figure 28.1 demonstrates, even on this basis the UK falls below countries with comparable incomes. The NHS in the UK, if nothing else, is relatively low cost.

28.3 Measuring the value

The increasing use of pharmaco-economic analyses as tools in health policy decision-making has highlighted the fact that the 'value' of a drug (or service) cannot be assessed solely on the basis of its acquisition cost. Rather, a drug's value should be considered relative to other therapies (or services) that are used for the same condition, and should include both the costs and clinical consequences associated with each. An important thing to remember when reading the following section is that all references to 'cost' refer to the total costs associated with a treatment pathway, and not solely the acquisition cost of the drug.

28.3.1 Types of analysis

The underlying premise of pharmaco-economic analyses is that fiscal resources are scarce and that there is a need to make decisions based on the relative value of different interventions in creating better health and/or longer life. There are five main analytical techniques used to evaluate the incremental value of products:[4]

1. Cost–consequence analysis (CCA);
2. Cost-effectiveness analysis (CEA);

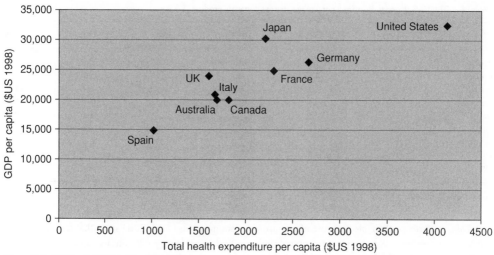

Figure 28.1 Relationship between total health spending per capita and gross domestic product per capita, 2006. Source: OECD Health Data 2008.

3. Cost–benefit analysis (CBA);
4. Cost-minimisation analysis (CMA); and
5. Cost–utility analysis (CUA).

Although the identification and valuation of the cost component (numerator) of these analyses are similar, it is the identification and valuation of the consequences (denominator) that truly differentiate these analytic techniques. A brief description of each of these techniques follows.

28.3.1.1 Cost–consequence analysis

The CCA is the most disaggregated of all the economic analyses and places the greatest interpretive burden on decision-makers. The incremental costs and clinical consequences of the drugs being compared are simply listed, with no indication of the relative importance of any of their components (e.g. a CCA involving drugs used in stroke prevention would include drug costs, hospital costs, other costs, such as those associated with any special monitoring necessary, number of strokes observed, the number of deaths observed and the rate of clinically meaningful side effects). CCAs are often presented alongside other analytical techniques, such as CEAs.

28.3.1.2 Cost-effectiveness analysis

In CEA, the total cost and the total benefits, measured in terms of an efficacy parameter, associated with two or more treatment pathways are added, and the increment is calculated. The incremental costs are then compared (in a ratio) with incremental outcomes (as measured in physical or natural units). Physical and natural units can include both intermediate (surrogate) clinical endpoints (e.g. millimetres of mercury blood pressure reduction, changes in FEV_1) or final endpoints (e.g. deaths averted or life-years gained). In a study that assessed the cost per deaths from pulmonary embolism averted, Hull et al.[5] reported that subcutaneous administration of low-dose heparin starting 2 hours before surgery was a cost-effective approach to prophylaxis compared with the four alternative regimens. It should be noted that although this study is somewhat dated, it was included because a critical assessment of this chapter can be found in Drummond et al.[6]

28.3.1.3 Cost–benefit analysis

In CBA, monetary values are assigned to the health consequences so that the overall ratio is expressed completely in financial terms (e.g. pounds, dollars, euros). In principle, CBA allows policy-makers and decision-makers to make allocative comparisons and decisions across divergent sectors (e.g. health care and transportation). Notwithstanding this advantage, the valuation of health outcomes can be problematic (e.g. what monetary value do you assign to a life-year gained?) and therefore CBAs tend to be performed less frequently than other analytic types. Trollfors[7] examined the cost–benefit of infant vaccination with a conjugated *Haemophilus influenzae* type b (HIB) vaccine versus no vaccination (i.e. the 'do nothing' option). After taking into account the value of lives lost, the study author concluded that the widespread vaccination of infants for HIB was cost-effective and that it saved lives and reduced human suffering.

28.3.1.4 Cost-minimisation analysis

Cost-minimisation analyses are performed when the clinical outcomes (e.g. efficacy and safety) of the comparator groups are virtually identical and for all practical purposes can be considered to be equal. Because no decision can be made based on differences in the clinical endpoints, decisions are based on the incremental costs of the treatment pathways. Such was the case in a study that assessed the cost-effectiveness of treating proximal deep vein thromboses (DVT) at home with low molecular weight heparin versus standard heparin therapy in hospital. A cost-minimisation approach was chosen for this analysis because the results from a comparative clinical trial confirmed that there were no statistically significant differences in safety or efficacy between the two treatment groups. The study authors concluded that for patients with acute proximal DVTs, treatment at home with low molecular weight heparin was less costly than hospital treatment with standard heparin.[8]

28.3.1.5 Cost–utility analysis

The CUA is a form of cost-effectiveness analysis in which the health outcomes are measured in terms of quality-adjusted life-years (QALYs) gained. The QALY is a measure that associates quantity of life (e.g. survival data and life expectancy) with quality of life, by amalgamating them into a single index. One QALY is equal to a year of full life quality. Because of its universal denominator that allows comparisons across divergent areas, CUA is a tool that can (in theory) be used by policy-makers to determine the best way to spend their limited resources.

In an attempt to assess the value of introducing a rehabilitation programme to the standard care of patients with chronic respiratory disease, Griffiths et al.[9] assessed the incremental cost utility of the rehabilitation programme versus standard care. The results of the analysis indicated that the incremental cost of adding rehabilitation to standard care was £152 and the incremental utility was 0.03 QALYs per patient. The study authors concluded that the pulmonary rehabilitation programme produced cost per QALY ratios within the bounds considered to be cost-effective and would probably result in financial benefits to the health service.

In summary, there are five types of analysis that can be used to assess the incremental cost-effectiveness of a drug or service. The type performed is generally predicated by the therapeutic area being evaluated, the research question being addressed and the clinical data available. For example, whereas a CBA (which converts clinical effect into monetary terms) may not be considered (for ethical reasons) to be the best choice for oncology or HIV-related evaluations, a CUA (which takes into account both quality of life and survival duration) may be considered appropriate.

28.3.2 Measuring the benefits

When used in an economic milieu, the term 'benefit' can mean different things to different groups, even when referring to the same drug or service. For a person with migraine the benefit of a new effective rapid-onset antimigraine therapy is that he or she may be able to alleviate the headaches more rapidly than with their current medication. Employers may benefit because their staff remain productive, and accident and emergency departments may benefit because migraineurs do not come to their waiting rooms seeking treatment.

The assessment of the clinical benefit of medicines is generally understood by clinicians, regulatory authorities and reimbursement authorities alike. Everyone instinctively understands the clinical benefit of decreasing a hypertensive patient's blood pressure to 130/90 mmHg or the benefit in reducing the number of strokes. However, in an era of increasing health care costs and funding decisions, there is a need not only to illustrate the clinical benefit of a drug, but to translate that clinical outcome into an economic benefit.

The actual acquisition cost of a drug or service should not be used in isolation to determine the value of a drug. Value should be assessed in an analysis that takes into account all consequences (both positive and negative) that result from use of the therapy. For example, if a therapy eliminates the need for surgery, the cost of the surgery would be eliminated from the overall treatment pathway. However, if the same therapy results in an adverse event that requires specific laboratory monitoring, the cost of the laboratory tests would be added into the treatment pathway. The accurate identification and valuation of resource items that result from the use of that therapy are extremely important components of economic analysis.

Cost identification often involves the development of a probability or decision tree of the therapeutic pathway that describes all relevant downstream events related to use of that therapy and its comparator(s). Once the relevant resources are identified, measured (e.g. number of physician visits, treatment of side effects, number and duration of hospital visits) and are determined to be representative of local treatment patterns, local costs/prices can be applied to those resources to determine the overall cost of that intervention. The scope of the resources (and costs) included in an analysis is determined by the perspective (or intended audience) of the study.

Perspectives can be very broad (i.e. societal) or extremely narrow (e.g. the casualty department in a particular hospital), depending on the analytical question posed (e.g. is drug W a cost-effective option to drug X, in the treatment of disease Y, in hospital Z?). It should be noted that an economic analysis may be performed using several different perspectives, and that a drug may be considered cost-effective from one perspective and not when assessed from a different perspective. For example, drugs or services that affect or influence a patient's ability to work may be cost-effective from a societal perspective owing to a reduction in productivity losses; however, these drugs may or may not be considered cost-effective from the perspective of a health care system.

When assessing a drug from the societal perspective, the following resource items should be included. This list is provided as an example only, and should not be considered exhaustive:

• Health system items (e.g. drugs, physicians and other health care workers, hospitalisations, laboratory tests, surgeries);
• Social services items (e.g. home help);
• Spillover costs on other sectors (e.g. additional educational costs related to the proportion of children who survive neonatal intensive care units with learning disabilities);
• Costs that fall on the patient and family (e.g. loss of wages, transportation).

Analyses from the health care system perspective (e.g. ministry or department of health) would include only those costs that are paid by that system.

Resource items can be identified and measured using several different techniques, each having both positive and negative attributes. These techniques include (but are not limited to) direct measurement in clinical trials,[10,11] direct measurement in activity-based costing exercises,[12] retrospective database assessment, direct measurement in disease registries and physician/health care professional estimation. The amount of economic data collected as part of clinical trials has increased substantially over the last few years, with a survey reporting the inclusion of pharmco-economics in up to 71% of both phase III

and IV studies.[13] It should be recognised that prior to regulatory authority approval, in most cases the only product-specific utilisation data available for inclusion in economic analyses are collected during the phase II and III clinical trials. Because of forced treatment compliance, protocol-driven physician visits and tests, and many clinical trials being conducted in multinational settings (many with quite diverse health care systems) such data may not necessarily reflect real-world resource utilisation patterns and real-world clinical benefit.

In summary, there is more to demonstrating the benefit of a drug than proving its clinical efficacy or looking at its acquisition cost. Such a demonstration involves translating both positive and negative clinical consequences into resource and/or fiscal consequences and then comparing these to other drugs or therapies commonly used for that indication. The identification, measurement and valuation of resource items associated with drug therapy are extremely important components of economic analysis, and attention should be paid to these areas when evaluating such studies. Economic analyses should be reported in such a manner that the reader can determine whether the treatment patterns and costs described are relevant to those in his or her country or area.

28.3.3 Evaluating economic analyses

In recent years there has been a dramatic increase in the number of studies published in the scientific literature that purport to be economic analyses. As with all areas of research, the quality of studies varies and care should be taken when reviewing published (and unpublished) economic analyses. Studies have shown that although improving over time, the general quality of many published economic analyses is still poor.[14,15]

As when evaluating the published medical literature, results from economic analyses should not be taken at face value. Claims of cost-effectiveness must be supported by assessments against appropriate comparators. Analyses comparing against placebo should be viewed with caution unless the drug or therapy in question is the very first treatment available for that disease or in the case of add-on therapy, if the placebo arm in the study actually represents current levels of usual care. Reports should be detailed, clear and transparent. It is crucial that readers are able to follow exactly what was carried out (with justification) throughout the analysis. Care should also be taken to determine that the type of analysis performed (e.g. CEA, CBA) corresponds with the analytical technique purported to be used in the study. Zarnke et al.[16] sampled the published literature to assess whether evaluations labelled as CBAs met the contemporary definition using CBA methodology. They reported that 53% of the 95 studies assessed were reclassified as cost comparisons because health outcomes were not appraised. Several authors have developed checklists that are useful when evaluating the overall quality of an economic analysis.[6,17] One of the best-known checklists is given in Box 28.1.

These checklists are useful tools that prompt the reader systematically to pose simple questions which aid in the critical assessment of the study. The first question prompts the reader to consider the overall validity of the research question. Did the investigators explain the problem and why it has not been adequately addressed? Are both the costs and the consequences of the drug under investigation included? Is the analysis incremental? Is the viewpoint (or perspective) of the analysis stated, and is it valid? The research question is well defined if it states the perspective and alternatives and makes it clear that both costs and consequences were to be compared.

The second question addresses the issue of relevant treatment comparators and the justification for those comparators. When discussing the issue of comparators, pharmaco-economic guidelines worldwide state that (at a minimum) the drug in question must be compared with the standard treatment or usual regimen. It should be noted that, unlike regulatory authorities, most decision-makers do not consider placebo to be a relevant comparator. When assessing the comprehensiveness of the description, the reader must decide whether the relevant alternatives have been compared. In order to do this, the reader must first identify the primary objective of the drug or service targeted for the evaluation.

An economic analysis does not measure the clinical effectiveness of a drug or its comparator: rather, it reports the fiscal consequences associated with their use. Question 3 serves as a reminder to the reader that the clinical data included in the economic analysis should be based on appropriately conducted clinical studies (considering both methodological rigour and generalisability), and that the study report should establish the clinical effectiveness of the treatments under investigation.

Question 4 addresses one of the most important issues in the critical assessment of economic analyses – the issue of identification and inclusion or exclusion of resources. The actual scope of the resources included should match the (stated) perspective of the analysis. It is important to note that it is not always possible to measure and value all the costs and consequences of the alternatives; however, a comprehensive list of the most important and relevant ones should be provided, along with justification for any major omissions. For example, a new drug has several side effects with similar rates of occurrence. One side effect results in a transient cough, another results in a gastrointestinal bleed. Given the scope of the total costs and/or resources involved, an economic analysis of this drug could probably justify non-inclusion of the treatment costs associated with the cough because such a cost would represent a very small percentage of overall costs and its exclusion would not change the overall conclusion of the analysis. However, because of the significant impact of even one hospitalisation, the costs associated with the gastrointestinal bleed must be included.

Questions 5 and 6 address the actual identification, quantification and valuation of resources and costs. Resources previously identified as being relevant to the analysis have to be collected, measured and reported in appropriate units. For example, if blood tests are determined to be a resource that is important to the analysis, the actual number of each specific test performed must be recorded (e.g. five complete blood

---

BOX 28.1 Ten questions to ask of any published study

1. Was a well-defined question posed in answerable form?
2. Was a comprehensive description of the competing alternatives given (i.e. can you tell who, did what, to whom, where and how often)?
3. Was the effectiveness of the programme of services established?
4. Were all the important and relevant costs and consequences for each alternative identified?
5. Were costs and consequences measured accurately in appropriate physical units (e.g. hours of nursing time, number of physician visits, lost workdays, gained life-years)?
6. Were costs and consequences valued credibly?
7. Were costs and consequences adjusted for differential timing?
8. Was an incremental analysis of costs and consequences of alternatives performed?
9. Was allowance made for the uncertainty in the estimates of costs and consequences?
10. Did the presentation and discussion of study results include all issues of concern to users?

After Drummond et al.[6]

cell counts). Because of differing treatment regimens across regions or countries, it is extremely important that there is full disclosure of each resource identified, along with the frequency of use. Such 'resource dictionaries' allow the person critically evaluating the analysis to determine whether the treatment patterns in the analysis accurately reflect treatment patterns in their area. In addition, the unit cost/price for each resource should be provided, along with the source of each value. The provision of unit prices/costs allows the reader to determine whether the relative costs shown in the analysis are similar to those found in his or her area.

Economic analyses may evaluate the effect of drugs or therapies over several years, and because economic analyses operate in the present, the costs and consequences that occur in the future have to be adjusted to reflect their present-day values. This process is called discounting – discounting basically assumes that one unit of monetary (or health outcome) value is worth more today than it will be worth in the future; therefore, future units have to be reduced to reflect this expected decrease in value.

Question 7 addresses the issue of differential timing and whether discounting of future costs and consequences has occurred. As a rule of thumb, economic analyses that are less than or equal to 1 year in duration are not discounted, as it is assumed that the relative value of items would not change within a year. It should also be noted that discount rates used in analyses vary from country to country. Justification should be provided for the rate used in the analysis.

Question 8 addresses another extremely important area in economic analysis – whether the analysis is incremental. For an analysis to be a truly meaningful comparison it is necessary to examine the additional costs that one drug or therapy imposes over another, compared with the additional effects or benefits it delivers. As with the issue of choice of the comparator drug, most economic guidelines worldwide stipulate that an economic analysis must be incremental.

Economic analyses (models) are only as good as their ability to represent reality at the level needed to draw useful conclusions. Because all economic evaluations contain some degree of imprecision, there is value in varying the parameters or estimates that have the greatest degree of uncertainty (i.e. perform a sensitivity analysis). Sensitivity analyses should be performed on the estimates that have the greatest degree of imprecision in order to see if the overall results are dependent on that parameter.

The final question asks about the 'validity' of the conclusions drawn by the study authors. Were the conclusions based on some overall index or ratio of costs to consequences, and was the index interpreted intelligently? Did the study authors provide benchmarks to aid in the interpretation of the study, and was the robustness of the conclusions discussed in light of results of the sensitivity and/or statistical analyses? Was subgroup analysis undertaken where relevant? Were the results compared with those of others who have investigated the same question? Were the limitations of the study and the generalisability of the results discussed? Were other relevant factors in the decision to adopt the intervention discussed (e.g. distribution, ethics)? And, finally, did the authors discuss implementation issues?

In summary, in a critical assessment of an economic analysis, careful attention should be paid to the choice of analytical technique, the relevance of the comparator and the identification, measurement and valuation of resources, ensuring that the latter components are relevant to the stated viewpoint of the analysis. Published checklists are useful tools that aid in the assessment of these analyses.

28.3.4 Interpreting cost-effectiveness ratios

Once the 'validity' of an analysis has been determined, it is up to the reader to decide whether or not the drug or service is a cost-effective treatment option in their setting. The fact that the majority of economic analyses (especially those found in the published literature) are performed in a setting that is different from that of the reader emphasises the need for transparency in reporting. Readers need to be able to assess whether the treatment patterns, the resources identified and the unit costs associated with those resources are applicable to their setting. Figure 28.2 provides a simple 'rule of thumb' reference as to whether a drug could potentially be considered to be a cost-effective option in therapy.

Drugs that are more (or equally) effective than the comparator drug (or service) and which have total costs that are either equal to or less than those of the comparator drug are generally considered to be a cost-effective option. It should be noted that if a drug is both more effective and has lower overall costs than the comparator, it is said to dominate the alternative. Readers should be aware that in cases of dominance some study authors will not provide the cost-effectiveness ratio: rather, they will simply state that the comparator drug was dominated.

Incremental cost* of drug A compared to drug B	Incremental effectiveness of drug A compared to drug B: More	Same	Less
More	??	XX	XX
Same	vv	??	XX
Less	vv	vv	??

* Cost refers to total expected expenditures that result from use of the drug.
vv Generally speaking, products fitting this profile would be considered cost-effective.
?? Products fitting this profile may be considered cost-effective, depending on the magnitude of the ratio.
XX Products fitting this profile are not considered to be cost-effective.

Figure 28.2 Assessment of the incremental cost-effectiveness of treatment options. After Drummond et al.[6]

This somewhat simplistic explanation becomes more complex when we consider drugs that are both more effective and more expensive, as is the case with many (most?) new therapies. Above or below what fiscal threshold are drugs considered cost-effective? There is no simple answer to this question because funding decisions are often made in response to fiscal (budgetary) realities at that point in time, even when considering drugs that are deemed to be cost-effective.

Notwithstanding these issues, attempts have been made to identify and quantify acceptability thresholds.[18,19] Laupacis et al.[18] proposed that new therapies be classified into one of five grades of recommendation based on the magnitude of their incremental benefits (Table 28.2).

Table 28.2 Proposed acceptability threshold

Grade	Description of incremental cost-effectiveness ratio	Recommendations
A	The new therapy is either equally or more effective and less costly than existing therapies (i.e. is dominant)	There is compelling evidence for adoption and appropriate utilisation of the new therapy
Ba	The new therapy is more effective than the existing one and costs less than $20,000 per QALY gained	There is strong evidence for adoption and appropriate utilisation of the new therapy
Bb	The new therapy is less effective than the existing one but its introduction would save more than $100,000 per QALY gained	
Ca	The new therapy is more effective than the existing one and costs $20,000–100,000 per QALY gained	There is moderate evidence for adoption and appropriate utilisation of the new therapy
Cb	The new therapy is less effective than existing one, but its introduction would save $20,000–100,000 per QALY gained	
Da	The new therapy is more effective than the existing one and costs more than $100,000 per QALY gained	There is weak evidence for adoption and appropriate utilisation of the new therapy
Db	The new therapy is less effective than existing one, but its introduction would save less than $20,000 per QALY gained	
E	The new therapy is less effective than or is as effective as the existing therapy and is more costly	Compelling evidence for rejection

After Laupacis et al.[18]

In summary, the assessment of whether or not a drug or therapy is cost-effective is often somewhat subjective, depending on the financial burden that the decision-maker is willing to assume. These decisions cannot and should not be made in isolation; rather, the costs and consequences of the therapy under investigation must be considered relative to existing usual or gold standard practices.

28.4 Compulsory economic evaluation: the ultimate measure

The most extreme way of ensuring that economic evaluations are undertaken and that the results affect service delivery is to make economic appraisal a compulsory part of the process of getting the intervention approved for practice. Several countries have made attempts to achieve this objective, with varying degrees of success. These countries include Australia, Canada, the Netherlands and the UK. For the purposes of this chapter we have chosen to focus on the approaches of the home countries of the two authors – Canada and the UK.

28.4.1 Canada

Formalized guidelines for the conduct and reporting of economic analyses have been in place in Canada since 1994 when the province of Ontario and the Canadian Agency for Drugs and Technologies in Health [CADTH, formerly known as the Canadian Coordinating Office of Health Technology Assessment (CCOHTA)] both issued guidelines regarding pharmaco-economic analyses.[20,21] As is the case with clinical treatment guidelines, these economic guidelines continue to evolve over time and have undergone several revisions since their initial issuance. Initially used as guidance for research, their role has expanded to a point where all provinces mandate that pharmaceutical manufacturers include economic evaluations based on the principles set out in these guidelines in their drug formulary submissions.[22]

Although economic analyses are not required to obtain regulatory approval for pharmaceutical products in Canada, they are required by all of the federal and provincial drug formularies and many private drug plan insurers as part of their formulary decision-making process. The importance of inclusion in a formulary (especially the federal and provincial formularies) to the uptake and utilization of new and existing drugs cannot be overstated. There is one basic 'truism' that exists in countries such as Canada, which

is that unless your drug is a so-called 'lifestyle' drug (i.e. one for which patients are willing to pay out of pocket), provincial formulary inclusion is essential for its overall (commercial) success. This is because most physicians (especially general and family practitioners) will not prescribe a drug until it is included in their local province's formulary.

Although the requirement for economic analyses may be seen by many to be 'another hurdle' used to reduce access to new medicines, it should also be viewed as a means to demonstrate the value of the new medicine. Prior to the requirement for economic analyses, the value of a drug was often solely determined by its potential impact on the decision-maker's drug budget. The net result of this method of decision-making was the non-reimbursement of many highly effective (albeit) expensive drugs. Since the introduction of economic requirements, it has become harder for formulary decision-makers to reject a drug solely because of its acquisition cost and potential budgetary impact.

28.4.1.1 Common drug review

The publicly funded federal, provincial and territorial drug formularies in Canada subsidise the cost of prescription drugs for individuals who are eligible for coverage under these programmes. With new drugs constantly emerging on the market, health policy-makers and drug plan managers need clear answers to the following questions. Does a new drug provide a clinical advantage over existing products? Is it cost-effective? Will it benefit certain patient groups?

Each province sought to answer these questions individually, using local expert formulary review committees that reviewed the clinical and cost-effectiveness evidence and made province-specific listing recommendations. In an attempt to reduce this duplication of effort, federal, provincial and territorial ministers of health (with the exception of the province of Quebec) formed an alliance that was tasked with solving this issue. The final recommendation of this alliance was the creation of a single entity that would perform these reviews – the Common Drug Review (CDR) directorate.

The CDR was established in March 2002 and formally started accepting drug reimbursement submissions in September 2003. It operates under the umbrella of Canada's health technology assessment organization, CADTH. Under the current CDR submission guidelines, pharmaceutical companies wishing to apply for reimbursement by federal, provincial and territorial drug formularies must submit a reimbursement dossier to the CDR. This mandatory submission applies to all new chemical entities (drugs), new combination products and (most recently) to drugs with new indications. The submission is evaluated in an approximately 6-month-long process by pharmacists, physicians and health economists. Results of these evaluations are then reviewed by the Canadian Expert Drug Advisory Committee (CEDAC). Based on this review, CEDAC provides a public recommendation regarding their listing recommendation for the drug under review. In addition to the 'list or do not list recommendation', the committee will make recommendations regarding reimbursement criteria and/or restrictions. These recommendations are then forwarded to each participating drug plan. It should be noted that a positive recommendation for listing from the CDR does not guarantee formulary listing as each province will then make a listing decision based on their plan's mandate, priorities and resources – the incremental cost impact on the drug formulary is an important component of this decision. The health ministers associated with each participating drug plan have publicly committed that they will not reimburse a drug that receives a negative review from the CDR – in other words, 'no means no, yes means maybe'.

To date, less than 50% of the drugs reviewed by the CDR have received positive listing recommendations and even less have been included on the drug formularies of participating federal, provincial and territorial drug plans. Although surrogate endpoints are accepted by regulatory authorities in many therapeutic areas, they are not always accepted by CEDAC. There has been a trend over the last couple of years to reject drugs in certain therapeutic areas (e.g. hypertension) that do not provide evidence of how those surrogate endpoints translate into clinically important outcomes.

More information about the CDR, including their submission requirements and listing recommendations can be found at http://www.cadth.ca/.

28.4.2 The UK

28.4.2.1 National Institute of Clinical Excellence

NICE was established as a Special Health Authority in April 1999. In establishing NICE, the Labour government hoped to improve standards of patient care and reduce inequalities in access to innovative treatments (i.e. postcode prescribing).

NICE was to achieve these aims by providing guidance to the NHS on the effectiveness and cost of clinical interventions. This would be performed by appraising new and existing technologies, developing disease-specific clinical guidelines and by supporting clinical audit. Perhaps unsurprisingly, it is the work of NICE in the technology appraisals arena that has dominated its work programme since 1999 and generated the most controversy both within and outside the UK.

For the purposes of this chapter the focus will be on the technology appraisals. However, for details of other aspects of the institute's work and their procedures, the NICE website is a useful source of material (http://www.nice.org.uk/). Since 2000, when NICE was accused of taking too long to appraise products, there have been two forms of technology appraisal: single technology appraisals (STA) and multiple technology appraisals (MTAs). STAs are especially for new products to market, the aim is that on assessment of the product it should be in the public domain within 6–13 weeks of launch, this it is hoped will avoid the 'NICE blight' phenomenon that was occurring with the MTAs. The MTAs have a much longer process and were appearing in public on average 18–24 months post-launch. These now tend to be measured for older products, where there are more than one treatment available for a condition and/or there are concerns over uptake.

The scope for the technology appraisals was set out in the Department of Health discussion paper *Faster Access to Modern Treatment: How NICE Appraisal will Work*. This document clearly states that it would be 'desirable to cover all kinds of clinical intervention on an equal basis', and in particular all medicines and medical devices; all therapeutic interventions and programmes of care; products and processes to diagnose and prevent disease and population screening programmes. In the discussion paper it is openly acknowledged that the principles of technology appraisal will be easier to implement in some areas than others and the example of the medical devices industry, where the evidence base in terms of randomised clinical trials may be more limited, is cited. However, this does not fully explain why the vast majority of technology appraisals carried out to date have been on pharmaceuticals. Ease of undertaking an appraisal should not be a requirement for an assessment to take place.

The selection of a technology for appraisal is undertaken by the Department of Health and the National Assembly of Wales. This selection is based upon one or more of the following criteria:

1. Is the technology likely to result in a significant health benefit, taken across the NHS as a whole, if given to all patients for whom it is indicated?

2. Is the technology likely to result in a significant impact on other health-related government policies (e.g. reduction in health inequalities)?

3. Is the technology likely to have a significant impact on NHS resources (financial or other) if given to all patients for whom it is indicated?

4. Is the institute likely to be able to add value by issuing national guidance? For instance, in the absence of such guidance is there likely to be significant controversy over the interpretation or significance of the available evidence on clinical and cost-effectiveness?

Details of both technology appraisal processes can be found on the website but, briefly, when a technology appraisal is referred from the Department of Health and the National Assembly of Wales all possible stakeholders are identified (stakeholders can be manufacturers, professional bodies and patient groups). They are then consulted on the scope of the appraisal. An independent review of the published literature is commissioned and submissions (both written and oral) are received from the stakeholders. The appraisal committee considers all this information and consults on its provisional views (appraisal consultation document) via the institute's website. The appraisal committee reconsiders it in the light of the comments and produces a final appraisal determination, which is again placed on the website. Stakeholders can appeal against it if they consider that the institute and the guidance have not fulfilled a number of criteria (details of the appeal process can be found on the website). Guidance is finally issued direct to the NHS.

The institute has set out quite clearly the data it wishes to see presented in a submission from a stakeholder. For each of the three main groups of stakeholders, patient/carer groups, health care professional groups, and manufacturers and sponsors, there is a separate set of guidelines. These may be accessed via the NICE website and should be essential reading for all those involved in the preparation of a submission.

Since the advent of NICE, evidence about cost-effectiveness is formally required to help determine whether new interventions should be made available at public expense. Currently, not all products are assessed by NICE but it is anticipated that in the foreseeable future, NICE's remit will be considerably extended. Decisions by NICE have major implications for future market access for all pharmaceuticals. Economic information available at launch can only provide initial guidance about value for money. Further evidence on cost-effectiveness in real-world use will also be required.

28.4.2.2 Scottish Medicines Consortium

The Scottish Medicines Consortium (SMC) was established in 2001 with the remit to provide advice to NHS boards and their area drug and therapeutics committees across Scotland about the status of all newly licensed medicines, all new formulations of existing medicines and any major new indications for established products. The SMC process (full details of which are available on their website http://www.scottishmedicines.org.uk/) requires pharmaceutical companies to complete a new product submission form. The aim is to make a recommendation soon after the launch of the product involved. The timescales involved usually require a submission to be made ahead of product launch. The entire process is extremely quick and it is possible for a decision to be made in 3 months from the manufacturer's submission. However, even a positive recommendation from SMC does not mean that the product will necessarily go on to formularies if other equivalent treatments already exist.

In 2007, the SMC made a total of 110 assessments of which 27 (25%) were considered 'acceptable for use', 29 (26%) were 'acceptable for restricted use' and 54 (49%) were 'not recommended for use'.[23]

28.4.2.3 All Wales Medicines Strategy Group

The remit of the All Wales Medicines Strategy Group (AWMSG) is similar to the SMC in that its function is to provide advice to the Minister for Health and Social Services (Wales) in 'an effective, efficient and transparent manner on strategic medicines management and prescribing' (AWMSG website). It currently differs from the SMC in that while it only reviews newly licensed medicines these products should not be assessed by NICE and should either be on oncology or cardiovascular product and/or cost over £2000 per patient per year. However, it is anticipated that in the near future the AWMSG will be moving to a process and review strategy which will be essentially the same as that of the SMC. Further information about the AWMSG process can be found on their website (www.wales.nhs.uk/awmsg/).

28.5 Conclusions

We live in an era in which the value of medicines can no longer be assumed and the phrase 'evidence-based' is no longer restricted to the realm of academics. The increasing financial burden on our health care systems has prompted decision-makers around the world to demand that the pharmaceutical industry provide proof of the value of new drugs being introduced into the market. Decision-makers in certain countries (e.g. Australia and Canada) have taken this requirement a step further by linking reimbursement approval to the provision of such evidence. Therefore, the provision of well-performed credible analyses is vital for the future of present and future pharmaceutical products.

Most (if not all) companies within the pharmaceutical industry have recognised that such requirements are now a permanent part of doing business, and have developed internal health economics expertise, both on a global (corporate) and on a country-specific level. It should be noted that because of the multidisciplinary nature of this area of research, pharmaceutical company-based health economists cannot operate in isolation from the other disciplines within the company. It is therefore vital that pharmaceutical physicians understand the basic principles and evidentiary needs of health economic evaluations in order to work with the health economists in the development of high-quality analyses.

References

1 Cohen D. The impact of health economics on health policy, health services and decision-making. In: Salek S, ed. *Pharmacoeconomics and Outcome Assessment – A Global Issue*. Haslemere: Euromed Communications, 1999.

2 Maynard A. NICE mess? *Pharm Times* 2001;22.

3 Abel-Smith B, Titmus R. *The Cost of the National Health Service in England and Wales*. Oxford: Oxford University Press, 1956.

4 Canadian Agency for Drugs and Technologies in Health. *Guidelines for the Economic Evaluation of Health Technologies: Canada*, 3rd edn. Ottawa: CADTH, 2006. http://www.cadth.ca/.

5 Hull RD, Hirsh J, Sackett DL, et al. Cost-effectiveness of primary and secondary prevention of fatal pulmonary embolism in high-risk surgical patients. *CMAJ* 1982; 127:990–5.

6 Drummond M, O'Brien B, Stoddart G, et al. *Methods for the Economic Evaluation of Health Care Programmes*, 3rd edn. Oxford: Oxford Medical Press, 2005.

7 Trollfors B. Cost–benefit analysis of general vaccination against *Haemophilus influenzae* type b in Sweden. *Scand J Infect Dis* 1994;26:611–4.

8 O'Brien B, Levine M, Willan A, et al. Economic evaluation of outpatient treatment with low-molecularweight heparin for proximal vein thrombosis. *Arch Intern Med* 1999;159:2298–304.

9 Griffiths TL, Phillips CJ, Burr SD, et al. Cost effectiveness of an outpatient multidisciplinary pulmonary rehabilitation programme. *Thorax* 2001;56:779–84.

10 Mauskopf J, Schulman K, Bell L, et al. A strategy for collecting pharmacoeconomic data during phase II/III clinical trials. *Pharmacoeconomics* 1996;264–77.

11 Coyle D, Drummond MF. Analyzing differences in the costs of treatment across centers within economic evaluations. *Int J Tech Assess Health Care* 2001;17:155–63.

12 Doyle JJ, Casciano JP, Arikian SR, et al. Full cost determination of different levels of care in the intensive care unit. *Pharmacoeconomics* 1996;10:395–408.

13 DiMasi JA, Caglarcan E, Wood-Armany M. Emerging role of pharmcoeconomics in the research and development decision making process. *Pharmacoeconomics* 2001; 19:753–66.

14 Bradley CA, Iskedjian M, Lanctôt KL, et al. Quality assessment of economic evaluations in selected pharmacy, medical, and health economics journals. *Ann Pharmacother* 1995;29:681–6.

15 Iskedjian M, Trakas K, Bradley CA, et al. Quality assessment of economic evaluations published in *Pharmacoeconomics*: the first four years (1992 to 1995). *Pharmacoeconomics* 1997;12:685–94.

16 Zarnke KB, Levine MA, O'Brien BJ. Cost–benefit analyses in the health care literature: don't judge a study by its label. *J Clin Epidemiol* 1997;50:813–22.

17 Sacristán JA, Soto J, Galende I. Evaluation of pharmacoeconomic studies: utilization of a checklist. *Ann Pharmacother* 1993;27:1126–33.

18 Laupacis A, Feeny D, Detsky A, et al. How attractive does a technology have to be to warrant adoption and utilization? Tentative guidelines for using clinical and economic evaluations. *CMAJ* 1992;146:473–81.

19 Holloway RG, Benesch CG, Rahilly CR, et al. A systematic review of cost-effectiveness research of stroke valuation and treatment. *Stroke* 1999;30:1340–9.

20 Canadian Coordinating Office for Health Technology Assessment (CCOHTA). *Guidelines for Economic Evaluation of Pharmaceuticals: Canada*. Ottawa: CCOHTA, 1997.

21 Ontario Ministry of Health. Ontario guidelines for economic analysis of pharmaceutical products. 1994: http://www.gov on.ca/health/english/pub/drugs/drugpro/economic.html.

22 Glennie JL, Torrance GW, Baladi JF, et al. The revised Canadian guidelines for the economic evaluation of pharmaceuticals. *Pharmacoeconomics* 1999;15:459–68.

23 NHS Scotland. Scottish Medicines consortium Annual Report 2007.

29 Controls on NHS medicines prescribing and expenditure in the UK (a historical perspective) with some international comparisons

John P. Griffin[1] and Jane R. Griffin[2]

[1] Asklepieion Consulting Ltd, Herts, UK
[2] Boehringer Ingelheim Ltd, Berks, UK

29.1 Introduction

The National Health Service (NHS), set up in 1948, achieved its 60th anniversary in 2008. What cost £276 million in its first year of operation is now costing £90 billion in 2008, and its cost is set to continue to rise. Since its inception there has been a dilemma expressed by Enoch Powell as the impossibility 'to reconcile the combination of unlimited demand and limited resources provided free'. Any move to change the principle of a service free at the point of need is one of great political sensitivity, as Nigel Lawson, a former Conservative Chancellor, expressed it, the NHS is 'the nearest thing the English have to a religion'. Sir Derek Wanless argued in 2001[1] that continuing to fund the health service through general taxation was the most cost-effective and fairest system for the future.

The medicines bill forms about £10 billion of the annual NHS expenditure. However, it is a component that, unlike other components of expenditure, is capable of being squeezed. There is a well-defined system of pharmaceutical distribution in the UK which is controlled by a licensing system covering manufacture, wholesale and retail supply. For every medicinal product there has to be a product licence or marketing authorisation, and the product may only be manufactured (or imported) and distributed for

sale in accordance with that licence. In addition, manufacturers are required to hold a manufacturer's licence and those who deal in medicines wholesale must hold a wholesale dealer's licence. An important factor in the control of the manufacture of human medicines in the UK is the activities of the Medicines Inspectorate of the Department of Health (DoH). Premises are inspected before a manufacturer's licence is granted, and at regular intervals thereafter. Withdrawal of licences and, rarely, prosecutions can result if standards are not maintained. In this respect the DoH gives detailed guidance regarding Good Manufacturing Practice (GMP).

The distribution of medicines from manufacturer to retailer is mainly a private function, the wholesaler covering their costs and earning their profit through the margin allowed in the retail price. The wholesale dealer's licence, among other things, seeks to ensure adequate record keeping, in case a batch of medicines has to be recalled.

In the UK, prescriptions are required for all medicines supplied under the NHS and for all prescription-only medicines. Prescriptions may only be written by a doctor or dentist registered in the UK. The UK NHS is financed primarily out of taxation and is available to all permanent residents. Most people are registered with a general medical practitioner (under contract with the NHS and paid mainly on a capitation basis), who provides primary care and is the normal route of referral to hospital and specialist services, whether in the NHS or the private sector. A small minority of the population obtain some or all

The Textbook of Pharmaceutical Medicine. Edited by John P. Griffin. © 2009, ISBN: 978-1-4051-8035-1.

of their medical treatment privately, mainly through insurance schemes.

As part of primary care, general practitioners (GPs) are free to prescribe virtually any medicine they consider desirable for the patient, with the exception of medicines in certain therapeutic categories covered by the 1985 and 1992 Selected List restrictions (see below).

In some, mainly rural, areas the doctor may also dispense the medicines prescribed, but more usually the patient takes the prescription to a community pharmacist, also under contract with the NHS, who dispenses the medicines and claims reimbursement at predetermined rates. Unless they are exempt, patients pay a prescription charge at the time of dispensing.

From April 1985, within certain therapeutic categories, GPs have been restricted in the medicines they may prescribe under the NHS to those included in a limited list. The excluded medicines are generally those that can be purchased directly by the patient without a prescription, (i.e. minor analgesics), but also include some prescription items, such as benzodiazepine sedatives and tranquillisers. The principle underlying this economy measure is that, in theory, for the therapeutic categories concerned, the only medicines prescribable at NHS expense should be those that meet a real clinical need at the lowest cost. The list will remain under review by an expert advisory committee, the Advisory Committee on National Health Services Drugs. For medicines no longer available under the NHS but for which a prescription is necessary, it is open to the doctor to prescribe these and to the patient to pay for them privately. These measures have, for all practical purposes, introduced a 'need clause' into the UK drug regulations.

The prescribing practices of GPs are monitored. After dispensing, the prescriptions are sent to one central point for authorisation of reimbursement, and thus it is possible to analyse each practitioner's prescribing habits and costs (PACT). A summary is sent to each practitioner, together with a note of the area and national averages. If a practitioner's costs are significantly different from the average this may be discussed with him or her by a doctor from the Regional Medical Service of the DoH.

29.2 NHS and Community Care Act 1990

Until 1 April 1991, the key features for the procurement of medicines in the Family Practitioner (GP) Service (FPS) were as follows: GPs were independent contractors to the Family Practitioner Committees (FPCs) with freedom to prescribe without cash constraints. The FPCs reported directly to the DoH and were responsible for paying GPs for the provision of primary health services. A small group of Regional Medical Services Officers (RMSOs) reported directly to the DoH and were responsible for ensuring economical prescribing of medicines by GPs. The non-dispensing GP was not involved in the procurement of medicines. The pharmacist bought and dispensed the product and was reimbursed by the Prescription Pricing Authority (PPA) on behalf of FPCs. The Regional Health Authority (RHA) had responsibility for the FPS.

Under the system introduced by the NHS and Community Care Act 1990, the government set an overall budget for GP prescribing, putting a cash restraint on the FPS medicines bill for the first time. The RHAs took over responsibility for the FPCs. Each RHA received a share of the overall drug budget and was responsible for allocating the budget to the newly named Family Health Service Authority (FHSA, formerly FPC). The FHSA set indicative amounts for medicines for each GP and was responsible for monitoring GPs' prescribing against that set amount.

In these circumstances, the main concern of FHSAs was to stay within their budget. They had little incentive to tackle the problem of under-prescribing, whereby GPs could give better patient care by spending more on medicines. Medical audit and FHSA visits were likely to be directed at high-spending practices rather than low-spending ones. After all, it must be borne in mind that one of the declared objectives of the original White Paper 'Working for Patients' was to exert 'downward pressure' on the NHS medicines bill. This Act operated in tandem with the other measures that have been taken since the inception of the NHS in 1948 to control NHS medicines expenditure.

29.3 Problem of the rising NHS medicines bill

The costs of health care are rising in all developed countries, and despite the fact that in the UK since the inception of the NHS in 1948, the cost of pharmaceuticals has been hovering at about 10% of the total, it has been the target of successive governments for savings. This is because health spending is made up of 70% fixed costs, which are difficult to change, and 30% variable costs. Pharmaceutical expenditure has historically been around one-third of the variable cost element and as such has been judged to be an obvious target for reduction and control. However, in the last few years there has been some increase in the proportion of the NHS budget spent on medicines, from 10.5% in 1990 to some 12% in 1998. Although there has been a significant increase in the average net ingredient cost of each prescription, the major cause of the rise has been an increase in the annual number of prescriptions, from some 500 million to 750 million for the UK over the last 10 years (*OHE Compendium of Health Statistics 2004–2005*, 16th edition). Much of this increase has been because of the demands of an ageing population.

The methods used to control NHS medicines expenditure have been on both the supply side, by attempting to reduce costs, and the demand side, by attempting to restrict volume. The 10 distinct measures taken by successive UK governments since 1948 to attempt to do this are reviewed in chronological order.

29.4 Prescription charges for NHS medicines

Prescription charges were first introduced in the UK in 1952, and are collected by the pharmacist when a doctor's prescription is dispensed. The money collected is not offset against the cost of the medicines prescribed but is allocated to the cost of running the pharmaceutical services. (The prescription charges levied in 1994 funded only 6% of the cost of pharmaceutical services.) Prescription charges should therefore be regarded as a revenue-raising exercise rather than a genuine co-payment for medicines dispensed.

In 1948, when the NHS was established by the then Minister of Health, Aneurin Bevan, during the Labour government of Clement Attlee, all prescriptions were supplied free of charge. A charge of 1s 0d (£0.05) per prescription, irrespective of the number of items, was eventually introduced in 1952. Shortly after this the charge was changed to 1s 0d (£0.05) per item on the prescription.[1,2]

For a short period between 1965 and 1968, under the Labour government of Harold Wilson, prescription charges were abolished. In 1968, however, charges were reintroduced and the concept of exemptions was introduced.

In 1971, when the prescription charge was £0.20, the proportion of prescriptions that were exempted was 52% of the total; of these, 32% were for the elderly

(men over 65 and women over 60) and 20% were for non-age-related reasons. In 1995, 89% of prescriptions were exempt from charge, 45% on grounds of age, which means that 44% of prescriptions were exempt from charge for non-age-related reasons.

The list of grounds for exemption from a prescription charge in the UK is extensive. The social grounds are low income, children below the age of 16 years, people in full-time education up to 19 years of age, pregnant women and women in the puerperium following either a live or still birth, old age (women over 60, men over 65, but since October 1995 men over 60) and war pensioners.

In addition, for social policy reasons, since July 1975 prescriptions for oral contraceptives have also been exempt from charges. The medical grounds for exemption from prescription charge are diabetes mellitus, diabetes insipidus, hypopituitarism, hypothyroidism, hypoparathyroidism, hypoadrenalism, myaesthenia gravis, epilepsy and permanent fistula (e.g. colostomy, ileostomy). In addition, police personnel can claim back from their employing authority any prescription charge they incur.

There are illogicalities in the system, as a patient who is exempt from paying a prescription charge gets all medicines free, even if the prescription is for the treatment of an illness unrelated to the medical condition for which the exemption has been allowed – for example, a millionaire with diabetes mellitus would be exempt from a prescription charge for a bottle of aspirin, whereas a parent with a chronic medical condition not on the exemption list would have to pay a charge for medicines prescribed for his or her chronic condition, such as rheumatoid arthritis, parkinsonism or hypertension. (This can to some extent be mitigated by purchase of an annual prescription season ticket, which for a flat sum covers the cost of all prescription charges for medicines and devices for the ensuing 12 months.)

In the 29 years from 1979 to 2008, there were annual increases in the prescription charge, from £0.20 per item to £7.10 per item. (In Wales the Welsh Assembly abolished the prescription charge which still continues to be levied in England, Scotland and Northern Ireland.) The government has attempted to use this tax to raise revenue and as an unsuccessful deterrent to patients demanding a prescription at each visit to their doctor. Because about 85% of prescriptions are exempt from charge, this latter objective has been deemed to be ineffective. This has been largely due at times to high levels of unemployment –

at times in excess of 3 million – during this period, which has also meant that the unemployed and their families have been exempt from prescription charges. In addition, unemployment also contributes to or is associated with ill health and demands for health care.[3]

In October 1995, the European Court of Justice in Luxembourg ruled on equal treatment for men and women regarding the age at which they should be exempted from paying an NHS prescription charge. Until then the exemption from the prescription charge had been linked to the state pensionable age of 60 years for women and 65 for men. Men are now exempt from the age of 60, at an estimated cost of £30 million per year in 1995 for lowering the age and £10 million for refunds for those men between 60 and 65 years who had paid for a prescription in the preceding 3 months.[4]

Another criticism of the current level of prescription charges is that in 1994, nearly 60% of prescribed medicines could either be purchased from a pharmacist for less than the prescription charge, or had a net ingredient cost less than the prescription charge.

Both physicians and economists have called for reform of the prescription charge exemptions for both social and medical conditions.[6-8] It has been pointed out that if the exemptions were reduced from 89% to 55% – the level that applied when they were first introduced – and the charge actually reduced to £2.50 per item, then £250 million per annum extra would have been collected at the 1995 prescribing level of 500 million items per year.[6] Changes in the current system would not only have to be logical but politically acceptable, and there is no indication that the political will to introduce changes is growing. Rationalisation of the exemptions from prescription charges and a variation of the current season ticket scheme linked to annual registration with a general practice have been proposed.[6,7]

In conclusion, charges for NHS prescriptions should be regarded as a tax rather than co-payment for the medicines prescribed. They have been inefficient as a deterrent on the demand side owing to the high level of exemptions. The application of the principle of exemption has led to legal action before the European courts on grounds of sex discrimination. Furthermore, a potential for a legal challenge exists on the grounds of social inequities and unfairness in selecting certain illnesses as worthy of exemption but not others, and has been considered by patient pressure groups.

29.5 Pharmaceutical Price Regulation Scheme

The prices of medicines sold to the NHS are controlled in the UK by the Pharmaceutical Price Regulation Scheme (PPRS),[8,9] negotiated periodically every 5–6 years by the DoH with the Association of the British Pharmaceutical Industry (ABPI), for example in 1979, 1986, 1993 and 1999. The PPRS controls the maximum – but not guaranteed – profits that pharmaceutical companies make on the capital they have invested in plant for research, development and manufacturing for sales made to the NHS. (Capital employed by the individual companies is allocated between that devoted to NHS sales and that for non-NHS sales and exports.)

The scheme was proposed in 1957, in an attempt by the pharmaceutical industry to stave off more draconian measures by the government of the day. It was known as the Voluntary Price Regulation Scheme but was neither voluntary nor a price regulation scheme. It was a profit regulation scheme. By the mid-1970s its name had been changed to the PPRS, but it still retained a level of inaccuracy even until the 1993 agreement. However, the most recent negotiation between the DoH and ABPI in 1999 was in effect no longer a voluntary agreement because of the statutory powers and penalties behind it. This leaves a lot less room for negotiation and flexibility. The 1999–2004 PPRS, which is in accordance with the provisions of the Health Act 1999 Section 33, leaves no room for uncertainty. It changes the status of the PPRS and makes it more formulaic.[11]

The scheme applies to all companies supplying NHS medicines prescribed by medical or dental practitioners or nurses qualified to prescribe. Generic medicines, whose price is determined by the Drug Tariff, are excluded, as are the over-the-counter (OTC) medicines, and sales of medicines derived from private (non-NHS) prescriptions.

29.5.1 Annual financial returns

Each company with sales to the NHS of more than £1 million per annum has to supply financial information and those with sales of between £1 million and £25 million have to supply full audited accounts. Companies with NHS sales greater than £25 million have to submit a full annual financial return (AFR). Products with NHS sales of greater than £100,000 and £500,000 have to be specifically identified. These annual returns cover the overall sales to the NHS and the costs incurred, such as research and development expenditure, manufacturing costs, general administrative costs, promotional expenditure and capital employed. (Details of specific produce costs or sales are not required.)

29.5.2 Profitability
The reasonableness of the maximum return on capital (ROC) earned by individual companies on home sales of NHS medicines is a matter for negotiation within a published range of 17% for level 1 and 21% for level 2, having regard to the nature and scale of the company's relevant investment and activities, and associated long-term risks.

29.5.3 Margin of tolerance
The allowable returns on capital will be associated with a margin of tolerance (MOT). Companies will be able to retain profits of up to 140% of the level 2 (21%) ROC target calculated by reference to level 2 allowances. Companies will not be granted price increases unless they are forecasting profits less than 50% of their level 1 (17%) ROC target calculated by reference to the level 1 allowances.

The MOT will not be available to a scheme member for any year in which it has had a price increase agreed by the department. Where a scheme member exceeds its level 1 target profit for a year in which it has received a price increase, all profits above the level 1 target will be repayable. Where a price increase is agreed by the department in the second half of a year, the department may decide that the MOT will not be available to a scheme member for the year following the increase.

If the department's assessment of an AFR shows profits in excess of the MOT, it will negotiate one or more of the following:
• Price reductions, during the accounting year following that covered by the return, to bring prospective profits down to an acceptable level, on the basis of available forecasts;
• Repayments of that amount of past profits that is agreed to exceed the MOT; or
• A delay or restriction of price increases agreed for the company, or both.

29.5.4 Profitability of companies with small capital base in UK
Prior to 1999, PPRS companies with a negligible capital base in the UK had their profits assessed on a return on sales basis, which ranged from 3.75 to 4.25%. Scheme members will now be able to include capital employed in their AFR on the basis of its inclusion in UK statutory accounts, by injection or by imputation in the transfer price. This will enable some companies that have been assessed as return on sales (ROS) companies under the 1993 scheme to be assessed as ROC companies under this agreement.

Alternatively, for scheme members whose AFR home sales exceed their average assessed home capital employed (excluding any capital imputation from the transfer price) by a factor of 3.5 or more, a target rate of profit will be set by dividing the ROC target rate by a factor of 3.5. The assessment of the returns of scheme members who elect for the ROS option will take account of the MOT on transfer price profit.

These changes in the 1999 PPRS have been introduced to enable the DoH to control transfer pricing arrangements, which the ABPI has long resisted.

29.5.5 Export disincentive
Profits allowed on sales of prescription medicines in the UK are limited to a target return on assets related to UK sales. Manufacturing assets used for NHS products are normally allocated between home sales to the NHS and exports pro rata to cost of sales. Costs must be computed on a fully allocated basis (i.e. overheads are spread on a consistent basis between home and export products).

The effect of an increased proportion of exports is to allocate an increased proportion of the manufacturing assets to exports and, by definition, a reduced share to the UK. Thus, the asset base on which target UK profit is computed is reduced. At the same time, an increased proportion of exports will allocate an increased proportion of annual fixed manufacturing overheads to export sales and hence a reduced proportion to UK NHS sales. The effect of this will be to reduce the cost of sales charged to the UK, with a consequent increase in profit.

The effect of these two factors constitutes a double disadvantage for any company wishing to increase its proportion of exports, as its UK NHS asset base is reduced and at the same time its national UK profits are increased. For a company below its target rate of return this will reduce the price increase it can apply for, and if it is over its target return it will increase the amount it pays back to the DoH or the amount by which it will have to reduce prices. This disincentive is particularly relevant for large tender business where multinationals typically have several manufacturing sources they can consider. Increasingly, they are placing the business in countries where the impact of the domestic market is either cost neutral or has a cost-positive impact. The export disincentive is becoming increasingly relevant in the context of the single European market, where the number of manufacturing facilities is being reduced by many multinationals and those that remain acquire substantial export business within the Community.

Under the most recent revision of the PPRS, the DoH will allocate 7.5% of the net value of each company's non-research and development fixed assets and its manufacturing infrastructure costs to its NHS sales before the balance is apportioned between home and export sales.[12]

29.5.6 Pricing of major new products

New products introduced following a major application for a product licence from the UK Licensing Authority may be priced at the discretion of the company on entering the market. This will have to take account of costs of research and development and the competition in the marketplace.

29.5.7 Promotional expenditure

Allocated expenditure by companies on product promotion is limited. The aggregate sales promotional allowance will be set as a percentage of total industry NHS sales. The distribution of the aggregate between individual companies is made on the basis of a formula agreed between the DoH and ABPI, for example, in the 1999 agreement promotional expenditure was allocated between three component parts:
1. Basic allowance of £464,000 per company.
2. A percentage of NHS sales allowance of 3% for level 1 and 6% for level 2.
3. An individual product servicing allowance of £58,000 for three products, £46,000 for a further three products, £35,000 for a further three products and a £23,000 allowance for the 10th and subsequent products. These allowances only apply to products with NHS sales greater than £100,000 per annum. These figures, agreed in October 1999, are subject to adjustment based on level of inflation.

29.5.8 Research and development expenditure

Under the 1999 revision of the PPRS, each company's research and development expenditure allowance will be 20% (level 2) of the company's sales to the NHS for assessing profitability under the scheme [however, a maximum of 17% (level 1) will be allowed for assessing applications from companies seeking a price increase].

For a maximum of 12 in-patent active substances, each with an individual sales level to the NHS of £500,000 or more, a company will be able to add 0.25% of total NHS turnover to their PPRS research and development allowance for each such active substance. Thus, a company could achieve a maximum allowance of 23% of NHS sales as its research and development allowance.[10]

29.5.9 2004 revision of the PPRS

In the summer of 2004 it was variously but widely rumoured that the pharmaceutical industry was facing a 6% price cut, or a 10% price cut phased over 10 years, or a 6% price cut over 2 years. In November 2004, when the details of the revised PPRS were announced for companies with sales to the NHS of over £10 million per annum there was to be a 7.0% price cut. The price cuts were graded so that smaller companies with annual turnover of less than £1 million were exempt from price cuts, those with an annual turnover of under £3.5 million had a 3.5% price cut enforced. Companies with annual turnover of under £9 million had to cut prices by 6.3%.

The threshold at which companies had to submit AFRs was increased from £1 million to £5 million annual sale of goods to the NHS. The allowable research and development allowance was increased by 5%.

The 2004 revision of the PPRS continued to allow companies launching a product that has been the subject of a major application for a marketing authorisation to be priced at the discretion of the company (see section 29.5.6). This freedom is cherished by the industry (see section 29.5.10).

29.5.10 Assessment of the PPRS

The weaknesses of the PPRS are clear from the above outline. These are first, the export disincentive, which discourages pharmaceutical companies from sourcing export orders from UK manufacturing sites, so that multinationals with several alternative sourcing arrangements will avoid using the UK. This is clearly disadvantageous for both jobs and UK balance of payments.

The promotional formula and the capping of allowable promotional expenses operate in favour of the pharmaceutical companies with large existing sales to the NHS, and to the disadvantage of small companies or companies wishing to start up business in the UK.

The cap on allowable research and development costs to 20% of NHS sales is a disincentive to conducting research in the UK at levels above this. Small and middle-sized companies are penalised more than the pharmaceutical giants by this provision. It also favours companies who have products in patent being sold to the NHS " 'but whose current pipeline may be weak, no financial provision is made to encourage companies with a strong pipeline to bring them forward more effectively other than an offer of 'jam tomorrow'." The position of companies marketing 'in-patent' products that have been licensed from other companies rather than their own research is unclear.

A number of non-UK European-based companies have criticised the rate of ROC on the basis that it favours companies with a large capital base in the UK and could therefore be regarded as an incentive to invest in the UK, which is contrary to European Union legislation.

The same group of companies have regarded the PPRS as discriminatory, as companies with a significant capital investment in the UK have their profits determined as return on capital base, whereas others that have a large investment in the European Union as a whole may operate in the UK as sales companies only. In this situation, these companies are treated on a percentage profit on sales, which are less favourable terms. Some US-owned companies with large UK operations have been particularly vociferous in their criticism of the PPRS.

In terms of curtailing NHS expenditure on medicines the effectiveness of the PPRS is more difficult to assess: it has the power to restrict price increases and 'claw back' excess profits, and the opportunities for the DoH to enforce these powers has been increased in the 1999 revision of the PPRS. The amount of money 'clawed back' from companies each year has been insignificant in the past compared to the overall medicines expenditure, but this will change.

In general, the pharmaceutical industry would regard the freedom to price new products without awaiting the outcome of protracted negotiations – that can delay marketing for months or even years in some European Union countries – as a major advantage that counterbalances the system's many faults. This freedom was maintained in the 1999 revision of the PPRS. In a recent assessment of various pricing and profit cost containment schemes, Scherer[3] in "Prescription Pricing Authority Annual Reports" 1994/5 makes the point that most such schemes are a disincentives for innovation; his view of the PPRS is less unfavourable: 'less impairment of such incentives would be expected with a system such as that used in Great Britain under which drug companies are allowed a generous profit rate of return on their assets, including capitalised research and development investments, even that system, however,

bases the results against smaller but innovative drug companies. . . . Achieving the best trade-off between technological progress and the affordability of drugs remains a challenging goal.'

29.6 Office of Fair Trading report on PPRS and its consequences

After the 2004 revision of the PPRS, intended to become operative in 2005 and extend up to 2010, a considerable outpouring of criticism of the scheme began to appear. In December 2005, Beale and Chard (lawyers with Burgess Salmon, a Bristol law firm),[29] in a review entitled 'Is the PPRS anti-competitive?', cited views gleaned from discussion with the Office of Fair Trading (OFT) who started an investigation into the PPRS in the autumn of 2005 with a view of producing a report by the end of 2006. The OFT were stated to be concerned that government procurement activities in this area in the form of the PPRS might have a negative impact on competition. This is related to the fact that the pharmaceutical market is characterised by a small number of very large companies from whom the government, through the NHS, makes a high proportion of government purchases. The OFT were stated to be concerned that under the 2004 PPRS, companies were allowed to generate profits from sales to the NHS of up to 21% of capital employed. The basic economic concern was that this measure encouraged inefficiency by allowing those companies with more capital employed to make higher profits under the PPRS. If economic efficiency were to be maximised, and minimal levels of capital were employed in producing existing drugs, this capital could be employed elsewhere, such as the development of new drugs. Another concern was that the PPRS favours companies with investments in the UK. This, according to Beale and Chard, is discriminatory, who refer to various US pharmaceutical companies who have expressed a view that the PPRS should be scrapped. Beale and Chard reported that the OFT had informed them that their final report would not be available before the end of 2006.

In February 2007 the OFT published its report into the PPRS which recommended that the scheme should be reformed. The OFT concluded that the pricing system should have a more value-based approach in order to deliver greater benefit to patients and reform could deliver better value for money for the NHS. A more value-based approach would also ensure that the production of clinically and cost-effective innovative products would be properly 'incentivised and rewarded'.

The government advised the ABPI in July 2007 of its intention to start renegotiations of the PPRS with a view of reaching agreement of a new voluntary scheme to start as early as possible in 2008.

In August 2007, the Department for Business Enterprise and Regulatory Reform published *Interim Government Response to Office of Fair Trading (OFT) market study on PPRS*.[30] This response picked up on the OFT recommendation that: 'Government should reform the PPRS, replacing current profit and price controls with a value based approach to pricing.' One major statement in this response was that 83% of prescriptions in 2007 were written generically as opposed to 51% in 1994, and this indicated a government commitment to cost-effective prescribing.

On 2 August 2007 it was publically announced that the Secretary of State for Health had decided that it was timely to enter into dialogue with industry to renegotiate the PPRS. A number of letters in the *British Medical Journal* reacted to the OFT recommendation of a shift to a 'value-based approach to pricing'. Timmins[31] stated 'a value-based' scheme would allow higher prices for drugs that were more effective – a move the OFT argued would stimulate innovation. Burnand,[32] of the BioIndustry Association, reacted to the proposal of the OFT, stating, 'Its proposals for introducing a value based system of drug pricing are inherently flawed and, if implemented, would lead to significant erosion of biopharmaceutical investment in the UK.' Messori,[33] from the Laboratory of Pharmacoeconomics based in Italy, stated that, 'From an ethical point of view, it is bad to use systems not based on clinical benefit' (such as the PPRS). Furness,[34] a former head of the PPRS Branch of the Department of Health, wrote, 'The PPRS is rooted in the past and fails to deliver its stated objectives and to reflect the realities of the modern NHS and the modern pharmaceutical industry.' Furness goes on to state 'the case for fundamental reform is now unanswerable'. All these letters express an inherent dislike for the PPRS but fail to advance any real positive solutions. Furness had plenty of opportunity to suggest changes while in his previous position at the Department of Health, but it is easier to criticise the PPRS for its obvious shortcomings than to create a viable and robust alternative.

On 29 February 2008, the DoH gave 6 months' notice to the ABPI and to PPRS scheme members in accordance with paragraph 5.1 of the 2004 PPRS negotiated scheme to terminate the current agreement. [Giving 6 months' notice to terminate the agreed scheme was necessary as a result of a High Court ruling in June 2007 that the PPRS was a contract. Previously it had been possible to terminate the PPRS agreements by mutual consent when agreement on a new or revised scheme had been reached (on the earlier assumption it was a non-contractual scheme)]. Therefore, the 2004 PPRS terminated on 31 August 2008. Without any control on the price of medicines companies would after this date have been free to increase prices, the DoH argued. Therefore, the DoH published on 18 June 2008 *Consultation on a Statutory Scheme to Control the Prices of Branded Medicines*.[35] These proposals can be summarised as follows:

• *Price freeze.* Subject to specific exceptions, no price increases will be permitted from 1 September 2008 and maximum prices will in effect be frozen at the reference price. The reference price is the NHS list price on 29 February 2008, the day that the DoH gave 6 months' notice of the termination of the 220 PPRS. For medicines placed on the market after 29 February, the reference price is the NHS list price on 31 August 2008. Freezing prices would not allow modulation, as occurs under the earlier voluntary scheme.

• *Price cut.* The government proposes to introduce a price cut of 3.9% from 1 January 2009 on all medicines covered by the new PPRS agreement.

• *Price fixing.* From 1 January 2009 where there is an equivalent generic, the price of out-of-patent branded medicines will be limited to a maximum price of 1.5 times the reimbursement price of the equivalent generic medicine as set out in Category M of the Drug Tariff. The prices of all products that lose patent protection after 1 January 2009 and for which there is a generic equivalent will also be limited to a maximum level that is 1.5 times the reimbursement price of the equivalent generic.

• *Discounts.* Traditionally, manufacturers of branded medicines offer discounts to wholesalers. The proposed price controls should take account of these discounts lest the value of price cut be jeopardised by reductions in discounts.

• *New products.* The government proposes that there should be controls on the maximum price of new products. New products that are new active substances would have freedom of pricing on entering the market. The Secretary of State for Health will be able to set the maximum price for products that are not new active substances.

The consultation document stated that the government would prefer to reach agreement on a voluntary scheme, but if it appears that a voluntary scheme would not be in place by 1 September 2008 the above statutory measures would replace the current PPRS. If agreement on a voluntary scheme were to be reached, the statutory scheme would still be introduced so that it could be applied to any company that did not sign up to the new PPRS agreement.

On 19 July 2008 the DoH published Statutory Instrument 2008 No 1938 which made regulations in exercise of powers in section 261(7), 262(1), 263–265, 266(1–2) and 272(7–8) of the National Health Service Act 2006(a). Essentially, the Statutory Instrument's content mirrored the Consultation Document. Under the entry Enforcement Section 6(1) there is the following statement: 'a price in excess of the maximum permitted by these Regulations shall be liable, on the demand of the Secretary of State, to pay him a recoverable sum calculated under the Schedule to these Regulations'. The schedule lays down escalating demands for the first, second and up to the fifth contravention.

29.7 2009 Pharmaceutical Price Regulation Scheme

In a joint letter from the DoH and the ABPI written on 19 November 2008 and a DoH press release, the terms of the renegotiated PPRS were announced. The new PPRS was to commence on 1 January 2009. The new scheme is to run for a minimum of 5 years and be non-contractual and voluntary.

The headline agreements were:
• A cut in the cost of drugs sold to the NHS by means of a 3.9% price cut to be introduced starting in February 2009.
• A further price cut of 1.9% to be introduced in January 2010.
• Subject to discussion with affected parties, the DoH is also to introduce generic substitution from January 2010. There would be further price adjustments in January of each year aimed as the proportion of savings from generic substitution varies with time.
• New and more flexible pricing arrangements that will enable drug companies to supply drugs to the NHS at lower initial prices, with the option of higher prices if value is proven at a later date.
• More systematic use of patient access schemes by drug companies to allow access to medicines that have not initially been assessed as cost or clinically effective by NICE.
Patient access schemes were agreed between the DoH and an individual pharmaceutical company for con-

sideration in the context of a NICE appraisal. These schemes are aimed at improving patient access to a medicine that has not initially been assessed as cost or clinically effective by NICE. The new PPRS sets out arrangements for patient access schemes (although subject to certain conditions to ensure that they are implemented sensibly and that the cumulative burden on the NHS is manageable). The Joint ABPI and DoH letter of 19 November 2008 states that: 'Full details of the arrangements on both flexible pricing and patient access schemes will be in the new PPRS agreement.' The ABPI and DoH have agreed that both the experience of both schemes will be reviewed by 2011:
• The 2009 PPRS will preserve companies' ability to set prices of new active substances as allowed under the present and previous schemes.
• An increase in the R&D allowance to a maximum of 30% of NHS sales for assessing AFRs including an increase of 10% of NHS sales for the variable rate of innovation.

It must be noted that although the documents issued on 19 November 2008 states that agreement has been reached, the DoH and ABPI are still finalising the text of the scheme as a result of which certain aspects of the 2009 PPRS may become clearer.

29.8 The Drug Tariff and reference pricing

The Drug Tariff operated by the DoH was the first reference price system. Introduced in the early 1950s, the tariff price represents the price that the PPA operates on when reimbursing pharmacists and dispensing doctors for the cost of materials dispensed, whether drugs, dressings or devices. The average price for each generic formulation is determined as an average of the prices of the largest four or five manufacturers for each generic formulation (generics in the UK being generally unbranded). The community pharmacist who dispenses the prescribed generic is reimbursed at the tariff price. The pharmacist therefore does not purchase generic preparations from manufacturers whose price is above the tariff price. This effectively forces a downward price spiral for generics, as their tariff price was originally determined on a yearly basis but is now done as frequently as each month.

The prices of generic medicines must inevitably rise in the near future as manufacturers move to produce patient packs, which will be required to contain patient information leaflets. Under EC legislation, bulk containers will almost inevitably be phased out of production (except perhaps for hospital use).

The concept of the UK's Drug Tariff has been adapted into the various European Reference Price models, namely the grouping together of similar products usually containing the same active substance – or members of the same therapeutic group (e.g. beta-adrenergic blocking agents) – and then setting a maximum cost that the payer will reimburse for any product in that group. In Germany there are 435 therapeutic groups of products covered by their reference price scheme. Reference pricing has already been introduced into France, the Netherlands, New Zealand and some provinces of Canada. Reference pricing fits well with the prevailing US belief that the key to capping health care expenditure is to offer financial incentives to patients. Reference pricing does just that, and in fact it has already been used in the states of Massachusetts and Delaware in their Medicaid programmes.

Wherever reference pricing in any form has been implemented, the reference price becomes the effective market price.

29.9 Contract purchase of medicines from cheap sources

In the early 1960s, when Enoch Powell was Minister of Health in Macmillan's Conservative government, the DoH bought large quantities of tetracycline from Poland for NHS hospital use. This was found to be clinically ineffective and of substandard quality; a public outcry in the medical press followed. The cheap drugs exercise was not repeated, but bulk hospital purchase at competitive contract prices continues, and this leads to wide discrepancies between the hospital price and the price charged to prescriptions written in the primary health care sector.

29.10 The MacGregor Committee

In the late 1960s, the DoH set up the Standing Committee on the Classification of Proprietary Preparations under the chairmanship of Professor Alastair Gould MacGregor. The committee became known as the MacGregor Committee.

The committee classified products subject to monographs in the British Pharmacopoeia (BP), the British Pharmaceutical Codex (BPC) and the British National Formulary (BNF) as Category M products.

Acceptable products other than monograph preparations were Category A products. All other products were Category B products; these were considered less effective or more toxic than those in Categories M or A or their efficacy was regarded as unproven. In practice, most combination products were regarded as undesirable and were relegated to Category B status. The deliberations of the MacGregor Committee were published as 'Proplist' that went through regular editions. The pages referring to Category B products had a black corner to the top of the page and they appeared in Proplist after Category M and A products. Pressure was exerted by local health authorities on doctors not to prescribe Category B preparations, and to use Category M products as a preference to both Category A and B preparations. Category A products were usually branded medicines and were more costly than the generic monographed preparations. Proplist was an early attempt to encourage doctors to prescribe generically and cheaply, thus exerting downward pressure on prescribing costs.

29.11 Generic substitution

In the UK, generic substitution was raised as a means of reducing the NHS medicines bill in the Greenfield Report of 1983, but was not implemented. However, generic substitution has been implemented by a number of reimbursement authorities, both insurance-based schemes as in the USA and nationally run health care schemes, for example, Sweden (introduced October 2002) and Finland (introduced 1 April 2003). Both countries' health care schemes claim very considerable savings of the order of 5% of national expenditure on medicines. Sweden is considering extending the scheme to lead to compulsory generic prescribing.

29.12 Enforced price reductions

In December 1983, the then Health Minister announced measures to cut industry profits and reduce the NHS medicines bill, then running at £1.3 billion per year, by £100 million. In November 1984, further measures were taken by reducing the ROC allowed under the PPRS from 25% to a range of 15–17%. ROC was raised to 17–21% in two stages under the 1986 renegotiation of the PPRS. In 1993, because of renegotiation of the PPRS, the ROC was left unchanged, but a price reduction of 2.5% on pharmaceuticals was enforced. This was negotiated by ABPI to be achieved by a 2.5% reduction overall on each company's products, but could be modulated by taking a larger reduction on some products than on others. The alternative to price reductions was for companies to present the DoH with a cheque equivalent to 2.5% of its sales to the NHS, a solution accepted but not favoured by the DoH, as the money disappeared into Treasury funds and so did not offer any real advantage to the department.

In the 1999 PPRS negotiations, as a part of the agreement, the DoH imposed a 4.5% price reduction on sales to the NHS. This was equivalent to a loss of sales by the industry of £200 million. Because the 1999 revision of the PPRS permits companies to modulate these enforced price reductions across their product range, it could be expected that companies would do so in such a way that competition from parallel-traded products would be reduced, maximum price reductions being applied to those products that were currently being most affected by parallel trade. The 2004 PPRS enforced a 7% price cut on the pharmaceutical industry.

29.13 Limited or selected lists

The first limited list proposals were announced in November 1984 and proposed that a list of 31 products was adequate to meet 'all clinical needs in the seven therapeutic areas of indigestion remedies, laxatives, analgesics, cold and cough remedies, vitamin preparations, tonics and benzodiazepines'. In the event, when the proposals became operational in April 1985, the initial list had been expanded to 129 products, and later to 160 products. The remaining products reimbursable on the NHS could only be dispensed if prescribed by their generic as opposed to their brand names.

The saving from the original limited list exercise in its first year of operation was claimed to be £75 million, and Ministers of Health over the next 10 years have been unable to quantify what, if any, the savings that took place in subsequent years, despite a series of parliamentary questions seeking this information.

If 10% of patients previously receiving prescriptions for an antacid were prescribed an H_2-receptor antagonist such as cimetidine or ranitidine, this claimed savings would not have been achieved. The growth in the H_2-receptor antagonist market was rapid at this time, and some of this growth must have been because of such escalation of prescribing.

In November 1992, the Secretary of State for Health announced the extension of the limited list procedure

to further 10 therapeutic categories: antidiarrhoeals; appetite suppressants; treatments for allergic disorders; hypnotics and anxiolytics; treatments for vaginal and vulval conditions; contraceptives; treatment for anaemia; topical antirheumatics; treatments for ear and nose conditions; and treatments for all skin conditions. These measures were announced despite repeated undertakings by a series of Conservative Secretaries of State for Health that the government had no intention of extending the limited list, and despite the fact that the DoH remains unable to quantify the savings achieved from the limited list exercise in the original seven categories.

The second limited list operation affecting 10 therapeutic categories, announced in November 1992, became an exercise to reduce the prices of products to preconceived 'reasonable levels', these being delegated by Health Ministers to the Advisory Committee on NHS Drugs chaired by a DoH official and having outside members from the medical and pharmaceutical professions. The achievement of this exercise has been to inveigle a number of companies into agreeing price reductions in exchange for their product's continuing to be presentable in the NHS. This exercise has therefore amounted to a reference price system with a non-transparent method of fixing the price. It is therefore probable that the second phase of the limited list operation was in breach of the Transparency Directive (89/105/EEC). (The price reductions achieved under this exercise were not permitted to be counted towards the 2.5% overall price reduction imposed as part of the 1993 PPRS agreement.)

The Advisory Committee on NHS Drugs, when examining oral contraceptives as one of the classes involved in the second phase of the limited list exercise, formed a preliminary position that the more expensive third-generation oral contraceptives should be precluded from availability on NHS prescription on grounds of cost. The outcry from women's groups, family planning practitioners and the medical profession was such that these proposals were never implemented.

29.14 Indicative prescribing scheme and GP fundholding

The indicative prescribing scheme (IPS) and GP fundholding were both introduced in 1991. These schemes were described by Whalley et al. in *Pharmacoeconomics* in 1992 and 1995, including the various incentives offered to both fundholders and non-fundholders to reduce their prescribing costs by allowing a proportion of the 'saving' to be used on other projects in the practice.[4,5] Their effects were summarised by Whalley as follows:

The IPS has generally failed to control the rise in drug costs because of unrealistic targets, organisational difficulties (inducing the lack of adequate data to set budgets properly) and because there was neither incentive nor penalty to encourage compliance on the part of the general practitioner (GP). The IPS stresses cost containment, and makes little allowance for the consideration of quality or appropriateness of prescribing.

GP fund holding, in contrast, has reduced the rate of rise of drug cost in participating GP practices, although it has not actually reduced drug costs ... Although there is a commitment on the part of the government to encourage and make use of data about economic evaluations of drug therapy and other medical interventions, so far the emphasis has been exclusively on cost containment.

29.15 Development of primary care groups

The Labour government elected in May 1997 committed itself to abolishing the concept of fundholding practices. This was not because of any fundamental disagreement with the concept of primary care commissioning per se, but rather because of the inevitable 'two-tierism' in service provision between fundholders and non-fundholders that resulted. In December 1997, the government produced its own White Paper, The New NHS: Modern, Dependable. When this document was first published it seemed to be signalling a new direction, but however much of the content could be described largely as a repackaging of existing (Conservative) policy, psychologically it felt different. The evolution of primary care groups (PCGs) can clearly be traced back to the fundholding initiative begun in 1991 (see Further Reading). Halpern expressed the opinion of many NHS commentators when be wrote:

The Government use of PCGs as a mechanism for managing primary care is no more than a continuation of the policies of the previous government. Although GP fundholders revelled in their initial freedoms, it is clear that the move towards total purchasing (in whatever guise) was a clear precursor of PCGs.

However, the Labour government has clearly stamped its mark on PCGs and essentially the changed philosophy behind them. The following quote from the White Paper summarises some of their thinking as follows:

[PCGs] will have control over resources but will have to account for how they have used them in improving efficiency and quality. The new role envisaged for GPs and community nurses will build on some of the most successful recent developments, in primary care. These professionals have seized opportunities to extend their role in recent years ... Despite its limitations, many innovative GPs and their fund managers have used the fundholding scheme to sharpen the responsiveness of some hospital services and to extend the range of services available in their own surgeries. But the fundholding scheme had also proved bureaucratic and costly. It has allowed development to take place in a fragmented way, outside a coherent strategic plan. It has artificially separated responsibility for emergency and planned care, and given advantage to some patients at the expense of others. So the government wants to keep what has worked about fundholding but discard what has not.

There are a couple of key differences between fundholding and PCGs. First, the unified budget. The White Paper did not set out much detail about the implications and consequences of a unified budget, but its importance should not be underestimated. Its implications for general practice and the NHS as a whole are probably only equalled by the clinical governance initiative (Royce). The government perceive the unified budget and clinical governance as the principal vehicle by which the long-standing problems of successive governments – cost constraint and medical practice variation – can be tackled. As Majeed and Malcolm (1999) writing in the *BMJ*, (see Further Reading) concluded:

The main factor behind the introduction of unified budgets is the belief that making general practitioners accountable for cost as well as the quality of health care will prove an effective method of tackling many of the problems facing the NHS.

Another key difference is that fundholding was always vulnerable to the charge that it was creating a two-tier NHS, but there is no opt out clause for general practices with the development of PCGs. Together with the unified budget, this means that resource decisions taken by one practice in a PCG have a direct impact on others. They are no longer islands, and practices have to be concerned with how well the PCG is doing as a whole and with any poorly performing practices within it, as the bottom line is that a PCG can be dragged down by them.

This helps to explain why GP involvement makes or breaks the Labour government's reforms. It boils down to simple economics: GPs, principally through their referral and prescribing decisions, commit the vast majority of PCGs' (and consequently NHS) resources. Ultimately, under the new NHS reforms, it is the GP who will have to take responsibility for limiting (and in many cases reversing) the growth in prescribing costs and hospital expenditure. In the ever-changing world of NHS organisation there is the opportunity for PCGs to apply to become primary care trusts (PCTs) which provides greater autonomy.

29.16　Changing the legal status of medicines from prescription only to over-the-counter availability

Speaking at the annual pharmaceutical conference on this matter in November 1993, Dr Brian Mawhinney, the UK Minister for Health, stated that self-medication 'encourages people to be more interested in and committed to their own health; [and] it empowers individuals with greater freedom to determine for themselves what medicines they will use'.

The theoretical advantages to the government are clear. First, by switching more medicines from being prescription only (POM) to over-the-counter (OTC) or pharmacy sale (P) and encouraging patients to self-medicate, it might be anticipated that the country's medicines bill would be reduced. Secondly, by encouraging patients to purchase their own medicine it obviates the need for a GP consultation, the main object of which was to obtain a prescription. However, although many items are available considerably cheaper than the prescription change, approximately 89% of prescription items were dispensed free. Thus, there is little incentive for most patients to purchase their medicines OTC.

In June 1997, DGIII of the European Commission circulated a consultation document, *A Guideline on Changing the Classification for the Supply of a Medicinal Product for Human Use*. The objective of this was to ensure that the route of sale will be the same in all Member States of the European Union. The grounds for making decisions on route of supply are based on safety considerations, and for medicines for purchase directly by the patient stringent requirements for information are proposed (the Commission document does not consider economic grounds for change of status).[16]

29.17　Encouragement to prescribe generically

A number of the above government initiatives have resulted in changing doctors' prescribing habits towards a greater use of generic formulations. Doctors are currently happier to prescribe generics as they have become more convinced of their quality. 'This was probably not unrelated to the fact that in the year ending August 1993, 80% of generic medicine sales in the United Kingdom originated from subsidiaries of the four multinational manufacturers Rhône Poulenc Rorer, Hoechst, Fisons and Ivax.'[17]

In 1993, the overall shape of the NHS market by value of products dispensed was as follows: generics accounted for 11% by value and over 41% by volume; prescriptions for medicines still within patent accounted for 26% by value but only 7% by volume. The bulk of the NHS prescription market, 63% by value and 52% by volume, was made up of active substances that were out of patent but still being prescribed by brand name.

In 1993, 7% of the 530 million prescriptions dispensed were for products in patent. On the basis of these products coming off patent, the DoH believed that by the year 2000, 60% of prescriptions would be dispensed generically. In a reply to a question in the House of Commons, the Minister of Health stated that for 1994–1995 more than 50% of GP prescriptions dispensed in England and Wales were written generically, with GP fundholders writing 55.3% by generic name and non-fundholders 50.5%. However, the highest figure recorded by the Office of Health Economics was 46% for the year 1998.

Overall, the government policies have been directed towards cheap drugs and a drive towards generic prescribing, and this has been successful to a very large extent. However, it is unfortunate that this policy has deterred doctors from prescribing newer in-patent products. In a study of the uptake of new chemical entities in 20 countries in 1993 a more rapid uptake expressed as percentage of all prescriptions filled with products marketed in the previous 5 years was seen in 17 countries compared with the UK.[18,19]

29.18　National Institute for Clinical Excellence

It was repeatedly claimed throughout the 1990s that the uptake of therapeutic advances in the UK was suboptimal.[20,21] In the year 1990, only 38% of the UK medicines bill was for products launched onto the market in the previous 20 years, thus 62% of medicines by value prescribed on the NHS were active substances introduced into the UK market earlier than 1970.[18] It was claimed that 'cost reducing philosophies and constraints have resulted in the under use of therapeutic advances in the United Kingdom'.[20]

In 1993, the Advisory Council on Science and Technology said 'that innovations, which are recognised as offering significant economic and/or quality of life advantages should be fully funded by the NHS'.[22] It was also pointed out that pressures by the DoH to prescribe cheaply was not the same as cost-effective prescribing.[23]

In 1997, the UK government proposed in the White Paper, The New NHS: Modern, Dependable, that the National Institute for Clinical Excellence (NICE) should be established,[23] a proposal endorsed by Griffin.[25]

NICE was established as a Special Health Authority in April 1999. In establishing NICE, the Labour government hoped to improve standards of patient care and reduce inequalities in access to innovative treatments ('postcode prescribing'). NICE was to achieve these aims by providing guidance to the NHS on the effectiveness and cost of clinical interventions. This would be done by the appraisal of new and existing technologies, and developing disease-specific clinical guidelines and supporting clinical audit. Perhaps unsurprisingly it is the work of NICE in the technology appraisal arena that has dominated its work programme since 1999 and generated most debate within and outside the UK.

Pharmaceuticals and other products and procedures are selected for appraisal by NICE, by the DoH and the National Assembly for Wales on the basis of the extent to which such technologies are likely to result in:

1. A significant health benefit, taken across the NHS as a whole, for example, might reduce hospital admissions or bed occupancy;

2. A significant impact on other health-related government policies, for example, a new approach to smoking cessation;

3. A significant impact on NHS resources, for example, in vitro fertilization.

NICE meets a medical need. If millions of patients are under-medicated something has to be done to rectify the situation. However, NICE guidance aimed at under-medication and 'postcode prescribing' has added some £700 million to the NHS bill for pharmaceuticals.[26] By the end of 2004, NICE had issued more than 250 appraisals and had announced the appointment of an executive director with the responsibility for implementing NICE appraisals.

It is inevitable that the increased cost of the NHS medicines bill will result in the introduction of measures elsewhere to curtail these rises. These measures undoubtedly influenced the changes to the PPRS agreement of 2004, that is, enforced price reductions, and possibly changes to the operation of the Drug Tariff.

The Labour Prime Minister, Mr Blair, gave an undertaking that the NHS would follow NICE guidance. Under the current rules, the DoH and the Welsh Assembly must make funding available for implementation of NICE appraisals within 3 months of their publication, unless instructed to the contrary.

NICE recommendations will have a major impact on the direction of industry research and development. It will also have major impact on politicians and civil servants who run the NHS, as NICE recommendations have already had considerable cost implications. The influence of the recommendations made by NICE are international and its decisions are closely monitored by other similar bodies [e.g. Canadian Agency for Drugs and Technologies in Health (CADTH) and Pharmaceutical Benefits Advisory Committee (PBAC)] across the world and as a consequence the NICE website is achieving around 35,000 hits per day.[26] The impact of their decisions can be seen most clearly in the uptake (or otherwise) in sales of appraised products and classes of drugs across the world.

29.19 European Transparency Directive

Under Directive 89/105/EEC 'relating to transparency of measures regulating the scope of national health insurance systems'[28] all measures introduced by national governments to control expenditure on medicines will have to be compatible with EU rules. The Directive applies to any national measures to control price or restrict the range of products covered by national health insurance systems. The specific articles of the Directive cover the various schemes operational within the Community and demands that objective and verifiable criteria are met in their implementation (see p. 532, Chapter 17.15.4) of 5th ed. Textbook of Pharmaceutical Medicine.

The Transparency Directive does not lay down a requirement for harmonisation of procedures, nor does it imply a need to harmonise prices within the Community, and even if harmonisation of prices were achieved the Directive does not mean that there would be harmonisation of health service reimbursement. As long as price differences exist between Member

States of the European Community, parallel importing or parallel trading of medicinal products from Member States with lower prices to those with higher prices will take place. In fact, parallel trading in medicinal products could be called importation of another Member State's price constraints. The European Commission and Member States' health authorities not only condone but covertly encourage parallel trading. This creates considerable problems for pharmaceutical companies. The UK's DoH claws back a percentage of the reimbursement due from the PPA to reduce the windfall profits made by pharmacists buying cheaply from parallel traders.

At present, health care systems remain a national prerogative and are subject to national rather than European controls, but operated within the broad scope of the Transparency Directive. However, future changes in the direction of greater pan-European harmonisation can be envisaged.

29.20 Supply of controlled drugs

Special arrangements apply to the prescribing of drugs of dependence in the UK under the provisions of the Misuse of Drugs Act 1971. Drugs controlled include cocaine, dipipanone, diamorphine (heroin), methadone, morphine, opium, pethidine, phencyclidine, lysergide (LSD), amphetamines, barbiturates, cannabis, codeine, pholcodine and certain drugs related to the amphetamines, such as chlorphentermine and diethylpropion.

For all controlled drugs, prescriptions must be signed and dated by the prescriber and the following particulars included in the prescriber's own handwriting: name and address of patient; form and strength of preparation as appropriate; total quantity in both words and figures, and dose.

Only medical practitioners who hold a special licence issued by the Home Secretary may prescribe diamorphine, dipipanone or cocaine for addicts; other practitioners must refer the addict to a treatment centre. This stipulation only applies to addicts and does not preclude the prescription of diamorphine or cocaine for the relief of pain caused by organic disease or injury (see p. 531 Chapter 17.15.3) of 5th ed. of *Textbook of Pharmaceutical Medicine*.

29.21 British National Formulary

The greatest influence on doctors to prescribe well is the provision of high quality information. This has been achieved over the last decades by the British National Formulary (BNF).

During the Second World War, 1939–1945, it was imperative to exercise strict economy in prescribing, and in 1941, the then Minister of Health, Dr Charles Hill, introduced the National War Formulary as 'a select range of medicaments sufficient in range to meet the ordinary requirements of therapeutics for doctors in the community and in hospital'. After the creation of the NHS in 1948, the BNF was published jointly by the British Medical Association (BMA) and the Pharmaceutical Society of Great Britain, appearing first in 1949 and then every 3 years until 1979.

In 1975, a paper was produced by the Professional Head of Medicines Division of the Department of Health and Social Security (DHSS; now DoH) for consideration by the Medicines Commission. It was proposed that a new style BNF should be produced because the DHSS was concerned that doctors were being unduly influenced by promotional material produced by the pharmaceutical industry that was leading to an escalating medicines bill for the NHS. It was suggested that the 'new style BNF' should fulfil the following criteria:

1. No longer be selective but give information on all medicines available for prescribing by doctors;
2. Give information on the price of medicines;
3. Draw attention to certain unsuitable products;
4. Be compact enough to fit into the pocket; and
5. Be kept up to date.

Initially, it was proposed that the Medicines Commission should publish this, but neither the BMA nor the Pharmaceutical Society were willing to surrender copyright. Negotiations between the DHSS, the BMA and the Pharmaceutical Society started in 1975, during which the DHSS gave an undertaking to produce a new edition of the BNF every 6 months that would be distributed free to all doctors and pharmacists. A Joint Formulary Committee (JFC) was set up under Professor Owen Wade as chairman with three members of the JFC appointed by the BMA, three by the Pharmaceutical Society and three by the DHSS. The role of the JFC was to commission therapeutic reviews of each body system disease areas from several experts and to produce an authoritative synthesis.

The first new style BNF appeared on 26 February 1981. It was comprehensive and drew attention to over 600 products in small print considered undesirable by the JFC. Pricing information was initially given in a price banding by letter – for example, A being 20p up to G for the most expensive course of treatment in excess of 450p. In later editions, actual prices were given in a format that allowed strict comparisons between treatments.

In the 24 years since it was first published in the current format, editions have appeared every 6 months and it has become generally regarded as the most influential guide to good prescribing practice. The BNF JFC as of May 2005 will publish a paediatric version annually. It will comprise monographs on safe and effective medicines for use in children, even if usage in children is not included in the summary of product characteristics. (Note: BNF is to come under auspices of NICE in 2009.)

29.22 International comparisons

The effectiveness of various measures to contain expenditure on medicines in the UK can only be assessed in the context of the situation in other European Union countries. Table 29.1 gives data for the total expenditure on health care as a percentage of gross domestic product (GDP), expenditure on medicines as a percentage of total health care spend, the national pharmaceutical industry's research and development expenditure in euro-millions, the general price index and the medicines price index nationally compared with a European price of 100, and the

Table 29.1 Health care expenditure and medicines expenditure as a percentage of gross domestic product (GDP). Source: Organisation for Economic Cooperation and Development Health Data 2007

Country	Spending on health care as percentage of GDP, in 2006	Spending on medicines and other medical durables as percentage of GDP
Austria	8.7	12.4
Belgium	10.3	16.9
Denmark	9.5	8.5
Finland	8.2	14.6
France	11.0	16.4
Germany	10.6	14.8
Greece	9.1	17.6
Italy	9.0	20.0
Japan	8.3	19.6
Netherlands	n/a	n/a
Norway	8.7	8.5
Portugal	10.2	–
Spain	8.4	29.7
Sweden	9.2	21.7
Switzerland	11.3	13.3
UK	8.4	–
USA	15.3	12.6

national pharmaceutical consumption per capita expressed as defined daily doses. These comparisons are based on Organisation for Economic Cooperation and Development (OECD) Health Data 2000.

From these figures the UK is seen as a country with a comparatively low per capita consumption of medicines, to have a high medicines price index and a strong pharmaceutical research base; therefore, the various measures to contain medicines expenditure would appear to have had their greatest impact on the demand side.

Three of the four countries with the highest industry research and development spend have the highest medicines price index. France is the exception in this respect but has the highest per capita level of medicine consumption. Expressed in another way, the three largest spenders on health care as a percentage of GDP are France, Switzerland and Germany, which are three of the four countries where the pharmaceutical industry invests most in research and development.

Conversely, in countries where the population is relatively small and where individual consumption of medicines is low and pharmaceutical industry investment is also low, the government is able to enforce low prices for medicines. These countries are typified by the Netherlands, Norway, Finland and Denmark. Sweden, where there is significant pharmaceutical research, is atypical of the rest of Scandinavia and the medicines price index and medicine consumption are approximately the European average.

It would appear that the national governments' desires to impose draconian measures to control pharmaceutical prices and/or consumption is modulated by financial/fiscal necessity not to damage its national researched-based industry. Balancing such conflicting demands has been the key to the strength of the PPRS scheme, as it was in its inception. It remains to be seen whether this has been retained or lost following the 2004 revision, which now has a legal basis.

The US government believes that the various European pharmaceutical pricing systems constitute barriers to free trade. The ambition of the US Trade Representative is to liberalise pharmaceutical pricing systems anywhere in the world. A provision in the newly enacted Medicare reform legislation requires the US Trade Representative to use trade negotiations – specifically those recently involving Australia –'as a way to achieve the elimination of Government measures such as price controls and reference pricing'. It is therefore paradoxical to see various US states' Medicaid systems adopting both generic substitution and Massachusetts and Delaware introducing reference price schemes. On 26 November 2003, Australia's

Minister for Trade, Mark Vaile, pointed out that Australia's Pharmaceutical Benefits Scheme negotiated prices with pharmaceutical companies, just as health plans do in the USA. Mr Vaile stated that such negotiations were 'fundamental policy of our government and consecutive governments in Australia'.

References

1 Wanless D. *Securing our Future Health: Taking a Long-Term View*. Interim Report. London: HM Treasury, 2001.
2 Office of Health Economics. *Compendium of Health Statistics*, 9th edn. London: Office of Health Economics, 1998.
3 Prescription Pricing Authority Annual Reports, 1994/5.
4 Griffin JR. *The Impact of Unemployment on Health*. Briefing No 29. London: Office of Health Economics, 1993.
5 Warden J. Men can have free prescriptions at 60. *BMJ* 1995;**311**:1118.
6 Griffin TD. Patient contribution to the cost of prescribed medicines in Europe. In: Griffin JP, O'Grady J, Wells FO, eds. *The Textbook of Pharmaceutical Medicine*, 2nd edn. Belfast: Queens University, 1995;581–94.
7 Griffin JP. Increasing cost of medicines. *Lancet* 1993; **341**:1156–7.
8 Green DG, Lucas DA. *Medicard: A Better Way to Pay for Medicines*. London: Institute of Economic Affairs Health and Welfare Unit, Choice in Welfare No 16, 1993.
9 Department of Health. *The Pharmaceutical Price Regulation Scheme*. London: HMSO, 1993. (Reference number Det DH 004643, 9/93.)
10 Association of the British Pharmaceutical Industry (ABPI). *A Guide to the Pharmaceutical Price Regulation Scheme (PPRS)*. London: ABPI, 1993.
11 *The Pharmaceutical Price Regulation Scheme*. ABPI and Department of Health. www.doh.gov.uk/pprs.htm.
12 Butler S. Will PPRS R&D benefits compensate for price cut in UK? *Scrip* 1999;**2457**:4.
13 Scherer FM. The pharmaceutical industry: prices and profits. *N Engl J Med* 2004;**351**:927–32.
14 Bligh J, Whalley T. The UK indicative prescribing scheme. *Pharmacoeconomics* 1992;**2**:137–52.
15 Whalley T, Wilson R, Bligh J. Current prescribing in primary care in the UK. *Pharmacoeconomics* 1995;**7**:320–31.
16 European Commission Director General III. *A Guideline on Changing the Classification for the Supply of a Medicinal Product for Human Use*. 12 July 1997.
17 Walker R. Generic medicines: reducing cost at the expense of quality? *Pharmacoeconomics* 1995;**7**:375–7.
18 Griffin JP. *Is therapeutic conservatism cost effective prescribing?* European Federation of Pharmaceutical Industries Associations, General Assembly 1993, 3rd session: Health Objectives and Cost Control.
19 Griffin JP. New drugs and their impact on health care. Report on the Workshop, New Provider Structures for Health insurance and Tax-based Health care Systems,

WHO Collaborating Centre for Public Health Research. Kiel 27–30 November 1995. Keil: WHO, 1996;71–83.
20 Griffin JP, Griffin TD. The economic implications of therapeutic conservatism. In: Teeling-Smith G, ed. *Innovative Competition in Medicine: a Schumpeterian Analysis of the Pharmaceutical Industry and the NHS*. London: Office of Health Economics, 1992;85–96.
21 Griffin JP, Griffin TD. The economic implications of therapeutic conservatism. *J R Coll Physicians Lond* 1993; **27**:121–6.
22 Griffin JP. Therapeutic conservatism: more costly in the long-term. *Pharmacoeconomics* 1995;**7**:378–87.
23 Advisory Council on Science and Technology. *A Report on Medical Research and Health*. London: HMSO, 1993;28.
24 Department of Health. *The New NHS: Modern, Dependable*. Cm 3807. London: Stationary Office Ltd., 1997.
25 Griffin JP. The need for pharmaco-economic evaluations in the NHS. *Pharmacoeconomics* 1998;**14**:241–50.
26 Brown PJ. NICE is here to stay. *Scrip* 2004;2917.
27 Rawlins M. Treading a fine line. *Scrip* 2003;65–7.
28 European Commission Directive 89/105 EEC. Relating to transparency of measures regulating the scope of national health insurance systems. *Official Journal of the European Communities* 1989.
29 Beale N, Chard J. Is the PPRS anti-competitive? *Scrip* 2005;18–19.
30 Department for Business Enterprise and Regulatory Reform. Pharmacutical Price Regulation Scheme – Interim Government response to the Office of Fair Trading (OFT) market study on PPRS. August 2007, URN 07/1247, London.
31 Timmins N. Government pushes ahead with plan for cheaper drugs deal for NHS. *BMJ* 2007;**335**:273.
32 Burnand A. Misconceptions about the PPRS. *BMJ* 2007; **335**;578.
33 Messori A. PPRS is not NICE. *BMJ* 2007;**335**;578.
34 Furniss J. PPRS: not dead yet. *BMJ* 2008;**336**; 406.
35 Department of Health. *Consulation on a Statutory Scheme to Control the Prices of Branded NHS Medicines*. London: HMSO, 18 June 2008.

Further reading

Brown PJ. Fiddling with prices. *Scrip* 2004;3–1.
Claxton K, Briggs A, Buxton MJ, Culyer A, McCabe C, Walker S, et al. Value based pricing for NHS drugs: an opportunity not to be missed? *BMJ* 2008;**336**;251–4.
Halpern S. Doctoring the truth? Milburn lets the cats out of the bag. *Br J Health Care Management* 1998;**4**:426.
Majeed A, Malcolm L. Unified budgets for primary care groups. *BMJ* 1999;**319**:772.
Moskowitz DB. Another rocky road for Pharma R&D. *Scrip* 2004;37–39.
Royce R. *Primary Care and the NHS Reforms: A Manager's View*. London: Office of Health Economics, 2000.

30 Due diligence and the role of the pharmaceutical physician

Geoffrey R. Barker

Duke University Medical Center, NC, USA

30.1 Introduction

Due diligence for a drug development project is usually understood to refer to an evaluation of data in anticipation of a proposed business deal. At the most basic level, it is the method whereby the potential buyer of a project (typically, an interested investor or corporate partner) attempts to assess the risks and future value-generating milestones, attendant to the transaction, looking both at the needs of the potential partner and the intended benefits of an anticipated partnering solution.

Often overlooked, however, is that the diligence process relies on the mutual exchange of information by the parties. For example, the seller simultaneously aims to ensure that the buyer has the appropriate financial resources to complete the transaction (and in a partnering situation that the buyer also has the wherewithal to maximize the future value of the asset) while also providing to the buyer all the available and relevant data and information that may have an effect on the perceived value and risk of the proposed transaction.

Due diligence is a complex process with interaction at different levels of information and also involving significant interpersonal skills. For the pharmaceutical physician charged with carrying out a diligence project it is important to feel that questions have been fully and frankly answered – and where the data are complete this can be a relatively straightforward process. In the more usual situation where the data are preliminary and are often presented as work in progress, this leads to grey areas, some of which can be resolved by understanding the specific molecule

The Textbook of Pharmaceutical Medicine. Edited by John P. Griffin. © 2009, ISBN: 978-1-4051-8035-1.

or drug properties and placing these alongside the current regulatory requirements.

Often, due diligence and commercial risk assessment is ultimately a judgement call which is based largely on past experience and personal intuition. In particular, the overall presentation of the data needs to be carefully considered to form an insight into possible weaknesses, bias and attendant risk (e.g. single spectacular results presented by an over-enthusiastic discoverer or founder will often need to be confirmed and validated).

By the nature of the businesses involved, due diligence is highly variable, hard work, time-consuming and frequently needs careful follow-up and revision before completion. Not every avenue can be fully explored and time spent determining the key issues are critical.

30.2 Role of the pharmaceutical physician

The role of the pharmaceutical physician in the diligence process depends on whether the physician is supplying data (i.e. representing the seller) or is reviewing the data on behalf of the buyer. In both scenarios, this multifaceted role can be as the leader, communicator and driver of the diligence, or as the clinical or medical support to the team. The physician may by seniority ultimately be the presenter of the final report to the governing board, or tasked subsequently with successfully carrying out of the board's decisions – which may require transmitting either a constructive negative or positive response.

The pharmaceutical physician will be used to evaluating small-molecule compounds but increasingly today more advanced therapeutics such as monoclonal antibodies or other biotechnology-derived products and technologies have reached advanced development stages and are on the table for potential marketing and licensing deals. These deals require the support of established identifiable data on quality, efficacy and safety sufficient to support an investigational new drug (IND) and/or later a new drug application (NDA) or marketing approval. Individual pharmaceutical physicians may themselves be categorized into one of the following roles:

• Pharmaceutical research and development (R&D) – drug discovery, biopharmaceuticals, vaccines and cell therapy;
• Pharmaceuticals – ethical, over-the-counter (OTC), generics;
• Consumer products – health, hygiene;
• Medical devices;
• Diagnostics and clinical measurements; and
• Food technology – nutraceuticals, minerals and vitamin supplements.

The situation is different for a pharmaceutical physician working within the venture capital (VC) arena from that for a physician working within an established pharmaceutical company. Most VC is undertaking a product-based investment so the physician, along with the diligence team, must also evaluate the findings, not only scientifically but also for their impact on the preliminary financial deal terms and how these terms may be amended to mitigate any increased exposure risk.

In a life science industry transaction, the seller who is anxious to achieve the optimal return has multiple options, such as mergers, acquisitions, sale of chosen assets or out-licensing of a technology. In addition, seeking VC funding or public offerings of equity are additional areas for the seller who will be anxious to achieve the best return. The buyer may be looking to invest, take over or otherwise acquire an interest in the seller and both parties may well have different agendas and time-lines.

Increasingly, smaller companies are turning to clinical research organisations to help them fund clinical development and thus offer evidence of human efficacy and greater value for their product. The pharmaceutical physician may therefore find involvement in so-called partnering solutions which seem to offer solutions previously available only within the pharmaceutical industry.

No matter what the specific context, due diligence is an ongoing review process leading to a final report to be used by management to support and understand the deal risks. For simple deals this can be the work of one or two individuals, but with more complex deals no single individual is able to cover all the necessary facts, and special teams supported by external experts will be needed. For example, deals may include stem cell therapy, gene therapy, proteomics and other personalised medicine products. The due diligence process and report writing can, if not carefully managed, considerably delay the deal process which carries significant financial penalties.

The reader and end user of the final report should be able to find a summary of the various specialized teams' findings and have adequate referencing to the source data. In addition, the risks identified by the teams in relation to the product should be highlighted – for example, potential delays in regulatory approval for insufficient or incomplete data should be highlighted. In particular, known regulatory areas of concern such as prolonged QT/QTc intervals with certain classes of antibiotics should be fully explored and explained along with estimates of additional data that might be needed.

30.3 Scope of due diligence

The timing and extent of the due diligence is defined by deal and the degree of risk aversion of the investor or buyer. The scope of the due diligence is defined by the parameters set for the final report and depends on the size of the proposed deal and the stage of preliminary discussions already undertaken by the business development teams of the parties concerned and the fit of the deal within the buyer's and seller's strategic business plans. Once the outline deal terms have been proposed the due diligence teams can be informed.

Drug discovery appears on the surface to be a straightforward process which begins with a concept, followed by designer molecules and screening of compound candidates to validate the underlying hypothesis. Optimized leads are generated, and preclinical evaluation and evidence of efficacy and safety in humans are developed through a structured process of clinical trials.

In the real world these activities often overlap each other, compete for funding and are sometimes merged together with important measurements such as absorption, distribution, metabolism, excretion and toxicology, or product development being delayed or overlooked – or are left incomplete in the rush to demonstrate human proof of concept and efficacy. This is where due diligence becomes a critical and logical step to track, review and verify the data available in the key areas required for commercial success.

30.4 Process of due diligence

The pharmaceutical physician must have, or have access to, adequate knowledge of the clinical features and mechanism of the relevant disease process. This may be achieved by first getting a general overview and then using key opinion leaders, discussing directly with the investigators and, possibly for biotech proposals, with the scientific advisory board members. Permission and direction is usually obtained from the seller as there could be significant commercial advantage and/or disadvantage to interested parties if any of these discussions were leaked to outsiders.

The physician may need, depending on circumstances, to undertake the clinical review away from the main review team and as such may require suitable facilities and relevant data in order to assess the safety and efficacy issues as well as subject risk and the relevance of the clinical application in the light of current practice and the known pathophysiology of the disease mechanism.

As a first step it is usual to appoint a leader or point person whose responsibility is to assess the proposal, and communicate and coordinate a logical evaluation from the initial data provided by the business development teams to determine the composition of the possible future due diligence teams.

Checklists should be developed and can be followed by a request for further information (RFI), which may require the signing of confidential disclosure agreements (CDAs) or increasing the scope of earlier versions if not already adequately covered as part of the initial business development team interactions.

Signing of CDAs should take place alongside legal consultation to determine any legal or commercial responsibilities arising from obtaining this data, especially for publicly traded companies.

At this stage in the due diligence process it should be possible to estimate the need for information on such areas as:
- Preclinical results;
- Toxicology;
- Chemistry;
- Manufacturing and controls;
- Regulatory;
- Clinical trial supplies;
- Clinical trials;
- Pharmacogenomic data;
- Thoughts from key opinion leaders;
- Statistical analysis;
- Sales and marketing;
- Labelling and leaflets;
- Distribution;
- Finance;
- Intellectual property;
- Legal;
- Product development; and
- Supply chains.

Budget, resource evaluation, availability of key personnel, an in-house secure document storage/tracking process and head count has to be determined in order to take the process forward.

Arrangements should be made to select and agree on the site where the data are to be made available as well as the availability of key personnel familiar with the data. Essential data includes the regulatory files, correspondence with the regulatory authorities, the product development plan, any clinical trial data and the proposed manufacturing process. Enquires should be made about the format of the data and requests for electronic copy for ease of use and search of key words. It may also be necessary to discuss and obtain consent for the removal of data from the data room for further analysis and agree on its subsequent destruction.

Other documents that should be requested for review may include:
- US Food and Drug Administation (FDA) or EU/Japanese agencies correspondence files and the availability of formal letters, meeting minutes, telephone logs and filing agreements.
- Any minutes and/or notes of planned pre-IND, or pre-investigational device exemption and end of phase II meetings and NDA discussions;
- All ongoing preclinical and clinical trials are reviewed and updated to determine their status and likely finish times;
- Any carcinogenicity assessment committee meetings completed or planned;
- Copies of all the clinical protocols and clinical monitor reports to assess the well-being of the trials and any investigator feedback;
- All information concerning reported adverse events and their analysis, periodic safety updates and internal safety summary data;
- Confirmation of regulatory reporting requirements to national agencies;
- Company drug product/device/technology development plans covering preclinical, clinical, chemistry manufacturing and control issues;
- Proposed marketing strategy plans;
- Associated drug master files and if so how this may be assessed.

The scope of the due diligence process may require discussion on the intellectual property rights, structure of the company and its previous corporate history, its financial solvency, manufacturing ability, research and development facilities and capabilities, reference checking on staffing and advisory board members.

Patentability and enforcement patents are essential elements of a proposed pharmaceutical business deal. Strong patent protection is a necessary part of drug development, especially for new chemical entities and specialty areas. It is important that only a patent attorney or patent agent experienced and currently up-to-date in the worldwide pharmaceutical patent laws, rules and regulations be in charge of the patenting process. The laws, rules and regulations vary on a country-by-country basis and are constantly changing. Case law continues to be developed in patentability and patent infringement. It is also important to consider at an early stage having access to team members with expertise in patent preparation and prosecution as well as patent infringement litigation. Information can be found on websites and from other sources that are useful for patentability, available patent protection, descriptions of the patent laws, rules and regulations and patent infringement litigation but it requires an experienced individual who is currently active and experienced in the scientific field of the therapeutic application and chemical entity of the drugs to apply this information to a successful business deal. It is not a role to be undertaken by the pharmaceutical physician.

It is possible that the deal can be completed solely on the information provided at this stage in the diligence process without more intensive due diligence because the team's overall findings support the deal. Conversely, the initial review may not support the deal and no further action may be required.

30.5 Writing and assembling the due diligence report

There is no uniformly accepted set of guidelines for the preparation of a due diligence report. The format chosen will reflect the style of the user company and should be presented in line with any approved in-house format. The specific contents vary on a case-by-case basis but should include information that can be conveniently assembled under the following headings:
• An executive summary;
• An overview of the due diligence process and findings in summary format;

• An assessment of the product under consideration;
• Current regulatory status;
• Desirable courses of action in relation to the product development;
• Market assessment opportunity of the product;
• A commercial review;
• Sales and marketing forecast;
• Any additional data that would be relevant to the decision-making process;
• The proposed investment memo and term sheet.

30.5.1 Executive summary
This needs to be brief and slanted to the needs of its audience and the end-user. Not everyone reading the report will have the same level of expertise, but all will want to see, in a well-presented and readily accessible format, the scope of the proposal and the relevant product information along with market analysis and projections. It is important to state clearly the risks and benefits of the proposal as identified by the due diligence process. Where possible, outline solutions should be offered to negative findings. Because users are involved at different levels in the decision process it is often helpful to offer the consensus view of the due diligence team because the members have been closely involved with the data and the members of the selling organisation and thus have a good idea of the ambience surrounding the deal and the scope for possible future successful collaboration.

30.5.2 Due diligence summary
The process of due diligence requires an assessment of a vast quantity of data and it is not appropriate to simply paginate and present these data. Data have to edited, summarized and put into perspective.

The reader wants to see the critical factors for and against the proposal and to be able to understand how these factors have been generated. Referenced access to the original data should be provided. Both the advantages and disadvantages of the new proposed product should be listed and some indication given as to where this product will fit into the current market and the possible competitors is helpful at this stage. The advantages and disadvantages of the new proposed product should be listed.

The key due diligence findings can be grouped under the general headings of quality/manufacturing and controls, efficacy, safety and intellectual property issues and should be presented with special reference to the proposed product profile. The current stage of clinical development should be summarized and a brief list of future studies thought to be necessary to achieve IND and or NDA/MA submission status. Timelines of proposed studies are critical. Potential delays should be clearly described.

30.5.3 Product assessment

This will depend on the stage of the product, and may be limited to animal data for proof-of-concept opportunities. Limited human data may be present and final study reports of these data are often not yet available. University academic institution development programmes do not always fulfil the full requirements of the regulatory authorities and care must be taken to ensure that data and study design has been interpreted and performed in an acceptable way.

Sometimes, the initial development and product profile have not been tailored to the potential marketing opportunity and as a result the studies provided may not yet adequately support the proposed indication or provide adequate competitor challenges. Early work is often carried out by a sub-contract organisation and the quality control needs to be carefully checked to ensure any data presented have come from validated sources and that work has been correctly carried out.

The final marketing locations will also necessitate reference to the European, Japanese and US regulatory requirements to ensure acceptance of product data. Not all countries in the world have agreed on a format for data and local country regulatory guidelines should be considered. However, many countries now accept the Common Technical Document (CTD) format.

The CTD is a convenient way of structuring the due diligence checklists. It has the important summary in section 2. A summary is intended to be a detailed factual summary of all the information provided for review. This is analogous to the results section of a scientific publication and is given to the health authority reviewers in those countries accepting the agreed CTD format as the basis for understanding the application; in the USA it may be given to FDA advisory committee members.

Efficacy requires the appropriate studies with adequate statistical power and, again, depending on the stage of the product development, such data may be available to a greater or lesser extent.

The summary should include pharmacokinetic and pharmacodynamic data and must support the next stage of development – for example, there must be adequate indication for the dosage selected for phase III. Endpoints, possible biomarkers and surrogate biomarkers (if chosen) must be representative of the current clinical and regulatory opinion for the indication for which the product has been developed. Safety should include all relevant animal toxicological findings and any adverse events should have been identified and explained. At the stage of development for which the due diligence is sought, the toxicology data may not yet be complete and care should be taken to ensure that what is available will support the next proposed/claimed human clinical development phase. Safety should have adequate data to support the writing of an investigators' brochure in relation to the metabolism, excretion, absorption, distribution plus preclinical assays if the product is claimed to be at IND level. If the product and or the disease process will require new diagnostic or treatment regimens, these must be justified and supported by expert opinion.

Quality includes chemistry, manufacturing and its associated controls. The new product must have information relevant to bulk drug supply and the presentation currently provided. Data should be forthcoming on the active pharmaceutical ingredients regarding batch scale, scalability, Good Manufacturing Practice (GMP) compliance and any specific handling requirements. The supply chain for drug substances, novel excipients and drug product as well as the availability of clinical trial supplies should be declared. Future pharmaceutical development of the presentation should be highlighted with appropriate staged progress to the final commercial form linked to the clinical program. For a drug product that is in later development, data should be available to indicate possible drug–drug interactions, the identification of all metabolites and data on dosing for special populations such as children or the elderly.

Often, the chemistry, manufacturing and controls (CMC) process is the rate-limiting factor in the development of a product and some agencies will not accept data until the CMC package is complete and signed off for GMP compliance; this is particularly the case for the advanced therapeutics where the product is essentially defined by the process. It is helpful to prepare a checklist based on the CMC section of the NDA/CTD to ensure that the major areas have been identified.

30.5.4 Regulatory review

The regulatory pathway is the key to successful submission of product data to the regulatory authorities. A seasoned team should be able to cover the USA, Europe and Japan with access to specific national agencies' experts to evaluate the submission history. An opinion on the content of the filing to date as to the reliability and ability of the data to support the proposed stage of development is essential. The precise extent of the regulatory opinion will vary with the deal and will differ for new chemical entities from that for established marketed products. This will require analysis of summary basis of approval of competitor products to place matters into context.

The regulatory review must assess the preclinical information for both content and result. Preclinical safety concerns must be adequately explained or researched. The clinical development pathway, study design and undertaking of Good Clinical Practice must support the proposed indications and these indications must be consistent with the thinking of the regulatory agencies for the different disease areas under study and conform to established labelling advice.

The presentation of the chemistry, manufacturing and controls data must satisfy GMP requirements as well as those associated with the product type and is another key area that is often overlooked in the rush to clear the animal data hurdle and find proof-of-concept plus human efficacy data. To ensure that delays are minimised the regulatory professional should check the data on:

- Purity/impurity profiles;
- Degradants;
- Analytical methods;
- Reference standards;
- The complete manufacturing process and any changes that have been introduced;
- Stability profiles.

It is essential that these checks ensure that the product profile is the same as or better than that of related material used in previous non-clinical and clinical programs in which relevant levels of related materials, etc. have been qualified.

30.5.5 Commercial review

There are several important aspects to commercial review. These involve the market opportunity for the product. In order to estimate this, it is often necessary to go directly to physicians to try to gauge their reception to the new product properties which have to be described in somewhat general terms in order to disguise it and prevent commercial advantage being lost.

Depending on the therapy area and the competitive marketplace, introducing a new product can be expensive and requires a dedicated team. For many small companies, their ability to compete is not sufficient to achieve optimal sales and revenue and often the strategy is to develop early products and sell them on later for clinical development and launch.

As part of the market opportunity, assessment experts are needed to cost out a launch and to confirm that the proposed product profile will be competitive and can be achieved by the proposed clinical development plan within the timespan needed for commercial success. The commercial view must also blend with the known findings of the regulatory, manufacturing, non-clinical and clinical efficacy experts. For example, if the product has a bitter taste or can only be made as an intravenous injection, the market projections will need careful appraisal and evaluation by both the sales forecast and commercial teams.

Depending on the life cycle stage of the product under consideration, it may be necessary to review all promotional material and important documents carefully, such as the investigators' brochure, to ensure accuracy with the available data sets. The impact of cautionary labelling based on observed adverse drug reactions or absence of specific subpopulations in trials must be carefully appraised with regards to decreased potential market share.

30.5.6 Pharmacogenomic data

The FDA and other national agencies are currently reviewing the data requirements for pharmacogenomics and biologics which are perceived to offer a platform for personalized medicine and their relevant publications should be studied. Any data that are to be part of the leaflet or label data relating to product claims, efficacy or safety will be reviewed in the usual way and so can be subject to the due diligence process. It is probable that data will also be available for due diligence from scientific research databases. This has to be submitted to the FDA via safe harbour but in the interest of full due diligence it should be explored and assessed.

30.5.7 Safety and subject risk

For an early product there may be very few safety data. The data may be limited to animal toxicology and so it is necessary to liaise with the regulatory team member to determine the relevance and completeness of data for an impending IND application.

The product may have been developed on a global pattern and will have data from countries other than the country for which the due diligence is being undertaken. Again, regulatory support is needed to ensure acceptability of, for example non-US studies for the FDA and the requirements of, say, the Japanese authorities for both preclinical and clinical studies.

Although the strict relevance of the preclinical (animal) data is open to mixed interpretation when extrapolated to human response, very early signals are critical and should be carefully identified. Such studies are the current expectation and absence of appropriate studies will halt progress and incur costs, both real and opportunity associated.

For the larger double-blind placebo-controlled randomised studies, the basic information to assess clinical safety requires access to the investigators' brochure, interim statistical data, clinical development program data, study reports and annual reporting data. A checklist should include:

- The incidence and type of adverse events;
- The number, type and relationship of serious adverse events reported in relation to the study products;
- The number of subject deaths and the final diagnosis;
- The number and reasons for subject withdrawal and the follow-up of these subjects;
- Laboratory values during the study;
- Subject vital signs data;
- ECG reports;
- Diagnostic and special imaging reports;
- *In vitro* test data;
- Microbiology and virology data;
- Quality of life assessments; and
- Relevant patient narratives for events.

30.5.7.1 For licensed products
- Access to MedWatch (US) and CIOMS (non-US);
- Periodic safety updates;
- Access to summary basis of approvals (SBAs);
- Access to regulatory agencies home pages;
- Internet search engines;
- Use of specialised data vendors for specific commercial product and clinical reviews.

30.5.8 Relevance of the product in the clinical setting
Access to scientists and physicians actively working in the proposed therapy area is a helpful way of assessing the relevance of the proposed product to current clinical practice. Using anonymised data, questions can be asked about:

- The need for the proposed new therapy and the idealised formulation;
- Ease of use (e.g. intravenous, topical or oral, once or twice daily dosing);
- Potential for drug–drug interactions;
- Suitable patient population;
- Adverse events for therapies for current treatment regimens;
- Impact of contraindications on prescribing preference; and

- Competitor environment and recent new scientific data presentations.

30.5.9 Product leaflet, labelling and literature review
Where this is available the clinical review needs to look closely at the proposed wording and assess the claims in the light of the available data. Again there may be differences in presentation and format between the differing national agencies. The physician can refer to the Physicians Drug Reference (PDR.com) and the FDA and/or regulatory agencies websites for further information on similar therapeutic products as well as other professional sites for specific prescribing guidelines for various indications. Specialist peer-group reviewed journals are important sources of information for both phase II and III clinical trials as are the websites listing ongoing clinical trials. Company websites are useful and can help the reader to understand novel developments. Care must be taken to recognize any potential bias contained in this information.

30.6 Due diligence in private equity and life science transactions

As interested parties such as private equity firms enter the health care field, buy-outs, mergers and acquisitions are becoming more frequent. Because these transactions come in a variety of different formats the pharmaceutical physician may find that the business and financial considerations dominate and may overshadow the due diligence process that has been outlined so far and which has been focused on a product acquisition. However, the basic tenet remains, that no sales or deal process is complete without pharmaceutical due diligence to assess the value of the assets.

The immediate problem is one of scale and to some extent cost for the hoard of due diligence niche specialist who will need to be on hand, not only to delve deeper but more extensively as the deal size grows – for example, the deal process will involve legal, taxation, general partner assessment, personnel, environmental, vendor, IT, pricing, marketing strategy in relation to the normal medical practice of the marketing country and sponsor due diligence.

All of these are only a step away from the role of a pharmaceutical physician who will need to remain focused on the efficacy, safety and quality of the pharmaceutical assets, yet remain cognizant of the findings in these niche areas. One significant worry is the regulatory environment and the challenges leading to overlap and perhaps competition between the different agencies in their efforts to ensure patient safety and the full and timely reporting of all adverse events. Special care needs to be taken to ensure that there are adequate procedures and paper trails in place to detect, passively and actively, adverse events and to take the necessary action to update the summary of product characteristics, patient leaflets and labelling for each agency where the product is marketed or under clinical trial evaluation. Close scrutiny of all regulatory agency inspections and letters is essential along with manufacturing and supply of drug substance, raw materials and finished drug product details, to ensure no unexpected surprises are awaiting which will reflect on the value of the asset.

30.7 Conclusions

The pharmaceutical physician is essential to the success of the due diligence process which requires a clear and precise assessment of the product(s) under consideration and its clinical risk–benefit as it relates to the proposed deal. This individual may be the team leader, the clinical reviewer, a member of the senior management assessment team or have the individual niche interests needed to support the deal process and provide an opinion for the future growth of the product(s).

In order to conduct a thorough investigation all the data, appropriate team members and the requisite environment must be in place and in order before the due diligence process begins. In fact, due diligence preparation and information gathering starts the moment it is decided that there is a commercial interest in a particular business and needs:
• A detailed listing of the exact due diligence steps to follow;
• A checklist of everything needed to to be done in each due diligence area;
• Specific due diligence tasks that need to be completed;
• All of the materials you need from the seller before you start.

Further reading

Hicks P, Huml RA, Howe K. Key items to consider for pharmaceutical due diligence from a nonclinical perspective. *Regulatory Affairs Focus* November 2006;32–43. [Prior to entering into any pharmaceutical or biotech partnership, it is fundamental to identify the potential partners' needs and any proposed partnering arrangements' risks and benefits.]

Huml RA, Barker GR. The process of due diligence from a clinical perspective. *Regulatory Affairs Focus* February/March 2004;44–6. [In order to enter into any partnering solution, it is important to identify the needs of the potential partner and the risks and benefits of proposed partnering solution.]

Huml RA, Barker GR, Cascade E, Fraser K. An outline for the final due diligence assessment report. *Regulatory Affairs Focus* August 2004;38–40. [Although every organization has its own process for assessing a partnering or licensing opportunity, best practice suggests that the evaluation of medical technologies should include an evaluation of product, market, legal, manufacturing and financial issues.]

Huml RA, Barker GR, Ryan RP. Pharmacogenomics role in drug development: a regulatory perspective. *Regulatory Affairs Focus* April 2004;51–4. [The FDA issued its first pharmacogenomics draft guidance in November 2003, and regulatory professionals are accelerating preparations to ensure that their companies, whether biotech, pharmaceutical or contract research, are poised to meet the challenges associated with pharmacogenomics during the drug development process.]

Huml RA, Barker GR, Tonkens RM, Hebert DA. An overview of the clinical and regulatory implications of QT interval prolongation. *Regulatory Affairs Focus* May 2004;40–3. [The QT interval measures the time it takes for the heart muscle to contract and relax. A QT interval lasts about four-tenths of a second.]

Huml RA, Bullard M. Partnering alternatives for biotechnology companies. *Regulatory Affairs Focus* November 2007;34–7. [The goal of every partnering deal, whether it involves co-development, co-promotion or strategic investing, should be to structure and plan for a long-term relationship that is beneficial to both parties from beginning to end (i.e. to get not only to Yes but past Yes).]

Huml RA, Tonkens RM, Tunnicliffe J. An overview of research and development due diligence. *Regulatory Affairs Focus* October 2005;24–8. [Venture capital equity investing and pharmaceutical product-based investing are risky business, requiring careful evaluation of the potential investment and/or prospective partner company.]

Huml RA, Zarcone D, Ryan RP. The process of due diligence from a regulatory perspective. *Regulatory Affairs Focus* November 2003;50–43. [In order to enter into any partnering solution, it is important to identify the needs of potential partner and the risks and benefits of a proposed partnering partner and the risks and benefits of a proposed partnering solution.]

Hurley ME, Mondabaugh SM. The business impact of regulatory affairs. *Regulatory Affairs Focus* March 2006. [Regulatory affairs professionals are expected to participate in multidisciplinary teams for due diligence of potential licensing opportunities.]

Merhr IJ. *A Guide to Due Diligence in Life Science Transactions.* D&MD Publications. ISBN 1-57936-218-4. September 2002. [Due diligence is a critical component of any major business transaction.]

Mitchell EJ. Pharmacogenomics and pharmaceutical development. *Regulatory Focus.* March 2008;36–9. [Will pharmacogenomics truly become part of a much larger paradigm of personalized medicine, predicting the best possible treatment option in a regulatory framework designed to pick up adverse reactions much earlier in the pharmaceutical life cycle?]

Rosania L. Due diligence: a regulatory perspective. *Regulatory Affairs Focus* May 2002. [Due diligence means different things depending on our perspective.]

Schomisch JW. Due diligence: assessing the regulatory risk. *Regulatory Affairs Focus* January 2002. [As the health care products industry evolves, more companies are faced with mergers, acquisitions, major joint ventures and marketing, distribution and product deals.]

www.acessdata.fda.gov/scripts/cder/drugsatfda/index.cfm [For USFDA reviews see Drugs@USA.]

www.emea.eu.int/index/indexh1.htlm. [For EMEA reviews see Human Medicines. List of Authorized Products (EPARS).]

Appendix 1
Declaration of Helsinki

The Declaration of Helsinki, one of the most significant documents on medical ethics, was adopted by the
World Medical Association (WMA) at its 18th General
Assembly in Helsinki in June 1964. The first revision
of the document was endorsed by the WMA at its
29th General Assembly in Tokyo in 1975. The most
significant addition in terms of the conduct of
medical research was the requirement that independent committees (ethics committees) review research
protocols. At the second revision adopted at the
35th WMA General Assembly in Venice in 1983 the
changes were fairly minor. The third revision was
adopted at the 48th WMA General Assembly in
Somerset West, South Africa in 1996, which was
amended at the 52nd WMA General Assembly held in
2000 at Edinburgh. This version introduced a number
of changes including reference to the vexed principle
of the use of placebos in therapeutic trials.

A very useful review of the history and development of the Declaration of Helsinki in the last four
decades from its evolution from the principles enunciated in the Nuremberg Code of 1947 to the current
version has been published in the *British Journal of
Clinical Pharmacology*[1] and is recommended reading,
it includes the texts of the various versions of the
Declaration.

The current version of the Declaration is reproduced below.

Reference

1 Carlson RV, Boyd KM, Webb D. The Revision of the
Declaration of Helsinki: past, present and future. *Br J Clin
Pharmacol* 2004;57:695–713.

The Textbook of Pharmaceutical Medicine. Edited by
John P. Griffin. © 2009, ISBN: 978-1-4051-8035-1.

Initiated: 1964
17.C Original: English

World Medical Association Declaration of Helsinki

Ethical Principles for Medical Research Involving Human Subjects

Adopted by the 18th WMA General Assembly
Helsinki, Finland, June 1964 and amended by the
29th WMA General Assembly, Tokyo, Japan, October
1975
35th WMA General Assembly, Venice, Italy, October
1983
41st WMA General Assembly, Hong Kong, September
1989
48th WMA General Assembly, Somerset West,
Republic of South Africa, October 1996 and the
52nd WMA General Assembly, Edinburgh, Scotland,
October 2000

A. Introduction

1. The World Medical Association has developed the
Declaration of Helsinki as a statement of ethical principles to provide guidance to physicians and other
participants in medical research involving human
subjects. Medical research involving human subjects
includes research on identifiable human material or
identifiable data.

2. It is the duty of the physician to promote and safeguard the health of the people. The physician's knowledge and conscience are dedicated to the fulfilment
of this duty.

3. The Declaration of Geneva of the World Medical
Association binds the physician with the words, 'The
health of my patient will be my first consideration,'
and the International Code of Medical Ethics declares
that: 'A physician shall act only in the patient's interest

when providing medical care which might have the effect of weakening the physical and mental condition of the patient.'

4. Medical progress is based on research which ultimately must rest in part on experimentation involving human subjects.

5. In medical research on human subjects, considerations related to the well-being of the human subject should take precedence over the interests of science and society.

6. The primary purpose of medical research involving human subjects is to improve prophylactic, diagnostic and therapeutic procedures and the understanding of the aetiology and pathogenesis of disease. Even the best proven prophylactic, diagnostic and therapeutic methods must continuously be challenged through research for their effectiveness, efficiency, accessibility and quality.

7. In current medical practice and in medical research, most prophylactic, diagnostic and therapeutic procedures involve risks and burdens.

8. Medical research is subject to ethical standards that promote respect for all human beings and protect their health and rights. Some research populations are vulnerable and need special protection. The particular needs of the economically and medically disadvantaged must be recognized. Special attention is also required for those who cannot give or refuse consent for themselves, for those who may be subject to giving consent under duress, for those who will not benefit personally from the research and for those for whom the research is combined with care.

9. Research investigators should be aware of the ethical, legal and regulatory requirements for research on human subjects in their own countries as well as applicable international requirements. No national ethical, legal or regulatory requirement should be allowed to reduce or eliminate any of the protections for human subjects set forth in this Declaration.

B. Basic principles for all medical research

10. It is the duty of the physician in medical research to protect the life, health, privacy and dignity of the human subject.

The WMA has initiated a review of the Declaration of Helsinki. The consultation period has ended and the working group is preparing a final draft for the October 2008 meeting of the Medical Ethics Committee Council and General Assembly in Seoul.

11. Medical research involving human subjects must conform to generally accepted scientific principles, be based on a thorough know ledge of the scientific literature, other relevant sources of information, and on adequate laboratory and, where appropriate, animal experimentation.

12. Appropriate caution must be exercised in the conduct of research which may affect the environment, and the welfare of animals used for research must be respected.

13. The design and performance of each experimental procedure involving human subjects should be clearly formulated in an experimental protocol. This protocol should be submitted for consideration, comment, guidance and, where appropriate, approval to a specially appointed ethical review committee, which must be independent of the investigator, the sponsor or any other kind of undue influence. This independent committee should be in conformity with the laws and regulations of the country in which the research experiment is performed. The committee has the right to monitor ongoing trials. The researcher has the obligation to provide monitoring information to the committee, especially any serious adverse events. The researcher should also submit to the committee, for review, information regarding funding, sponsors, institutional affiliations, other potential conflicts of interest and incentives for subjects.

14. The research protocol should always contain a statement of the ethical considerations involved and should indicate that there is compliance with the principles enunciated in this Declaration.

15. Medical research involving human subjects should be conducted only by scientifically qualified persons and under the supervision of a clinically competent medical person. The responsibility for the human subject must always rest with a medically qualified person and never rest on the subject of the research, even though the subject has given consent.

16. Every medical research project involving human subjects should be preceded by careful assessment of predictable risks and burdens in comparison with foreseeable benefits to the subject or to others. This does not preclude the participation of healthy volunteers in medical research. The design of all studies should be publicly available.

17. Physicians should abstain from engaging in research projects involving human subjects unless they are confident that the risks involved have been adequately assessed and can be satisfactorily managed. Physicians should cease any investigation if the risks are found to outweigh the potential benefits

or if there is conclusive proof of positive and beneficial results.

18. Medical research involving human subjects should only be conducted if the importance of the objective outweighs the inherent risks and burdens to the subject. This is especially important when the human subjects are healthy volunteers.

19. Medical research is only justified if there is a reasonable likelihood that the populations in which the research is carried out stand to benefit from the results of the research.

20. The subjects must be volunteers and informed participants in the research project.

21. The right of research subjects to safeguard their integrity must always be respected. Every precaution should be taken to respect the privacy of the subject, the confidentiality of the patient's information and to minimize the impact of the study on the subject's physical and mental integrity and on the personality of the subject.

22. In any research on human beings, each potential subject must be adequately informed of the aims, methods, sources of funding, any possible conflicts of interest, institutional affiliations of the researcher, the anticipated benefits and potential risks of the study and the discomfort it may entail. The subject should be informed of the right to abstain from participation in the study or to withdraw consent to participate at any time without reprisal. After ensuring that the subject has understood the information, the physician should then obtain the subject's freely-given informed consent, preferably in writing. If the consent cannot be obtained in writing, the non-written consent must be formally documented and witnessed.

23. When obtaining informed consent for the research project the physician should be particularly cautious if the subject is in a dependent relationship with the physician or may consent under duress. In that case the informed consent should be obtained by a well-informed physician who is not engaged in the investigation and who is completely independent of this relationship.

24. For a research subject who is legally incompetent, physically or mentally incapable of giving consent or is a legally incompetent minor, the investigator must obtain informed consent from the legally authorized representative in accordance with applicable law. These groups should not be included in research unless the research is necessary to promote the health of the population represented and this research cannot instead be performed on legally competent persons.

25. When a subject deemed legally incompetent, such as a minor child, is able to give assent to decisions about participation in research, the investigator must obtain that assent in addition to the consent of the legally authorized representative.

26. Research on individuals from whom it is not possible to obtain consent, including proxy or advance consent, should be done only if the physical/mental condition that prevents obtaining informed consent is a necessary characteristic of the research population. The specific reasons for involving research subjects with a condition that renders them unable to give informed consent should be stated in the experimental protocol for consideration and approval of the review committee. The protocol should state that consent to remain in the research should be obtained as soon as possible from the individual or a legally authorized surrogate.

27. Both authors and publishers have ethical obligations. In publication of the results of research, the investigators are obliged to preserve the accuracy of the results. Negative as well as positive results should be published or otherwise publicly available. Sources of funding, institutional affiliations and any possible conflicts of interest should be declared in the publication. Reports of experimentation not in accordance with the principles laid down in this Declaration should not be accepted for publication.

C. Additional principles for medical research combined with medical care

28. The physician may combine medical research with medical care, only to the extent that the research is justified by its potential prophylactic, diagnostic or therapeutic value. When medical research is combined with medical care, additional standards apply to protect the patients who are research subjects.

29. The benefits, risks, burdens and effectiveness of a new method should be tested against those of the best current prophylactic, diagnostic and therapeutic methods. This does not exclude the use of placebo, or no treatment, in studies where no proven prophylactic, diagnostic or therapeutic method exists.

30. At the conclusion of the study, every patient entered into the study should be assured of access to the best proven prophylactic, diagnostic and therapeutic methods identified by the study.

31. The physician should fully inform the patient which aspects of the care are related to the research. The refusal of a patient to participate in a study must never interfere with the patient–physician relationship.

32. In the treatment of a patient, where proven pro-phylactic, diagnostic and therapeutic methods do not exist or have been ineffective, the physician, with informed consent from the patient, must be free to use unproven or new prophylactic, diagnostic and therapeutic measures, if in the physician's judgement it offers hope of saving life, re-establishing health or alleviating suffering. Where possible, these measures should be made the object of research, designed to evaluate their safety and efficacy. In all cases, new information should be recorded and, where appro-priate, published. The other relevant guidelines of this Declaration should be followed.

Appendix 2
Guidelines and Documentation for Implementation of Clinical Trials

Clinical trial agreement for pharmaceutical industry sponsored research in NHS Trusts

This agreement dated   day of   20..
is between
[. . . insert name . . .] NHS TRUST, of [. . . insert address . . .]
(Hereinafter known as the 'NHS Trust')
AND
[. . . insert name . . .], of [. . . insert address . . .]
(Hereinafter known as the 'Sponsor')
NOW

WHEREAS the Sponsor is a pharmaceutical company involved in the research, development, manufacture and sale of medicines for use in humans
WHEREAS the Sponsor is developing new treatments for patients with [. . . insert disease . . .]
WHEREAS the NHS Trust is concerned with the diagnosis, treatment and prevention of disease and clinical research for the improvement of health care
WHEREAS the NHS Trust has a particular interest and expertise in [. . . insert disease . . .]
WHEREAS the Sponsor wishes to contract with the NHS Trust to undertake a sponsored clinical trial entitled:
[. . . insert title . . .]
It is agreed that the NHS Trust and Sponsor shall participate in the aforementioned clinical trial in accordance with this Agreement.

The Textbook of Pharmaceutical Medicine. Edited by
John P. Griffin. © 2009, ISBN: 978-1-4051-8035-1.

1 Definitions

1.1 The following words and phrases have the following meanings:
'Clinical Trial' means the investigation to be conducted at the Trial Site in accordance with the Protocol numbered [. . . insert identification number . . .].
'Clinical Trial Subject' means a person recruited to participate in the Clinical Trial.
'Confidential Information' means in the case of obligations imposed upon the NHS Trust under clauses 6.2 and 12.8 any and all information relating to the Clinical Trial including the Investigational Medicinal Product and in the case of obligations imposed upon the Parties under clause 6.2 all information concerning the arrangements contemplated by this Agreement or the business affairs of one Party that it discloses to the other Party pursuant to or in connection with this Agreement.
'ICH GCP' means the ICH Harmonised Tripartite Guideline for Good Clinical Practice (CPMP/ICH/ 135/95) together with such other good clinical practice requirements as are specified in Directive 2001/ 20/EC of the European Parliament and the Council of 4 April 2001 relating to medicinal products for human use and in guidance published by the European Commission pursuant to such Directive.
'Intellectual Property Rights' means patents, trademarks, copyrights, rights to extract information from a database, design rights and all rights or forms of protection of a similar nature or having equivalent or

the similar effect to any of them which may subsist anywhere in the world, whether or not any of them are registered and including applications for registration of any of them.

'Investigational Medicinal Product' means [. . . insert details of study drug/control material . . .] as defined in the Protocol.

'Know How' means all technical and other information which is not in the public domain, including but not limited to information comprising or relating to concepts, discoveries, data, designs, formulae, ideas, inventions, methods, models, procedures, designs for experiments and tests and results of experimentation and testing, processes, specifications and techniques, laboratory records, clinical data, manufacturing data and information contained in submissions to regulatory authorities.

'Monitor' means one or more persons appointed by the Sponsor to monitor compliance of the Clinical Trial with ICH GCP and to conduct source data verification.

'NHS Trust' means the [. . . insert name . . .] NHS Trust that is a signatory to this Agreement.

'Party' means the Sponsor, or the NHS Trust and 'Parties' shall mean both of them.

'Protocol' means the description of the Clinical Trial and all amendments thereto as the Parties may from time to time agree. Such amendments will be signed by the Parties and form a part of this Agreement.

'R&D Office' means the NHS Trust department responsible for the administration of this Clinical Trial on behalf of the NHS Trust.

'Site File' means the file maintained by the Site Principal Investigator containing the documentation specified in section 8 of ICH GCP (edition CPMP/ICH/135/95).

'Site Principal Investigator' means the person who will lead and coordinate the work of the Clinical Trial at the Trial Site on behalf of the NHS Trust or any other person as may be agreed from time to time between the Parties as a replacement.

'Sponsor' means the corporate entity that is a signatory to this Agreement.

'Timelines' means the dates set out in Appendix 2.2 hereto as may be amended by agreement between the Parties and Timeline shall mean any one of such dates.

'Trial Site(s)' means any premises occupied by the NHS Trust.

1.2 Any reference to a statutory provision shall be deemed to include reference to any statutory modification or re-enactment of it.

2 Site Principal Investigator

2.1 The NHS Trust represents that it is entitled to procure and the NHS Trust will procure the Services of [. . . insert name of investigator . . .] to act as Site Principal Investigator and shall ensure the performance of the obligations of the Site Principal Investigator set out in this Agreement.

2.2 The NHS Trust represents that the Site Principal Investigator has the necessary expertise to perform the Clinical Trial and that the Site Principal Investigator meets and will continue to meet the conditions set out at Appendix 2.6 to this Agreement.

2.3 The NHS Trust shall notify the Sponsor if [. . . insert name of investigator . . .] ceases to be employed by or associated with the NHS Trust, and shall use its best endeavours to find a replacement acceptable to both the Sponsor and the NHS Trust. If no mutually acceptable replacement can be found the Sponsor may terminate this Agreement pursuant to clause 12.3 below.

3 Clinical Trial Governance

3.1 The Sponsor shall inform the NHS Trust and the Site Principal Investigator of the name and telephone number of the Monitor and the name of the person who will be available as a point of contact. The Sponsor shall also provide the Site Principal Investigator with an emergency number to enable adverse event reporting at any time.

3.2 The Parties shall comply with all laws and statutes applicable to the performance of the Clinical Trial including, but not limited to, the Human Rights Act 1998, the Data Protection Act 1998, the Medicines Act 1968, and with all relevant guidance relating to medicines and clinical trials from time to time in force including, but not limited to the ICH GCP, the World Medical Association Declaration of Helsinki, entitled 'Ethical Principles for Medical Research Involving Human Subjects' (1996 version) and the NHS Research Governance Framework for Health and Social Care of March 2001, as amended from time to time.

3.3 The Sponsor shall comply with all guidelines from time to time in force and published by the Association of the British Pharmaceutical Industry in relation to clinical trials and in particular those entitled 'Clinical Trial Compensation Guidelines' (1991) a copy of which is set out in Appendix 2.3.

3.4 The Sponsor shall not commit (and warrants that in entering into the Agreement it has not committed) any of the following facts:

3.4.1 Provide or offer to provide to any person in the employment of the NHS Trust any gift or consideration not contemplated by the financial arrangements set out at clause 10 below in relation to the negotiation or performance of this Agreement or any other contract with the NHS Trust.

3.4.2 Make payment or agree to make payment of any commission to any person in the employment of the NHS Trust whether in relation to this Agreement or any other contract with the NHS Trust.

3.5 If the Sponsor or any of his employees, agents or sub-contractors, or any person acting on their behalf, commits any of the acts referred to in clause 3.4 above or commits any offence under the Prevention of Corruption Acts 1889 to 1916, in relation to this or any other agreement with the NHS Trust or an authority that is a health service body within the meaning given by Section 4(2) of the National Health Service and Community Care Act 1990, the NHS Trust shall be entitled, in addition to any other remedy available, to terminate this Agreement with immediate effect.

3.6 Should there be any inconsistency between the Protocol and the other terms of this Agreement the terms of the Protocol shall prevail to the extent of such inconsistency.

4 Obligations of the Parties

4.1 The Site Principal Investigator shall be responsible for obtaining and maintaining all approvals from the relevant local research ethics committee for the conduct of the Clinical Trial and the Site Principal Investigator shall keep the Sponsor fully apprised of the progress of ethics committee submissions and shall upon request provide the Sponsor with all correspondence relating to such submissions. The Site Principal Investigator shall not consent to any change in the Protocol requested by a relevant ethics committee without the prior written consent of the Sponsor.

4.2 The Parties shall conduct the Clinical Trial in accordance with:

(i) the Protocol a copy of which for the purposes of identification appears at Appendix 2.1 to this Agreement;

(ii) the current marketing authorisation for the Investigational Medicinal Product or, as the case may be, Clinical Trial Certificate or Clinical Trial Exemption Certificate applicable to the Clinical Trial; and

(iii) the terms and conditions of the approval of the relevant [. . . insert name . . .] Ethics Committee(s)

and the NHS Trust shall ensure that neither administration of the Investigational Medicinal Product to any Clinical Trial Subject nor any other clinical intervention mandated by the Protocol takes place in relation to any such Clinical Trial Subject until it is satisfied that all relevant regulatory and ethics committee approvals have been obtained.

4.3 The Sponsor shall make available to the Site Principal Investigator copies of the documentation referred to in sub-paragraphs (i) and (ii) of clause 4.2 above and the Site Principal Investigator shall include such documents together with the Ethics Committee approvals in the Site File.

4.4 The Site Principal Investigator shall inform the Sponsor immediately upon learning of the existence of any of financial arrangement or interest between the Site Principal Investigator and the Sponsor of the type described at paragraph (f) of Appendix 2.6 hereto and for the purposes of the obligation contained in such paragraph the Sponsor shall advise the Site Principal Investigator in writing of the completion date of the Clinical Trial.

4.5 Neither the NHS Trust nor the Site Principal Investigator shall permit the Investigational Medicinal Product to be used for any purpose other than the conduct of the Clinical Trial and upon termination or expiration of this Agreement all unused Investigational Medicinal Product shall, at the Sponsor's option, either be returned to the Sponsor or disposed of in accordance with the Protocol.

4.6 The NHS Trust shall recruit [. . . insert number . . .] Clinical Trial Subjects to participate in the Clinical Trial and the Parties shall conduct the Clinical Trial in accordance with the Timelines.

4.7 In the event that the Clinical Trial is part of a multicentre clinical trial (which for the purposes of this Agreement shall mean that at least one other institution is taking part) the Sponsor may amend the number of Clinical Trial Subjects to be recruited pursuant to clause 4.6 above as follows:

4.7.1 if in the reasonable opinion of the Sponsor recruitment of Clinical Trial Subjects is proceeding at a rate below that required to enable the relevant Timeline to be met the Sponsor may by notice to the NHS Trust require recruitment at the Trial Site to cease and the terms of the Agreement shall relate thereafter to the number of Clinical Trial Subjects who have been accepted for treatment in the Clinical Trial at the date of such notice; or

4.7.2 if recruitment of Clinical Trial Subjects is proceeding at a rate above that required to meet the relevant Timeline the Sponsor may with the agreement of the NHS Trust increase the number of Clinical Trial Subjects to be recruited.

4.8 The NHS Trust shall permit the Monitor access to the records of Clinical Trial Subjects for monitoring and source data verification, such access to be arranged at mutually convenient times and on reasonable notice. The Sponsor will report on the Clinical Trial activity to the NHS Trust R&D Office, the frequency of reports to be [. . . insert period as appropriate to the Protocol . . .]. The Sponsor will alert the R&D Director of the NHS Trust promptly to significant issues (in the opinion of the Monitor) relating to the conduct of the Clinical Trial. In the event that the Sponsor reasonably believes there has been any research misconduct in relation to the Clinical Trial the NHS Trust and the Site Principal Investigator shall provide all reasonable assistance to any investigation into any alleged research misconduct undertaken by or on behalf of the Sponsor. At its conclusion, the Sponsor and the R&D Director of the NHS Trust shall review the conduct of the Clinical Trial at the Trial Site, such review to take place within 3 months of Trial Site close-out.

4.9 The NHS Trust shall ensure that any clinical samples required to be tested during the course of the Clinical Trial are tested in accordance with the Protocol and at a laboratory approved by the Sponsor.

4.10 Upon completion of the Clinical Trial (whether prematurely or otherwise) the Site Principal Investigator shall [provide the Sponsor with/cooperate with the Sponsor in producing] a report of the Clinical Trial detailing the methodology, results and containing an analysis of the results and drawing appropriate conclusions.

4.11 Neither the NHS Trust nor the Site Principal Investigator shall during the term of this Agreement conduct any other trial which might adversely affect the NHS Trust's ability to perform its obligations under this Agreement.

5 Liabilities and indemnity

5.1 In the event of any claim or proceeding in respect of personal injury made or brought against the NHS Trust by a Clinical Trial Subject, the Sponsor shall indemnify the NHS Trust, its servants, agents and employees in accordance with the terms of the indemnity set out at Appendix 2.4 hereto.

5.2 The Sponsor shall indemnify the NHS Trust, its servants, agents and employees against all claims, proceedings, costs and expenses (including reasonable legal costs) in respect of loss of or damage to property which is the result of negligence on the part of the Sponsor or of a breach by the Sponsor of any of its obligations under this Agreement, save to the extent that any such loss or damage is the result of negligence on the part of the NHS Trust, its servants, agents or employees or of a breach of the obligations of the NHS Trust under this Agreement.

5.3 The NHS Trust shall indemnify the Sponsor, its servants, agents and employees against all claims, proceedings, costs and expenses (including reasonable legal costs) in respect of loss of or damage to property which is the result of negligence on the part of the NHS Trust or of a breach by the NHS Trust of its obligations under this Agreement, save to the extent that any such loss or damage is the result of negligence on the part of the Sponsor, its servants, agents or employees or of a breach of the obligations of the Sponsor under this Agreement.

5.4 Where a Party is required to provide an indemnity under clause 5.2 or (as the case may be) clause 5.3 above, that Party shall have the right to take over full care and control of the defence to any claim or proceeding by a third party, said defence to be at the sole expense of the indemnifying Party. The indemnifying Party shall be entitled to use legal counsel of his choice. The indemnifying Party shall keep the other Party fully informed of the progress of any such claim or proceeding, will consult fully with the other Party on the nature of any defence to be advanced, and will not compromise or settle any such claim or proceeding (whether by admission, statement or payment) nor will it conduct itself in such a way as could prejudice the defence of any such claim or proceeding without the written approval of the other Party, such approval not to be unreasonably withheld. Each Party will give the other written notice of any claim or proceeding brought against it with respect to any matter to which it may be entitled to indemnification under clause 5.2 or (as the case may be) clause 5.3 above and each Party will also use its best endeavours to inform the other Party promptly of any circumstances thought likely to give rise to any such claim or proceeding. Each Party will give to the other Party such help as may reasonably be required for the conduct and prompt handling of any such claim or proceeding.

5.5 In no circumstances shall either Party be liable to the other in contract, tort (including negligence or breach of statutory duty) or otherwise howsoever arising or whatever the cause thereof, for any loss of profit, business, reputation, contracts, revenues or anticipated savings for any special, indirect or consequential damage of any nature, which arises directly or indirectly from any default on the part of either Party. Nothing in this clause shall affect the responsibility of either Party in relation to death or personal injury caused by the negligence of that Party or its servants, agents or employees.

5.6 For the purpose of the indemnity provided in clause 5.2 above, the expression 'agents' shall include, but shall not be limited to, any person providing services to the NHS Trust under a contract for services or otherwise.

5.7 The Sponsor will take out appropriate insurance cover or will provide evidence to the satisfaction of the NHS Trust of self-insurance in respect of its potential liability under clauses 5.1 and 5.2 above and such cover shall be for a minimum of £ [. . . insert amount . . .] in respect of any one occurrence or series of occurrences arising from one event. The Sponsor shall produce to the NHS Trust, on request, copies of insurance policies or other evidence thereof together with evidence that such policies remain in full force and effect. The terms of any insurance or the amount of cover shall not relieve the Sponsor of any liabilities under this Agreement.

6 Confidentiality

6.1 Medical confidentiality

The Parties agree to adhere to the principles of medical confidentiality in relation to Clinical Trial Subjects involved in the Clinical Trial. Personal data shall not be disclosed to the Sponsor by the NHS Trust save where this is required directly or indirectly to satisfy the requirements of the Protocol or for the purpose of monitoring or adverse event reporting. The Sponsor shall not disclose the identity of Clinical Trial Subjects to third parties without prior written consent of the Clinical Trial Subject, in accordance with the requirements of the Data Protection Act 1998 and the principles set out in the Report of the Caldicott Committee on the review of patient identifiable information dated December 1997, a copy of which the NHS Trust shall supply to the Sponsor on request.

6.2 Confidential information

6.2.1 The NHS Trust and the Sponsor shall ensure that only those of its officers and employees directly concerned with the carrying out of this Agreement have access to the Confidential Information and each Party undertakes to treat as strictly confidential and not to disclose to any third party any Confidential Information save where disclosure is required by a

regulatory authority or by law and not to make use of any Confidential Information other than in accordance with this Agreement without the prior written consent of the other Party.

6.2.2 In the event of a Party visiting the establishment of the other Party, the visiting Party undertakes that any further information relating to other clinical trials which may come to the visiting Party's knowledge as a result of any such visit, shall be kept strictly confidential and that any such information will not be disclosed to any third party or made use of in any way by the visiting Party without prior written permission of the other Party.

6.2.3 The obligations of confidentiality set out in this clause 6.2 shall not apply to Confidential Information which is (i) published or generally available to the public through no fault of the receiving Party, (ii) in the possession of the receiving Party prior to the date of this Agreement and is not subject to a duty of confidentiality, (iii) independently developed by the receiving Party and is not subject to a duty of confidentiality, (iv) obtained by the receiving Party from a third party not subject to a duty of confidentiality.

6.3 This clause 6 shall continue to apply after the expiry or termination of this Agreement.

7 Publicity

The Sponsor will not use the name of the NHS Trust, nor of any member of the NHS Trust's staff, in any publicity, advertising or news release without the prior written approval of an authorised representative of the NHS Trust, such approval not to be unreasonably withheld. The NHS Trust will not use the name of the Sponsor nor of any of its employees, in any publicity without the prior written approval of the Sponsor.

8 Publication

8.1 The Sponsor recognises that the NHS Trust and Site Principal Investigator have a responsibility under the Research Governance Framework for Health and Social Care to ensure that results of scientific interest arising from the Clinical Trial are appropriately published and disseminated. The Sponsor agrees that employees of the NHS Trust shall be permitted to present at symposia, national or regional professional meetings, and to publish in journals, theses or dissertations, or otherwise of their own choosing, methods and results of the Clinical Trial subject to the publication policy described in the Protocol. If the Clinical Trial is multicentred (as defined in clause 4.7 above), any publication based on the results obtained at the Trial Site (or a group of sites) shall not be made before the first multicentre publication. If a publication concerns the analyses of sub-sets of data from a multicentred Clinical Trial the publication shall make reference to the relevant multicentre publication(s).

8.2 Upon completion of the Clinical Trial, and any prior publication of multicentre data, or when the Clinical Trial data are adequate (in Sponsor's reasonable judgement), the NHS Trust may prepare the data deriving from the Clinical Trial for publication. Such data will be submitted to the Sponsor for review and comment prior to publication. In order to ensure that the Sponsor will be able to make comments and suggestions where pertinent, material for public dissemination will be submitted to the Sponsor for review at least sixty (60) days (or the time limit specified in the Protocol if longer) prior to submission for publication, public dissemination, or review by a publication committee.

8.3 The NHS Trust agrees that all reasonable comments made by the Sponsor in relation to a proposed publication by the NHS Trust will be incorporated by the NHS Trust into the publication.

8.4 During the period for review of a proposed publication referred to in clause 8.2 above, the Sponsor shall be entitled to make a reasoned request to the NHS Trust that publication be delayed for a period of up to six (6) months from the date of first submission to the Sponsor in order to enable the Sponsor to take steps to protect its proprietary information and the NHS Trust shall not unreasonably withhold its consent to such a request.

9 Intellectual Property

9.1 All Intellectual Property Rights and Know How owned by or licensed to NHS Trust prior to and after the date of this Agreement other than any Intellectual Property Rights and Know How arising from the Clinical Trial is and shall remain the property of the NHS Trust.

9.2 All Intellectual Property Rights and Know How owned by or licensed to the Sponsor prior to and after the date of this Agreement other than any Intellectual Property Rights and Know How arising out of the Clinical Trial is and shall remain the property of the Sponsor.

9.3 All Intellectual Property Rights and Know How arising from the Clinical Trial shall vest in or be exclusively licensed to the Sponsor in accordance with clauses 9.4 and 9.5 below.

9.4 The NHS Trust hereby assigns its rights in all Intellectual Property Rights and, to the extent possible in all Know How, arising out of the Clinical Trial to the Sponsor and at the request and expense of the Sponsor, the NHS Trust and the Site Principal Investigator shall execute all such documents and do all such other acts and things as the Sponsor may reasonably require in order to vest fully and effectively all such Intellectual Property Rights and Know How in the Sponsor or its nominee.

9.5 NHS Trust and Site Principal Investigator shall promptly disclose to the Sponsor any and all Know How generated pursuant to this Agreement and undertake not to use such Know How other than for the purposes of this Agreement without the prior written consent of the Sponsor, such consent not to be unreasonably withheld. NHS Trust hereby grants to the Sponsor an exclusive, worldwide, irrevocable, fully paid up royalty free licence under such Know How (to the extent such Know How is not assigned pursuant to clause 9.4 above) to exploit the same for any purpose whatsoever.

10 Financial arrangements

10.1 Arrangements relating to the financing of this Clinical Trial by the Sponsor are set out in Appendix 2.5 hereto.

10.2 All payments will be made according to the schedule contained in Appendix 2.5 on presentation of a VAT invoice to the Sponsor by the NHS Trust.

10.3 The Sponsor shall make payment within thirty (30) days of the date of receipt of the invoice mentioned in clause 10.2 above.

10.4 Any delay in the payment of the payee invoices by the Sponsor will incur an interest charge on any amounts overdue of 2% per month above the National Westminster Bank plc base rate prevailing on the date the payment is due.

11 Term

This Agreement will remain in effect until completion of the Clinical Trial, close-out of the Trial Site and completion of the obligations of the Parties under this Agreement or earlier termination in accordance with this Agreement.

12 Early termination

12.1 Either the Sponsor or the NHS Trust (the Terminating Party) may terminate this Agreement with immediate effect at any time if the other Party (the Defaulting Party) is:

12.1.1 in breach of any of the Defaulting Party's obligations hereunder (including a failure without just cause to meet a Timeline) and fails to remedy such breach where it is capable of remedy within 28 days of a written notice from the Terminating Party specifying the breach and requiring its remedy;

12.1.2 declared insolvent or has an administrator or receiver appointed over all or any part of its assets or ceases or threatens to cease to carry on its business.

12.2 A Party may terminate this Agreement on notice to the other Party with immediate effect if it is reasonably of the opinion that the Clinical Trial should cease in the interests of the health of Clinical Trial Subjects involved in the Clinical Trial.

12.3 The Sponsor may terminate this Agreement on notice to the NHS Trust if [. . . insert name of investigator . . .] is no longer able (for whatever reason) to act as Site Principal Investigator and no replacement mutually acceptable to the NHS Trust and the Sponsor can be found.

12.4 The Sponsor may terminate this Agreement immediately upon notice in writing to the NHS Trust for reasons not falling within clauses 12.1, 12.2 or 12.3 above, save that in such circumstances the provisions of clause 12.6 below shall also apply. In all such circumstances the Sponsor shall confer with the Site Principal Investigator and use its best endeavours to minimise any inconvenience or harm to Clinical Trial Subjects caused by the premature termination of the Clinical Trial.

12.5 In the event of early termination of this Agreement by the Sponsor, pursuant to clauses 12.2, 12.3 and 12.4 and subject to an obligation on the NHS Trust and the Site Principal Investigator to mitigate any loss, the Sponsor shall pay all costs incurred and falling due for payment up to the date of termination, and also all expenditure falling due for payment after the date of termination which arises from commitments reasonably and necessarily incurred by the NHS Trust for the performance of the Clinical Trial prior to the date of termination, and agreed with the Sponsor.

12.6 In the event of early termination pursuant to clause 12.4 above the Sponsor shall make a compensatory payment in accordance with Appendix 2.5.

12.7 In the event of early termination if payment (whether for salaries or otherwise) has been made by the Sponsor to the NHS Trust in advance for work not completed such monies shall be applied to termination related costs and in the case of termination pursuant to clause 12.4 above towards the compensatory payment payable pursuant to clause 12.6 and the remainder of the monies shall be returned forthwith to the Sponsor.

12.8 At close-out of the Trial Site following termination or expiration of this Agreement the NHS Trust shall immediately deliver to the Sponsor all Confidential Information and any other unused materials provided to the NHS Trust pursuant to this Agreement.

12.9 Termination of this Agreement will be without prejudice to the accrued rights and liabilities of the Parties under this Agreement.

13 Relationship between the Parties

13.1 Neither Party may assign its rights under this Agreement or any part thereof without the prior written consent of the other Party and neither Party may sub-contract the performance of all or any of its obligations under this Agreement without the prior written consent of the other Party. Any party who so sub-contracts shall be responsible for the acts and omissions of its sub-contractors as though they were its own.

13.2 Nothing shall be construed as creating a partnership, contract of employment or relationship of principal and agent between the Parties.

14 Agreement and modification

14.1 Any change in the terms of this Agreement shall be valid only if the change is made in writing, agreed and signed by the Parties.

14.2 This Agreement including its Appendices contains the entire understanding between the Parties and supersedes all other negotiations representations and undertakings whether written or oral of prior date between the Parties relating to the Clinical Trial which is the subject of this Agreement.

15 *Force majeure*

Neither Party shall be liable to the other Party or shall be in default of its obligations hereunder if such default is the result of war, hostilities, revolution, civil commotion, strike, epidemic, accident, fire, wind, flood or because of any act of God or other cause beyond the reasonable control of the Party affected. The Party affected by such circumstances shall promptly notify the other Party in writing when such circumstances cause a delay or failure in performance ('a Delay') and where they cease to do so. In the event of a Delay lasting for [. . . insert number . . .] weeks or more the non-affected Party shall have the right to terminate this Agreement immediately by notice in writing to the other Party.

16 Notices

Any notices under this Agreement shall be in writing, signed by the relevant Party to this Agreement and delivered personally, by courier or by recorded delivery post.

Notices to the Sponsor shall be addressed to: [. . . insert address . . .]

Notices to the NHS Trust shall be addressed to: [. . . insert address . . .]

17 Rights of Third Parties

Nothing in this Agreement is intended to confer on any person any right to enforce any term of this Agreement which that person would not have had but for the Contracts (Rights of Third Parties) Act 1999.

18 Waiver

No failure, delay, relaxation or indulgence by any Party in exercising any right conferred on such Party by this Agreement shall operate as a waiver of such right, nor shall any single or partial exercise of any such right nor any single failure to do so, preclude any other or future exercise of it, or the exercise of any other right under this Agreement.

19 Dispute resolution

19.1 In the event of a dispute the Parties agree to attempt to settle it by mediation in accordance with the Centre for Effective Dispute Resolution Model Mediation Procedure. To initiate a mediation a Party must give notice in writing (ADR Notice) to the other Party requesting mediation in accordance with this clause. The Parties shall seek to agree the nomination of the mediator, but in the absence of agreement he shall be nominated by the President for the time being of the British Medical Association. The mediation will start no later than [20] days after date of the ADR Notice. If the dispute is not resolved within [30] days of the ADR Notice a Party may by written notice to the other refer the dispute to arbitration in accordance with clause 19.2 below.

19.2 If the Parties are unable to settle a dispute arising out of or in connection with this Agreement by mediation the dispute shall be finally settled by arbitration in accordance with the UNCITRAL Arbitration Rules as at present in force (the 'UNCITRAL Rules'). The Notice of Arbitration shall be served in accordance with Article 3 of the UNCITRAL Rules and a single arbitrator shall be appointed by agreement of the Parties or in the absence of agreement, by the President for the time being of the British Medical Association. The seat of arbitration shall be London and the language of the arbitral proceedings shall be English. All and any awards of the arbitrators shall be made in accordance with the UNCITRAL Rules in writing and shall be binding on the Parties who expressly exclude all and any rights of appeal from all and any awards to the extent that such exclusion may be validly made.

20 Governing law

This Agreement shall be interpreted and governed by English Law.

Signed on behalf of the:

SPONSOR: . . . .

. . . . Date: . . . .

(Print name and position)

Signed on behalf of the:

NHS TRUST . . . .

. . . . Date: . . . .

(Print name and position)

Authorised signatory (Chief Executive, Director of R&D, or Finance Director)

Appendix 2.1

The Protocol

Appendix 2.2

Timelines for Parties

Milestone	Sponsor responsibility	Site responsibility	Target date
Provision of materials for Ethics Committee submission	X		
Ethics Committee submission	[X]	X	
Trial Site initiation visit	X	X	
First Clinical Trial Subject recruited		X	
Last Clinical Trial Subject recruited		X	
All CRF queries submitted	X		
All CRF queries completed		X	

Appendix 2.3

Clinical Trial Compensation Guidelines

Appendix 2.4

Form of Indemnity

1. The Sponsor indemnifies and holds harmless the NHS Trust and its employees and agents against all claims and proceedings (to include any settlements or ex gratia payments made with the consent of the Parties hereto and reasonable legal and expert costs and expenses) made or brought (whether successfully or otherwise):

1.1 by or on behalf of Clinical Trial Subjects and (or their dependants) against the NHS Trust or any of its employees or agents for personal injury (including death) to Clinical Trial Subjects arising out of or relating to the administration of the product(s) under investigation or any clinical intervention or procedure provided for or required by the Protocol to which the Clinical Trial Subjects would not have been exposed but for their participation in the Clinical Trial;

1.2 by the NHS Trust its employees or agents or by or on behalf of a Clinical Trial Subject for a declaration concerning the treatment of a Clinical Trial Subject who has suffered such personal injury.

2. The above indemnity by the Sponsor shall not apply to any such claim or proceeding:

2.1 to the extent that such personal injury (including death) is caused by the negligent or wrongful acts or omissions or breach of statutory duty of the NHS Trust, its employees or agents;

2.2 to the extent that such personal injury (including death) is caused by the failure of the NHS Trust, its employees, or agents to conduct the Clinical Trial in accordance with the Protocol;

2.3 unless as soon as reasonably practicable following receipt of notice of such claim or proceeding, the NHS Trust shall have notified the Sponsor in writing of it and shall, upon the Sponsor's request, and that the Sponsor's cost, have permitted the Sponsor to have full care and control of the claim or proceeding using legal representation of its own choosing;

2.4 If the NHS Trust, its employees, or agents shall have made any admission in respect of such claim or proceeding or taken any action relating to such claim or proceeding prejudicial to the defence of it without the written consent of the Sponsor such consent not to be unreasonably withheld provided that this condition shall not be treated as breached by any statement properly made by the NHS Trust, its employees or agents in connection with the operation of the NHS Trust's internal complaint procedures, accident reporting procedures or disciplinary procedures or where such a statement is required by law.

3. The Sponsor shall keep the NHS Trust and its legal advisors fully informed of the progress of any such claim or proceeding, will consult fully with the NHS Trust on the nature of any defence to be advanced and will not settle any such claim or proceeding without the written approval of the NHS Trust (such approval not to be unreasonably withheld).

4. Without prejudice to the provisions of paragraph 2.3 above, the NHS Trust will use its reasonable endeavours to inform the Sponsor promptly of any circumstances reasonably sought likely to give rise to any such claim or proceeding of which it is directly aware and shall keep the Sponsor reasonably informed of developments in relation to any such claim or proceeding even where the NHS Trust decides not to make a claim under this indemnity. Likewise, the Sponsor shall use its reasonable endeavours to inform the NHS Trust or any circumstances and shall keep the NHS Trust reasonably informed of developments in relation to any such claim or proceeding made or brought against the Sponsor alone.

5. The NHS Trust and the Sponsor will each give to the other such help as may reasonably be required for the official conduct and prompt handling of any claim or proceeding by or on behalf of Clinical Trial Subjects (or their dependants) or concerning such a declaration as is referred to in paragraph 1.2 above.

6. Without prejudice to the foregoing if injury is suffered by a Clinical Trial Subject while participating in the Clinical Trial, the Sponsor agrees to operate in good faith the guidelines published in 1991 by the Association of the British Pharmaceutical Industry and entitled 'Clinical Trial Compensation Guidelines' and shall request the Site Principal Investigator to make clear to the Clinical Trial Subjects that the Clinical Trial is being conducted subject to the Association guidelines.

7. For the purpose of this indemnity, the expression 'agents' shall be deemed to include without limitation any nurse or other health professional providing services to the NHS Trust under a contract for services or otherwise and any person carrying out work for the NHS Trust under such a contract connected with such of the NHS Trust's facilities and equipment as are made available for the Clinical Trial.

Appendix 2.5

Financial Arrangements

Appendix 2.6

Conditions Applicable to the Site Principal Investigator

(a) He is free to participate in the Clinical Trial and there are no rights which may be exercised by or obligations owed to any third party which might prevent or restrict his performance of the obligations detailed in this Agreement.

(b) He is not involved in any regulatory or misconduct litigation or investigation by the Food and Drug Administration, the Medicines Control Agency, the European Medicines Evaluation Agency, the General Medical Council or other regulatory authorities. No data produced by him in any previous clinical study has been rejected because of concerns as to its accuracy or because it was generated by fraud.

(c) He has considered, and is satisfied that, facilities appropriate to the Clinical Trial are available to him at the Trial Site and that he is supported, and will continue to be supported, by medical and other staff of sufficient number and experience to enable the NHS Trust to perform the Clinical Trial efficiently and in accordance with its obligations under the Agreement.

(d) He carries medical liability insurance (or the NHS Trust carries medical liability insurance covering him) and details and evidence of the coverage will be provided to Sponsor upon request.

(e) during the Clinical Trial, he will not serve as an investigator or other significant participant in any clinical trial for another sponsor if such activity might adversely affect his ability to perform his obligations under this Agreement.

(f) Neither he, nor his spouse nor any dependent children, have entered into and will not enter into any financial arrangements with the Sponsor to hold financial interests in the Sponsor that are required to be disclosed pursuant to the US Code of Federal Regulations Title 21, Part 54, namely (i) any financial arrangement whereby the value of the compensation paid in respect of the performance of the Clinical Trial could be influenced by the outcome of the Clinical Trial (as defined in 21 CFR 54.2(a)), (ii) any proprietary interest in the product being tested (as defined in 21 CFR 54.2(c)), (iii) any significant equity interest in the Sponsor (as defined in 21 CFR 54.2(b)) and (iv) any significant payments from the Sponsor such as grants to fund ongoing research, compensation in the form of equipment, retainers for ongoing consultation or honoraria (as defined in 21 CFR 54.2(f)). In the case of subparagraphs (iii) and (iv) the Site Principal Investigator understands that such prohibitions relate to the period that the Site Principal Investigator is carrying out the Clinical Trial and for 1 year following completion of the Clinical Trial.

Form of Indemnity for Clinical Studies

To: [Name and address of sponsoring company] ('the Sponsor')
From: [Name and address of health authority/health board/NHS Trust] ('the Authority')
Re: Clinical study No ( ) with [name of product]

1. It is proposed that the Authority should agree to participate in the above sponsored study ('the Study') involving [patients of the Authority] [non-patient volunteers] ('the Subjects') to be conducted by [name of investigator(s)] ('the Investigator') in accordance with the protocol annexed, as amended from time to time with the agreement of the Sponsor and the Investigator ('the Protocol'). The Sponsor confirms that it is a term of its agreement with the Investigator that the Investigator shall obtain all necessary approvals of the applicable Local Research Ethics Committee and shall resolve with the Authority any issues of a revenue nature.

2. The Authority agrees to participate by allowing the Study to be undertaken on its premises utilising such facilities, personnel and equipment as the Investigator may reasonably need for the purpose of the Study.

3. In consideration of such participation by the Authority, and subject to paragraph 4 below, the Sponsor indemnifies and holds harmless the Authority and its employees and agents against all claims and proceedings (to include any settlements or ex gratia payments made with the consent of the parties hereto and reasonable legal and expert costs and expenses) made or brought (whether successfully or otherwise).

(a) by or on behalf of Subjects taking part in the Study (or their dependants) against the Authority or any of its employees or agents for personal injury (including death) to Subjects arising out of or relating to the administration of the product(s) under investigation or any clinical intervention or procedure provided for or required by the Protocol to which the Subjects would not have been exposed but for their participation in the Study.

(b) by the Authority, its employees or agents or by or on behalf of a Subject for a declaration concerning the treatment of a Subject who has suffered such personal injury.

4. The above indemnity by the Sponsor shall not apply to any such claim or proceeding:

4.1 to the extent that such personal injury (including death) is caused by the negligent or wrongful acts or omissions or breach of statutory duty of the Authority, its employees or agents.

4.2 to the extent that such personal injury (including death) is caused by the failure of the Authority, its employees, or agents to conduct the Study in accordance with the Protocol.

4.3 unless as soon as reasonably practicable following receipt of notice of such claim or proceeding, the Authority shall have notified the Sponsor in writing of it and shall, upon the Sponsor's request, and at the Sponsor's cost, have permitted the Sponsor to have full care and control of the claim or proceeding using legal representation of its own choosing.

4.4 if the Authority, its employees, or agents shall have made any admission in respect of such claim or proceeding or taken any action relating to such claim or proceeding prejudicial to the defence of it without the written consent of the Sponsor such consent not to be unreasonably withheld provided that this condition shall not be treated as breached by any statement properly made by the Authority, its employees or agents in connection with the operation of the Authority's internal complaint procedures, accident reporting procedures or disciplinary procedures or where such statement is required by law.

5. The Sponsor shall keep the Authority and its legal advisers fully informed of the progress of any such claim or proceeding, will consult fully with the Authority on the nature of any defence to be advanced and will not settle any such claim or proceeding without the written approval of the Authority (such approval not to be unreasonably withheld).

6. Without prejudice to the provisions of paragraph 4.3 above, the Authority will use its reasonable endeavours to inform the Sponsor promptly of any circumstances reasonably thought likely to give rise to any such claim or proceeding of which it is directly aware and shall keep the Sponsor reasonably informed of developments in relation to any such claim or proceeding even where the Authority decides not to make a claim under this indemnity. Likewise, the Sponsor shall use its reasonable endeavours to inform the Authority of any such circumstances and shall keep the Authority reasonably informed of developments in relation to any such claim or proceeding made or brought against the Sponsor alone.

7. The Authority and the Sponsor will each give to the other such help as may reasonably be required for the efficient conduct and prompt handling of any claim or proceeding by or on behalf of Subjects (or their dependants) or concerning such a declaration as is referred to in paragraph 3(b) above.

8. Without prejudice to the foregoing if injury is suffered by a Subject while participating in the Study, the Sponsor agrees to operate in good faith the Guidelines published in 1991 by The Association of the British Pharmaceutical Industry and entitled 'Clinical Trial Compensation Guidelines' (where the Subject is a patient) and the Guidelines published in 1988 by the same Association and entitled 'Guidelines for Medical Experiments in non-patient Human Volunteers' (where the subject is not a patient) and shall request the Investigator to make clear to the Subjects that the Study is being conducted subject to the applicable Association Guidelines.

9. For the purpose of this indemnity, the expression 'agents' shall be deemed to include without limitation any nurse or other health professional providing services to the Authority under a contract for services or otherwise and any person carrying out work for the Authority under such a contract connected with such of the Authority's facilities and equipment as are made available for the Study under paragraph 2 above.

10. This indemnity shall be governed by and construed in accordance with English/Scots* law.

SIGNED on behalf of the Health Authority/Health Board/NHS Trust

....

Chief Executive/District General Manager

SIGNED on behalf of the Company

....

Dated ....

* Delete as appropriate.

Form of Indemnity for Clinical Studies

From:　('the Sponsor')
To:　　('the Trust') Re:

1. It is proposed that the Trust should agree to participate in the above sponsored study ('the Study') involving patients of the Trust ('the Subjects') to be conducted by .... ('the Investigator') in accordance with the protocol annexed, as amended from time to time with the agreement of the Sponsor and the Investigator ('the Protocol'). The Sponsor confirms that it is a term of its agreement with the Investigator that the Investigator shall obtain all necessary approvals of the applicable Local Research Ethics Committee and shall resolve with the Trust any issues of a revenue nature.

2. The Trust agrees to participate by allowing the Study to be undertaken on its premises utilising such facilities, personnel and equipment as the Investigator may reasonably need for the purpose of the Study.

3. In consideration of such participation by the Trust and subject to paragraph 4 below, the Sponsor indemnifies and holds harmless the Trust and its employees and agents against all claims and proceedings (to include any settlements or ex gratia payments made with the consent of the parties hereto and reasonable legal and expert costs and expenses) made or brought (whether successfully or otherwise):

(a) by or on behalf of Subjects taking part in the Study (or their dependants) against the Trust or any of its employees and agents for personal injury (including death) to Subjects arising out of or relating to the administration of the product(s) under investigation or any clinical intervention or procedure provided for or required by the Protocol to which the Subjects would not have been exposed but for their participation in the Study.

(b) by the Trust, its employees or agents or by or on behalf of a Subject for a declaration concerning the treatment of a Subject who has suffered such personal injury.

4. The above indemnity by the Sponsor shall not apply to any such claim or proceeding:

(a) to the extent that such personal injury (including death) is caused by the negligent or wrongful acts or omissions or breach of statutory duty of the Trust, its employees, or any agents;

(b) to the extent that such personal injury (including death) is caused by the failure of the Trust, its employees, or any agents to conduct the Study within the NHS in accordance with the Protocol;

(c) unless as soon as reasonably practicable following receipt of notice of such claim or proceeding, the Trust shall have notified the Sponsor in writing of it and shall, upon the Sponsor's request, and at the Sponsor's cost, have permitted the Sponsor to have full care and control of the claim or proceeding using legal representation of its own choosing;

(d) if the Trust, its employees, or agents shall have made any admission in respect of such claim or proceeding or taken any action relating to such claim or proceeding prejudicial to the defence of it without the written consent of the Sponsor such consent not to be unreasonably withheld provided that this condition shall not be treated as breached by any statement properly made by the Trust, its employees or agents in connection with the operation of the Trust's internal complaint procedures, accident reporting procedures or disciplinary procedures or where such statement is required by law.

5. The Sponsor shall keep the Trust and its legal advisers fully informed of the progress of any such claim or proceeding, will consult fully with the Trust on the nature of any defence to be advanced and will not settle any such claim or proceeding without the written approval of the Trust (such approval not to be unreasonably withheld).

6. Without prejudice to the provisions of paragraph 4(c) above, the Trust will use its reasonable endeavours to inform the Sponsor promptly of any circumstances reasonably thought likely to give rise to any such claim or proceeding of which it is directly aware and shall keep the Sponsor reasonably informed of developments in relation to any such claim or proceeding even where the Trust decides not to make a claim under this indemnity. Likewise, the Sponsor shall use its reasonable endeavours to inform the Trust of any such circumstances and shall keep the Trust reasonably informed of developments in relation to any such claim or proceeding made or brought against the Sponsor alone.

7. The Trust and the Sponsor will each give to the other such help as may reasonably be required for the efficient conduct and prompt handling of any claim

or proceeding by or on behalf of Subjects (or their dependants) or concerning such a declaration as is referred to in paragraph 3(b) above.

8. Without prejudice to the foregoing if injury is suffered by a Subject while participating in the study, the Sponsor agrees to operate in good faith the Guidelines published in 1991 by The Association of the British Pharmaceutical Industry and entitled 'Clinical Trial Compensation Guidelines' (where the subject is a patient) and the 'Guidelines for Medical Experiments on Non-Patient Human Volunteers' (where the Subject is not a patient) and shall request the Investigator to make clear to the Subjects that the Study is being conducted subject to the applicable Association Guidelines.

9. For the purpose of this indemnity, the expression 'agents' shall be deemed to include without limitation any nurse or other health professional providing services to the Trust under a contract for services or otherwise and any person carrying out work for the Trust under such a contract connected with such of the Trust's facilities and equipment as are made available for the study under paragraph 2 above.

10. This indemnity shall be governed by and construed in accordance with Scots law.

SIGNED for and on behalf of the NHS Trust

SIGNED ....

PRINTED ....

Chief Executive

DATED ....

SIGNED for and on behalf of the Sponsor

SIGNED ....

PRINTED ....

DATED ....

ABPI Guideline on Advertising for Subjects for Clinical Trials

As a result of a number of enquiries to the Medical Affairs Department of the Association of the British Pharmaceutical Industry (ABPI) and the recognition that the media was being increasingly used to advertise for subjects for clinical trials, the ABPI Medical Committee set up a Task Group to develop these guidelines.

Recently, the European Commission (EC) have included an appendix on advertising for trial subjects in the detailed guidance on the application to be submitted for an ethics committee opinion on a clinical trial on a medicinal product for human use. The ABPI guideline set out below takes into account the views of the Medical Committee and additional guidance from the EC guideline. Research Ethics Committees (RECs) should be invited to review all materials used to recruit subjects for all phases of clinical trials, including, but not limited to:

1. Television and radio advertisements.
2. Letters, posters, newsletters, etc.
3. Newspaper advertisements.
4. Internet web sites.

1 Essential Information for an Advertisement

1. A statement indicating that the study involves research.
2. A contact name and phone number for the subject to contact.
3. Some of the eligibility criteria.

4. The likely duration of the subject's participation for a specific study.
5. That the advertisement has been approved by an ethics committee.
6. That your general practitioner will be informed that you are taking part in the clinical trial.
7. That any response to the advertisement will be recorded but will not indicate any obligation.

2 Additional Permitted Content

1. The purpose of the research may be described.
2. The location of the research.
3. The company or institution involved may be named if appropriate.

3 Statements That Should Not Be Used

1. Implied or expressed claims of safety or efficacy.
2. Undue emphasis on reimbursement but mention of reimbursement is permitted.
3. Any express or implied claim that the research is FDA or MCA approved.
4. Use of the term 'new' unless qualified, i.e. 'new research medicine', 'new investigational medicine'.
5. The compound's name.
6. Care should be taken to ensure that advertisements are in no way promotional for the medicine concerned. The ethics committee approval of any advertising material should be kept with the master study file.

Guidelines for company-sponsored Safety Assessment of Marketed Medicines (SAMM)

Introduction

It is well-recognised that there is a continuous need to monitor the safety of medicines as they are used in clinical practice. Spontaneous reporting schemes (e.g. the UK yellow card system) provide important early warning signals of potential drug hazards and also provide a means of continuous surveillance. Formal studies to evaluate safety may also be necessary, particularly in the confirmation and characterisation of possible hazards identified at an earlier stage of drug development. Such studies may also be useful in identifying previously unsuspected reactions.

Scope of guidelines

These guidelines apply to the conduct of all company-sponsored studies which evaluate the safety of marketed products. They take the place of previous guidelines on post-marketing surveillance which were published in 1988 (*BMJ* 1998;296:399–400). Studies performed under those guidelines were found to have some notable limitations (*BMJ* 1992;304:1470–2) and these new guidelines have been prepared in response to the problems identified. The major changes may be summarised as follows:

1. The scope of the guidelines has been expanded to include all company-sponsored studies which are carried out to evaluate safety of marketed medicines. It should be emphasised that this includes both studies conducted in general practice and in the hospital setting. The name of the guidelines has been changed to reflect the emphasis on safety assessment rather than merely surveillance.

2. The guidelines have been developed to provide a framework on which a variety of data collection methods can be used to improve the evaluation of the safety of marketed medicines. Whilst it is recognised that the design used needs to be tailored to particular drugs and hazards, the guidelines define the essential principles which may be applied in a variety of situations. The study methods in this field continue to develop and therefore there will be a need to review regularly these guidelines to ensure that they reflect advances made in the assessment of drug safety.

The guidelines have been formulated and agreed by a Working Party which includes representation from the Medicines Control Agency (MCA), Committee on Safety of Medicines (CSM), Association of the British Pharmaceutical Industry (ABPI), British Medical Association (BMA) and the Royal College of General Practitioners (RCGP). Other guidelines exist for the conduct of 'Phase IV clinical trials' where the medication is provided by the sponsoring company (see section 2(b) below). Some of these studies will also meet the definition of a SAMM study (see below) and should therefore also comply with the present guidelines.

1 Definition of Safety Assessment of Marketed Medicines

(a) Safety assessment of marketed medicines (SAMM) is defined as 'a formal investigation conducted for the purpose of assessing the clinical safety of marketed medicine(s) in clinical practice'.

(b) Any study of a marketed drug which has the evaluation of clinical safety as a specific objective should be included. Safety evaluation will be a specific objective in post-marketing studies either when there is a known safety issue under investigation and/or when the numbers of patients to be included will add significantly to the existing safety data for the product(s). Smaller studies conducted primarily for other purposes should not be considered as SAMM studies. However, if a study which is not conducted for the purpose of evaluating safety unexpectedly identifies a hazard, the manufacturer would be expected to inform the MCA immediately and the section of these guidelines covering liaison with regulatory authorities would thereafter apply.

In cases of doubt as to whether or not a study comes under the scope of the guidelines the sponsor should discuss the intended study plan with the MCA.

2 Scope and objectives of SAMM

(a) SAMM may be conducted for the purpose of identifying previously unrecognised safety issues (hypothesis-generation) or to investigate possible hazards (hypothesis-testing).

(b) A variety of designs may be appropriate including observational cohort studies, cas–surveillance or case–control studies. Clinical trials may also be used to evaluate the safety of marketed products, involving systematic allocation of treatment (e.g. randomisation). Such studies must also adhere to the current guidelines for Phase IV clinical trials.

(c) The design to be used will depend on the objectives of the study, which must be clearly defined in the study plan. Any specific safety concerns to be investigated should be identified in the study plan and explicitly addressed by the proposed methods.

3 Design of studies

Observational cohort studies

(a) The population studied should be as representative as possible of the general population of users, and be unselected unless specifically targeted by the objectives of the study (e.g. a study of the elderly). Exclusion criteria should be limited to the contraindications stated in the data sheet or summary of product characteristics (SPC). The prescriber should be provided with a data sheet or SPC for all products to be used. Where the product is prescribed outside the indications on the data sheet, such patients should be included in the analysis of the study findings.

(b) Observational cohort studies should normally include appropriate comparator group(s). The comparator group(s) will usually include patients with the disease/indication(s) relevant to the primary study drug and such patients will usually be treated with alternative therapies.

(c) The product(s) should be prescribed in the usual manner, for example on an FP10 form written by the general practitioner or through the usual hospital procedures.

(d) Patients must not be prescribed particular medicines in order to include them in observational cohort studies since this is unethical (see section 15 of the 'Guidelines on the Practices of Ethics Committees in Medical Research involving Human Subjects', Royal College of Physicians, 1990).

(e) The prescribing of a drug and the inclusion of the patient in a study are two issues which must be clearly separated. Drugs must be prescribed solely as a result of a normal clinical evaluation, and since such indications may vary from doctor to doctor a justification for the prescription should be recorded in the study documents. In contrast, the inclusion of the patient in the study must be solely dependent upon the criteria for recruitment which have been specifically identified in the study procedures. Any deviation from the study criteria for recruitment could lead to selection bias.

(f) The study plan should stipulate the maximum number of patients to be entered by a single doctor. No patient should be prospectively entered into more than one study simultaneously.

Case–control studies

(g) Case–control studies are usually conducted retrospectively. In case–control studies comparison is made between the history of drug exposure of cases with the disease of interest and appropriate controls without the disease. The study design should attempt to account for known sources of bias and confounding.

Case–surveillance

(h) The purpose of case–surveillance is to study patients with diseases which are likely to be drug-related and to ascertain drug exposure. Companies who sponsor such studies should liaise particularly closely with the MCA in order to determine the most appropriate arrangements for the reporting of cases.

Clinical trials

(i) Large clinical trials are sometimes useful in the investigation of post-marketing safety issues and these may involve random allocation to treatment. In other respects, an attempt should be made to study patients under as normal conditions as possible. Exclusion criteria should be limited to the contraindications in the data sheet or SPC unless they are closely related to the particular objectives of the study. Clinical trials must also adhere to the current guidelines for Phase IV clinical trials (see 2(b) above). Studies which fulfil the definition of SAMM but are performed under a clinical trial exemption (CTX) or under the clinical trial on a marketed product (CTMP) scheme are within the scope of these guidelines.

4 Conduct of studies

(a) Responsibility for the conduct and quality of company-sponsored studies shall be vested in the company's medical department under the supervision of a named medical practitioner registered in the UK, and whose name shall be recorded in the study documents.

(b) Where a study is performed for a company by an agent, a named medical practitioner registered in the UK shall be identified by the agent to supervise the study and liaise with the company's medical department.

(c) Consideration should be given to the appointment of an independent advisory group(s) to monitor the safety information and oversee the study.

5 Liaison with regulatory authorities

(a) Companies proposing to perform a SAMM study are encouraged to discuss the draft study plan with the Medicines Control Agency (MCA) at an early state. Particular consideration should be given to specific safety issues which may require investigation.

(b) Before the study commences a study plan should be finalised which explains the aims and objectives of the study, the methods to be used (including statistical analysis) and the record keeping which is to be maintained. The company shall submit the study plan plus any pro posed initial communications to doctors to the MCA at least 1 month before the planned start of the study. The MCA will review the proposed study and may comment. The responsibility for the conduct of the study will, however, rest with the sponsoring pharmaceutical company.

(c) The company should inform the MCA when the study has commenced and will normally provide a brief report on its progress at least every 6 months, or more frequently if required by MCA.

(d) The regulatory requirements for reporting of suspected adverse reactions must be fulfilled. Companies should endeavour to ensure that they are notified of serious suspected adverse reactions and should report these to the MCA within 15 days of receipt. Events which are not suspected by the investigator to be adverse reactions should not be reported individually as they occur. These and minor adverse reactions should be included in the final report.

(e) A final report on the study should be sent to the MCA within 3 months of follow-up being completed. Ideally, this should be a full report but a brief report within 3 months followed by a full report within 6 months of completion of the study would normally be acceptable. The findings of the study should be submitted for publication.

(f) Companies are encouraged to follow MCA guidelines on the content of progress reports and final reports.

6 Promotion of medicines

(a) SAMM studies should not be conducted for the purposes of promotion.

(b) Company representatives should not be involved in SAMM studies in such a way that it could be seen as a promotional exercise.

7 Doctor participation

(a) Subject to the doctor's terms of service, payment may be offered to the doctor in recompense for his time and any expenses incurred according to the suggested scale of fees published by the BMA.

(b) No inducement for a doctor to participate in a SAMM study should be offered, requested or given.

8 Ethical issues

(a) The highest possible standards of professional conduct and confidentiality must always be maintained. The patient's right to confidentiality is paramount. The patient's identity in the study documents should be codified and only his or her doctor should be capable of decoding it.

(b) Responsibility for the retrieval of information from personal medical records lies with the consultant or general practitioner responsible for the patient's care. Such information should be directed to the medical practitioner nominated by the company or agent, who is thereafter responsible for the handling of such information.

(c) Reference to a Research Ethics Committee is required if patients are to be approached for information, additional investigations are to be performed or if it is proposed to allocate patients systematically to treatments.

9 Procedure for complaints

A study which gives cause for concern on scientific, ethical or promotional grounds should be referred to the MCA, ABPI and the company concerned. Concerns regarding possible scientific fraud should be referred to the ABPI. They will be investigated and, if appropriate, referred to the General Medical Council.

10 Review of Guidelines

The Working Party will review these guidelines as necessary.

Association of the British Pharmaceutical Industry (ABPI)
British Medical Association (BMA)
Committee on Safety of Medicines (CSM)
Medicines Control Agency (MCA)
Royal College of General Practitioners (RCGP)

Reporting of suspected adverse drug reactions: the role of the medical representative

What are a company's responsibilities in respect of safety information it receives back on its medicines?
The ABPI Code of Practice, in line with European Directive 75/319/EEC, calls for an efficient transfer of information on adverse drug reactions. In the case of defective medicines, an ABPI 'Batch Recall of Pharmaceutical Products' system is in operation. In the ABPI Expanded Syllabus, batch recall is referred to in the 'Pharmaceutical Technology' section and adverse drug reactions in the 'Pharmacology and Classification of Medicines' and the 'Pharmaceutical Industry and the NHS' sections.

Relevant sections of the ABPI Code of Practice are:
Clause 13 *Scientific Service Responsible for Information*
Companies must have a scientific service to compile and collate all information, whether received from medical representatives or from any other source, about the medicines which they market.
Clause 15.6 *Representatives*
Representatives must transmit forthwith to the scientific service referred to in clause 13 any information which they receive in relation to the use of the medicines which they promote, particularly reports of side effects.

What is an adverse drug reaction?
A reaction which is harmful and unintended and which occurs at doses normally used in humans for the prophylaxis, diagnosis, or treatment of disease or the modification of physiological function.

What is your own responsibility?
As the company's representative you have an important role in the process of collecting information on possible adverse reactions and quality defects to the products we market. You will often be the only contact that a health care professional has with the company, and it is known that some health care staff report suspected adverse reactions only to the representative.

Your involvement in this reporting process will help to emphasise the importance of your role in providing a service to medicine and patient care.

Why collect information on suspected adverse drug reactions?
There are two main reasons why a company needs to collect this information:
1. The company requires information in order to establish and monitor the safety profile of a product. At the time a new product is first marketed its efficacy

has been well defined. As a relatively small number of patients will have taken part in clinical trials during the development of a new medicine, it is likely that only the more common side effects will have been identified. It is only after larger scale use of the product in normal clinical practice that less common reactions may be detected and an indication of the more common side effects determined.
2. The company has a legal obligation to report all suspected serious adverse drug reactions (ADRs) occurring in the European Union to the Licensing Authority within 15 days of the receipt from any health professional. Serious and unexpected suspected ADRs are required to be reported from outside the EU within 15 days of receipt from health professionals. All other ADRs should be reported in the periodic safety updates.

Reporting of ADRs
The detection and recording of ADRs is of vital importance and doctors are urged to report adverse reactions direct to the Committee on Safety of Medicines (CSM) as follows:
• For medicines introduced recently – as indicated by an inverted black triangle (▼) in the product entry in the British National Formulary, MIMS and the ABPI Data Sheet Compendium – doctors and hospital pharmacists are asked to report *all* suspected reactions. This includes any adverse or any unexpected event, however minor, which could conceivably be attributed to the medicine. Reports should be made despite uncertainty about a cause or relationship, irrespective of whether or not the reaction is well recognised and even when other medicines have been taken concurrently. (The legal position for the pharmaceutical industry requires the reporting of all serious ADRs from the UK or other EU countries, and of all serious and unexpected ADRs from countries outside the EU.)

The CSM decides when the black triangle can be removed (usually after 2 years), the decision being based on experience in use. Note that references to new formulations or presentations of an established medicine will not usually require a black triangle.
• For established medicines, doctors and hospital pharmacists are asked to report serious suspected reactions including those that are fatal, life-threatening, disabling, incapacitating or which result in hospital admission or prolong hospitalisation for in-patients. They should be reported even if the effect is well recognised.

What is a 'yellow card'?

Yellow prepaid letter cards for reporting adverse reactions are available from the CSM at a Freepost address.

'Yellow cards' are also found in the back of the British National Formulary, with the ABPI Data Sheet Compendium, and interleaved with National Health Service General Practitioner FP10 prescription forms.

What company action is taken on reports of suspected ADRs?

All reports on suspected ADRs are co-ordinated and assessed in the company's Medical Department and/or Pharmacovigilance Unit. As much relevant information as possible is obtained from the doctor concerned to enable physicians and scientists to assess the case and determine whether the reaction was caused by the product. A special company ADR card which is often similar to the CSM 'yellow card' may be sent to the doctor to be completed with the required details.

Pharmaceutical companies are now required to report all serious suspected ADRs to the CSM within 15 calendar days of receipt of the original information by the representative or other appropriate employee. Companies are also now obliged to submit reports received from 'all health professionals (doctors, dentists, coroners, pharmacists and nurses)' (ref: The

Medicines for Human Use (Marketing Authorisations, etc,) Regulations 1994). All reports are retained by the company and the information used to build up a well-defined safety profile of a medicine so the company can advise prescribing doctors as necessary.

What is the doctor's responsibility?

Some reports of suspected ADRs come directly to the Medical Department from doctors, and other health professionals (e.g. pharmacists, dentists and nurses). Doctors are requested to report suspected ADRs to the CSM on 'yellow cards', as described above.

However, it is known that many suspected ADRs are not reported by doctors – some estimates put the proportion notified to the CSM as only 1–25% of total 'reportable' reactions.

The CSM issues a briefing sheet on Adverse Drug Reaction reporting to all prescribing doctors and a section on Adverse Reactions to Drugs is contained in the Section of the British National Formulary relating to 'Guidance on Prescribing'.

What if a doctor mentions a suspected ADR?

When a doctor or hospital pharmacist tells you of a suspected ADR to a company product there is a recommended course of action to follow:

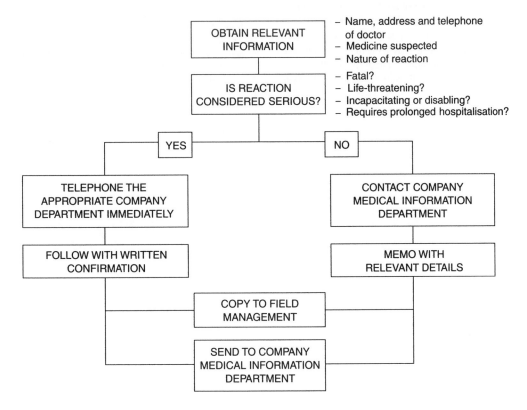

Note: It is as well to inform doctors who report ADRs to medical representatives that the company is legally obliged to report the ADR to the CSM in 15 calendar days, and that a rapid reply would be appreciated if further information is required.

Committee on Safety of Medicines

The Committee on Safety of Medicines (CSM) was established in 1970 under section 4 of the Medicines Act 1968. Its Terms of Reference are:

• To give advice with respect to safety, quality and efficacy in relation to human use of any substance or article (not being an instrument, apparatus or appliance) to which any provision of the Medicines Act 1968 is applicable.

• To promote the collection and investigation of information relating to adverse reactions for the purpose of enabling such advice to be given.

The work of the CSM involves:

(i) Advising the Licensing Authority (UK Health Ministers) of whether on the grounds of safety, quality, and efficacy, medicinal products should be allowed to enter or remain upon the market – the authority is statutorily required to consult the Committee where for example it is minded to refuse the grant of a marketing authorisation on these grounds.

(ii) A statutory responsibility for collecting and investigating information on adverse drug reactions.

The CSM has 30 members and meets fortnightly, but by using a pairing system members are only asked to attend once a month. The term of office of the current Committee will expire on 31 December 1998.

There are three sub-committees of the CSM: Biologicals; Chemistry, Planning and Standards; and Pharmacovigilance.

There is a 24-hour Freephone service available to all parts of the UK for advice and information on suspected adverse drug reactions: contact the National Yellow Card Information Service at the MCA on 0800 731 6789.

The following addresses and phone numbers may be useful:

Medicines Control Agency, CSM Freepost, London SW8 5BR (0800 731 6789).

Regional Centres:

CSM Mersey, Freepost, Liverpool, L3 3AB (0151 794 8113)

CSM Northern, Freepost 1085, Newcastle upon Tyne, NE1 1BR (0191 2321525)

CSM Wales, Freepost, Cardiff, CF4 1ZZ (01222 744181)

CSM West Midlands, Freepost SW2991, Birmingham, B18 7BR (no phone number)

Further reading

British National Formulary published every 6 months by the British Medical Association and the Royal Pharmaceutical Society of Great Britain.

Reporting Adverse Drug Reactions – A BMA Policy Document. British Medical Association, 1996. Price £5.95.

British Recall of Pharmaceutical Products, 2nd edn. Association of the British Pharmaceutical Industry (ABPI), 1994.

Code of Practice for the Pharmaceutical Industry. ABPI for the Prescription Medicines Code of Practice Authority, 1998.

Appendix 3
Directive 2001/20/EC of the European Parliament and of the Council of 4 April 2001

on the approximation of the laws, regulations and administrative provisions of the Member States relating to the implementation of good clinical practice in the conduct of clinical trials on medicinal products for human use.

Only European Community legislation printed in the paper edition of the *Official Journal of the European Union* is deemed authentic.

The European Parliament and the Council of the European Union

Having regard to the Treaty establishing the European Community, and in particular Article 95 thereof,

Having regard to the proposal from the Commission,[1]

Having regard to the opinion of the Economic and Social Committee,[2]

Acting in accordance with the procedure laid down in Article 251 of the Treaty.[3]

Whereas:

1. Council Directive 65/65/EEC of 26 January 1965 on the approximation of provisions laid down by law, regulation or administrative action relating to medicinal products[4] requires that applications for authorisation to place a medicinal product on the market should be accompanied by a dossier containing particulars and documents relating to the results of tests and clinical trials carried out on the product. Council Directive 75/318/EEC of 20 May 1975 on the approx-

imation of the laws of Member States relating to analytical, pharmacotoxicological and clinical standards and protocols in respect of the testing of medicinal products[5] lays down uniform rules on the compilation of dossiers including their presentation.

2. The accepted basis for the conduct of clinical trials in humans is founded in the protection of human rights and the dignity of the human being with regard to the application of biology and medicine, as for instance reflected in the 1996 version of the Helsinki Declaration. The clinical trial subject's protection is safeguarded through risk assessment based on the results of toxicological experiments prior to any clinical trial, screening by Ethics Committees and Member States' competent authorities, and rules on the protection of personal data.

3. Persons who are incapable of giving legal consent to clinical trials should be given special protection. It is incumbent on the Member States to lay down rules to this effect. Such persons may not be included in clinical trials if the same results can be obtained using persons capable of giving consent. Normally these

---

[1] OJ C 306, 8.10.1997, p. 9 and OJ C 161, 8.6.1999, p. 5.

[2] OJ C 95, 30.3.1998, p. 1.

[3] Opinion of the European Parliament of 17 November 1998 (OJ C 379, 7.12.1998, p. 27). Council Common Position of 20 July 2000 (OJ C 300, 20.10.2000, p. 32) and Decision of the European Parliament of 12 December 2000. Council Decision of 26 February 2001.

[4] OJ 22, 9.2.1965, p. 1/65. Directive as last amended by Council Directive 93/39/EEC (OJ L 214, 24.8.1993, p. 22).

[5] OJ L 147, 9.6.1975, p. 1. Directive as last amended by Commission Directive 1999/83/EC (OJ L 243, 15.9.1999, p. 9).

The Textbook of Pharmaceutical Medicine. Edited by John P. Griffin. © 2009, ISBN: 978-1-4051-8035-1.

persons should be included in clinical trials only when there are grounds for expecting that the administering of the medicinal product would be of direct benefit to the patient, thereby outweighing the risks. However, there is a need for clinical trials involving children to improve the treatment available to them. Children represent a vulnerable population with developmental, physiological and psychological differences from adults, which make age- and development-related research important for their benefit. Medicinal products, including vaccines, for children need to be tested scientifically before widespread use. This can only be achieved by ensuring that medicinal products which are likely to be of significant clinical value for children are fully studied. The clinical trials required for this purpose should be carried out under conditions affording the best possible protection for the subjects. Criteria for the protection of children in clinical trials therefore need to be laid down.

4. In the case of other persons incapable of giving their consent, such as persons with dementia, psychiatric patients, etc., inclusion in clinical trials in such cases should be on an even more restrictive basis. Medicinal products for trial may be administered to all such individuals only when there are grounds for assuming that the direct benefit to the patient outweighs the risks. Moreover, in such cases the written consent of the patient's legal representative, given in cooperation with the treating doctor, is necessary before participation in any such clinical trial.

5. The notion of legal representative refers back to existing national law and consequently may include natural or legal persons, an authority and/or a body provided for by national law.

6. In order to achieve optimum protection of health, obsolete or repetitive tests will not be carried out, whether within the Community or in third countries. The harmonisation of technical requirements for the development of medicinal products should therefore be pursued through the appropriate fora, in particular the International Conference on Harmonisation.

7. For medicinal products falling within the scope of Part A of the Annex to Council Regulation (EEC) No 2309/93 of 22 July 1993 laying down Community procedures for the authorisation and supervision of medicinal products for human and veterinary use and establishing a European Agency for the Evaluation of Medicinal Products,[6] which include products intended for gene therapy or cell therapy, prior scientific evaluation by the European Agency for the Evaluation of Medicinal Products (hereinafter referred to as the 'Agency'), assisted by the Committee for Proprietary Medicinal Products, is mandatory before the Commission grants marketing authorisation. In the course of this evaluation, the said Committee may request full details of the results of the clinical trials on which the application for marketing authorisation is based and, consequently, on the manner in which these trials were conducted and the same Committee may go so far as to require the applicant for such authorisation to conduct further clinical trials. Provision must therefore be made to allow the Agency to have full information on the conduct of any clinical trial for such medicinal products.

8. A single opinion for each Member State concerned reduces delay in the commencement of a trial without jeopardising the well-being of the people participating in the trial or excluding the possibility of rejecting it in specific sites.

9. Information on the content, commencement and termination of a clinical trial should be available to the Member States where the trial takes place and all the other Member States should have access to the same information. A European database bringing together this information should therefore be set up, with due regard for the rules of confidentiality.

10. Clinical trials are a complex operation, generally lasting one or more years, usually involving numerous participants and several trial sites, often in different Member States. Member States' current practices diverge considerably on the rules on commencement and conduct of the clinical trials and the requirements for carrying them out vary widely. This therefore results in delays and complications detrimental to effective conduct of such trials in the Community. It is therefore necessary to simplify and harmonise the administrative provisions governing such trials by establishing a clear, transparent procedure and creating conditions conducive to effective coordination of such clinical trials in the Community by the authorities concerned.

11. As a rule, authorisation should be implicit, i.e. if there has been a vote in favour by the Ethics Committee and the competent authority has not objected within a given period, it should be possible to begin the clinical trials. In exceptional cases raising especially complex problems, explicit written authorisation should, however, be required.

12. The principles of good manufacturing practice should be applied to investigational medicinal products.

---

[6] OJ L 214, 24.8.1993, p.1. Regulation as amended by Commission Regulation (EC) No 649/98 (OJ L 88, 24.3.1998, p. 7).

13. Special provisions should be laid down for the labelling of these products.

14. Non-commercial clinical trials conducted by researchers without the participation of the pharmaceuticals industry may be of great benefit to the patients concerned. The Directive should therefore take account of the special position of trials whose planning does not require particular manufacturing or packaging processes, if these trials are carried out with medicinal products with a marketing authorisation within the meaning of Directive 65/65/EEC, manufactured or imported in accordance with the provisions of Directives 75/319/EEC and 91/356/EEC, and on patients with the same characteristics as those covered by the indication specified in this marketing authorisation. Labelling of the investigational medicinal products intended for trials of this nature should be subject to simplified provisions laid down in the good manufacturing practice guidelines on investigational products and in Directive 91/356/EEC.

15. The verification of compliance with the standards of good clinical practice and the need to subject data, information and documents to inspection in order to confirm that they have been properly generated, recorded and reported are essential in order to justify the involvement of human subjects in clinical trials.

16. The person participating in a trial must consent to the scrutiny of personal information during inspection by competent authorities and properly authorised persons, provided that such personal information is treated as strictly confidential and is not made publicly available.

17. This Directive is to apply without prejudice to Directive 95/46/EEC of the European Parliament and of the Council of 24 October 1995 on the protection of individuals with regard to the processing of personal data and on the free movement of such data.[7]

18. It is also necessary to make provision for the monitoring of adverse reactions occurring in clinical trials using Community surveillance (pharmacovigilance) procedures in order to ensure the immediate cessation of any clinical trial in which there is an unacceptable level of risk.

19. The measures necessary for the implementation of this Directive should be adopted in accordance with Council Decision 1999/468/EC of 28 June 1999 laying down the procedures for the exercise of implementing powers conferred on the Commission,[8]

---

[7] OJ L 281, 23.11.1995, p. 31.
[8] OJ L 184,17.7.1999, p. 23.

Have adopted this directive

Article 1
Scope

1. This Directive establishes specific provisions regarding the conduct of clinical trials, including multicentre trials, on human subjects involving medicinal products as defined in Article 1 of Directive 65/65/EEC, in particular relating to the implementation of good clinical practice. This Directive does not apply to non-interventional trials.

2. Good clinical practice is a set of internationally recognised ethical and scientific quality requirements which must be observed for designing, conducting, recording and reporting clinical trials that involve the participation of human subjects. Compliance with this good practice provides assurance that the rights, safety and well-being of trial subjects are protected, and that the results of the clinical trials are credible.

3. The principles of good clinical practice and detailed guidelines in line with those principles shall be adopted and, if necessary, revised to take account of technical and scientific progress in accordance with the procedure referred to in Article 21(2).

These detailed guidelines shall be published by the Commission.

4. All clinical trials, including bioavailability and bioequivalence studies, shall be designed, conducted and reported in accordance with the principles of good clinical practice.

Article 2
Definitions

For the purposes of this Directive the following definitions shall apply:

(a) *Clinical trial:* any investigation in human subjects intended to discover or verify the clinical, pharmacological and/or other pharmacodynamic effects of one or more investigational medicinal product(s), and/or to identify any adverse reactions to one or more investigational medicinal product(s) and/or to study absorption, distribution, metabolism and excretion of one or more investigational medicinal product(s) with the object of ascertaining its (their) safety and/or efficacy.

This includes clinical trials carried out in either one site or multiple sites, whether in one or more than one Member State.

(b) *Multicentre clinical trial:* a clinical trial conducted according to a single protocol but at more than one site, and therefore by more than one investigator, in which the trial sites may be located in a single

Member State, in a number of Member States and/or in Member States and third countries.

(c) *Non-interventional trial:* a study where the medicinal product(s) is (are) prescribed in the usual manner in accordance with the terms of the marketing authorisation. The assignment of the patient to a particular therapeutic strategy is not decided in advance by a trial protocol but falls within current practice and the prescription of the medicine is clearly separated from the decision to include the patient in the study. No additional diagnostic or monitoring procedures shall be applied to the patients and epidemiological methods shall be used for the analysis of collected data.

(d) *Investigational medicinal product:* a pharmaceutical form of an active substance or placebo being tested or used as a reference in a clinical trial, including products already with a marketing authorisation but used or assembled (formulated or packaged) in a way different from the authorised form, or when used for an unauthorised indication, or when used to gain further information about the authorised form.

(e) *Sponsor:* an individual, company, institution or organisation which takes responsibility for the initiation, management and/or financing of a clinical trial.

(f) *Investigator:* a doctor or a person following a profession agreed in the Member State for investigations because of the scientific background and the experience in patient care it requires. The investigator is responsible for the conduct of a clinical trial at a trial site. If a trial is conducted by a team of individuals at a trial site, the investigator is the leader responsible for the team and may be called the principal investigator.

(g) *Investigator's brochure:* a compilation of the clinical and non-clinical data on the investigational medicinal product or products which are relevant to the study of the product or products in human subjects.

(h) *Protocol:* a document that describes the objective(s), design, methodology, statistical considerations and organisation of a trial. The term protocol refers to the protocol, successive versions of the protocol and protocol amendments.

(i) *Subject:* an individual who participates in a clinical trial as either a recipient of the investigational medicinal product or a control.

(j) *Informed consent:* decision, which must be written, dated and signed, to take part in a clinical trial, taken freely after being duly informed of its nature, significance, implications and risks and appropriately documented, by any person capable of giving consent or, where the person is not capable of giving consent, by his or her legal representative; if the person concerned is unable to write, oral consent in the presence of at least one witness may be given in exceptional cases, as provided for in national legislation.

(k) *Ethics Committee:* an independent body in a Member State, consisting of health care professionals and non-medical members, whose responsibility it is to protect the rights, safety and well-being of human subjects involved in a trial and to provide public assurance of that protection, by, among other things, expressing an opinion on the trial protocol, the suitability of the investigators and the adequacy of facilities, and on the methods and documents to be used to inform trial subjects and obtain their informed consent.

(l) *Inspection:* the act by a competent authority of conducting an official review of documents, facilities, records, quality assurance arrangements and any other resources that are deemed by the competent authority to be related to the clinical trial and that may be located at the site of the trial, at the sponsor's and/or contract research organisation's facilities, or at other establishments which the competent authority sees fit to inspect.

(m) *Adverse event:* any untoward medical occurrence in a patient or clinical trial subject administered a medicinal product and which does not necessarily have a causal relationship with this treatment.

(n) *Adverse reaction:* all untoward and unintended responses to an investigational medicinal product related to any dose administered.

(o) *Serious adverse event or serious adverse reaction:* any untoward medical occurrence or effect that at any dose results in death, is life-threatening, requires hospitalisation or prolongation of existing hospitalisation, results in persistent or significant disability or incapacity, or is a congenital anomaly or birth defect.

(p) *Unexpected adverse reaction:* an adverse reaction, the nature or severity of which is not consistent with the applicable product information (e.g. investigator's brochure for an unauthorised investigational product or summary of product characteristics for an authorised product).

Article 3
Protection of clinical trial subjects
1. This Directive shall apply without prejudice to the national provisions on the protection of clinical trial subjects if they are more comprehensive than the provisions of this Directive and consistent with the procedures and timescales specified therein. Member States shall, insofar as they have not already done so, adopt detailed rules to protect from abuse individuals who are incapable of giving their informed consent.

2. A clinical trial may be undertaken only if, in particular:

(a) the foreseeable risks and inconveniences have been weighed against the anticipated benefit for the individual trial subject and other present and future patients. A clinical trial may be initiated only if the Ethics Committee and/or the competent authority comes to the conclusion that the anticipated therapeutic and public health benefits justify the risks and may be continued only if compliance with this requirement is permanently monitored;

(b) the trial subject or, when the person is not able to give informed consent, his legal representative has had the opportunity, in a prior interview with the investigator or a member of the investigating team, to understand the objectives, risks and inconveniences of the trial, and the conditions under which it is to be conducted and has also been informed of his right to withdraw from the trial at any time;

(c) the rights of the subject to physical and mental integrity, to privacy and to the protection of the data concerning him in accordance with Directive 95/46/EC are safeguarded;

(d) the trial subject or, when the person is not able to give informed consent, his legal representative has given his written con sent after being informed of the nature, significance, implications and risks of the clinical trial; if the individual is unable to write, oral consent in the presence of at least one witness may be given in exceptional cases, as provided for in national legislation;

(e) the subject may without any resulting detriment withdraw from the clinical trial at any time by revoking his informed consent;

(f) provision has been made for insurance or indemnity to cover the liability of the investigator and sponsor.

3. The medical care given to, and medical decisions made on behalf of, subjects shall be the responsibility of an appropriately qualified doctor or, where appropriate, of a qualified dentist.

4. The subject shall be provided with a contact point where he may obtain further information.

Article 4
Clinical trials on minors

In addition to any other relevant restriction, a clinical trial on minors may be undertaken only if:

(a) The informed consent of the parents or legal representative has been obtained; consent must represent the minor's presumed will and may be revoked at any time, without detriment to the minor.

(b) The minor has received information according to its capacity of understanding, from staff with experience with minors, regarding the trial, the risks and the benefits.

(c) The explicit wish of a minor who is capable of forming an opinion and assessing this information to refuse participation or to be withdrawn from the clinical trial at any time is considered by the investigator or where appropriate the principal investigator.

(d) No incentives or financial inducements are given except compensation.

(e) Some direct benefit for the group of patients is obtained from the clinical trial and only where such research is essential to validate data obtained in clinical trials on persons able to give informed consent or by other research methods; additionally, such research should either relate directly to a clinical condition from which the minor concerned suffers or be of such a nature that it can only be carried out on minors.

(f) The corresponding scientific guidelines of the Agency have been followed.

(g) Clinical trials have been designed to minimise pain, discomfort, fear and any other foreseeable risk in relation to the disease and developmental stage; both the risk threshold and the degree of distress have to be specially defined and constantly monitored.

(h) The Ethics Committee, with paediatric expertise or after taking advice in clinical, ethical and psychosocial problems in the field of paediatrics, has endorsed the protocol.

(i) The interests of the patient always prevail over those of science and society.

Article 5
Clinical trials on incapacitated adults not able to give informed legal consent

In the case of other persons incapable of giving informed legal consent, all relevant requirements listed for persons capable of giving such consent shall apply. In addition to these requirements, inclusion in clinical trials of incapacitated adults who have not given or not refused informed consent before the onset of their incapacity shall be allowed only if:

(a) The informed consent of the legal representative has been obtained; consent must represent the subject's presumed will and may be revoked at any time, without detriment to the subject.

(b) The person not able to give informed legal consent has received information according to his/her capacity of understanding regarding the trial, the risks and the benefits.

(c) The explicit wish of a subject who is capable of forming an opinion and assessing this information to refuse participation in, or to be withdrawn from, the clinical trial at any time is considered by the investigator or where appropriate the principal investigator.

(d) No incentives or financial inducements are given except compensation.

(e) Such research is essential to validate data obtained in clinical trials on persons able to give informed consent or by other research methods and relates directly to a life-threatening or debilitating clinical condition from which the incapacitated adult concerned suffers.

(f) Clinical trials have been designed to minimise pain, discomfort, fear and any other foreseeable risk in relation to the disease and developmental stage; both the risk threshold and the degree of distress shall be specially defined and constantly monitored.

(g) The Ethics Committee, with expertise in the relevant disease and the patient population concerned or after taking advice in clinical, ethical and psychosocial questions in the field of the relevant disease and patient population concerned, has endorsed the protocol.

(h) The interests of the patient always prevail over those of science and society.

(i) There are grounds for expecting that administering the medicinal product to be tested will produce a benefit to the patient outweighing the risks or produce no risk at all.

Article 6
Ethics Committee

1. For the purposes of implementation of the clinical trials, Member States shall take the measures necessary for establishment and operation of Ethics Committees.

2. The Ethics Committee shall give its opinion, before a clinical trial commences, on any issue requested.

3. In preparing its opinion, the Ethics Committee shall consider, in particular:

(a) the relevance of the clinical trial and the trial design;

(b) whether the evaluation of the anticipated benefits and risks as required under Article 3(2)(a) is satisfactory and whether the conclusions are justified;

(c) the protocol;

(d) the suitability of the investigator and supporting staff;

(e) the investigator's brochure;

(f) the quality of the facilities;

(g) the adequacy and completeness of the written information to be given and the procedure to be followed for the purpose of obtaining informed consent and the justification for the research on persons incapable of giving informed consent as regards the specific restrictions laid down in Article 3;

(h) provision for indemnity or compensation in the event of injury or death attributable to a clinical trial;

(i) any insurance or indemnity to cover the liability of the investigator and sponsor;

(j) the amounts and, where appropriate, the arrangements for rewarding or compensating investigators and trial subjects and the relevant aspects of any agreement between the sponsor and the site; and

(k) the arrangements for the recruitment of subjects.

4. Notwithstanding the provisions of this Article, a Member State may decide that the competent authority it has designated for the purpose of Article 9 shall be responsible for the consideration of, and the giving of an opinion on, the matters referred to in paragraph 3(h), (i) and (j) of this Article.

When a Member State avails itself of this provision, it shall notify the Commission, the other Member States and the Agency.

5. The Ethics Committee shall have a maximum of 60 days from the date of receipt of a valid application to give its reasoned opinion to the applicant and the competent authority in the Member State concerned.

6. Within the period of examination of the application for an opinion, the Ethics Committee may send a single request for information supplementary to that already supplied by the applicant. The period laid down in paragraph 5 shall be suspended until receipt of the supplementary information.

7. No extension to the 60-day period referred to in paragraph 5 shall be permissible except in the case of trials involving medicinal products for gene therapy or somatic cell therapy or medicinal products containing genetically modified organisms. In this case, an extension of a maximum of 30 days shall be permitted. For these products, this 90-day period may be extended by a further 90 days in the event of consultation of a group or a committee in accordance with the regulations and procedures of the Member States concerned. In the case of xenogenic cell therapy, there shall be no time limit to the authorisation period.

Article 7
Single opinion

For multicentre clinical trials limited to the territory of a single Member State, Member States shall establish a procedure providing, notwithstanding the number of Ethics Committees, for the adoption of a single opinion for that Member State.

In the case of multicentre clinical trials carried out in more than one Member State simultaneously, a single opinion shall be given for each Member State concerned by the clinical trial.

Article 8
Detailed guidance

The Commission, in consultation with Member States and interested parties, shall draw up and publish detailed guidance on the application format and documentation to be submitted in an application for an Ethics Committee opinion, in particular regarding the information that is given to subjects, and on the appropriate safeguards for the protection of personal data.

Article 9
Commencement of a clinical trial

1. Member States shall take the measures necessary to ensure that the procedure described in this Article is followed for commencement of a clinical trial. The sponsor may not start a clinical trial until the Ethics Committee has issued a favourable opinion and inasmuch as the competent authority of the Member State concerned has not informed the sponsor of any grounds for non-acceptance. The procedures to reach these decisions can be run in parallel or not, depending on the sponsor.

2. Before commencing any clinical trial, the sponsor shall be required to submit a valid request for authorisation to the competent authority of the Member State in which the sponsor plans to conduct the clinical trial.

3. If the competent authority of the Member State notifies the sponsor of grounds for non-acceptance, the sponsor may, on one occasion only, amend the content of the request referred to in paragraph 2 in order to take due account of the grounds given. If the sponsor fails to amend the request accordingly, the request shall be considered rejected and the clinical trial may not commence.

4. Consideration of a valid request for authorisation by the competent authority as stated in paragraph 2 shall be carried out as rapidly as possible and may not exceed 60 days. The Member States may lay down a shorter period than 60 days within their area of responsibility if that is in compliance with current practice. The competent authority can nevertheless notify the sponsor before the end of this period that it has no grounds for non-acceptance.

No further extensions to the period referred to in the first sub-paragraph shall be permissible except in the case of trials involving the medicinal products listed in paragraph 6, for which an extension of a maximum of 30 days shall be permitted. For these products, this 90-day period may be extended by a further 90 days in the event of consultation of a group or a committee in accordance with the regulations and procedures of the Member States concerned. In the case of xenogenic cell therapy there shall be no time limit to the authorisation period.

5. Without prejudice to paragraph 6, written authorisation may be required before the commencement of clinical trials for such trials on medicinal products which do not have a marketing authorisation within the meaning of Directive 65/65/EEC and are referred to in Part A of the Annex to Regulation (EEC) No 2309/93, and other medicinal products with special characteristics, such as medicinal products the active ingredient or active ingredients of which is or are a biological product or biological products of human or animal origin, or contains biological components of human or animal origin, or the manufacturing of which requires such components.

6. Written authorisation shall be required before commencing clinical trials involving medicinal products for gene therapy, somatic cell therapy including xenogenic cell therapy and all medicinal products containing genetically modified organisms. No gene therapy trials may be carried out which result in modifications to the subject's germ line genetic identity.

7. This authorisation shall be issued without prejudice to the application of Council Directives 90/219/EEC of 23 April 1990 on the contained use of genetically modified micro-organisms[9] and 90/220/EEC of 23 April 1990 on the deliberate release into the environment of genetically modified organisms.[10]

8. In consultation with Member States, the Commission shall draw up and publish detailed guidance on:

(a) the format and contents of the request referred to in paragraph 2 as well as the documentation to be submitted to support that request, on the quality and manufacture of the investigational medicinal product, any toxicological and pharmacological tests, the protocol and clinical information on the investigational medicinal product including the investigator's brochure;

(b) the presentation and content of the proposed amendment referred to in point (a) of Article 10 on substantial amendments made to the protocol;

(c) the declaration of the end of the clinical trial.

Article 10
Conduct of a clinical trial

Amendments may be made to the conduct of a clinical trial following the procedure described hereinafter.

---

[9] OJ L 117, 8.5.1990, p. 1. Directive as last amended by Directive 98/81/EC (OJ L 330, 5.12.1998, p. 13).

[10] OJ L 117, 8.5.1990, p. 15. Directive as last amended by Commission Directive 97/35/EC (OJ L 169, 27.6.1997, p. 72).

(a) After the commencement of the clinical trial, the sponsor may make amendments to the protocol. If those amendments are substantial and are likely to have an impact on the safety of the trial subjects or to change the interpretation of the scientific documents in support of the conduct of the trial, or if they are otherwise significant, the sponsor shall notify the competent authorities of the Member State or Member States concerned of the reasons for, and content of, these amendments and shall inform the ethics committee or committees concerned in accordance with Articles 6 and 9.

On the basis of the details referred to in Article 6(3) and in accordance with Article 7, the Ethics Committee shall give an opinion within a maximum of 35 days of the date of receipt of the proposed amendment in good and due form. If this opinion is unfavourable, the sponsor may not implement the amendment to the protocol. If the opinion of the Ethics Committee is favourable and the competent authorities of the Member States have raised no grounds for non-acceptance of the abovementioned substantial amendments, the sponsor shall proceed to conduct the clinical trial following the amended protocol. Should this not be the case, the sponsor shall either take account of the grounds for non-acceptance and adapt the proposed amendment to the protocol accordingly or withdraw the proposed amendment.

(b) Without prejudice to point (a), in the light of the circumstances, notably the occurrence of any new event relating to the conduct of the trial or the development of the investigational medicinal product where that new event is likely to affect the safety of the subjects, the sponsor and the investigator shall take appropriate urgent safety measures to protect the subjects against any immediate hazard. The sponsor shall forthwith inform the competent authorities of those new events and the measures taken and shall ensure that the Ethics Committee is notified at the same time.

(c) Within 90 days of the end of a clinical trial the sponsor shall notify the competent authorities of the Member State or Member States concerned and the Ethics Committee that the clinical trial has ended. If the trial has to be terminated early, this period shall be reduced to 15 days and the reasons clearly explained.

Article 11
Exchange of information

1. Member States in whose territory the clinical trial takes place shall enter in a European database, accessible only to the competent authorities of the Member States, the Agency and the Commission:

(a) extracts from the request for authorisation referred to in Article 9(2);

(b) any amendments made to the request, as provided for in Article 9(3);

(c) any amendments made to the protocol, as provided for in point a of Article 10;

(d) the favourable opinion of the Ethics Committee;

(e) the declaration of the end of the clinical trial; and

(f) a reference to the inspections carried out on conformity with Good Clinical Practice.

2. At the substantiated request of any Member State, the Agency or the Commission, the competent authority to which the request for authorisation was submitted shall supply all further information concerning the clinical trial in question other than the data already in the European database.

3. In consultation with the Member States, the Commission shall draw up and publish detailed guidance on the relevant data to be included in this European database, which it operates with the assistance of the Agency, as well as the methods for electronic communication of the data. The detailed guidance thus drawn up shall ensure that the confidentiality of the data is strictly observed.

Article 12
Suspension of the trial or infringements

1. Where a Member State has objective grounds for considering that the conditions in the request for authorisation referred to in Article 9(2) are no longer met or has information raising doubts about the safety or scientific validity of the clinical trial, it may suspend or prohibit the clinical trial and shall notify the sponsor thereof.

Before the Member State reaches its decision it shall, except where there is imminent risk, ask the sponsor and/or the investigator for their opinion, to be delivered within 1 week.

In this case, the competent authority concerned shall forthwith inform the other competent authorities, the Ethics Committee concerned, the Agency and the Commission of its decision to suspend or prohibit the trial and of the reasons for the decision.

2. Where a competent authority has objective grounds for considering that the sponsor or the investigator or any other person involved in the conduct of the trial no longer meets the obligations laid down, it shall forthwith inform him thereof, indicating the course of action which he must take to remedy this state of affairs. The competent authority concerned shall forthwith inform the Ethics Committee, the other competent authorities and the Commission of this course of action.

Article 13
Manufacture and import of investigational medicinal products

1. Member States shall take all appropriate measures to ensure that the manufacture or importation of investigational medicinal products is subject to the holding of authorisation.

In order to obtain the authorisation, the applicant and, subsequently, the holder of the authorisation, shall meet at least the requirements defined in accordance with the procedure referred to in Article 21(2).

2. Member States shall take all appropriate measures to ensure that the holder of the authorisation referred to in paragraph 1 has permanently and continuously at his disposal the services of at least one qualified person who, in accordance with the conditions laid down in Article 23 of the second Council Directive 75/319/EEC of 20 May 1975 on the approximation of provisions laid down by law, regulation or administrative action relating to proprietary medicinal products,[11] is responsible in particular for carrying out the duties specified in paragraph 3 of this Article.

3. Member States shall take all appropriate measures to ensure that the qualified person referred to in Article 21 of Directive 75/319/EEC, without prejudice to his relationship with the manufacturer or importer, is responsible, in the context of the procedures referred to in Article 25 of the said Directive, for ensuring:

(a) in the case of investigational medicinal products manufactured in the Member State concerned, that each batch of medicinal products has been manufactured and checked in compliance with the requirements of Commission Directive 91/356/EEC of 13 June 1991 laying down the principles and guidelines of good manufacturing practice for medicinal products for human use,[12] the product specification file and the information notified pursuant to Article 9(2) of this Directive;

(b) in the case of investigational medicinal products manufactured in a third country, that each production batch has been manufactured and checked in accordance with standards of good manufacturing practice at least equivalent to those laid down in Commission Directive 91/356/EEC, in accordance with the product specification file, and that each production batch has been checked in accordance

with the information notified pursuant to Article 9(2) of this Directive;

(c) in the case of an investigational medicinal product which is a comparator product from a third country, and which has a marketing authorisation, where the documentation certifying that each production batch has been manufactured in conditions at least equivalent to the standards of good manufacturing practice referred to above cannot be obtained, that each production batch has undergone all relevant analyses, tests or checks necessary to confirm its quality in accordance with the information notified pursuant to Article 9(2) of this Directive.

Detailed guidance on the elements to be taken into account when evaluating products with the object of releasing batches within the Community shall be drawn up pursuant to the Good Manufacturing Practice guidelines, and in particular Annex 13 to the said guidelines. Such guidelines will be adopted in accordance with the procedure referred to in Article 21(2) of this Directive and published in accordance with Article 19a of Directive 75/319/EEC.

Insofar as the provisions laid down in (a), (b) or (c) are complied with, investigational medicinal products shall not have to undergo any further checks if they are imported into another Member State together with batch release certification signed by the qualified person.

4. In all cases, the qualified person must certify in a register or equivalent document that each production batch satisfies the provisions of this Article. The said register or equivalent document shall be kept up to date as operations are carried out and shall remain at the disposal of the agents of the competent authority for the period specified in the provisions of the Member States concerned. This period shall in any event be not less than 5 years.

5. Any person engaging in activities as the qualified person referral to in Article 21 of Directive 75/319/EEC as regards investigational medicinal products at the time when this Directive is applied in the Member State where that person is, but without complying with the conditions laid down in Articles 23 and 24 of that Directive, shall be authorised to continue those activities in the Member State concerned.

Article 14
Labelling

The particulars to appear in at least the official language(s) of the Member State on the outer packaging of investigational medicinal products or, where there is no outer packaging, on the immediate packaging,

---

[11] OJ L 147, 9.6.1975, p. 13. Directive as last amended by Council Directive 93/39/EC (OJ L214,24.8.1993, p. 22).
[12] OJ L 193, 17.7.1991, p. 30.

shall be published by the Commission in the Good Manufacturing Practice guidelines on investigational medicinal products adopted in accordance with Article 19a of Directive 75/319/EEC.

In addition, these guidelines shall lay down adapted provisions relating to labelling for investigational medicinal products intended for clinical trials with the following characteristics:

• the planning of the trial does not require particular manufacturing or packaging processes;

• the trial is conducted with medicinal products with, in the Member States concerned by the study, a marketing authorisation within the meaning of Directive 65/65/EEC, manufactured or imported in accordance with the provisions of Directive 75/319/EEC; and

• the patients participating in the trial have the same characteristics as those covered by the indication specified in the abovementioned authorisation.

Article 15
Verification of compliance of investigational medicinal products with good clinical and manufacturing practice

1. To verify compliance with the provisions on Good Clinical and Manufacturing Practice. Member States shall appoint inspectors to inspect the sites concerned by any clinical trial conducted, particularly the trial site or sites, the manufacturing site of the investigational medicinal product, any laboratory used for analyses in the clinical trial and/or the sponsor's premises. The inspections shall be conducted by the competent authority of the Member State concerned, which shall inform the Agency; they shall be carried out on behalf of the Community and the results shall be recognised by all the other Member States. These inspections shall be coordinated by the Agency, within the framework of its powers as provided for in Regulation (EEC) No 2309/93. A Member State may request assistance from another Member State in this matter.

2. Following inspection, an inspection report shall be prepared. It must be made available to the sponsor while safeguarding confidential aspects. It may be made available to the other Member States, to the Ethics Committee and to the Agency, at their reasoned request.

3. At the request of the Agency, within the framework of its powers as provided for in Regulation (EEC) No 2309/93, or of one of the Member States concerned, and following consultation with the Member States concerned, the Commission may request

a new inspection should verification of compliance with this Directive reveal differences between Member States.

4. Subject to any arrangements which may have been concluded between the Community and third countries, the Commission, upon receipt of a reasoned request from a Member State or on its own initiative, or a Member State may propose that the trial site and/or the sponsor's premises and/or the manufacturer established in a third country undergo an inspection. The inspection shall be carried out by duly qualified Community inspectors.

5. The detailed guidelines on the documentation relating to the clinical trial, which shall, constitute the master file on the trial, archiving, qualifications of inspectors and inspection procedures to verify compliance of the clinical trial in question with this Directive shall be adopted and revised in accordance with the procedure referred to in Article 21(2).

Article 16
Notification of adverse events

1. The investigator shall report all serious adverse events immediately to the sponsor except for those that the protocol or investigator's brochure identifies as not requiring immediate reporting. The immediate report shall be followed by detailed written reports. The immediate and follow-up reports shall identify subjects by unique code numbers assigned to the latter.

2. Adverse events and/or laboratory abnormalities identified in the protocol as critical to safety evaluations shall be reported to the sponsor according to the reporting requirements and within the time periods specified in the protocol.

3. For reported deaths of a subject, the investigator shall supply the sponsor and the Ethics Committee with any additional information requested.

4. The sponsor shall keep detailed records of all adverse events which are reported to him by the investigator or investigators. These records shall be submitted to the Member States in whose territory the clinical trial is being conducted, if they so request.

Article 17
Notification of serious adverse reactions

1. (a) The sponsor shall ensure that all relevant information about suspected serious unexpected adverse reactions that are fatal or life-threatening is recorded and reported as soon as possible to the competent authorities in all the Member States concerned, and to the Ethics Committee, and in any case no later than 7 days after knowledge by the sponsor of such a case,

and that relevant follow-up information is subsequently communicated within an additional 8 days.

(b) All other suspected serious unexpected adverse reactions shall be reported to the competent authorities concerned and to the Ethics Committee concerned as soon as possible but within a maximum of 15 days of first knowledge by the sponsor.

(c) Each Member State shall ensure that all suspected unexpected serious adverse reactions to an investigational medicinal product which are brought to its attention are recorded.

(d) The sponsor shall also inform all investigators.

2. Once a year throughout the clinical trial, the sponsor shall provide the Member States in whose territory the clinical trial is being conducted and the Ethics Committee with a listing of all suspected serious adverse reactions which have occurred over this period and a report of the subjects' safety.

3. (a) Each Member State shall see to it that all suspected unexpected serious adverse reactions to an investigational medicinal product which are brought to its attention are immediately entered in a European database to which, in accordance with Article 11(1), only the competent authorities of the Member States, the Agency and the Commission shall have access.

(b) The Agency shall make the information notified by the sponsor available to the competent authorities of the Member States.

Article 18
Guidance concerning reports

The Commission, in consultation with the Agency, Member States and interested parties, shall draw up and publish detailed guidance on the collection, verification and presentation of adverse event/reaction reports, together with decoding procedures for unexpected serious adverse reactions.

Article 19
General provisions

This Directive is without prejudice to the civil and criminal liability of the sponsor or the investigator. To this end, the sponsor or a legal representative of the sponsor must be established in the Community.

Unless Member States have established precise conditions for exceptional circumstances, investigational medicinal products and, as the case may be, the devices used for their administration shall be made available free of charge by the sponsor. The Member States shall inform the Commission of such conditions.

Article 20
Adaptation to scientific and technical progress

This Directive shall be adapted to take account of scientific and technical progress in accordance with the procedure referred to in Article 21(2).

Article 21
Committee procedure

1. The Commission shall be assisted by the Standing Committee on Medicinal Products for Human Use, set up by Article 2b of Directive 75/318/EEC (hereinafter referred to as the Committee).

2. Where reference is made to this paragraph, Articles 5 and 7 of Decision 1999/468/EC shall apply, having regard to the provisions of Article 8 thereof.

The period referred to in Article 5(6) of Decision 1999/468/EC shall be set at 3 months.

3. The Committee shall adopt its rules of procedure.

Article 22
Application

1. Member States shall adopt and publish before 1 May 2003 the laws, regulations and administrative provisions necessary to comply with this Directive. They shall forthwith inform the Commission thereof.

They shall apply these provisions at the latest with effect from 1 May 2004.

When Member States adopt these provisions, they shall contain a reference to this Directive or shall be accompanied by such reference on the occasion of their official publication. The methods of making such reference shall be laid down by Member States.

2. Member States shall communicate to the Commission the text of the provisions of national law which they adopt in the field governed by this Directive.

Article 23
Entry into force

The Directive shall enter into force on the day of its publication in the *Official Journal of the European Communities*.

Article 24
Addresses

This Directive is addressed to the Member States. Done at Luxembourg, 4 April 2001.

For the European Parliament	For the Council
The President	The President
N. FONTAINE	B. ROSENGREN

Appendix 4
The Syllabus for Pharmaceutical Medicine

The original syllabus of 14 sections, each containing key topics in pharmaceutical medicine, was approved in 1975. These sections of the syllabus were expanded in 1983 by the Joint Advisory Committee (JAC), which also oversaw the Postgraduate Course in Pharmaceutical Medicine (UWIST, now Cardiff University) curriculum. Teachers on the course, who judged the level of knowledge of the attendees, were constantly expanding the taught curriculum in order to meet their real needs. The JAC and the Board of Examiners for the Diploma in Pharmaceutical Medicine monitored this dynamic process and the 1983 review of the syllabus consolidated these revisions.

In 1989, the Faculty of Pharmaceutical Medicine of the Royal Colleges of Physicians of the UK was established but the Board of Examiners was maintained as a separate entity, under the aegis of the Edinburgh College, during the Faculty's formative years. A Curriculum Working Party was formed in 1989 by the Board of Examiners and reported to a joint meeting of the Board and the Faculty's Qualifications and Examinations Committee. The proposals were endorsed and the Working Party was asked to develop a comprehensive syllabus and a related modular training programme suitable for tuition on approved courses. Its second report in November 1990 presented a proposed revision of the syllabus, which would comprise 18 sections, and these also provided for the curricula of suitable training modules that could be 'mixed and matched' into training blocks. In fact, the revised syllabus was edited into 12 sections by amalgamating those on drug development and those on clinical trials. The new syllabus was agreed in December 1990 and became effective for the Diploma examination held in November 1992.

In 1994, the Diploma in Pharmaceutical Medicine was transferred from the Edinburgh College to the Faculty. The Board of Examiners for the Diploma created Working Parties to formalise its operational procedures (1995) and to issue guidance notes for candidates (1996).

In 1995 the Syllabus for Pharmaceutical Medicine (the Faculty's syllabus for its Diploma in Pharmaceutical Medicine) was adopted by the International Federation of Associations of Pharmaceutical Physicians (IFAPP), to provide a unified Syllabus for Pharmaceutical Medicine from which to derive core curricula for courses in pharmaceutical medicine in its member associations in Europe and around the world.

The syllabus for the UK Diploma in Pharmaceutical Medicine was revised in 1998, 2003 and in 2006 (current version); with revision in 2003 of the regulations, operational procedures and guidance notes. The Syllabus for Pharmaceutical Medicine is now separated into eight sections, an integration which required the 12 sections operational since 1992 being coalesced into seven sections and a new section, Therapeutics, being added.

The Syllabus for Pharmaceutical Medicine, 2008, is produced below. It also serves as the syllabus for the UK Diploma in Pharmaceutical Medicine.

Syllabus for Pharmaceutical Medicine

Introduction
The content of the syllabus is listed under the separate sections below. There is a considerable degree of overlap. Some topics appear in more than one section and it is not intended to imply that any topic is restricted only to those sections under which it is listed. The order of listing does not reflect importance.

The Syllabus for Pharmaceutical Medicine is composed of eight sections:

The Textbook of Pharmaceutical Medicine. Edited by John P. Griffin. © 2009, ISBN: 978-1-4051-8035-1.

1. Medicines regulation
2. Clinical pharmacology
3. Statistics and data management
4. Clinical development
5. Health care marketplace
6. Drug safety and pharmacovigilance
7. Discovery of new medicines
8. Therapeutics

Section 1. Medicines regulation
• The general principles of medicines regulation
• Medicines regulation in the UK, European Union (EU), USA, Japan
• Activities and contribution of International Conference on Harmonisation (ICH)
• Good Manufacturing Practices, Good Laboratory Practices, Good Clinical Practices
• Clinical trials regulations – investigational new drug (IND), clinical trial authorisation (CTA), EU Directives, etc.
• Common technical document, overviews
• Key pharmacovigilance regulations including reporting of adverse drug reactions, periodic safety update reports
• Product information – summary of product characteristics, prescribing information/package insert, patient information leaflets
• Licensing – MAA, NDA, abridged applications, updating and maintaining licences
• Orphan drugs
• Provisions for and use of unlicensed medicines
• Drug abuse and dependence
• Non-prescription drugs and reclassification of prescription only and pharmacy only medicines
• Medical device regulations
• Fraud and professional misconduct
• Product defects and recall
• Ethics and ethics committees
• Pharmacopoeias

Section 2. Clinical pharmacology
Non-clinical development to support testing in humans
• Safety testing – acute, subacute toxicology, genotoxicology, reproductive toxicology, local tolerance, safety pharmacology, hypersensitivity and immunotoxicology, carcinogenicity
• Small molecules and biologicals
• Pharmacokinetics; *in vitro* and *in vivo* study of metabolism; absorption, distribution, metabolism and elimination (ADME)
• Pharmaceutical development of drug substance and drug product: formulations, manufacture and supply of materials, labelling and presentation, stability and storage, purity, compatibility, disposal

Exploratory clinical development
• Assessment of non-clinical data
• Planning of studies in exploratory development
• Populations for exploratory studies – healthy volunteers and patients
• Dose selection
• Ethics – principles, peer review, informed consent, Declaration of Helsinki, protection of research subjects, minimising risk
• Regulation
• Studies – objectives, design, conduct and analysis, choice of site
• Tolerability and safety
• Use of biomarkers and pharmacodynamic endpoints, imaging, dose–response, proof-of-concept, disease models
• Pharmacokinetics, ADME and pharmacokinetic/pharmacodynamic models
• Interpretation of study design, analysis and results

Clinical pharmacokinetics
• Concepts – half-life, volume of distribution, clearance
• Bioavailability and bioequivalence
• Drug–drug and drug–disease interactions (extrinsic factors)
• Studies in different populations (intrinsic factors)
• Pharmacogenetics
• Population pharmacokinetics
• Applicability of pharmacokinetics to dosage regimen and study design

Section 3. Statistics and data management
The purpose and fundamentals of statistics
Trial design, hypothesis testing, power
• Pre-trial decisions and specification
• Risk factors, confounding variables
• The null hypothesis, type I and II errors, significance, power
• Minimising bias

Measurement and types of data
• Standardisation
• Variations in biometry in population, in disease
• Patient instruments

Data collection and management
• Options for data collection (manual and electronic)
• Creation, maintenance and security of databases, software validation and archiving

- Data management from clinical trials: source documents, corrections, computer capture, verifications and extraction, coding
- Within-trial decisions, data management, extraction and manipulation

Types of analysis
- Analysis of efficacy endpoints and of safety
- Interim analysis
- Paired and non-paired tests, parametric and non-parametric tests, confidence limits
- Handling of rating and visual analogue scales, patient diaries and laboratory values
- Sensitivity and specificity of indices
- True and apparent incidence and prevalence data

Interpretation of study design, analysis and results
- Assessment of violations, withdrawals, errors, bias
- Statistical principles and issues in report writing: data manipulation, transposition, merging
- Clinical interpretation of trial results
- Final report writing and formatting for registration dossier and publications

Section 4. Clinical development
Planning and organisation
- Organisation and operation of project teams
- Target product profile, target label, clinical development plans
- Integrated project planning
- Expanded access programmes
- Paediatric programme planning
- Requirements for licensing of new medicines
- Budgeting and costs control

Regulation and ethics
- In UK, EU, USA, Japan to include:
EU Directives and guidances
ICH – Good Clinical Practices
- Ethics – principles, peer review, Declaration of Helsinki, informed consent
- Regulatory review
- Indemnity and compensation
- Confidentiality and data protection

Interventional and non-interventional clinical trials
- Planning of pre-licensing and post-licensing clinical trial programmes – use of non-clinical and existing clinical trial data
- Study types and designs; choice of comparator

- Documentation – writing and reviewing protocol and reports, source document review, case report form design and review, study master file preparation
- Investigator's brochure content, review and maintenance
- Contractual arrangements with investigators and contract research organisations
- Study conduct
- Quality control and quality assurance
- Adverse events and serious adverse events – definitions, collection, reporting, reconciliation, assessment and coding review
- Aggregate clinical trial report reviews, including annual reports and common technical document summaries
- Interpretation of study design, analysis and results
- Formulations, manufacture and supply of materials, labelling and presentation, stability and storage, purity, compatibility, disposal
- Data management and statistical analysis

Section 5. Health care marketplace
- Quality of life
- Intellectual property, legal issues, parallel imports
- Marketing structure and competition, price negotiations
- National and local formularies
- Product information, advertising and claims
- Product support and promotion
- Product life-cycle management
- Product liability and compensation
- Legal and regulatory framework and industry self-regulation; codes of practice covering advertising including those of the Medicines and Healthcare products Regulatory Agency (MHRA) (Advertising and Promotion of Medicines in the UK, the 'Blue Guide'), the Association of the British Pharmaceutical Industry (ABPI) and the European Federation of Pharmaceutical Industries and Associations (EFPIA)
- Principles and practice of marketing
- Measurement of health care, governmental policy and third-party reimbursement
- Principles of health economics
- Pharmaco-epidemiology
- Competition, in-licensing, co-marketing

Section 6. Drug safety and pharmacovigilance
Pharmacovigilance
- The role of the pharmaceutical physician in pharmacovigilance and drug safety
- Periodic safety update reports

- Main sources of epidemiological pharmacovigilance information
- Signal detection, interpretation and management
- Post-authorisation safety studies
- Benefit–risk assessment
- Issue and crisis management

Adverse events and adverse drug reactions
- Mechanisms and classification of adverse events and adverse reactions
- Collection of adverse events in clinical trials
- Spontaneous reporting post-marketing
- Role of sponsors and investigators in reporting and regulatory requirements [European Medicines Agency (EMEA) Guidance]
- Predisposing factors in health and disease
- Dosage, accumulation, medication errors and interactions
- Assessment of evidence for causality and association
- Product labelling including summary of product characteristics/prescribing information/package insert and patient information leaflets

Managing risk
- Risk management
- Safety specification
- 'Dear Health Care Professional' communication
- Product withdrawal procedures
- Drug abuse and dependence
- Off-label use and misuse

Section 7. Discovery of new medicines
- The philosophy behind and organisation of research
- Disease target identification and selection
- Patenting new active substances
- Natural products; novel indications
- Receptor-based approaches, agonists, antagonists, enzyme inhibitors, genomics, proteomics
- Lead optimisation and candidate selection of molecules for exploratory human investigation
- *In vitro* and *in vivo* testing of new compounds
- Relationship between animal and human pharmacology

Section 8. Therapeutics
- Major drug classes (including biologicals): mode of action, use, safety
- Measurement of drug effects
- Adverse drug reactions
- Benefit–risk
- Drug interactions
- Prescribing for particular populations (e.g. children, elderly, pregnant and breastfeeding women, patients with renal or hepatic impairment)
- Controlled drugs and drug dependence
- Overdosage and treatment of poisoning
- Patient compliance and information
- Therapeutic drug monitoring

Index

abciximab 57, 58, 66
absorption 95, 96
ACE inhibitors 10, 46–8
acetylcholinesterase inhibitors 6
adalimumab (Humira) 63, 66
addiction 3–4
ADME (absorption, distribution, metabolism and
    excretion) 29–30, 102, 141–2, 167, 349, 501–2
adolescents, major depressive disorder 393
α- and β-adrenergic receptors 13, 14, 32
ADROIT (Adverse Drug Reactions On-line Information
    Tracking) 432
advanced therapies 459–60, 518–19
adverse events 372–409
  in Australia 634
  causality 226–7
  clinical trials 191–2, 225, 226–7
  formulation and 87
  frequency 102
  information and 322–3, 326
  medical devices 519
  prescription event monitoring 391–2
  profile 272
  rare 398
  rechallenge 227
  reporting in Japan 611–12
  serious (SAE) 226, 611–12
  spontaneous event reporting 379–88, 421–2
  unlicensed medicines 342
  volunteer studies 347
adverse reactions 372–409
  in Australia 614, 634
  clinical trials 225–6
  CSM and monitoring 428–32
  FDA's system 572
  information and 322–3, 326
  mechanisms involved 404
  negligence 370
  predictability 108
  risk 374–5
  Salvarsan 416

suspected serious (SSAR) 226
suspected unexpected serious (SUSAR) 226, 227–8, 449
Types A to F 225–6
voluntary reporting 421–2
volunteer studies 150, 347–8
Adverse Reaction Series leaflets 422, 430, 431
advertisements
  in Australia 638
  direct to consumer 305, 320, 593
  EU controls 311, 361–2, 440, 448, 493–4
  of prescription medicines 317
  and promotion 310–13
  self-regulation 313–17
  for subject recruitment 223–4
  in UK 416, 425, 433
  unlicensed medicines 336–7
  in US 546, 556, 593
Advertising Action Group (UK) 433
Advertising Standards Authority (ASA, UK) 312, 316
Advisory Committee on NHS Drugs (UK) 675, 684
AIDS crisis 560, 571
alemtuzumab 66
aliskirin 50
allergic contact dermatitis 125
All Wales Medicines Strategy Group (AWMSG) 300, 306–7,
    308, 327, 672
Ames test 143
amiodarone 104
analysis of covariance (ANCOVA) 263–4
analytical development 83–4
angiotensin agonists/antagonists 10, 37–8
angiotensin-converting enzyme (ACE) inhibitors 6
animal drugs 543–4
Animal and Scientific Procedures Act (1986, UK) 352
animal studies
  genomics 17, 18
  human experimentation and 347
  juvenile toxicity 119
  legislation and ethical issues 351–2, 448
  numbers used 132
  preclinical safety testing 101–36